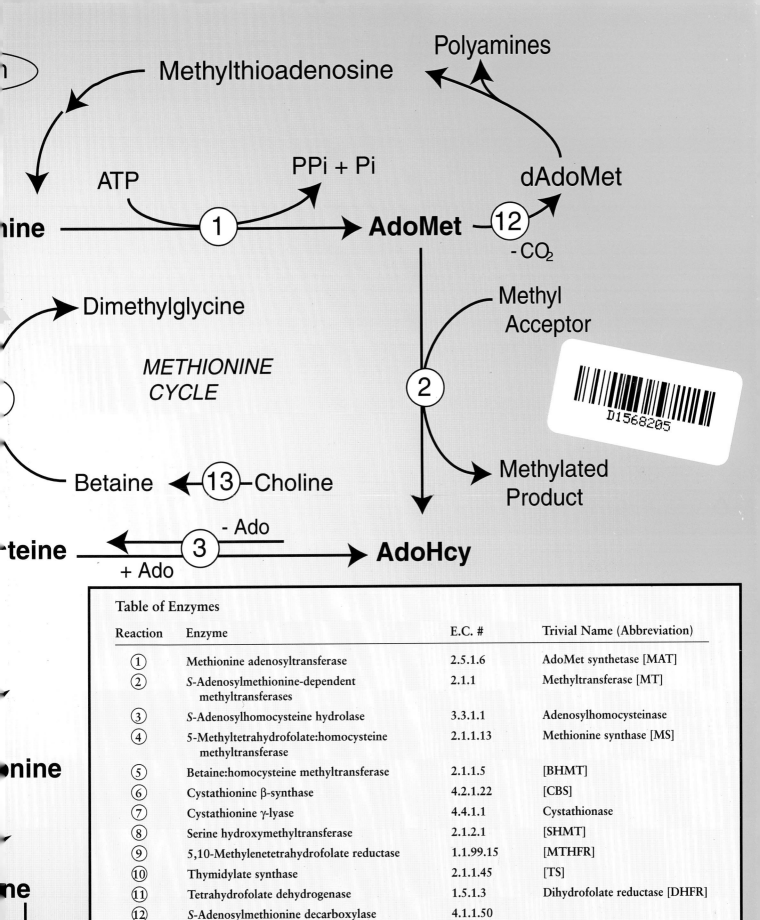

Polyamines

Methylthioadenosine

PPi + Pi

ATP

dAdoMet

ine ——(1)—→ **AdoMet** —(12)—→ dAdoMet
- CO$_2$

Dimethylglycine

METHIONINE CYCLE

Methyl Acceptor

(2)

Betaine ←(13)— Choline

Methylated Product

- Ado

teine ←(3)— + Ado —→ **AdoHcy**

ine

ne

SO$_4^{2-}$

Reaction	Enzyme	E.C. #	Trivial Name (Abbreviation)
(1)	Methionine adenosyltransferase	2.5.1.6	AdoMet synthetase [MAT]
(2)	S-Adenosylmethionine-dependent methyltransferases	2.1.1	Methyltransferase [MT]
(3)	S-Adenosylhomocysteine hydrolase	3.3.1.1	Adenosylhomocysteinase
(4)	5-Methyltetrahydrofolate:homocysteine methyltransferase	2.1.1.13	Methionine synthase [MS]
(5)	Betaine:homocysteine methyltransferase	2.1.1.5	[BHMT]
(6)	Cystathionine β-synthase	4.2.1.22	[CBS]
(7)	Cystathionine γ-lyase	4.4.1.1	Cystathionase
(8)	Serine hydroxymethyltransferase	2.1.2.1	[SHMT]
(9)	5,10-Methylenetetrahydrofolate reductase	1.1.99.15	[MTHFR]
(10)	Thymidylate synthase	2.1.1.45	[TS]
(11)	Tetrahydrofolate dehydrogenase	1.5.1.3	Dihydrofolate reductase [DHFR]
(12)	S-Adenosylmethionine decarboxylase	4.1.1.50	
(13)	Choline dehydrogenase	1.1.99.1	
(14)	Methionyl-tRNA synthetase	6.1.1.10	[AARS]
(15)	Paraoxonase	3.1.1.2	[PON1]

Table of Enzymes

HOMOCYSTEINE IN HEALTH AND DISEASE

High levels of homocysteine have recently been identified as an important risk factor in cardiovascular disease. Homocysteine-related abnormalities are also thought to contribute to birth defects and dementia; and many common acquired diseases, drugs, and genetic disorders adversely affect the metabolism of homocysteine. In this book a multidisciplinary team of the world's experts in the field give a clear, up-to-date analysis of the biochemistry and metabolism of homocysteine and the genetics, epidemiology, clinical settings, causes, impact, and treatment of homocysteine disorders. This is a uniquely comprehensive account of the broad range of medical, nutritional, and methodological implications of homocysteine for health and disease.

Ralph Carmel is Director of Research in the Department of Medicine of the New York Methodist Hospital and Professor of Medicine at Weill Medical College of Cornell University. He has published widely in the field of vitamin B_{12} metabolism and disorders as they relate to homocysteine, aging, neurological disorders, absorptive disorders, and inborn errors of metabolism and has clinical interests in vitamin B_{12} and folate deficiency and hyperhomocysteinemia.

Donald W. Jacobsen is a member of the Professional Staff in the Department of Cell Biology, Lerner Research Institute, of the Cleveland Clinic Foundation, and Director of the Laboratory for Homocysteine Research at the Cleveland Clinic Foundation. He is CCF Professor of Chemistry and CCF Professor of Biology at Cleveland State University. He has published broadly in the area of homocysteine, vitamin B_{12}, folate, and related issues and has an interest in the management of patients with hyperhomocysteinemia.

Homocysteine in Health and Disease

Edited by

RALPH CARMEL
New York Methodist Hospital

DONALD W. JACOBSEN
Cleveland Clinic Foundation

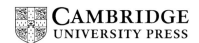

PUBLISHED BY THE PRESS SYNDICATE OF THE UNIVERSITY OF CAMBRIDGE
The Pitt Building, Trumpington Street, Cambridge, United Kingdom

CAMBRIDGE UNIVERSITY PRESS
The Edinburgh Building, Cambridge CB2 2RU, UK
40 West 20th Street, New York, NY 10011-4211, USA
10 Stamford Road, Oakleigh, Melbourne 3166, Australia
Ruiz de Alarcón 13, 28014 Madrid, Spain
Dock House, The Waterfront, Cape Town 8001, South Africa

http://www.cambridge.org

First published 2001

Printed in the United Kingdom at the University Press, Cambridge

Typefaces Sabon 10/12 and Franklin Gothic   *System* Quark XPress™   [HT]

A catalog record for this book is available from the British Library

Library of Congress Cataloging in Publication data

Homocysteine in health and disease / edited by Ralph Carmel, Donald W. Jacobsen.
     p. ; cm
   Includes bibliographical references and index.
   ISBN 0-521-65319-3 (hardback)
     1. Homocysteine—Pathophysiology. 2. Homocysteine—Metabolism—Disorders. 3. Homocysteine—
   Physiological effect. I. Carmel, Ralph. II. Jacobsen, Donald W. (Donald Weldon), 1939–
   [DNLM: 1. Hyperhomocysteinemia—physiopathology. 2. Cardiovascular Diseases—etiology.
   3. Homocysteine—metabolism. 4. Hyperhomocysteinemia—complications. WD 205.5.A5 H768 2001]
   RC632.H65 H66 2001
   616.1′071—dc21   00-46795

ISBN 0 521 65319 3 hardback

To our wives, Martha and Lolly

Contents

Contributors

John T. Brosnan
Department of Biochemistry
Memorial University of Newfoundland
St. John's, Newfoundland, Canada

Ralph Carmel
Department of Medicine
New York Methodist Hospital
Brooklyn, New York

Peter K. Chiang
Division of Experimental Therapeutics
Walter Reed Army Institute of Research
Washington, D.C.

Robert Clarke
Clinical Trial Service Unit
Radcliffe Infirmary
University of Oxford
Oxford, United Kingdom

Steven G. Clarke
Department of Chemistry and Biochemistry
University of California, Los Angeles
Molecular Biology Institute
Los Angeles, California

Fred Cobb
Duke Center for Living
Duke University Medical Center
Durham, North Carolina

Robert J. Cook
Department of Biochemistry
Vanderbilt University Medical School
Nashville, Tennessee

Fernando J. Corrales
Faculdad de Medicina
Universidad de Navarra
Pamplona, Spain

Armando D'Angelo
Coagulation Service
IRCCS H.San. Raffaele
Milano, Italy

Nicholas Dudman (deceased)
University of New South Wales
Prince Henry Hospital
Little Bay, Australia

T.K.A.B. Eskes
Department of Obstetrics and Gynecology
University Hospital Nijmegen
Nijmegen, The Netherlands

Margret Arnadottir
Department of Medicine
Landspitali University Hospital Hringbraut
Reykjavik, Iceland

Matías A. Avila
Faculdad de Medicina
Universidad de Navarra
Pamplona, Spain

Ruma Banerjee
Department of Biochemistry
University of Nebraska
Lincoln, Nebraska

Kelley Banfield
Department of Chemistry and Biochemistry
University of California, Los Angeles
Molecular Biology Institute
Los Angeles, California

Chiara Beltrametti
Coagulation Service
IRCCS H.San Raffaele
Milano, Italy

Henk J. Blom
Laboratory of Pediatrics and Neurology
University Hospital Nijmegen
Nijmegen, The Netherlands

Godfried Boers
Department of Internal Medicine
University Hospital Nijmegen
Nijmegen, The Netherlands

James D. Finkelstein
VA Medical Center
Washington, D.C.

Brian Fowler
Metabolic Unit
University Children's Hospital Basel
Basel, Switzerland

Timothy A. Garrow
Department of Food Science and Human Nutrition
University of Illinois
Urbana, Illinois

Andrew J. Gow
Department of Medicine
Duke University Medical Center
Durham, North Carolina

Jesse F. Gregory III
Food Science and Human Nutrition Department
University of Florida
Gainesville, Florida

Katherine A. Hajjar
Departments of Pediatrics and Medicine
Weill Medical College of Cornell University
New York, New York

Jay W. Heinecke
Division of Lipid Research
Washington University School of Medicine
St. Louis, Missouri

Björn Hultberg
Department of Clinical Chemistry
University Hospital in Lund
Lund, Sweden

Donald W. Jacobsen
Department of Cell Biology
Lerner Research Institute
Cleveland Clinic Foundation
Cleveland, Ohio

Hieronim Jakubowski
Department of Microbiology and Molecular Genetics
UMDNJ- New Jersey Medical School
Newark, New Jersey

Viktor Kožich
Institute of Inherited Metabolic Disorders
First Faculty of Medicine, Charles University
Prague, Czech Republic

Jan P. Kraus
Departments of Pediatrics and Cellular and
    Structural Biology
University of Colorado Health Sciences Center
Denver, Colorado

Warren D. Kruger
Division of Popular Science
Fox Chase Cancer Center
Philadelphia, Pennsylvania

Steven R. Lentz
Veterans Affairs Medical Center
Department of Internal Medicine
University of Iowa College of Medicine
Iowa City, Iowa

Martha L. Ludwig
Biophysics Research Division
Department of Biological Chemistry
University of Michigan
Ann Arbor, Michigan

José M. Mato
Faculdad de Medicina
Universidad de Navarra
Pamplona, Spain

Rowena G. Matthews
Biophysics Research Division
Department of Biological Chemistry
University of Michigan
Ann Arbor, Michigan

Jan Møller
University Department of Biochemistry
Aarhus University Hospital at Skejby
Aarhus, Denmark

Anne M. Molloy
Department of Biochemistry
Trinity College
Dublin, Ireland

Ottar Nygård
LOCUS for Homocysteine and Related Vitamins
Armauer Hansens hus
University of Bergen
Bergen, Norway

Horatiu Olteanu
Department of Biochemstry
University of Nebraska
Lincoln, Nebraska

Sean T. Prigge
Division of Experimental Therapeutics
Walter Reed Army Institute of Research
Washington, D.C.

Karsten Rasmussen
University Department of Clinical Biochemistry
Aarhus University Hospital at Skejby
Aarhus, Denmark

Helga Refsum
LOCUS for Homocysteine and Related Vitamins
Armauer Hansens hus
University of Bergen
Bergen, Norway

Killian Robinson
Department of Internal Medicine
Wake Forest University School of Medicine
Winston-Salem, North Carolina

David S. Rosenblatt
Division of Medical Genetics
McGill University Health Centre
Montreal, Quebec, Canada

Rima Rozen
Department of Human Genetics, Pediatrics and Biology
Montreal Children's Hospital
Montreal, Quebec, Canada

John M. Scott
Department of Biochemistry
Trinity College
Dublin, Ireland

Jonathan Silberberg
Cardiovascular Unit
John Hunter Hospital
Newcastle, Australia

J. David Spence
Stroke Prevention and Atherosclerosis Research
  Centre
Robarts Research Institute
London, Ontario, Canada

Jonathan S. Stamler
Department of Medicine
Duke University Medical Center
Durham, North Carolina

Meir Stampfer
Channing Laboratory
Harvard Medical School
Boston, Massachusetts

James F. Toole
Stroke Research Center
Wake Forest University School of Medicine
Winston-Salem, North Carolina

Johan B. Ubbink
Department of Chemical Pathology
University of Pretoria
Pretoria, South Africa

Per Magne Ueland
LOCUS for Homocysteine and Related Vitamins
Armauer Hansens hus
University of Bergen
Bergen, Norway

Petra Verhoef
Wageningen Centre for Food Science and
  Division of Human Nutrition and Epidemiology
Wageningen University
Wageningen, The Netherlands

Stein Emil Vollset
Section for Medical Statistics
Department of Public Health and Primary
  Health Care
University of Bergen
Bergen, Norway

Donald G. Weir
Department of Clinical Medicine
Trinity College Centre
St. James Hospital
Dublin, Ireland

Bridget Wilcken
New South Wales Biochemical Genetics Service
The New Children's Hospital
Sydney, Australia

David E. L. Wilcken
Cardiovascular Genetics Laboratory
Prince of Wales Hospital
Randwick, Australia

Preface

The study of obscure subjects has a way of generating ultimately important intellectual ideas and practical advances. Homocysteine is a recent example of this regular, yet somehow always surprising, phenomenon in science. For decades, its study was the province of a few investigators and physicians who were interested in a rare inborn error of metabolism and a small corner of amino acid biochemistry. Thanks in great part to their efforts, it is now a burgeoning field of research with important medical implications spanning many disciplines. The study of homocysteine promises to continue to provide new insights and new surprises.

Information about homocysteine and its associations has now matured enough to warrant its comprehensive compilation into a book, indeed into a book of some size. Interest in the clinical problems associated with high levels of homocysteine and their possible amelioration by therapy, especially vitamin therapy, has been grasped eagerly not only by scientists and clinicians but also by the lay public. Homocysteine has now become a rather famous amino acid.

The first half of the book is devoted to the biochemistry and physiology of homocysteine, which sits at a critical branch point between the remethylation and transsulfuration pathways. Here, the book presents the chemistry of homocysteine, the pathways, enzymes, and cofactors that govern its metabolism, the important intermediates that are active in so many biochemical processes, the distribution and metabolism in cells and specific tissues, and the methodology of the measurement of homocysteine. A detailed examination of the methionine cycle and the biochemistry of S-adenosylmethionine is included. Attention is also devoted to the metabolic cycles of folic acid, cobalamin, and vitamin B_6, which intersect with homocysteine metabolism so intimately and influence homocysteine status so strongly.

Brief mention must be made here of terminology, more fully discussed in Chapter 2. The name homocysteine is specific for the thiol-containing amino acid. However, tissues and especially plasma contain related disulfides that are usually measured together with homocysteine. Common usage has given the sum of reduced and oxidized species the name *total homocysteine* or, more often, simply the imprecise, generic designation of *homocysteine*. We have generally allowed these commonly used names to stand.

The second half of the book concerns, first, the clinical disorders that alter homocysteine status. These conditions include the major genetic disorders of homocysteine metabolism, the genetic disorders of cobalamin and folate metabolism, and the growing variety of gene polymorphisms that directly or indirectly affect homocysteine metabolism. An even longer roster of chapters presents the many acquired disorders, such as the three major vitamin deficiencies and renal failure, as well as other diseases, drugs and conditions, such as lifestyle factors, that produce or contribute to hyperhomocysteinemia.

Next are those conditions that appear to follow from the altered homocysteine status. The vascular, thrombotic, and obstetrical disorders for which hyperhomocysteinemia constitutes a risk factor and which may actually result from it are addressed individually. Given the large potential stakes in this clinical area and the wealth of information that has appeared during the last decade, their epidemiology, manifestations, and possible mechanisms are discussed from several perspectives. The final chapters are devoted to issues of intervention and therapy. Attention is also given to the rationales and goals of the homocysteine-lowering trials that have just begun but whose outcome will not be known for several years. These trials will help to resolve a major question by distinguishing between hyperhomocysteinemia as a cause and hyperhomocysteinemia as a marker for the many serious sequelae with which it is associated.

This book was written with clinicians and scientists of a wide range of disciplines in mind. We hope each will be able to derive useful information from all its facets, biochemical, epidemiological, genetic, nutritional, and clinical. We have tried to steer a course between offering a systematic "textbook" and giving the authors, all of whom have been deeply involved in creating the existing body of knowledge, leeway to develop and present their own individual perspectives.

Although the latter approach risks occasional repetition and in a few places even differences in emphasis or opinion, we deemed this to be a price worth paying even as we and the authors strove to keep it at a minimum. We leave it to the reader to judge the result.

We feel honored to have edited this book, a role we embraced despite the knowledge of what such an undertaking can do to one's normal work and family life. For the book's successful completion, we thank Dr. Donald K. Briggs for first encouraging the undertaking; Martha Carmel for her tireless, good humored, and effective handling of many of the details surrounding the manuscripts; Pat DiBello for editorial assistance; and the editors and staff of Cambridge University Press for their expertise and advice. We were aware that prefaces to books often include thanks to spouses for their support and understanding; we have come to fully understand the reasons for this practice, and indeed to appreciate more fully our wives' tolerance for the many years before this project ever began.

Most of all, however, we thank all the investigators who contributed the chapters that comprise the book and gave enthusiastically of their time and talents. Sadly, we give special remembrance to Dr. Nicholas Dudman who succumbed to his illness shortly after completing his chapter, created under such difficult and grievous circumstances.

Ralph Carmel, M.D.
Donald W. Jacobsen, Ph.D.

1

Historical Overview and Recent Perspectives

DAVID E.L. WILCKEN
BRIDGET WILCKEN

This book provides a comprehensive account of current knowledge about the place of the sulfur-containing amino acid, homocysteine, in health and disease. Markedly elevated levels of homocysteine in human plasma and urine were first described in certain rare inborn errors of metabolism. More recently, mild elevations have been found to be associated with coronary, cerebral, and peripheral vascular disease, renal disease, dementia, neural tube defects, and other disorders. As an introduction, it may be appropriate to review briefly how knowledge about this amino acid has evolved.

Homocysteine Metabolism

Homocysteine occupies a pivotal position in the metabolism of the essential amino acid, methionine. It is at the junction point of the transsulfuration pathway and the formation of cysteine and excretion of sulfur on the one hand and the remethylation of homocysteine to methionine with conservation of the carbon skeleton on the other (22). These findings followed the identification in 1932 by Butz and du Vigneaud of homocysteine as a biologically important amino acid (5). With a clearer picture of methionine metabolism and the various cofactors involved came the realization that an elevation of homocysteine could reflect deficiencies of the various vitamins of functional relevance in the pathway — vitamin B_6, cobalamin, and

folic acid. It later became evident that renal function was an important contributor to homocysteine homeostasis. The discovery of the inborn error of metabolism, homocystinuria, initiated the upsurge of interest in homocysteine because of the precocious vascular disease, which was one of the major clinical features associated with the disorder.

Discovery of the Homocystinurias and Development of the Homocysteine Theory of Vascular Disease

The inborn errors leading to homocystinuria involve one of two pathways, transsulfuration or remethylation. In the transsulfuration pathway, there is a deficiency of cystathionine β-synthase, the enzyme mediating the transformation of homocysteine to cystathionine. Defects in remethylation result from inborn errors of metabolism or transport of cobalamin or folic acid, which affect the remethylation of homocysteine to methionine (Metabolic Diagram, Reaction 4). These are rare disorders, but the least rare is cystathionine β-synthase deficiency, cases of which were first reported in 1962. Two of the earliest described patients are shown in Figure 1.1 (7). Additional cases were quickly identified, and by 1965 the principal clinical features had been described (24). The first studies identified high concentrations of homocystine, the oxidized form of homocysteine, in the urine of some children with mental retardation. These children also had high circulating concentrations of homocysteine, measured as the oxidized compound, homocystine, and the mixed disulfide, cysteine-homocysteine. Methionine was also increased. In 1964 Mudd and colleagues identified the enzyme defect and established that this form of homocystinuria was due to a deficiency of cystathionine β-synthase (22). This provided the explanation for the elevations of both homocysteine and methionine found in this disorder.

Four major clinical hallmarks were frequently present in the disorder: dislocation of the ocular lens, a marfanoid habitus and other skeletal abnormalities, a degree of mental retardation, and most important, thromboembolic disease, which was the usual cause of premature death (22). Severe cases may have all of these features, but mild cases may have few or none. In 1969, Mudd and colleagues described a case of a different kind in which homocystinuria was combined with methylmalonic aciduria, but plasma methionine was low (23). This first case of a remethylating disorder was in an infant who died at 7 weeks of age. This case prompted the postulation by McCully that the vascular complications were a consequence of the ele-

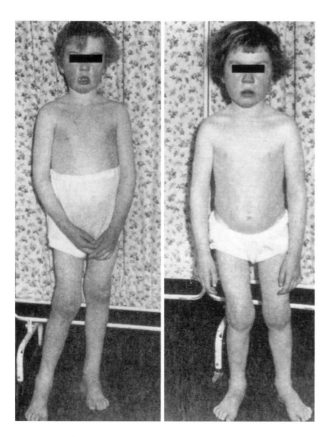

Fig. 1.1. The two homocystinuric sisters identified by Carson et al. (7) in the early 1960s (6-year-old sister on the left and 4-year-old on the right). The abnormalities included mental retardation, seizures, and dislocation of ocular lenses. Visible features include mottled skin and "knock knees." (Reproduced from Carson et al. [7], with permission.)

vated homocysteine rather than the result of any of the other complex metabolic changes occurring in cystathionine β-synthase deficiency (19).

At autopsy on the infant, McCully documented the presence of widespread vascular lesions. It was known at this time that cystathionine β-synthase-deficient patients also had precocious vascular disease but that their markedly elevated circulating levels of homocysteine were associated with increased circulating methionine as would be predicted with diminished cystathionine β-synthase activity. McCully noted that in two discrete disorders of metabolism associated with vascular disease, elevated homocysteine was common to both. He suggested that the elevated homocysteine was responsible for the vascular changes (19).

To establish that the increased homocysteine was responsible for the vascular changes, it was necessary to show that lowering the elevated levels would reduce the associated cardiovascular risk. It was soon established that in a proportion of patients with cystathionine β-synthase deficiency, the elevated homocysteine levels could be markedly reduced with large doses of

pyridoxine (vitamin B_6) (24). In 1985, a landmark review by Mudd and colleagues of more than 600 patients showed that about half the patients were responsive to treatment with pharmacological doses of pyridoxine and were subsequently referred to as pyridoxine-responsive cystathionine β-synthase-deficient patients. The remaining patients had little or no response to pyridoxine (25). Although there is some overlap between these two groups, in general this distinction remains true and reflects, in part, the presence or absence of some residual cystathionine β-synthase activity (24). In this major review, Mudd and colleagues showed that after the age of about 10 years, the risk of a vascular event progressively increased. By the age of 30 years, approximately 50% of untreated cystathionine β-synthase-deficient patients had had either a cerebral thrombosis, a venous thrombosis, or a myocardial infarction. Mudd and colleagues were able to establish that this risk was reduced in treated pyridoxine-responsive patients (25).

Pyridoxine-responsive patients also require folic acid (37) and cobalamin (43) to maintain maximal lowering of homocysteine levels. A low methionine diet plus methionine-free amino acid supplementation is effective treatment for pyridoxine nonresponsive patients, but is usually tolerated only if introduced in infancy (24). However, homocysteine levels in patients diagnosed later can be lowered by the addition of betaine to the other therapies (42). Betaine enhances the remethylation of homocysteine to methionine by an alternative pathway (Metabolic Diagram, Reaction 5). By using this combined therapy, we were able to establish that treatment in patients not responsive to pyridoxine also reduced cardiovascular risk strikingly, even though this regimen frequently increased circulating methionine to quite high levels (43). The most recent analysis of the effect of long-term treatment in altering the natural history of vascular events in 84 cystathionine β-synthase-deficient patients attending centers in Australia ($n = 32$), the Netherlands ($n = 28$), and Ireland ($n = 24$) involved a total of 1,314 patient years of treatment. This shows quite unequivocally that treatment to lower the high homocysteine levels in these patients dramatically reduced cardiovascular risk (46). Nevertheless, in all these studies, total homocysteine levels achieved with treatment remained much higher than those seen in what is now known as "mild hyperhomocysteinemia."

Mild Homocysteine Elevation (Hyperhomocysteinemia) and Cardiovascular Risk

The accepted risk factors — elevated lipids, smoking, hypertension, diabetes, gender, and age — do not explain the occurrence and severity of a sizable proportion of cases of vascular disease, particularly coronary disease, in the general population. The recognition that untreated young homocystinuric patients develop aggressive vascular disease, resulting in a high mortality rate, led us to consider the possibility that even a very modest elevation of homocysteine could itself be a risk factor; or that it could amplify the effects of other risk factors to produce early onset vascular disease.

To explore this possibility we studied a group of patients with early onset (< 50 years) coronary disease established by coronary angiography and measured cysteine-homocysteine as a reflection of circulating homocysteine before and after the challenge of a methionine load (100 mg/kg) (44). The findings were compared with those in a normal age-matched control group known to be free of coronary artery disease. The approach of a methionine challenge had already been used by Sardharwalla and colleagues for the detection of heterozygotes for homocystinuria resulting from cystathionine β-synthase deficiency (29). We found significant increases in cysteine-homocysteine 4 hours after the load in coronary patients compared with the control group, results consistent with a reduced ability to metabolize homocysteine in some patients with premature coronary artery disease when this pathway is stressed. In another study, total free homocysteine measurements showed that 2 of 20 patients with premature coronary artery disease (identical twins) had elevated fasting and postmethionine load homocysteine levels and that these were normalized by oral folic acid (41).

These early findings have been confirmed in numerous subsequent studies, and it is now firmly established that 20% to 30% of patients with coronary, cerebrovascular, and peripheral vascular disease have mild homocysteine elevation, either in the fasting state or after a methionine load (28). Most heterozygotes for cystathionine β-synthase deficiency had been shown to exhibit abnormalities of methionine metabolism (29, 41). It had been recognized that heterozygotes could occur with a frequency of up to 1% in the general population (24); therefore, it had been postulated that patients with vascular disease who had mild hyperhomocysteinemia might include considerable numbers of cystathionine β-synthase heterozygotes. However, this was investigated further by Mudd and colleagues, who reviewed a large number of obligate heterozygotes and could not find definite evidence for increased risk. They concluded that if there was any increased risk, it would have to be small (24). Recent studies have not found any evidence of mutations in the cystathionine β-synthase gene in patients with vascular disease and mild hyperhomocysteinemia (13).

In 1995, an important meta-analysis of 27 studies in more than 4,000 subjects concluded that homocys-

teine elevation was an independent risk factor for vascular disease in the coronary, cerebral, and peripheral circulation (3). This finding has been confirmed in most of the prospective studies conducted so far (28).

Notwithstanding the clear-cut association between the modest homocysteine elevation and vascular disease, whether these small increases do of themselves confer vascular risk or are secondary phenomena is still to be determined. Mildly increased levels of plasma homocysteine are strongly associated with some of the standard risk factors, and there is the need to control for these to determine any independent homocysteine contribution. The large population-based Hordaland study showed that elevated plasma homocysteine was also associated positively with male sex, age, smoking, blood pressure, elevated total cholesterol, and lack of exercise (27). This relationship has been further investigated by a multicenter case-control study that showed that elevations of homocysteine interacted with conventional risk factors, but conferred a similar but independent effect on vascular disease (15). Another study by Nygård and colleagues showed that the risk appeared dose-related, even within the normal range, although the numbers were small in some of the outcome groups (26). Among the large number of recently reported studies, an interesting new one showed a significant and positive relationship between homocysteine levels and increased carotid artery wall thickness in a large randomly selected sample from the general population (20).

A finding that could cast doubt on the direct cause-and-effect aspect relates to a mutation in the 5,10-methylenetetrahydrofolate reductase (MTHFR) gene, a thermolabile variant (14). About 11% to 12% of the white population is homozygous for this variant, which is associated with a modest homocysteine elevation when folate levels are below the population median. A meta-analysis of the results of studies of the distribution of this variant revealed that homozygosity does not confer enhanced cardiovascular risk (4) even though the levels of homocysteine were mildly increased in the 13 studies in which it had been measured. There is a possibility that these surprising results could be explained if the MTHFR mutation conferred protection by another mechanism related to thymidine and DNA synthesis (see Metabolic Diagram). Also arguing somewhat against a direct cause-and-effect relationship of homocysteine in the pathogenesis of vascular disease is the apparently small vascular risk in cystathionine β-synthase-deficient patients during treatment, even when their homocysteine levels, although lowered, are still very high. However, in these studies (43, 46) only 19 of 84 patients were 40 years old or older.

The mechanism for an effect of homocysteine has remained elusive, but recent interesting data showed that small increases in circulating homocysteine are associated with reduced endothelial-dependent vasodilatation (32), and that this may also occur transiently when homocysteine levels are increased after a methionine load (8). These effects may result from homocysteine-induced oxidative stress as supported by the finding by Kanani et al., that oral ascorbic acid prevented the endothelial dysfunction associated with a twofold to threefold rise in homocysteine after a standard methionine load (18). Usui et al. suggested that homocysteine-induced oxidative changes affected endothelial nitric oxide-dependent vasodilatation and that there was an antioxidant effect of folic acid (33). They showed that a single large dose of folic acid prevented impairment of nitric oxide-mediated vasodilatation following a methionine load without altering the associated acute increase in homocysteine levels. An antioxidant effect of folate could also explain the increase in endothelial-dependent brachial artery dilatation found in 18 healthy adults after 6 weeks of oral folate, which lowered the plasma homocysteine levels significantly (1). It is also well known that B-vitamin deficiencies occur frequently in the older age group among whom mild homocysteine elevation and vascular disease are prevalent (6, 30).

The effect of lowering homocysteine levels on cardiovascular risk should be resolved within the next few years by the results of the seven major folate (± cobalamin) trials currently under way in patients with vascular disease (9). These trials will show whether folate medication, which lowers homocysteine levels in most people (28), is protective; but they will not address the issue of whether there is a direct effect on vascular disease of mildly elevated homocysteine levels.

Renal Disease

Also relevant to the homocysteine hypothesis is the possible contribution of elevated plasma homocysteine to the greatly enhanced cardiovascular risk seen in patients with chronic renal failure. In chronic renal failure, vascular risk is increased 20-fold (36) for reasons that are by no means clear. The notion that homocysteine elevation may contribute to renal failure came from the knowledge that the kidneys metabolize homocysteine and are responsible for about 70% of plasma homocysteine clearance under physiological conditions. We reasoned that the plasma homocysteine concentration would be increased when clearance is reduced. To explore this possibility, in the late 1970s we measured homocysteine levels in patients with chronic renal failure and transplant recipients with mildly impaired renal function; homocysteine levels were significantly elevated (39, 40). These increased

levels were markedly reduced by oral folate, and their decline was positively and linearly related to the extent of renal function impairment (38). These findings have been confirmed in many subsequent studies. The recent demonstration that in end-stage renal failure it is remethylation, rather than transsulfuration, that is impaired is in agreement with the homocysteine-lowering effect of folate but not pyridoxine in this situation (34). It remains a strong possibility that elevated homocysteine levels, which are generally of much greater magnitude than the elevation usually found in patients with vascular disease, contribute to vascular disease in patients with renal insufficiency. Data from prospective studies are consistent with this notion (2, 21).

Neural Tube Defects and Other Adverse Pregnancy Outcomes

The pioneering work of Smithells and colleagues has clearly established that preconceptional folate supplementation prevents more than 50% of all neural tube defects (31). This suggested that modest homocysteine elevation might be a marker for an increased risk of neural tube defect. The possibility that the 11% to 12% of women homozygous for the MTHFR mutation are at increased risk of having children with neural tube defects when their folate intake is below the population median has been explored by van der Put and colleagues (35). Their data show that homozygosity for this common 667C→T mutation confers about a twofold increase in neural tube defect risk in the Dutch population.

Preliminary studies have suggested that other adverse pregnancy events and fetal malformations could be associated with elevated homocysteine levels. These include recurrent early pregnancy loss, abruptio placenta, early-onset preeclampsia (11), and nonsyndromic orofacial clefts (45). The mechanisms in clefting and neural tube defect may well be more related to DNA synthesis, whereas abruptio placenta and other pregnancy problems could be a manifestation of placental vasculopathy.

Alzheimer's Disease, Vascular Dementia, and Hyperhomocysteinemia

Evidence has recently been accumulating that patients with histologically confirmed Alzheimer's disease have significantly higher circulating levels of homocysteine and lower levels of folate and cobalamin than control subjects. The stability of the findings over time makes it unlikely that the elevated homocysteine levels are a consequence of the disease (10). This was a well-designed study by the Oxford group, whose study had large numbers and involved long follow-up evaluation. The findings have been confirmed by another rather different approach (17). In addition, hyperhomocysteinemia has been associated with subcortical vascular encephalopathy secondary to small vessel disease (12). If treatment to lower the elevated homocysteine levels prevented or delayed onset of Alzheimer's disease or some forms of vascular dementia, this would be a most significant discovery that would have considerable public health significance.

Conclusion

Lessons learned from the uncommon inborn errors of metabolism resulting in markedly elevated circulating homocysteine have led to the acquisition of new knowledge in many areas. These new insights have set in motion a reappraisal of the etiology and diverse manifestations of cardiovascular risk, in particular the relevance of mild homocysteine elevation to thrombogenesis and endothelial dysfunction. Studies of patients with homocystinuria have provided further insights into methionine metabolism and the relevance of the B vitamins to modest homocysteine elevation, particularly in the elderly. There has also been greater understanding of the role of the kidney in homocysteine homeostasis, as well as its possible contribution to the pathogenesis of the vascular disease frequently seen in renal insufficiency. The common MTHFR gene variant affecting folate metabolism and thus the remethylation of homocysteine to methionine, has been identified. As a result, we have become aware of the increased folate requirements of the 11% of Caucasians who are homozygous for this polymorphism, as well as the concomitant increased risk of offspring with neural tube defect, which is largely preventable by folate supplementation. A number of other disorders that may be associated with mild hyperhomocysteinemia, including dementia, were discussed at the recent conference in Nijmegen (16). The mechanisms are not yet established with certainty. Different mechanisms may be involved for the different associations, and the key issue of cause and effect is yet to be resolved. The role of folate supplementation in the prevention of the increased risks of vascular disease is being actively explored. This book deals with these and other issues that define the role of homocysteine homeostasis in health and disease.

REFERENCES

1. Bellamy, MF, McDowell, IF, Ramsey, MW, Brownlee, M, Newcombe, RG, Lewis, MJ. Oral folate enhances endothelial function in hyperhomocysteinaemic subjects. *Eur J Clin Invest* 1999; 29: 659–62.
2. Bostom, AG, Shemin, D, Verhoef, P, Nadeau, MR, Jacques, PF, Selhub, J, Dworkin, L, Rosenberg, IH. Elevated fasting total plasma homocysteine levels and cardiovascular disease outcomes in maintenance dialysis patients: A prospective study. *Arterioscler Thromb Vasc Biol* 1997; 17: 2554–58.
3. Boushey, CJ, Beresford, SAA, Omenn, GS, Motulsky, AG. A quantitative assessment of plasma homocysteine as a risk factor for vascular disease: Probable benefits of increasing folic acid intakes. *JAMA* 1995; 274: 1049–57.
4. Brattström, L, Wilcken, DEL, Öhrvick, J, Brudin, L. The common methylenetetrahydrofolate reductase gene mutation leads to hyperhomocysteinemia but not to vascular disease—the result of a meta-analysis. *Circulation* 1998; 98: 2520–26.
5. Butz, LW, du Vigneaud, V. The formation of a homologue of cystine by the decompensation of methionine with sulfuric acid. *J Biol Chem* 1932; 99: 135–42.
6. Carmel, R, Green, R, Jacobsen, DW, Rasmussen, K, Florea, M, Azen, C. Serum cobalamin, homocysteine, and methylmalonic acid concentrations in a multiethnic elderly population: Ethnic and sex differences in cobalamin and metabolite abnormalities. *Am J Clin Nutr* 1999; 70: 904–10.
7. Carson, NAJ, Cusworth, DC, Dent, CE, Field, CMB, Neill, DW, Westall, RG. Homocystinuria: A new inborn error of metabolism associated with mental deficiency. *Arch Dis Child* 1963; 38: 425–36.
8. Chambers, JC, McGregor, A, Jean-Marie, J, Obeid, OA, Kooner, JS. Demonstration of rapid onset vascular endothelial dysfunction after hyperhomocysteinaemia: An effect reversible with vitamin C therapy. *Circulation* 1999; 99: 1156–60.
9. Clarke, R, Collins, R. Can dietary supplements with folic acid or vitamin B$_6$ reduce cardiovascular risk? Design of clinical trials to test the homocysteine hypothesis of vascular disease. *J Cardiovasc Risk* 1998; 5: 249–55.
10. Clarke, R, Smith, AD, Jobst, KA, Refsum, H, Sutton, L, Ueland, PM. Folate, vitamin B$_{12}$, and serum total homocysteine levels in confirmed Alzheimer disease. *Arch Neurol* 1998; 55: 1449–55.
11. Eskes, TKAB, Steegers, EAP, Merkus, HMWM. Hyperhomocysteinemia in obstetrics and gynecology: A unifying concept. *Neth J Med* 1998; 52: S16–7.
12. Fassbender, K, Mielke O, Bertsch, T, Nafe B, Fröschen, S, and Hennerici, M. Homocysteine in cerebral macroangiography and microangiopathy. *Lancet* 1999; 353: 1586–1587.
13. Fowler, B. Disorders of homocysteine metabolism. *J Inherit Metab Dis* 1997; 20: 270–85.
14. Frosst, P, Blom, HJ, Milos, R, Goyette, P, Sheppard, CA, Matthews, RG, Boers, GJH, Den Heijer, M, Kluijtmans, LAJ, van den Heuvel, LP, and Rozen, R. A candidate genetic risk factor for vascular disease: a common mutation in methylenetetrahydrofolate reductase. *Nature Genet.* 1995; 10: 111–113.
15. Graham, IM, Daly, LE, Refsum, HM, Robinson, K, Brattström, L, Ueland, PM, Palma-Reis, RJ, Boers, GHJ, Sheahan, RG, Israelsson, B, Uiterwaal, CS, Meleady, R, McMaster, D, Verhoef, P, Witteman, J, Rubba, P, Bellet, H, Wautrecht, JC, De Valk, HW, Lúis, ACS, Parrot-Roulaud, FM, Tan, KS, Higgins, I, and Garcon, D. Plasma homocysteine as a risk factor for vascular disease—The European concerted action project. *J. Am. Med. Assoc.* 1997; 277: 1775–1781.

16. Homocysteine metabolism. Second International Conference. *Neth J Med* 1998; 52: S1–S64.

17. Joosten, E, Lesaffre, E, Riezler, R, Ghekiere, V, Dereymaeker, L, Pelenans, W, Dejaejer, E. Is metabolic evidence for vitamin B$_{12}$ and folate deficiency more frequent in elderly patients with Alzheimer's disease? *J Gerontol Series A* 1997; 52: M76–9.

18. Kanani, PM, Sinkey, CA, Browning, GRL, Allaman, M, Knapp, HR, Haynes, WG. . Role of oxidant stress in endothelial dysfunction produced by experimental hyperhomocyst(e)inemia in humans. *Circulation* 1999; 100: 1161–68.

19. McCully, KS. Vascular pathology of homocysteinemia: Implication for the pathogenesis of arteriosclerosis. *Am J Pathol* 1969; 56: 111–28.

20. McQuillan, BM, Beilby, JP, Nidorf, M, Thompson, PL, Hung, J. Hyperhomocysteinaemia but not the C677T mutation of methylenetetrahydrofolate reductase is an independent risk determinant of carotid wall thickening. *Circulation* 1999; 99: 2383–88.

21. Moustapha, A, Naso, A, Nahlawi, M, Gupta, A, Arheart, KL, Jacobsen, DW, Robinson, K, Dennis, VW. Prospective study of hyperhomocysteinemia as an adverse cardiovascular risk factor in end-stage renal disease. *Circulation* 1998; 97: 138–41.

22. Mudd, SH, Finkelstein, JD, Irreverre, F, Laster, L. Homocystinuria: An enzymatic defect. *Science* 1964; 143: 1443–45.

23. Mudd, SH, Levy, HL, Abeles, RH. A derangement in B$_{12}$ metabolism leading to homocystinemia: Cystathioninemia and methylmalonic aciduria. *Biochem Biophys Res Commun* 1969; 35: 121–26.

24. Mudd, SH, Levy, HL, Skovby, F. Disorders of transsulfuration. In *The Metabolic and Molecular Basis of Inherited Disease*, 7th ed. (Scriver, CR, Beaudet, AL, Sly, WS, Valle, D, eds.). McGraw-Hill, New York, 1995; pp. 1279–1327.

25. Mudd, SH, Skovby, F, Levy, HL, Pettigrew, KD, Wilcken, B, Pyeritz, RE, Andria, G, Boers, GHJ, Bromberg, IL, Cerone, R, Fowler, B, Grobe, H, Schmidt, H, Schweitzer, L. The natural history of homocystinuria due to cystathionine β-synthase deficiency. *Am J Hum Genet* 1985; 37: 1–31.

26. Nygård, O, Nordrehaug, H, Refsum, HM, Ueland, PM. Farstad. M. Vollset, SE. Plasma homocysteine levels and mortality in patients with coronary disease. *N Engl J Med* 1997; 337: 230–36.

27. Nygård, O, Vollset, SE, Refsum, H, Stensvold, I, Tverdazl, A, Nordrehaug, J, Ueland, P, Kvale, G. Total plasma homocysteine and cardiovascular risk factor profile. The Hordaland Homocysteine Study. *JAMA* 1995; 274: 1526–33.

28. Refsum, H, Ueland, PM, Nygård, O, Vollset, SE. Homocysteine and cardiovascular disease. *Annu Rev Med* 1998; 49: 31–62.

29. Sardharwalla, IB, Fowler, B, Robins, AJ, Komrower, GM. Detection of heterozygotes for homocystinuria: Study of sulphur-containing amino acids in plasma and urine after L-methionine loading. *Arch Dis Child* 1974; 49: 553–56.

30. Selhub, J, Jacques, PF, Bostom, AG, D'Agostino, RB, Wilson, PWF, Belanger, AJ, O'Leary, DH, Wolf, PA, Schaefer, EJ, Rosenberg, IH. Association between plasma homocysteine concentrations and extracranial carotid-artery stenosis. *N Engl J Med* 1995; 332: 286–91.

31. Smithells, RW, Sheppard, S, Schorah, CJ, Seller, MJ, Nevin, NC, Harris, R, Read, AP, and Fielding, DW. Possible prevention of neural-tube defects by periconceptional vitamin supplementation. *Lancet*, 1980; i: 339–340.

32. Tawakol, A, Omland, T, Gerhard, M, Wu, JT, Creager, MA. Hyperhomocyst(e)inemia is associated with impaired endothelium-dependent vasodilatation in humans. *Circulation* 1997; 95: 1119–21.

33. Usui, M, Matsuoka, H, Miyazaki, H, Ueda, S, Okuda, S, Imaizumi, T. Endothelial dysfunction by acute hyperhomocyst(e)inaemia: Restoration by folic acid. *Clin Sci* 1999; 96: 235–39.

34. van Guldener, C, Kulik, W, Berger, R, Dijkstra, DA, Jakobs, J, Reijngoud, D-J, Donker, AJM, Stehouwer, CDA, de Meer, K. Homocysteine and methionine metabolism in ESRD: A stable isotope study. *Kidney Int* 1999; 56: 1064–71.

35. van der Put, NMJ, Eskes, TKAB, Blom, HJ. Is the common 677C→T mutation in the methylenetetrahydrofolate reductase gene a risk factor for neural tube defects? A meta-analysis. *Q J Med* 1997; 90: 111–115.

36. Wheeler, DC. Cardiovascular disease in patients with chronic renal failure. *Lancet* 1996; 348: 1673–74.

37. Wilcken, B, Turner, B. Homocystinuria: Reduced folate levels during pyridoxine treatment. *Arch Dis Child* 1973; 48: 58–62.

38. Wilcken, DEL, Dudman, NPB, Tyrrell, PA, Robertson, MR. Folic acid lowers elevated plasma homocyst(e)ine in chronic renal insufficiency: Possible implications for prevention of vascular disease. *Metabolism* 1988; 37: 697–701.

39. Wilcken, DEL, Gupta, VJ, Reddy, SG. Accumulation of sulphur-containing amino acids including cysteine-homocysteine in patients on maintenance haemodialysis. *Clin Sci* 1980; 58: 427–30.

40. Wilcken, DEL, Gupta, VJ. Sulphur containing amino acids in chronic renal failure with particular reference to homocystine and cysteine-homocysteine mixed disulphide. *Eur J Clin Invest* 1979; 9: 301–07.

41. Wilcken, DEL, Reddy, SG, Gupta, VJ. Homocysteinemia, ischaemic heart disease, and the carrier state for homocystinuria. *Metabolism* 1983; 32: 363–70.

42. Wilcken, DEL, Wilcken, B, Dudman, NPB, Tyrrell, PA. Homocystinuria—the effects of betaine in the treatment of patients not responsive to pyridoxine. *N Engl J Med* 1983; 309: 448–53.

43. Wilcken, DEL, Wilcken, B. The natural history of vascular disease in homocystinuria and the effects of treatment. *J Inherit Metab Dis* 1997; 20: 295–300.

44. Wilcken, DEL, Wilcken, B. The pathogenesis of coronary artery disease: A possible role for methionine metabolism. *J Clin Invest* 1976; 57: 1079–82.

45. Wong, WY, Eskes, TKAB, Kuijpers-Jagtman, AM, Spauwen, PHM, Steegers, EAP, Thomas, CMG, Hamel, BCJ, Blom, HJ, and Steegers-Theunissen, RPM. Nonsyndromic orofacial clefts: Association with maternal hyperhomocysteinemia. *Teratology*, 1999; 60: 253–57.

46. Yap, S, Boers, GHJ, Wilcken, B, Wilcken, DEL, Naughten, ER. A three-center study of the effects of long-term treatment of patients with homocystinuria due to cystathionine β-synthase deficiency. *J Inherit Metab Dis* (in press).

PART ONE

BIOCHEMISTRY AND PHYSIOLOGY

2

Practical Chemistry of Homocysteine and Other Thiols

DONALD W. JACOBSEN

The sulfhydryl-containing amino acids, or aminothiols, maintain intracellular and extracellular redox homeostasis and are part of the armamentarium of antioxidant defense systems. They are also precursors and intermediates in numerous metabolic pathways and facilitate the removal of noxious compounds. The "good thiols," glutathione and cysteine, are well known and abundant. The intracellular concentration of glutathione is usually in the 1 to 10 mmol/L range, and plasma total cysteine ranges from 200 to 300 μmol/L. Homocysteine is perhaps less well known because it is normally found at relatively low concentrations within the cell (≤ 1 μmol/L) and in the circulation (5 to 15 μmol/L). However, elevated plasma total homocysteine (hyperhomocysteinemia) has acquired the reputation as the "not-so good thiol" because of its association with cardiovascular disease (6, 54), end-stage renal disease (4, 13), hypothyroidism (25, 46), neural tube defects (16, 63), and cognitive dysfunction including Alzheimer's disease (8, 34).

This chapter focuses on the structure and physiological chemistry of homocysteine and closely related thiols, with special emphasis on the circulating forms of homocysteine. How homocysteine reacts with intracellular constituents is largely unknown, but the forms of homocysteine found in plasma and serum are now well characterized and offer clues to possible reaction mechanisms that could occur within the cell. Other chapters in this book describe specialized chemically related topics such as homocysteine thiolactone (see Chapter 3), homocysteine and lipid oxidation (see Chapter 4), and nitrosothiols (see Chapter 5).

Discovery of Homocysteine

Homocysteine was discovered 70 years ago by Butz and du Vigneaud at the University of Illinois (5). By heating methionine in sulfuric acid, a compound was isolated and crystalized that had chemical properties similar to those of cysteine and cystine. Using elemental analysis data and other chemical properties, the investigators concluded that they had synthesized "*bis*-(γ-amino-γ-carboxypropyl) disulfide" and suggested that it be called homocystine since it had the structure of the "next higher symmetrical homolog of cystine." They also suggested that homocystine might support growth on cysteine-deficient diets in advance of the discovery of the transsulfuration pathway.

Homocysteine thiolactone was first prepared from methionine by Baernstein (2) in 1934 and further characterized by the du Vigneaud group (14, 56). L-homocysteine thiolactone, a very stable form of homocysteine, can be converted to L-homocysteine by alkaline hydrolysis (2, 43). L-homocysteine is thus available for cell culture and other studies. Although racemic D,L-homocysteine is commercially available and is widely used for in vivo, ex vivo, in situ, and in vitro studies, the presence of the unnatural D-isomer of homocysteine may complicate the interpretation of experimental results.

Structure of Homocysteine and Related Thiols

Homocysteine is a key branch-point intermediate in the ubiquitous four-step methionine cycle (see Metabolic Diagram), the function of which is to generate one-carbon methyl groups for transmethylation reactions essential to all life forms. In mammals homocysteine can be diverted from the methionine cycle into the two-step transsulfuration pathway to generate the nonessential aminothiol cysteine. The essential amino acid methionine, therefore, is the precursor of homocysteine and cysteine, and all three compounds have structural similarities (Figure 2.1).

Methionine contains a sulfide sulfur, the general structure of which can be designated R-S-R′. Homocysteine and cysteine are sulfhydryl compounds (R-SH), and the words *homocysteine* and *cysteine* have precise chemical meanings, referring only to the R-SH forms shown in Figure 2.1. However, in recent years,

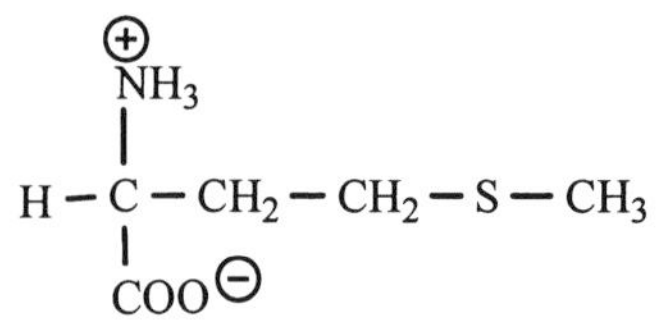

Methionine

MW 149.21

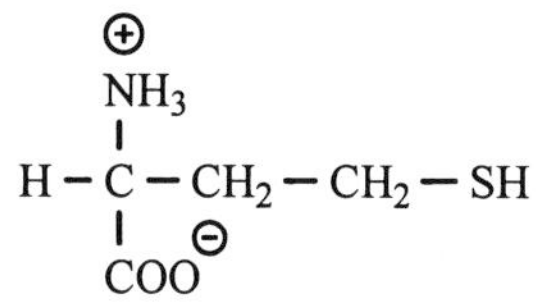

Homocysteine

MW 135.19

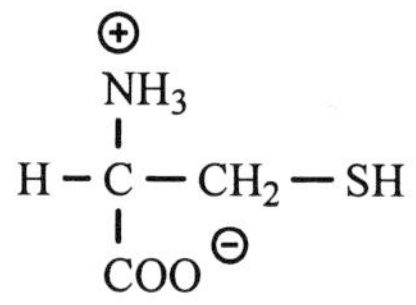

Cysteine

MW 121.16

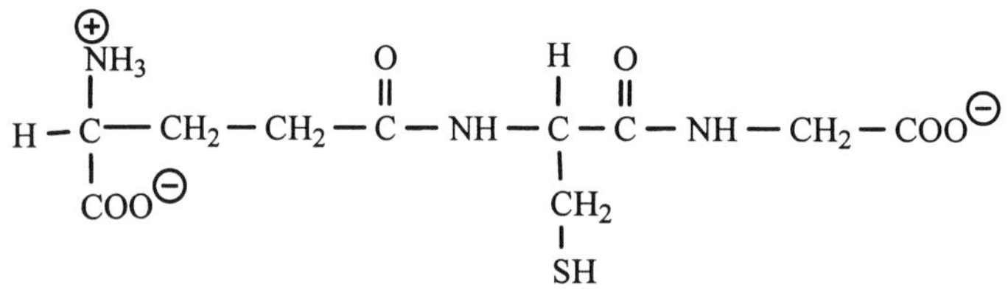

Glutathione

MW 306.32

Fig. 2.1. The structures of methionine, homocysteine, cysteine, and glutathione.

these words have taken on generic meaning as well; and it is common, particularly in the clinical literature, to use the word *homocysteine* when referring to all circulating forms of homocysteine. In this book the term *plasma total homocysteine* refers to all circulating forms of homocysteine (*vide infra*).

Compounds that contain a free sulfhydryl group are known as "thiols." Other low-molecular-weight biological thiols include glutathione (Figure 2.1), coenzyme A, and the dithiol, dihydrolipoic acid. Glutathione, a tripeptide-containing glutamic acid, cysteine, and glycine, is the most abundant intracellular thiol and is utilized in a number of host defense systems including protection against reactive oxygen species and xenobiotics.

A general chemical property of thiols is their ability to oxidize in the presence of an electron acceptor such as molecular oxygen to form disulfides (-S-S-) (*vide infra*). Thus, homocysteine will autooxidize to form homocystine and cysteine will autooxidize to form cystine (Figure 2.2). Glutathione will also undergo autooxidation to form oxidized glutathione (Figure 2.2). The latter is formed intracellularly as a result of glutathione peroxidase activity during breakdown of reactive oxygen species. But in the reducing environment of the cell and the presence of glutathione reductase, oxidized glutathione is converted back to glutathione.

Homocysteine can oxidize with other thiols such as cysteine and glutathione to form mixed disulfides, and

these compounds are referred to as "homocysteine-cysteine mixed disulfide" and "homocysteine-glutathione mixed disulfide" (Figure 2.3).

The other major class of thiols and disulfides consists of those found in peptides and proteins that contain cysteine. The intramolecular disulfide bonds formed by the oxidation of cysteine residues in peptides and proteins are primary structural elements (covalent bonds) that contribute to the final three-dimensional conformations. Peptides and proteins may also contain "free cysteine residues" that can autooxidize (e.g., serum albumin, to form disulfide dimers,) or can react with low molecular thiols to form stable disulfide bond complexes. Thus, > 70% of the homocysteine and approximately 50% of the cysteine in the circulation are bound to plasma protein cysteine residues through disulfide bonds (Figure 2.4).

Homocysteine thiolactone, the product of aminoacyl tRNA synthetase editing reactions (see Chapter 3), is the five-membered condensed ring form of homocysteine. Although this compound may be exported to the circulation, there is no reliable evidence for its existence in human plasma, perhaps because of nonspecific esterase activity found in plasma and on the surface of the vascular endothelium (15). Also, it was recently reported that human serum paraoxonase hydrolyzes homocysteine thiolactone as well (29a).

Nomenclature

Homocysteine and homocystine refer to the reduced and oxidized forms of homocysteine, respectively, and likewise for cysteine and cystine. Other oxidized forms of homocysteine include the mixed disulfides with free

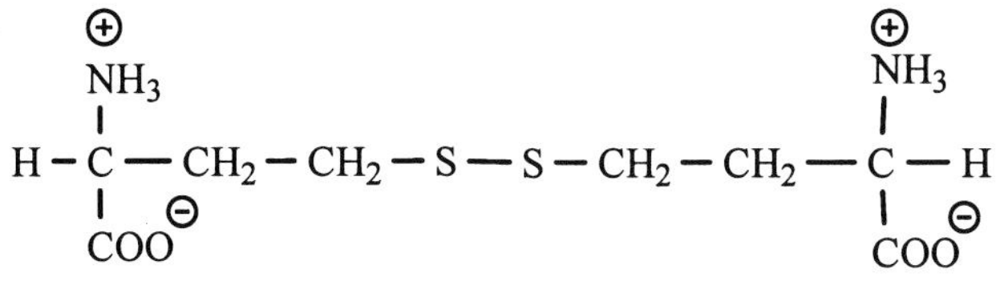

Homocystine

MW 268.36

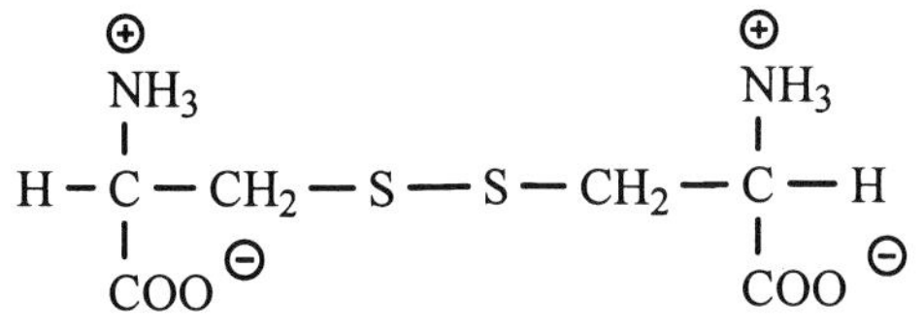

Cystine

MW 240.30

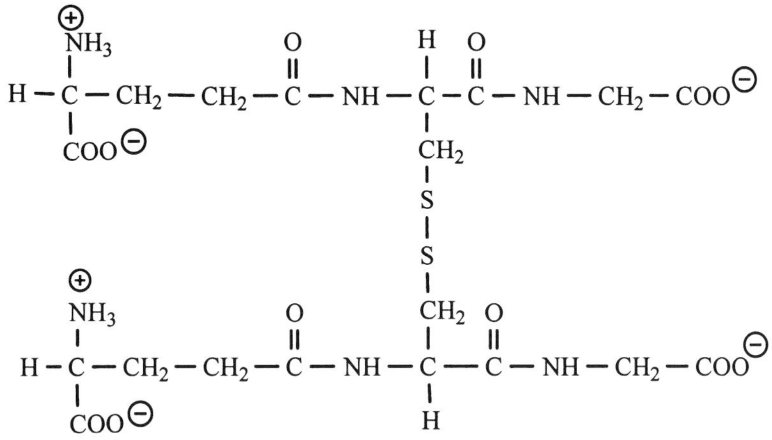

Oxidized glutathione

MW 610.62

Fig. 2.2. The structures of the oxidized forms of homocysteine, cysteine, and glutathione: homocystine, cystine, and oxidized glutathione.

Fig. 2.3. The structures of homocysteine-cysteine mixed disulfide and homocysteine-glutathione mixed disulfide.

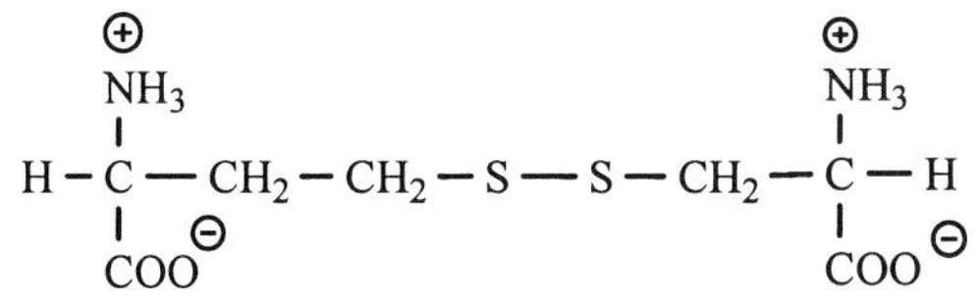

Homocysteine-cysteine mixed disulfide

MW 254.33

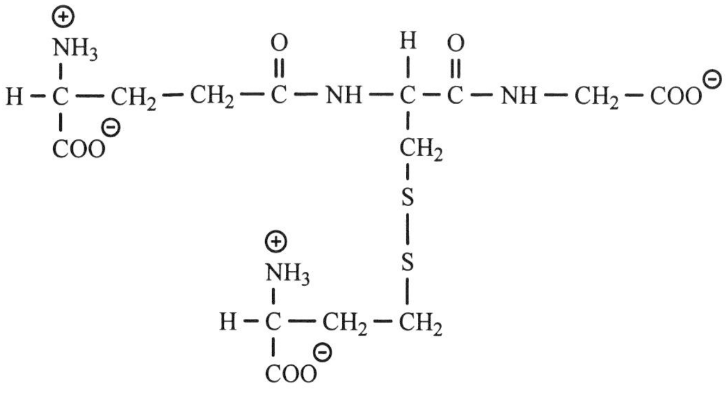

Homocysteine-glutathione mixed disulfide

MW 439.49

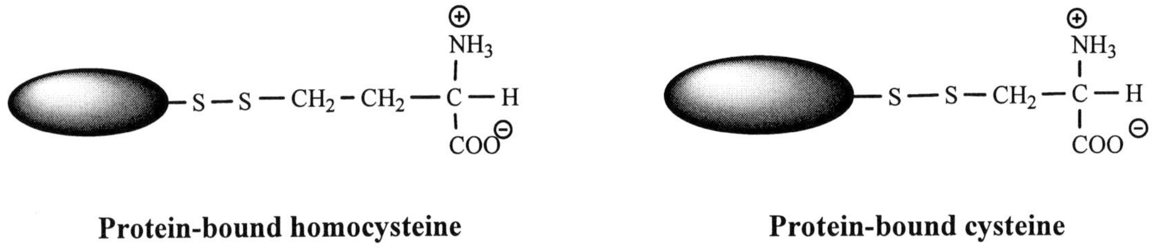

$$\text{Protein} - S - S - CH_2 - CH_2 - \underset{\underset{COO^{\ominus}}{|}}{\overset{\overset{\oplus}{NH_3}}{\underset{|}{C}}} - H$$

Protein-bound homocysteine

$$\text{Protein} - S - S - CH_2 - \underset{\underset{COO^{\ominus}}{|}}{\overset{\overset{\oplus}{NH_3}}{\underset{|}{C}}} - H$$

Protein-bound cysteine

Fig. 2.4. The structures of protein-bound homocysteine and protein-bound cysteine.

cysteine and cysteine residues found in protein. As previously mentioned, the sum of reduced and oxidized forms of homocysteine in the circulation is known as plasma (serum) total homocysteine (also, total plasma [serum] homocysteine). Likewise, plasma total cysteine and plasma total glutathione refer to the combined sum of reduced and oxidized forms of cysteine and glutathione. The word *homocyst(e)ine* has also been used for unspecified forms of homocysteine and plasma total homocysteine (44). However, since the parentheses cannot be pronounced in speech, the use of the word *homocyst(e)ine* is becoming less popular.

Although the use of abbreviations in the field is commonplace, until recently there has been no standardization of an abbreviation system. Thus, Hcy, Hcy-SH, and HSH have all been used for homocysteine. Plasma total homocysteine is often abbreviated tHcy. This text does not use abbreviations for homocysteine. Instead words with precise chemical definitions are used to avoid confusion. However, the word *homocysteine* is used generically, particularly when referring to it as a risk factor. *Hyperhomocysteinemia* is another word that is almost always used in a generic sense. *Hyperhomocyst(e)inemia* is also used to indicate multiple unspecified forms of homocysteine in circulation. A recent consensus statement on nomenclature and the use of abbreviations has appeared (45a). This will help to standardize nomenclature and meaning in the homocysteine field.

Chemical Reactivity of Homocysteine in the Circulation

The plasma of healthy individuals has finite concentrations of reduced and oxidized forms of homocysteine. Plasma total homocysteine concentrations appear to increase with age throughout life. Reported reference ranges are as follows: newborns and young children, 3 to 6 µmol/L (24, 64); adolescents, 5 to 8 µmol/L (55, 62); younger and middle age adults, 5 to 13 µmol/L (54); and elderly individuals usually > 10 µmol/L (9). An interesting study from France showed that cente-

narians had plasma total homocysteine concentrations between 25 and 27 µmol/L (17).

The cellular origins of circulating homocysteine in healthy individuals, and for that matter hyperhomocysteinemics, are unclear. Because the methionine cycle is ubiquitous, perhaps all cells make a small but finite contribution to plasma total homocysteine. Also, the precise chemical form that is exported and whether there may be cellular differences in the forms exported are not known. Because the intracellular environment is a reducing one, it is likely that reduced homocysteine is transported into circulation.

The amount of homocysteine exported to the circulation depends on metabolic capacity. Intracellular homocysteine is remethylated back to methionine in most cells by cobalamin-dependent methionine synthase (Metabolic Diagram, Reaction 4). The efficiency of the remethylation process depends on several factors: 1) availability of the cosubstrate 5-methyltetrahydrofolate, 2) adequate levels of the micronutrients that drive the production of 5-methyltetrahydrofolate (vitamins B_1, B_2, and B_6), and 3) availability of the cobalamin cofactor methylcobalamin. In the liver and kidney, homocysteine can also be metabolized through the transsulfuration pathway by cystathionine β-synthase (Metabolic Diagram, Reaction 6). The efficiency of the transsulfuration pathway is, in part, determined by the availability of the cofactor pyridoxal 5'-phosphate. Liver and kidney also have an alternative remethylation pathway that utilizes betaine as the methyl-group donor substrate, (Metabolic Diagram, Reaction 5). Thus, micronutrient deficiencies, particularly of folate, cobalamin, and vitamin B_6, will impair the metabolic capacity for homocysteine, resulting in greater export to the blood.

Redox Status of Homocysteine and Other Aminothiols in Plasma

The chemistry of homocysteine in the circulation is governed by its reactive sulfhydryl group. In healthy individuals, less than 1% of plasma total homocysteine is found as free reduced homocysteine. Mansoor et al. (39) collected venous blood from healthy male and female donors into tubes containing the anticoagulant heparin and monobromobimane, a sulfhydryl-trapping reagent. The concentrations of free reduced homocysteine, cysteine, cysteinylglycine (a by-product of glutathione degradation), and glutathione were determined by reverse-phase high-performance liquid chromatography with fluorescence detection. The mean concentration of free reduced homocysteine was < 0.3 μmol/L compared with ~ 9, 4.5, and 3 μmol/L for cysteine, cysteinylglycine, and glutathione, respectively (Table 2.1) (39).

The same study also determined the levels of the free oxidized forms of homocysteine, cysteine, cysteinylglycine, and glutathione to be ~ 2, 83, 8, and 1 μmol/L, respectively. For homocysteine, the free oxidized forms included primarily homocystine and the mixed disulfide with cysteine. Traces of homocysteine mixed disulfides with cysteinylglycine and glutathione, although not determined directly, may have been present also. The protein-bound forms of homocysteine, cysteine, cysteinylglycine, and glutathione were found at mean concentrations of ~ 10, 165, 17, and 1.5 μmol/L, respectively (39). This study was one of the earliest to accurately assess the redox status of homocysteine and other low molecular weight aminothiols in the circulation.

The percent distribution of reduced and oxidized forms of homocysteine in plasma is shown in Table 2.2. The oxidized forms of homocysteine clearly make up the bulk of circulating homocysteine, with protein-bound homocysteine accounting for > 70% of plasma total homocysteine. Homocystinuric patients have significantly higher concentrations of free reduced homocysteine, where values approaching 100 μmol/L have been reported (40). These patients have higher levels of free reduced cysteine, but in some patients the concentration of free reduced homocysteine actually exceeds that of free reduced cysteine. The concentrations of free oxidized cysteine and protein-bound cysteine are significantly below values seen in healthy individuals (40).

Table 2.2. Percent Distribution of Reduced and Oxidized Homocysteine in Human Plasma

Reduced:

Homocysteine	≤ 1%

Oxidized:

Homocystine	5–15%
Mixed disulfides:	
Cysteine-homocysteine	5–15%
Protein-bound homocysteine	>70%

Table 2.1. Redox Status of Homocysteine and Other Aminothiols in Normal Human Plasma

Concentration, μmol/L

Aminothiol	Reduced	Free Oxidized	Protein-bound	Total
Homocysteine	< 0.3	2	10	~ 12
Cysteine	9	83	165	257
Cysteinylglycine	3	8	17	28
Glutathione	4.5	1	1.5	6

Data from Mansoor et al. (39), average mean values from healthy females (*n* = 10) and males (*n* = 8).

Chemical Reactivity of Plasma Homocysteine after Methionine Loading

Administration of L-methionine perorally, usually 100 mg/kg (670 μmol/kg) body weight, is frequently used to assess the body's overall capacity to metabolize homocysteine (see Chapter 19). The so-called methionine-loading study is used to identify individuals who have normal basal plasma total homocysteine, but who develop abnormally elevated transient hyperhomocysteinemia with prolonged clearance after the methionine challenge. The kinetics of the reduced, oxidized, and protein-bound forms of homocysteine, cysteine, and cysteinylglycine have been examined in healthy men and provide information on the dynamic redox equilibria that exist between the aminothiols in circulation (38). After an oral methionine load, all forms of homocysteine increase in concentration within the first 8 hours. Free-reduced homocysteine increases twofold to threefold within 2 to 3 hours and then falls to preload values within 24 hours. The twofold to threefold increase in protein-bound homocysteine reaches a peak within 6 to 8 hours and then declines to preload values within 24 to 48 hours. Free oxidized homocysteine consisting of homocystine and low molecular weight mixed disulfides also increases approximately twofold within 4 to 6 hours and then falls to preload values within 24 to 48 hours. In contrast there are dramatic decreases in the concentrations of both protein-bound cysteine and protein-bound cysteinylglycine (38). These observations suggest that free reduced homocysteine is displacing protein-bound cysteine and protein-bound cysteinyl-glycine during the transient hyperhomocysteinemia that occurs following a methionine load. Mechanisms to account for these observations are discussed below.

Chemical Reactivity of Plasma Homocysteine after Homocysteine Loading

The entry of free reduced homocysteine into the circulation after methionine loading as described above (38), or after direct homocysteine loading (37), can alter the redox status of other aminothiols. L-homocysteine (67 µmol/kg body weight) was administered to healthy subjects perorally (37). There was a rapid increase in free reduced homocysteine concentration, reaching twentyfold above baseline in 15 minutes, which then declined to basal levels within 2 hours. There was a similar increase in free reduced cysteine. The concentration of protein-bound homocysteine increased more slowly, reaching peak values that were fourfold to fivefold above baseline within 1 to 2 hours. This was paralleled by a decrease in protein-bound cysteine suggesting that homocysteine was displacing cysteine from plasma protein (37). Kinetic analysis of the peroral homocysteine loading study revealed that the elimination of plasma homocysteine was first order with a half-life of 223 ± 45 minutes (21). Less than 2% of the administered homocysteine was recovered in the urine.

The methionine and homocysteine loading studies provide important clues to the possible chemical mechanisms involving homocysteine in circulation. These mechanisms, based largely on in vitro studies, are discussed in the following sections.

Chemical Properties of Homocysteine and Other Thiols

Sulfur is the eighth most abundant element in the human body. It resides in Group 16 of the periodic table between oxygen and selenium, and is followed by tellurium and polonium. However, there are, great differences between the chemistries of oxygen and sulfur, owing in large part to the lower electronegativity of sulfur, a lesser tendency of hydrogen bond formation with sulfur, the ability of sulfur to form hexacoordinate compounds through *d*-orbital bonding, and the ability of sulfur to catenate, forming Sn^{2-} structures (10). The disulfide bond (-S-S-) bond, a primary structural element of peptides and proteins, is much more stable than the peroxide bond (-O-O-).

Thiols undergo facile oxidation to disulfides. They also oxidize to sulfenic (RSOH), sulfinic (RSO$_2$H), and sulfonic (RSO$_3$H) acids. It is beyond the scope of this chapter to present an in depth account of the known physical and chemical properties of homocysteine and other thiols with respect to these higher oxidation states. The reader is referred to excellent monographs and reviews for more detailed information (10, 19, 26, 29, 30, 47, 48).

Thiolate Anion Formation

A fundamental property of a biological thiol is the ability of its sulfhydryl group hydrogen to dissociate. Thus, biological thiols are weak acids, and the general

reaction for hydrogen ion dissociation can be written as RSH $\leftrightarrows$ RS$^-$ + H$^+$. The negative log of the dissociation constant Ka (pKa) and the negative log of the hydrogen ion concentration (pH) are related in the Henderson-Hasselbalch equation:

$$pH = pKa + \log([RS^-]/[RSH])$$

When the concentration of the conjugate base [RS$^-$] equals the concentration of the weak acid [RSH], the pK_a of the weak acid is equal to the pH of the solution. Stated another way, the pK_a represents the pH at which the sulfhydryl group is half-titrated. The pK_as for biological and commonly used nonbiological thiols are shown in Table 2.3. The pK_a for the sulfhydryl group of free cysteine is approximately 8.5. This means that at physiological pH, slightly less than 10% of the free cysteine molecules are in the thiolate anion form. The pK_a of the sulfhydryl group of cysteine when incorporated into polypeptides or proteins can change by up to 3 to 4 orders of magnitude owing to the charge effects of surrounding amino acid residues. Thus, the pK_a of Cys$_{34}$ in albumin is approximately 5 (35, 49), suggesting that in the circulation the unoccupied Cys$_{34}$ residue exists as a thiolate anion.

The dissociation of the sulfhydryl group for homocysteine is shown in Reaction 1. As can be seen in Table 2.3, estimates of the pK_a for the homocysteine sulfhydryl group range from 8.7 to 10. If we assume an average pK_a of approximately 9.5, then at physiological pH, slightly less than 1% of the homocysteine molecules will be in the thiolate anion form. What does this mean in terms of a normal concentration of plasma total homocysteine of, for example, 10 µmol/L? The concentration of free reduced homocysteine in this example would be

Table 2.3. Acidic Dissociation Constants for the Sulfhydryl Group of Biological and Nonbiological Thiols

Compound	pK_a	Reference
L-Cysteine	8.5	Benesch, Benesch (3)
D,L-Homocysteine	8.7	Friedman et al. (18)
D,L-Homocysteine	10.0	Benesch, Benesch (3)
Glutathione	8.6	Friedman et al. (18)
Penicillamine	7.9	Friedman et al. (18)
N-Acetylcysteine	9.5	Friedman et al. (18)
2-Mercaptoethanol	9.5	Danehy, Noel (11)
1,4-Dithioerythritol	9.0 (pK_{a1}) 9.9 (pK_{a2})	Zahler, Cleland (69)
1,4-Dithiothreitol	8.3 (pH$_{a1}$) 9.5 (pK_{a2})	Zahler, Cleland (69)

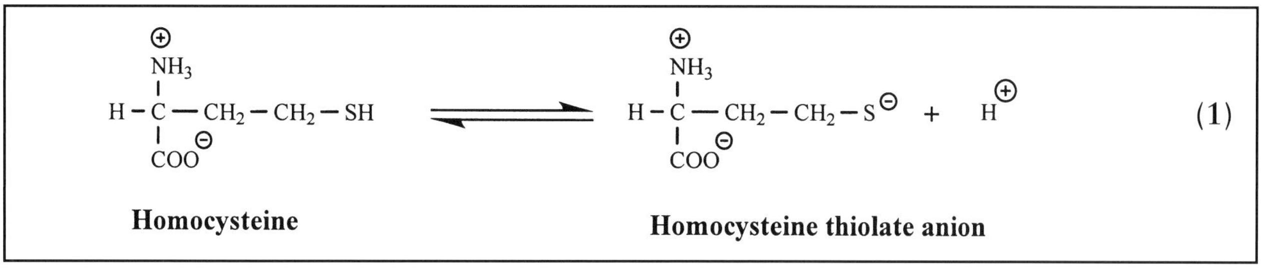

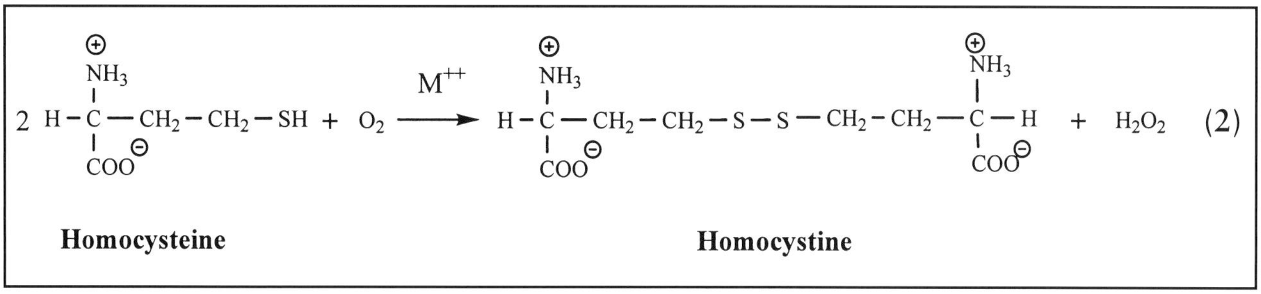

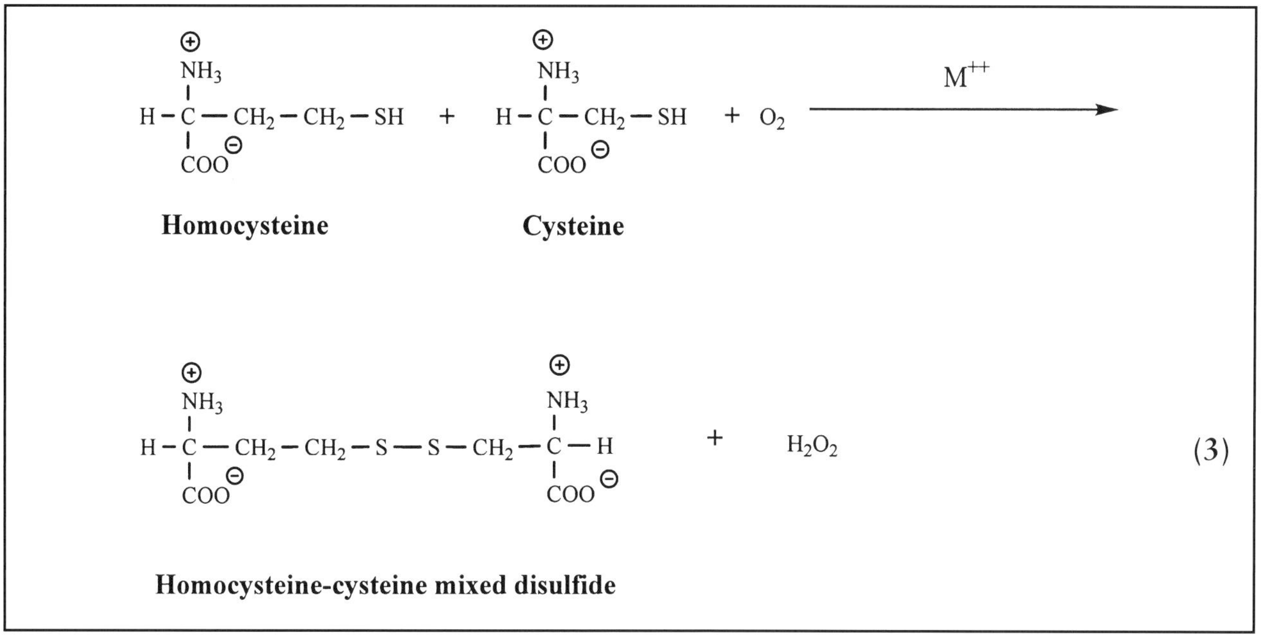

(1)

Homocysteine   **Homocysteine thiolate anion**

(2)

Homocysteine   **Homocystine**

(3)

Homocysteine   **Cysteine**

Homocysteine-cysteine mixed disulfide

approximately 0.1 μmol/L, of which 1% would be in the thiolate anion form, which is equivalent to 0.001 μmol/L (1 nmol/L). Even though the concentration of homocysteine thiolate anion is low at physiological pH, its increased nucleophilicity with respect to the cysteine thiolate anion is likely to result in enhanced thiol/disulfide exchange activity, as described later.

Autooxidation and Oxidation of Homocysteine

Biological and nonbiological thiols undergo autooxidation in the presence of molecular oxygen at physiological pH according to the general reaction $2\ RSH +$

$O_2 \leftrightarrows RSSR + H_2O_2$. The reaction is catalyzed by transition metals such as copper and cobalt, and the products include the disulfide plus hydrogen peroxide and other reactive oxygen species (7, 12, 28, 31, 42, 60). The autooxidation of homocysteine is shown in Reaction 2. Although the product homocystine has been detected in human serum (50) and human urine (45), its mechanism of formation in vivo, whether by autooxidation or by other mechanisms, is poorly understood. Homocysteine can also oxidize with other compounds containing sulfhydryl groups, such as free cysteine (Reaction 3) and proteins that have exposed cysteine residues (Reaction 4). With the use of conven-

Homocysteine + **Protein**—SH + O_2 $\xrightarrow{M^{++}}$

$$\text{H}-\overset{\overset{\oplus}{\text{NH}_3}}{\underset{\text{COO}^{\ominus}}{\text{C}}}-\text{CH}_2-\text{CH}_2-\text{SH} \;+\; \text{Protein}-\text{SH} \;+\; O_2$$

Protein-bound homocysteine

$$\text{Protein}-\text{S}-\text{S}-\text{CH}_2-\text{CH}_2-\overset{\overset{\oplus}{\text{NH}_3}}{\underset{\text{COO}^{\ominus}}{\text{C}}}-\text{H} \;+\; H_2O_2 \qquad (4)$$

Cysteinylglycine

$$2\;\;\overset{\oplus}{\text{NH}_3}-\overset{\overset{\text{H}}{|}}{\underset{\underset{\text{SH}}{\overset{|}{\text{CH}_2}}}{\text{C}}}-\overset{\overset{\text{O}}{\|}}{\text{C}}-\text{NH}-\text{CH}_2-\text{COO}^{\ominus} \;+\; O_2 \;\;\xrightarrow{M^{++}}$$

Cystinyl-*bis*-(diglycine)

$$\begin{array}{c}\overset{\oplus}{\text{NH}_3}-\overset{\overset{\text{H}}{|}}{\underset{\text{CH}_2}{\text{C}}}-\overset{\overset{\text{O}}{\|}}{\text{C}}-\text{NH}-\text{CH}_2-\text{COO}^{\ominus}\\ |\\ \text{S}\\ |\\ \text{S}\\ |\\ \overset{\oplus}{\text{NH}_3}-\underset{\text{H}}{\overset{\overset{\text{CH}_2}{|}}{\text{C}}}-\overset{\overset{\text{O}}{\|}}{\text{C}}-\text{NH}-\text{CH}_2-\text{COO}^{\ominus}\end{array} \;+\; H_2O_2 \qquad (5)$$

tional ion-exchange chromatography, homocysteine-cysteine mixed disulfide was one of the first forms of homocysteine detected in plasma from healthy donors (20, 59, 65). Homocysteine-cysteine mixed disulfide is also elevated in the plasma of patients with end-stage renal disease (57, 61, 66, 67). It was the first form of homocysteine identified in plasma from nonhomocystinuric patients as a possible risk factor for cardiovascular disease (68).

The autooxidation of cysteinylglycine in the circulation (Reaction 5) may explain the presence of cystinyl-*bis*-(diglycine) in human plasma (1, 51). Cysteinylglycine is produced during the metabolism of glutathione by membrane-bound γ-glutamyl transpeptidase (41).

The mechanisms of metal-catalyzed thiol autooxidation and oxidation reactions are complex, involving metal-thiol complexes, nucleophilic attack, and thiyl and oxygen radicals (23, 31). In the case of cobalamin and cobinamide-mediated thiol autooxidation, the mechanism probably involves the formation of a thiolate anion-cobalamin/cobinamide complex followed by the attack of a second thiolate anion to give a 2-electron reduced cobalamin/cobinamide and the disulfide (28). The reduced cobalamin/cobinamide is then oxidized by molecular oxygen yielding Co^{3+}-cobalamin/cobinamide and hydrogen peroxide. Evidence has also been obtained for the formation superoxide anion radical during cobalamin-catalyzed thiol oxidation (27).

Thiolate/Disulfide Exchange

The major form of homocysteine in the circulation, accounting for > 70% plasma total homocysteine, is covalently bound to protein cysteine residues as a mixed disulfide. Albumin, which contains 35 cysteine residues, 34 of which are in the form of intrachain disulfide bonds, appears to be a carrier of homocysteine in circulation (53). Human serum albumin contains a single free cysteine residue in the N-terminal portion of the molecule at position 34 (22). Cysteine and glutathione are carried as disulfides at this site on albumin (52).

During methionine (38) and homocysteine (21, 37) loading in healthy subjects, plasma protein-bound cysteine is displaced by homocysteine. The mechanism is likely to involve a thiolate/disulfide exchange reaction in which a homocysteine thiolate anion attacks protein-bound cysteine to form protein-bound homocysteine mixed disulfide and free cysteine thiolate anion (Reaction 6). Because the homocysteine thiolate anion has greater nucleophilicity than the cysteine thiolate anion, the equilibrium constant for the reaction favors the formation of protein-bound homocysteine. This is

apparently the case under physiological conditions since the predominate species of homocysteine in circulation is protein-bound mixed disulfide despite a relatively high concentration of free reduced cysteine (Table 2.1). In a series of model studies using purified human serum albumin–S_{34}-S-cysteine, L-homocysteine rapidly displaced protein-bound cysteine to form protein-bound homocysteine mixed disulfide (Sengupta, Chen, and Jacobsen, unpublished observations).

A significant fraction of circulating human serum albumin exists as mercaptalbumin (i.e., with a free sulfhydryl group at position Cys_{34}). At physiological pH, most of the Cys_{34} sulfur exists as a thiolate anion owing to its abnormally low pK_a (35, 49). Again in model studies using purified human mercaptalbumin, it can be shown that the albumin thiolate anion can attack homocystine (or homocysteine-cysteine mixed disulfide) to form protein-bound homocysteine (Reaction 7) (Sengupta, Chen, and Jacobsen, unpublished observations). Prior blockage of the albumin thiolate anion with N-ethylmaleimide prevented the formation of protein-bound homocysteine.

Thiolate/disulfide exchange can explain the formation of homocysteine-cysteine mixed disulfide as an alternative mechanism to trace-metal catalyzed oxidation (Reaction 3). In Reaction 8, homocysteine thiolate anion attacks cystine with the formation of the mixed disulfide and free cysteine thiolate anion.

Significance of Protein-bound Homocysteine

It is now well established that > 70% of the homocysteine in the plasma of healthy individuals and mildly hyperhomocysteinemic subjects circulates as a mixed disulfide with protein. This was first observed in homocystinuric patients (33, 36), normal individuals (33), and patients receiving hemodialysis for end-stage-renal disease (32). It was reported that obligate heterozygotes for cystathionine β-synthase deficiency had higher concentrations of protein-bound homocysteine than normal individuals (58), but there was too much overlap between normal subjects and heterozygotes to be of diagnostic value. In homocystinuric patients, with much larger fractions of free reduced homocysteine, the concentration of protein-bound cysteine is greatly reduced compared with that in normal individuals (36, 40).

When plasma or serum is stored frozen for prolonged periods, the fractions of free reduced homocysteine and free oxidized species decrease and become protein-bound via disulfide linkages. Because current assays for plasma total homocysteine use reducing agents to break disulfide bonds (see Chapter 18), all forms of homocysteine, except possible trace amounts of homocystamide, are determined.

As discussed in Chapter 35, the forms of homocysteine that may be atherogenic have not been identified. Thus, a mechanistic understanding of the formation of homocysteine, homocysteine-cysteine mixed disulfide, and protein-bound homocysteine mixed disulfide remains an important issue. In addition, approximately 66% of the total exchangeable albumin pool resides outside the arteriovenous circulatory system in the extravascular space. The transport of homocysteine between the vascular and extravascular spaces and the effect that it might have on nonvascular cells and tissues are largely unknown. Chemistry will eventually provide us with an understanding of why homocysteine is a major independent risk factor for cardiovascular disease.

REFERENCES

1. Armstrong, MD. The occurrence of cystinylglycine in blood plasma. *Biochim Biophys Acta* 1979; 584: 542–44.
2. Baernstein HD. A modification of the method for determining methionine in proteins. *J Biol Chem* 1934; 106: 451–56.
3. Benesch, RE, Benesch, R. The acid strength of the -SH group in cysteine and related compounds. *J Am Chem Soc* 1955; 77: 5877–81.
4. Bostom, AG, Lathrop, L. Hyperhomocysteinemia in end-stage renal disease: Prevalence, etiology, and potential

relationship to arteriosclerotic outcomes. *Kidney Int* 1997; 52: 10–20.

5. Butz, LW, du Vigneaud, V. The formation of a homologue of cystine by the decomposition of methionine with sulfuric acid. *J Biol Chem* 1932; 99: 135–42.

6. Cattaneo, M. Hyperhomocysteinemia, atherosclerosis and thrombosis. *Thromb Haemost* 1999; 81: 165–76.

7. Cavallini, D, De Marco, C, Dupre, S, Rotilio, G. The copper catalyzed oxidation of cysteine to cystine. *Arch Biochem Biophys* 1969; 130: 354–61.

8. Clarke, R, Smith, AD, Jobst, KA, Refsum, H, Sutton, L, Ueland, PM. Folate, vitamin B_{12}, and serum total homocysteine levels in confirmed Alzheimer disease. *Arch Neurol* 1998; 55: 1449–55.

9. Clarke, R, Woodhouse, P, Ulvik, A, Frost, C, Sherliker, P, Refsum, H, Ueland, PM, Khaw, KT. Variability and determinants of total homocysteine concentrations in plasma in an elderly population. *Clin Chem* 1998; 44: 102–07.

10. Cotton, FA, Wilkinson, G, Murillo, CA, Bochmann, M. *Advanced Inorganic Chemistry.* John Wiley and Sons, Inc., New York, 1999.

11. Danehy, JP, Noel, CJ. The relative nucleophilic character of several mercaptans toward ethylene oxide. *J Am Chem Soc* 1960; 82: 2511–15.

12. De Marco, C, Dupre, S, Crifo, C, Rotilio, G, Cavallini, D. Copper-catalyzed oxidation of thiomalic acid. *Arch Biochem Biophys* 1971; 144: 496–502.

13. Dennis, VW, Robinson, K. Homocysteinemia and vascular disease in end-stage renal disease. *Kidney Int* 1996; 50 Suppl. 57: S11–S17.

14. du Vigneaud, V, Patterson, WI, Hunt, M. Opening of the ring of the thiolactone of homocysteine. *J Biol Chem* 1938; 126: 217–31.

15. Dudman, NPB, Hicks, C, Lynch, JF, Wilcken, DEL, Wang, J. Homocysteine thiolactone disposal by human arterial endothelial cells and serum in vitro. *Arterioscler Thromb* 1991; 11: 663–70.

16. Eskes, TKAB. Open or closed? A world of difference: A history of homocysteine research. *Nutr Rev* 1998; 56: 236–44.

17. Faure-Delanef, L, Quéré, I, Chasse, JF, Guerassimenko, O, Lesaulnier, M, Bellet, H, Zittoun, J, Kamoun, P, Cohen, D. Methylenetetrahydrofolate reductase thermolabile variant and human longevity. *Am J Hum Genet* 1997; 60: 999–1001.

18. Friedman, M, Cavins, JF, Wall, JS. Relative nucleophilic reactivities of amino groups and mercaptide ions in addition to reactions with *a,b*-unsaturated compounds. *J Am Chem Soc* 1965; 87: 3672–82.

19. Friedman, M. *The Chemistry and Biochemistry of the Sulfhydryl Group in Amino Acids, Peptides and Proteins.* Pergamon Press, New York, 1973.

20. Gupta, VJ, Wilcken, DEL. The detection of cysteine-homocysteine mixed disulphide in plasma of normal fasting man. *Eur J Clin Invest* 1978; 8: 205–7.

21. Guttormsen, AB, Mansoor, AM, Fiskerstrand, T, Ueland, PM, Refsum, H. Kinetics of plasma homocysteine in healthy subjects after peroral homocysteine loading. *Clin Chem* 1993; 39: 1390–97.

22. He, XM, Carter, DC. Atomic structure and chemistry of human serum albumin. *Nature* 1992; 358: 209–15.

23. Hogg, N. The effect of cyst(e)ine on the auto-oxidation of homocysteine. *Free Radic Biol Med* 1999; 27: 28–33.

24. Hongsprabhas, P, Saboohi, F, Aranda, JV, Bardin, CL, Kovacs, LB, Papageorgiou, AN, Hoffer, LJ. Plasma homocysteine concentrations of preterm infants. *Biol Neonate* 1999; 76: 65–71.

25. Hussein, WI, Green, R, Jacobsen, DW, Faiman, C. Normalization of hyperhomocysteinemia with L-thyroxine in hypothyroidism. *Ann Intern Med* 1999; 131: 348–51.

26. Huxtable, RJ. *Biochemistry of Sulfur.* Plenum Press, New York, 1986,

27. Jacobsen, DW, Pezacka, EH, Brown, KL. The inhibition of corrinoid-catalyzed oxidation of mercaptoethanol by methyl iodide: Mechanistic implications. *J Inorg Biochem* 1993; 50: 47–63.

28. Jacobsen, DW, Troxell, LS, Brown, KL. Catalysis of thiol oxidation by cobalamins and cobinamides: Reaction products and kinetics. *Biochemistry* 1984; 23: 2017–25.

29. Jakoby, WB, Griffith, OW (eds.). *Methods in Enzymology,* Vol. 143. *Sulfur and Sulfur Amino Acids.* Academic Press, Inc., San Diego, 1987.

29a. Jakubowski, H. Calcium-dependent human serum homocysteine thiolactone hydrolase – A protective mechanism against protein N-homocysteinylation. *J Biol. Chem.,* 2000; 275: 3957–3962.

30. Jocelyn, PC. *Biochemistry of the SH Group.* Academic Press, New York, 1972.

31. Kachur AV, Koch CJ, Biaglow JE. Mechanism of copper-catalyzed autoxidation of cysteine. *Free Radic Res* 1999; 31: 23–34.

32. Kang, S-S, Wong, PVK, Bidani, A, Milanez, S. Plasma protein-bound homocyst(e)ine in patients requiring chronic haemodialysis. *Clin Sci* 1983; 65: 335–36.

33. Kang, S-S, Wong, PWK, Becker, N. Protein-bound homocyst(e)ine in normal subjects and in patients with homocystinuria. *Pediatr Res* 1979; 13: 1141–43.

34. Lehmann, M, Gottfries, CG, Regland, B. Identification of cognitive impairment in the elderly: Homocysteine is an early marker. *Dementia* 1999; 10: 12–20.

35. Lewis, SD, Misra, DC, Shafer, JA. Preparation and properties of serum and plasma proteins. XXX. Crystalline derivatives of human serum albumin and of certain other proteins. *Biochemistry* 1980; 19: 6129–37.

36. Malloy, MH, Rassin, DK, Gaull, GE. Plasma cysteine in homocysteinemia. *Am J Clin Nutr* 1981; 34: 2619–21.

37. Mansoor, MA, Guttormsen, AB, Fiskerstrand, T, Refsum, H, Ueland, PM, Svardal, AM. Redox status and protein binding of plasma aminothiols during the transient hyperhomocysteinemia that follows homocysteine administration. *Clin Chem* 1993; 39: 980–85.

38. Mansoor, MA, Svardal, AM, Schneede, J, Ueland, PM. Dynamic relation between reduced, oxidized, and protein-bound homocysteine and other thiol components in plasma during methionine loading in healthy men. *Clin Chem* 1992; 38: 1316–21.

39. Mansoor, MA, Svardal, AM, Ueland, PM. Determination of the in vivo redox status of cysteine, cysteinylglycine, homocysteine, and glutathione in human plasma. *Anal Biochem* 1992; 200: 218–29.

40. Mansoor, MA, Ueland, PM, Aarsland, A, Svardal, AM. Redox status and protein binding of plasma homocysteine and other aminothiols in patients with homocystinuria. *Metabolism* 1993; 42: 1481–85.

41. Meister, A. Glutathione metabolism. *Methods Enzymol* 1995; 251: 3–7.

42. Misra, HP. Generation of superoxide free radical during the autoxidation of thiols. *J Biol Chem* 1974; 249: 2151–55.

43. Mudd, SH, Finkelstein, JD, Irreverre, F, Laster, L. Transsulfuration in mammals. Microassays and tissue distribution of three enzymes of the pathway. *J Biol Chem* 1965; 240: 4382–92.

44. Mudd, SH, Levy, HL. Plasma homocyst(e)ine or homocysteine? *N Engl J Med* 1995; 333: 325.

45. Mudd, SH, Levy, HL, Skovby, F. Disorders of transsulfuration. In *The Metabolic and Molecular Bases of Inherited Disease* (Scriver, CR, Beaudet, AL, Sly, WS, Valle, D (eds.). McGraw-Hill, Inc, New York, 1995; pp. 1279–1327.

45a. Mudd, SH, Finkelstein, JD, Refsum, H, Ueland, PM, Malinow, MR, Lentz, SR, Jacobsen, DW, Brattström, L, Wilcken, B, Wilcken, DEL, Blom, HJ, Stabler, SP, Allen, RH, Selhub, J, and Rosenberg, IH. Homocysteine and its disulfide derivatives. A suggested consensus terminology. *Arterioscler. Thromb. Vasc. Biol.,* 2000; 20: 1704–1706.

46. Nedrebo, BG, Ericsson, UB, Nygård, O, Refsum, H, Ueland, PM, Aakvaag, A, Aanderud, S, Lien, EA. Plasma total homocysteine levels in hyperthyroid and hypothyroid patients. *Metabolism* 1998; 47: 89–93.

47. Packer, L (ed.). *Methods in Enzymology,* Vol. 252. *Biothiols.* Part B. *Glutathione and Thioredoxin: Thiols in Signal Transduction and Gene Regulation.* Academic Press, Inc., San Diego, 1995.

48. Packer, L (ed). *Methods in Enzymology,* Vol. 251. *Biothiols,* Part A. *Monothiols and Dithiols, Protein Thiols, and Thiyl Radicals.* Academic Press, Inc., San Diego, 1995.

49. Pedersen, AO, Jacobsen, J. Reactivity of the thiol group in human and bovine albumin at pH 3–9, as measured by exchange with 2,2′-dithiodipyridine. *Eur J Biochem* 1980; 106: 291–95.

50. Perry TL, Hansen, S. Technical pitfalls leading to errors in the quantitation of plasma amino acids. *Clin Chim Acta* 1969; 25: 53–8.

51. Perry, TL, Hansen, S. Cystinylglycine in plasma: Diagnostic relevance for pyroglutamic acidemia, homocystinuria, and phenylketonuria. *Clin Chim Acta* 1981; 117: 7–12.

52. Peters T Jr. Serum albumin. *Adv Protein Chem* 1985; 37: 161–245.

53. Refsum, H, Helland, S, Ueland, PM. Radioenzymic determination of homocysteine in plasma and urine. *Clin Chem* 1985; 31: 624–28.

54. Refsum, H, Ueland, P, Nygård, O, Vollset, SE. Homocysteine and cardiovascular disease. *Annu Rev Med* 1998; 49: 31–62.

55. Refsum, H, Wesenberg, F, Ueland, PM. Plasma homocysteine in children with acute lymphoblastic leukemia: Changes during a chemotherapeutic regimen including methotrexate. *Cancer Res* 1991; 51: 828–35.

56. Riegel, B, du Vigneaud, V. The isolation of homocysteine and its conversion to a thiolactone. *J Biol Chem* 1935; 112: 149–54.

57. Robins, AJ, Milewczyk, BK, Booth, EM, Mallick, NP. Plasma amino acid abnormalities in chronic renal failure. *Clin Chim Acta* 1972; 42: 215–17.

58. Sartorio, R, Carrozzo, R, Corbo, L, Andria, G. Protein-bound plasma homocyt(e)ine and identification of heterozygotes for cystathionine-synthase deficiency. *J Inherit Metab Dis* 1986; 9: 25–9.

59. Schneider, JA, Bradley, KH, Seegmiller, JE. Identification and measurement of cysteine-homocysteine mixed disulfide in plasma. *J Lab Clin Med* 1968; 71: 122–125.

60. Slater, EC. Role of sulphydryl groups in the oxidation of pyruvate. *Nature* 1952; 170: 970–971.

61. Smolin, LA, Laidlaw, SA, Kopple, JD. Altered plasma free and protein-bound sulfur amino acid levels in patients undergoing maintenance hemodialysis. *Am J Clin Nutr* 1987; 45: 737–43.

62. Tonstad, S, Refsum, H, Ueland, PM. Association between plasma total homocysteine and parental history of cardiovascular disease in children with familial hypercholesterolemia. *Circulation* 1997; 96: 1803–08.

63. VanAerts, LAGJM, Blom, HJ, Deabreu, RA, Trijbels, FJM, Eskes, TKAB, Peereboom-Stegeman, JHJC, Noordhoek, J. Prevention of neural tube defects by and toxicity of L-homocysteine in cultured postimplantation rat embryos. *Teratology* 1994; 50: 348–60.

64. Vilaseca MA, Moyano, D, Ferrer, I, Artuch, R. Total homocysteine in pediatric patients. *Clin Chem* 1997; 43: 690–92.

65. Wilcken, DEL, Gupta, VJ. Cysteine-homocysteine mixed disulphide: Differing plasma concentrations in normal men and women. *Clin Sci* 1979; 57: 211–15.

66. Wilcken, DEL, Gupta, VJ. Sulphur containing amino acids in chronic renal failure with particular reference to homocystine and cysteine-homocysteine mixed disulphide. *Eur J Clin Invest* 1979; 9: 301–7.

67. Wilcken, DEL, Gupta, VJ, Reddy, SG. Accumulation of sulphur-containing amino acids including cysteine-homocysteine in patients on maintenance haemodialysis. *Clin Sci* 1980; 58: 427–30.

68. Wilcken, DEL, Wilcken, B. The pathogenesis of coronary artery disease; A possible role for methionine metabolism. *J Clin Invest* 1976; 57: 1079–82.

69. Zahler, WL, Cleland, WW. A specific and sensitive assay for disulfides. *J Biol Chem* 1968; 243: 716–19.

3

Biosynthesis and Reactions of Homocysteine Thiolactone

HIERONIM JAKUBOWSKI

Although homocysteine thiolactone was obtained by chemical synthesis in the 1930s, the first indication of its biological significance came almost 50 years later with the discovery of the enzymatic conversion of homocysteine (Hcy) to homocysteine thiolactone in error editing reactions of some aminoacyl-tRNA synthetases (AARSs) (reviewed in [21, 23, 28]). The nonprotein amino acid homocysteine is misactivated by several AARSs and forms an AARS-bound homocysteinyl~adenosine monophosphate (homocysteinyl~AMP). Subsequent rejection of the homocysteinyl~AMP intermediate involves an intramolecular reaction in which the side chain thiolate of homocysteine displaces the AMP group from the activated homocysteine, forming thiolactone as a product. The energy of the anhydride bond of homocysteinyl~AMP is conserved in an intramolecular thioester bond of homocysteine thiolactone. Consequently, homocysteine thiolactone is chemically reactive and easily acylates any free amino groups, such as side chain lysine groups in proteins. Thiolactone is present in all cell types examined from bacterial to human, and its synthesis is greatly enhanced under conditions of elevated homocysteine levels. Specific calcium-dependent homocysteine thiolactonase, a component of high-density lipoproteins, is involved in detoxification of homocysteine thiolactone in human serum.

Chemical Synthesis and Properties of Homocysteine Thiolactone

Homocysteine thiolactone is an intramolecular thioester of homocysteine. The thiolactone is prepared by boiling either 1) homocysteine for 10 minutes with 6 N HCl (37) (Reaction 1), or (2) methionine for 4 hours with hydriodic acid (2) (Reaction 2).

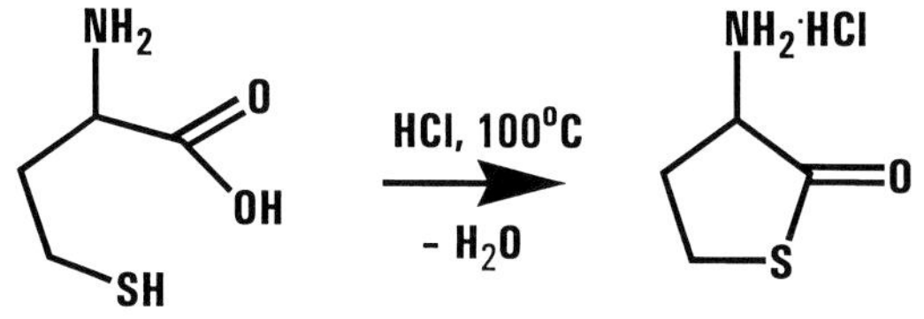

(1)

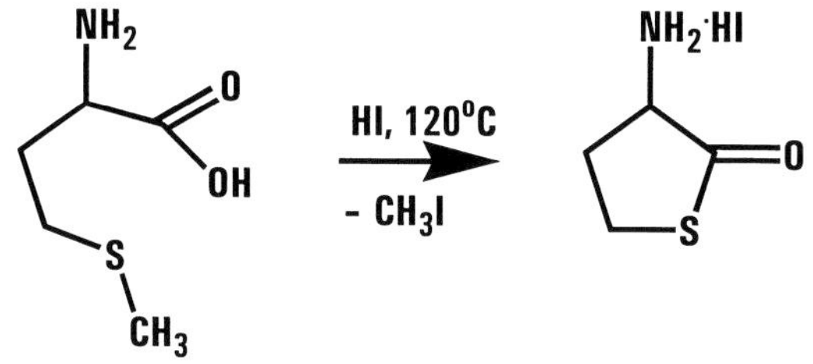

(2)

The hydrochloric acid salt of thiolactone is stable indefinitely at room temperature. Under physiological conditions (pH 7.4, 37°C), homocysteine thiolactone (half-life of ~25 h, refs. 5, 19) is more stable than intermolecular aminoacyl-thioesters (e.g., methionyl-S-CoA hydrolyzes with a half life of 2.2 h, ref. 22). In 0.1 mol/L NaOH, hydrolysis of the thiolactone is completed in 15 min at room temperature (19). Like all thioesters (36), homocysteine thiolactone absorbs ultraviolet light with a maximum at 240 nm and ε = 3,500 $M^{-1}cm^{-1}$ in water (16). The pK_a of its amino group is unusually low at 7.1 (1). Thus, under physiological conditions, the thiolactone is neutral and freely diffuses through cell membranes (10, 14–16, 19, 30).

Biological Formation of Homocysteine Thiolactone

Aminoacyl-tRNA Synthetases Convert Homocysteine to Thiolactone

The nonprotein amino acid homocysteine, an obligatory precursor of methionine in all cells, poses an accuracy problem for the protein biosynthetic apparatus (21, 23, 28). Several AARSs, such as MetRS, IleRS, LeuRS, ValRS, and LysRS, misactivate homocysteine and form an AARS-bound homocysteinyl~AMP according to Reaction 3 (Table 3.1).

Ralph Carmel and Donald W. Jacobsen, eds. *Homocysteine in Health and Disease*.
Printed in the United States of America.

$$\text{AARS} + \text{Hcy} + \text{ATP} \Leftrightarrow \text{AARS} \bullet \text{Hcy}{\sim}\text{AMP} + \text{PPi} \quad (3)$$
$$\downarrow$$
$$\text{Hcy thiolactone}$$

However, misactivated homocysteine is not transferred to tRNA by any of these enzymes (9, 22, 23). Instead, Hcy~AMP is efficiently rejected or edited (23, 24, 28) (Table 3.1) as indicated by the side reaction in equation 3. Editing of Hcy~AMP involves an intramolecular reaction in which the side chain thiolate of homocysteine displaces the AMP group from the carboxylate of the activated homocysteine, forming thiolactone as a product (Reaction 4). The energy of the anhydride bond of Hcy~AMP is conserved in an intramolecular thioester bond of homocysteine thiolactone. Consequently, homocysteine thiolactone is chemically reactive and easily acylates any nucleophile (e.g., side chain amino groups of protein lysine residues) (19, 25, 27).

(4)

The formation of homocysteine thiolactone is abolished by the presence of an excess of a cognate amino acid (20, 28). This suggests that homocysteine thiolactone is synthesized at the site that catalyzes the aminoacylation of tRNA with a cognate amino acid. The ratio of AMP to thiolactone formed during homocysteine editing by AARSs is 1.0, which indicates that there is no hydrolysis of Hcy~AMP to homocysteine + AMP (20). The formation of homocysteine thiolactone occurs on the enzyme and is mediated by a thiol-binding subsite to which the side chain of homocysteine binds (17, 18, 20, 24). Because homocysteine thiolactone forms at the active site of MetRS, the synthesis of the thiolactone increases with an increase in the homocysteine/methionine ratio.

Synthesis of Homocysteine Thiolactone is Governed by the Competition Between Homocysteine and Methionine for the Active Site of MetRS

Because homocysteine thiolactone is formed at the active site of an AARS (17, 18, 20, 24, 28, 32), specificity of an AARS is a major determinant of its formation. A biologically relevant definition of specificity refers to the discrimination between a cognate amino acid and homocysteine (Table 3.1) in a mixture of the two substrates (8). For example, specificity of MetRS refers to the discrimination between the cognate methionine and a noncognate homocysteine in a mixture of methionine and homocysteine,

as is the case in vivo. Specificity is a function of both substrate binding (K_m) and catalytic rate (k_{cat}). If methionine and homocysteine compete for MetRS, then the rates, v, of methionine and homocysteine activation are:

$$\text{d}[\text{Met}]/\text{d}t = v_{\text{Met}} = (k_{cat}/K_m)_{\text{Met}}[\text{MetRS}][\text{Met}]$$

$$\text{d}[\text{Hcy}]/\text{d}t = v_{\text{Hcy}} = (k_{cat}/K_m)_{\text{Hcy}}[\text{MetRS}][\text{Hcy}]$$

and the specificity is

$$v_{\text{Met}}/v_{\text{Hcy}} = (k_{cat}/K_m)_{\text{Met}}[\text{Met}]/(k_{cat}/K_m)_{\text{Hcy}}[\text{Hcy}].$$

Thus, specificity of MetRS, in the sense of discrimination between methionine and homocysteine, is determined by the ratios of k_{cat}/K_m and of concentrations of methionine [Met] and homocysteine [Hcy]. Competition between methionine and homocysteine for the active site of MetRS occurs in vivo; the synthesis of homocysteine thiolactone increases with an increase in the [Hcy]/[Met] ratio (10, 14–16, 19, 30, 31).

Homocysteine Thiolactone Formation Occurs at the Active Site of MetRS

A fundamental question is how the structure of the active site of an AARS determines the accuracy of the aminoacylation reaction and prevents incorporation of homocysteine to tRNA. Are the synthetic and editing sites physically separated, or are they subsites of a single active site? What structural elements are responsible for editing of homocysteine? What are the features of the active site that prevent a cognate amino acid, such as methionine, from being edited and a noncognate substrate, such as homocysteine, from becoming attached to tRNA? Two powerful techniques, namely, crystallography and site-directed mutagenesis, are being used to answer these questions.

Editing is triggered by weak interactions of the side chain of a misactivated homocysteine with the specificity pocket of the active site. This has been demonstrated with bacterial MetRS (17, 32). IleRS and ValRS also use a similar editing mechanism for rejecting homocysteine and cysteine (18). The active site of MetRS directs methionine and homocysteine into the synthetic and editing pathways, respectively, by employing three subsites (Figure 3.1):

1. A subsite containing Asp52 and Arg233, which bind α-amino and carboxyl groups, respectively, of the amino acid substrates
2. The specificity subsite, containing Trp305, Phe197, and Tyr15, which preferentially binds the side chain of the cognate substrate methionine

Table 3.1.   Misactivation of Homocysteine and Synthesis of Homocysteine Thiolactone by *E. coli* Aminoacyl-tRNA Synthetases (AARSs)

| AARS | Misactivation of Homocysteine | | | Homocysteine Thiolactone Synthesis |
	k_{cat} (S^{-1})	K_m (mmol/L)	Selectivity[a]	k_{cat} (S^{-1})
MetRS[b]	87	5.2	0.0054	1.2
IleRS[b]	14	1.5	0.0025	1.5
LeuRS[c]	6	2.1	0.0083	2.0
ValRS[b]	1.6	10	0.0002	0.2
LysRS[d]				1.2

[a] Selectivity is a relative rate of activation of homocysteine versus a cognate amino acid. It is derived from a catalytic efficiency (k_{cat}/K_m) for homocysteine divided by catalytic efficiency for a cognate amino acid in the ATP/PP$_i$ exchange reaction (28).
[b] Data from Jakubowski and Fersht (28).
[c] Data from Englisch et al. (6).
[d] Data from Jakubowski (20).

3. The thiol-binding subsite, which interacts specifically with the side chain thiol of homocysteine.

In the synthetic pathway, intermolecular reaction of the activated carboxyl group of methionine with the 2′-hydroxyl of the terminal adenosine of tRNA^{Met} yields Met-tRNA^{Met}. In the editing pathway, intramolecular reaction of the activated carboxyl group of homocysteine with the sulfur of its side chain yields homocysteine thiolactone (Reaction 4).

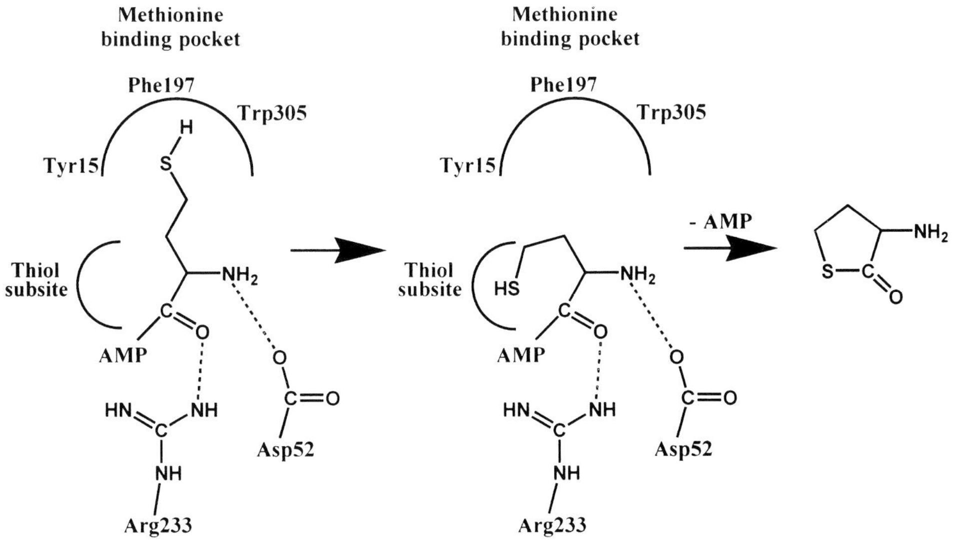

Fig. 3.1.   Editing of homocysteine by MetRS. (Adapted from Jakubowski [17, 18, 23] and Kim et al. [30].) The MetRS-catalyzed cyclization of homocysteinyl~AMP to form homocysteine thiolactone and AMP, which are subsequently released from the synthetic/editing active site of MetRS, is shown. (Reproduced from Jakubowski [24], with permission.)

Whether an amino acid completes the synthetic or editing pathway is determined by the competition for its activated carboxyl group between the side chain of the amino acid and the terminal adenosine of tRNA^{Met}. Methionine completes the synthetic pathway because its side chain is firmly bound in the active site by hydrophobic and hydrogen bonding interactions with Trp305 and Tyr15, respectively, preventing the sulfur atom of methionine from competing with the 3′-terminal adenosine of tRNA^{Met} for the carboxyl carbon of methionine. Consistent with these functions, side chains of Trp305 and Tyr15 are located on opposite sides of the cavity forming a putative methionine binding pocket observed in the crystallographic structure of MetRS (32). The side chain of homocysteine, missing the methyl group of methionine, cannot interact with Trp305, Phe197, and Tyr15 as strongly as the side chain of methionine does. Therefore, the activated carboxyl of homocysteine reacts intramolecularly with the side chain of homocysteine (Figure 3.1), instead of reacting intermolecularly with the 3′-terminal adenosine of tRNA^Met. This reaction is facilitated by specific binding of the side chain of homocysteine to the thiol-binding subsite. Because intramolecular reactions are more favored than intermolecular reactions, homocysteine is not transferred to tRNA but is cyclized to homocysteine thiolactone. The editing pathway is a default pathway. As expected from this model, methionine enters the editing pathway when its side chain cannot firmly bind to the specificity subsite, as is the case with W305A, Y15F, and Y15A MetRS mutants. Met can also enter the editing pathway when the thiol subsite is occupied by a thiol mimicking the side chain of homocysteine. Residues Arg233 and Asp52 of MetRS, essential for catalysis of the synthetic reaction, are also involved in catalysis of editing.

Homocysteine Thiolactone is Synthesized in vivo by MetRS

A simple two-dimensional thin layer chromatographic system separates homocysteine thiolactone from other cellular sulfur-containing compounds present in [^35S] labeled cell cultures (14). Because homocysteine thiolactone absorbs ultraviolet light with a maximum at 240 nm, it is possible to follow the formation of homocysteine thiolactone in cultures (incubated with homocysteine) by spectrometry (10, 16). These two assays, combined with other biochemical and genetic approaches, demonstrated that in all cell types examined, homocysteine is metabolized to homocysteine thiolactone by MetRS. IleRS and LeuRS can also convert homocysteine to the thiolactone in vivo under some conditions (14) (Figure 3.2).

Homocysteine thiolactone is a component of sulfur amino acid pools in cultured human endothelial cells (31) (Table 3.2). Homocysteine thiolactone is also synthesized by human fibroblasts (19), breast cancer cells (19) (Table 3.3), HeLa cells, and normal BALB/c 3T3 and transformed RAG mouse cells (30). Genetic evidence indicates that MetRS is involved in synthesis of homocysteine thiolactone in Chinese hamster ovary cells (30). Because of its mostly neutral character at physiological pH (pK_a of homocysteine thiolactone is 7.1 [1]), the thiolactone accumulates in culture medium.

Homocysteine thiolactone is also a component of sulfur amino acid pools in *Escherichia coli* and the yeast *Saccharomyces cerevisiae* (Table 3.2); however, most of the thiolactone (> 99%) accumulates in culture medium. Microbial synthesis of homocysteine thiolactone from endogenous homocysteine in vivo is inhibited by methionine, but not by any other amino acid (14,

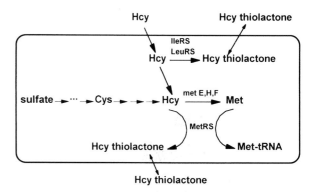

Fig. 3.2. Channeling of homocysteine (Hcy) in *Escherichia coli*. Exogenous homocysteine (supplied in the media) is edited by MetRS, IleRS, and LeuRS (16, 24). Endogenous homocysteine (produced from sulfate in the methionine biosynthetic pathway) is edited exclusively by MetRS (14). (Reproduced from Jakubowski [24], with permission.)

15); the in vitro synthesis of the thiolactone by bacterial MetRS is also specifically inhibited by methionine (28). In the yeast *S. cerevisiae,* both cytoplasmic (15) and mitochondrial MetRSs (Fasiolo and Jakubowski, unpublished data) convert homocysteine to thiolactone.

MetRS mutants defective in the methionine binding site of the enzyme, in *E. coli* (14), yeast (15), and Chinese hamster ovary cells (30), are also defective in homocysteine thiolactone synthesis. In addition, overproduction of MetRS in *E. coli* and yeast leads to proportional overproduction of the thiolactone. These observations demonstrate that MetRS is responsible for thiolactone synthesis from endogenous homocysteine, in all cell types. In fact, it is unlikely that any other enzyme makes the thiolactone from endogenous homocysteine in vivo. The C-terminal domain of MetRS is essential for editing of endogenous homocysteine (10), most likely by allowing interaction of MetRS with a component of the methionine biosynthetic pathway. Thus, any fraction of cellular homocysteine that cannot be metabolized to methionine is channeled to MetRS for editing.

In cultures of *E. coli,* exogenous homocysteine (taken up from the medium) is metabolized to the thiolactone by two other synthetases, IleRS and LeuRS, in addition to MetRS (16) (Figure 3.2). This indicates that the extent of homocysteine editing in bacterial cells is governed by compartmentation or channeling of homocysteine (Figure 3.2), an important factor in maintaining accuracy of amino acid selection by AARSs in vivo (16). Because the three AARSs contribute about equally to metabolic conversion of exogenous homocysteine to thiolactone in *E. coli,* the synthesis of thiolactone from exogenous homocysteine is only partially inhibited by either methionine, isoleucine, or leucine; complete inhibition is observed

Table 3.2.   Intracellular Levels of Homocysteine Thiolactone, Homocysteine, and Methionine in Various Cells

Organism	Intracellular Concentration (pmol/10^7 cells)		
	Thiolactone	Homocysteine	Methionine
E. coli[a]			
Wild type	0.12	0.66	0.49
metE(MS$^-$)	0.42	0.10	<0.01
metG146(MetRS$^-$)	0.04	1.12	0.26
S. cerevisiae[b]			
Wild type	<0.3	<4	80
cys2cys4(CBS$^-$)	40	275	92
met6(MS$^-$)	175	360	0
mes1 (MetRS$^-$)	<0.3	2	87
met6mes1	<2	65	0
Homo sapiens			
Endothelial cells[c]			
5 µmol/L Met	5	30	160
5 µmol/L Met + 10 µmol/L folic acid	<1	<6	150
2 µmol/L Hcy	<5	84 (170)	23 (2,000)
8 µmol/L Hcy	25	520 (760)	75 (5,600)
8 µmol/L Hcy + 10 µmol/L folic acid	<1	260 (2.0)	280 (52,000)

[a] Data from Jakubowski (14).
[b] Data from Jakubowski (15).
[c] Data from Jakubowski et al. (31) Human umbilical vein endothelial cells grown to confluence in M199 medium supplemented with 15% fetal bovine serum, endothelial cells growth factor, heparin, and antibiotics were labeled with [^{35}S]methionine or [^{35}S]homocysteine for 24 hours in the presence of methionine-free M199 medium supplemented with dialyzed 15% fetal bovine serum, endothelial cells growth factor, and heparin. The M199 medium contains physiological levels (27 nmol/L) of folic acid. Values in parentheses indicate cellular levels of protein-Hcy or protein-Met. Protein-Hcy and protein-Met denote homocysteine and methionine, respectively, recovered after acid hydrolysis of dithiothreitol-treated proteins.

only when methionine, isoleucine, and leucine are added together to bacterial cultures.

Elevation of Homocysteine Levels Leads to Enhanced Synthesis of Thiolactone

Under normal metabolic conditions, synthesis of homocysteine thiolactone is low because intracellular concentrations of homocysteine are relatively low (Table 3.2). However, the synthesis of homocysteine thiolactone is enhanced when homocysteine levels are increased owing to reduction in its transmethylation and/or transsulfuration (Figure 3.3; see also Metabolic Diagram). For example, methionine synthase mutants of *E. coli* (14) and yeast (15), cystathionine β-synthatse mutants of yeast (15) and human fibroblasts (19), as well as normal human fibroblasts (19) and endothelial cells (27, 31) maintained in folic acid-limited medium accumulate homocysteine and synthesize large amounts of thiolactone. Millimolar concentrations of the thiolactone are produced in cultures of methionine synthase mutants of *E. coli* and yeast maintained on homocysteine. As much as 60% of the metabolized homocysteine is converted into thiolactone in cultures of human vascular endothelial cells maintained on homocysteine in methionine-free

M199 medium (Table 3.3). Endothelial cells synthesize high levels of homocysteine thiolactone because physiological levels of folic acid (27 nmol/L) present in M199 medium are not sufficient to support transmethylation of homocysteine to methionine by methionine synthase (see Metabolic Diagram) in these cells (31). Supplementation of M199 media with 30 nmol/L 5-methyltetrahydrofolate, a main form of folate in blood, is also insufficient to support transmethylation of homocysteine to methionine (41). Because of this, homocysteine does not support growth of endothelial cells in methionine-free media (Jakubowski, unpublished data).

Metabolism of Homocysteine Thiolactone in Human Cell Cultures and Serum

Homocysteine thiolactone undergoes two major reactions in human cells and serum in vitro: protein homocysteinylation at lysine residues (19, 25–27) and enzymatic hydrolysis to homocysteine (4, 19, 25–27) by calcium-dependent homocysteine thiolactonase, a component of high-density lipoprotein (26, 27) (Figure 3.3). Homocysteine produced in serum by enzymatic hydrolysis of the thiolactone forms a serum albumin-S-S-homocysteine adduct (Figure 3.4B); free homocysteine is

Table 3.3.   Metabolic Conversion of Endogenous and Exogenous Homocysteine into Thiolactone in Various Organisms[a]

Organism	Endogenous Hcy → Thiolactone (%)	Exogenous Hcy → Thiolactone (%)
E. coli[b]		
wild type (strain K38)	1.0	15
metE (MS⁻)	100	100
S. cerevisae[b]		
wild type (strain S288C)	0.2	0.6
met6 (MS⁻)	70	79
cys2cys4 (CBS⁻)	13	34
Homo sapiens[c]		
endothelial cells[d]	36	63
+ μmol/L folic acid	<0.3	
normal fibroblasts (GM1126)[e]	0.2	
+ aminopterin	2.7	
CBS⁻ fibroblasts (GM1128)[e]	0.7	0.2
+ aminopterin	10	0.6
breast cancer (HTB132)[e]	2	5
+ aminopterin	16	44

[a] Endogenous homocysteine (Hcy) is made in the methionine biosynthetic pathway. Exogenous homocysteine is supplied to culture media. Each number represents % metabolized homocysteine that was recovered as the thiolactone. For example, in endothelial cells incubated with exogenous homocysteine, 63% of metabolized homocysteine was recovered as thiolactone.

[b] Data from Jakubowski (14, 15). Microorganisms were grown on minimal media. The precursor of endogenous homocysteine is sulfate.

[c] Methionine is a precursor of endogenous homocysteine. 90% of methionine is incorporated directly into proteins and 10% is converted to endogenous homocysteine which can be subsequently remethylated to methionine or converted to homocysteine thiolactone.

[d] Endothelial cells were cultured and labeled with [³⁵S]methionine or [³⁵S]homocysteine in methionine-free M199 media, described in the legend to Table 3.1 (31).

[e] Data from Jakubowski (19).

released from the adduct by treatment with dithiothreitol. Enzymatic hydrolysis of the thiolactone to homocysteine also occurs in vivo, as shown by means of dietary supplementation or injection of homocysteine thiolactone as a source of homocysteine in laboratory animals. Homocysteine thiolactone is rapidly eliminated from blood and cells (3–5, 19, 25–27, 33). For instance, the half-life of exogenous homocysteine thiolactone in human serum is ~ 1 hour (4, 25–27). This might be the reason that thiolactone could not be detected in vivo (3, 4, 35). In human serum, about half the thiolactone incorporated into protein is released as free homocysteine after reduction with dithiothreitol (19, 25–27). The other half represents homocysteine attached via an amide bond between its carboxyl group and the amino group of a protein lysine residue (25–27) (Figure 3.4A).

Protein Homocysteinylation

After acid hydrolysis, a small amount of [³⁵S]homocysteine was recovered from protein of cultured cells incubated with [³⁵S]methionine. More homocysteine was recovered from proteins when human cells were treated with aminopterin, an antifolate drug that indirectly inhibits methionine synthase (19). In recent experiments

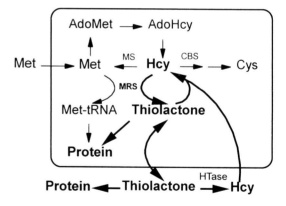

Fig. 3.3.   Schematic representation of the metabolism of homocysteine thiolactone in a human cell. When the functions of methionine synthase (MS) or cystathionine β-synthase (CBS) are limited or prevented, homocysteine is mostly converted into homocysteine thiolactone by methionyl-tRNA synthetase (MRS) (30). Homocysteine thiolactone acylates lysine residues of cellular and extracellular proteins (19, 25–27) or is hydrolyzed to homocysteine by a calcium-dependent homocysteine thiolactonase (HTase), which is tightly associated with HDL in serum (26, 27). (Reproduced from Jakubowski [27], with permission.)

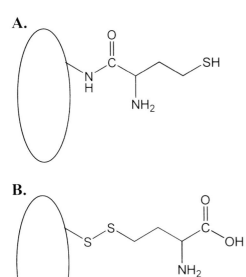

Fig. 3.4. Schematic structures of protein-N-Hcy and protein-S-S-Hcy. (A) In protein-N-Hcy the carboxyl group of homocysteine forms an amide bond with the side chain amino group of protein lysine residue. (B) In protein-S-S-Hcy the thiol of homocysteine forms a disulfide bond with the side chain thiol of protein cysteine residue. The ovals represent protein molecules (26). (Reproduced from Jakubowski [26], with permission.)

with [^{35}S]methionine-labeled human umbilical vein artery endothelial cells in which methionine synthase was severely inhibited by deprivation of folic acid, homocysteine incorporation into protein represented up to 36% of the incorporation of methionine (27, 31). When these endothelial cells were labeled with [^{35}S]homocysteine, incorporation of homocysteine into intracellular protein represented up to 15% of the incorporation of methionine; more homocysteine (65%) was incorporated into extracellular protein (Table 3.2) (27, 31). Cellular levels of protein-homocysteine are greater than the levels of free homocysteine (Table 3.2). Data suggest that homocysteine incorporation into protein is post-translational, reflecting facile homocysteinylation of protein lysine residues by homocysteine thiolactone (Figure 3.4A). Indeed, phenylthiohydantoin-(S-carboxymethyl)-homocysteine can be recovered from tissue culture proteins subjected to carboxymethylation and Edman degradation (31).

Reactions of homocysteine thiolactone with protein lysine residues are robust under physiological conditions (25) (Table 3.4). In human serum incubated with thiolactone, protein homocysteinylation is a major reaction that could be observed with as little as 10 nmol/L thiolactone. Individual proteins are homocysteinylated at rates proportional to their lysine contents (Figure

3.5). Homocysteinylation results in protein damage, manifested as loss of function, multimerization, and precipitation of extensively modified proteins (25).

Model enzymes, such as methionyl-tRNA synthetase and trypsin (Figure 3.6), were inactivated by homocysteinylation (25). Lysine oxidase, an important enzyme responsible for post-translational modification essential for the biogenesis of connective tissue matrices, is irreversibly inactivated by homocysteine thiolactone, which derivatizes the active site tyrosinequinone cofactor (33). In addition to a loss of function, protein homocysteinylation can also generate modified proteins that are physiologically detrimental in other ways. For example, homocysteinylated-low density lipoprotein elicits immune response in rabbits (7). Rabbit antiserum against homocysteinylated-low density lipoprotein adduct was also shown to react with homocysteinylated-protein adducts of albumin, hemoglobin, and serum proteins. This antigen specificity suggests that the rabbit antiserum reacts with εN-(Hcy)-Lys epitopes.

Small amounts of homocysteine are present in acid hydrolysates of dithiothreitol-treated human serum proteins. More homocysteine is present in acid hydrolysates of dithiothreitol-treated serum proteins from subjects with elevated homocysteine levels (Table 3.5) (27).

High-Density Lipoprotein-Associated Homocysteine Thiolactonase in Human Serum

Homocysteine thiolactone is hydrolyzed to homocysteine in human serum by a single specific enzyme, homocysteine thiolactonase, which is present at a concentration of ~50 µg/mL or ~1 µmol/L (25–27). Human vascular endothelial cells have been reported to possess a vigorous thiolactone-hydrolyzing activity (4). However, we were not able to detect any enzy-

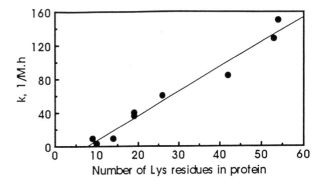

Fig. 3.5. Relationship between lysine (Lys) contents of proteins and second order rate constants, k, of their modification by homocysteine thiolactone [25]. (Reproduced from Jakubowski [25], with permission.)

Table 3.4.   Second Order Rate Constants for Reactions of Homocysteine Thiolactone with Proteins and Other Compounds[a]

Protein (mol wt in kDa) or Other Compound	k at 25°C (L/mol/hr)	k at 37°C (L/mol/hr)
Albumin (68)	128	466
Transferrin (80)	150	560
γ-Globulin (140)	112	280
Fibrinogen (340)	101	
Low density lipoprotein (500)	150	
α₂-Macroglobulin (725)	400	
Hemoglobin (64)	84	600
Myoglobin (16)	40	
Cytochrome C (12.5)	36	150
α-Crystalline	10	
Trypsin (24)	9	
RNase A (12.5)	3	
DNase I (37)	9	
MetRS (64)	60	
Poly-Lys (150)		6,700
LysLys		26
LysAla		3.0
Lysine	1.0	5.0
α-N-Acetyl-Lysine		3.8
ε-N-Acetyl-Lysine		1.2
Streptomycin[b]		2,000

[a] Second order rate constants, k, were calculated from homocysteinylation rates obtained with 5 to 10 mg/ml protein or 10 to 20 mmol/L lysine and 5 μmol/L-10 mmol/L-[35S]homocysteine thiolactone (25). (Reproduced from Jakubowski [25], with permission.
[b] Data from Jakubowski, (31).

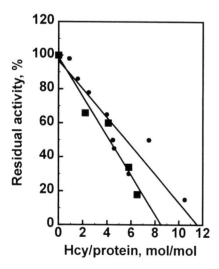

Fig. 3.6.   Homocysteinylation results in inactivation of MetRS and trypsin. Residual enzymatic activities of MetRS (■) and trypsin (•) are plotted as a function of a number of homocysteine (Hcy) molecules incorporated per molecule of protein (25). (Reproduced from Jakubowski [25], with permission.)

matic hydrolysis of thiolactone to homocysteine by endothelial cells (31). A possible explanation for the activity described by Dudman et al. (4) is provided by our observation that streptomycin, present in endothelial cell culture media used by Dudman et al., vigorously reacts with homocysteine thiolactone. A second-order reaction of homocysteine thiolactone with streptomycin (k = 2,000 $M^{-1}h^{-1}$, Table 3.4) (31) is 400 times faster than with lysine (k = 5 $M^{-1}h^{-1}$, Table 3.4). Efficient synthesis of thiolactone by endothelial cells (Tables 3.2 and 3.3) (31) also indicates that thiolactonase activity is absent in these cells.

The serum thiolactonase is present in mammals but absent in birds (Table 3.6). The human serum enzyme requires calcium for activity and stability, is inhibited noncompetitively by isoleucine (K_i = 2 mmol/L) and penicillamine (K_i = 0.2 mmol/L), and is associated with high-density lipoprotein fraction of lipoproteins. When human lipoproteins are fractionated in the presence of calcium, the thiolactonase activity is present in high-density lipoproteins and absent in low-density lipoproteins. In the absence of detergents, the thiolactonase copurifies with apolipoprotein AI. Purification to homogeneity can be achieved only in the presence of nonionic detergents, such as Igepal C-630. Purified homocysteine thiolactonase migrates as a protein of molecular weight of 45 kDa on denaturing polyacrylamide gels. The enzyme exhibits a remarkable degree of substrate specificity toward homocysteine thiolactone. Although homoserine lactone is a substrate, it is not known to occur in human cells. Other related thioesters, such as N-acetyl-homocysteine thiolactone and acetyl-S-coenzyme A, or esters, such as O-acetyl-serine, methyl and ethyl esters of methionine, phenylalanine, alanine, β-alanine, and cysteine are not substrates. However, the thiolactonase also hydrolyzes nonnatural aryl esters phenyl acetate and p-nitrophenol acetate, as well as the organophosphate paraoxon. Extensive research has focused on serum paraoxonase, an organophosphate-detoxifying enzyme whose natural substrate and function remained heretofore unknown (34). The thiolactonase and PON1 activities comigrate at all steps of purification and have identical N-terminal amino acid sequences. Sera from *PON1*-knockout mice are also deficient in homocysteine thiolactonase activity (Table 3.6). Taken together, these data indicate that paraoxonase is in fact homocysteine thiolactonase, and its likely natural function is to detoxify homocysteine thiolactone and, therefore, to protect proteins against homocysteinylation.

Serum homocysteine thiolactonase activity varies 5-fold between different ethnic groups (Jakubowski and Pratt, unpublished data). There is a strong association between *PON1* genotype and homocysteine thiolactonase activity in human populations: high thiolactonase activity is associated with L55 and R192 alleles; low thiolactonase activity is associated with M55 and Q192 alleles. Frequencies of high activity homocysteine thiolactonase/paraoxonase alleles are higher in blacks (0.82 L55 and 0.64 R192) than in whites (0.64 L55 and 0.39 R192). This results in 67% and 39% of black individuals being homozygous for the L55 and R192 high activity forms, respectively, compared with 47% and 3%, respectively, of white individuals. Conversely, only 3% and 12% of blacks are homozygous for the M55 and Q192 low activity forms, respectively, compared with 15% and 44% of whites (Jakubowski and Pratt, unpublished data). It remains to be determined whether these genetic and biochemical differences contribute to a risk for homocysteine-induced cardiovascular disease.

Homocysteine Thiolactone Toxicity and the Protective Role of Thiolactonase

The toxicity of homocysteine thiolactone and the protective role of homocysteine thiolactonase in vivo have been demonstrated in some studies, or can be inferred from other studies. For example, chronic infusions of baboons with homocysteine thiolactone (12) or homocysteine (13) cause atherosclerosis. Similar infusions of rabbits, which have much higher serum levels of thiolactonase than primates (Table 3.7), failed to produce atherosclerosis (3). L-Homocysteine, but not the D- form, is toxic to rat embryos (40). However, both L- and D-forms of homocysteine thiolactone are toxic (40). The stereospecific embryotoxicity of L-homocysteine is consistent with the stereospecificity of methionyl-tRNA synthetase, which converts L-homocysteine, but not D-homocysteine to thiolactone (9, 28). In contrast, embryotoxicity of both L- and D-forms of thiolactone is consistent with identical chemical reactivities of the two stereoisomers of thiolactone toward proteins. Metabolic conversion of homocysteine to thiolactone can also account for the toxicity of homocysteine to chicken embryos (38). This suggestion is supported by the observation that homocysteine thiolactone, which cannot be converted to homocysteine in the chicken owing to the lack of thiolactonase (Table 3.7), is toxic to chicken embryos (38).

Human genetic epidemiological studies suggest that reduced paraoxonase activity may support the development of atherosclerosis (34). To examine a role of paraoxonase (PON1) in vivo, PON1-deficient mice were created (39). Compared with their wild-type littermates, *PON1*-knockout mice were extremely sensitive to organophosphates, as expected. Unexpectedly, the deficient mice were also more susceptible to ather-

Table 3.5. Levels of Protein-Homocysteine and Homocysteine in Samples of Human Sera[a]

Source of serum	Protein-homocysteine (μmol/L)	Homocysteine (μmol/L)
Normal subjects (n = 4)	1.2 ± 0.3	10.3 ± 4.4
Homocystinuric subjects		
Subject 1	3.0	49
Subject 2	4.5	111
Subject 3	7.0	144

[a] Samples of human sera containing indicated levels of homocysteine were obtained from the late Dr. Lindenbaum. Protein-homocysteine, released by acid hydrolysis of dithiothreitol-treated serum proteins (19) was determined by high-performance liquid chromatography. (Reproduced from Jakubowski [27], with permission.)

Table 3.6. Homocysteine (Hcy) Thiolactonase is Absent in PON1-Knockout Mice[a]

Genotype	Relative Hcy Thiolactonase Activity (%)	Relative PON1 Activity (%)
Female		
PON1[+/+]	100	100
PON1[+/−]	51	50
PON1[−/−]	0	0
Male		
PON1[+/+]	73	70
PON1[+/−]	30	40
PON1[−/−]	0	0

[a] Sera from PON1-deficient mice were kindly provided by Diana M. Shih and Aldons J. Lusis (UCLA) (39) and assayed as described in Jakubowski (26).

Table 3.7.   Relative Levels of Serum Homocysteine Thiolactonase Activity in Various Organisms[a]

Organism	Relative Homocysteine Thiolactonase Activity (%)
Human (n = 10)	100 ± 50
Bovine (n = 2)	100 ± 10
Horse (n = 1)	100
Rabbit (n = 3)	600 ± 90
Mouse (n = 4)	500 ± 80
Chicken (n = 2)	0

[a] Homocysteine thiolactonase levels were determined by following the formation of homocysteine from homocysteine thiolactone. (Data from Jakubowski [26].)
n = number of subjects.

osclerosis than their wild-type littermates. The finding that paraoxonase is in fact thiolactonase (Table 3.6) (26) may explain a protective role of paraoxonase in preventing atherosclerosis (39). Results of a recent clinical trial (11), showing that low activity of paraoxonase is associated with the extent of coronary artery disease in human subjects homozygous for the 5,10-methylenetetrahydrofolate reductase 677C→T genotype (i.e., having elevated homocysteine levels), are consistent with the proposed homocysteine thiolactone-detoxifying role of thiolactonase/paraoxonase. These observations underline the importance of examining variability of thiolactonase/paraoxonase in future studies of associations between homocysteine and vascular diseases.

Clinical Correlation: Role of Homocysteine Thiolactone in Human Disease

Elevated levels of homocysteine can lead to cardiovascular diseases and neural tube defects in humans. However, it is not known why homocysteine is harmful. Homocysteine is metabolically converted to homocysteine thiolactone, a reactive thioester. This conversion occurs in all human cell types, including vascular endothelial cells. Because homocysteine is a by-product of methylation reactions, synthesis of homocysteine thiolactone in human cells is inadvertent; however, the extent of thiolactone synthesis depends on specific genetic and metabolic conditions. When methionine synthase activity is inhibited by folate deprivation, almost all homocysteine is converted to thiolactone. Subsequent inadvertent homocysteinylation of cellular and extracellular proteins by homocysteine thiolactone may lead to impaired function. The metabolic conversion of homocysteine to homocysteine thiolactone, the reactivity of the thiolactone toward proteins, and result-

ing protein damage may explain some pathological consequences of elevated homocysteine levels including atherosclerosis. The tight association of homocysteine thiolactonase with high-density lipoproteins in serum could contribute to the protective role of high-density lipoproteins in the human vascular system.

REFERENCES

1. Anderson, RF, Packer, JE. The radiolysis of aqueous solutions of homocysteine thiolactone. *Int J Radiat Phys Chem* 1974; 6: 33–46.
2. Baernstein, HD. A modification of the method for determining methionine in proteins. *J Biol Chem* 1934; 106: 451–56.
3. Donahue, S, Sturman, JA, Gaul, G. Arteriosclerosis due to homocysteinemia: Failure to reproduce the model in weaning rabbits. *Am J Pathol* 1974; 77: 167–74.
4. Dudman, NPB, Hicks, C, Lynch, JF, Wilcken, DEL, Wang, J. Homocysteine thiolactone disposal by human arterial endothelial cells and serum in vitro. *Arterioscler Thromb* 1991; 11: 663–70.
5. Dudman, NPB, Wilken, DEL. Homocysteine thiolactone in experimental homocysteinemia. *Biochem Med* 1981; 27: 244–53.
6. Englisch, S, Englisch, U, von der Haar, F, Cramer, F. The proofreading of hydroxy analogues of leucine and isoleucine by leucyl-tRNA synthetases from *Escherichia coli* and yeast. *Nucleic Acids Res* 1986; 14: 7529–39.
7. Ferguson, E, Parthasarathy, S, Joseph, J, Kalyanaraman, B. Generation and initial characterization of a novel polyclonal antibody directed against homocysteine thiolactone-modified low density lipoprotein. *J Lipid Res* 1998; 39: 925–33.
8. Fersht, A. *Enzyme Structure and Mechanism.* WH. Freeman & Co., Riding and San Francisco, 1977; pp. 97: 275–87.
9. Fersht, AR, Dingwall, C. An editing mechanism for the methionyl-tRNA synthetase in the selection of amino acids in protein synthesis. *Biochemistry* 1979; 18: 1250–56.
10. Gao, W, Goldman, E, Jakubowski, H. Role of carboxy terminal region in proofreading function of methionyl-tRNA synthetase in *Escherichia coli*. *Biochemistry* 1994; 33: 11528–35.
11. Gardemann, A, Wiedemann, H, Philipp, M, Katz, N, Tillmanns, H, Hehrlein, FW, Haberbosch, W. The TT genotype of the methylenetetrahydrofolate reductase C677T gene polymorphism is associated with the extent of coronary arteriosclerosis in patients at high risk for coronary artery disease. *Eur Heart J* 1999; 20: 584–92.
12. Harker, LA, Slichter, SJ, Scott, CR, Ross, R. Homocystinemia: Vascular injury and arterial thrombosis. *N Engl J Med* 1974; 291: 537–41.
13. Harker, LA, Harlan, JM, Ross, R. Effect of sulfinpyrazone on homocysteine-induced injury and atherosclerosis in baboons. *Circ Res* 1983; 53: 731–38.
14. Jakubowski, H. Proofreading in vivo: Editing of homocysteine by methionyl-tRNA synthetase in *Escherichia coli. Proc Natl Acad Sci USA* 1990; 87: 4504–08.

15. Jakubowski, H. Proofreading in vivo: Editing of homo-cysteine by methionyl-tRNA synthetase in the yeast *Saccharomyces cerevisiae*. *EMBO J* 1991; 10: 593–98.

16. Jakubowski, H. Proofreading in vivo: Editing of homo-cysteine by aminoacyl-tRNA synthetases in *Escherichia coli*. *J Biol Chem* 1995; 270: 17672–73.

17. Jakubowski, H. The synthetic/editing site of an aminoa-cyl-tRNA synthetase: Evidence for binding of thiols in the editing subsite. *Biochemistry* 1996; 35: 8252–59.

18. Jakubowski, H. Proofreading in trans by an aminoacyl-tRNA synthetase: A model for single site editing by isoleucyl-tRNA synthetase. *Nucleic Acids Res* 1996; 24: 2505–10.

19. Jakubowski, H. Metabolism of homocysteine thiolactone in human cell cultures: Possible mechanism for pathologi-cal consequences of elevated homocysteine levels. *J Biol Chem* 1997; 272: 1935–42.

20. Jakubowski, H. Aminoacyl thioester chemistry of class II aminoacyl-tRNA synthetases. *Biochemistry* 1997; 36: 11077–85.

21. Jakubowski, H. Synthesis of homocysteine thiolactone in normal and malignant cells. In *Homocysteine Metabo-lism: From Basic Science to Clinical Medicine*. (Graham, I, Refsum, H, Rosenberg, IH, Ueland, PM, eds.). Kluwer Academic Publishers. Boston, Dordrecht, London, 1997; pp. 157–65.

22. Jakubowski, H. Aminoacylation of coenzyme A and pan-tetheine by aminoacyl-tRNA synthetases: Possible link between noncoded and coded peptide synthesis. *Biochemistry* 1998; 37: 5147–53.

23. Jakubowski, H. Misacylation of tRNA^Lys with noncog-nate amino acids by lysyl-tRNA synthetase. *Biochemistry* 1999; 38: 8088–93.

24. Jakubowski, H. tRNA synthetase proofreading of amino acids. In *Encyclopedia of Life Sciences*, Nature Publishing Group, London. 2000. Available at: http://www.els.ne

25. Jakubowski, H. Protein homocysteinylation: Possible mechanism underlying pathological consequences of ele-vated homocysteine levels. *FASEB J* 1999; 13: 2277–82.

26. Jakubowski, H. Calcium-dependent human serum homo-cysteine thiolactone hydrolase: A protective mechanism against protein N-homocysteinylation. *J Biol Chem* 2000; 275: 3957–62.

27. Jakubowski, H. Homocysteine thiolactone: Metabolic origin and protein homocysteinylation in the human. *J Nutr* 2000; 130: 377S–81S.

28. Jakubowski, H, Fersht, A. Alternative pathways of rejec-tion of noncognate amino acids by aminoacyl-tRNA syn-thetases. *Nucleic Acids Res* 1981; 9: 3105–17.

29. Jakubowski, H, Goldman, E. Editing of errors in selection of amino acids for protein synthesis. *Microbiol Rev* 1992; 56: 412–29.

30. Jakubowski, H, Goldman, E. Synthesis of homocysteine thiolactone by methionyl-tRNA synthetase in cultured mammalian cells. *FEBS Lett* 1993; 317: 593–98.

31. Jakubowski, H, Zhang, L, Bardeguez, A, Jakubowski, H. Homocysteine thiolactone and protein homocysteinyla-tion in human endothelial cells: Implications for athero-sclerosis. *Circ Res* 2000; 87: 45–51.

32. Kim, HY, Ghosh, G, Schulman, LH, Brunie, S, Jakubowski, H. The relationship between synthetic and editing functions of the active site of an aminoacyl-tRNA synthetase. *Proc Natl Acad Sci USA* 1993; 90: 11553–57.

33. Liu, G, Nellaiappan, K, Kagan, HM. Irreversible inhibi-tion of lysyl oxidase by homocysteine thiolactone and its selenium and oxygen analogues. *J Biol Chem* 1997; 272: 32370–77.

34. Mackness, B, Durrington, PN, Mackness, MI. Human serum paraoxonase. *Gen Pharmacol* 1998; 31: 329–36.

35. Mudd, HS, Matorin, AI, Levy, HL. Homocysteine thiolac-tone: Failure to detect in human serum or plasma. *Res Commun Chem Pathol Pharmacol* 1989; 63: 297–300.

36. Racker, E. Glutathione-homocysteine transhydrogenase. *J Biol Chem* 1955; 217: 867–74.

37. Riegel, B, Du Vigneaud, V. The isolation of homocysteine and its conversion to a thiolactone. *J Biol Chem* 1935; 112: 149–54.

38. Rosenquist, TH, Ratashak, SA, Selhub, J. Homocysteine induces congenital defects of the heart and neural tube: Effect of folic acid. *Proc Natl Acad Sci USA* 1996; 93: 15227–32.

39. Shih, DM, Gu, L, Navab, M, Li, WF, Hama, S, Castellani, LW, Furlong, CE, Costa, LG, Fogelman, AM, Lusis, AJ. Mice lacking serum paraoxonase are susceptible to organophosphate toxicity and atherosclerosis. *Nature* 1998; 394: 284–87.

40. van Aerts, LAGJM, Klaasboer, HH, Postma, NS, Pertijs, JCLM, Copius Peereboom, JHJ, Eskes, TKAB, Noordhoek, J. Stereospecific in vitro embryotoxicity of L-homocys-teine in pre- and post-implantation rodent embryos. *Toxic. In Vitro* 1993; 7: 743–49.

41. Van der Molen, EF, van der Huevel, LPWJ, Te Poele Pothoff, MTWB, Monnens, LAH, Eskes, TKAB, Blom, HJ. The effect of folic acid on the homocysteine metabo-lism in human umbilical vein endothelial cells (HUVECs). *Eur J Clin Invest* 1996; 26: 304–09.

4

Unique Aspects of Sulfur Chemistry: Homocysteine and Lipid Oxidation

JAY W. HEINECKE

Atherosclerotic vascular disease remains the leading cause of death in the Western world despite the dietary changes, exercise regimens and cholesterol-lowering medications that have decreased the myocardial infarction rate in recent years. To make further progress, we must improve our understanding of the biochemical and physiological changes that encourage plaque formation in the artery wall. Then we can develop therapies that specifically target those causal factors.

Hypercholesterolemia is a well-known risk factor for atherosclerosis (5). However, high cholesterol levels and other traditional factors such as hypertension affect only a fraction of those who develop atherosclerosis. A lesser known contributor is elevated blood levels of homocysteine. More than 25 years ago, McCully (24) concluded from the widespread arterial thrombosis and atherosclerosis in infants suffering from homocystinuria that even moderately elevated blood levels of homocysteine might be one potential cause of thrombosis and atherosclerosis in individuals without homocystinuria. As discussed extensively in other chapters in this book, subsequent epidemiological and clinical studies have strongly supported this hypothesis.

The molecular mechanisms that accelerate atherosclerosis in hyperhomocysteinemia likely differ from those that damage the artery wall in homocystinuria, but they remain poorly understood. One potential pathway involves the generation of reactive intermediates that damage the endothelium and promote thrombus formation. In this chapter, we review the oxidation chemistry of homocysteine and its potential to damage lipids. We also evaluate the evidence that oxidation contributes to the pathogenesis of homocysteine-induced vascular disease.

Homocysteine, Homocystine, and Protein-Disulfide-Linked Homocysteine

Homocysteine is formed during methionine metabolism (reviewed in Chapters 6 through 8). As a free amino acid, it exists in either a reduced (homocysteine, a thiol RSH) or oxidized (homocystine, a disulfide RSSR) form. Its redox chemistry is dominated by its thiol group (SH), which in contrast to most nucleophiles is readily oxidized (6, 19). Oxidation of two homocysteine molecules yields the disulfide, two protons (H^+), and two electrons (e^-):

$$2 \ RSH = RSSR + 2 \ H^+ + 2 \ e^-$$

These electrons then can react singly or in pairs. When oxygen is the electron acceptor, the products are superoxide (the one-electron form of reduced molecular oxygen) or hydrogen peroxide (the two-electron form of reduced molecular oxygen). Other reactive compounds, such as hypochlorous acid and reactive nitrogen species, also can be reduced by thiols, although at very different rates (6).

In biological systems, homocystine is present as the disulfide homocysteine (RSSR), as a mixed disulfide with other low-molecular-weight thiols (homocysteine-cysteine and homocysteine-glutathione mixed disulfides, RSSR′), and as homocysteine disulfide cross-linked to proteins (RSS-Protein). This distinction among the various forms is important because the oxidation chemistry of homocysteine depends on the presence of the thiol group (6, 19). In normal individuals, the free, reduced form of the amino acid represents less than 2% of plasma total homocysteine, whereas low-molecular-weight disulfides and mixed disulfides account for about 30% and protein-disulfide-linked homocysteine for about 70% (30, 46). In subjects with genetic disorders of homocysteine metabolism, the concentration of free homocysteine increases exponentially as plasma total homocysteine levels rise (30).

Thiol Chemistry

Glutathione is the major intracellular thiol and is present at mmol/L concentrations (25). Because it can

Ralph Carmel and Donald W. Jacobsen, eds. *Homocysteine in Health and Disease*. © Cambridge University Press 2001. All rights reserved. Printed in the United States of America.

scavenge reactive intermediates, it plays an important role in protecting cells from oxidative stress. However, thiols such as glutathione and homocysteine have a dark side that makes them potentially deleterious to cells. In the presence of metal ions and oxygen, they can autooxidize, generating highly reactive partially reduced oxygen species (27, 38). Thiols also can initiate lipid peroxidation (36, 43), produce hydroxyl radical (35, 44), and oxidatively cleave proteins in a reaction that requires iron (20). Thus, regulating the oxidation state of sulfur-containing amino acids is an important strategy for curbing cellular damage.

The rates at which various metal ions oxidize thiol depend on both the metal and chemical structure of the thiol (19). Copper oxidizes glutathione more efficiently than iron; the reverse is true for cysteine. Metal-catalyzed oxidation of thiols can be stimulated, inhibited, or unaffected by metal chelators.

Another important factor controlling thiol oxidation is pH (19). The pK_a of thiol groups is generally ~ 8.4; therefore, at neutral pH (7.4), approximately 10% of a thiol will be present as its thiolate anion (the deprotonated thiol, RS^-). Because this anion is the reactive moiety, the rate of oxidation and of thiyl radical ($RS\bullet$) generation is strongly dependent on pH.

$$RSH - RS^- + H^+$$

$$RS^- \rightarrow RS^\bullet + e^-$$

Reactions of thiols therefore are generally inhibited by acidic conditions but promoted at alkaline pH.

The thiyl radical generated by the one-electron oxidation of a thiol reacts rapidly with another thiol (most efficiently the thiolate anion) to yield the radical disulfide anion ($RSSR^{\bullet-}$).

$$RS^- + RS^\bullet \rightarrow RSSR^{\bullet-}$$

The radical disulfide anion is a strongly reducing species that reacts with both metal ions and oxygen (6). When oxygen is the reactant, the product is superoxide ($O_2^{\bullet-}$).

$$RSSR^{\bullet-} + O_2 \rightarrow O_2^{\bullet-} + RSSR$$

The potential toxicity of superoxide has led to the proposal that glutathione must function in concert with superoxide dismutase to protect cells against oxidative stress (47).

Vascular Pathology of Homocystinuria

Patients with homocystinuria and massive elevations of plasma total homocysteine typically exhibit endothelial denudation and both arterial and venous thrombosis. As noted previously, their plasma levels of homocysteine increase from less than 2% to more than 10% to 20% of their plasma total homocysteine levels (30). Harker et al. (11) demonstrated that nonhuman primates continuously infused with homocysteine develop all of the pathological hallmarks of homocystinuria. This observation strongly supports the hypothesis that homocysteine directly mediates vascular injury in this genetic disorder.

The exact mechanisms are unknown. One possible mediator is reactive intermediates generated by homocysteine oxidation. Thus, homocysteine is highly toxic to cultured endothelial cells by a reaction that requires copper ions (38). The ability of redox-active metal ions such as copper to promote thiol autooxidation raises the possibility that the cytotoxic effects are mediated by reactive intermediates such as superoxide or its dismutation product, hydrogen peroxide (H_2O_2).

$$O_2^{\bullet-} + O_2^{\bullet-} + 2H^+ \rightarrow H_2O_2 + O_2$$

Indeed, the peroxide scavenger catalase completely protects endothelial cells from homocysteine, indicating that hydrogen peroxide may be the cytotoxic agent (38). Collectively, these observations suggest that reactive intermediates generated by homocysteine may be important in endothelial dysfunction in homocystinuria. Subsequent loss of endothelium would expose the intimal matrix, triggering platelet activation and thrombus formation.

Pathophysiology of Atherosclerosis

Unlike patients with homocystinuria, those with atherosclerotic vascular disease rarely develop endothelial denudation (3). Instead, they have artery wall lesions characterized by the presence of cholesterol-laden macrophages, smooth muscle cells, and extracellular lipid. When these lesions rupture, they can trigger thrombus formation. The thrombi can obstruct blood flow and precipitate a myocardial infarction.

One important risk factor for atherosclerosis is an elevated level of low-density lipoprotein, the major carrier of blood cholesterol (5). Paradoxically, low-density lipoprotein fails to exert potentially atherogenic effects in vitro (8, 9). However, oxidation of its lipid moieties renders low-density lipoprotein atherogenic, and a wealth of evidence indicates that low-density lipoprotein must be oxidized to promote vascular disease (reviewed in Heinecke [17] and Wood and Graham [49]). Immunohistochemical studies with monoclonal antibodies that specifically recognize protein-bound lipid oxidation products provide direct evidence for low-density lipoprotein oxidation in the artery wall. Low-density lipoprotein with indications of oxidative damage also has been isolated from human and animal atherosclerotic lesions. Moreover, several chemically unrelated lipid-soluble antioxidants retard or inhibit atherosclerosis in hypercholesterolemic animals, and epidemiological studies suggest that a high dietary intake of antioxidants is associated with a decreased risk for coronary artery disease. Most significantly, vitamin E prevents acute coronary events in patients with established atherosclerotic vascular disease (41), suggesting that oxidative damage plays a causal role in atherogenesis.

Cultured Arterial Cells Promote Low-Density Lipoprotein Oxidation

One important pathway for low-density lipoprotein oxidation in vitro involves redox-active transition metal ions. Increasing concentrations of iron or copper modify low-density lipoproteins incubated with smooth muscle cells (15) or even low-density lipoproteins alone if the metals are present at sufficiently high concentrations (15, 39). Also, metal chelators inhibit low-density lipoprotein oxidation by cultured artery wall cells (15, 28, 39). Moreover, protein-bound metal ions in ceruloplasmin (31) and hemin (1) promote low-density lipoprotein oxidation, although the mechanisms may differ from those involving free metal ions.

Despite extensive study, the mechanisms by which metal ions stimulate low-density lipoprotein oxidation are poorly understood. Reduced metal ions (M^{n+}) catalyze the decomposition of lipid peroxides (LOOH) into alkoxyl radical (LO•), a potent oxidizing species (6, 34, 42).

$$M^{n+} + LOOH \rightarrow LO• + HO^- + M^{n+ -1}$$

If the hydroperoxide-derived radicals are not scavenged by antioxidants, they can attack polyunsaturated fatty acids (LH) to form carbon-centered radicals (L•) that initiate the radical chain reaction of lipid peroxidation.

$$LO• + LH \rightarrow LOH + L•$$

The reaction cycle continues until antioxidants or reactions that cross-link radicals terminate lipid peroxidation.

The relevance of this mechanism is uncertain because it is unclear whether free metal ions are available in vivo and because low-density lipoprotein isolated from plasma contains extremely low levels of hydroperoxides (4). It is important to note, however, that levels of lipid oxidation products are elevated in a small fraction of plasma low-density lipoprotein termed LDL⁻ (18). This suggests that further oxidation

of preformed hydroperoxides might be physiologically relevant. LDL⁻ is of uncertain origin, but it may be generated in blood or arise from the oxidation of low-density lipoprotein in peripheral tissue.

Several cellular pathways promote low-density lipoprotein oxidation, including the enzymatic systems lipoxygenase and myeloperoxidase and reactive oxygen species such as superoxide (reviewed in Heinecke [17]). We have shown that cultured human and monkey arterial smooth muscle cells produce extracellular superoxide and oxidize low-density lipoprotein by a pathway that requires metal ions and is inhibited by superoxide dismutase (12). Similar results have been reported for rabbit endothelial cells, rabbit arterial smooth muscle cells, activated human monocytes, and human skin fibroblasts (7, 40).

Sulfur-containing amino acids represent one potential pathway for superoxide production because they can cycle between their thiol and disulfide forms and are known to enter and leave cells by specialized transport pathways (2, 27, 38). Thus, when L-cystine, the disulfide form of L-cysteine, was omitted from the incubation medium of arterial smooth muscle cells, superoxide production was inhibited (16). It was restored when L-cysteine was added back. Neither cyanide nor uncouplers of oxidative phosphorylation blocked superoxide production in this system, indicating that mitochondrial electron transport was not directly involved. Both superoxide production and low-density lipoprotein modification were L-cystine-dependent. Low-density lipoprotein oxidation also required redox-active transition metal ions, such as copper, in the incubation medium.

Based on these observations, we have proposed that one mechanism for superoxide production and low-density lipoprotein modification by cells involves the uptake of L-cystine from the medium (16). After intracellular reduction, L-cysteine, or a thiol derived from it, leaves the cell. The thiol then is reoxidized extracellularly with the concomitant reduction of oxygen to superoxide. Studies of cultured macrophages, endothelial cells, and THP-1 cells, a human macrophage cell line, strongly support this proposed mechanism (10, 37). All three cell types produced extracellular thiol, and they all oxidized low-density lipoprotein by an L-cystine-dependent pathway. Moreover, both thiol production and low-density lipoprotein oxidation by macrophages and endothelial cells were inhibited by L-glutamate, which blocks the cellular uptake of L-cystine by a specific membrane-associated transport system (2). Low-density lipoprotein incubated with thiols in a cell-free system also undergoes lipid peroxidation and is converted to a form that exerts atherogenic effects in vitro (14, 32, 37). These observations are consistent with the proposal that low-density lipoprotein can be oxidized by thiols excreted from cells (Figure 4.1).

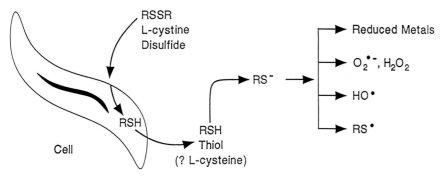

Fig. 4.1. Proposed role of cellular thiols (RSH) in promoting low-density lipoprotein lipid oxidation. Cells take up L-cystine (RSSR) and reduce it intracellularly to a thiol. The thiol then leaves the cell, undergoes deprotonation to form the sulfhydryl anion (RS⁻), and autooxidizes in the presence of metal ions with the concomitant generation of a variety of intermediates that can promote lipid peroxidation. These include reduced metal ions, reactive oxygen species, such as superoxide anion radical ($O_2^{\bullet-}$), hydrogen peroxide (H_2O_2) and hydroxyl radical ($HO^\bullet$), and thiyl radical ($RS^\bullet$).

Thiols Promote Low-Density Lipoprotein Lipid Peroxidation

To explore the possibility that thiols promote low-density lipoprotein oxidation, the ability of cysteine, glutathione, and homocysteine to promote low-density lipoprotein lipid peroxidation was examined in vitro (14). All three thiols modified low-density lipoprotein by reactions requiring redox-active transition metal ions. Two different lipid-soluble antioxidants inhibited these reactions, implicating lipid oxidation in the pathway. Moreover, low-density lipoprotein modified by thiols and copper contained high levels of lipid peroxidation products, confirming that thiols promote low-density lipoprotein modification by a pathway involving lipid peroxidation.

Scavengers of reactive species were used to investigate the mechanism (14). Superoxide dismutase inhibited low-density lipoprotein modification by copper and cysteine, suggesting that metal ions and superoxide were generating thiyl radical. This species would then react with thiolate anion to form the disulfide radical anion, which is oxidized by oxygen to yield superoxide and the disulfide (6).

Superoxide might promote low-density lipoprotein lipid peroxidation by several additional mechanisms. One pathway involves the generation of hydroxyl radical via metal-catalyzed Fenton chemistry (35, 36, 43). First, superoxide reduces a redox-active metal ion (6). The latter then reacts with hydrogen peroxide, which can be produced by the dismutation of superoxide, to generate hydroxyl radical ($HO^\bullet$).

$$M^{n+} + O_2^{\bullet-} \rightarrow M^{n+-1} + O_2$$

$$O_2^{\bullet-} + O_2^{\bullet-} + 2H^+ \rightarrow H_2O_2 + O_2$$

$$M^{n+-1} + H_2O_2 \rightarrow M^{n+} + HO^\bullet + HO^-$$

Hydroxyl radical is an extremely oxidizing intermediate that readily abstracts a hydrogen atom from polyunsaturated fatty acids (6). The products are carbon-centered radicals ($L^\bullet$) that initiate the radical chain reaction of lipid peroxidation (6, 34). The Fenton pathway does not appear to operate when thiols peroxidize low-density lipoprotein lipids, because both the peroxide scavenger catalase and the hydroxyl radical scavenger mannitol failed to inhibit lipid peroxidation (14). However, we cannot exclude the possibility that the metal catalysts were protein-bound and therefore insensitive to catalase and mannitol (20, 44).

In contrast to cysteine, glutathione and homocysteine promoted low-density lipoprotein lipid peroxidation by pathways that were not inhibited by superoxide dismutase (14). Similar results have been reported by Wood and Graham, who also showed that the rate of low-density lipoprotein lipid peroxidation correlated strongly with that of thiol autooxidation (49). Stimulation of lipid peroxidation of liposomes by thiols and by ADP-chelated iron also are independent of superoxide because lipid peroxidation was insensitive to superoxide dismutase and oxygen (26, 43). As noted previously, thiol oxidation can generate thiyl radicals. These species abstract hydrogen atom from polyunsaturated fatty acids at a constant rate in the range of 10^7 $dm^3mol^{-1}sec^{-1}$ (36). Therefore, thiols may form sulfur-centered radicals that directly oxidize low-density lipoprotein lipids.

Thiols also may be able to oxidize low-density lipoprotein through other reactions. For example, peroxidation of brain synaptosomes and phospholipid liposomes requires both oxidized and reduced iron (26). Observing that the optimal ratio of Fe^{3+} to Fe^{2+} is ~ 1, Minotti and Aust proposed that a Fe^{3+}-O-O-Fe^{2+} complex initiates lipid peroxidation (26). This may explain the decreased peroxidation sometimes observed at high concentrations of thiol; under these conditions, most of the metal ion may be present in reduced form, inhibiting lipid peroxidation.

Copper itself promotes low-density lipoprotein oxidation in the absence of exogenous reducing agents because it is reduced by the vitamin E that is carried in low-density lipoprotein (23). In the absence of ethylenediaminetetraacetic acid (EDTA), thiols inhibit this copper-mediated, low-density lipoprotein oxidation, which suggests they act as antioxidants to inhibit lipid peroxidation (21). However, the disulfide forms of certain thiols and the S-methylated form of homocysteine also are inhibitory, strongly suggesting that the effect is independent of the thiol group. Because amino acids chelate metal ions and because thiol oxidation can be inhibited by chelation, the likely mechanism involves amino acid-metal chelates that are unable to promote lipid peroxidation (19, 21).

The vitamin E in low-density lipoprotein fails to reduce iron (23). Moreover, iron requires an exogenous reductant such as superoxide to stimulate low-density lipoprotein oxidation (12, 23); this is consistent with the proposed role of metal reduction in low-density lipoprotein lipid peroxidation. Thiols also promote iron-dependent, low-density lipoprotein lipid peroxidation in the absence of EDTA (21). Thus, the effects of thiols on low-density lipoprotein oxidation in vitro are complex. Thiols can promote lipid peroxidation by both superoxide-dependent and independent pathways. They also inhibit copper-promoted oxidation, apparently by chelating the metal ion. The mechanism likely depends on the metal ion and its chelation state, the reduction potential of the thiol, and the substrate for oxidation.

Homocysteine-Induced Endothelial Dysfunction in Atherogenesis

As well as promoting low-density lipoprotein oxidation, reactive species generated by homocysteine may induce endothelial dysfunction and promote atherosclerosis by other mechanisms (reviewed in 46). Vasomotor relaxation is impaired in humans and in primates with hyperhomocysteinemia, perhaps reflecting the interaction of homocysteine with nitric oxide. Homocysteine also impairs endothelial anticoagulant function, induces the expression of tissue factor, activates the nuclear transcription factor NF-κB, and promotes smooth muscle cell proliferation. The biochemical mechanisms underlying these effects are unknown, but they may involve oxidative damage of cellular lipids, proteins, and nucleic acids.

Hyperhomocysteinemia and Lipid Peroxidation Products In Vivo

Gas chromatography/mass spectrometry has been used to explore lipid peroxidation in vivo (29, 33). This highly sensitive and specific analytical method uses a stable, isotopically labeled internal standard that, apart from its heavy isotope, is structurally identical to the target analyte and therefore exhibits nearly identical behavior during extraction, processing, and chromatographic analyses (13). Including such a standard corrects for analyte loss during processing and increases the precision of quantitative measurements. Using isotope dilution gas chromatography/mass spectrometry, it is possible to unambiguously quantify trace amounts of analyte in a complex biological mixture.

This method can detect F_2-isoprostanes in lipids. In vitro, this family of prostaglandin F_2-like compounds arises from oxidation of arachidonic acid (reviewed in 29, 33). Isotope dilution gas chromatography/mass spectrometry measurements of these compounds in plasma and urine of both animal models and humans provide strong evidence that F_2-isoprostanes are reliable markers of lipid peroxidation in vivo.

A recent study examined the relationship between F_2-isoprostanes and plasma total levels of homocysteine in humans (45). The samples came from a subset of men enrolled in a trial of antioxidant supplementation and the risk of atherosclerosis. The mean F_2-isoprostane level of the men whose plasma total homocysteine levels fell into the highest quintile was 50% higher than that of the men in the lowest quintile; a linear regression model revealed that the level of homocysteine was the strongest predictor of plasma F_2-isoprostane levels. These observations provide the first tantalizing evidence that hyperhomocysteinemia promotes lipid peroxidation in vivo. In future studies, it will be important to further examine the relationship between homocysteine levels and oxidation products in vivo.

Future Directions

Homocysteine may promote vascular disease by a number of different mechanisms, and it likely acts through different pathways in homocystinuria and hyperhomocysteinemia. Links between hyperhomocysteinemia and lipid peroxidation suggest that reactive intermediates resulting from thiol oxidation may play an important role in the development of atherosclerosis in the 5% to 7% of the population that suffers from hyperhomocysteinemia. This raises the exciting possibility that antioxidants might constitute a powerful weapon in our therapeutic armamentarium to inhibit vascular disease in these individuals.

REFERENCES

1. Balla, G, Eaton, JW, Belcher, JD, Vercellotti, GM. Hemin. A possible physiological mediator of low density lipoprotein oxidation and endothelial injury. *Arterioscler Thromb* 1991; 11: 1700–11.

2. Bannai, S, Kitamura, E. Transport interaction of cystine and L-glutamate in human diploid fibroblasts in culture. *J Biol Chem* 1980; 255: 2372–76.

3. Berliner, JA, Heinecke, JW. The role of oxidized lipoproteins in atherogenesis. *Free Radic Biol Med* 1996; 20: 707–27.

4. Bowry, VW, Stanley, KK, Stocker, R. High density lipoprotein is the major carrier of lipid hydroperoxides in human blood plasma of fasting donors. *Proc Natl Acad Sci USA* 1992; 89: 10316–19.

5. Brown, MS, Goldstein, JL. Koch's postulates for cholesterol. *Cell* 1992; 71: 187–88.

6. Buettner, GR. The pecking order of free radicals and antioxidants: Lipid peroxidation, α-tocopherol, and ascorbate. *Arch Biochem Biophys* 1993; 300: 535–43.

7. Cathcart, MK, McNally, AK, Morel, DW, Chisolm, GM. Superoxide anion participation in human monocyte-mediated oxidation of low-density lipoprotein and conversion of low-density lipoprotein to a cytotoxin. *J Immunol* 1989; 142: 1963–69.

8. Fogelman, AM, Shechter, I, Seager, J, Hokom, M, Child, JS, Edwards, PA. Malondialdehyde alteration of low density lipoproteins leads to cholesterol ester accumulation in human monocyte-macrophages. *Proc Natl Acad Sci USA* 1980; 77: 2214–17.

9. Goldstein, JL, Ho, YK, Basu, SK, Brown, MS. Binding site on macrophages that mediates uptake and degradation of acetylated low density lipoprotein, producing massive cholesterol deposition. *Proc Natl Acad Sci USA* 1979; 76: 333–36.

10. Graham, A, Wood, JL, O'Leary, VJ, Stone, D. Human (THP-1) macrophages oxidize LDL by a thiol-dependent mechanism. *Free Radic Res* 1996; 25: 181–82.

11. Harker, LA, Ross, R, Slichter, SJ, Scott, CR. Homocystine-induced arteriosclerosis: The role of endothelial cell injury and platelet response in its genesis. *J Clin Invest* 1976; 58: 731–41.

12. Heinecke, JW, Baker, L, Rosen, H, Chait, A. Superoxide-mediated modification of low density lipoprotein by arterial smooth muscle cells. *J Clin Invest* 1986; 77: 757–61.

13. Heinecke, JW, Hsu, FF, Crowley, JR, Hazen, SL, Leeuwenburgh, C, Mueller, DM, Rasmussen, JE, Turk, J. Detecting oxidative modification of biomolecules with isotope dilution mass spectrometry: Sensitive and quantitative assays for oxidized amino acids in proteins and tissues. *Methods Enzymol* 1998; 300: 124–44.

14. Heinecke, JW, Kawamura, M, Suzuki, L, Chait, A. Oxidation of low density lipoprotein by thiols: Superoxide-dependent and -independent mechanisms. *J Lipid Res* 1993; 34: 2051–61.

15. Heinecke, JW, Rosen, H, Chait, A. Iron and copper promote modification of low density lipoprotein by human arterial smooth muscle cells in culture. *J Clin Invest* 1984; 74: 1890–94.

16. Heinecke, JW, Rosen, H, Suzuki, LA, Chait, A. The role of sulfur-containing amino acids in superoxide production and modification of low density lipoprotein by arterial smooth muscle cells. *J Biol Chem* 1987; 262: 10098–103.

17. Heinecke, JW. Oxidant and antioxidants in the pathogenesis of atherosclerosis: Implications for the oxidized low

18. Hodis, HN, Kramsch, DM, Avogaro, P, Bittolo-Bon, G, Cazzolato, G, Hwang, J, Peterson, H, Sevanian, A. Biochemical and cytotoxic characteristics of an in vivo circulating oxidized low density lipoprotein (LDL⁻). *J Lipid Res* 1994; 35: 669–77.

19. Jocelyn, PC. *Biochemistry of the SH Group: The Occurrence, Chemical Properties Metabolism and Biological Function of Thiols and Disulphides.* Academic Press, New York. 1972; 95–136.

20. Kim, K, Rhee, SG, Stadtman, ER. Nonenzymatic cleavage of proteins by reactive oxygen species generated by dithiothreitol and iron. *J Biol Chem* 1985; 260: 15394–98.

21. Lynch, S, Frei, B. Physiological thiol compounds exert pro- and anti-oxidant effects, respectively, on iron- and copper-dependent oxidation of human low-density lipoprotein. *Biochem Biophys Acta* 1997; 1345: 215–21.

22. Lynch, SM, Frei, B. Mechanisms of copper- and iron-dependent oxidative modification of human low density lipoprotein. *J Lipid Res* 1993; 34: 1745–53.

23. Lynch, SM, Frei, B. Reduction of copper, but not iron, by human low density lipoprotein. *J Biol Chem* 1995; 270: 5155–63.

24. McCully, KS. Vascular pathology of hyperhomocysteinemia: Implications for the pathogenesis of atherosclerosis. *Am J Pathol* 1969; 56: 111–28.

25. Meister, A. Glutathione metabolism and its selective modification. *J Biol Chem* 1988; 263: 17205–208.

26. Minotti, G, Aust, SD. Redox cycling of iron and lipid peroxidation. *Lipids* 1992; 27: 219–26.

27. Misra, HP. Generation of superoxide free radical during the autooxidation of thiols. *J Biol Chem* 1974; 249: 2151–55.

28. Morel, DW, DiCorleto, PE, Chisolm, GM. Endothelial and smooth muscle cells alter low density lipoprotein in vitro by free radical oxidation. *Arteriosclerosis* 1984; 4: 357–64.

29. Morrow, JD, Roberts, LJ. The isoprostanes: Current knowledge and directions for future research. *Biochem Pharmacol* 1996; 51: 1–9.

30. Mudd, SH, Levy, HL. Plasma homocyst(e)ine or homocysteine? *N Engl J Med* 1995; 333: 325.

31. Mukhopadhyay, CK, Ehrenwald, E, Fox, PL. Ceruloplasmin enhances smooth muscle cell- and endothelial cell-mediated low density lipoprotein oxidation by a superoxide-dependent mechanism. *J Biol Chem* 1996; 271: 14773–78.

32. Parthasarathy, S. Oxidation of low-density lipoprotein by thiol compounds leads to its recognition by the acetyl LDL receptor. *Biochim Biophys Acta* 1987; 917: 337–40.

33. Patrono, C, FitzGerald, GA. Isoprostanes: Potential markers of oxidant stress in atherothrombotic disease. *Arterioscler Thromb Vasc Biol* 1997; 17: 2309–15.

34. Porter, NA. Chemistry of lipid peroxidation. *Methods Enzymol* 1984; 105: 273–82.

35. Rowley, DA, Halliwell, B. Superoxide-dependent formation of hydroxyl radicals in the presence of thiol compounds. *FEBS Lett* 1982; 138: 33–6.

36. Schoneich, C, Dillinger, U, von Bruchhausen, F, Asmus, K-D. Oxidation of polyunsaturated fatty acids and lipids through thiyl and sulfonyl radicals: Reaction kinetics, and

influence of oxygen and structure of thiyl radicals. *Arch Biochem Biophys* 1992; 292: 456–67.

37. Sparrow, CP, Olszewski, J. Cellular oxidation of low density lipoprotein is caused by thiol production in media containing transition metal ions. *J Lipid Res* 1993; 34: 1219–28.

38. Starkebaum, G, Harlan, JM. Endothelial cell injury due to copper-catalyzed hydrogen peroxide generation from homocysteine. *J Clin Invest* 1986; 77: 1370–76.

39. Steinbrecher, UP, Parthasarathy, S, Leake, DS, Witztum, JL, Steinberg, D. Modification of low density lipoprotein by endothelial cells involves lipid peroxidation and degradation of low density lipoprotein phospholipids. *Proc Natl Acad Sci USA* 1984; 81: 3883–87.

40. Steinbrecher, UP. Role of superoxide in endothelial cell modification of low-density lipoproteins. *Biochim Biophys Acta* 1988; 959: 20–30.

41. Stephens, NG, Parsons, A, Schofield, PM, Kelly, F, Cheeseman, K, Mitchinson, MJ, Brown, MJ. Randomised controlled trial of vitamin E in patients with coronary disease: Cambridge Heart Antioxidant Study (CHAOS). *Lancet* 1996; 347: 781–86.

42. Thomas, JP, Kalyanaraman, B, Girotti, W. Involvement of preexisting lipid hydroperoxides in Cu^{2+}-stimulated oxi-

dation of low-density lipoprotein. *Arch Biochem Biophys* 1994; 315: 244–54.

43. Tien, M, Bucher, JR, Aust, SD. Thiol-dependent lipid peroxidation. *Biochem Biophys Res Commun* 1982; 107: 279–85.

44. Van Steveninck, J, van der Zee, J, Dubbelman, TMAR. Site-specific and bulk-phase generation of hydroxyl radicals in the presence of cupric ions and thiol compounds. *Biochem J* 1985; 232: 309–11.

45. Voutilainen, S, Morrow, J, Roberts, LJ, Alfthan, G, Alho, H, Nyyssonen, K, Salonen, JT. Enhanced in vivo lipid peroxidation at elevated total plasma homocysteine levels. *Arterioscler Thromb Vasc Biol* 1999; 19: 1263–66.

46. Welch, GN, Loscalzo, J. Mechanisms of disease: Homocysteine and atherothrombosis. *N Engl J Med* 1998; 338: 1042–50.

47. Winterbourn, CC. Superoxide as an intracellular radical sink. *Free Radic Biol Med* 1993; 14: 85–90.

48. Witztum, JL, Steinberg, D. Role of oxidized low density lipoprotein in atherogenesis. *J Clin Invest* 1991; 88: 1785–92.

49. Wood, JL, Graham, A. Structural requirements for oxidation of low density lipoprotein by thiols. *FEBS Lett* 1995; 366: 75–80.

5

Homocysteine, Nitric Oxide, and Nitrosothiols

ANDREW J. GOW
FRED COBB
JONATHAN S. STAMLER

Although epidemiological studies have shown that mild to moderate hyperhomocysteinemia increases the risk for developing atherosclerosis, the molecular mechanisms have not been clearly defined (3, 19, 21). A prevailing viewpoint has linked homocysteine to oxidative stress. The principle is that the SH group of homocysteine is oxidized to a disulfide bond (-S-S-) in a reaction that is coupled to the formation of reactive oxygen species, such as superoxide and hydrogen peroxide. Reactive oxygen species, in turn, cause endothelial dysfunction, decrease nitric oxide production, and thereby accelerate atherosclerosis (14). Inasmuch as nitric oxide (and related molecules) can directly scavenge superoxide and/or react with the thiol of homocysteine to block the generation of reactive oxygen species, they are believed to counter homocysteine-induced injury. Moreover, the S-nitrosothiol that is formed in the reaction between nitric oxide and homocysteine has a broad spectrum of antiatherogenic properties, including antiplatelet activity, inhibitory effects on smooth muscle cell proliferation, prevention of white blood cell adhesion, and protection against endothelial cell apoptosis.

Is this model relevant and does this oxidative mechanism contribute to the growing body of data identifying hyperhomocysteinemia with oxidative stress? The answer may be no. Direct generation of reactive oxygen species by homocysteine seems unlikely to have physiological relevance. Rather, it is probable that the oxidative stress is a secondary effect, which may be subject to regulation by nitric oxide. In making this case, properties of homocysteine that may differentiate it from other biological thiols and specific molecular mechanisms that may contribute to its unique cellular toxicities must be considered. This chapter provides a brief overview of reactions between thiols and nitric oxide. We favor the notion that homocysteine-induced toxicity results mainly from effects on the methyl cycle that perturb methylation reactions and that the balance between nitric oxide and homocysteine may be a key to whether the response is physiological or maladaptive.

Plasma Total Homocysteine

The reduced thiol residue of homocysteine is capable of undergoing the same oxidation and reduction reactions as cysteine, glutathione, and cysteinylglycine; however, it is unlikely to function as a major oxidant or antioxidant because its concentration is too low. In plasma, the concentration of homocysteine-free thiol is nanomolar, whereas albumin (thiol) is 400 to 600 µmol/L, cysteine is 10 to 20 µmol/L, and glutathione is 3 to 5 µmol/L. Homocysteine is primarily found in its oxidized states, homocystine, homocysteine mixed disulfide, and protein-bound homocysteine. Homocysteine thiolactone (see Chapter 3), which is formed from an intramolecular condensation reaction between the thiol and the carboxylic acid (acyclic thioester), may also occur in plasma in submicromolar concentrations (4). Thiolactone formation is unique to homocysteine owing to the extra carbon atom within the side chain (cysteine has only a single carbon within its side chain, whereas homocysteine has two). One molecular mechanism that may be involved in homocysteine-mediated injury involves direct modification of proteins by thiolactone (8). This compound contains an activated carboxyl group, which can react readily with primary amines, such as lysine, to form a homocystamide adduct (4). Homocysteine thiolactone reacts readily with low-density lipoprotein and can inhibit lysyl oxidase (5, 8, 15). It has even been suggested that homocysteine thiolactone might disrupt mitochondrial function (12).

Total (reduced + oxidized) homocysteine is in the low micromolar range in the average person. The concentration of total homocysteine is thus similar to that of plasma S-nitrosothiols, which circulate at low micromolar concentrations. S-nitrosohomocysteine has not been detected in vivo, but it must exist in dynamic equilibrium with other S-nitrosothiols that are present in proportion to the concentration of free thiol: *S*-nitrosoalbumin (~6 μmol/L [6, 24]) > *S*-nitrosocysteine (~250 nmol/L [18, 22]) ≥ *S*-nitrosoglutathione (~180 nmol/L; A Leone, personal communication) and potentially other low molecular weight thiols (16). Homocysteine is thus the most likely of the biological thiols to be subject to regulation by nitric oxide. *S*-nitrosohomocysteine is less susceptible than native homocysteine to oxidation and thiolactone formation (25).

Thiol and Nitric Oxide Reactions

Nitric oxide and its higher oxides can react with thiols to produce *S*-nitrosothiols and higher oxides of sulfur (23). From a mechanistic standpoint, the formation of nitrosothiol (SNO) involves either a direct reaction between nitric oxide (NO) and thiol in the presence of an electron acceptor (Reaction 1) (7) or a reaction of the nitrosonium cation (NO$^+$) (Reaction 2) (23).

$$R\text{-}SH + NO \rightarrow R\text{-}SNO + H^+ + e^- \qquad (1)$$

$$R\text{-}S^- + NO^+ \rightarrow R\text{-}SNO \qquad (2)$$

Transition metals and oxygen facilitate and may even catalyze the interconversion of nitric oxide to NO$^+$ equivalents in biological systems (Figure 5.1) (23, 26, 28). In the case of the reaction of nitric oxide with vicinal thiols or where thiol is in high excess over nitric

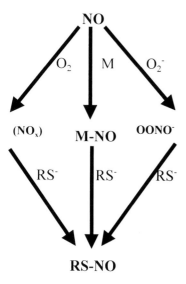

Fig. 5.1. Framework of nitric oxide (NO) responses in biological systems. Nitric oxide reactions in the presence of oxygen, superoxide, or transition metals (M) form products that support additional nitrosative reactions with thiols; nitrite + nitrate (NO$_x$) need not form as an intermediate in these *S*-nitrosothiol (SNO)-generating reactions, and peroxynitrite (OONO$^-$) may generate other nitrosative species when produced in nonstoichiometric amounts.

oxide (> 1,000:1), disulfide is formed with the concomitant generation of nitroxyl anion (NO$^-$) (23). Thus *S*-nitrosylation may accelerate disulfide formation (Reaction 3). Nitroxyl can also be generated from a reaction producing sulfenic acids (Reaction 4).

$$RS(NO)\text{-}R'SH \rightarrow RSSR' + H^+ + NO^- \qquad (3)$$

$$R\text{-}SNO + H_2O \rightarrow R\text{-}SOH + H^+ + NO^- \qquad (4)$$

Some of these reactions can result in the generation of reactive oxygen species (e.g., superoxide from the direct reaction of nitric oxide with a thiol) (Figure 5.2) (7). Generally, however, production of reactive oxygen species is low and superoxide will be readily scavenged, if not by thiols themselves then by ascorbate and superoxide dismutase. Moreover, these reactions need to be put into physiological context. The superoxide generation reaction, for example, actually generates *S*-nitrosothiols that are resistant to reactions with superoxide, whereas nitric oxide reacts readily with superoxide to form the powerful oxidant peroxynitrite. That is, *S*-nitrosothiol formation is a way of protecting nitric oxide from reactions with superoxide that may enhance toxicity. In addition, *S*-nitrosation of homocysteine prevents it from generating reactive oxygen species and from cyclizing to form thiolactone.

Nitrosation of the thiol also dramatically changes its biological activity, endowing the amino acid, peptide, or protein with vasodilatory, antiplatelet, and even antioxidant properties. *S*-nitrosylation of proteins may also alter protein function. That is, *S*-nitrosylation is a post-translational modification that has been adapted as a biological signal to regulate protein function. Ion channels, enzymes, receptors, G proteins, and transcription factors can all be regulated in this manner (6). In particular, p21^{ras} is activated by *S*-nitrosylation (11) and hepatic methionine adenosyltransferase is inhibited (see Chapter 6) (20). The following sections consider the potential ramifications of such regulation with respect to the mechanism by which homocysteine mediates toxicity.

Oxidative Stress

Hyperhomocysteinemia has been associated with endothelial dysfunction (1, 2). This has led a number of investigators to examine the effects of homocysteine on endothelial cells in culture (see Chapter 35). Homocysteine exposure in vitro results in endothelial cell damage most likely through the production of reactive oxygen species such as hydrogen peroxide (27, 32). It has been proposed that the generation of reactive oxygen species results in the consumption of endothelial-derived nitric oxide and that this loss of

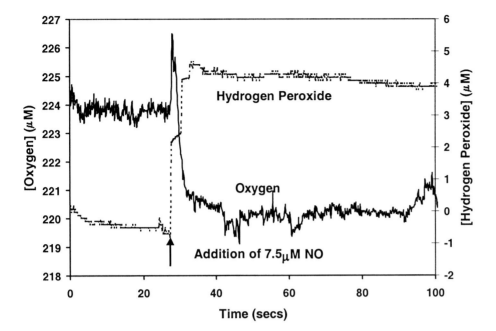

Fig. 5.2. Oxygen consumption and production of reactive oxygen species as a result of nitric oxide (NO) addition to buffer in the presence of cysteine. Oxygen and hydrogen peroxide were monitored by electrodes equilibrated in 1 mL of phosphate buffered saline, 100 μmol/L diethylenetriaminepentaacetic acid, and 2,400 units of superoxide dismutase. 5 μL of 1.5 mmol/L NO was added at the indicated time. Hydrogen peroxide generation was dependent on the presence of both superoxide dismutase and cysteine, indicating superoxide was the product of the reaction of NO with cysteine.

bioavailable nitric oxide is a major cause of endothelial dysfunction. This viewpoint is supported by studies showing that inhibition of endothelial nitric oxide synthase, scavenging of endothelial-derived relaxing factor, or exposure to agents that increase endothelial reactive oxygen species induce apoptosis (see Chapters 35 and 36 for additional details of homocysteine and vascular production of nitric oxide).

Indeed, incubation of confluent endothelial cells with homocysteine, but less so with cysteine, results in a concentration-dependent loss of nitric oxide-related activity. That endothelial cells may be less susceptible to cysteine-induced injury (31) is difficult to reconcile with the idea of thiol-mediated reactive oxygen species generation because the thiol group of cysteine readily participates in such redox reactions. Moreover, it appears that contaminant copper is a required cofactor in this process (whereas free copper is not readily available in vivo) and very high (nonphysiological) concentrations (27) of homocysteine are typically used to generate reactive oxygen species. Cells cannot be killed even with millimolar concentrations of homocysteine when it is added in complex buffers that would scavenge reactive oxygen species and chelate

contaminant-free metals (J. Stamler, unpublished observation). It seems improbable that endothelial exposure to circulating levels of homocysteine would be capable of producing an oxidative injury or a nitric oxide deficiency. The question arises, however, as to what the relationship is between plasma homocysteine and the intracellular thiol/redox state.

Inhibition of Methyltransferase

S-adenosylmethionine (AdoMet) is formed by the addition of the adenosyl adduct of ATP to methionine (Metabolic Diagram, Reaction 1). Because of the high transfer potential stored during this process, AdoMet is a potent donor of activated methyl groups and has been implicated in a number of cellular regulatory processes. Upon donation of a methyl group, AdoMet forms S-adenosylhomocysteine (AdoHcy), which is the precursor of homocysteine. Hepatic methionine adenosyltransferase, the rate-limiting enzyme in the methyl cycle, is regulated by S-nitrosylation of a conserved cysteine that conforms to the "nitrosylation motif" (20). The enzyme is kept partly nitrosylated in resting cells by constitutive nitric oxide synthase activity and is completely inhibited by stoichiometric S-nitrosylation (see Chapter 6 for details). Steady-state nitrosylation of methionine adenosyltransferase is exquisitely sensitive to both the redox state and nitric oxide synthase activity: either depletion of glutathione or upregulation of nitric oxide synthase potentiates the inhibition. As AdoMet is a precursor of homocysteine, the implication is that nitric oxide may dictate levels of homocysteine in cells by regulating its synthesis in the liver. Conversely, nitric oxide deficits may lead to hyperhomocysteinemia.

AdoHcy is a potent inhibitor of methyltransferases and, as such, can inhibit processes controlled by methylation. Homocysteine is in equilibrium with AdoHcy (Metabolic Diagram, Reaction 3). High homocysteine, therefore, may result in inhibition of methylation reactions. As methylation is a key component of a number of signal transduction pathways and regulates transcription, hypomethylation could result in alterations in protein expression and activity (13). p21ras is a case in point. Hypomethylation of p21ras has been shown to decrease its membrane association and activity (13, 33). In this way, hyperhomocysteine-

mia may cause endothelial dysfunction. S-nitrosylation of p21ras activates the protein (10). Nitric oxide may thereby counter homocysteine-induced hypomethylation and preserve endothelial integrity.

Homocysteine has been shown to upregulate DNA synthesis, in particular the transcription of cyclin A, an important cell cycle regulator in the G_1-S phase transit (30). An increase in cyclin A expression has been proposed as a mechanism for the stimulation of smooth muscle cell proliferation, which has been observed on homocysteine exposure (29). Another potential mechanism for this proliferation is the effect of homocysteine on collagen. Polymerized collagen antagonizes smooth muscle cell proliferation. One of the key enzymes in the polymerization process is lysyl oxidase, which is inhibited by homocysteine (possibly via the formation of the thiolactone) (15). In addition, homocysteine increases the synthesis of collagen by smooth muscle cells in culture (17). By increasing collagen synthesis and decreasing its polymerization, homocysteine increases the concentration of collagen monomer, a strong stimulus for smooth muscle cell proliferation. Nitric oxide may inhibit collagen synthesis, although the mechanism is not understood (9).

As well as increasing the expression of proteins such as cyclin A, homocysteine exposure has been

Fig. 5.3. Detection of S-nitrosylhomocysteine formation from endogenous nitrites and nitrates (NOx). Endothelial cells were stimulated by high shear stress forces to secrete nitric oxide for 15 minutes in the presence (A, B) or absence of (C, D) of 1 mmol/L homocysteine. Effluent was then transferred within 10 minutes for analysis by chemiluminesence. B and D are paired samples of A and C, respectively, after their pretreatment with HgCl₂, which displaces nitric oxide selectively from thiol adducts. HgCl₂ is shown to attenuate significantly the signal from homocysteine-exposed cells (A vs. B) but has little effect on the signal in the absence of homocysteine (C vs. D). The signal is also greatly reduced in the absence of added thiol (A vs. C). Note that the relative gain in B, C, and D is twice that in A. (Reproduced from Stamler et al. [25], with permission.)

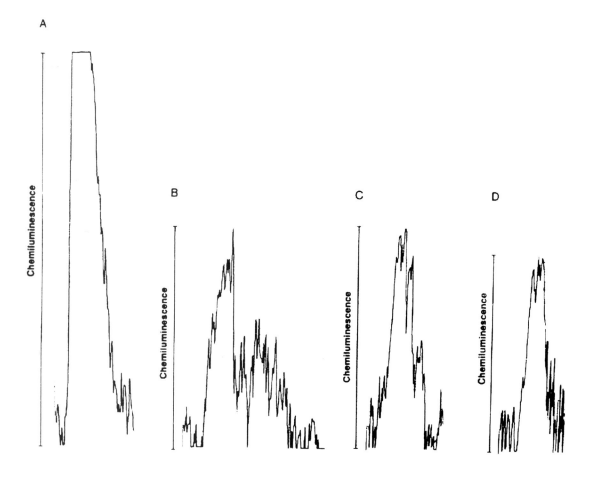

shown to decrease the expression of others. At least in culture, homocysteine exposure decreases the activity of endothelial glutathione peroxidase, a major intracellular defense against reactive oxygen species, at the level of mRNA (31). This reduction in peroxidase expression can be seen with as little as 50 µmol/L homocysteine. Clearly a reduction in glutathione peroxidase activity would result in increased reactive oxygen species, as the defense system against such species would be compromised.

Nitrosation of Homocysteine

An overriding theme in the mechanisms of homocysteine-mediated injury is the reliance on a reactive thiol. This brings to mind the possibility that the reactivity of homocysteine may be regulated by nitric oxide. S-nitrosohomocysteine has been shown to form in biological systems (25), and endothelial cells can support the reaction (Figure 5.3). How might the nitrosation of homocysteine affect its potential pathological activities?

It has already been mentioned that nitric oxide might inhibit the oxidative reactions of homocysteine (physiological relevance notwithstanding). Homocysteine can also alter the expression of critical proteins at the level of transcription and nitric oxide counters this effect. The precise mechanism in the case of enzymes such as glutathione peroxidase is unknown, but, more generally, methylation has been implicated. Ultimately, methylation is regulated at the level of AdoHcy, which inhibits AdoMet formation. S-nitrosylation may inhibit these effects by 1) changing the structural form of the homocysteine substrate (S-nitrosohomocysteine will not form AdoHcy, 2) activating p21^{ras}, and 3) inhibiting methionine adenosyltransferase. Nitric oxide may also regulate the level of homocysteine through additional effects on methyl cycle enzymes.

S-nitrosation of homocysteine prevents thiolactone formation. This would effectively abolish the atherogenicity of homocysteine mediated by lysyl oxidase-induced smooth muscle cell proliferation. In addition, S-nitrosothiols (such as S-nitrosohomocysteine) have antiproliferative effects in their own right.

Indeed, S-nitrosothiols are known to have a number of beneficial vascular effects including vasodilatation, inhibition of smooth muscle cell proliferation, prevention of leukocyte attachment, and inhibition of platelet aggregation. In particular, nanomolar concentrations of S-nitrosohomocysteine have been shown to inhibit ADP- and collagen-induced aggregation of platelets (25), whereas homocysteine and homocysteine thiolactone have no effect on platelets at concentrations lower than 10 mmol/L. One of the potential effects of S-nitrosothiol is to activate guanylate cyclase and thereby increase the intracellular concentration of cyclic guanosine monophosphate (cGMP). Incubation of platelets with 100 µmol/L S-nitrosohomocysteine for 1 minute results in a threefold to fourfold increase in the concentration of cGMP. Presumably, this increase in cGMP forms a major part of the antiaggregatory effect of S-nitrosohomocysteine (25).

Administration of S-nitrosohomocysteine to precontracted vessel rings in a bioassay chamber results in vasorelaxation. The half-maximal inhibitor concentration of this effect is approximately 250 nmol/L, which is 16-fold lower than that of S-nitrosocysteine (Figure 5.4) (25). This vasorelaxing effect of S-nitrosohomocysteine is presumably a cGMP-mediated process, as it can be inhibited by the guanylate cyclase inhibitor, methylene blue.

Incubation of endothelial cells activated to produce nitric oxide by shear stress with 1 mmol/L homocysteine results in the formation of bioactive S-nitrosohomocysteine (25) (Figure 5.3). These observations raise the intriguing possibility that homocysteine and nitric oxide exist in a balance within the vascular system. In other words, the effects of homocysteine may be tightly regulated by production of nitric oxide from the endothelium, which converts it to S-nitrosohomocysteine. Conversely, homocysteine may serve to

Fig. 5.4. S-nitrosohomocysteine-induced vasorelaxation. Deendothelialized rabbit aortas were contracted with 1 µmol/L epinephrine (E) and relaxations were induced with S-nitrosohomocysteine in a dose-dependent manner. The inset provides a time scale and contraction force scale. (Reproduced from Stamler et al. [25], with permission.

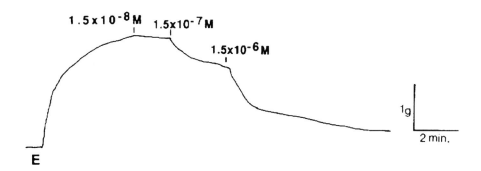

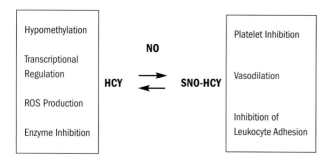

Fig. 5.5. A diagrammatic model of the potential pathological and physiological effects of homocysteine and *S*-nitrosohomocysteine. (ROS, reactive oxygen species; NO, nitric oxide; Hcy, homocysteine; SNO, *S*-nitrosothiol.)

potentiate the effects of nitric oxide by stabilizing it as a *S*-nitrosothiol.

An imbalance may be caused either by increased homocysteine or decreased nitric oxide. Overproduction of homocysteine relative to nitric oxide may predispose to thiolactone formation (perhaps resulting in lysyl oxidase inhibition and modification of low-density lipoprotein), inhibition of AdoMet synthesis, and transcriptional modulation (increasing cyclin A and decreasing glutathione peroxidase expression). Ultimately, the consequence is oxidative stress, which typifies endothelial dysfunction irrespective of the cause. The reactive oxygen species will scavenge nitric oxide and thereby accentuate the initial imbalance between nitric oxide and homocysteine, resulting in further uncontrolled homocysteine production and decreased *S*-nitrosohomocysteine. The end result would be a spiral into worsening injury of the vessel wall.

Nitric oxide-related molecules convert homocysteine from a pathological mediator to a physiological weapon against atherosclerosis, and homocysteine protects the bioactivity of nitric oxide from reactive oxygen species that could otherwise consume it. *S*-nitrosothiols such as *S*-nitrosohomocysteine may also be endowed with activity distinct from nitric oxide itself. This proposal is summarized in Figure 5.5. It may be that the ratio of nitric oxide to homocysteine provides a better marker of atherogenic risk than plasma total homocysteine.

REFERENCES

 1. Chambers, JC, McGregor, A, Jean-Marie, J, Kooner, JS. Acute hyperhomocysteinaemia and endothelial dysfunction. *Lancet* 1998; 351: 36–7.
 2. Chambers, JC, McGregor, A, Jean-Marie, J, Obeid, OA, Kooner, JS. Demonstration of rapid onset vascular endothelial dysfunction after hyperhomocysteinemia: An effect reversible with vitamin C therapy. *Circulation* 1999; 99: 1156–60.
 3. Domagala, TB, Undas, A, Libura, M, Szczeklik, A. Pathogenesis of vascular disease in hyperhomocysteinaemia. *J Cardiovasc Risk* 1998; 5: 239–47.
 4. Ferguson, E, Hogg, N, Antholine, WE, Joseph, J, Singh, RJ, Parthasarathy, S, Kalyanaraman, B. Characterization of the adduct formed from the reaction between homocysteine thiolactone and low-density lipoprotein: Antioxidant implications. *Free Radic Biol Med* 1999; 26: 968–77.
 5. Ferguson, E, Parthasarathy, S, Joseph, J, Kalyanaraman, B. Generation and initial characterization of a novel polyclonal antibody directed against homocysteine thiolactone-modified low density lipoprotein. *J Lipid Res* 1998; 39: 925–33.
 6. Gaston, B. Nitric oxide and thiol groups. *Biochim Biophys Acta* 1999; 1411: 323–33.
 7. Gow, AJ, Buerk, DG, Ischiropoulos, H. A novel reaction mechanism for the formation of *S*-nitrosothiol in vivo. *J Biol Chem* 1997; 272: 2841–45.
 8. Jakubowski, H. Metabolism of homocysteine thiolactone in human cell cultures. Possible mechanism for pathological consequences of elevated homocysteine levels. *J Biol Chem* 1997; 272: 1935–42.
 9. Lafont, A, Durand, E, Samuel, JL, Besse, B, Addad, F, Lévy, BI, Desnos, M, Guérot, C, Boulanger, CM. Endothelial dysfunction and collagen accumulation: Two independent factors for restenosis and constrictive remodeling after experimental angioplasty. *Circulation* 1999; 100: 1109–15.
10. Lander, HM, Hajjar, DP, Hempstead, BL, Mirza, UA, Chait, BT, Campbell, S, Quilliam, LA. A molecular redox switch on p21(ras). Structural basis for the nitric oxide-p21(ras) interaction. *J Biol Chem* 1997; 272: 4323–26.
11. Lander, HM, Jacovina, AT, Davis, RJ, Tauras, JM. Differential activation of mitogen-activated protein kinases by nitric oxide-related species. *J Biol Chem* 1996; 271: 19705–709.
12. Lash, LH, Anders, MW. Mechanism of *S*-(1, 2-dichlorovinyl)-L-cysteine and *S*-(1, 2-dichlorovinyl)-L-homocysteine-induced renal mitochondrial toxicity. *Mol Pharmacol* 1987; 32: 549–56.
13. Lee, ME, Wang. H. Homocysteine and hypomethylation. A novel link to vascular disease. *Trends Cardiovasc Med* 1999; 9: 49–54.
14. Lentz, SR. Homocysteine and vascular dysfunction. *Life Sci* 1997; 61: 1205–15.
15. Liu, G, Nellaiappan, K, Kagan, HM. Irreversible inhibition of lysyl oxidase by homocysteine thiolactone and its selenium and oxygen analogues. Implications for homocystinuria. *J Biol Chem* 1997; 272: 32370–77.
16. MacMicking, JD, North, RJ, LaCourse, R, Mudgett, JS, Shah, SK, Nathan, CF. Identification of nitric oxide synthase as a protective locus against tuberculosis. *Proc Natl Acad Sci USA* 1997; 94: 5243–48.
17. Majors, A, Ehrhart, LA, Pezacka, EH. Homocysteine as a risk factor for vascular disease. Enhanced collagen production and accumulation by smooth muscle cells. *Arterioscler Thromb Vasc Biol* 1997; 17: 2074–81.
18. Marzinzig, M, Nussler, AK, Stadler, J, Marzinzig, E, Barthlen, W, Nussler, NC, Beger, HG, Morris, Jr., SM,

Bruckner, UB. Improved methods to measure end products of nitric oxide in biological fluids: Nitrite, nitrate, and *S*-nitrosothiols. *Nitric Oxide* 1997; 1: 177–89.

19. McCully, KS. Chemical pathology of homocysteine. I. Atherogenesis. *Ann Clin Lab Sci* 1993; 23: 477–93.

20. Perez-Mato, I, Castro, C, Ruiz, FA, Corrales, FJ, Mato, JM. Methionine adenosyltransferase *S*-nitrosylation is regulated by the basic and acidic amino acids surrounding the target thiol. *J Biol Chem* 1999; 274: 17075–79.

21. Refsum, H, Ueland, PM, Nygård, O, Vollset, SE. Homocysteine and cardiovascular disease. *Annu Rev Med* 1998; 49: 31–62.

22. Scharfstein, JS, Keaney, Jr, JF, Slivka, A, Welch, GN, Vita, JA, Stamler, JS, Loscalzo, J. In vivo transfer of nitric oxide between a plasma protein-bound reservoir and low molecular weight thiols. *J Clin Invest* 1994; 94: 1432–39.

23. Stamler, JS, Hausladen, A. Oxidative modifications in nitrosative stress. *Nature Struct Biol* 1998; 5: 247–49.

24. Stamler, JS, Jaraki, O, Osborne, J, Simon, DI, Keaney, J, Vita, JXSD, Valeri, CR, Loscalzo, J. Nitric oxide circulates in mammalian plasma primarily as an *S*-nitroso adduct of serum albumin. *Proc Natl Acad Sci USA* 1992; 89: 7674–77.

25. Stamler, JS, Osborne, JA, Jaraki, O, Rabbani, LE, Mullins, M, Singel, D, Loscalzo, J. Adverse vascular effects of homocysteine are modulated by endothelium-derived relaxing factor and related oxides of nitrogen. *J Clin Invest* 1993; 91: 308–18.

26. Stamler, JS, Singel, DJ, Loscalzo, J. Biochemistry of nitric oxide and its redox-activated forms. *Science* 1992; 258: 1898–1902.

27. Starkebaum, G, Harlan, JM. Endothelial cell injury due to copper-catalyzed hydrogen peroxide generation from homocysteine. *J Clin Invest* 1986; 77: 1370–76.

28. Stubauer, G, Giuffre, A, Sarti, P. Mechanism of *S*-nitrosothiol formation and degradation mediated by copper ions. *J Biol Chem* 1999; 274: 28128–33.

29. Tsai, JC, Perrella, MA, Yoshizumi, M, Hsieh, CM, Haber, E, Schlegel, R, Lee, ME. Promotion of vascular smooth muscle cell growth by homocysteine: A link to atherosclerosis. *Proc Natl Acad Sci USA* 1994; 91: 6369–73.

30. Tsai, JC, Wang, H, Perrella, MA, Yoshizumi, M, Sibinga, NE, Tan, LC, Haber, E, Chang, TH, Schlegel, R, Lee, ME. Induction of cyclin A gene expression by homocysteine in vascular smooth muscle cells. *J Clin Invest* 1996; 97: 146–53.

31. Upchurch, GR, Jr, Welch, GN, Fabian, AJ, Freedman, JE, Johnson, JL, Keaney, JF, Jr, Loscalzo, J. Homocyst(e)ine decreases bioavailable nitric oxide by a mechanism involving glutathione peroxidase. *J Biol Chem* 1997; 272: 17012–17.

32. Wall, RT, Harlan, JM, Harker, LA, Striker, GE. Homocysteine-induced endothelial cell injury in vitro: A model for the study of vascular injury. *Thromb Res* 1980; 18: 113–21.

33. Wang, H, Yoshizumi, M, Lai, K, Tsai, JC, Perrella, MA, Haber, E, Lee, ME. Inhibition of growth and p21ras methylation in vascular endothelial cells by homocysteine but not cysteine. *J Biol Chem* 1997; 272: 25380–85.

6

Biosynthesis of S-Adenosylmethionine

JOSÉ M. MATO
MATÍAS A. AVILA
FERNANDO J. CORRALES

S-Adenosylmethionine Formation

In mammals, *S*-adenosylmethionine (AdoMet) serves as the methyl donor for many biological methylation reactions (such as cytidylylguanylate [CpG] islands in DNA, proteins, phospholipids, adrenergic, dopaminergic, and serotoninergic molecules) and provides the propylamino group for the synthesis of polyamines (20, 76, 92). AdoMet is synthesized from L-methionine and ATP in a two-step reaction catalyzed by methionine adenosyltransferase (AdoMet synthetase, or MAT; Metabolic Diagram, Reaction 1) (19, 80). The formation of AdoMet has been best studied by Markham et al. (88) using AdoMet synthetase purified from *Escherichia coli* (88). In the first step, AdoMet is formed by direct attack of the sulfur atom of methionine on the C5′ atom of ATP, with cleavage of the complete tripolyphosphate moiety from ATP. In the second reaction, the tripolyphosphate thus generated is hydrolyzed asymmetrically to form inorganic phosphate and pyrophosphate. The three products of the reaction are released simultaneously. Two Mg^{2+} ions and one K^+ ion are required for optimal enzyme activity. The cloning and sequencing of the structural genes or cDNAs encoding for a large variety of AdoMet synthetases, including *Mycoplasma genitalium*; *E. coli*; *Saccharomyces cerevisiae*; *Arabidopsis thaliana*; human, rat, and mice liver; and human and rat kidney, show that AdoMet synthetase is an exceptionally well-conserved enzyme through evolution (92). Therefore, although the catalytic mechanism of the enzyme has

been studied in detail only in *E. coli*, all existing AdoMet synthetases are thought to work similarly.

AdoMet synthetase from *E. coli* has been crystallized and the structure solved with a resolution of 3 Å (125). The active enzyme exists as a tetramer of a single subunit of 383 amino acids. Each subunit consists of three structural domains related to each other by a pseudo threefold symmetry. Pairs of subunits form dimers. Each dimer is a tight complex, with a wide interface area between subunits that accommodates two active sites. Each active site is made by both subunits. Tetramers are formed by two dimers with a rather small interface area between them. The high equilibrium constant of *E. coli* AdoMet synthetase tetramer (about 10^{10} L/mol) agrees with the enzyme existing only as a tetramer.

Rat liver AdoMet synthetase exists in two forms, as a tetramer (MAT I) and as a dimer (MAT III) of the same α1 subunit of 43.7 kDa (5). Figure 6.1 shows a model structure of rat liver AdoMet synthetase. Studies carried out with recombinant rat liver enzyme indicate that the equilibrium constant of the tetramer

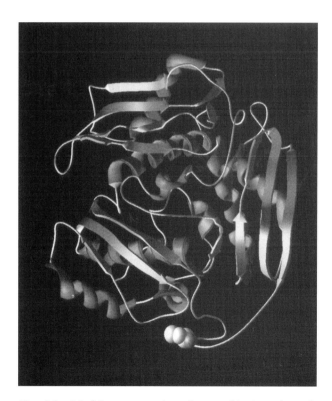

Fig. 6.1. Model structure of rat liver methionine adenosyltransferase. The model structure for the rat liver AdoMet synthetase α subunit has been obtained using the data available for the *E. coli* enzyme. For cysteine residue 121 a space-filling representation was used.

is about 5×10^5 L/mol (94). This value is well within the range reported for other proteins (45) and much lower than the value reported for the *E. coli* enzyme (see previously). It is clear that if the enzyme exists in the liver also as a dimer, its equilibrium constant must be much lower than that of *E. coli,* which exists only as a tetramer. The fact that rat liver tetramer and dimer can be purified from the liver as stable forms, which are not in equilibrium, suggests that regulation of the levels of both enzyme pools in this organ might be due to some post-translational modification. Nothing is known, however, about how the relative amount of each oligomeric form of AdoMet synthetase is regulated in vivo by the liver.

Both liver isoforms differ in kinetic parameters and in their regulatory properties (16, 82, 102, 104, 121). The K_m for methionine is lowest for MAT I (23 µmol/L to 1 mmol/L) and highest for MAT III (215 µmol/L to 7 mmol/L), with different reported values depending on the methods used to purify the enzymes (16, 82, 102, 104, 121). Because the hepatic concentration of methionine is approximately 50 to 80 µmol/L (15, 37), the specific activity of MAT I is likely to be 10-fold higher than that of MAT III under physiological conditions (15). MAT I and MAT III also differ in their response to dimethylsulfoxide. Whereas MAT III is activated by dimethylsulfoxide about 50-fold at low concentration of methionine, MAT I increases its activity only slightly in the presence of dimethylsulfoxide (14). The function of MAT III, which is not saturated under physiological conditions, is to clear methionine from the blood when there is a load of this amino acid as after feeding a meal rich in protein. This agrees with data showing that both in humans and rats, the liver is the organ where the majority of methionine is metabolized (37, 99).

The liver also contains glycine *N*-methyltransferase, a liver-specific enzyme that accounts for approximately 1% of hepatic cytosolic protein and whose main function is to remove the excess of AdoMet synthesized during a methionine load (136). In this way, when large amounts of AdoMet are being synthesized by the liver, the excess of this molecule is not used to hypermethylate DNA or proteins, or to increase the synthesis of polyamines, which could be harmful to the hepatic cells. In contrast, the function of MAT I seems to be to supply the liver with sufficient AdoMet to maintain essential cellular processes, such as DNA, protein and lipid methylation, and polyamine synthesis, even under conditions, such as during fasting, where the serum blood levels of methionine are low. Studies in which the kinetic constants are well determined using pure hepatic AdoMet synthetase isoforms are needed.

Extrahepatic tissues have only one AdoMet synthetase (MAT II), which has a low K_m for methionine (approximately 4 to 10 µmol/L) (76). AdoMet strongly inhibits MAT II (50% inhibitory concentration = 60 µmol/L, which is close to the normal intracellular AdoMet concentration (37, 40). MAT II appears to be a heterotetramer of two α2 and two β subunits (76, 78). The sequence similarity between the hepatic and extrahepatic α subunits is high. Thus, liver and kidney α subunits (from human or rat) display a sequence similarity of around 84% (92). The α subunit is unrelated to the β subunit by peptide mapping and immunoreactivity (77, 79), and the β subunit may have a regulatory function (76). The fact that the expression of the extrahepatic α subunit in *E. coli* yields an active enzyme (33) indicates that the β subunit is not necessary for activity. Moreover, because the α subunit of AdoMet synthetase is remarkably well conserved and, as shown for *E. coli,* the active site is accommodated between two α subunits, it is unlikely that the extrahepatic AdoMet synthetase is a heterotetramer formed of two α 2 and two β subunits. Alternatively, MAT II may be a homotetramer of the same α subunit, and the β subunit may interact with this oligomeric form regulating its kinetic constants. Cloning and sequencing of the β subunit has been recently achieved, (1) and there is no sequence homology between α1 or α2 and β. Coexpression of the α and β subunits and crystalization of the native and recombinant enzymes are needed to understand the molecular nature of MAT II and its regulation.

Two Genes Coding for AdoMet Synthetase in Mammals

As previously mentioned, three forms of AdoMet synthetase have been found in mammalian tissues (16, 79, 102, 121). MAT I and MAT II are present primarily in adult liver (16, 62), and MAT II is responsible for AdoMet synthesis in fetal liver as well as in kidney, brain, lymphocytes, testis, and to a lesser extent adult liver (76, 96). As already noted, the different enzyme isoforms have distinct kinetic and regulatory properties (reviewed in 92). The cloning and sequencing of the structural genes and cDNAs encoding for AdoMet synthetase helped to explain the tissue differences in AdoMet synthesis. The two native MAT I and MAT III isozymes are a homotetramer and a homodimer, respectively, of the same 43.7 kDa polypeptide, derived from a 3.4 kb mRNA, the α1 subunit (5, 68). In human and mouse tissues, α1 is the product of the single copy *MAT1A* gene (4, 113, 133) that maps to chromosome 10q22 in humans (23). The major start site of transcription in the rat was located 29 nucleotides downstream of the putative TATA sequence (3), the same position as that described for the mouse *MAT1A* gene (113). The human and mouse genes have been isolated from genomic libraries using the corresponding cDNAs as probes. (113, 133). Both genes contain nine exons and eight introns spanning ~20 and 18 kb, respectively. Exons 1 and 9 code for the entire 5′ and 3′ untranslated regions, respectively. *MAT1A* is expressed only in the adult liver, predominantly in parenchymal cells, although liver endothelial cells and Kupffer's cells have been recently reported to express this gene (54, 113, 117, 133).

In fetal hepatocytes and other tissues, AdoMet synthetase activity derives from the expression of a separate *MAT2A* gene (33, 67, 79, 96). This gene, recently isolated in the rat, spans approximately 7 kb and consists of nine exons interrupted by eight introns. Exon 1 contains the entire 5′-noncoding region and translation start codon; exon 9 contains the translation stop codon and the long 3′-noncoding region. The transcription initiation site is located 123 base pairs upstream of the translation start codon (61). Comparison of the rat *MAT2A* gene to that of the mouse *MAT1A* gene (113) shows that the exon structure of the two genes is very similar, with identical insertion sites of all corresponding introns (61). *MAT2A* expression results in two mRNA species of 3.8 and 3.4 kb, probably derived from the two distinct initiation sites present in the promoter (87). This gene encodes for a catalytic subunit (α2), which, as mentioned, in the native MAT II isozyme has been proposed to be associated with a regulatory (β) subunit in the form of a tetramer (1, 31, 32, 79, 96). *MAT2A* cDNA has been cloned from human and rat kidney (66, 67), and the human gene has been mapped to chromosome 2p11.2 (33). As for the β subunit, it is present in various tissues such as human lymphocytes, erythrocytes, and bovine brain (1, 33, 79, 87, 96).

As previously mentioned, there is no sequence homology between α1 or α2 and β subunits (1). However, the sequence similarity between the kidney α2 and liver α1 subunits is high, reaching 84% in human enzymes and comparable values between rat liver and kidney α subunits. When rat and human α1 subunits are compared, a sequence similarity of 95% is observed (3, 4). Comparative analysis along the evolutionary scale shows that AdoMet synthetase is an exceptionally well-conserved enzyme (92). The fact that its gene is among the 482 genes found in *M. genitalium*, a bacteria with one of the smallest genomes for a self-replicating organism (42), supports a critical role for this enzyme in cell function.

Regulation of AdoMet Synthetase Gene Expression

Early studies described that liver AdoMet synthetase activity varied during development, being almost undetectable in the mouse fetal liver until the last days of gestation (59). In the rat, AdoMet synthetase activity is also very low in the fetal liver, increasing progressively toward the end of gestation (24, 103). After birth, AdoMet synthetase activity is constant, showing a slight decrease in adult animals (41). Based on the differential effect of dimethylsulfoxide on different AdoMet synthetase isozymes, it was originally proposed that hepatic enzyme activity during fetal life was derived from MAT II, and that the MAT I/III isozyme was induced later in development and significantly at birth (103). Immunohistochemical studies using antibodies specific for the isozymes supported this view (65).

As molecular tools became available, the differential expression of *MAT1A* and *MAT2A* genes has been characterized in human and rat liver at different developmental stages. Both *MAT1A* and *MAT2A* mRNAs were detected by reverse transcriptase polymerase chain reaction (PCR) in human fetal liver, whereas only *MAT1A* mRNA was expressed in adult liver (67). In the developing rat liver *MAT1A* mRNA was first detected by gestational day 19, and its levels increased sharply at birth (54). This response is probably triggered by the perinatal rise in glucagon levels and the concomitant stimulation of cAMP production (54). The mechanisms behind *MAT1A* silencing in the developing rat hepatocyte are beginning to be elucidated and may involve the hypermethylation of its promoter region (127). *MAT2A* mRNA was expressed in the rat fetal liver throughout development; it was still detectable up to day 20 of the postnatal period, although at much lower levels than in the fetal period (54).

The rat, murine, and human *MAT1A* 5′ regions have been cloned and sequenced (6, 113, 139). The rat and murine *MAT1A* promoters share limited similarity to the human promoter (139). Functional analysis by transient transfection has shown that the rat promoter is active not only in liver-type cells such as HepG2 and H35, but also in a nonhepatic cell such as Chinese hamster ovary cells (6). This finding raises the possibility that the liver-restricted expression of the endogenous gene is not mediated by tissue-specific factors. In this regard, other mechanisms involved in transcriptional silencing of tissue-specific genes have been evaluated recently. The *MAT1A* promoter is hypermethylated at CpG sites in extrahepatic tissues, whereas in the liver where the gene is actively transcribed, the levels of promoter methylation are low (Figure 6.2) (127). It has been demonstrated that increased histone acetylation is critical to maintaining a decondensed and active state of chromatin and that the underlying pattern of CpG methylation modulates histone acetylation (101). Interestingly, the degree of acetylation of histones associated with the *MAT1A*

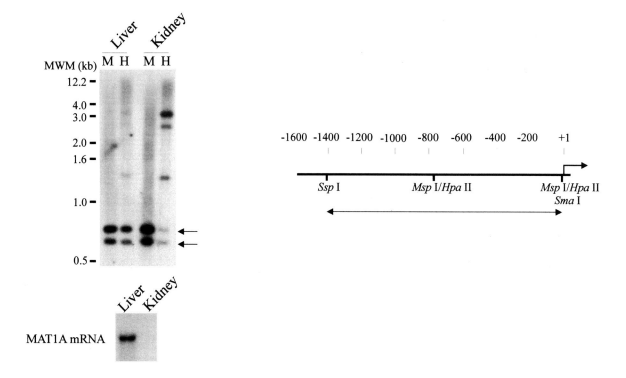

Fig. 6.2. Analysis of the methylation status of the 5′ region of *MAT1A* gene in rat liver and kidney. Genomic DNA from both tissues was digested with *Ssp*I and with either *Msp*I or *Hpa*II. *Msp*I and *Hpa*II recognize the same sequence in DNA (CCGG); however, *Hpa*II cannot cut if the internal C is methylated, but *Msp*I is not inhibited by this modification. After digestion, the samples were analyzed by Southern blotting (left panel). The probe is indicated in the right panel, along with a restriction map of *MAT1A* promoter. *Hpa*II treatment of kidney DNA (left panel, lane H) generated much less of the two 0.64 and 0.75 kb bands (marked by arrows) than present in *Hpa*II-treated liver DNA. This indicates that the *MAT1A* promoter is hypermethylated in kidney and hypomethylated in liver, correlating with the pattern of expression of this gene (as shown by Northern blotting in the lower part of left panel). (Adapted from Torres et al. [127], with permission.)

promoter is about 15-fold higher in the liver than in the kidney (Figure 6.3) (127). All these observations suggest that mechanisms involving DNA methylation and histone acetylation may be responsible for the liver-restricted expression of *MAT1A*.

The rat and human *MAT2A* promoters have been cloned and sequenced (61, 87). The sequence of the human *MAT2A* 5′-flanking region shares little similarity to its rat counterpart, and no similarity to the rat or murine *MAT1A* promoters. Interestingly, when constructs carrying a reporter gene downstream of the rat *MAT2A* promoter were transfected into rat hepatocytes, very low transcriptional activity was observed, but the same constructs drove reporter gene expression in cultured kidney fibroblasts and rat hepatocellular carcinoma cells (61).

Of interest, the rat *MAT2A* gene was hypermethylated in the liver but hypomethylated outside this organ, and the histones associated with this gene were hyperacetylated in the kidney and hypoacetylated in the liver (128). However, when the methylation pattern of the 5′ region of *MAT2A* was analyzed, no differences were observed between the liver and other tissues such as kidney and spleen, all of which showed the same degree of hypomethylation (Avila, Torres, Mato, unpublished data). This observation probably indicates that the differences in the methylation pattern for this gene among tissues could derive from the transcribed region. It is interesting that the differential histone acetylation pattern observed for *MAT2A* was preserved at the promoter level, being hyperacetylated in kidney and hypoacetylated in liver (Avila, Torres, Mato, unpublished data).

AdoMet synthetase gene expression in regenerating rat liver after partial hepatectomy has been characterized (64, 70). DNA synthesis begins in the remaining liver mass within 12 to 16 hours, and complete restoration of the liver mass is achieved within 7 to 10 days (81). Under these conditions, a switch in AdoMet synthetase gene expression was observed; *MAT2A* was induced and *MAT1A* mRNA levels decreased (70). This pattern of gene expression is reminiscent of that found in the developing hepatocyte, where *MAT2A* predominates over the liver-specific *MAT1A*. It is interesting that in rat and human-derived cancer cell lines and hepatoma tissues *MAT2A* is induced and *MAT1A* is expressed at reduced or undetectable levels (17, 18).

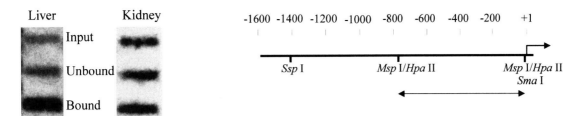

Fig. 6.3. In vivo acetylation pattern of histones associated with *MAT1A* promoter in rat liver and kidney tissue. Mononucleosomes from both tissues were prepared and immunoprecipitated with an antibody specific to acetylated histone H4. DNA was extracted from the input, antibody-bound and unbound fractions were generated in the immunoprecipitation procedure, and equal amounts were slot-blotted onto nitrocellulose filters. Filters were hybridized with a probe derived from rat *MAT1A* promoter close to the transcription initiation site, indicated in the right panel of the figure. The intensity of signal from the antibody-bound slot relative to the input slot gives the enrichment generated by the antibody selection. Quantitation of this signal indicates a strong enrichment (10- to 15-fold) in the bound fraction compared with the input fraction in liver, where the gene is actively transcribed, and no enrichment in kidney. (Adapted from Torres et al. [127], with permission.)

These observations suggest that the type of AdoMet synthetase expressed in the hepatocyte may be related to the proliferative state of the cell. Furthermore, it has been shown that the type of AdoMet synthetase expressed by the cell strongly influences the rate of cell growth and DNA synthesis. *MAT2A* gene expression is associated with more rapid cell growth, but the opposite is true for *MAT1A* expression (17). *MAT2A* expression in lymphocytes is also induced in response to proliferative signals (126). These changes may help to meet the increased demand of AdoMet utilization in the proliferating cell. Regarding the mechanisms behind the silencing of *MAT1A* expression during liver neoplastic transformation, it has been found that *MAT1A* is hypermethylated in the HepG2 human hepatoma cell line (127). In addition, treatment of these cells with the demethylating agent 5′-aza-2 deoxycytidine (140) induces *MAT1A* expression (127). This finding is consistent with a role for CpG methylation in *MAT1A* silencing not only in transformed cells but also in extrahepatic tissues. In addition, reduced levels of histone acetylation seem to be involved in the silencing of *MAT1A* expression in transformed hepatic cells, as shown by the reinduction of *MAT1A* expression in HepG2 cells after treatment with the histone deacetylase inhibitor, trichostatin (127).

Regarding the hormonal regulation of *MAT1A* expression, previous studies in adrenalectomized rats showed that glucocorticoids stimulate liver AdoMet synthetase activity (105, 106, 118). Glucocorticoids, such as triamcinolone, have a direct effect on the expression of the liver-specific gene (55). Treatment of adrenalectomized rats, whose liver *MAT1A* expression is reduced, with triamcinolone significantly induces *MAT1A* mRNA levels. Furthermore, incubation of cultured rat hepatocytes or the H35 rat hepatoma cell line with triamcinolone results in a dose- and time-dependent induction of *MAT1A* mRNA (55). The human gene is also responsive to glucocorticoids (139). Insulin modulates the stimulatory effect of glucocorticoids on *MAT1A* expression, a situation commonly found for genes that respond to both types of hormones. Nuclear run on studies and transient transfection experiments in H35 cells using constructs of *MAT1A* promoter coupled to reporter genes demonstrated a direct stimulatory effect of these hormones on *MAT1A* transcription (55); a similar response was observed in the human *MAT1A* promoter (139). *MAT2A* mRNA levels were downregulated in H35 rat hepatoma cells in response to triamcinolone, resulting in a differential regulation of both genes by glucocorticoids in the same cell (Mato & Alvarez, unpublished data).

Finally, *MAT1A* expression in liver is modulated when rats are exposed to low oxygen concentrations (25, 27). Rats kept in hypoxic conditions for 9 days showed reduced levels of *MAT1A* mRNA in the liver; consequently liver AdoMet content was decreased and overall DNA methylation was reduced. The mechanisms involved in oxygen regulation of liver *MAT1A* expression have been studied in primary cultures of rat hepatocytes (7), and the effects of hypoxia were reproduced. This finding suggests that the downregulation of liver *MAT1A* expression in rats during hypoxia is a direct response of the hepatocyte to low oxygen levels. Hypoxia decreased *MAT1A* transcription and reduced *MAT1A* mRNA stability in cultured hepatocytes. These responses may represent an adaptive mechanism of the hepatic cell to downregulate AdoMet synthetase activity when ATP levels are compromised during hypoxia. A similar situation has been described for other ATP-consuming liver enzymes, such as phosphoenolpyruvate carboxykinase, whose expression is limited by low oxygen levels (73). In contrast, a chronically limited oxygen supply to the hepatic parenchyma, as found in liver cirrhosis, may compromise AdoMet synthesis and promote cell injury. This hypothesis is supported by the beneficial effect of

AdoMet administration to cirrhotic patients reported in a clinical trial (93).

Regulation of AdoMet Synthetase Activity

AdoMet synthetase is a central enzyme in the hepatic catabolism of methionine (92). This essential enzyme must be regulated precisely to ensure the cellular requirements of AdoMet and polyamines but prevent unnecessary consumption of ATP, which could compromise the viability of the cell. As previously discussed, different subunit composition and/or oligomeric states account for the kinetic differences between AdoMet synthetase subspecies (16, 78, 85, 104, 121). The cellular factors regulating the activity of AdoMet synthetase are beginning to be defined. Apart from the proposed regulatory capacity of the β subunit, little is known about the post-translational regulation of MAT II activity. However, MAT I and MAT III, which play a central role in methionine catabolism in the liver, have developed a specific regulatory mechanism controlled by the redox state of the cell. No other AdoMet synthetase so far described has been shown to be regulated by this mechanism.

Under oxidative/nitrosative stress, liver AdoMet synthetase activity is markedly decreased. Inhibition of glutathione synthesis in rats by the administration of L-buthionine-(S,R)-sulfoximine (29), a specific inhibitor of γ-glutamylcysteine synthetase, or the depletion of glutathione levels by carbon tetrachloride treatment (28) leads to a marked reduction of liver AdoMet synthetase activity. In addition, increased production of nitric oxide in the liver during septic shock or hypoxia is associated with the inactivation of hepatic AdoMet synthetase, whereas inhibition of nitric oxide synthase, by N^G-nitro-L-arginine methylester, prevented AdoMet synthetase inactivation in response to hypoxia (7–9). Alcoholic cirrhosis in humans, which is accompanied by the formation of free radicals and glutathione depletion (84), is also associated with reduced liver AdoMet synthetase activity (15, 89) and impaired methionine metabolism (69, 75). The correlation between both the formation of free radicals and a depletion of glutathione levels and liver AdoMet synthetase inactivation agrees with the finding that different thiol-reacting compounds, including fumarylacetoacetate (11), p-chloromercuribenzoate (102), oxidized glutathione, (104) and nitric oxide (9), reduce AdoMet synthetase activity.

All this evidence suggests that the redox state of the cysteine residues plays a key role in the control of liver AdoMet synthetase activity. Although the hepatic AdoMet synthetase subunit contains 10 cysteine residues, reactive oxygen and nitrogen species, including hydroxyl radical, nitric oxide, and peroxynitrite, inactivate the enzyme by specific interaction with one of these cysteines at position 121, which is conserved in rat, mouse, and human liver AdoMet synthetase (3, 4, 63). All other known sequences of AdoMet synthetase contain a glycine instead of a cysteine residue at this position (46). Site-directed mutagenesis studies demonstrate that the enzymatic activity of a recombinant hepatic AdoMet synthetase in which cysteine 121 was substituted by a serine residue was not decreased by hydrogen peroxide or by the nitric oxide donors, S-nitroso-N-acetyl-penicillamine and S-nitrosoglutathione (9, 115). Furthermore replacement of cysteine 121 by serine had no effect on AdoMet synthetase activity (95), indicating that this residue is not essential for enzyme catalysis. Inactivation, however, was not prevented by replacement by serine of any of the other nine cysteine residues of the liver AdoMet synthetase subunit (9, 115).

Purified MAT I and MAT III are inactivated by hydrogen peroxide by covalently modifying cysteine 121 (115). Although cysteine 121 may be oxidized to a sulfinic or sulfonic acid, no direct evidence of this modification is yet available. Kinetic studies indicate that MAT I and MAT III have a similar 50% inhibitory concentration of 160 μmol/L and that the effect of hydrogen peroxide is on the V_{max}, with no alteration of the K_m for the substrates methionine or ATP (115). Glutathione reverses the inactivation by hydrogen peroxide of both oligomeric forms of liver AdoMet synthetase. However, whereas 3 mmol/L glutathione is enough to reverse the inactivation of MAT III, the concentration required to completely reactivate MAT I is 25 mmol/L (115). Because the intracellular concentration of glutathione in mammalian liver is 5 to 10 mmol/L and decreases to 1 mmol/L under oxidative stress, physiological glutathione levels can reactivate MAT III. However, it is unlikely that MAT I could be reactivated after oxidation. This difference in sensitivity to reactivation by glutathione might be the reason for the reduced MAT I activity found in patients with alcoholic liver cirrhosis (15), a condition known to be accompanied by decreased glutathione levels and increased generation of reactive oxygen species (84).

Hepatic AdoMet synthetase is regulated by S-nitrosylation through a mechanism similar to that demonstrated for hemoglobin, cardiac calcium release channel, and caspase 3 (86, 120, 138). MAT I and MAT III, purified from rat liver, were inactivated by nitric oxide donors such as S-nitroso-N-acetyl-penicillamine (9) and S-nitrosoglutathione (112). Substitution of cysteine 121 by a serine residue protected liver AdoMet synthetase from inactivation by these nitric oxide donors (9, 112). Incubation with 100 μmol/L S-nitrosoglutathione inactivates MAT I and MAT III about 70%. However, whereas MAT I incorporates one nitric oxide per subunit, in MAT III three *S*-nitroso groups per enzyme subunit are formed (112). Different accessibility to *S*-nitrosylation of cysteine residues that are located in the interaction surfaces between dimers and are thus inaccessible in the tetrameric form might account for the different number of the *S*-nitroso groups formed. Incubation with saturating (millimolar) concentrations of *S*-nitrosoglutathione leads to the formation of eight *S*-nitroso groups per subunit in both AdoMet synthetase isoforms (112). This finding agrees with the observation that liver AdoMet synthetase contains 10 cysteine residues, two of which form an intrasubunit disulfide bridge, probably between cysteine residues 35 and 67 (90). *S*-nitrosylation of both MAT I and MAT III is reversed by intracellular concentrations of glutathione (9, 112).

This observation might raise doubts about the implication of *S*-nitrosylation on the regulation of AdoMet synthetase activity in vivo. However, intraperitoneal injection of lipopolysaccharide into rats resulted in the accumulation of nitrites and nitrates in serum and in the inactivation of hepatic AdoMet synthetase (112). The analysis of MAT III purified from lipopolysaccharide-treated animals revealed a marked increase in its *S*-nitrosylation in the presence of normal concentrations of glutathione and oxidized glutathione (112). In addition, incubation of isolated rat hepatocytes with *S*-nitrosoglutathione monoethyl ester, a nitric oxide donor permeable to the cell membrane, induced a fivefold to eightfold increase in the hepatocyte nitric oxide content, which promotes AdoMet synthetase *S*-nitrosylation and inactivation (112). Inactivation of AdoMet synthetase by *S*-nitrosylation induced a fivefold reduction of the AdoMet content of hepatocytes within 15 minutes (110), which agrees with the observation that the half-life of hepatic AdoMet is only about 5 minutes (37). Removal of the nitric oxide donor from the incubation medium led to the denitrosylation and reactivation of AdoMet synthetase and to the rapid recovery of the cellular AdoMet levels (110).

Reversible inactivation of liver AdoMet synthetase by *S*-nitrosylation arises then as a mechanism to regulate the hepatic content of AdoMet. Recent data also demonstrate that incubation of isolated rat hepatocytes with buthionine-S,R-sulfoximine or its intraperitoneal injection into rats induces a reduction of hepatic glutathione and leads to the *S*-nitrosylation and inactivation of hepatic AdoMet synthetase (30). Restoration of glutathione levels in hepatocytes and rats by treatment with the monoethyl ester of glutathione reversed AdoMet synthetase *S*-nitrosylation and inactivation (30). These observations suggest that AdoMet synthetase can exist as active and inactive forms in equilibrium in the cell. This equilibrium can be modified by alteration of the nitric oxide levels or by a depletion of intracellular glutathione. Therefore, an increase in nitric oxide levels or depletion of cellular glutathione will shift the equilibrium toward the inactive, nitrosylated form, whereas a reduction of nitric oxide content or replenishment of glutathione levels results in the denitrosylation and reactivation of liver AdoMet synthetase.

As indicated previously, inactivation of liver AdoMet synthetase by oxidation or nitrosylation occurs by the specific and covalent modification of cysteine (121). According to the structural model of hepatic AdoMet synthetase (115), based on the crystal structure of the *E. coli* enzyme (124, 125), this cysteine is located at a flexible loop over the active site cleft of the enzyme (124, 125) (Figure 6.1). The loop can adopt two different conformations, open and closed, and it has been proposed that access of the substrates to the active site is prevented in the closed conformation (46). Nitrosylation or oxidation of cysteine 121 may induce a conformational change in the flexible loop, making the active site less accessible, probably by switching the loop into the closed conformation.

It has been proposed that protein *S*-nitrosylation involves an acid-base-catalyzed nitrosothiol/thiol exchange reaction, where the target cysteine residue is next to basic and acidic amino acids that reduce the pK_a of the thiol group (120). In hepatic AdoMet synthetase, cysteine 121 is not flanked by acidic and basic amino acids. However, arginine residues 357 and 363, as well as aspartic acid 355, configure the tridimensional microenvironment of cysteine 121 (110). Replacement of these residues by serine markedly reduces the capacity of *S*-nitrosoglutathione to *S*-nitrosylate and inactivates liver AdoMet synthetase (110). According to these observations, the guanidino groups of arginine 357 and 363 may facilitate the deprotonation of the sulfur group of cysteine 121. This would increase the nucleophilicity of this residue (by lowering its pK_a) and consequently would facilitate the nitrosylation of its sulfur group. The function of the γ-COOH group of the aspartic acid 355 may be to facilitate the protonation of *S*-nitrosoglutathione and, accordingly, facilitate the donation of the nitric oxide group (Figure 6.4).

Recognition of this topology is likely to prove useful in identifying new targets of protein *S*-nitrosylation. In addition, the definition of this structural motif might facilitate the design of new *S*-nitrosylation sites in proteins that are not regulated by nitric oxide. As previously mentioned, cysteine 121 is specific to human, rat, and mouse liver AdoMet synthetase, whereas all other known sequences of this enzyme contain a glycine instead of a cysteine residue at this position (46).

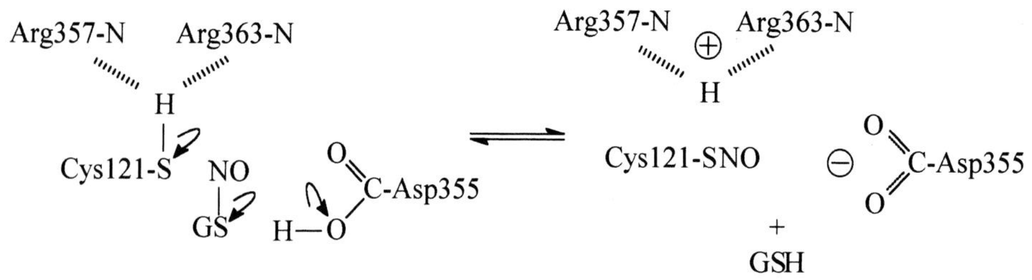

Fig. 6.4. Hypothesis for *S*-nitrosylation reaction of cysteine 121 of rat liver AdoMet synthetase by *S*-nitrosoglutathione. The guanidino groups of arginine residues 357 and 363 increase the nucleophilicity of the thiol group of cysteine 121, thus favoring its nitrosylation. The γ-COOH group of aspartic acid 355 transfers a proton to *S*-nitrosoglutathione (GSNO), thereby enhancing the donation of its nitric oxide (NO) group (GSH, glutathione; looping arrows indicate movement of electron pairs).

However, arginine 357, arginine 363, and aspartic acid 355, which facilitate the *S*-nitrosylation of cysteine 121 in liver AdoMet synthetase, are conserved in MAT II. Replacement of glycine 120 by cysteine results in a MAT II mutant protein that incorporates about 1 mol of nitrosothiol/mol of AdoMet synthetase subunit and is 80% inactivated after incubation with micromolar concentrations of *S*-nitrosoglutathione. The wild-type enzyme is not similarly affected. As observed with the liver enzyme, nitrosylation and inactivation of the MAT II mutant by *S*-nitrosoglutathione is reversed by 2 mmol/L glutathione (21).

Hepatic AdoMet synthetase is responsible for the catabolism of as much as 48% of ingested methionine, which is converted to AdoMet at the expense of ATP. Regulation of the synthetase by oxidation or nitrosylation of cysteine residue 121 might have important pathophysiological consequences. With hypoxia or septic shock, the hepatic production of nitric oxide and/or reactive oxygen species increases, switching AdoMet synthetase into its less active conformation. In this state, the consumption of ATP by AdoMet synthetase would be reduced. This would help regulate the hepatic utilization of ATP and thus prevent nicotinamide adenine dinucleotide depletion and down regulation of mitochondrial energy production during the stress imposed by either oxygen- or nitrogen-reactive species. Indeed, overexpression of rat liver AdoMet synthetase cDNA in Chinese hamster ovary cells led to ATP and nicotinamide adenine dinucleotide depletion and increased the sensitivity of the cells to oxidative stress (114, 115).

Hepatic AdoMet Synthetase Deficiency

Recent studies suggest that deficiency of hepatic AdoMet synthetase leads to brain demyelinization, neurological symptoms, or mental deficits. The screening of newborns for high levels of serum methionine is done routinely in testing for cystathionine β-synthase deficiency. From these tests, a subset of children have been found to have isolated persistent hypermethioninemia without any other metabolic abnormalities (97, 98). Liver biopsy specimens of seven such patients revealed a deficiency of hepatic AdoMet synthetase (39, 47, 48, 52, 53, 57). However, AdoMet synthetase activity was normal in erythrocytes, lymphocytes, or fibroblasts (39, 48, 51). Chronic hypermethioninemia, associated with a deficiency of hepatic AdoMet synthetase activity, has long been considered a benign disorder because the patients lacked clinical symptoms. However, two patients with isolated hypermethioninemia have displayed neurological deficits, including brain demyelinization (98, 123).

The elucidation of the genomic organization of the *MAT1A* gene (113, 133) allowed the molecular basis of hepatic AdoMet synthetase deficiency to be established in patients with isolated hypermethioninemia, including the two with brain demyelinization (23, 133). Analysis of the *MAT1A* gene from 34 patients identified thus far has defined 11 amino acid substitutions in the α1 subunit: A55D, 185stop, R199C, R264H, L305P, 1322M, 350stop, 351stop, R356Q, P357L, and G378S. Although all of them abolish or reduce hepatic AdoMet synthetase activity, only two patients have had neurological abnormalities (23).

It can be hypothesized that a complete lack of hepatic AdoMet synthetase activity and the subsequent impairment of hepatic synthesis of phosphatidylcholine and creatine may be responsible for the neurological symptoms (reviewed in 122). The *MAT1A* gene in the two neurologically impaired patients contains mutations that result in truncated AdoMet synthetase α1 subunits of 350 (351stop) and 349 (350stop) amino acids, respectively. The finding that the 349- and 350-truncated forms of liver AdoMet synthetase expressed in bacteria are devoid of enzyme activity supports this proposal. In contrast, two patients who expressed a truncated α1 subunit of only 184 amino acids (23, 60) had no evident neurological abnormalities. This apparent discrepancy might be explained by considering that the residual activity of the mutated forms of hepatic AdoMet synthetase and/or the low levels of MAT II expressed in the liver may be sufficient to prevent severe clinical manifestations (23, 60, 133). In addition, the neurological abnormalities might be attributable to insults other than the patients' *MAT1A* mutations (98). Nevertheless, considerable evidence remains that links presumably low AdoMet concentrations with demyelinization. Administration of cycloleucine, an inhibitor of AdoMet synthetase activity, to rats induced abnormalities of myelin in rats that were prevented, at least in part, by the administration of AdoMet (12). Moreover, the demyelinization in one patient was reversed by administration of AdoMet (123).

Hypermethioninemia associated with most of these mutations behaves as an autosomal recessive trait (23, 133). Chamberlin (22), however, described two cases of persistent hypermethioninemia inherited in a dominant fashion. Their hypermethioninemia was probably caused by a single allelic *MAT1A* mutation, R264H, in the α subunit with a predicted retention of about 30% of normal MAT I/III activity in the liver (13, 22). This residual activity might explain the absence of clinical abnormalities in these hypermethioninemic individuals. Mudd's group proposed a threshold of 50% to 60% liver AdoMet synthetase activity, below which hypermethioninemia results (23, 98). The dominant effect of the R264H mutation suggests that the mutant R264H α subunits form heterodimers with wild-type subunits, resulting in an inactive enzyme.

Site-directed mutagenesis and crystallographic studies with the *E. coli* enzyme support this hypothesis. Replacement of arginine 264 by noncharged residues or by histidine, which is weakly basic, diminished the ability of mutant subunits to dimerize and resulted in an almost complete loss of enzymatic activity (22). However, substitution of arginine 264 by lysine resulted in a mutant α1 subunit maintaining a strong positive charge at position 264, which forms dimers and retains more that 20% of wild-type enzyme activity (22). Cotransfection studies suggest that R264 wild-type α1 subunits can dimerize with R264H mutant subunits, although the heterodimer retains some enzymatic activity (22) Analysis of the crystal structure of *E. coli* AdoMet synthetase revealed that AdoMet synthetase subunits interact to form dimers through polar interactions involving a salt bridge between R244 of one subunit and E42 and T242 of the other (124, 125). These three amino acids are conserved across species (113) and human α1 subunits correspond to R264, E57, and T262. It seems likely that R264 and E57/T262 are involved in a salt bridge that stabilizes human AdoMet synthetase α1 dimers; accordingly, replacement of R264 will abolish the R264-E57/T262 salt bridge between subunits, resulting in a diminished capacity to dimerize and decreased catalytic activity.

Although the molecular basis for persistent hypermethioninemia has been established, how a deficiency of hepatic AdoMet synthetase can induce neurological abnormalities requires further study. Moreover, it would be of interest to analyze whether a deficiency of hepatic AdoMet synthetase increases susceptibility to insults such as alcohol or viral infections. This might be especially relevant to the dominant R264H mutation, which presumably is more prevalent in the population than are the recessive mutations.

Clinical Use of S-Adenosylmethionine

Patients with cirrhosis of different causes, including alcohol, often have hypermethioninemia and delayed plasma clearance of methionine after intravenous injection or oral administration of this amino acid (69, 75). The hypermethioninemia can be attributed to a 50% to 60% decrease in the activity of the liver-specific AdoMet synthetase (15, 89). This probably contributes to the decreased hepatic glutathione level in patients with alcoholic liver disease, which can be prevented by AdoMet administration (35), and to the reduced urinary excretion of sulfate (69). The fall in hepatic glutathione level in liver disease can further contribute to inactivation of liver-specific AdoMet synthetase since a 30% reduction in hepatic glutathione levels resulted in a 60% reduction in hepatic AdoMet synthetase activity and a 40% reduction in AdoMet levels (29).

The decrease in AdoMet synthetase activity in liver disease occurred without any significant change in the *MAT1A* mRNA level, and a post-translational mechanism was postulated (4). A fall in the enzyme activity can be the result of a decrease in the ratio of tetramer to dimer or of a covalent modification of the enzyme without a change in the oligomeric equilibrium. As mentioned in the section on regulation of AdoMet synthetase activity, the liver enzyme contains a critical cysteine 121 residue. Modification of this critical cysteine residue by nitric oxide or other oxidative agents inactivates the enzyme (9, 95, 104, 110, 112, 115). In end-stage liver disease, the decrease in AdoMet synthetase activity affected the tetramer more selectively (15). Part of the selective loss of the tetramer may be due to a reduction in the glutathione/oxidized glutathione ratio (91). Oxidative stress may contribute to the inactivation of liver-specific AdoMet synthase.

Although liver-specific AdoMet synthetase is inactivated in end-stage alcoholic liver injury in humans, changes in the enzyme and in AdoMet in animal models of ethanol-induced liver injury are far from clear. In rats given 50% ethanol by gavage and low protein diet for up to 10 days, Finkelstein et al. (38) showed induction of hepatic AdoMet synthetase activity. No other study has examined changes in AdoMet synthetase after alcohol administration. Changes in AdoMet level have been variable. Despite a 50% decrease in AdoMet synthetase activity, cirrhotic patients did not have a lower hepatic AdoMet level (15). In the baboon model, both decreased AdoMet and glutathione levels occurred, and AdoMet treatment ameliorated alcohol-induced liver injury (83). AdoMet levels were unchanged at 4 weeks in rats fed an ethanol liquid diet, but the levels declined at 8 weeks (10). Trimble et al. (129) showed decreased hepatic AdoMet levels after 3 weeks of similar ethanol feeding (129). However, micropigs exhibited no change in the hepatic AdoMet level after 12 months of ethanol intake (58). The reasons for these discrepancies are unclear. After 9 weeks of intragastric ethanol infusion, the relative expression of non-liver-specific AdoMet synthetase increased, the hepatic AdoMet level fell, and global DNA hypomethylation was observed (Lu, Tsukamoto, and Mato, unpublished data). This model has the advantage of absolute control over nutrient and ethanol intake, resulting in excellent reproducibility (74, 130–132).

Küpffer's cells express both genes of AdoMet synthetase, *MAT1A* and *MAT2A* (117). It will be important to determine if oxidative stress inactivates liver-specific AdoMet synthetase in Küpffer's cells of ethanol-fed animals. If AdoMet is decreased in Küpffer's cells of alcoholic livers, this may be an important signaling mediator in the induction of tumor necrosis factor, which is released by Küpffer's cells and promotes alcoholic liver injury (26, 72, 131). Rats with decreased hepatic AdoMet levels are known to be predisposed to liver injury caused by lipopolysaccharide, which can be prevented with exogenous AdoMet treatment (26, 36). This is important because bacterial endotoxemia has been implicated in the activation of Küpffer's cells (2, 100, 116). Furthermore, rats with deficient hepatic AdoMet levels had much higher basal serum tumor necrosis factor levels and secreted much more tumor necrosis factor after lipopolysaccharide challenge (26). Incubation of murine macrophage cells with AdoMet downregulated tumor necrosis factor mRNA and protein synthesis on stimulation by lipopolysaccharide (137).

Carbon tetrachloride-induced liver fibrosis in rats has been accompanied by a reduction in hepatic AdoMet synthesis, total DNA methylation, and glutathione content; and AdoMet treatment prevented carbon tetrachloride-induced liver injury (28, 50, 134). AdoMet treatment prevents experimental hepatotoxic effects of a variety of agents, such as galactosamine, paracetamol, cytokines, thioacetamide, methadone, heroin, and lead (reviewed in 92). The efficacy of AdoMet has also been demonstrated in

other types of liver cell injury (35, 92). The efficacy of AdoMet has been shown in clinical trials of patients with cholestasis of pregnancy or chronic liver disease (43, 44, 56). With respect to alcohol-induced liver damage, AdoMet administration increased the hepatic glutathione level in patients with alcoholic and nonalcoholic liver disease (135) and decreased blood levels of ethanol and acetaldehyde in healthy volunteers after the administration of ethanol (34). After these encouraging results, a 24-month, double-blind, randomized, placebo-controlled trial examined the effects of AdoMet treatment in alcoholic liver cirrhosis. The results indicate that long-term treatment with AdoMet (1,200 mg/day orally) improves survival or delays liver transplantation, especially in less advanced liver disease (93) (Figure 6.5). The overall morbidity and mortality were significantly smaller in the AdoMet group than in the placebo group (29% vs. 12%, $p = 0.025$).

The type of AdoMet synthetase expressed by the cell influences the cellular AdoMet level and the extent of DNA methylation (17, 70, 71). The authors also found a switch in gene expression from *MAT1A* to *MAT2A* in liver cancer (18), which may be pathogenetically important because cells that express *MAT2A* grow more rapidly than cells that express *MAT1A* (17). The liver cancer cells, which express mainly *MAT2A*, had lower cellular AdoMet content and overall DNA hypomethylation. Treatment of rats with thioacetamide, a hepatic carcinogen, also increased the expression of *MAT2A* and reduced the

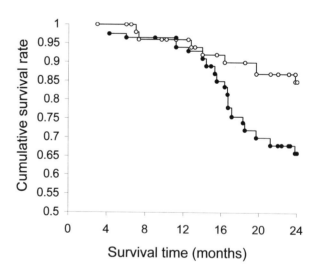

Fig. 6.5. Cumulative survival of alcoholic cirrhotic patients treated with 1,200 mg/day of oral AdoMet ($n = 57$; open circles) or with placebo ($n = 58$; closed circles). The difference between the groups is statistically significant by the log rank test ($p = 0.046$). Survival is described as the time to death or liver transplantation. (Adapted from Mato et al. [93], with permission.)

activity of liver-specific AdoMet synthetase, although it did not change the *MAT1A* mRNA level (71). The AdoMet content, AdoMet to AdoHcy ratio, and DNA methylation all decreased during treatment with thioacetamide (71). Feo and colleagues reported similar changes, along with an increased expression of protooncogenes, such as c-*myc*, c-Ha-*ras*, and C-Ki-*ras*, during the early stages of diethylnitrosamine-induced rat liver carcinogenesis (49, 108, 109, 119). Moreover, diets deficient in methyl groups (restricted intake of methionine, choline, folates, and cobalamin) led to spontaneous formation of hepatocarcinoma in rats. The rats showed a decrease in AdoMet content and overall DNA hypomethylation with breaks in genomic DNA and within the *p53* gene (111).

The mechanisms controlling the silencing of *MAT1A* in liver cancer cells is beginning to be characterized. Silencing of *MAT1A* follows hypermethylation of the promoter and association of the gene with nonacetylated histones; in HepG2 human hepatoma cells that normally express the *MAT2A* gene isoform, inhibition of DNA methylation or inhibition of histone deacetylation leads to *MAT1A* gene expression (127). Increased methylation of the promoter of *MAT1A* and a reduction of the hepatic AdoMet synthetase mRNA have been observed in carbon tetrachloride-induced liver fibrosis in rats (127). Hypermethylation of the liver *MAT1A* promoter accompanied by a reduction in *MAT1A* expression has also been observed in patients with alcoholic and hepatitis C-induced cirrhosis (Avila et al., unpublished data). In addition, the expression of the main enzymes of methionine metabolism was impaired in the liver of cirrhotic patients (Avila et al., unpublished).

The important question is whether such changes contribute to the increased risk of developing hepatocarcinoma in cirrhosis and, if so, whether AdoMet administration can reduce this risk. Of interest, AdoMet administration has been shown to prevent the formation of hepatocarcinoma induced chemically in rats (107). The mechanism underlying the induction of *MAT2A* gene expression in cancer cells is less clear, but the possibility that its expression is activated by changes in chromatin conformation at the promoter level associated with enhanced histone acetylation should be investigated.

REFERENCES

1. Halim, A-B, LeGros, L, Geller, A, Kotb, M. Expression and functional interaction of the catalytic and regulatory subunits of human methionine adenosyltransferase in mammalian cells. *J Biol Chem* 1999; 274: 29720–25.
2. Adachi, Y, Moore, LE, Bradford, BU, Gao, W, Thurman, RG. Antibiotics prevent liver injury in rats following long-term exposure to ethanol. *Gastroenterology* 1995; 108: 218–24.
3. Alvarez, L, Asunción, M, Corrales, F, Pajares, MA, Mato, JM. Analysis of the 5′ non-coding region of rat liver S-adenosylmethionine synthetase mRNA and comparison of the Mr deduced from the cDNA sequence and the purified enzyme. *FEBS Lett* 1991; 290: 142–46.
4. Alvarez, L, Corrales, F, Martin-Duce, A, Mato, JM. Characterization of a full-length cDNA encoding human liver S-adenosylmethionine synthetase: Tissue-specific gene expression and mRNA levels in hepatopathies. *Biochem J* 1993; 293: 481–86.
5. Alvarez, L, Mingorance, J, Pajares, MA, Mato, JM. Expression of rat liver S-adenosylmethionine synthetase in *Escherichia coli* results in two active oligomeric forms. *Biochem J* 1994; 301: 557–61.
6. Alvarez, L, Sánchez-Góngora, E, Mingorance, J, Pajares, MA, Mato, JM. Characterization of rat liver-specific methionine adenosyltransferase gene promoter. Role of distal upstream cis-acting elements in the regulation of the transcriptional activity. *J Biol Chem* 1997; 272: 22875–83.
7. Avila, MA, Carretero, MV, Rodriguez, EN, Mato, JM. Regulation by hypoxia of methionine adenosyltransferase activity and gene expression in rat hepatocytes. *Gastroenterology* 1998; 114: 364–71.
8. Avila, MA, Corrales, FJ, Ruiz, F, Sánchez-Góngora, E, Mingorance, J, Carretero, MV, Mato, IM. Specific interaction of methionine adenosyltransferase with free radicals. *Biofactors* 1998; 8: 27–32.
9. Avila, MA, Mingorance, J, Martinez-Chantar, ML, Casado, M, Martin-Sanz, P, Bosca, L, Mato, JM. Regulation of rat liver S-adenosylmethionine synthetase during septic shock: Role of nitric oxide. *Hepatology* 1997; 25: 391–96.
10. Barak, AJ, Beckenhauer, HC, Junnila, M, Tuma, DJ. Dietary betaine promotes generation of hepatic S-adenosylmethionine and protects the liver from ethanol induced fatty infiltration: Alcoholism. *Clin Exp Res* 1993; 17: 552–55.
11. Berger, R, Van Faassen, H, Smith GP. Biochemical studies on the enzymatic deficiencies in hereditary tyrosinemia. *Clin Chim Acta* 1983; 134: 129–41.
12. Bianchi, R, Calzi, F, Bellasio, R, Savaresi, S, Galbete, JL, Tsankova, V, Tacconi, MT. Role of methyl groups in myelinization. *J Peripheral Nerv Syst* 1997; 2: 84–7.
13. Blom, HJ, Davidson, AJ, Finkelstein, JD, Luder, AS, Bernardini, I, Martin, JJ, Tangerman, A, Trijbels, JM, Mudd, SH, Goodman, SI, Gahl, WA. Persistent hypermethioninaemia with dominant inheritance. *J Inherit Metab Dis* 1992; 15: 188–97.
14. Cabrero, C, Alemany, S. Conversion of rat liver S-adenosyl-L-methionine synthetase from high-Mr form to low-Mr form by LiBr. *Biochim Biophys Acta* 1988; 952: 277–81.
15. Cabrero, C, Duce, AM, Ortiz, P, Alemany, S, Mato, JM. Specific loss of the high-molecular-weight form of S-adenosyl-L-methionine synthetase in human liver cirrhosis. *Hepatology* 1988; 8: 1530–34.

16. Cabrero, C, Puerta, J, Alemany, S. Purification and comparison of two forms of S-adenosyl-L-methionine synthetase from rat liver. *Eur J Biochem* 1987; 170: 299–304.

17. Cai, J, Mao, Z, Hwang, JJ, Lu, SC. Differential expression of methionine adenosyltransferase genes influences the rate of growth of human hepatocellular carcinoma cells. *Cancer Res* 1998; 58: 1444–50.

18. Cai, J, Sun, WM, Hwang, JJ, Stain, SC, Lu, SC. Changes in S-adenosylmethionine synthetase in human liver cancer: Molecular characterization and significance. *Hepatology* 1996; 24: 1090–97.

19. Cantoni, G. S-adenosylmethionine: A new intermediate form enzymatically from L-methionine and adenosine triphosphate. *J Biol Chem* 1953; 204: 403–16.

20. Cantoni, GL. Biochemical methylations: Selected aspects. *Annu Rev Biochem* 1975; 44: 435–41.

21. Castro, C, Ruiz, FA, Pérez-Mato, I, Sánchez del Pino, MM, LeGros, L, Geller, AM, Kotb, M, Corrales, FJ, Mato, JM. Creation of a functional S-nitrosylation site in vitro by single point mutation. *FEBS Lett* 1999; 459: 319–322.

22. Chamberlin, ME, Ubagai, T, Mudd, SH, Levy, HL, Chou, JY. Dominant inheritance of isolated hypermethioninemia is associated with a mutation in the human methionine adenosyltransferase 1A gene. *Am J Hum Genet* 1997; 60: 540–46.

23. Chamberlin, ME, Ubagai, T, Mudd, SH, Wilson, WG, Leonard, JV, Chou, JY. Demyelination of the brain is associated with methionine adenosyltransferase I/III deficiency. *J Clin Invest* 1996; 98: 1021–27.

24. Chase, HP, Volpe, JJ, Laster, L. Transsulfuration in mammals: Fetal and early development of methionine-activating enzyme and its relation to hormonal influences. *J Clin Invest* 1968; 47: 2099–2108.

25. Chawla, RK, Jones, DP. Abnormal metabolism of S-adenosyl-L-methionine in hypoxic rat liver. Similarities to its abnormal metabolism in alcoholic cirrhosis. *Biochim Biophys Acta* 1994; 1199: 45–51.

26. Chawla, RK, Watson, WH, Easting, CE, Lee, EY, Schmidt, J, McClain, CJ. S-adenosylmethionine deficiency and TNF-alfa in lipopolysaccharide-induced hepatic injury. *Am J Physiol* 1998; 38: G125–29.

27. Chawla, RK, Watson, WH, Jones, DP. Effect of hypoxia on hepatic DNA methylation and tRNA methyltransferase in rat: Similarities to effects of methyl-deficient diets. *J Cell Biochem* 1996; 61: 72–80.

28. Corrales, F, Gimenez, A, Alvarez, L, Caballeria, J, Pajares, MA, Andreu, H, Pares, A, Mato, JM, Rodes, J. S-adenosylmethionine treatment prevents carbon tetrachloride-induced S-adenosylmethionine synthetase inactivation and attenuates liver injury. *Hepatology* 1992; 16: 1022–27.

29. Corrales, F, Ochoa, P, Rivas, C, Martin-Lomas, M, Mato, JM, Pajares, MA. Inhibition of glutathione synthesis in the liver leads to S-adenosyl-L-methionine synthetase reduction. *Hepatology* 1991; 14: 528–33.

30. Corrales, FJ, Ruiz, FA, Mato, JM. In vivo regulation by glutathione of methionine adenosyltransferase S-nitrosylation in rat liver. *J Hepatol* 1999; 31: 887–94.

31. De La Rosa, J, Geller, AM, LeGros, Jr, HL, Kotb, M. Induction of interleukin 2 production but not methionine adenosyltransferase activity or S-adenosylmethionine turnover in Jurkat T-cells. *Cancer Res* 1992; 52: 3361–66.

32. De La Rosa, J, LeGros, Jr, HI, Geller, AM, Kotb, M. Changes in the relative amount of subunits of methionine adenosyltransferase in human lymphocytes upon stimulation with a polyclonal T cell mitogen. *J Biol Chem* 1992; 267: 10699–704.

33. De La Rosa, J, Ostrowski, J, Hryniewicz, MM, Kredich, NM, Kotb, M, LeGros, Jr, HI, Valentine, M, Geller, AM. Chromosomal localization and catalytic properties of the recombinant alpha subunit of human lymphocyte methionine adenosyltransferase. *J Biol Chem* 1995; 270: 21860–68.

34. DiPadova, C, Tritapepe, R, Rovagnati, P, Pozzoli, M, Stramentinoli, G. Decreased blood levels of ethanol and acetaldehyde by S-adenosyl-L-methionine in humans. *Arch Toxicol* 1984; 7: 240–42.

35. Dunne, JB, Davenport, M, Williams, R, Tredger, JM. Evidence that S-adenosylmethionine and N-acetylcysteine reduce injury from sequential cold and warm ischaemia in the isolated perfused rat liver. *Transplantation* 1994; 57: 1161–68.

36. Easting, CE, McClain, CJ, Lee, EY, Bagby, GJ, Chawla, RK. Choline deficiency augments and antibody to tumour necrosis factor α attenuates endotoxin-induced hepatic injury. *Alcohol* 1997; 21: 1037–41.

37. Finkelstein, JD. Methionine metabolism in mammals. *J Nutr Biochem* 1990; 1: 228–37.

38. Finkelstein, JD, Cello, JP, Kyle, WE. Ethanol-induced changes in methionine metabolism in rat liver. *Biochem Biophys Res Commun* 1974; 61: 525–31.

39. Finkelstein, JD, Kyle, WE, Martin, JJ. Abnormal methionine adenosyltransferase in hypermethioninemia. *Biochem Biophys Res Commun* 1975; 66: 1491–97.

40. Finkelstein, JD, Martin, JJ. Methionine metabolism in mammals. Adaptation to methionine excess. *J Biol Chem* 1986; 261: 1582–87.

41. Finkelstein, JD, Mudd, SH. Transsulfuration in mammals: The methionine sparing effect of cystine. *J Biol Chem* 1967; 242: 873–80.

42. Fraser, CM, Gocayne, JD, White, O, Adams, MD, Clayton, RA, Fleischmann, RD, Bult, CJ, Kerlavage, AR, Sutton, G, Kelley, JM, Fritchman, JL, Weidman, JF, Small, KV, Sandusky, M, Fuhrmann, J, Nguyen, D, Utterback, TR, Saudek, DM, Phillips, CA, Merrick, JM, Tomb, JF, Dougherty, BA, Bott, KF, Hu, PC, Lucier, TS, Peterson, SN, Smith, HO, Hutchison, CA, Venter, JC. The minimal gene complement of *Mycoplasma genitalium*. *Science* 1995; 270: 397–403.

43. Frezza, M, Surrenti, C, Manzillo, G, Fiaccadori, F, Bortolini, M, DiPadova, C. Oral S-adenosylmethionine in the symptomatic treatment of intrahepatic cholestasis: A double-blind, placebo controlled study. *Gastroenterology* 1990; 99: 211–15.

44. Frezza, M, Tritapepe, R, Pozzato, G, DiPadova, C. Prevention by S-adenosylmethionine of estrogen-induced hepatobiliary toxicity in women. *Am J Gastroenterol* 1988; 83: 1098–102.

45. Friedman, FK, Beychok, S. Probes of subunit assembly and reconstitution pathways in multisubunit proteins. *Annu Rev Biochem* 1979; 48: 217–50.

46. Fu, Z, Hu, Y, Markham, GD, Takusagawa, F. Flexible loop in the structure of *S*-adenosylmethionine synthetase crystallized in the tetragonal modification. *J Biomol Struct Dyn* 1996; 13: 727–39.

47. Gahl, WA, Bernardini, I, Finkelstein, JD, Tangerman, A, Martin, JJ, Blom, HJ, Mullen, KD, Mudd, SH. Transsulfuration in an adult with hepatic methionine adenosyltransferase deficiency. *J Clin Invest* 1988; 81: 390–97.

48. Gahl, WA, Finkelstein, JD, Mullen, KD, Bernardini, I, Martin, JJ, Backlund, P, Ishak, KG, Hoofnagle, JH, Mudd, SH. Hepatic methionine adenosyltransferase deficiency in a 31-year-old man. *Am J Hum Genet* 1987; 40: 39–49.

49. Garcea, R, Pascale, R, Daino, L, Frassetto, S, Cozzolina, P, Ruggio, ME, Vannini, MG, Gaspa, L, Feo, F. Variations of ornithine decarboxylase activity and *S*-adenosyl-L-methionine and 5′-methylthioadenosine contents during the development of diethylnitrosamine-induced liver hyperplastic nodules and hepatocellular carcinoma. *Carcinogenesis* 1987; 8: 653–58.

50. Gassó, M, Rubio, M, Varela-Moreiras, G, Cabré, M, Caballería, J, Alonso Aperte, E, Deulofeu, R, Camps, J, Giménez, A, Pajares, MA, Pares, A, Mato, JM, Rodes, J. Effects of *S*-adenosylmethionine on lipid peroxidation and liver fibrogenesis in carbon tetrachloride-induced cirrhosis. *J Hepatol* 1996; 25: 200–205.

51. Gaull, GE, Bender, AN, Vulovic, D, Tallan, HH, Schaffner, F. Methioninemia and myopathy: A new disorder. *Ann Neurol* 1981; 9: 423–32.

52. Gaull, GE, Tallan, HH. Methionine adenosyltransferase deficiency: New enzymatic defect associated with hypermethioninemia. *Science* 1974; 186: 59–60.

53. Gaull, GE, Tallan, HH, Lonsdale, D, Przyrembel, H, Schaffner, F, von Bassewitz, DB. Hypermethioninemia associated with methionine adenosyltransferase deficiency: Clinical, morphologic, and biochemical observations on four patients. *J Pediatr* 1981; 98: 734–41.

54. Gil, B, Casado, M, Pajares, MA, Bosca, L, Mato, JM, Martin-Sanz, P, Alvarez, L. Differential expression pattern of *S*-adenosylmethionine synthetase isoenzymes during rat liver development. *Hepatology* 1996; 24: 876–81.

55. Gil, B, Pajares, MA, Mato, JM, Alvarez, L. Glucocorticoid regulation of hepatic *S*-adenosylmethionine synthetase gene expression. *Endocrinology* 1997; 138: 1251–58.

56. Giudici, GA, LeGrazie, C, DiPadova, C. The use of ademethionine (SAMe) in the treatment of cholestatic liver disorders. Meta-analysis of clinical trials., pp. 67–79. In *Methionine Metabolism: Molecular Mechanisms and Clinical Implications* (Mato, JM, Lieber, C, Kaplowitz, N, Caballero, A, eds.). C.S.I.C. Press, Madrid, 1992; pp. 67–79.

57. Gout, JP, Serre, JC, Dieterlen, M, Antener, I, Frappat, P, Bost, M, Beaudoing, A. [Still another cause of hypermethioninemia in children: *S*-adenosylmethionine synthetase deficiency]. *Arch Fr Pediatr* 1977; 34: 416–23.

58. Halsted, CH, Villanueva, J, Chandler, CJ, Stabler, SP, Allen, RH, Muskhelishvili, L, James, SJ, Poirier, L. Ethanol feeding of micropigs alters methionine metabo-

lism and increases hepatocellular apoptosis and proliferation. *Hepatology* 1996; 23: 497–505.

59. Hancock, RL. *S*-adenosylmethionine-synthesizing activity of normal and neoplastic mouse tissue. *Cancer Res* 1966; 26: 2425–30.

60. Hazelwood, S, Bernardini, I, Shotelersuk, V, Tangerman, A, Guo, J, Mudd, H, Gahl, WA. Normal brain myelination in a patient homozygous for a mutation that encodes a severely truncated methionine adenosyltransferase I/III. *Am J Med Genet* 1998; 75: 395–400.

61. Hiroki, T, Horikawa, S, Tsukada, K. Structure of the rat methionine adenosyltransferase 2A gene and its promoter. *Eur J Biochem* 1997; 250: 653–60.

62. Hoffman, JL. Fractionation of methionine adenosyltransferase isozymes (rat liver). *Methods Enzymol* 1983; 94: 223–28.

63. Horikawa, S, Ishikawa, M, Ozasa, H, Tsukada, K. Isolation of a cDNA encoding the rat liver *S*-adenosylmethionine synthetase. *Eur J Biochem* 1989; 184: 497–501.

64. Horikawa, S, Ozasa, H, Ito, K, Katsuyama, I, Tsukada, K, Sugiyama, T. Expression of *S*-adenosylmethionine synthetase isozyme genes in regenerating rat liver after partial hepatectomy. *Biochem Mol Biol Int* 1996; 40: 807–14.

65. Horikawa, S, Ozasa, H, Ota, K, Tsukada, K. Immunohistochemical analysis of rat *S*-adenosylmethionine synthetase isozymes in developmental liver. *FEBS Lett* 1993; 330: 307–11.

66. Horikawa, S, Sasuga, J, Shimizu, K, Ozasa, H, Tsukada, K. Molecular cloning and nucleotide sequence of cDNA encoding the rat kidney *S*-adenosylmethionine synthetase. *J Biol Chem* 1990; 265: 13683–86.

67. Horikawa, S, Tsukada, K. Molecular cloning and developmental expression of a human kidney *S*-adenosylmethionine synthetase. *FEBS Lett* 1992; 312: 37–41.

68. Horikawa, S, Tsukada, K. Molecular cloning and nucleotide sequence of cDNA encoding the human liver *S*-adenosylmethionine synthetase. *Biochem Int* 1991; 25: 81–90.

69. Horowitz, JH, Rypins, EB, Henderson, JM, Heymsfield, SB, Moffitt, SD, Bain, RP, Chawla, RK, Bleier, JC, Rudman, D. Evidence for impairment of transsulfuration pathway in cirrhosis. *Gastroenterology* 1981; 81: 668–75.

70. Huang, ZZ, Mao, Z, Cai, J, Lu, SC. Changes in methionine adenosyltransferase during liver regeneration in the rat. *Am J Physiol* 1998; 275: G14–21.

71. Huang, ZZ, Mato, JM, Kanel, G, Lu, SC. Differential effect of thioacetamide on hepatic methionine adenosyltransferase expression in the rat. *Hepatology* 1999; 29: 1471–78.

72. Iimuro, Y, Gallucci, RM, Luster, MI, Kono, H, Thurman, RG. Antibodies to tumour necrosis factor α attenuate hepatic necrosis and inflammation caused by chronic exposure to ethanol in the rat. *Hepatology* 1997; 26: 1530–37.

73. Jungermann, K, Kietzmann, T. Zonation of parenchymal and nonparenchymal metabolism in liver. *Annu Rev Nutr* 1996; 16: 179–203.

74. Kamimura, S, Gaal, K, Briton, RS, Bacon, BR, Triadafilopoulos, G, Tsukamoto, H. Increased 4-hydroxynonenal levels in experimental alcoholic liver disease:

Association of lipid peroxidation with liver fibrosis. *Hepatology* 1992; 16: 448–53.

75. Kinsell, LW, Harper, HA, Barton, HC, Michaels, GD, Weiss, HA. Rate of disappearance from plasma of intravenously administered methionine in patients with liver damage. *Science* 1947; 106: 589–94.

76. Kotb, M, Geller, AM. Methionine adenosyltransferase: Structure and function. *Pharmacol Ther* 1993; 59: 125–43.

77. Kotb, M, Geller, AM, Markham, GD, Kredich, NM, De La Rosa, J, Beachey, EH. Antigenic conservation of primary structural regions of S-adenosylmethionine synthetase. *Biochim Biophys Acta* 1990; 1040: 137–44.

78. Kotb, M, Kredich, NM. Regulation of human lymphocyte S-adenosylmethionine synthetase by product inhibition. *Biochim Biophys Acta* 1990; 1039: 253–60.

79. Kotb, M, Kredich, NM. S-Adenosylmethionine synthetase from human lymphocytes. Purification and characterization. *J Biol Chem* 1985; 260: 3923–30.

80. Kotb, M, Mudd, SH, Mato, JM, Geller, AM, Kredich, NM, Chou, JY, Cantoni, GL. Consensus nomenclature for the mammalian methionine adenosyltransferase genes and gene products [letter]. *Trends Genet* 1997; 13: 51–2.

81. LaBrecque, D. Liver regeneration: A picture emerges from the puzzle. *Am J Gastroenterol* 1994; 89: S86–S96.

82. Liau, MC, Chang, CF, Belanger, L, Grenier, A. Correlation of isozyme patterns of S-adenosylmethionine synthetase with fetal stages and pathological states of the liver. *Cancer Res* 1979; 39: 162–69.

83. Lieber, CS, Casini, A, DeCarli, LM, Kim, C, Lowe, N, Sasaki, R, Leo, MA. S-adenosyl-L-methionine attenuates alcohol-induced liver injury in the baboon. *Hepatology* 1990; 11: 165–72.

84. Lieber, CS, Leo, MA. Alcohol and the liver. In *Medical and Nutritional Complications of Alcoholism: Mechanisms and Management.* (Lieber, CS, ed.). Plenum Press, New York, 1992; pp. 185–239.

85. Lombardini, JB, Chou, TC, Talalay, P. Regulatory properties of adenosine triphosphate-L-methionine S-adenosyltransferase of rat liver. *Biochem J* 1973; 135: 43–57.

86. Mannick, JB, Hausladen, A, Liu, L, Hess, DT, Zeng, M, Miao, QX, Kane, LS, Gow, AJ, Stamler, JS. Fas-induced caspase denitrosylation. *Science* 1999; 284: 651–53.

87. Mao, Z, Liu, S, Cai, J, Huang, ZZ, Lu, SC. Cloning and functional characterization of the 5′-flanking region of human methionine adenosyltransferase 2A gene. *Biochem Biophys Res Commun* 1998; 248: 479–84.

88. Markham, GD, Hafner, EW, Tabor, CW, Tabor, H. S-Adenosylmethionine synthetase from *Escherichia coli. J Biol Chem* 1980; 255: 9082–92.

89. Martín-Duce, A, Ortiz, P, Cabrero, C, Mato, JM. S-Adenosyl-L-methionine synthetase and phospholipid methyltransferase are inhibited in human cirrhosis. *Hepatology* 1988; 8: 65–8.

90. Martínez-Chantar, ML, Pajares, MA. Assignment of a single disulfide bridge in rat liver methionine adenosyltransferase. *Eur J Biochem* 1999; 267: 1–8.

91. Mato, JM, Alvarez, L, Ortiz, P, Mingorance, J, Duran, C, Pajares, MA. S-adenosyl-L-methionine synthetase and

methionine metabolism deficiencies in cirrhosis. *Adv Exp Med Biol* 1994; 368: 113–17.

92. Mato, JM, Alvarez, L, Ortiz, P, Pajares, MA. S-adenosylmethionine synthesis: Molecular mechanisms and clinical implications. *Pharmacol Ther* 1997; 73: 265–80.

93. Mato, JM, Cámara, J, Fernández de Paz, J, Caballería, L, Coll, S, Caballero, A, García-Buey, L, Beltrán, J, Benita, V, Caballería, J, Solà, R, Moreno-Otero, R, Barrao, F, Martín-Duce, A, Correa, JA, Parés, A, Barrao, E, García-Magaz, I, Puerta, JL, Moreno, J, Boissard, G, Ortiz, P, Rodés, J. S-adenosylmethionine in alcoholic liver cirrhosis: A randomized, placebo-controlled, double-blind, multicentre clinical trial. *J Hepatol* 1999; 30: 1081–89.

94. Mingorance, J, Alvarez, L, Pajares, MA, Mato, JM. Recombinant rat liver S-adenosyl-L-methionine synthetase tetramers and dimers are in equilibrium. *Int J Biochem Cell Biol* 1997; 29: 485–91.

95. Mingorance, J, Alvarez, L, Sánchez-Góngora, E, Mato, JM, Pajares, MA. Site-directed mutagenesis of rat liver S-adenosylmethionine synthetase. Identification of a cysteine residue critical for the oligomeric state. *Biochem J* 1996; 315: 761–66.

96. Mitsui, K, Teraoka, H, Tsukada, K. Complete purification and immunochemical analysis of S-adenosylmethionine synthetase from bovine brain. *J Biol Chem* 1988; 263: 11211–16.

97. Mudd, SH, Levy, HL, Skovby, F. Disorders of transsulfuration. In *The Metabolic Bases of Inherited Disease.* Scriver, CR, Beaudet, AL, Charles, L, Sly, WS, Valle, D. (eds.). McGraw Hill Inc., New York, 1994; pp. 1279–1327.

98. Mudd, SH, Levy, HL, Tangerman, A, Boujet, C, Buist, N, Davidson-Mundt, A, Hudgins, L, Oyanagi, K, Nagao, M, Wilson, WG. Isolated persistent hypermethioninemia. *Am J Hum Genet* 1995; 57: 882–92.

99. Mudd, SH, Poole, JR. Labile methyl balances for normal humans on various dietary regimens. *Metabolism* 1975; 29: 707–20.

100. Nanji, AA, Griniuviene, B, Yacoub, LK, Fogt, F, Tahan, SR. Intercellular adhesion molecule-1 expression in experimental alcoholic liver disease: Relationship to endotoxemia and TNF α messenger RNA. *Exp Mol Pathol* 1995; 62: 42–51.

101. Ng, HH, Bird, A. DNA methylation and chromatin modification. *Curr Opin Genet Dev* 1999; 9: 158–63.

102. Okada, G, Teraoka, H, Tsukada, K. Multiple species of mammalian S-adenosylmethionine synthetase. Partial purification and characterization. *Biochemistry* 1981; 20: 934–40.

103. Okada, G, Watanabe, Y, Tsukada, K. Changes in patterns of S-adenosylmethionine synthetases in fetal and postnatal rat liver. *Cancer Res* 1980; 40: 2895–97.

104. Pajares, MA, Duran C, Corrales, F, Pliego, MM, Mato, JM. Modulation of rat liver S-adenosylmethionine synthetase activity by glutathione. *J Biol Chem* 1992; 267: 17598–605.

105. Pan, F, Chang, GG, Lee, SC, Tang, MS. Induction of methionine adenosyltransferase in rat liver by corticosteroids. *Proc Soc Exp Biol Med USA* 1968; 128: 611–16.

106. Pan, F, Tarver, H. Effects of diet and other factors on methionine adenosyltransferase levels in rat liver. *J Nutr* 1967; 92: 274–80.

107. Pascale, RM, Simile, MM, De Miglio, MR, Nufris, A, Daino, L, Seddaiu, MA, Rao, PM, Rajalakshmi, S, Sarma, DS, Feo, F. Chemoprevention by S-adenosyl-L-methionine of rat liver carcinogenesis initiated by 1,2-dimethylhydrazine and promoted by orotic acid. *Carcinogenesis* 1995; 16: 427–30.

108. Pascale, RM, Simile, MM, Ruggio, ME, Seddaiu, MA, Satta, G, Sequenza, MJ, Daino, L, Vannini, MG, Lai, P, Feo, F. Reversal by 5-azacytidine of the S-adenosyl-L-methionine-induced inhibition of the development of putative preneoplastic foci in rat liver carcinogenesis. *Cancer Lett* 1991; 56: 259–65.

109. Pascale, RM, Simile, MM, Satta, G, Seddaiu, MA, Daino, L, Pinna, G, Vinci, MA, Gaspa, L, Feo, F. Comparative effects of L-methionine, S-adenosyl-L-methionine and 5′-methylthioadenosine on the growth of preneoplastic lesions and DNA methylation in rat liver during the early stages of hepatocarcinogenesis. *Anticancer Res* 1991; 11: 617–24.

110. Pérez-Mato, I, Castro, C, Ruiz, FA, Corrales, FJ, Mato, JM. Methionine adenosyltransferase S-nitrosylation is regulated by the basic and acidic amino acids surrounding the target thiol. *J Biol Chem* 1999; 274: 17075–80.

111. Pogribny, IP, Basnakian, AG, Miller, BJ, Lopatina, NG, Poirier, LA, James, SJ. Breaks in genomic DNA and within the p53 gene are associated with hypomethylation in livers of folate/methyl-deficient rats. *Cancer Res* 1995; 55: 1894–901.

112. Ruiz, F, Corrales, FJ, Miqueo, C, Mato, JM. Nitric oxide inactivates rat hepatic methionine adenosyltransferase in vivo by S-nitrosylation. *Hepatology* 1998; 28: 1051–57.

113. Sakata, SF, Shelly, LL, Ruppert, S, Schutz, G, Chou, JY. Cloning and expression of murine S-adenosylmethionine synthetase. *J Biol Chem* 1993; 268: 13978–86.

114. Sánchez-Góngora, E, Pastorino, JG, Alvarez, L, Pajares, MA, Garcia, C, Vina, JR, Mato, JM, Farber, JL. Increased sensitivity to oxidative injury in Chinese hamster ovary cells stably transfected with rat liver S-adenosylmethionine synthetase cDNA. *Biochem J* 1996; 319: 767–73.

115. Sánchez-Góngora, E, Ruiz, F, Mingorance, J, An, W, Corrales, FJ, Mato, JM. Interaction of liver methionine adenosyltransferase with hydroxyl radical. *FASEB J* 1997; 11: 1013–9.

116. Schonker, S, Bay, MK. Alcohol and endotoxin: Another path to alcoholic liver injury. *Alcohol Clin Exp Res* 1995; 19: 1364–66.

117. Shimizu-Saito, K, Horikawa, S, Kojima, N, Shiga, J, Senoo, H, Tsukada, K. Differential expression of S-adenosylmethionine synthetase isozymes in different cell types of rat liver. *Hepatology* 1997; 26: 424–31.

118. Shou, L, Pan, F, Chin, SF. Pancreatic hormones and hepatic methionine adenosyltransferase in the rat. *Proc Soc Exp Biol Med USA* 1969; 131: 1012–18.

119. Simile, MM, Pascale, RM, De Miglio, MR, Nufris, A, Daino, L, Seddaiu, MA, Gaspa, L, Feo, F. Correlation between S-adenosyl-L-methionine content and produc-tion of c-myc, c-Ha-ras, and c-Ki-ras mRNA transcripts in the early stages of rat liver carcinogenesis. *Cancer Lett* 1994; 79: 9–16.

120. Stamler, JS, Toone, EJ, Lipton, SA, Sucher, NJ. (S)NO signals: Translocation, regulation, and a consensus motif. *Neuron* 1997; 18: 691–6.

121. Sullivan, DM, Hoffman, JL. Fractionation and kinetic properties of rat liver and kidney methionine adenosyl-transferase isozymes. *Biochemistry* 1983; 22: 1636–41.

122. Surtees, R. Demyelination and inborn errors of the single carbon transfer pathway. *Eur J Pediatr* 1998; 157(Suppl 2): S118–21.

123. Surtees, R, Leonard, J, Austin, S. Association of demyeli-nation with deficiency of cerebrospinal-fluid S-adenosyl-methionine in inborn errors of methyl-transfer pathway. *Lancet* 1991; 338: 1550–54.

124. Takusagawa, F, Kamitori, S, Markham, GD. Structure and function of S-adenosylmethionine synthetase: Crystal structures of S-adenosylmethionine synthetase with ADP, BrADP, and PPi at 28 angstroms resolution. *Biochemistry* 1996; 35: 2586–96.

125. Takusagawa, F, Kamitori, S, Misaki, S, Markham, GD. Crystal structure of S-adenosylmethionine synthetase. *J Biol Chem* 1996; 271: 136–47.

126. Tobena, R, Horikawa, S, Calvo, V, Alemany, S. Interleukin-2 induces γ-S-adenosyl-L-methionine syn-thetase gene expression during T-lymphocyte activation. *Biochem J* 1996; 319: 929–33.

127. Torres, L, Avila, MA, Carretero, MV, Latasa, MU, Caballería, J, López-Rodas, G, Boukaba, A, Lu, SC, Franco, L, Mato, JM. Liver-specific methionine adeno-syltransferase MAT1A gene expression is associated with a specific pattern of promoter methylation and histone acetylation: Implications for MAT1A silencing during transformation. *FASEB J* 2000; 14: 95–102.

128. Torres, L, López-Rodas, G, Latasa, MU, Carretero, MV, Boukaba, A, Rodríguez, JL, Franco, L, Mato, JM, Avila, MA. DNA methylation and histone acetylation of rat methionine adenosyltransferase 1A and 2A genes is tis-sue-specific. *Int J Biochem Cell Biol* 2000; 34: 397–404.

129. Trimble, KC, Molloy, AM, Scott, JM, Weir, DG. The effect of ethanol on one-carbon metabolism: Increased methionine catabolism and lipotrope methyl-group wastage. *Hepatology* 1993; 18: 984–89.

130. Tsukamoto, H, French, SW, Benson, N, Delgado, G, Rao, GA, Larkin, EC, Largman, C. Severe and progres-sive steatosis and focal necrosis in rat liver induced by continuous intragastric infusion of ethanol and low fat diet. *Hepatology* 1985; 5: 224–32.

131. Tsukamoto, H, Gaal, K, French, SW. Insights into the pathogenesis of alcoholic liver necrosis and fibrosis: Status report. *Hepatology* 1990; 13: 599–608.

132. Tsukamoto, H, Towner, SJ, Ciofalo, LM, French, SW. Ethanol-induced liver fibrosis in rats fed high fat diet. *Hepatology* 1986; 6: 814–22.

133. Ubagai, T, Lei, KJ, Huang, S, Mudd, SH, Levy, HL, Chou, JY. Molecular mechanisms of an inborn error of methionine pathway. Methionine adenosyltransferase deficiency. *J Clin Invest* 1995; 96: 1943–47.

134. Varela-Moreiras, G, Alonso-Aperte, E, Rubio, M, Gassó, M, Deulofeu, R, Alvarez, L, Caballería, J, Rodés, J, Mato, JM. Carbon tetrachloride-induced hepatic injury is associated with global DNA hypomethylation and homocysteinemia: Effect of S-adenosylmethionine treatment. *Hepatology* 1995; 22: 1310–15.

135. Vendemiale, G, Altomare, E, Trizio, T, Le Grazie, C, Di Padova, C, Salerno, MT, Carrieri, V, Albano, O. Effect of oral S-adenosyl-L-methionine on hepatic glutathione in patients with liver disease. *Scand J Gastroenterol* 1989; 24: 407–15.

136. Wagner, C, Pattaneyek, R, Newcomer, M, Krupenko, N. Glycine N-methyltransferase: structure and function. In *Methionine Metabolism: Molecular Mechanisms and Clinical Implications.* (Mato, JM, Caballero, A, eds.). C.S.I.C., Madrid, 1998; pp. 35–43.

137. Watson, WH, Zhao, Y, Chawla, RK. S-adenosylmethionine attenuates the lipopolysaccharide-induced expression of the gene for tumour necrosis factor alpha. *Biochem J* 1999; 342: 21–5.

138. Xu, L, Eu, JP, Meissner, G, Stamler, JS. Activation of the cardiac calcium release channel (ryanodine receptor) by poly-S-nitrosylation. *Science* 1998; 279: 234–47.

139. Zeng, Z, Huang, Z-Z, Chen, C, Yang, H, Mao, Z, Lu, SC. Cloning and functional characterization of the 5′-flanking region of human methionine adenosyltransferase 1A gene. *Biochem J* 2000; 14: 95–102.

140. Zingg, JM, Jones, PA. Genetic and epigenetic aspects of DNA methylation on genome expression, evolution, mutation and carcinogenesis. *Carcinogenesis* 1997; 18: 869–82.

7

S-Adenosylmethionine-dependent Methyltransferases

STEVEN CLARKE
KELLEY BANFIELD

Mammalian *S*-adenosylmethionine-dependent methyltransferases each catalyze a reaction, giving rise to two products — *S*-adenosylhomocysteine and one of a variety of methylated biomolecules including nucleic acids, proteins, lipids, and small molecules. *S*-adenosylhomocysteine is subsequently broken down to adenosine and homocysteine by *S*-adenosylhomocysteine hydrolase (Figure 7.1). The homocysteine formed can be either remethylated to methionine or converted to cysteine via cystathionine (30, 72). As such, these methyltransferases are bifunctional; they make up an essential part of the conduit for the conversion of methionine to cysteine in addition to generating methylated products.

Recent attention has been drawn to methyltransferases to understand how elevated plasma total homocysteine levels are connected to disease. This is because higher intracellular homocysteine levels are expected to correlate with lower methyltransferase activities as described later. The inhibition of these enzymes may represent a specific biochemical mechanism that may explain at least some of the cellular toxicity associated with homocysteine accumulation. This chapter reviews the data on mammalian methyltransferases, allowing us to

identify enzymes that might be particularly sensitive to inhibition and thus may be prime targets for homocysteine-associated effects.

Why would elevated intracellular free homocysteine levels necessarily result in the inhibition of cellular *S*-adenosylmethionine-dependent methyltransferases? This effect comes from two linked reactions. First, higher levels of homocysteine result in higher levels of *S*-adenosylhomocysteine by mass action effects on the *S*-adenosylhomocysteine hydrolase reaction, where the equilibrium favors the conversion of homocysteine and adenosine to *S*-adenosylhomocysteine (22). Second, *S*-adenosylhomocysteine is a potent product inhibitor of most *S*-adenosylmethionine-dependent methyltransferases, with K_i values in the submicromolar to low micromolar range (Figure 7.1). In fact, the K_i value for *S*-adenosylhomocysteine is often less than the K_m value for *S*-adenosylmethionine (10, 11, 46, 67, 97, 112). The potential loss of the body's ability to efficiently catalyze methyltransfer reactions thus may be linked to the higher risk of premature cardiovascular disease and the other clinical features, including neurological impairment, that results from total homocysteine accumulation in plasma and urine (52, 84).

The specific questions to be addressed are these: How many different types of *S*-adenosylmethionine-dependent methyltransferases occur in mammals? What reactions do they catalyze? How sensitive is each reaction to inhibition by *S*-adenosylhomocysteine? Are the known increases in plasma total homocysteine actually correlated with increases in intracellular *S*-adenosylhomocysteine? Can we begin to correlate the

Fig. 7.1. Metabolic relationships between *S*-adenosylmethionine, *S*-adenosylhomocysteine, and homocysteine in mammalian cells. *S*-adenosylmethionine-dependent methyltransferases using various methyl-accepting substrates (designated X) are inhibited by the product, *S*-adenosylhomocysteine, which can accumulate in the presence of homocysteine because the equilibrium of the *S*-adenosylhomocysteine hydrolase reaction favors *S*-adenosylhomocysteine formation.

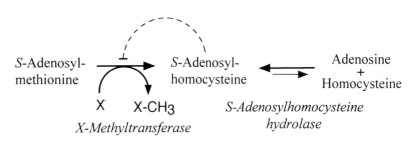

effects of their inhibition with the specific pathologies seen with elevated homocysteine levels?

Mechanistic Links Between Homocysteine Accumulation, Methyltransferase Inhibition, and Disease

The possible connection between elevated plasma total homocysteine and methyltransferase inhibition was apparent to the biochemists who first characterized homocystinuria (28, 29). Evidence was presented early on that elevated plasma total homocysteine can result in the appearance of S-adenosylhomocysteine in the urine, where it is otherwise not found (83). This hypothesis has only recently begun to be experimentally tested.

The clearest demonstration of a mechanistic connection between homocysteine accumulation, S-adenosylhomocysteine accumulation, and the inhibition of methyltransferases has been made by Perna and co-workers (77–82). Their interest has been in the mechanism of cellular injury in patients with chronic renal failure. Previously, investigators demonstrated that plasma total homocysteine is mildly elevated and may be associated with the premature occlusive arterial disease seen in these patients (14, 15). Perna and co-workers showed that erythrocyte S-adenosylhomocysteine levels are fourfold to eightfold higher in patients with renal failure, whereas little change in S-adenosylmethionine levels was observed (77). This change is accompanied by an up to 50% inhibition in the activity of the erythrocyte repair protein L-isoaspartate (D-aspartate) O-methyltransferase (77, 79, 80). Recently, it has been found that the plasma ratio of S-adenosylmethionine/S-adenosylhomocysteine (presumably reflecting the intracellular situation) is lowered in patients with end-stage renal failure (66). Additionally, a stable isotope study has shown that whole body transmethylation rates are decreased about 24% in these individuals (99).

In a second type of approach, Wang and co-workers used a cell culture system to provide evidence that increased homocysteine concentrations in the medium in the physiological range may specifically inhibit the methyltransferase that catalyzes the "capping" of protein C-terminal isoprenylcysteine residues (62, 107). Wang et al. (107) reported that the incubation of human aortic endothelial cells with 50 µmol/L homocysteine resulted in an eightfold decrease in the ratio of S-adenosylmethionine to S-adenosylhomocysteine. This decrease was accompanied by the inhibition of DNA synthesis and a 50% inhibition in the C-terminal methylation of one or more members of the small G-protein ras family, presumably as a result of the inhibition of isoprenylcysteine methyltransferase.

It is clear that a similar mechanism of inhibition can generally take place with other types of methyltransferases, and it would be expected that increased S-adenosylhomocysteine would affect many of these enzymes in the cell (8). It is therefore useful to briefly examine some of the relevant features of these enzymes. However, much more must be learned about the correlation of levels of extracellular total homocysteine and intracellular S-adenosylhomocysteine in different tissues. Indeed, it has been pointed out that elevated plasma total homocysteine may be a result of the *increased* activity of intracellular methyltransferases (D. E. Vance, personal communication). Additionally, the intracellular concentration of adenosine will also affect the position of equilibrium between homocysteine and S-adenosylhomocysteine, and it is important to know how these adenosine levels change under various physiological conditions.

Mammalian Methyltransferases Catalyze a Variety of Reactions

Table 7.1 shows all of the known types of mammalian S-adenosylmethionine-dependent methyltransferases. These 39 species were identified by selecting AdoMet-dependent mammalian species from the Enzyme Commission list (E.C. 2.1.1.XX) using the "Enzyme" database of the Swiss Institute for Bioinformatics (http://www.expasy.ch/enzyme/) as well as literature searches using the Medline data base from 1966 to the present. We have also been aided by the recent compilation of methyltransferases prepared by Blumenthal (5).

Table 7.1 lists a total of two DNA methyltransferases, 10 RNA methyltransferases, 3 lipid methyltransferases, 11 protein methyltransferases, and 13 small molecule methyltransferases. In many cases, the gene and enzyme have been well described. In other cases, the presence of a methyltransferase is only inferred from the presence of a well-characterized methylated product. Variants created by RNA splicing reactions and other processes further enlarge the diversity of these methyltransferases. Although Table 7.1 aims to include all well-characterized enzymes, new methyltransferases will certainly be added as more is learned about methylation pathways. Efforts have been made previously to use conserved sequence motifs in a large family of these methyltransferases to identify new methyltransferases in the output of genomic sequencing projects (54, 73). In the yeast *Saccharomyces cerevisiae*, where the complete genome sequence is known, it has been possible to identify 26 potentially novel methyltransferases (73). With a nearly complete sequence of the human genome released in the year 2000, it will be possible to extend this approach to identify new human methyltrans-

Table 7.1 Mammalian S-Adenosylmethionine-dependent Methyltransferases

E. C. #	Enzyme Name	Gene Designation	Methyl-accepting Substrate	Function	Notes	Reference
DNA						
2.1.1.37	DNA (cytosine-5-)-methyltransferase 1	DNMT1	DNA	Regulation of gene expression, chromosome inactivation, genomic imprinting	Major activity	50, 101
2.1.1.37	DNA (cytosine-5-)-methyltransferase 3	DNMT3	DNA		Minor activity	50, 101
RNA						
2.1.1.56	mRNA (guanine-N 7-)-methyltransferase	RNMT	$GpppN_1N_2$	mRNA capping	Three alternatively spliced forms	6
	Cap I-mRNA 2'-O-methyltransferase		$N7mGpppN_1N_2$	mRNA capping	Nuclear enzyme	6
	Cap II-mRNA 2'-O-methyltransferase (2'-O-methyladenosine-N 6-)-methyltransferase		$N7mGppp^mN_1N_2$	mRNA capping	Cytoplasmic enzyme	6
			$N7mGppp^mA_1^mN_2$	mRNA capping	Cytoplasmic enzyme	6
	mRNA N 6-adenosine methyltransferase		Internal adenosine residues	Affects efficiency of pre-mRNA splicing or transport to cytoplasm		6
2.1.1.29	tRNA (cytosine-5-)-methyltransferase		tRNA	Alters flexibility of tRNA for codon recognition		47
2.1.1.31	tRNA (guanine-N 1-)-methyltransferase		tRNA	Alters flexibility of tRNA for codon recognition		47
2.1.1.32	tRNA (guanine-N 2-)-methyltransferase		tRNA	Alters flexibility of tRNA for codon recognition		47
2.1.1.36	tRNA (adenine-N 1-)-methyltransferase		tRNA	Alters flexibility of tRNA for codon recognition		47
	rRNA (2'-ribose-O)-methyltransferase		Internal adenosine residues in rRNA	rRNA maturation and ribosome assembly?		26
LIPIDS						
2.1.1.17	Phosphatidylethanolamine N-methyltransferase	PEMPT	Phosphatidyl-ethanolamine	Phosphatidylcholine synthesis	PEMT1, PEMT2 splice variants	98, 105
	Dihydroxynonaprenylbenzoate O-methyltransferase	COQ3	Pathway precursors	Ubiquinone synthesis	Rat gene cloned, human ESTs* present	69, 53a
	COQ5 C-methyltransferase	COQ5	Pathway precursors	Ubiquinone synthesis	Yeast gene cloned, human ESTs* present	3
PROTEIN **Carboxyl**						
2.1.1.77	Protein L-isoaspartate (D-aspartate) O-methyltransferase	PCMT1	L-isoaspartate, D-aspartate residues	Protein repair		20

(continues)

Table 7.1 *Continued*

E. C. #	Enzyme Name	Gene Designation	Methyl-accepting Substrate	Function	Notes	Reference
2.1.1.100	Protein S-isoprenylcysteine O-methyltransferase	ICMT	C-terminal isoprenyl cysteine residues	Protein stability? G-proteins and Ras processing and localization		115, 3a
	Protein phosphatase 2a O-methyltransferase	LCMT	C-terminal leucine residues on PP2A	Regulation of metabolism?		114, 21a
Lysine						
2.1.1.43	Histone-lysine N-methyltransferase		Histones	Unknown		65
2.1.1.60	Calmodulin-lysine N-methyltransferase	CLNMT	Calmodulin	Unknown		113
Arginine						
2.1.1.126	[Myelin basic protein]-arginine N-methyltransferase		Arginine residues on myelin basic protein	Unknown		59
	Protein arginine N-methyltransferase 1	PRMT1	Arginine residues	Signal transduction, nuclear transport?		64
	Protein arginine N-methyltransferase 3	PRMT3	Arginine residues	Signal transduction, nuclear transport?		92
	Coactivator-associated arginine methyltransferase-1	CARM1	Arginine residues	Transcriptional control?		16
Histidine						
	Protein histidine N-methyltransferase		Histidine residues on actin and myosin			76
Other						
	Diphthine synthase	DPR5(Y)	α-Amino group of a modified histidine residue	Diphthamide synthesis in EF-2	Homologous human ESTs* of yeast DPH5 enzyme	70

SMALL MOLECULES

N-Methyltransferases

2.1.1.1	Nicotinamide N-methyltransferase	NNMT	Nicotinamide and other pyridines	Metabolism of nicotinamide and other pyridines		91
2.1.1.2	Guanidinoacetate N-methyltransferase	GAMT	Guanidinoacetate	Creatine synthesis		51, 74
2.1.1.8	Histamine N-methyltransferase	HNMT	Histamine	Histamine inactivation		100
2.1.1.20	Glycine N-methyltransferase	GNMT	Glycine	Sarcosine synthesis, regulation of homocysteine pathway		41, 17a
2.1.1.28	Phenylethanolamine N-methyltransferase	PNMT	Phenylethanol-amine	Epinephrine synthesis		63
	β-Carboline-2-N-methyltransferase	β C-2-NMT	β-carbolines (norharman and harman)	Unknown	Similar to INMT but highly expressed in brain	35
	Indolethylamine N-methyltransferase	INMT	Tryptamine, others	Unknown	Similar to βC-2-NMT but expressed in non-neural tissue	94

O-Methyltransferases

2.1.1.4	Hydroxyindole O-methyltransferase	HIOMT	Serotonin	Melatonin synthesis		23
2.1.1.6	Catechol O-methyltransferase	COMT	Catechols (epinephrine, norepinephrine, dopamine and others)	Epinephrine, norepinephrine and dopamine inactivation		102

S- and As-Methyltransferases

2.1.1.9	Thiol S-methyltransferase	TMT	Thiols	Metabolism of endogenous and xenobiotic compounds		9
2.1.1.67	Thiopurine S-methyltransferase	TPMT	Thiopurines	Metabolism of endogenous and xenobiotic compounds		27
	Thioether S-methyltransferase		Thioethers (sulfur, selenium, tellurium)	Metabolism of endogenous and xenobiotic compounds		108
	Arsenite methyltransferase		Arsenite	Metabolism of endogenous and xenobiotic compounds		93

*EST, expressed sequence tag.

Table 7.2   Possible Mammalian Methyltransferases

	Enzyme Name	Gene	Substrate	Source	Notes	Ref.
DNA						
	DNA (cytosine-5-)-methyltransferase 2	*DNMT2*	DNA	Human	No enzymatic activity demonstrated	50
RNA						
	tRNA 2′-O-ribose methyltransferase		Ribose of tRNA	Yeast	Human homolog identified	12
PROTEIN						
Arginine						
	Protein arginine *N*-methyltransferase 2	*PRMT2*	Arginine residues	Human	No enzymatic activity demonstrated	34
Lysine						
	Hsp68, Hsc70 and BiP protein lysine *N*-methyltransferase		Hsp68, Hsc70, BiP	Mouse	Distinct enzyme not identified	106
	Myosin lysine *N*-methyltransferase		Myosin lysine residues	Rabbit	Distinct enzyme not identified	96
	EF-1α lysine *N*-methyltransferase		EF-1α	Rabbit	Distinct enzyme not identified	24
	Citrate synthase lysine *N*-methyltransferase		Lysine residues	Pig	Distinct enzyme not identified	4
	Myosin N-terminal alanine *N*-methyltransferase		N-terminal alanine residue of myosin	Human	Distinct enzyme not identified	48

ferases as well as to link newly described genes to known methyltransferases.

There are cases where the presence of a mammalian methyltransferase is either less certain or where it is unclear which enzyme catalyzes the reaction. Table 7.2 includes potential methyltransferases encoded by genes with amino acid sequence homology to other methyltransferases but where no enzyme activity has yet been demonstrated. Also included are species where the methylation chemistry is well established, but it is unknown whether a distinct enzyme is involved or the reaction can be catalyzed by a previously known methyltransferase. With further research, some of these species can be added to the group in Table 7.1, whereas others may turn out not to be *S*-adenosylmethionine-dependent methyltransferases at all.

Functions of S-Adenosylmethionine-dependent Methyltransferases

From the data in Table 7.1, we can divide the known or postulated functions of most of these enzymes into five broad and sometimes overlapping categories: small molecule biosynthesis; inactivation and elimination of small molecules and xenobiotics; stabilization of DNA, RNA, and proteins; cellular signaling pathways; and protein synthesis. It is notable that several

of these enzymes have been shown to be involved with neurochemical processes.

Small Molecule Biosynthesis

Six methyltransferases from Table 7.1 catalyze biosynthetic steps. The phosphatidylethanolamine *N*-methyltransferase catalyzes the conversion of phosphatidylethanolamine to phosphatidylcholine in the liver in an alternate pathway of phosphatidylcholine synthesis and is responsible for about 15% of the total biosynthesis of this major membrane structural building block (104). In mice whose gene encoding this activity is disrupted, their overall physiology is not apparently affected (103); however, when the animals were stressed by a choline-deficient diet, their liver function was severely compromised (104). This pathway may thus be important when organisms are under nutritional deprivation or are pregnant (104).

Two methyltransferases are involved in the synthesis of coenzyme Q or ubiquinone, the COQ3 O-methyltransferase and COQ5 C-methyltransferase (3, 18, 53a, 69). Ubiquinone is an essential electron carrier in mitochondrial oxidative phosphorylation and has antioxidant roles as well (18). The loss of ubiquinone would be expected to severely impact the ability of cells to produce adenosine triphosphate (ATP) for their energy needs. Another enzyme, the guanidinoacetate methyltransferase, catalyzes a crucial step in the biosynthesis of creatine phosphate, which serves as a buffer for ATP and an additional source of cellular energy. Loss of this activity might also be reflected in diminished cellular energy metabolism. The reaction may account for the bulk of hepatic S-adenosylmethionine use and thus represents a major potential source of homocysteine for cysteine biosynthesis (72).

Two distinct methyltransferases, the hydroxyindole and the phenylethanolamine methyltransferases, catalyze steps in the biosynthesis of the neurotransmitter/hormones melatonin and epinephrine. The loss of activity of these methyltransferases might be expected to result in abnormal neurotransmitter levels and aberrant neurological function. As discussed later, at least two methyltransferases are also involved in inactivation pathways of neurotransmitters, and the loss of these activities would also be expected to affect the function of the brain.

Inactivation and Elimination of Small Molecules and Xenobiotics

Seven methyltransferases listed in Table 7.1 have crucial roles in inactivating hormones and neurotransmitters and in preparing other types of endogenous and xenobiotic small molecules for elimination from the body. These enzymes can be characterized by their ability to remove molecules that have served their function or may be intrinsically toxic to the body.

Two methyltransferases catalyze the inactivation of neurotransmitters/hormones. The catechol O-methyltransferase acts on dopamine, norepinephrine, and epinephrine; the histamine N-methyltransferase acts on histamine (111). Knockout mice with a homozygous disruption in the gene for catechol O-methyltransferase display some behavioral changes but otherwise appear to be fairly normal (40).

The nicotinamide methyltransferase appears to be involved in the elimination of excess pyridine compounds from cells by fixing a positive charge on its aromatic ring (1, 88). Four other methyltransferases in Table 7.1 appear to be involved in the metabolism of sulfur, selenium, and arsenic compounds in the cell. The methyl acceptors for these enzymes can either represent normal products of metabolism (such as hydrogen sulfide) or xenobiotic compounds. The membrane-bound thiol methyltransferase and the soluble thiopurine methyltransferase recognize a variety of sulfhydryl-containing species (37, 111). The thioether products of these enzymes can then be recognized by the thioether methyltransferase that methylates these products as well as selenoethers to generate positively charged molecules that can be more readily excreted in the urine (108). A related species can also methylate arsenite and represents a detoxification pathway for this toxin (116).

Finally, two similar methyltransferases are present that modify tryptamine and related compounds and may serve similar functions. One of these enzymes is most active in non-neuronal tissues (94, 95), and a second activity from brain appears to activate the precursor form of neurotoxins such as the β-carbolines (35). It will be of interest to see if endogenous substrates for these enzymes exist.

Stabilization of DNA, RNA, and Proteins

At least seven types of methyltransferases appear to function in ensuring nucleic acid and protein stability. In humans, two genes have been described that catalyze the methylation of cytidine residues in CpG contexts in reactions that appear to both activate and inactivate transcription (Table 7.1). Null mutants have been prepared of the DNMT1 gene encoding the major mammalian activity in mouse embryonic stem cells (17). These cells have elevated mutation rates, suggesting the importance of the methylation reaction in maintaining the genome. RNA molecules are also modified by a variety of methyltransferases, as described in the section on protein synthesis. One of these enzymes, the mRNA cap methyltransferase that forms 7-methylguanine, is essential to yeast cells and may stabilize mRNAs against exonucleolytic degradation in addition to playing roles in translation initiation and efficiency (6, 68).

Protein stability also appears to be dependent on methyltransferase action. The widely distributed protein L-isoaspartyl (D-aspartyl) methyltransferase specifically recognizes polypeptides that have been spontaneously damaged in the aging process by the conversion of normal L-aspartyl and L-asparaginyl residues to L-isoaspartyl and D-aspartyl residues (20). The methylation of theses species can initiate a pathway that leads to their reconversion to L-aspartate residues (20). This pathway has been specifically studied in relation to the elevated homocysteine levels in patients with renal disease, as discussed earlier (77–82). The elevated homocysteine levels are directly correlated with elevated erythrocyte S-adenosylhomocysteine levels and the inhibition of the protein L-isoaspartate (D-aspartate) methyltransferase. Notably, it has been demonstrated that increased plasma total homocysteine is a general feature of aging (42).

Knockout mice that totally lack the protein L-isoaspartate (D-aspartate) methyltransferase demonstrated both a slow growth phenotype and a fatal seizure phenotype that resulted in death at 20 to 60 days after birth (58). The seizure phenotype was characterized as a persistent defect in the electrical activity of the brain and led directly to the slow growth phenotype (57). Interestingly, seizures are found in some patients with homocystinuria, although it is possible that these can result from homocysteine or one of its metabolites acting directly as an excitatory amino acid (2).

Proteins can also be stabilized by methylation reactions against untimely proteolytic degradation. The best example of this is the action of the protein isoprenylcysteine methyltransferase that "caps" the C-terminal isoprenylcysteine residue of a class of proteins including the small and large G proteins involved in signal transduction, the cGMP phosphodiesterase involved in visual information processing in the retina, and the nuclear lamins (19, 49, 115). Another possible set of examples are the two known methyltransferases that catalyze the sequential trimethylation of lysine residues to give species more resistance to proteolysis (113), but may affect the functions of the proteins as well (21). Other proteins contain trimethyllysine residues at specific sites and at least one protein contains an N-terminal trimethylalanine residue, but the methyltransferase or methyltransferases responsible for these modifications have not been identified (Table 7.2) (4, 24, 48, 96, 106).

Cellular Signaling

Four of the methyltransferases in Table 7.1 appear to be involved in signal transduction pathways. The catalytic subunit of protein phosphatase 2A is carboxyl methylated at its C-terminal leucine residue in a reversible reaction that may control the activity of this enzyme (21a, 60). This phosphatase is a major player in the regulation of amino acid and lipid metabolism by reversible protein phosphorylation/dephosphorylation reactions (21a, 60).

Recently, mammalian genes encoding the three type I protein arginine N-methyltransferases have been described that appear to be involved in the modulation of cellular metabolism (16, 34, 92). These enzymes all catalyze the asymmetrical dimethylation of the side chain guanidino group nitrogen atoms of a variety of eukaryotic proteins. Several roles have been described for them including modulating the interaction of proteins with RNA, regulation of signaling pathways, and the regulation of nuclear protein transport.

Protein Synthesis

The modification of a histidine residue in elongation factor 2 to diphthamide includes the trimethylation of an α-amino group (70). This modification is apparently crucial for the function of this factor because the ADP-ribosylation of this residue by diphtheria toxin inhibits protein synthesis. There are also a variety of methylation reactions to the sugars and bases of ribosomal, messenger, and transfer RNA. The function of these modifications is poorly understood, but it has been hypothesized that they are important in the processing and transport of these species to the cytosol (6,47).

Methyltransferases with Other Types of Functions

Methyltransfer reactions offer an opportunity to expand the pool of amino acids that can be incorporated into proteins. Here, post-translational methylation can create new amino acid residues that can endow proteins with new functions. The role of methyltransferases in diphthamide synthesis was discussed previously. In many cases, however, the role of the modification is not so clear.

The type II protein, arginine methyltransferase, specifically catalyzes the symmetrical dimethylation of arginine-107 of myelin basic protein (59). Although the precise role for the latter enzyme is unknown, it is interesting to note that demyelination in brain is associated with depletion of S-adenosylmethionine (13). Another highly specific protein methyltransferase modifies the histidine-73 residue on actin and possibly myosin. Interestingly, this modification is present in actins from lower eukaryotes to vertebrates with the notable exception of the yeasts (55).

Finally, the glycine methyltransferase appears to have multiple roles in the cell. It appears to be the species responsible for allowing the pathway from methionine to cysteine to occur even when the rate of the other methyltransferases is insufficient to provide adequate levels of S-adenosylhomocysteine. The conversion of glycine to sarcosine and the subsequent oxidative metabolism of sarcosine in the mitochondrial electron transport pathway can effectively remove excess methyl groups from the cell and in the process control the ratio of S-adenosylmethionine to S-adenosylhomocysteine (72). This function requires that it be relatively resistant to product inhibition by S-adenosylhomocysteine and this is reflected in the relatively high K_i value of 35 μmol/L in Table 7.3.

Assessment of the Inhibition of Specific Methyltransferases by Elevated S-Adenosylhomocysteine Levels

Table 7.3 shows the values for the kinetic constants (K_m value for S-adenosylmethionine and K_i value for S-adenosylhomocysteine) that are known for the mammalian methyltransferases described in Table 7.1. It is immediately clear that there is a range of these values such that some methyltransferases will be much more susceptible to the inhibitory effect of S-adenosylhomocysteine than others. Because S-adenosylhomocysteine is generally a competitive inhibitor, the catalytic activity of these methyltransferases in vivo is also a function of the concentration of S-adenosylme-

Table 7.3 Sensitivity of Methyltransferases to Inhibition by *S*-Adenosylhomocysteine

Methyltransferase	K_m for AdoMet (μmol/L)	K_i for AdoHcy (μmol/L)	Source	Fraction of Maximal Methyltransferase Activity			Percentage of activity at 100 μmol/L relative to 1 μmol/L AdoHcy	Fraction of Maximal Methyltransferase Activity		Percentage activity at 6.7 μmol/L relative to 0.8 μmol/L AdoHcy	Reference
				AdoMet 30 μmol/L AdoHcy 1 μmol/L	AdoMet 30 μmol/L AdoHcy 10 μmol/L	AdoMet 30 μmol/L AdoHcy 100 μmol/L		Control AdoMet 2.7 μmol/L AdoHcy 0.8 μmol/L	Uremic AdoMet 2.7 μmol/L AdoHcy 6.7 μmol/L		
DNA											
DNA (cytosine-5-) 1	1.4	1.4	Mouse erythroleukemia cells	0.93	0.72	0.23	25%	0.55	0.25	45%	32
RNA											
tRNA (cytosine-5-)	0.5	0.9	Human HeLa cell	0.97	0.83	0.35	36%	0.74	0.39	53%	56
tRNA (guanine-N 1-)	3	0.11	Rat liver	0.50	0.10	0.01	2%	0.10	0.01	15%	38
tRNA (guanine-N 2-)	2	23	Rat liver	0.93	0.91	0.74	79%	0.57	0.51	90%	38
tRNA (adenine-N 1-)	0.3	0.85	Rat liver	0.98	0.89	0.46	47%	0.82	0.50	61%	39
rRNA (2'-ribose-O)	0.24 (K_d AdoMet)	0.17 (K_d AdoHcy)	Mouse nucleoli	0.95	0.68	0.18	18%	0.66	0.22	33%	26
LIPIDS											
Phosphatidylethanolamine	18.2	3.8	Rat liver	0.57	0.31	0.06	10%	0.11	0.05	47%	43, 44, 45
PROTEIN											
Carboxyl											
Protein-L-isoaspartate (D-aspartate)	2	0.08	Bovine brain	0.53	0.11	0.01	2%	0.11	0.02	14%	53
Protein S-isoprenylcysteine	2.1	9.2	Rat liver	0.93	0.87	0.55	59%	0.54	0.43	79%	90
Lysine											
Calmodulin-lysine N-	2	15.2 (IC_{50} value)	Rat testes	0.93	0.90	0.66	71%	0.56	0.48	86%	113

(continues)

Table 7.3 *Continued*

Methyltransferase	Source	K_m for AdoMet (μmol/L)	K_i for AdoHcy (μmol/L)	Fraction of Maximal Methyltransferase Activity				Fraction of Maximal Methyltransferase Activity			Reference
				AdoMet 30 μmol/L AdoHcy 1 μmol/L	AdoMet 30 μmol/L AdoHcy 10 μmol/L	AdoMet 30 μmol/L AdoHcy 100 μmol/L	Percentage of activity at 100 μmol/L relative to 1 μmol/L AdoHcy	Control AdoMet 2.7 μmol/L AdoHcy 0.8 μmol/L	Uremic AdoMet 2.7 μmol/L AdoHcy 6.7 μmol/L	Percentage activity at 6.7 μmol/L relative to 0.8 μmol/L AdoHcy	
Histone-lysine N-Arginine	Rat brain nuclei	12.5	5.9	0.67	0.47	0.12	18%	0.16	0.09	57%	25
[Myelin basic protein]-arginine	Calf brain	4.4	1.8	0.81	0.51	0.11	13%	0.30	0.12	39%	36
Protein arginine I	Calf brain	8	2.3	0.72	0.41	0.08	11%	0.20	0.08	40%	36
SMALL MOLECULES **N-Methyltransferases**											
Guanidinoacetate	Pig liver	49	16	0.37	0.27	0.08	21%	0.05	0.04	75%	51
Histamine	Mouse kidney	1.7	11.8 (IC$_{50}$ value)	0.94	0.91	0.65	69%	0.60	0.50	84%	89
Glycine	Rabbit liver	100	35	0.23	0.19	0.07	32%	0.03	0.02	86%	41
Phenylethanolamine	Rabbit liver	10	1.4	0.64	0.27	0.04	6%	0.15	0.04	30%	23
β-Carboline-2	Bovine brain	81	14.8 (IC$_{50}$ value)	0.26	0.18	0.05	18%	0.03	0.02	73%	35
Indolethylamine	Rabbit lung	54.3	8.65	0.33	0.20	0.04	13%	0.04	0.03	63%	7
O-Methyltransferases											
Hydroxyindole	Rabbit liver	14	2.1	0.59	0.27	0.04	7%	0.12	0.04	36%	23
Catechol	Human brain	3.1	1	0.83	0.47	0.09	11%	0.33	0.10	31%	87
S-Methyltransferases											
Thiopurine	Mouse Liver	3	5.8 (IC$_{50}$ value)	0.90	0.79	0.35	40%	0.44	0.29	67%	75
Thioether	Mouse lung	1	40 (IC$_{50}$ value)	0.97	0.96	0.90	93%	0.73	0.70	96%	71

thionine (11). Assuming competitive inhibition, the Michaelis-Menton expression for the rate of the transmethylation reaction is:

$$\text{Fraction of maximal velocity} = \frac{[\text{AdoMet}]}{(K_m + K_m [\text{AdoHcy}]/K_i + [\text{AdoMet}])}$$

Here, [AdoMet] and [AdoHcy] are the concentrations of S-adenosylmethionine and S-adenosylhomocysteine, respectively, K_i is the inhibition constant for S-adenosylhomocysteine, and K_m is the Michaelis constant for S-adenosylmethionine. Cantoni et al. (11) initially made calculations for a group of 10 methyltransferases and calculated the percentage of maximal activity at ratios of AdoMet/AdoHcy of 4 and 1.6 and assumed concentrations of AdoMet and AdoHcy. Those enzymes with low K_i values relative to K_m values were more markedly inhibited at the lower AdoMet/AdoHcy ratio. In Table 7.3, we calculated relative enzyme activities using the preceding equation, assuming an approximate physiological level of 30 μmol/L S-adenosylmethionine and 1 μmol/L S-adenosylhomocysteine in nonliver cells (46). These values are also calculated for 10-fold and 100-fold increased concentrations of S-adenosylhomocysteine, which represent approximate concentrations that may occur in mild and severe homocystinuria, respectively. In the calculations for nonliver cells, the level of S-adenosylmethionine is assumed to stay constant at about 30 μmol/L (46).

In nucleated mammalian cells, there is little information on the actual levels of intracellular S-adenosylmethionine and S-adenosylhomocysteine as a function of plasma total homocysteine. However, Perna and co-workers have shed light on the situation in human red blood cells (78). They correlated changes in control patients and patients with chronic renal disease of plasma total homocysteine concentrations with changes in red cell adenosine, S-adenosylmethionine, and S-adenosylhomocysteine levels (78). Plasma total homocysteine was 12 μmol/L in the control group and 41 μmol/L in the patient group. This difference was also reflected in the erythrocyte levels of 8 and 32 μmol/L, respectively (78). Adenosine levels were about 1 μmol/L in each group. If the portion of the total homocysteine in the free state was known, the erythrocyte concentration of S-adenosylhomocysteine could be calculated from the equilibrium constant of the S-adenosylhomocysteine hydrolase reaction of 1.4×10^{-6} (22). However, the direct measurement of the S-adenosylhomocysteine concentration revealed values of 0.8 μmol/L in the control group and 6.7 μmol/L in the uremic patient group, whereas the concentration of S-adenosylmethionine was about 2.7 μmol/L in both groups (78). These

results suggest that the concentration of S-adenosylhomocysteine, at least in erythrocytes, may be a linear function of plasma total homocysteine, a result consistent with the equilibrium relationship given the unchanging adenosine concentration. Table 7.3 shows data for the level of inhibition expected for each of the methyltransferases under the conditions of mildly elevated plasma total homocysteine found in patients with chronic renal disease.

There may be significant tissue differences in the way in which S-adenosylhomocysteine levels respond to increases in plasma total homocysteine. Cell culture experiments have shown that 50 μmol/L homocysteine has little or no effect in vascular smooth muscle cells or fibroblasts while dramatically increasing the concentration of S-adenosylhomocysteine in vascular endothelial cells (107). Additionally, increased extracellular homocysteine resulted in a parallel increase in S-adenosylmethionine and S-adenosylhomocysteine concentrations in liver (31, 44), lessening the potential degree of inhibition of methyltransferases.

More Likely and Less Likely Targets for Homocysteine-linked Methyltransferase Inhibition and Pathogenesis: Comparing the Clinical Features of Homocysteine Accumulation with Effects of Methyltransferase Loss

The results of the calculations in Table 7.3 make clear that even at relatively high levels of intracellular S-adenosylhomocysteine, some methyltransferases can retain most of their activity. The function of these species, therefore, would not be expected to be markedly changed by elevated plasma total homocysteine. By contrast, several other methyltransferases appear to be particularly sensitive to S-adenosylhomocysteine inhibition. At the mildly elevated homocysteine levels seen in uremic patients, the guanine-N-1 tRNA methyltransferase and the protein repair L-isoaspartate (D-aspartate) methyltransferase are inhibited more than 70% (15% and 14% residual activity, respectively) (Table 7.3). At higher levels, significant inhibition is also seen with two protein arginine methyltransferases and three enzymes involved in the metabolism of neurotransmitters and related compounds — phenylethanolamine N-methyltransferase involved in the synthesis of epinephrine, catechol O-methyltransferase involved in its degradation (as well as that of dopamine and norepinephrine), and the β-carboline-2-N-methyltransferase with an unknown physiological function (Table 7.3). Because mice totally deficient in the catechol O-methyltransferase show only mild behavioral effects (40), this activity may not be important with respect to possible homocysteine-induced methyltransferase inhibition. However, it is possible that an additive effect of the inhibition of multiple enzyme activities drives the phenotypic expression of the pathology.

It will be interesting to see if the inhibition of any of these latter enzymes in humans with elevated homocysteine levels may be correlated with seizures and types of disturbances linked to altered brain metabolism (33, 61). In at least one case study, homocystinuria and schizophrenic behavior have been tightly linked (33), and in a more recent study it has been reported that hyperhomocysteinemia can often be found in schizophrenic patients (86). However, as mentioned previously, homocysteine has neuromodulator properties itself (2). These studies suggest that homocysteine-induced loss of these methyltransferase activities may result in an abnormal balance of these neurotransmitters. The knowledge that deficiency of the protein L-isoaspartate (D-aspartate) methyltransferase can lead to seizures in mice (57, 58), and that limitation of the type II protein arginine methyltransferase action resulting from S-adenosylmethionine-depletion may be linked to demyelinization (13), strengthens the possible link between homocysteine-induced methylation loss and neurological pathology.

It will also be of interest to examine the role of the protein repair methyltransferase in relation to vascular disease. This enzyme has been shown to be trapped in the extracellular space when blood vessels are injured and may play a role in the repair of damaged collagen molecules (109, 110).

Conclusion

The clinical features resulting from homocysteine accumulation may be linked, at least in part, to the inhibition of cellular methyltransferases by changes in the cellular ratio of S-adenosylmethionine and S-adenosylhomocysteine. To begin to address this problem, this chapter has detailed the present state of knowledge of mammalian methyltransferases and the effects of inhibiting their activities. Humans have at least 39 distinct methyltransferases that catalyze a broad range of reactions for a broad range of cellular functions. Although it is difficult at this point to specifically link the inhibition of any one of the methyltransferases to the pathology resulting from homocysteine buildup, the partial loss of many of these enzymes and the cumulative effect of the loss of function of this large group of enzymes may in fact be reflected in cardiovascular damage, neurological pathology, and the other clinical features that are described elsewhere in this book. Further work is war-

ranted to study the function of individual methyltransferases and to identify new methyltransferases.

REFERENCES

1. Aksoy, S, Brandriff, BF, Ward, A, Little, PF, Weinshilboum, RM. Human nicotinamide N-methyltransferase gene. Molecular cloning, structural characterization and chromosomal localization. *Genomics* 1995; 29: 555–61.

2. Allen, IC, Grieve, A, Griffiths, R. Differential changes in the content of amino acid neurotransmitters in discrete regions of the rat brain prior to the onset and during the course of homocysteine-induced seizures. *J Neurochem* 1986; 46: 1582–92.

3. Barkovich, RJ, Shtanko, A, Shepherd, JA, Lee, PT, Myles, DC, Tzagoloff, A, Clarke, CF. Characterization of the COQ5 gene from *Saccharomyces cerevisiae*. Evidence for a C-methyltransferase in ubiquinone biosynthesis. *J Biol Chem* 1997; 272: 9182–28.

3a. Bergo, MO, Leung, GK, Ambroziak, P, Otto, JC, Casey, PJ, Young, SG. Targeted inactivation of the isoprenylcysteine carboxyl methyltransferase gene causes mislocalization of K-ras in mammalian cells. *J Biol Chem* 2000; 275: 17605–10.

4. Bloxham, DP, Parmelee, DC, Kumar, S, Wade, RD, Ericsson, LH, Neurath, H, Walsh, KA, Titani K. Primary structure of porcine heart citrate synthase. *Proc Natl Acad Sci USA* 1981; 78: 5381–85.

5. Blumenthal, R. Appendix I—AdoMet-Dependent MTases in E. C. Database. In *S-Adenosylmethionine-dependent Methyltransferases: Structures and Function.* (Cheng, X, Blumenthal, RM, eds.). World Scientific Publishing Company, Singapore, 1999; pp. 393–400.

6. Bokar, JA, Rottman, FM. Nucleoside methylation in eukaryotic mRNA: HeLa mRNA (N6-adenosine)methyltransferase. In *S-Adenosylmethionine-dependent Methyltransferases: Structures and Function.* (Cheng, X, Blumenthal, RM, eds.). World Scientific Publishing Company, Singapore, 1999; pp. 227–53.

7. Borchardt, RT. The inhibition of indolethylamine-N-methyltransferase by analogs of S-adenosylhomocysteine. *Biochem Pharmacol* 1975; 24: 1542–44.

8. Borchardt, RT. S-Adenosyl-L-methionine-dependent macromolecule methyltransferases. Potential targets for the design of chemotherapeutic agents. *J Med Chem* 1980; 23: 347–57.

9. Borchardt, Rt, Cheng, CF. Purification and characterization of rat liver microsomal thiol methyltransferase. *Biochim Biophys Acta* 1978; 522: 340–53.

10. Cantoni, GL, Chiang, PK. The role of S-adenosylhomocysteine and S-adenosylhomocysteine hydrolase in the control of biological methylations. In *Natural Sulfur Compounds.* (Cavallini, D, Gaull, GE, Zappia, V, eds.). Plenum Press, New York, 1980; pp. 67–80.

11. Cantoni, GL, Richards, HH, Chiang, PK. Inhibitors of S-adenosylhomocysteine hydrolase and their role in the regulation of biological methylation. In *Transmethylation. Proceedings of the Conference on Transmethylation, Bethesda, Maryland, U.S.A. on October 16–19, 1978.*

(Usdin, E, Borchardt, RT, Creveling, CR, eds.). Elsevier/North-Holland, New York, 1979; pp. 155–64.

12. Cavaille, J, Chetouani, F, Bachellerie, JP. The yeast *Saccharomyces cerevisiae* YDL112w ORF encodes the putative 2′-O-ribose methyltransferase catalyzing the formation of Gm18 in tRNAs. *RNA* 1999; 5: 66–81.

13. Chamberlin, ME, Ubagai, T, Mudd, SH, Wilson, WG, Leonard, JV, Chou, JY. Demyelination of the brain is associated with methionine adenosyltransferase I/III deficiency. *J Clin Invest* 1996; 98: 1021–27.

14. Chauveau, P, Chadefaux, B, Coudé, M, Aupetit, J, Hannedouche, T, Kamoun, P, Jungers, P. Increased plasma total homocysteine concentration in patients with chronic renal failure. *Miner Electrolyte Metab* 1992; 18: 196–98.

15. Chauveau, P, Chadefaux, B, Coudé, M, Aupetit, J, Hannedouche, T, Kamoun, P, Jungers, P. Hyperhomocysteinemia, a risk factor for atherosclerosis in chronic uremic patients. *Kidney Int* 1993; Supplement 41: S72–7.

16. Chen, D, Ma, H, Hong, H, Koh, SS, Huang, SM, Schurter, BT, Aswad, DW, Stallcup, MR. Regulation of transcription by a protein methyltransferase. *Science* 1999; 284: 2174–77.

17. Chen, RZ, Pettersson, U, Beard, C, Jackson-Grusby, L, Jaenisch, R. DNA hypomethylation leads to elevated mutation rates. *Nature* 1998; 395: 89–93.

17a. Chen, YM, Chen, LY, Wong, FH, Lee, CM, Chang, IJ, Yang-Feng, TL. Genomic structure, expression, and chromosomal localization of the human glycine *N*-methyltransferase gene. *Genomics* 2000; 66: 43–47.

18. Clarke, CF. New advances in Coenzyme Q biosynthesis. *Protoplasma*. In press, 2000.

19. Clarke, S. Protein isoprenylation and methylation at carboxyl-terminal cysteine residues. *Annu Rev Biochem* 1992; 61: 355–386.

20. Clarke, S. A protein carboxyl methyltransferase that recognizes age-damaged peptides and proteins and participates in their repair. In *S-Adenosylmethionine-dependent Methyltransferases: Structures and Function*. (Cheng, X, Blumenthal, RM, eds.). World Scientific Publishing Company, Singapore, 1999; pp. 123–48.

21. Cobb, JA, Han, CH, Wills, DM, Roberts, DM. Structural elements within the methylation loop (residues 112–117) and EF hands III and IV of calmodulin are required for Lys(115) trimethylation. *Biochem J* 1999; 340: 417–24.

21a. De Baere, I, Derua, R, Janssens, V, Van Hoof, C, Waelkens, E, Merlevede, W, Goris, J. Purification of porcine brain protein phosphatase 2A leucine carboxyl methyltransferase and cloning of the human homologue. *Biochemistry* 1999; 38: 16539–47.

22. de la Haba, G, Cantoni, GL. The enzymatic synthesis of S-adenosyl-L-homocysteine from adenosine and homocysteine. *J Biol Chem* 1959; 234: 603–8.

23. Deguchi, T, Barchas, J. Inhibition of transmethylations of biogenic amines by S-adenosylhomocysteine. *J Biol Chem* 1971; 246: 3175–81.

24. Dever, TE, Costello, CE, Owens, CL, Rosenberry, TL, Merrick, WC. Location of seven post-translational modifications in rabbit elongation factor 1 alpha including dimethyllysine, trimethyllysine, and glycerylphosphorylethanolamine. *J Biol Chem* 1989; 264: 20518–25.

25. Duerre, JA, Wallwork, JC, Quick, DP, Ford, KM. In vitro studies on the methylation of histones in rat brain nuclei. *J Biol Chem* 1977; 252: 5981–85.

26. Eichler, DC. Characterization of nucleolar 2′-O-methyltransferase and its involvement in the methylation of mouse precursor ribosomal RNA. *Biochimie* 1994; 76: 1115–22.

27. Fessing, MY, Belkov, VM, Krynetski, EY, Evans, WE. Molecular cloning and functional characterization of the cDNA encoding the murine thiopurine S-methyltransferase (TPMT). *FEBS Lett* 1998; 424: 143–45.

28. Finkelstein, JD. Methionine metabolism in mammals. In *Inherited Disorders of Sulfur Metabolism* (Carson, NAJ, Raine, DN, eds.). Williams and Wilkins, Baltimore, 1971; pp. 1–13.

29. Finkelstein, JD. Methionine metabolism in mammals. The biochemical basis for homocystinuria. *Metabolism* 1974; 23: 387–98.

30. Finkelstein, JD. The metabolism of homocysteine. Pathways and regulation. *Eur J Pediatr* 1998; 157 Suppl 2: S40–44.

31. Finkelstein, JD, Martin, JJ. Methionine metabolism in mammals. Adaptation to methionine stress. *J Biol Chem* 1986; 261: 1582–87.

32. Flynn, J, Reich, N. Murine DNA (cytosine-5-)methyltransferase. Steady-state and substrate trapping analyses of the kinetic mechanism. *Biochemistry* 1998; 37: 15162–69.

33. Freeman, JM, Finkelstein, JD, Mudd, SH. Folate-responsive homocystinuria and schizophrenia: A defect in methylation due to deficient 5,10-methylenetetrahydrofolate reductase activity. *N Engl J Med* 1975; 292: 491–96.

34. Gary, JD, Clarke, S. Modulation of RNA and protein interactions by protein arginine methylation. *Prog Nucl Acids Res Mol Biol* 1998; 61: 65–131.

35. Gearhart, DA, Neafsey, EJ, Collins, MA. Characterization of brain beta-carboline-2-N-methyltransferase: An enzyme that may play a role in idiopathic Parkinson's disease. *Neurochem Res* 1997; 22: 113–21.

36. Ghosh, SK, Paik, WK, Kim, S. Purification and molecular identification of two protein methylases I from calf brain. Myelin basic protein- and histone-specific enzyme. *J Biol Chem* 1988; 263: 19024–33.

37. Glauser, TA, Nelson, AN, Zemboer, DE, Lipsky, JJ, Wienshilboum, RM. Diethyldithiocarbamate S-methylation. Evidence for catalysis by human liver thiol methyltransferase and thiopurine methyltransferase. *J Pharmacol Exp Ther* 1993; 266: 23–32.

38. Glick, JM, Averyhart, VM, Leboy, PS. Purification and characterization of two tRNA-(guanine)-methyltransferases from rat liver. *Biochim Biophys Acta* 1978; 518: 158–71.

39. Glick, JM, Leboy, PS. Purification and properties of tRNA (adenine-1)-methyltransferase from rat liver. *J Biol Chem* 1977; 252: 4790–95.

40. Gogos, JA, Morgan, M, Luine, V, Santha, M, Ogawa, S, Pfaff, D, Karayiorgou, M. Catechol-O-methyltransferase-deficient mice exhibit sexually dimorphic changes

in catecholamine levels and behavior. *Proc Natl Acad Sci USA* 1998; 95: 9991–96.

41. Heady, JE, Kerr, SJ. Purification and characterization of glycine N-methyltransferase. *J Biol Chem* 1973; 248: 69–72.

42. Herrmann, W, Quast, S, Ullrich, M, Schultze, H, Bodis, M, Geisel, J. Hyperhomocysteinemia in high-aged subjects. Relation of B-vitamins, folic acid, renal function and the methylenetetrahydrofolate reductase mutation. *Atherosclerosis* 1999; 144: 91–101.

43. Hoffman, DR, Cornatzer, WE. Microsomal phosphatidylethanolamine methyltransferase. Some physical and kinetic properties. *Lipids* 1981; 16: 533–40.

44. Hoffman, DR, Cornatzer, WE, Duerre, JA. Relationship between tissue levels of S-adenosylmethionine, S-adenosylhomocysteine, and transmethylation reactions. *Can J Biochem* 1979; 57: 56–65.

45. Hoffman, DR, Haning, JA, Cornatzer, WE. Microsomal phosphatidylethanolamine methyltransferase. Inhibition by S-adenosylhomocysteine. *Lipids* 1981; 16: 561–67.

46. Hoffman, DR, Marion, DW, Cornatzer, WE, Duerre, JA. S-Adenosylmethionine and S-adenosylhomocysteine metabolism in isolated rat liver. Effects of L-methionine, L-homocysteine, and adenosine. *J Biol Chem* 1980; 255: 10822–27.

47. Holmes, WM. tRNA Methyltransferases. In *S-Adenosylmethionine-dependent Methyltransferases: Structures and Function.* (Cheng, X, Blumenthal, RM, eds.). World Scientific Publishing Company, Singapore, 1999; pp. 185–98.

48. Holt, JC, Caulfield, JB, Norton, P, Chantler, PD, Slayter, HS, Margossian, SS. Human cardiac myosin light chains. Sequence comparisons between myosin LC1 and LC2 from normal and idiopathic dilated cardiomyopathic hearts. *Mol Cell Biochem* 1995; 145: 89–96.

49. Hrycyna, CA, Clarke, S. Modification of eucaryotic signaling proteins by C-terminal methylation reactions. *Pharmacol Ther* 1993; 59: 281–300.

50. Hsu, DW, Lin, MJ, Lee, TL, Wen, SC, Chen, X, Shen, CK. Two major forms of DNA (cytosine-5) methyltransferase in human somatic tissues. *Proc Natl Acad Sci USA* 1999; 96: 9751–56.

51. Im, YS, Chiang, PK, Cantoni, GL. Guanidoacetate methyltransferase. Purification and molecular properties. *J Biol Chem* 1979; 254: 11047–50.

52. Jacobsen DW. Homocysteine and vitamins in cardiovascular disease. *Clin Chem* 1998; 44: 1833–43.

53. Johnson, BA, Aswad, DW. Kinetic properties of bovine brain protein L-isoaspartyl methyltransferase determined using a synthetic isoaspartyl peptide substrate. *Neurochem Res* 1993; 18: 87–94.

53a. Jonassen, T, Clarke, CF. Isolation and functional expression of human COQ3, a gene encoding a methyltransferase required for ubiquinone biosynthesis. *J Biol Chem* 2000; 275: 12381–12387.

54. Kagan, RM, Clarke, S. Widespread occurrence of three sequence motifs in diverse S-adenosylmethionine-dependent methyltransferases suggests a common structure for these enzymes. *Arch Biochem Biophys* 1994; 310: 417–27.

55. Kalhor, HR, Niewmierzycka, A, Faull, KF, Yao, X, Grade, S, Clarke, S, Rubenstein, PA. A highly conserved 3-methylhistidine modification is absent in yeast actin. *Arch Biochem Biophys* 1999; 370: 105–111.

56. Keith, JM, Winters, EM, Moss, B. Purification and characterization of a HeLa cell transfer RNA (cytosine-5-)-methyltransferase. *J Biol Chem* 1990; 255: 4636–44.

57. Kim, E, Lowenson, JD, Clarke, S, Young, SG. Phenotypic analysis of seizure-prone mice lacking L-isoaspartate (D-aspartate) O-methyltransferase. *J Biol Chem* 1999; 274: 20671–78.

58. Kim, E, Lowenson, JD, MacLaren, DC, Clarke, S, Young, SG. Deficiency of a protein-repair enzyme results in the accumulation of altered proteins, retardation of growth, and fatal seizures in mice. *Proc Natl Acad Sci USA* 1997; 94: 6132–37.

59. Kim, S, Lim, IK, Park, GH, Paik, WK. Biological methylation of myelin basic protein. Enzymology and biological significance. *Int J Biochem Cell Biol* 1997; 29: 743–51.

60. Kowlura, A, Seavey, SE, Rabaglia, ME, Nesher, R, Metz, SA. Carboxylmethylation of the catalytic subunit of protein phosphatase 2A in insulin-secreting cells. Evidence for functional consequences on enzyme activity and insulin secretion. *Endocrinology* 1996; 137: 2315–23.

61. Laster, L, Mudd, SH, Finkelstein, JD, Irreverre, F. Homocystinuria due to cystathionine synthase deficiency. The metabolism of L-methionine. *J Clin Invest* 1965; 44: 1708–19.

62. Lee, ME, Wang, H. Homocysteine and hypomethylation. A novel link to vascular disease. *Trends Cardiovasc Med* 1999; 9: 49–54.

63. Lew, JY, Matsumoto, Y, Pearson, J, Goldstein, M, Hokfelt, T, Fuxe, K. Localization and characterization of phenylethanolamine N-methyltransferase in the brain of various mammalian species. *Brain Res* 1977; 119: 199–210.

64. Lin, WJ, Gary, JD, Yang, MC, Clarke, S, Herschman, HR. The mammalian immediate-early TIS21 protein and the leukemia-associated BTG1 protein interact with a protein-arginine N-methyltransferase. *J Biol Chem* 1996; 271: 15034–44.

65. Lobet, Y, Lhoest, J, Colson, C. Partial purification and characterization of the specific protein-lysine N-methyltransferase of YL32, a yeast ribosomal protein. *Biochim Biophys Acta* 1989; 997: 224–31.

66. Loehrer, FM, Angst, CP, Brunner, FP, Haefeli, WE, Fowler, B. Evidence for disturbed S-adenosylmethionine: S-adenosylhomocysteine ratio in patients with end-stage renal failure—a cause for disturbed methylation reactions? *Nephrol Dial Transplant* 1998; 13: 656–61.

67. Mann, JD, Mudd, SH. Alkaloids and plant metabolism. IV. The tyramine methylpherase of barley roots. *J Biol Chem* 1963; 238: 381–85.

68. Mao, X, Schwer, B, Shuman, S. Yeast mRNA cap methyltransferase is a 50-kilodalton protein encoded by an essential gene. *Mol Cell Biol* 1995; 15: 4167–74.

69. Marbois, BN, Hsu, A, Pillai, R, Colicelli, J, Clarke, CF. Cloning of a rat cDNA encoding dihydroxypolyprenylbenzoate methyltransferase by functional complementa-

tion of a *Saccharomyces cerevisiae* mutant deficient in ubiquinone biosynthesis. *Gene* 1994; 138: 213–17.

70. Mattheakis, LC, Shen, WH, Collier, RJ. DPH5: A methyltransferase gene required for diphthamide biosynthesis in *Saccharomyces cerevisiae*. *Mol Cell Biol* 1992; 12: 4026–37.

71. Mozier, NM, McConnell, KP, Hoffman, JL. S-adenosyl-L-methionine:thioether S-methyltransferase, a new enzyme in sulfur and selenium metabolism. *J Biol Chem* 1988; 263: 4527–31.

72. Mudd, SH, Levy, HL, Skovby, F. Disorders of transulfuration. In *The Metabolic Basis of Inherited Disease*, 7th ed (Scriver, CR, Beaudet, AL, Sly, WS, Valle, D, eds.). McGraw Hill, New York, 1995; pp. 1279–1318.

73. Niewmierzycka, A, Clarke, S. S-Adenosylmethionine-dependent methylation in *Saccharomyces cerevisiae*. Identification of a novel protein arginine methyltransferase. *J Biol Chem* 1999; 274: 814–22.

74. Ogawa, H, Ishiguro, Y, Fujioka, M. Guanidoacetate methyltransferase from rat liver: Purification, properties, and evidence for the involvement of sulfhydryl groups for activity. *Arch Biochem Biophys* 1983; 226: 265–75.

75. Otterness, DM, Weinshilboum, RM. Mouse thiopurine methyltransferase pharmacogenetics: Biochemical studies and recombinant inbred strains. *J Pharmacol Exp Ther* 1987; 243: 180–86.

76. Paik, WK, Kim, S. Protein methylation. *Science* 1971; 174: 114–19.

77. Perna, AF, Ingrosso, D, Zappia, V, Galletti, P, Capasso, G, De Santo, NG. Enzymatic methyl esterification of erythrocyte membrane proteins is impaired in chronic renal failure. Evidence for high levels of the natural inhibitor S-adenosylhomocysteine. *J Clin Invest* 1993; 91: 2497–503.

78. Perna, AF, Ingrosso, D, De Santo, NG, Galletti, P, Zappia, V. Mechanism of erythrocyte accumulation of methylation inhibitor S-adenosylhomocysteine in uremia. *Kidney Int* 1995; 47: 247–53.

79. Perna, AF, D'Aniello, A, Lowenson, JD, Clarke, S, De Santo, NG, Ingrosso, D. D-aspartate content of erythrocyte membrane proteins is decreased in uremia. Implications for the repair of damaged proteins. *J Am Soc Nephrol* 1997; 8: 95–104.

80. Perna, AF, Ingrosso, D, De Santo, NG, Galletti, P, Brunone, M, Zappia, V. Metabolic consequences of folate-induced reduction of hyperhomocysteinemia in uremia. *J Am Soc Nephrol* 1997; 8: 1899–1905.

81. Perna, AF, Ingrosso, D, Castaldo, P, De Santo, NG, Galletti, P, Zappia, V. Homocysteine, a new crucial element in the pathogenesis of uremic cardiovascular complications. *Miner Electrolyte Metab* 1999; 25: 95–9.

82. Perna, AF, Castaldo, P, Ingrosso, D, De Santo, NG. Homocysteine, a new cardiovascular risk factor, is also a powerful uremic toxin. *J Nephrol* 1999; 12: 230–240.

83. Perry, TL, Hansen, S, MacDougall, L, Warrington, PD. Sulfur-containing amino acids in the plasma and urine of homocystinurics. *Clin Chem Acta* 1967; 15: 409–20.

84. Perry, TL. Homocystinuria. In *Heritable Disorders of Amino Acid Metabolism: Patterns of Clinical Expression and Genetic Variation* (Nyhan WL, ed.). John Wiley and Sons, New York, 1974; pp. 395–428.

85. Raha, A, Wagner, C, MacDonald, RG, Bresnick, E. Rat liver cytosolic 4 S polycyclic aromatic hydrocarbon-binding protein is glycine N-methyltransferase. *J Biol Chem* 1994; 269: 5750–56.

86. Regland, B, Johansson, BV, Grenfeldt, B, Hjelmgren, LT, Medhus, M. Homocysteinemia is a common feature of schizophrenia. *J Neural Transm* 1995; 100: 165–69.

87. Rivett, AJ, Roth, JA. Kinetic studies on the O-methylation of dopamine by human brain membrane-bound catechol O-methyltransferase. *Biochemistry* 1982; 21: 1740–42.

88. Scheller, T, Orgacka, H, Szumlanski, CL, Weinshilboum, RM. Mouse liver nicotinamide N-methyltransferase pharmacogenetics. Biochemical properties and variation in activity among inbred strains. *Pharmacogenetics* 1996; 6: 43–53.

89. Scott, MC, Guerciolini, R, Szumlanski, C, Weinshilboum, RM. Mouse kidney histamine N-methyltransferase: Assay conditions, biochemical properties and strain variation. *Agents Actions* 1991; 32: 194–202.

90. Stephenson, RC, Clarke, S. Identification of a C-terminal protein carboxyl methyltransferase in rat liver membranes utilizing a synthetic farnesyl cysteine-containing peptide substrate. *J Biol Chem* 1990; 265: 16248–54.

91. Swiatek, KR, Simon, LN, Chao, KL. Nicotinamide methyltransferase and S-adenosylmethionine: 5'-methylthioadenosine hydrolase. Control of transfer ribonucleic acid methylation. *Biochemistry* 1973; 12: 4670–74.

92. Tang, J, Gary, JD, Clarke, S, Herschman, HR. PRMT 3, a type I protein arginine N-methyltransferase that differs from PRMT1 in its oligomerization, subcellular localization, substrate specificity, and regulation. *J Biol Chem* 1998; 273: 16935–45.

93. Thompson, DJ: A chemical hypothesis for arsenic methylation in mammals. *Chem Biol Interact* 1993; 88: 89–114.

94. Thompson, MA, Weinshilboum, RM. Rabbit lung indolethylamine N-methyltransferase. cDNA and gene cloning and characterization. *J Biol Chem* 1998; 273: 34502–10.

95. Thompson, MA, Moon, E, Kim, U-J, Xu, J, Siciliano, MJ, Weinshilboum, RM. Human indolethylamine N-methyltransferase. cDNA cloning and expression, gene cloning, and chromosomal localization. *Genomics* 1999; 61: 285–297.

96. Tong, SW, Elzinga, M. Amino acid sequence of rabbit skeletal muscle myosin. 50-kDa fragment of the heavy chain. *J Biol Chem* 1990; 265: 4893–901.

97. Ueland, PM. Pharmacological and biochemical aspects of S-adenosylhomocysteine and S-adenosylhomocysteine hydrolase. *Pharmacol Rev* 1982; 34: 223–52.

98. Vance, DE, Walkey, CJ, Cui, Z. Phosphatidylethanolamine N-methyltransferase from liver. *Biochim Biophys Acta* 1997; 1348: 142–50.

99. Van Guldener, C, Kulik, W, Berger, R, Dijkstra, DA, Jakobs, C, Reijngoud, D-J, Donker, AJM, Stehouwer, CDA, De Meer, K. Homocysteine and methionine

netabolism in ESRD: A stable isotope study. *Kidney Int* 1999; 56: 1064–71.

100. Van Loon, JA, Pazmino, PA, Weinshilboum, RM. Human erythrocyte histamine *N*-methyltransferase: Radiochemical microassay and biochemical properties. *Clin Chim Acta* 1985; 149: 237–51.

101. Vertino, PM. Eucaryotic DNA methyltransferases. In *S-Adenosylmethionine-dependent Methyltransferases: Structures and Function*. (Cheng, X, Blumenthal, RM, eds.). World Scientific Publishing Company, Singapore, 1999; pp. 341–72.

102. Vidgren, J, Ovaska, M, Tenhunen, J, Tilgmann, C, Lotta, T, Mannisto, P. Catechol O-methyltransferase. In *S-Adenosylmethionine-dependent Methyltransferases: Structures and Function*. (Cheng, X, Blumenthal, RM, eds.). World Scientific Publishing Company, Singapore, 1999; pp. 55–91.

103. Walkey, CJ, Donohue, LR, Bronson, R, Agellon, LB, Vance, DE. Disruption of the murine gene encoding phosphatidylethanolamine *N*-methyltransferase. *Proc Natl Acad Sci USA* 1997; 94: 12880–85.

104. Walkey, CJ, Yu, L, Agellon, LB, Vance, DE. Biochemical and evolutionary significance of phospholipid methylation. *J Biol Chem* 1998; 273: 27043–46.

105. Walkey, CJ, Shields, DJ, Vance, DE. Identification of three novel cDNAs for human phosphatidylethanolamine *N*-methyltransferase and localization of the human gene on chromosome 17p11.2. *Biochim Biophys Acta* 1999; 1436: 405–12.

106. Wang, C, Lin, JM, Lazarides, E. Methylations of 70,000-Da heat shock proteins in 3T3 cells: Alterations by arsenite treatment, by different stages of growth and by virus transformation. *Arch Biochem Biophys* 1992; 297: 169–75.

107. Wang, H, Yoshizumi, M, Lai, K, Tsai, JC, Perrella, MA, Haber, E, Lee, ME. Inhibition of growth and p21[ras] methylation in vascular endothelial cells by homocysteine but not cysteine. *J Biol Chem* 1997; 272: 25380–9⁻ ̄

108. Warner, DR, Mozier, NM, Pearson, JD, Hoffman, JL. Cloning and base sequence analysis of a cDNA encoding mouse lung thioether-*S*-methyltransferase. *Biochim Biophys Acta* 1995; 1246: 160–66.

109. Weber, DJ, McFadden, PN. Detection and characterization of a protein isoaspartyl methyltransferase which becomes trapped in the extracellular space during blood vessel injury. *J Protein Chem* 1997; 16: 257–67.

110. Weber, DJ, McFadden, PN. Injury-induced enzymatic methylation of aging collagen in the extracellular matrix of blood vessels. *J Protein Chem* 1997; 16: 269–81.

111. Weinshilboum, RM, Otterness, DM, Szumlanski, CL. Methylation pharmacogenetics: Catechol O-methyltransferase, thiopurine methyltransferase, and histamine *N*-methyltransferase. *Annu Rev Pharmacol Toxicol* 1999; 39: 19–52.

112. Wolfe, MS, Borchardt, RT. *S*-Adenosyl-L-homocysteine hydrolase as a target for antiviral chemotherapy. *J Med Chem* 1991; 34: 1521–30.

113. Wright, LS, Bertics, PJ, Siegel, FL. Calmodulin *N*-methyltransferase. Kinetics, mechanism, and inhibitors. *J Biol Chem* 1996; 271: 12737–43.

114. Xie, H, Clarke, S. Protein phosphatase 2A is reversibly modified by methyl esterification at its C-terminal leucine residue in bovine brain. *J Biol Chem* 1994; 269: 1981–84.

115. Young, SG, Ambroziak, P, Kim, E, Clarke, S. Post-prenylation protein processing: CXXX (CaaX) endoproteases and isoprenylcysteine carboxyl methyltransferase. In *The Enzymes*, Vol 21. (Tamanoi, F, Sigman, DS, eds.). Academic Press, New York, pp. 155–213, 2000.

116. Zakharyan, RA, Ayala-Fierro, F, Cullen, WR, Carter, DM, Aposhian, HV. Enzymatic methylation of arsenic compounds. VII. Monomethylarsonous acid (MMAIII) is the substrate for MMA methyltransferase of rabbit liver and human hepatocytes. *Toxicol Appl Pharmacol* 1999; 158: 9–15.

8

S-Adenosylhomocysteine Hydrolase

SEAN T. PRIGGE
PETER K. CHIANG

In biological systems, *S*-adenosylmethionine (AdoMet) is the most widely used methyl donor. A multitude of methylases transfer the methyl group from AdoMet to their respective biological acceptors, forming *S*-adenosylhomocysteine (AdoHcy), which in turn is hydrolyzed by *S*-adenosylhomocysteine hydrolase (12, 15). AdoHcy hydrolase (Metabolic Diagram, Reaction 3) is a popular pharmacological target because its inhibition can affect the methylation status of nucleic acids, phospholipids, proteins, and small molecules (15, 18). Among the many biological correlates with the inhibition of AdoHcy hydrolase, some permanent and some transient, are the modulation of gene expression, induction of cellular differentiation, regulation of transcription factors, and cellular mobility. Furthermore, inhibitors of this enzyme have impressive antiviral, antiparasitic, antiarthritic, and immunosuppressive activities.

The reaction catalyzed by AdoHcy hydrolase requires nicotinamide adenine dinucleotide (NAD$^+$) as a cofactor, and is reversible, with an equilibrium constant (K_{eq}) of about 1 μmol/L, favoring the synthetic direction [adenosine + homocysteine $\rightleftarrows$ *S*-adenosylhomocysteine]. The equilibrium can be shifted further in the synthetic direction by phosphate ions (52). Under physiological conditions, the reaction proceeds in the hydrolytic direction owing to the rapid removal and metabolism of the hydrolysis products, adenosine and

homocysteine. Adenosine is metabolized by adenosine kinase and adenosine deaminase, whereas homocysteine is used for the synthesis of methionine and cysteine. AdoHcy hydrolase is the only enzyme involved in mammalian AdoHcy metabolism and is the sole source of homocysteine in mammals. Because elevated homocysteine levels are a risk factor in vascular disease, AdoHcy hydrolase may play a role in the disease process (66). The homeostatic levels of AdoHcy are also of critical importance because AdoHcy is a potent inhibitor of AdoMet-dependent methylases. The key role of AdoHcy hydrolase in mammalian survival is showcased by the fact that the deletion of the gene is associated with embryo lethality in mice (63).

AdoHcy hydrolase has broad substrate specificity and can substitute adenosine with a number of other nucleosides to form the corresponding *S*-nucleosidyl-homocysteine [3-deaza-adenosine + homocysteine $\rightleftarrows$ 3-deaza-*S*-adenosylhomocysteine] (14). Likewise, it can substitute cysteine for homocysteine to form *S*-nucleosidylcysteine [adenosine + cysteine $\rightleftarrows$ *S*-adenosylcysteine] (36). AdoHcy hydrolase also reacts with a number of mechanistic inhibitors, some of which covalently modify the active site residues and are time-dependent inactivators.

The reaction mechanism of AdoHcy hydrolase involves oxidation-reduction cycling of enzyme-bound NAD (71, 72). An oxidation of the 3′-hydroxyl group of AdoHcy sugar moiety by enzyme-bound NAD$^+$ gives the corresponding 3′-keto derivative which after the β-elimination of homocysteine, yields 3′-keto-4′,5′-didehydro-5′-deoxyadenosine. Michael addition of water to the 4′,5′-double bond yields 3′-keto-adenosine, and a subsequent reduction of the latter by NADH generates adenosine. Dissociation of adenosine completes the reaction cycle.

Several forms of AdoHcy hydrolase have been isolated. The enzyme exists as a dimer in some plants and as a tetramer in mammals. The AdoHcy hydrolase of the prokaryote *Alcaligenes faecalis* contains six subunits and is immunologically distinct from the mammalian AdoHcy hydrolases (84). Two forms of AdoHcy hydrolase were identified in bovine liver, one containing four NAD$^+$ molecules/tetramer, and the other only two NAD$^+$ molecules/tetramer (73). Both forms are enzymatically active, but there are significant differences in terms of kinetic parameters (74). The AdoHcy hydrolase from *A. faecalis* may also exist in a form with two subunits per NAD$^+$ (three NAD$^+$ molecules/hexamer). When this AdoHcy hydrolase is inactivated with neplanocin A, only three NAD$^+$ molecules are reduced to NADH per hexamer (59). Half-site reactivity has been proposed for this kind of inactivation.

By using Western blots, it was estimated that mouse liver contains about twelve times more AdoHcy hydrolase than the kidney, which in turn contains five times more than the brain. The liver AdoHcy hydrolase binds one atom of copper per subunit of the enzyme (5). The hepatic level of AdoHcy hydrolase was decreased by 45% in copper-deficient mice, and the binding of copper by the enzyme suggests a role in regulating tissue copper levels and the distribution of intracellular copper.

Pathological Correlates

Pathological conditions are associated with elevated AdoHcy in tissues. The most interesting case is found in mice that are genetically engineered for adenosine deaminase deficiency, the symptom of which is combined immunodeficiency. These mice have a drastic reduction of AdoHcy hydrolase and a pronounced accumulation of 2′-deoxyadenosine and 2′-deoxyadenosine triphosphate (dATP) in the thymus and spleen (9). Adenosine is markedly increased in all tissues examined and the adenosine deaminase-deficient mice also exhibit severe pulmonary insufficiency and bone and kidney abnormalities. The observation that a striking deficiency of AdoHcy hydrolase is found in some patients with adenosine deaminase deficiency supports these findings (41). Despite the reduction in AdoHcy hydrolase levels, it has been suggested that dATP accumulation in the T lymphocytes is probably more important in the genesis of lymphocyte toxicity than AdoHcy hydrolase inactivation (106).

Elevated plasma levels of homocysteine are found in patients with renal failure. The high concentration of homocysteine may lead to increased AdoHcy synthesis by AdoHcy hydrolase, which in turn would inhibit methylase activity and increase AdoMet levels. The ratio of plasma AdoMet/AdoHcy in these patients is 0.36, compared with 2.7 for healthy volunteers (56). Hemodialysis fails to restore the normal levels of AdoMet and AdoHcy. Thus, these patients' renal failure is associated with the reduction in the ratio of AdoMet/AdoHcy, which is a reflection of impaired methylation.

In the brain of genetically epileptic E1 mice, AdoHcy hydrolase is downregulated, and leads to a higher than normal accumulation of AdoHcy (69). The epileptic mice are characterized by disordered feedback regulation of the AdoMet-dependent methyl transfer pathway. Interestingly, AdoHcy inhibits the binding of the antiseizure drug flunitrazepam to rat brain membranes with a K_i of 8 μmol/L. This observation indicates that AdoHcy may interact with endogenous benzodiazepine receptors (93).

Both cell cycle and cellular differentiation modulate AdoHcy hydrolase activity. In mastocytoma cells, levels of AdoHcy hydrolase reach a maximum when cells change from the G1/S phase to the G2 phase (45). In contrast, a decrease of AdoHcy hydrolase activity is specifically associated with the G1 phase of the cell cycle in HL-60 leukemia cells (20). When HL-60 cell differentiation is induced by dimethyl sulfoxide, both AdoMet and AdoHcy levels decrease rapidly without affecting the AdoMet/AdoHcy ratio (21). AdoHcy hydrolase activity in human red blood cells undergoes a threefold to fourfold decrease as the cells age (11). These observations can have important implications when studying the modulation of AdoHcy hydrolase activity and its biochemical or biological correlates, especially when inhibitors are used.

AdoHcy Hydrolase Genes

AdoHcy hydrolase genes are well represented among eukaryotes, bacteria, and archaea. A search of complete microorganism genomes, however, shows that some bacteria and archaea lack identifiable AdoHcy hydrolase genes. A comparison of the AdoHcy hydrolase genes of 35 species (Figure 8.1) shows that their sequences range from 399 (Aeropyrum pernix) to 527 (Drosophila melanogaster) residues in length, out of which 44 residues are conserved across all 35 sequences. Many of these conserved residues are in or around the substrate and cofactor binding sites (see next section) including a glycine-rich hexapeptide, GXGXXG, which is thought to bind NAD (33, 39, 68). Pairwise sequence identity between AdoHcy hydrolase genes ranges from 34% to 98%.

Two cDNA clones of human AdoHcy hydrolase have been isolated from a placental cDNA library, and each is comprised of 1,299 bp of DNA encoding a 432 amino-acid protein of 47.7 kDa. The clones contain minor sequence differences, but more significantly, one clone contains a 101 bp intron, but the other does not (24). There is only a single gene locus for the human AdoHcy hydrolase, and it is located in chromosome 20 (7, 40). However, polymorphisms of AdoHcy hydrolase exist in human populations. There are two common alleles in Germany, AdoHcyH*1 and AdoHcyH*2, with frequencies of 0.96 and 0.04, respectively (6). In Italy, three common alleles are found, AdoHcyH*1, AdoHcyH*2, and AdoHcyH*3; the gene frequencies are 0.968, 0.023, and 0.009, respectively (23).

Transcriptional regulation of rat AdoHcy hydrolase was studied by cloning the DNA upstream of the transcription start into a luciferase reporter plasmid (62). This upstream region contained sites for AP-2, SP-1,

```
  1    MSDKLPYKVADIGLAAWGRKALDIAENEMPGLMRMRERYSASKPLKGARI

 51    AGCLHMTVETAVLIETLVTLGAEVQWSSCNIFSTQDHAAAAIAKAGIPVY

101    AWKGETDEEYLWCIEQTLYFKDGPLNMILDDGGDLTNLIHTKYPQLLPGI

151    RGISEETTGVHNLYKMMANGILKVPAINVNDSVTKSKFDNLYGCRESLI

201    DGIKRATDVMIAGKVAVVAGYGDVGKGCAQALRGFGARVIITEIDPINAL

251    QAAMEGYEVTTMDEACQEGNIFVTTTGCIDIILGRHFEQMKDDAIVCNIG

301    HFDVEIDVKWLNENAVEKVNIKPQVDRYRLKNGRRIILLAEGRLVNLGCA

351    MGHPSFVMSNSFTNQVMAQIELWTHPDKYPVGVHFLPKKLDEAVAEAHLG

401    KLNVKLTKLTEKQAQYLGMSCDGPFKPDHYRY
```

Fig. 8.1. Primary and secondary structure of human AdoHcy hydrolase. The sequence of human AdoHcy hydrolase is shown with α-helical residues highlighted in dark gray shading and β-sheet residues highlighted in light gray shading (94). Residues that are identical among 35 AdoHcy hydrolase sequences are underlined.

glucocorticoid-responsive element, and a TATA-like sequence. Promoter activity was measured in Chinese hamster ovary cells transiently infccted with the reporter plasmid. Mutational analysis showed that the SP-1 site was predominantly responsible for promoter activity, whereas the other sites had little effect on promoter activity.

Structure and Mechanism

The three-dimensional structures of rat and human AdoHcy hydrolase have been solved by x-ray crystallography (43, 94). The two enzymes share 96% sequence identity and a high degree of structural similarity. Both enzymes are homotetramers composed of ~48 kDa subunits, each of which contains one molecule of NAD (Figure 8.2A). The AdoHcy hydrolase monomers have three domains. The NAD domain (residues 193–346) exhibits a core of parallel α/β structure and binds the NAD^+ cofactor. The catalytic domain (residues 1–190 and 355–402) also contains parallel α/β structure and forms the putative binding pocket for AdoHcy. The carboxy terminal residues (403–431) form an extended dimerization domain that binds to the NAD domain of the adjacent monomer and interacts with the adenine end of the NAD found on the adjacent monomer. In the AdoHcy hydrolase tetramer, the NAD domains and the dimerization domains form almost all of the interdomain contacts, potentially allowing the catalytic domains some degree of flexibility relative to the rest of the tetramer.

Binding of the NAD cofactor is typical of NAD-dependent dehydrogenases, using a GXGXXG motif (Figure 8.1) to form hydrogen bonds with NAD. The bound conformations of NAD in the structures of rat and human AdoHcy hydrolase are almost identical, highlighting the similarity between the two structures. The most significant difference between the rat and human AdoHcy hydrolase structures can be seen when the two structures are superimposed. The root mean square distance between the α carbons of both monomers is 1.5Å, whereas the root mean square distance is 0.3Å for the catalytic domains alone and 0.2Å for the NAD domains alone. A hingelike conformational shift brings the catalytic domain closer to the NAD domain in the human AdoHcy hydrolase structure, perhaps as a result of binding the inhibitor (1′R,2′S,3′R)-9-(2′,3′-dihydroxycyclopentan-1′-yl) adenine (DHCeA; Figure 8.2B). This inhibitor is an adenosine analog presumed to mimic the binding of the adenosyl moiety of AdoHcy (94).

The structures of rat and human AdoHcy hydrolase provide valuable insight into the reaction mechanism proposed by Palmer and Abeles (71, 72). The AdoHcy hydrolase mechanism requires transfer of hydride, addition of water, and proton transfer by two active site residues (Figure 8.3). Based on the AdoHcy hydrolase structures, two mechanisms have been proposed that include these steps (43, 94). However, the two suppositions disagree on the identity of the two active site residues (see Figure 8.2B for a view of active site residues) that act as acid-base catalysts (B_1 and B_2 in Figure 8.3) in the proton transfer steps. Turner and co-workers (94) proposed that K186 acts as B_1 because K186 is closest to the site of proton extraction in the inhibitor, DHCeA (analogous to the 3′-hydroxyl in AdoHcy). Hu and co-workers (43) proposed that nearby E156 acts as B_1. They also propose that H55 or D131 acts as B_2, whereas Turner and co-workers (94) argue that H55 and D131 activate a water molecule that is well positioned to act as B_2. They further suggest that this water molecule is the one that is subsequently added to the 5′-carbon of AdoHcy during the hydrolysis step. The notion that this water can act as B_2 is strengthened by the evidence that 4′-carbon of AdoHcy exchanges with solvent (72).

Inhibitors

Many adenosine analogs and derivatives are potent inhibitors of AdoHcy hydrolase. The inhibition by nucleosides can be achieved either by steady-state kinetics or time-dependent inactivation (14, 36, 54). In general, there are two types of mechanism-based, time-dependent inhibitors. Type I inactivators mimic step 1 of the AdoHcy hydrolase reaction (Figure 8.3) by reducing enzyme-bound NAD^+ to NADH; the reduced NADH remains noncovalently bound to the enzyme, thus disabling catalytic cycling. Type II inactivators are catalytically activated and become covalently bound to the enzyme. Step 3 of the AdoHcy hydrolase reaction (Figure 8.3) is thought to proceed through the formation of an intermediate with a 4′,5′-double bond, which is then hydrolyzed by water. Type II inactivators are activated through the addition of water to generate electrophilic species that undergo nucleophilic attack by protein residues (100).

The nucleoside inhibitors of AdoHcy hydrolase have been reviewed by Chiang (15). The bulk of the work on AdoHcy hydrolase inhibitors and on the biological effects of these inhibitors (see next section) centers around four compounds. The first potent inhibitor of AdoHcy hydrolase was 3-deaza-adenosine (Figure

8.4) (19). After the discovery that aristeromycin [carbocyclic adenosine] was also a potent inhibitor (37), 3-deaza-(±)aristeromycin (Figure 8.4) was synthesized. Montgomery and co-workers (64) found that 3-deaza-(±)aristeromycin was not only a more potent inhibitor of AdoHcy hydrolase, but it was also resistant to degradation by adenosine deaminase. So far, the most potent inhibitor of AdoHcy hydrolase is 3-deaza-neplanocin (Figure 8.4), which is a modification of the natural product neplanocin-A (10, 92, 105).

Although they are potent AdoHcy hydrolase inhibitors, neplanocin A and 3-deaza-neplanocin are cytotoxic to host cells (32, 42, 46). Cytotoxicity is thought to result from the phosphorylation of the 6′-hydroxyl group by adenosine kinase and subsequent metabolism by cellular enzymes. Recent attempts to synthesize less cytotoxic neplanocin analogs have focused on substitutions at the 2-position of the adenosine ring and the 6′-position of the cyclopentenyl ring (corresponds to the 5′-position of adenosine) (27). Obara and co-workers (67) showed that 2-flourone-planocin is not a substrate for adenosine deaminase, yet it retains the antiviral activity of neplanocin. Substitutions at the 6′-position yield AdoHcy hydrolase inhibitors such as (6′R)-6′-C-methylneplanocin (Figure 8.4), which are poor substrates of adenosine deaminase and adenosine kinase, but are still AdoHcy

Fig. 8.3. AdoHcy hydrolase reaction mechanism. A five-step reaction mechanism for AdoHcy hydrolase (adapted from Palmer and Abeles [71, 72]) is shown. Recent mechanistic proposals (43, 94) disagree on the identity of the two active-site, acid-base catalysts (B_1 and B_2).

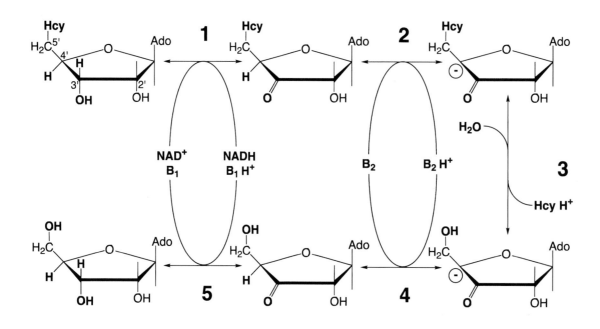

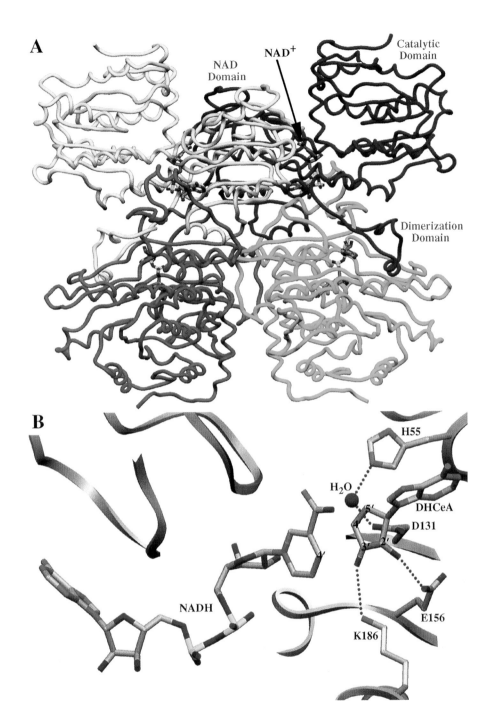

Fig. 8.2. AdoHcy hydrolase structure. (**A**) Rat AdoHcy hydrolase tetramer (43). The α carbon trace of the rat AdoHcy hydrolase tetramer is shown. Each monomer is a different color (red, yellow, blue, and green) and the four bound NAD cofactors are colored by atom type (carbon is gray, oxygen is red, nitrogen is blue, and phosphorus is green). The three AdoHcy hydrolase domains of the red monomer are labeled in red. (**B**) Human AdoHcy hydrolase active site (94). The active site of human AdoHcy hydrolase is shown with bound NADH, inhibitor (DHCeA or (1′R,2′S,3′R)-9-(2′,3′-dihydroxycyclopentan-1′-yl) adenine) and water (red sphere). The inhibitor, NADH and key active site residues, are colored by atom type.

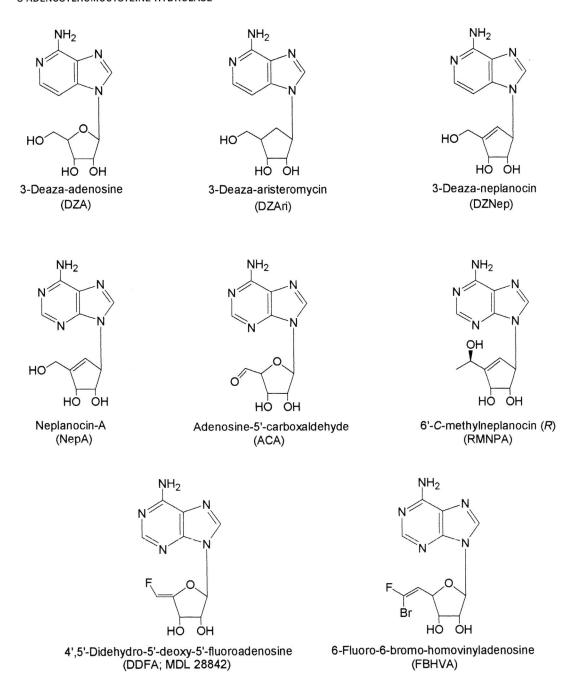

Fig. 8.4. Structures of eight nucleoside inhibitors of AdoHcy hydrolase.

hydrolase inhibitors (85–87). Some of these compounds have recently been shown to be active against the human immunodeficiency virus (26).

Most of the adenosine analog inhibitors of AdoHcy hydrolase are type I inactivators, which are substrates for the 3′-oxidative activity of AdoHcy hydrolase (Figure 8.3, Step 1), but are not further catalyzed by the 5′-hydrolytic activity (Figure 8.3, Step 3). It was

found that NAD-depleted AdoHcy hydrolase converted 4′,5′-didehydro-5′-deoxy-5′-fluoroadenosine (DDFA; Figure 8.4) (61) into adenosine-5′-carboxaldehyde (Figure 8.4) through 5′-hydrolysis (107). The hydrolysis product, adenosine-5′-carboxaldehyde, is a type I inhibitor and is subject to the 3′-oxidative activity of AdoHcy hydrolase (55). Recent work with vinylhalide derivatives of adenosine (100) and aristeromycin (102) showed that these and similar compounds (65, 77, 95, 101) are also prodrug inhibitors of AdoHcy hydrolase and are activated by 5′-hydrolysis. Activated inhibitors can show type I or type II inhibition. Dihalohomovinyl nucleoside analogs derived from adenosine were activated by hydrolysis without subsequent 3'-oxidation (100). Addition of water is thought to generate electrophilic acyl halides or α-halo ketone species that could undergo nucleophilic attack by nearby active site amino acids. Tritium labeling demonstrated that the 6'-fluoro-6'-bromo analog (Figure 8.4) covalently modifies AdoHcy hydrolase (100).

Biological Effects of AdoHcy Hydrolase Inhibitors

The biological and biochemical effects of AdoHcy hydrolase inhibitors are myriad. Administration of these compounds has profound consequences on mammalian cells, ranging from the induction of cellular differentiation to the regulation of gene expression and apoptosis. The biological effects of the inhibitors of AdoHcy hydrolase have been reviewed (15).

Antiviral Effects

After the initial report of Bader and co-workers (3), remarkable antiviral effects were demonstrated for the inhibitors of AdoHcy hydrolase in vitro and in vivo, for both the DNA and RNA viruses (15, 27). Despite many impressive antiviral effects, the precise mode of action of these inhibitors remains controversial (15).

The adenosine analogs neplanocin A and 3-deaza-neplanocin exhibit the most potent antiviral activities, as well as inhibition of AdoHcy hydrolase (10, 22, 44, 60, 96, 104). Many AdoHcy hydrolase inhibitors block human immunodeficiency virus replication (25–27), but neplanocin A and 3-deaza-neplanocin induced a 3- to 18-fold increase in potency against azidothymidine-resistant human immunodeficiency virus isolates (60). Among other viruses, African swine fever virus was very sensitive to 3-deaza-neplanocin, which showed the largest therapeutic index among a large number of AdoHcy inhibitors tested (96). In vivo, 3-deaza-(±)aristeromycin suppressed the formation of tail lesions in mice infected with vaccinia virus (28) and, in a separate study, cured mice infected with Ebola virus (44).

The possible inhibition of viral methylation has long been an attractive hypothesis to explain the antiviral effect of AdoHcy hydrolase inhibitors (64). However, Stoltzfus and Montgomery (90) showed that the antiviral effect of 3-deaza-adenosine was not due to an inhibition of viral methylation because 3-deaza-adenosine did not inhibit N^7-methylguanosine methylation in cellular poly(A)$^+$ RNA isolated from cells infected with avian sarcoma virus. The antiviral effects of neplanocin A may not involve methylation either. Neplanocin A blocks the replication of influenza virus

only in methionine-depleted medium. Because neplanocin A caused large increases in the cellular AdoHcy levels regardless of the medium used, it was concluded that the antiviral effect of neplanocin A was not due to the accumulation of AdoHcy (104).

There are several other possible explanations for the antiviral effects of AdoHcy hydrolase inhibitors. One hypothesis follows from the observation that late influenza mRNAs are not transported from the nucleus to the cytoplasm in the presence of 3-deaza-adenosine (97). It was concluded that inhibition of the synthesis of a viral protein may act as a transportation barrier (31). Other hypotheses touch on the metabolic effects of AdoHcy hydrolase inhibitors. Nucleotide derivatives of 3-deaza-adenosine, 3-deaza-(±)aristeromycin, neplanocin A, and 3-deaza-neplanocin have been isolated from several cell lines after treatment with these inhibitors (4, 32, 60, 79). The derivatives of these compounds can be incorporated into AdoMet analogs (e.g., S-neplanocylmethionine) in lieu of adenosine [50, 98, 109]. It is not clear which of these inhibitor metabolites is responsible for the observed antiviral activity or what the specific mechanism of inactivation is. Nevertheless, the inhibitory effect of 3-deaza-neplanocin on the long terminal repeat of the human immunodeficiency virus has been confirmed (25, 60).

Cellular Differentiation

Administration of AdoHcy hydrolase inhibitors arrests the growth of many cell types and can induce cellular differentiation. The reversibility and duration of the induced changes, and the specific effects of different inhibitors vary considerably depending on the cell type and the nature of the inhibitor. When 3T3-L1 fibroblasts are treated with 3-deaza-adenosine or 3-deaza-(±)aristeromycin, they differentiate into adipocytes (13, 108). The induced differentiation is not reversed by the absence of the inhibitor. Human promyelocytic leukemia cells (HL-60) treated with 3-deaza-adenosine, 3-deaza-(±)aristeromycin or 3-deaza-neplanocin undergo functional and morphological differentiation into cells more like that of normal leukocytes. However, unlike the effect on 3T3-L1 fibroblasts, the continuous presence of the compounds is required to maintain the morphological change (1, 58).

The effects of AdoHcy hydrolase inhibitors on cellular differentiation, whether to induce differentiation or to inhibit it, can be potentiated by homocysteine thiolactone. Myoblast cells differentiate into multinucleated myofibers after treatment with 50 μmol/L 3-deaza-adenosine, but differentiation is triggered by 10-fold less 3-deaza-adenosine in the presence of 100 μmol/L homocysteine thiolactone (80). 3-Deaza-adenosine repressed the differentiation of murine erythroleukemia cells induced by various agents (83). The inhibition was potentiated by homocysteine thiolactone, was reversible, and was accompanied by a 71% decrease in the AdoMet/AdoHcy ratio (83). Of interest, 3-deaza-(±)aristeromycin altered AdoHcy levels in myoblast cells (10-fold increase), but did not induce differentiation into multinucleated myofibers (80).

The ratio of AdoMet to AdoHcy varies dramatically during the normal developmental cycle of the primitive eukaryote *Dictyostelium discoideum*. These changes are not related to changes in AdoHcy hydrolase because constant levels of both the protein and its activity were observed over the course of differentiation (35). The effects of AdoHcy hydrolase inhibitors on cellular differentiation may be linked to their ability to perturb the AdoMet/AdoHcy ratio. Keratinocyte differentiation was increased after treatment with DDFA along with a decrease in the AdoMet/AdoHcy ratio (70). Undifferentiated keratinocytes treated with DDFA also displayed a decreased AdoMet/AdoHcy ratio, indicating that the perturbation of the AdoMet/AdoHcy ratio was due to the inhibitor (70).

Gene Expression

The ability of the AdoHcy inhibitors, 3-deaza-adenosine, 3-deaza-(±)aristeromycin, and 3-deaza-neplanocin, to activate gene expression was demonstrated in F9 teratocarcinoma cells (16). The activation of the collagen IV gene was quantitated by monitoring mRNA levels and by measuring the activity of collagen IV promoter-enhancer-CAT constructs in transfected cells (16). There was a dose-dependent effect and it required 48 hours before the activation effect became apparent.

The activation of the collagen IV gene was not due to methylation of the gene since digestion with *Hpa*II and *Msp*I demonstrated no observable change in collagen IV gene methylation. Similarly, a transient increase in the expression of c-*myc* mRNA in HL-60 cells was observed after treatment with 3-deaza-(±)aristeromycin. However, no difference in the methylation pattern of the c-*myc* DNA sequence was found, as determined by digestion with *Hpa*II and *Msp*I. (57).

Treatment with AdoHcy hydrolase inhibitors can, in some cases, lead to an inhibition of gene expression. 3-Deaza-adenosine, 3-deaza-(±)aristeromycin, and 3-deaza-neplanocin inhibited the production of tumor necrosis factor-α in mouse macrophage cells stimulated with lipopolysaccharide. 3-Deaza-adenosine reduced the level of tumor necrosis factor mRNA, but 3-deaza-(±)aristeromycin and 3-deaza-neplanocin did not, implying that 3-deaza-(±)aristeromycin and 3-deaza-neplanocin inhibit a post-transcriptional step of tumor necrosis factor production (48). In a later study,

Jeong and co-workers (47) demonstrated that 3-deaza-adenosine inhibited the transcriptional activity of nuclear factor-κB.

The production of other proteins is also inhibited by 3-deaza-adenosine. For example, when human aortic endothelial cells were treated with 3-deaza-adenosine, thrombin-stimulated platelet-derived growth factor production was abolished (81). 3-Deaza-adenosine also reduced the steady-state levels of mRNAs of platelet-derived growth factor-A chain, platelet-derived growth factor-B chain, and E-selectin in cells stimulated by thrombin or phorbol ester. Similarly, 3-deaza-adenosine prevented the upregulation of intercellular adhesion molecule-1 in stimulated human umbilical vein endothelial cells (49).

Inhibition of Phospholipid Methylation

3-Deaza-adenosine drastically inhibits phospholipid methylation in rat liver tissue, in *Tetrahymena,* and in various cultured cells (17, 75, 88, 99). An accelerated cytidine 5′-diphosphate-choline pathway in all these observations, excepting human platelets (82) and A2058 human melanoma cells (53), accompanies the inhibition.

Antiparasitic Effects

The antimalarial activity of AdoHcy hydrolase inhibitors was demonstrated for 3-deaza-adenosine and neplanocin A in vitro (91, 98). DDFA inhibited the in vitro growth of the human malaria parasite *Plasmodium falciparum* and the in vivo growth of the mouse malaria parasite *Plasmodium berghei* (8). Inhibition of *P. berghei* growth was accompanied by an increase in AdoHcy levels in the mouse erythrocyte. It was not clear whether the antiparasitic effects of DDFA were due to direct inhibition of malarial AdoHcy hydrolase, or due to indirect effects stemming from the inhibition of the mouse AdoHcy hydrolase (8). The growth of *Leishmania donovani* was arrested by 3-deaza-(±)aristeromycin and was abrogated partially by exogenous AdoMet (39). 3-Deaza-neplanocin inhibited the in vitro growth of all 23 strains of the American *Leishmania* parasite (*L. mexicana* and *L. brasiliensis*) (2). Similarly, the in vivo administration of 3-deaza-neplanocin significantly reduced the development of cutaneous leishmaniasis in mice (2).

Apoptosis

High doses of 3-deaza-adenosine caused apoptosis in HL-60 cells (76). Homocysteine (1 mmol/L) partially abrogated 3-deaza-adenosine-induced apoptosis in HL-60 cells (29). Pretreatment of the cells incubated with 3-deaza-adenosine plus 1 mmol/L homocysteine with 3-deaza-(±)aristeromycin diminished 3-deaza-S-adenosylhomocysteine and almost completely abrogated apoptosis (30). Additionally, exposure of the cells to a high dose of 3-deaza-(±)aristeromycin alone resulted in an increase in AdoHcy to 8.4-fold control levels, without changes in AdoMet and no initiation of apoptosis. These results, combined with the fact that 3-deaza-(±)aristeromycin does not induce apoptosis, suggest that 3-deaza-adenosine exerts its apoptosis-initiating effect through the elevation of cellular 3-deaza-S-adenosylhomocysteine.

The apoptotic effect was studied further by Kim and co-workers (51) who found that 3-deaza-adenosine, 3-deaza-(±)aristeromycin, and 1-β-D-arabinofuranosyl-1H-imidazo[4,5-c]pyridine (DZAra-A) induced DNA fragmentation in a dose-dependent and time-dependent manner. Cycloheximide completely blocked the DNA fragmentation induced by each of the analogs. In contrast to the partial effect observed with HL-60 cells (29), 0.1 mmol/L homocysteine thiolactone did not abrogate the DNA fragmentation caused by 3-deaza-adenosine, but did so for 3-deaza-(±)aristeromycin and DZAra-A in the L1210 murine leukemia cells (51). Flow cytometry analysis revealed that 3-deaza-adenosine arrested the cells in the G2/M phase, compared with the blockade of S phase by 3-deaza-(±)aristeromycin. 3-Deaza-adenosine induced a decrease in the expression of c-*myc* within minutes, followed by an elevated expression of nuclear factor-κB DNA binding activity. The latter binding activity became more pronounced after 24 hours, along with a disappearance of AP-1 binding activity. 3-Deaza-adenosine most likely inhibited the RNA synthesis of c-*myc*, the reduction of which could trigger a cascade of gene transcription leading to apoptosis in L1210 cells. Whether 3-deaza-(±)aristeromycin or DZAra-A could also trigger the same pattern of molecular events awaits further investigation.

Rounds and co-workers (78) linked the intracellular metabolism of adenosine to apoptosis in endothelial cells. They found that the AdoHcy hydrolase inhibitor DDFA caused apoptosis, and it decreased the ratio of AdoMet to AdoHcy compared with untreated control cells. Because DNA fragmentation in apoptotic cells was potentiated by coincubation with 0.1 mmol/L homocysteine, it was speculated that the mechanism of inducing apoptosis in endothelial cells involves inhibition of AdoHcy hydrolase.

Sodium Transport

A recent and provocative observation has shown that aldosterone-induced sodium transport is mediated by the activity of AdoHcy hydrolase in A6 toad kidney epithelial cells (89). Aldosterone seems to induce AdoHcy hydrolase activity that in turn is necessary for aldosterone-induced sodium reabsorption. The inhibitor 3-deaza-adenosine decreased sodium reabsorption. When the cells were treated with antisense, but not sense, oligonucleotides of AdoHcy hydrolase, both aldosterone-induced enzyme activity and sodium current were decreased, indicating that the AdoHcy hydrolase activity is linked to sodium reabsorption. Additionally, overexpression of AdoHcy hydrolase potentiated the aldosterone-induced sodium current. Aldosterone may increase AdoHcy hydrolase activity through a post-translational modification of the enzyme, possibly via phosphorylation or acylation.

Mechanisms of Inhibitor Resistance

The physiological level of AdoHcy hydrolase is regulated by glucocorticoids in concert with that of AdoMet synthetase (103). Coregulation of both enzymes is a mechanism for maintaining a homeostatic AdoMet/AdoHcy ratio. Two resistant cell lines were developed from C1300 murine neuroblastoma tumor cells, one resistant to 3-deaza-neplanocin and one to DDFA (38). These resistant cell lines showed cross-resistance to both of these inhibitors, without changes in AdoHcy hydrolase activity. Nor was there a difference in AdoHcy concentration when the cell lines were treated with 3-deaza-neplanocin or DDFA. In contrast, cellular AdoMet increased fivefold and AdoMet synthetase activity also increased significantly. Thus, these cells adapted to the inhibitors by elevating intracellular AdoMet.

Elevated levels of AdoMet also appear to be involved in the mechanism of resistance in 3-deaza-(±)aristeromycin-resistant human B-lymphocytes that are deficient in nucleoside kinase (34). The resistant cells have normal AdoHcy hydrolase activity and do not block the uptake of 3-deaza-(±)aristeromycin. However, they possess highly elevated AdoMet level and they rapidly export AdoHcy. As a result, the intracellular AdoMet/AdoHcy ratio is higher than it is in normal human B-lymphocytes. The AdoMet synthetase activity is not altered in these cells as it is in the inhibitor-resistant murine neuroblastoma cells. Hence, the metabolic adaptation in the 3-deaza-(±)aristeromycin-resistant cells is to overcome the inhibition of methylation reactions by a much higher AdoMet/AdoHcy ratio.

The recent elucidation of the rat and human AdoHcy hydrolase structures (43, 94) coupled with the discovery of dozens of AdoHcy hydrolase genes in diverse organisms has rapidly expanded our understanding of this enzyme. These insights into the structure and mechanism of AdoHcy hydrolases should aid the efforts to develop specific inhibitors. The nucleoside inhibitors of AdoHcy hydrolase have proven to be valuable tools in probing the physiology of mammalian cells. In many cases, the mode of action responsible for their biological effects still awaits biochemical elaboration, especially regarding their antiviral effects, induction of genes, and cellular differentiation.

REFERENCES

1. Aarbakke, J, Miura, GA, Prytz, PS, Bessesen, A, Slordal, L, Gordon, RK, Chiang, PK. Induction of HL-60 cell differentiation by 3-deaza-(+/−)-aristeromycin, an inhibitor of S-adenosylhomocysteine hydrolase. *Cancer Res* 1986; 46: 5469–72.

2. Avila, JL, Avila, A, Polegre, MA, Marquez, VE. Specific inhibitory effect of 3-deazaneplanocin A against several *Leishmania mexicana* and *L. braziliensis* strains. *Am J Trop Med Hyg* 1997; 57: 407–12.

3. Bader, JP, Brown, NR, Chiang, PK, Cantoni, GL. 3-Deazaadenosine, an inhibitor of adenosylhomocysteine hydrolase, inhibits reproduction of Rous sarcoma virus and transformation of chick embryo cells. *Virology* 1978; 89: 494–505.

4. Bennett, LL Jr, Allan, PW, Rose, LM, Comber, RN, Secrist, JA 3d. Differences in the metabolism and metabolic effects of the carbocyclic adenosine analogs, neplanocin A and aristeromycin. *Mol Pharmacol* 1986; 29: 383–90.

5. Bethin, KE, Cimato, TR, Ettinger, MJ. Copper binding to mouse liver S-adenosylhomocysteine hydrolase and the effects of copper on its levels. *J Biol Chem* 1995; 270: 20703–11.

6. Bissbort, S, Bender, K, Wienker, TF, Grzeschik, KH. Genetics of human S-adenosylhomocysteine hydrolase. A new polymorphism in man. *Hum Genet* 1983; 65: 68–71.

7. Bissbort, S, Hitzeroth, HW, van den Berg, CT, Wienker, TF. Linkage relationship between the genes for adenosine deaminase and S-adenosyl-homocysteine hydrolase on human chromosome 20. *Hum Genet* 1987; 77: 277–79.

8. Bitonti, AJ, Baumann, RJ, Jarvi, ET, McCarthy, JR, McCann, PP. Antimalarial activity of a 4′,5′-unsaturated 5′-fluoroadenosine mechanism-based inhibitor of S-adenosyl-L-homocysteine hydrolase. *Biochem Pharmacol* 1990; 40: 601–6.

9. Blackburn, MR, Datta, SK, Kellems, RE. Adenosine deaminase-deficient mice generated using a two-stage genetic engineering strategy exhibit a combined immunodeficiency. *J Biol Chem* 1998; 273: 5093–100.

10. Borchardt, RT, Keller, BT, Patel-Thombre, U, Neplanocin, A. A potent inhibitor of S-adenosylhomocysteine hydrolase and of vaccinia virus multiplication in mouse L929 cells. *J Biol Chem* 1984; 259: 4353–8.

11. Bozzi, A, Furciniti-La Chiusa, B, Strom, R, Crifo, C. S-adenosylhomocysteine hydrolase and adenosine deaminase activities in human red cell ageing. *Clin Chim Acta* 1990; 189: 81–6.

12. Cantoni, GL. Biological methylation: Selected aspects. *Annu Rev Biochem* 1975; 44: 435–51.

13. Chiang, PK. Conversion of 3T3-L1 fibroblasts to fat cells by an inhibitor of methylation: Effect of 3-deaza-adenosine. *Science* 1981; 211: 1164–66.

14. Chiang, PK. S-Adenosylhomocysteine hydrolase: Measurement of activity and use of inhibitors. In *Methods in Pharmacology: Methods Used in Adenosine Research*, vol. 6 (Paton, OM, ed.). Plenum Press, New York, 1985; pp. 127–45.

15. Chiang, PK. Biological effects of inhibitors of S-adenosylhomocysteine hydrolase. *Pharmacol Ther* 1998; 77: 115–34.

16. Chiang, PK, Burbelo, PD, Brugh, SA, Gordon, RK, Fukuda, K, Yamada, Y. Activation of collagen IV gene expression in F9 teratocarcinoma cells by 3-deazaadenosine analogs. Indirect inhibitors of methylation. *J Biol Chem* 1992; 267: 4988–91.

17. Chiang, PK, Cantoni, GL. Perturbation of biochemical transmethylations by 3-deazaadenosine in vivo. *Biochem Pharmacol* 1979; 28: 1897–902.

18. Chiang, PK, Gordon, RK, Tal, J, Zeng, GC, Doctor, BP, Pardhasaradhi, K, McCann, PP. S-Adenosylmethionine and methylation. *FASEB J* 1996; 10: 471–80.

19. Chiang, PK, Richards, HH, Cantoni, GL. S-Adenosyl-L-homocysteine hydrolase: Analogues of S-adenosyl-L-homocysteine as potential inhibitors. *Mol Pharmacol* 1977; 13: 939–47.

20. Chiba, P, Plas, A, Wessels, JM, De Bruyn, CH. S-adenosylhomocysteine hydrolase activity during differentiation of HL-60 cells. *Biosci Rep* 1984; 4: 687–94.

21. Chiba, P, Wallner, C, Kaiser, E. S-adenosylmethionine metabolism in HL-60 cells: Effect of cell cycle and differentiation. *Biochim Biophys Acta* 1988; 971: 38–45.

22. Cools, M, de Clercq, E. Correlation between the antiviral activity of acyclic and carbocyclic adenosine analogues in murine L929 cells and their inhibitory effect on L929 cells S-adenosylhomocysteine hydrolase. *Biochem Pharmacol* 1989; 38: 1061–67.

23. Corbo, RM, Palmarino, R, Schiattarella, E, Giannini, MA, Scacchi, R. Polymorphism of S-adenosylhomocysteine hydrolase in Italy. *Hum Hered* 1987; 37: 186–89.

24. Coulter-Karis, DE, Hershfield, MS. Sequence of full length cDNA for human S-adenosylhomocysteine hydrolase. *Ann Hum Genet* 1989; 53: 169–75.

25. Daelemans, D, Esté, JA, Witvrouw, M, Pannecouque, C, Jonckheere, H, Aquaro, S, Perno, CF, Clercq, ED, Vandamme, AM. S-adenosylhomocysteine hydrolase inhibitors interfere with the replication of human immunodeficiency virus type 1 through inhibition of the LTR transactivation. *Mol Pharmacol* 1997; 52: 1157–63.

26. Daelemans, D, Vandamme, AM, Shuto, S, Matsuda, A, De Clercq, E. Stereospecificity of 6′-C-neplanocin A analogues as inhibitors of S-adenosylhomocysteine hydrolase activity and human immunodeficiency virus replication. *Nucleosides Nucleotides* 1998; 17: 479–86.

27. De Clercq, E. Carbocyclic adenosine analogues as S-adenosylhomocysteine hydrolase inhibitors and antiviral agents: Recent advances. *Nucleosides Nucleotides* 1998; 17: 625–34.

28. De Clercq, E, Bergstrom, DE, Holy, A, Montgomery, JA. Broad-spectrum antiviral activity of adenosine analogues. *Antiviral Res* 1984; 4: 119–33.

29. Endresen, PC, Eide, TJ, Aarbakke, J. Cell death initiated by 3-deazaadenosine in HL-60 cells is apoptosis and is partially inhibited by homocysteine. *Biochem Pharmacol* 1993; 46: 1893–901.

30. Endresen, PC, Loennechen, T, Kildalsen, H, Aarbakke, J. Apoptosis and transmethylation metabolites in HL-60 cells. *J Pharmacol Exp Ther* 1996; 278: 1318–24.

31. Fischer, AA, Muller, K, Scholtissek, C. Specific inhibition of the synthesis of influenza virus late proteins and stimulation of early, M2, and NS2 protein synthesis by 3-deazaadenosine. *Virology* 1990; 177: 523–31.

32. Glazer, RI, Knode, MC. Neplanocin, A. A cyclopentenyl analog of adenosine with specificity for inhibiting RNA methylation. *J Biol Chem* 1984; 259: 12964–69.

33. Gomi, T, Date, T, Ogawa, H, Fujioka, M, Aksamit, RR, Backlund, PS Jr, Cantoni, GL. Expression of rat liver *S*-adenosylhomocysteinase cDNA in *Escherichia coli* and mutagenesis at the putative NAD binding site. *J Biol Chem* 1989; 264: 16138–42.

34. Greenberg, ML, Chaffee, S, Hershfield, MS. Basis for resistance to 3-deazaaristeromycin, an inhibitor of *S*-adenosylhomocysteine hydrolase, in human B-lymphoblasts. *J Biol Chem* 1989; 264: 795–803.

35. Guitton, MC, Keller, BT, Part, D, De Gunzburg, J, Borchardt, RT, Veron, M. *S*-adenosylmethionine, *S*-adenosylhomocysteine and *S*-adenosylhomocysteine hydrolase variations during differentiation of *Dictyostelium discoideum*. *Cell Differ* 1988; 22: 203–10.

36. Guranowski, A, Jakubowski, H. Substrate specificity of *S*-adenosylhomocysteinase. Cysteine is a substrate of the plant and mammalian enzymes. *Biochim Biophys Acta* 1983; 742: 250–56.

37. Guranowski, A, Montgomery, JA, Cantoni, GL, Chiang, PK. Adenosine analogues as substrates and inhibitors of *S*-adenosylhomocysteine hydrolase. *Biochemistry* 1981; 20: 110–15.

38. Hamre, MR, Clark, SH, Mirkin, BL. Resistance to inhibitors of *S*-adenosyl-L-homocysteine hydrolase in C1300 murine neuroblastoma tumor cells is associated with increased methionine adenosyltransferase activity. *Oncol Res* 1995; 7: 487–92.

39. Henderson, DM, Hanson, S, Allen, T, Wilson, K, Coulter-Karis, DE, Greenberg, ML, Hershfield, MS, Ullman, B. Cloning of the gene encoding *Leishmania donovani S*-adenosylhomocysteine hydrolase, a potential target for anti-parasitic chemotherapy. *Mol Biochem Parasitol* 1992; 53: 169–83.

40. Hershfield, MS, Francke, U. The human genes for *S*-adenosylhomocysteine hydrolase and adenosine deaminase are syntenic on chromosome 20. *Science* 1982; 216: 739–42.

41. Hershfield, MS, Kredich, NM, Ownby, DR, Ownby, H, Buckley, R. In vivo inactivation of erythrocyte *S*-adenosylhomocysteine hydrolase by 2′-deoxyadenosine in adenosine deaminase-deficient patients. *J Clin Invest* 1979; 63: 807–11.

42. Hoshi, A, Yoshida, M, Iigo, M, Tokuzen, R, Fukukawa, K, Ueda, T. Antitumor activity of derivatives of

neplanocin A in vivo and in vitro. *J Pharmacobiodyn* 1986; 9: 202–6.

43. Hu, Y, Komoto, J, Huang, Y, Gomi, T, Ogawa, H, Takata, Y, Fujioka, M, Takusagawa, F. Crystal structure of *S*-adenosylhomocysteine hydrolase from rat liver. *Biochemistry* 1999; 38: 8323–33.

44. Huggins, J, Zhang, ZX, Bray, M. Antiviral drug therapy of filovirus infections: *S*-adenosylhomocysteine hydrolase inhibitors inhibit Ebola virus in vitro and in a lethal mouse model. *J Infect Dis* 1999; 179 Suppl 1: S240–74.

45. Ichikawa, A, Sato, S, Tomita, K. Purification and characterization of *S*-adenosylhomocysteine hydrolase from mouse mastocytoma P-815 cells. Evidence for cell cycle-specific fluctuation of the enzyme activity. *J Biochem (Tokyo)* 1985; 97: 189–97.

46. Inaba, M, Nagashima, K, Tsukagoshi, S, Sakurai, Y. Biochemical mode of cytotoxic action of neplanocin A in L1210 leukemic cells. *Cancer Res* 1986; 46: 1063–67.

47. Jeong, SY, Ahn, SG, Lee, JH, Kim, HS, Kim, JW, Rhim, H, Jeong, SW, Kim, IK. 3-Deazaadenosine, a *S*-adenosylhomocysteine hydrolase inhibitor, has dual effects on NF-kappaB regulation. Inhibition of NF-kappaB transcriptional activity and promotion of Ikappa Balpha degradation. *J Biol Chem* 1999; 274: 18981–88.

48. Jeong, SY, Lee, JH, Kim, HS, Hong, SH, Cheong, CH, Kim, IK. 3-Deazaadenosine analogues inhibit the production of tumour necrosis factor-alpha in RAW264.7 cells stimulated with lipopolysaccharide. *Immunology* 1996; 89: 558–62.

49. Jurgensen, CH, Huber, BE, Zimmerman, TP, Wolberg, G. 3-Deazaadenosine inhibits leukocyte adhesion and ICAM-1 biosynthesis in tumor necrosis factor-stimulated human endothelial cells. *J Immunol* 1990; 144: 653–61.

50. Keller, BT, Borchardt, RT. Metabolic conversion of neplanocin A to *S*-neplanocylmethionine by mouse L 929 cells. *Biochem Biophys Res Commun* 1984; 120: 131–37.

51. Kim, IK, Li, CH, Young, HA, Lee, JH, Kim, HS, Pardhasaradhi, K, Garcia, GE, Chiang, PK. Apoptosis of L1210 cells induced by 3-deazaadenosine analogs: Differential expression of c-*myc* and NF-*k*B and molecular events. *J Biomed Sci* 1997; 4: 83–90.

52. Kloor, D, Fuchs, S, Petroktistis, F, Delabar, U, Muhlbauer, B, Quast, U, Osswald, H. Effects of ions on adenosine binding and enzyme activity of purified *S*-adenosylhomocysteine hydrolase from bovine kidney. *Biochem Pharmacol* 1998; 56: 1493–6.

53. Liotta, LA, Mandler, R, Murano, G, Katz, DA, Gordon, RK, Chiang, PK, Schiffmann, E. Tumor cell autocrine motility factor. *Proc Natl Acad Sci USA* 1986; 83: 3302–6.

54. Liu, S, Wolfe, MS, Borchardt, RT. Rational approaches to the design of antiviral agents based on *S*-adenosyl-L-homocysteine hydrolase as a molecular target. *Antiviral Res* 1992; 19: 247–65.

55. Liu, S, Wnuk, SF, Yuan, C, Robins, MJ, Borchardt, RT. Adenosine-5′-carboxaldehyde: A potent inhibitor of *S*-adenosyl-L-homocysteine hydrolase. *J Med Chem* 1993; 36: 883–87.

56. Loehrer, FM, Angst, CP, Brunner, FP, Haefeli, WE, Fowler, B. Evidence for disturbed *S*-adenosylmethionine:

S-adenosylhomocysteine ratio in patients with end-stage renal failure: A cause for disturbed methylation reactions? *Nephrol Dial Transplant* 1998; 13: 656–61.

57. Loennechen, T, Nilsen, IW, Moens, U, Andersen, A, Aarbakke, J. Is there an association between an increase in c-myc RNA steady state levels and c-myc methylation in HL-60 cells treated with 3-deaza-(+/–)-aristeromycin, an indirect inhibitor of methylation? *Biochem Pharmacol* 1992; 44: 1283–89.

58. Loennechen, T, Prytz, PS, Aarbakke, J. DNA-methylation in HL-60 cells treated with 3-deaza-(+/–)-aristeromycin and 3-deazaadenosine. *Biochem Pharmacol* 1989; 38: 2748–51.

59. Matuszewska, B, Borchardt, RT. The mechanism of inhibition of *Alcaligenes faecalis* S-adenosylhomocysteine hydrolase by neplanocin A. *Arch Biochem Biophys* 1987; 256: 50–5.

60. Mayers, DL, Mikovits, JA, Bharat, H, Hewlett, IK, Estrada, JS, Wolfe, AD, Garcia, GE, Doctor, BP, Burke, DS, Gordon, RK, Lane, JR, and Chiang, PK.: Anti-Human immunodeficiency virus 1 (HIV-1) activities of 3-deazaadenosine analogs: increased potency against 3′-azido-3′-deoxythymidine-resistant HIV-1 strains. *Proc Natl Acad Sci USA*, 1995; 92: 215–219.

61. McCarthy, JR, Jarvi, ET, Matthews, DP, Edwards, ML, Prakash, NJ, Bowlin, IL, Mehdi, S, Sunkara, PS, Bey, P. 4′,5′-Unsaturated 5′-fluoroadenosine nucleosides: Potent mechanism-based inhibitors of *S*-adenosylhomocysteine hydrolase. *J Am Chem Soc* 1989; 111: 1127–28.

62. Merta, A, Aksamit, RR, Cantoni, GL. The rat S-adenosylhomocysteine hydrolase promoter. *Biochem Biophys Res Commun* 1997; 240: 580–85.

63. Miller, MW, Duhl, DM, Winkes, BM, Arredondo-Vega, F, Saxon, PJ, Wolff, GL, Epstein, CJ, Hershfield, MS, Barsh, GS. The mouse lethal nonagouti (a(x)) mutation deletes the *S*-adenosylhomocysteine hydrolase (Ahcy) gene. *EMBO J* 1994; 13: 1806–16.

64. Montgomery, JA, Clayton, SJ, Thomas, HJ, Shannon, WM, Arnett, G, Bodner, AJ, Kim, IK, Cantoni, GL, Chiang, PK. Carbocyclic analogue of 3-deazaadenosine: A novel antiviral agent using *S*-adenosylhomocysteine hydrolase as a pharmacological target. *J Med Chem* 1982; 25: 626–29.

65. Muzard, M, Vandenplas, C, Guillerm, D, Guillerm, G. The mechanism of inactivation of *S*-adenosylhomocysteine hydrolase by fluorinated analogs of 5′-methylthioadenosine. *J Enzyme Inhib* 1998; 13: 443–56.

66. Nygård, O, Nordrehaug, JE, Refsum, H, Ueland, PM, Farstad, M, Vollset, SE. Plasma homocysteine levels and mortality in patients with coronary artery disease. *N Engl J Med* 1997; 337: 230–36.

67. Obara, T, Shuto, S, Saito, Y, Snoeck, R, Andrei, G, Balzarini, J, De Clercq, E, Matsuda, A. New neplanocin analogues. 7. Synthesis and antiviral activity of 2-halo derivatives of neplanocin A. *J Med Chem* 1996; 39: 3847–52.

68. Ogawa, H, Gomi, T, Mueckler, MM, Fujioka, M, Backlund, PS Jr, Aksamit, RR, Unson, CG, Cantoni, GL. Amino acid sequence of *S*-adenosyl-L-homocysteine

hydrolase from rat liver as derived from the cDNA sequence. *Proc Natl Acad Sci USA* 1987; 84: 719–23.

69. Ohmori, O, Hirano, H, Ono, T, Abe, K, Mita, T. Down-regulation of *S*-adenosylhomocysteine hydrolase in the active methyl transfer system in the brain of genetically epileptic El mice. *Neurochem Res* 1996; 21: 1173–80.

70. Paller, AS, Arnsmeier, SL, Clark, SH, Mirkin, BL. Z-4′,5′-didehydro-5′-deoxy-5′-fluoroadenosine (MDL 28,842), an irreversible inhibitor of *S*-adenosylhomocysteine hydrolase, suppresses proliferation of cultured keratinocytes and squamous carcinoma cell lines. *Cancer Res* 1993; 53: 6058–60.

71. Palmer, JL, Abeles, RH. Mechanism for enzymatic thioether formation. Mechanism of action of *S*-adenosylhomocysteinase. *J Biol Chem* 1976; 251: 5817–19.

72. Palmer, JL, Abeles, RH. The mechanism of action of *S*-adenosylhomocysteinase. *J Biol Chem* 1979; 254: 1217–26.

73. Parry, RJ, Muscate, A, Askonas, LJ. 9-(5′,6′-dideoxy-beta-D-ribo-hex-5′-ynofuranosyl)adenine, a novel irreversible inhibitor of *S*-adenosylhomocysteine hydrolase. *Biochemistry* 1991; 30: 9988–97.

74. Parry, RJ, Muscate, A, Hertel, LW. Comparison of the inhibition of type A and type B *S*-adenosylhomocysteine hydrolase: Effects of cofactor content on inhibition behavior and nucleoside binding. *J Enzyme Inhib* 1995; 8: 243–53.

75. Pritchard, PH, Chiang, PK, Cantoni, GL, Vance, DE. Inhibition of phosphatidylethanolamine *N*-methylation by 3-deazaadenosine stimulates the synthesis of phosphatidylcholine via the CDP-choline pathway. *J Biol Chem* 1982; 257: 6362–67.

76. Prytz, PS, Aarbakke, J. Differential cell cycle perturbation by transmethylation inhibitors. *Biochem Pharmacol* 1990; 39: 203–6.

77. Robins, MJ, Wnuk, SF, Yang, X, Yuan, CS, Borchardt, RT, Balzarini, J, De Clercq, E. Inactivation of *S*-adenosyl-L-homocysteine hydrolase and antiviral activity with 5′,5′,6′,6′-tetradehydro-6′-deoxy-6′-halohomoadenosine analogues (4′-haloacetylene analogues derived from adenosine). *J Med Chem* 1998; 41: 3857–64.

78. Rounds, S, Yee, WL, Dawicki, DD, Harrington, E, Parks, N, Cutaia, MV. Mechanism of extracellular ATP- and adenosine-induced apoptosis of cultured pulmonary artery endothelial cells. *Am J Physiol* 1998; 275: L379–88.

79. Saunders, PP, Tan, MT, Robins, RK. Metabolism and action of neplanocin A in Chinese hamster ovary cells. *Biochem Pharmacol* 1985; 34: 2749–54.

80. Scarpa, S, Strom, R, Bozzi, A, Aksamit, RR, Backlund, PS Jr, Chen, J, Cantoni, GL. Differentiation of myoblast cell lines and biological methylation: 3-Deazaadenosine stimulates formation of multinucleated myofibers. *Proc Natl Acad Sci USA* 1984; 81: 3064–68.

81. Shankar, R, de la Motte, CA, DiCorleto, PE. 3-Deazaadenosine inhibits thrombin-stimulated platelet-derived growth factor production and endothelial-leukocyte adhesion molecule-1-mediated monocytic cell adhesion in human aortic endothelial cells. *J Biol Chem* 1992; 267: 9376–82.

82. Shattil, SJ, Montgomery, JA, Chiang, PK. The effect of pharmacologic inhibition of phospholipid methylation on human platelet function. *Blood* 1982; 59: 906–12.

83. Sherman, ML, Shafman, TD, Spriggs, DR, Kufe, DW. Inhibition of murine erythroleukemia cell differentiation by 3-deazaadenosine. *Cancer Res* 1985; 45: 5830–34.

84. Shimizu, S, Shiozaki, S, Ohshiro, T, Yamada, H. Occurrence of *S*-adenosylhomocysteine hydrolase in prokaryote cells. Characterization of the enzyme from *Alcaligenes faecalis* and role of the enzyme in the activated methyl cycle. *Eur J Biochem* 1984; 141: 385–92.

85. Shuto, S, Obara, T, Saito, Y, Andrei, G, Snoeck, R, De Clercq, E, Matsuda, A. New neplanocin analogues. 6. Synthesis and potent antiviral activity of 6'-homoneplanocin A1. *J Med Chem* 1996; 39: 2392–99.

86. Shuto, S, Obara, T, Saito, Y, Yamashita, K, Tanaka, M, Sasaki, T, Andrei, G, Snoeck, R, Neyts, J, Padalko, E, Balzarini, J, De Clercq, E, Matsuda, A. New neplanocin analogues. VIII. Synthesis and biological activity of 6'-C-ethyl, -ethenyl, and -ethynyl derivatives of neplanocin A. *Chem Pharm Bull (Tokyo)* 1997; 45: 1163–68.

87. Shuto, S, Obara, T, Toriya, M, Hosoya, M, Snoeck, R, Andrei, G, Balzarini, J, De Clercq, E. New neplanocin analogues. I. Synthesis of 6'-modified neplanocin A derivatives as broad-spectrum antiviral agents. *J Med Chem* 1992; 35: 324–31.

88. Smith, JD, Ledoux, DN. Effect of the methylation inhibitors 3-deazaadenosine and 3-deazaaristeromycin on phosphatidylcholine formation in *Tetrahymena*. *Biochim Biophys Acta* 1990; 1047: 290–93.

89. Stockand, JD, Al-Baldawi, NF, Al-Khalili, OK, Worrell, RT, Eaton, DC. *S*-adenosyl-L-homocysteine hydrolase regulates aldosterone-induced Na+ transport. *J Biol Chem* 1999; 274: 3842–50.

90. Stoltzfus, CM, Montgomery, JA. Selective inhibition of avian sarcoma virus protein synthesis in 3-deazaadenosine-treated infected chicken embryo fibroblasts. *J Virol* 1981; 38: 173–83.

91. Trager, W, Tershakovec, M, Chiang, PK, Cantoni, GL. *Plasmodium falciparum*: Antimalarial activity in culture of sinefungin and other methylation inhibitors. *Exp Parasitol* 1980; 50: 83–9.

92. Tseng, CKH, Marquez, VE, Fuller, RW, Goldstein, BM, Haines, DR, McPherson, H, Parsons, JL, Shannon, WM, Arnett, G, Hollingshead, M, and Driscoll, JS. Synthesis of 3-deazaneplanocin A, a powerful inhibitor of *S*-adenosylhomocysteine hydrolase with potent and selective in vitro and in vivo antiviral activities. *J Med Chem* 1989; 32: 1442–1446.

93. Tsvetnitsky, V, Campbell, IC, Gibbons, WA. *S*-adenosyl-L-homocysteine and 5'-methylthioadenosine inhibit binding of [3H]flunitrazepam to rat brain membranes. *Eur J Pharmacol* 1995; 282: 255–58.

94. Turner, MA, Yuan, CS, Borchardt, RT, Hershfield, MS, Smith, GD, Howell, PL. Structure determination of selenomethionyl *S*-adenosylhomocysteine hydrolase using data at a single wavelength. *Nat Struct Biol* 1998; 5: 369–76.

95. Vandenplas, C, Guillerm, D, Guillerm, G. A new series of mechanism-based inhibitors of *S*-adenosyl-L-homocysteine hydrolase from beef liver. *Nucleosides Nucleotides* 1999; 18: 569–70.

96. Villalon, MD, Gil-Fernandez, C, De Clercq, E. Activity of several *S*-adenosylhomocysteine hydrolase inhibitors against African swine fever virus replication in Vero cells. *Antiviral Res* 1993; 20: 131–44.

97. Vogel, U, Kunerl, M, Scholtissek, C. Influenza A virus late mRNAs are specifically retained in the nucleus in the presence of a methyltransferase or a protein kinase inhibitor. *Virology* 1994; 198: 227–33.

98. Whaun, JM, Miura, GA, Brown, ND, Gordon, RK, Chiang, PK. Antimalarial activity of neplanocin A with perturbations in the metabolism of purines, polyamines and *S*-adenosylmethionine. *J Pharmacol Exp Ther* 1986; 236: 277–83.

99. Wiesmann, WP, Johnson, JP, Miura, GA, Chaing, PK. Aldosterone-stimulated transmethylations are linked to sodium transport. *Am J Physiol* 1985; 248: F43–7.

100. Wnuk, SF, Mao, Y, Yuan, CS, Borchardt, RT, Andrei, G, Balzarini, J, De Clercq, E, Robins, MJ. Discovery of type II (covalent) inactivation of *S*-adenosyl-L-homocysteine hydrolase involving its "hydrolytic activity": Synthesis and evaluation of dihalohomovinyl nucleoside analogues derived from adenosine. *J Med Chem* 1998; 41: 3078–83.

101. Wnuk, SF, Yuan, CS, Borchardt, RT, Balzarini, J, De Clercq, E, Robins, MJ. Anticancer and antiviral effects and inactivation of *S*-adenosyl-L-homocysteine hydrolase with 5'-carboxaldehydes and oximes synthesized from adenosine and sugar-modified analogues. *J Med Chem* 1997; 40: 1608–18.

102. Wnuk, SF, Yuan, CS, Borchardt, RT, Robins, MJ. Synthesis of homologated halovinyl derivatives from aristeromycin and their inhibition of human placental *S*-adenosyl-L-homocysteine hydrolase. *Nucleosides Nucleotides* 1998; 17: 99–113.

103. Wong, DL, Hayashi, RJ, Ciaranello, RD. Regulation of biogenic amine methyltransferases by glucocorticoids via *S*-adenosylmethionine and its metabolizing enzymes, methionine adenosyltransferase and *S*-adenosylhomocysteine hydrolase. *Brain Res* 1985; 330: 209–16.

104. Woyciuk, P, Linder, M, Scholtissek, C. The methyltransferase inhibitor Neplanocin A interferes with influenza virus replication by a mechanism different from that of 3-deazaadenosine. *Virus Res* 1995; 35: 91–9.

105. Yaginuma, S, Muto, N, Tsujino, M, Sudate, Y, Hayashi, M, Otani, M. Studies on neplanocin A, new antitumor antibiotic. I. Producing organism, isolation and characterization. *J Antibiot (Tokyo)* 1981; 34: 359–66.

106. Young, GJ, Hallam, LJ, Jack, I, Van Der Weyden, MB. *S*-adenosylhomocysteine hydrolase inactivation and purine toxicity in cultured human T- and B-lymphoblasts. *J Lab Clin Med* 1984; 104: 86–95.

107. Yuan, CS, Yeh, J, Liu, S, Borchardt, RT. Mechanism of inactivation of *S*-adenosylhomocysteine hydrolase by

(Z)-4′,5′-didehydro-5′-deoxy-5′-fluoroadenosine. *J Biol Chem* 1993; 268: 17030–37.

108. Zeng, G, Dave, JR, Chiang, PK. Induction of proto-oncogenes during 3-deazaadenosine-stimulated differentiation of 3T3-L1 fibroblasts to adipocytes: Mimicry of insulin action. *Oncol Res* 1997; 9: 205–11.

109. Zimmerman, TP, Deeprose, RD, Wolberg, G, Duncan, GS. Metabolic formation of nucleoside-modified analogues of *S*-adenosylmethionine. *Biochem Biophys Res Commun* 1979; 91: 997–1004.

9

Regulation of Homocysteine Metabolism

JAMES D. FINKELSTEIN

Methionine metabolism in mammalian cells is a summation of two major reaction sequences: the methionine cycle, which is ubiquitous, and the transsulfuration pathway, which has a more limited distribution. Furthermore these pathways intersect with those necessary for the synthesis and utilization of other significant metabolites including folic acid, choline, the polyamines, and cysteine and its derivatives. Consequently, the goal of metabolic regulation is to ensure the appropriate distribution of metabolites among these pathways while preventing the accumulation of homocysteine, S-adenosylhomocysteine (AdoHcy), and other potentially toxic intermediates. This chapter summarizes the current knowledge, with particular reference to areas of active investigation.

The Metabolic Pathways

Methionine Cycle

The methionine cycle appears to be present in all normal mammalian cells (10). Other chapters in this volume describe the individual, component reactions. Thus, Chapter 6 provides a comprehensive review of the methionine adenosyltransferases. Every cell has the ability to synthesize S-adenosylmethionine (AdoMet) (Metabolic Diagram, Reaction 1); however, only liver possesses the high K_m methionine adenosyltransferase-III that allows increased AdoMet synthesis in response to excessive methionine. In contrast, the concentration of AdoMet in extrahepatic tissues varies within a more restricted range. Once synthesized, AdoMet can move between intracellular compartments and most appears to be retained within the cell of origin. Newly developed techniques for the measurement of plasma AdoMet (4), as well as studies of patients lacking methionine adenosyltransferase-III (5, 37), should help to clarify the significance of intercellular transfer. AdoMet can serve as the methyl donor in any one of numerous transmethylation reactions (Metabolic Diagram, Reaction 2). Alternatively, following decarboxylation (Metabolic Diagram, Reaction 12), the propylamine moiety can be used in the sequential syntheses of the polyamines spermidine and spermine. Despite the essential biological functions of the polyamines, their synthesis affects only minimally the total cellular metabolism of methionine. It is estimated that less than 10% of the available AdoMet is utilized in this process (33). Furthermore, 5-methylthioadenosine, the product after propylamine transfer, can be recycled to methionine (2).

Chapter 7 emphasizes the array of essential biological functions that require AdoMet-dependent transmethylation reactions. Despite both the specificity of these enzymes and the diversity of their methyl acceptors, all produce AdoHcy, which is a potent inhibitor of most of the enzymes (3). Normal metabolism requires the removal of AdoHcy and three processes exist for this purpose. AdoHcy can be bound by specific, saturable, intracellular sites (39) or may be transported to the extracellular space from which it can be removed primarily by the kidney (8, 22). Lastly, all cells possess AdoHcy hydrolase (Metabolic Diagram, Reaction 3) (see Chapter 8) and changes in the tissue content of this enzyme or its inhibition may change the tissue concentration of AdoHcy (10). Furthermore, the equilibrium of this reaction favors AdoHcy synthesis and both products, adenosine and homocysteine, must be removed to direct flow in the hydrolytic direction (7).

The adenosine deaminase reaction removes adenosine and three mechanisms exist for the disposition of homocysteine. As with AdoHcy, homocysteine may be bound to protein or may be transported from the cell (38). The latter may be a common means for detoxification because many tissues extract homocysteine from the extracellular compartment. Indeed the "normal" concentration of plasma total homocysteine is likely to represent the transfer of the metabolite from sites of synthesis to the liver and other sites of catabolism.

Three enzymes utilize homocysteine as a substrate. One enzyme diverts the homocysteine to the irreversible transsulfuration pathway, and the other two resynthesize methionine and thus conserve the homocysteine within the methionine cycle. All normal mammalian cells appear able to synthesize 5-methyltetrahydrofolate (Metabolic Diagram, Reaction 9) and to utilize this substrate as the methyl donor in the methionine synthase reaction (Metabolic Diagram, Reaction 4) (10). This is the only reaction that recycles this folate form. Because methylcobalamin is an essential coenzyme, methionine synthase is the point of intersection for folate and cobalamin metabolism. The second homocysteine methyltransferase uses betaine, the obligatory product of choline oxidation, as the methyl donor. Unlike methionine synthase, betaine homocysteine methyltransferase (Metabolic Diagram, Reaction 5) has a limited distribution. It is present in mammalian livers and primate kidneys (10, 29). The finding of the enzyme in monkey lens (34), as well as in kidney, suggests a possible linkage to the osmoregulatory functions of betaine.

Transsulfuration

Cystathionine β-synthase (CBS) (Metabolic Diagram. Reaction 6), the third enzyme that utilizes homocysteine, is the first unique and biologically irreversible reaction in the transsulfuration pathway from methionine to cysteine. This pyridoxal phosphate requiring enzyme has a heme prosthetic group, and activity is related to the redox state, being greater when the heme iron is in the ferric form (25, 40). The irreversibility of the CBS reaction explains the inability of cysteine to serve as a precursor for methionine in animal tissues. Cystathionine γ-lyase (Metabolic Diagram, Reaction 7) completes the transsulfuration sequence. This enzyme also requires pyridoxal phosphate but appears to have a lesser affinity for the cofactor. Consequently impairment of cystathionine γ-lyase precedes impairment of CBS in the evolution of pyridoxine deficiency.

There are significant differences in the distribution of the transsulfuration enzymes in rat tissues (10). Neither enzyme is present in heart, lung, testes, adrenal, or spleen. Brain and adipose tissue contain CBS, but cystathionine γ-lyase is barely detectable. Cysteine must be an essential nutrient in these seven tissues. In addition, the anticipated accumulation of cystathionine in mammalian brain does occur; however, the physiological significance remains undefined. Only four tissues — liver, kidney, small intestine, and pancreas — possess both transsulfuration enzymes. It is interesting that these same tissues have the most rapid turnover rate for glutathione (30), and the hypothesis that the synthesis of this important metabolite is linked to the transsulfuration pathway merits further study (20, 41).

The further metabolism of cysteine is beyond the scope of this chapter. Suffice it to say that, in addition to glutathione, these reaction sequences produce taurine, sulfate, and other physiologically significant metabolites.

Alternate and Minor Pathways

The Metabolic Diagram in the endplate is a simplification. It fails to include several additional pathways that utilize metabolites of methionine. Because choline can be synthesized by the methylation of phosphatidylethanolamine, there is a second methyl group cycle comprised of methionine — AdoMet –choline – betaine – methionine. Similarly, the figure does not show that, owing to the production of 5,10-methylenetetrahydrofolate, the sequential oxidative demethylation of dimethylglycine and sarcosine constitutes an intersection of folate and choline metabolism (for more details, see Chapter 11). Subsequently, the methyl groups formed by the methylenetetrahydrofolate reductase reaction are incorporated into methionine by means of the methionine synthase reaction. The net result is the conservation of the three methyl groups of betaine.

Methionine transamination does occur but only at abnormally high concentrations of the amino acid (10, 36). Patients with genetic defects in methionine adenosyltransferase-III with a resultant impaired synthesis of AdoMet are one example (32). Even under these circumstances, only a limited fraction of the methionine is metabolized by transamination, and this must be considered a minor pathway for methionine metabolism.

Both free methionine and methionine incorporated into protein may be oxidized to methionine sulfoxide in reactions involving exogenous or endogenous oxidants and catalyzed by flavin monooxygenases (35). Methionine sulfoxide reductases may catalyze the resynthesis of the amino acid (26), and this cyclical process may represent an important means for the protection of proteins from oxidant stress (28). In addition, the progressive increase in oxidized residues may constitute one form for the biological aging of proteins. Despite this potential physiological relevance, the oxidation of methionine involves only a small fraction of the metabolically active amino acid.

Chapter 3 discusses the erroneous synthesis of homocysteine-tRNA from intracellular homocysteine. The subsequent release of homocysteine thiolactone (23) or methionine (1) corrects this error. The thiolactone, a highly reactive compound, may homocysteinylate proteins. Because the rate of thiolactone formation appears to be a function of homocysteine accumulation, this process may be significant in the pathochemistry of the disorders of homocysteine metabolism (23); however, it is less likely to be significant in normal tissues.

Metabolic Regulation

Studies in experimental animals and observations in patients with rare genetically determined enzyme defects resulted in the concept that methionine metabolism was a cycle with three potential outlets formed by the synthesis of protein, AdoMet decarboxylase, and the CBS reaction (21). Each of these outlets depends on the distribution of substrate between competing reactions at the three metabolic sites. An earlier section of this chapter discussed the basis for discounting the polyamine pathway. Similarly the regulatory significance of the competition for methionine between protein synthesis and the synthesis of AdoMet was minimized because an equilibrium between protein synthesis and catabolism should characterize a biological steady state. (Reevaluation of this assumption is necessary, as it is likely to be inconsistent with the metabolic patterns characteristic of growth, aging, and disease.) Thus most research has focused on the third site, the CBS reaction. This simplified formulation, that regulation of methionine metabolism is based on either the rate of cycling or the percentage of the homocysteine that is converted to cystathionine during each cycle, was tested in animal experiments and in studies with human subjects.

Direct evidence for regulation derived from studies in which isolated rat livers were perfused with [3H]methyl-[35S]methionine, or [14C]methyl-methionine (10). The radioisotope disappearance curves allowed the determination of both the half-life of the methyl group of methionine and the fraction of homocysteine diverted to transsulfuration during each cycle. The values for rats fed a chow diet were 5.5 minutes and 45%. Subsequently the metabolic patterns were studied with donor livers from rats fed diets that differed in protein content. The change from 3.5% casein to 55% casein caused a marked shortening of the methyl group half-life from 9.3 to 4.8 minutes. Concurrently, the percentage transsulfuration rose from 10% to 70%. In a remarkable series of balance studies with normal male subjects, Mudd and Poole (33) determined that the percentage transsulfuration declined from 53% to 20% with the restriction of dietary methionine and choline.

Subsequent studies in patients with sarcosinemia resulting from deficiency of sarcosine dehydrogenase provided an estimate of 2.4 to 4.9 minutes for the half-life of the methyl group of methionine (31). Thus the human studies validated the relevance of the in vitro animal investigations.

Two mechanisms regulate the distribution of homocysteine among the competing reactions — the inherent kinetic properties of the relevant enzymes and alterations in the tissue content of these enzymes.

Tissue Content of Enzymes

The variation of the enzyme patterns between tissues is the most obvious example of this means for metabolic regulation (10). In an earlier section I noted the absence of CBS in heart, lung, spleen, testes, and adrenal; the unique ability of the liver to synthesize AdoMet in response to a methionine load; and the restricted occurrence of betaine methyltransferase. Age, diet, and endocrine status are among the other factors that affect the tissue content of the enzymes. These share several characteristics. The stimuli are sustained over a prolonged period of time, and the effects may be specific to both tissue and enzyme. Table 9.1 illustrates the relationship between age and the specific activities of the enzymes in rat livers. The values for CBS and cystathionine-γ-lyase increase with age. In contrast the specific activity of AdoHcy hydrolase is constant and those for methionine adenosyltransferase, betaine methyltransferase, methionine synthase, and methylenetetrahydrofolate reductase decline significantly. The metabolic pattern appears to shift with aging from methionine conservation to transsulfuration.

The studies of the effects of the protein content of the diet (Table 9.2) on the content of the enzymes in rat livers demonstrate a different pattern. CBS, cystathionine γ-lyase, AdoHcy hydrolase, and betaine

Table 9.1.   Effects of Age on Enzymes of Methionine Metabolism in Rat Liver

Weight (g)	MAT	SAHH	CBS	CGL	BHMT	MS	MTHFR
14	165	118	43	63	150	284	282
46	153	106	87	83	114	173	129
134	124	96	88	116	109	108	80
276	100	100	100	100	100	100	100

The table presents the specific activity of each enzyme as a percentage of the specific activity of that enzyme in the livers of the oldest animals (9, 12, 13, 16).
MAT, methionine adenosyltransferase; SAHH, adenosylhomocysteine hydrolase; CBS, cystathionine β-synthase; CGL, cystathionine γ-lyase; BHMT, betaine homocysteine methyltransferase; MS, methionine synthase; MTHFR, methylenetetrahydrofolate reductase.

Table 9.2. Effects of Dietary Protein on Enzymes of Methionine Metabolism in Rat Liver

Protein (%)	MAT	SAHH	CBS	CGL	BHMT	MS	MTHFR
3.5	100	100	100	100	100	100	100
26	67	120	390	351	153	56	112
55	142	206	452	290	182	27	89

Results for the specific activity of each enzyme are expressed as the percentage of the value for the specific activity of that enzyme in the livers of rats fed the 3.5% casein diet. (9, 12, 13, 16). MAT, methionine adenosyltransferase; SAHH, adenosylhomocysteine hydrolase; CBS, cystathionine β-synthase; CGL, cystathionine γ-lyase; BHMT, betaine homocysteine methyltransferase; MS, methionine synthase; MTHFR, methylenetetrahydrofolate reductase.

methyltransferase all increase with increasing dietary protein. Simultaneously, methionine synthase decreases markedly, methylenetetrahydrofolate reductase is not affected, and methionine adenosyltransferase shows a biphasic response, increasing with both severe protein restriction and dietary protein excess. In other studies, the dietary content of methionine, cysteine, and choline were important determinants of the content of enzymes in liver and extrahepatic tissues.

Table 9.3 summarizes the studies of the effects of various endocrine manipulations on the enzyme activities in rat liver. It is apparent that no two enzymes respond similarly to all treatments, although at least one treatment caused a significant change in the hepatic content of each enzyme, with the exception of methionine synthase. Furthermore the enzyme changes in extrahepatic tissues did not necessarily correspond to the changes in liver. For example, thyroxine treatment caused a 40% increase in renal cystathionine γ-lyase in contrast to the 73% reduction in the hepatic enzyme. Similarly treatment with thyroxine, testosterone, alloxan, and glucagon all resulted in a reduction of renal CBS. Thus the effects of hormone administration are specific for hormone, tissue, and enzyme.

Kinetic Properties of the Enzymes

The regulatory mechanism that is inherent in the kinetic properties of the enzymes allows an immediate response to metabolic perturbations. It derives from the affinity for substrates, product inhibition, and the allosteric effector properties of the various metabolites. Based on these characteristics, together with the response of the hepatic content of each of the enzymes to the methionine content of the diet, we defined two classes of enzymes (10). The "methionine conserving" enzymes have relatively low Michaelis constants for their sulfur-containing substrates; are inhibited by their products; and are impaired by AdoMet and possibly AdoHcy. Their hepatic content decreases with increased dietary methionine. As shown in Table 9.4, the conserving enzymes include methionine adenosyltransferases I and II, AdoHcy hydrolase, and methionine synthase. Although AdoMet is essential for the reductive methylation required to maintain methionine synthase in its active form, this enzyme is included in the conserving group because AdoMet also inhibits methylenetetrahydrofolate reductase and thus the formation of substrate for methionine synthase (24, 27). In all likelihood, the net effect of AdoMet on methionine synthase activity is negative. With the addition of one or more of the numerous AdoMet-dependent methyltransferases, the identity of the conserving enzymes and the methionine cycle is apparent. The classification of betaine homocysteine methyltransferase is ambiguous. This enzyme possesses the kinetic properties of the conserving group; however, the hepatic content is increased both by methionine restriction and methionine supplementation (10).

The enzymes of the "methionine catabolyzing" group have relatively high K_m values for their sulfur-containing substrates, are not inhibited by their products, and are activated or facilitated by AdoMet and AdoHcy. Their hepatic content increases in response to increased dietary methionine. Methionine adenosyltransferase III, CBS, and cystathionine γ-lyase fulfill these criteria. To make up the transsulfuration pathway, this group requires a methyltransferase that has a high K_m for AdoMet, is relatively insensitive to inhibition by AdoHcy, increases with increased dietary methionine, and utilizes an available substrate to produce a nontoxic product that can be recycled to the substrate form. Glycine methyltransferase, which has these characteristics, is included in the table (10). It is notable that the tissue distribution of glycine methyltransferase parallels that for the other transsulfuration enzymes (43).

Table 9.4 illustrates the two mechanisms of regulation inherent in the kinetic properties of the enzymes that provide the basis for the distribution of homocysteine between remethylation and transsulfuration. The first is the difference in the affinity for this substrate. The K_{Hcy} values for methionine synthase and betaine homocysteine methyltransferase are at least one order of magnitude lower than the value for CBS. Thus the fraction of homocysteine diverted to transsulfuration

Table 9.3. Effects of Hormones on Enzymes of Methionine Metabolism in Rat Liver

	MAT	SAHH	CBS	CGL	BHMT	MS	MTHFR
Hydrocortisone	158*	124*	151*	84	300*	96	112*
Thyroxine	83	84*	101	27*	35*	78	148*
Growth hormone	160	99	100	120	77	98	120*
Estradiol	176*	120*	104	145*	91	82	116*
Testosterone	123*		98	109	115	78	119
Alloxan	298*		141*	115	170*	75	85
Glucagon	99	95	195*	180*	110	100	105

Each control and treatment group contained at least five rats. The values represent the mean of the individual specific activities of the enzymes in the livers of treated animals as a percentage of the value for simultaneously treated, control rats (9, 12, 13, 16).
*Change is statistically significant, $p < 0.05$
MAT, methionine adenosyltransferase; SAHH, adenosylhomocysteine hydrolase; CBS, cystathionine β-synthase; CGL, cystathionine γ-lyase; BHMT, betaine homocysteine methyltransferase; MS, methionine synthase; MTHFR, methylenetetrahydrofolate reductase.

should increase as the concentration of the substrate increases (18).

The effector properties of three metabolites — AdoMet, AdoHcy, and methyltetrahydrofolate — provide the basis for additional metabolic regulation. In normal animals, methionine excess is the usual basis for increased tissue AdoMet. As shown in Table 9.4, this metabolite inhibits methionine synthase by inhibiting the synthesis of methyltetrahydrofolate (24, 27), inactivates the betaine enzyme (17), and activates CBS (15). These properties provide the basis for an "AdoMet switch"; high levels enhancing flow of homocysteine out of the methionine cycle and into the transsulfuration sequence (Figure 9.1). The switch, which requires the presence of both remethylation and CBS, can occur only in liver, kidney, pancreas, intestine, brain, and adipose tissue. In addition, we must consider whether concentrations of AdoMet necessary to activate this switch may occur only in liver, or in kidney after the administration of exogenous AdoMet (11). It is not clear that increasing concentrations of AdoMet will lead to a progressive and absolute reduction in homocysteine methylation in the absence of the competing CBS.

Owing to these theoretical limitations to the regulatory potential of AdoMet, we must consider the possibility that AdoHcy may be a more significant effector, particularly in extrahepatic tissues. The dominant regulatory property of this metabolite is the inhibition of transmethylation reactions. However, additional effects include the activation of CBS and the inhibition of betaine homocysteine methyltransferase (14). The net effect of AdoHcy on methionine synthase is unpredictable. It is an inhibitor of the enzyme but, by releasing methylenetetrahydrofolate reductase from inhibition by AdoMet, it may enhance the synthesis of the substrate (27). In vitro studies suggest that increasing concentrations of AdoHcy facilitates transsulfuration in liver (18).

Table 9.4 does not show the regulatory potential of methyltetrahydrofolate, which is an inhibitor of the glycine methyltransferase reaction (42). Tissue concentrations of methyltetrahydrofolate vary inversely with the availability of methionine, presumably reflecting the modulation of methylenetetrahydrofolate reductase by AdoMet. Thus a low concentration of methyltetrahydrofolate, corresponding to methionine excess, would tend to facilitate the utilization of surplus S-adenosylmethionine in the glycine methyltransferase reaction. Conversely, high concentrations of methyltetrahydrofolate, usually an

Table 9.4. Kinetic Properties of the Enzymes of Methionine Metabolism

Enzyme	K_s	Effect of Metabolites		
		Met	AdoMet	AdoHcy
Methionine conserving				
Methionine adenosyltransferase				
I	23–43 µmol/L	S	P,I	
II	4–10 µmol/L	S	P,I	
Adenosylhomocysteinase				
Hydrolysis	8–60 µmol/L			S
Synthesis	160 µmol/L			P,I
Betaine methyltransferase	4–60 µmol/L	P,I	I	I
Methionine synthase	2–60 µmol/L	P,I	A	I
MTHFR	NA		I	A
Methionine catabolizing				
Methionine adenosyltransferase III	0.2–7 mmol/L	S	P,A	
Cystathionine β-synthase	1–25 mmol/L		A	A
Cystathionine γ-lyase	0.5–3.5 mmol/L			
Glycine methyltransferase	50–320 µmol/L		A	I

K_s = Michaelis constant for sulfur-containing substrate; S, substrate; P, product; A, activator or positive effector; I, inhibitor or inactivator; MTHFR, methylenetetrahydrofolate reductase.

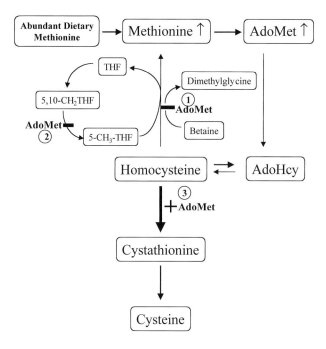

Fig. 9.1. Allosteric regulation of homocysteine metabolism by *S*-adenosylmethionine (AdoMet). Under conditions of abundant dietary methionine, intracellular concentrations of methionine and AdoMet will increase. AdoMet is a positive allosteric effector for cystathionine-β-synthase (Reaction 3) and a negative effector for both betaine:homocysteine methyltransferase (Reaction 1) and methylenetetrahydrofolate reductase (Reaction 2). Thus, AdoMet serves as a switch to divert homocysteine into the transsulfuration pathway.

index of limited availability of methionine, would inhibit glycine methyltransferase and would conserve AdoMet. This inverse relationship of methyltetrahydrofolate and methionine (or AdoMet) is vulnerable to disruption by nutritional deficiencies and genetic disorders.

Relative Contributions to Metabolic Regulation

To define the contributions of the several mechanisms to the regulation of methionine metabolism in mammalian liver, investigators routinely extrapolated from studies of the factors affecting the tissue content of the relevant enzymes, often without regard to either the kinetics of the enzymes or the concentrations of the regulatory metabolites. To address this limitation, we developed an in vitro model of the regulatory site formed by the three enzymes that metabolize homocysteine. This method allowed us to vary independently the concentrations of enzymes, substrates, and other effectors. All of the enzymatic reactions proceed simultaneously under conditions that simulate the in vivo situation rather than conditions optimal for any one enzyme. Indeed the ability to measure competition for

substrate between the enzymes was an important dimension of the model. Another significant difference from standard enzyme assays was our use of the high enzyme concentrations found in vivo.

Using this technique, we studied simulations of metabolism in livers of rats fed a standard laboratory ration and purified diets containing graded amounts of methionine. The results for the distribution of homocysteine between remethylation and transsulfuration were consistent with our previous determinations in the isolated perfused livers. The percentage transsulfuration in the model for the chow diet was 46% with both the betaine enzyme and methionine synthase contributing equally to the remethylation (18). Similarly, we found that a marked, 12-fold increase in transsulfuration was the basis for the adaptation to dietary methionine excess. Furthermore, this change derived primarily from changes in the concentrations of metabolites rather than from the increase in content of enzyme. The role of competition between enzymes was evident (19). Lastly, we studied the mechanism for the methionine-sparing effect of cystine (20). Cystine can replace methionine in only one biological function — the synthesis of cysteine. Compared with the pattern in the rats fed methionine, homocysteine metabolism in livers of the rats fed cystine declined from 60% to 15% in the fraction transsulfurated, together with a reduction of 60% in total homocysteine metabolized. Product formation decreased in all three reactions, despite an increase in the content of both homocysteine methyltransferases. Again the contributions to regulation of the concentrations of both metabolic effectors and substrates were highly significant (20).

Regulation by Oxidation/Reduction State

Recent studies provide the basis for a third mechanism that regulates the distribution of homocysteine between transsulfuration and remethylation. In this case, the driving force is the differential effect on methionine synthase and CBS of the oxidation/reduction state of the intracellular environment. Chapter 12 details the relevant characteristics of methionine synthase. The enzyme is vulnerable to oxidation and maintenance of activity requires periodic reductive methylation. It is likely that the system for reductive methylation of mammalian methionine synthase utilizes either recently cloned methionine synthase reductase (27a) or cytochrome b$_5$ and cytochrome P450 reductase together with NADPH and AdoMet (6) (see Chapter 12). In contrast, CBS is a heme protein (25) and activity increases in an oxidative environment (40). Taken together these observations, largely by Banerjee and colleagues, may represent the first demonstration that increased transsulfuration is a metabolic response to oxidative stress.

This is teleologically attractive because it is consistent with the hypothesis that a major function of the transsulfuration sequence is the synthesis of glutathione.

REFERENCES

1. Antonio, CM, Nunes, MC, Refsum, H, Abraham, AK. A novel pathway for the conversion of homocysteine to methionine in eukaryotes. *Biochem J* 1997; 328: 165–70.
2. Backlund, PS Jr, Smith, RA. Methionine synthesis from 5′-methylthioadenosine in rat liver, *J Biol Chem* 1981; 256: 1533–35.
3. Cantoni, GL, Richards, HH, Chiang, PK. Inhibitors of S-adenosylhomocysteine hydrolase and their role in the regulation of biological methylation. In *Transmethylation* (Usdin, E, Borchardt, RT, Creveling, CR, eds.). Elsevier, New York, 1978; 155–64.
4. Capdelia, A, Wagner, C. Measurement of plasma S-adenosylmethionine and S-adenosylhomocysteine as their fluorescent isoindoles. *Anal Biochem* 1998; 264: 180–84.
5. Chamberlin, ME, Ubagai, T, Mudd, SH, Wilson, WG, Leonard, JV, Choi, JY. Demyelination of the brain is associated with methionine adenosyltransferase I/III deficiency. *J Clin Invest* 1996; 98: 1021–27.
6. Chen, Z, Banerjee, R. Purification of soluble cytochrome b_5 as a component of the reductive activation of porcine methionine synthase. *J Biol Chem* 1998; 273: 26248–55.
7. De la Haba, G, Cantoni, GL. The enzymatic synthesis of S-adenosyl-L-homocysteine from adenosine and homocysteine. *J Biol Chem* 1959; 234: 603–8.
8. Duerre, JA, Miller, CH, Reams, GG. Metabolism of S-adenosyl-L-homocysteine in vivo by the rat. *J Biol Chem* 1969; 244: 107–11.
9. Finkelstein, JD. Methionine metabolism in mammals: Effects of age, diet and hormonal therapy on three enzymes of the pathway in rat tissues. *Arch Biochem Biophys* 1967; 122: 583–590.
10. Finkelstein, JD. Methionine metabolism in mammals. *J Nutr Biochem* 1990; 1: 228–37.
11. Finkelstein, JD. Transmethylation in liver diseases. In *Cholestasis* (Gentilini, P, Arias, IM, McIntyre, N, Rodes, J, eds.). Elsevier Science, Amsterdam, 1994; 273–81.
12. Finkelstein, JD, Harris, B. Methionine metabolism in mammals. Synthesis of S-adenosylhomocysteine in rat tissues. *Arch Biochem Biophys* 1973; 159: 160–65.
13. Finkelstein, JD, Kyle, WE, Harris, BJ. Methionine metabolism in mammals. Regulation of homocysteine methyltransferases in rat tissues. *Arch Biochem Biophys* 1971; 146: 84–92.
14. Finkelstein, JD, Kyle, WE, Harris, B. Methionine metabolism in mammals: Regulatory effects of S-adenosylhomocysteine. *Arch Biochem Biophys* 1974; 165: 774–79.
15. Finkelstein, JD, Kyle, WE, Martin, JJ, Pick, A. Activation of cystathionine synthase by adenosylmethionine and adenosylethionine, *Biochem Biophys Res Commun* 1975; 66: 81–7.
16. Finkelstein, JD, Martin, JJ, Kyle, WE, Harris, BJ. Methionine metabolism in mammals. Regulation of

17. Finkelstein, JD, Martin, JJ. Inactivation of betaine-homocysteine methyltransferase by adenosylmethionine and adenosylethionine. *Biochem Biophys Res Commun* 1984; 118: 14–9.
18. Finkelstein, JD, Martin, JJ. Methionine metabolism in mammals. Distribution of homocysteine between competing pathways. *J Biol Chem* 1984; 259: 9508–13.
19. Finkelstein, JD, Martin, JJ. Methionine metabolism in mammals. Adaptation to methionine excess. *J Biol Chem* 1986; 261: 1582–87.
20. Finkelstein, JD, Martin, JJ, Harris, BJ. Methionine metabolism in mammals: The methionine-sparing effect of cystine. *J Biol Chem* 1988; 263: 11750–54.
21. Finkelstein, JD, Mudd, SH. Transsulfuration in mammals. The methionine sparing effect of cystine. *J Biol Chem* 1967; 242: 873–80.
22. Hoffman, DR, Cornatzer, WE, Duerre, JA. Relationship between tissue levels of S-adenosylmethionine, S-adenosylhomocysteine and transmethylation reactions. *Can J Biochem* 1979; 57: 56–65.
23. Jakubowski, H. Metabolism of homocysteine thiolactone in human cell cultures. *J Biol Chem* 1997; 272: 1935–42.
24. Jencks, DA, Matthews, RG. Allosteric inhibition of methylenetetrahydrofolate reductase by adenosylmethionine. *J Biol Chem* 1987; 262: 2485–93.
25. Kery, V, Bukovska, G, Kraus, JP. Transsulfuration depends on heme in addition to pyridoxal 5′-phosphate. *J Biol Chem* 1994; 269: 25283–88.
26. Kuschel, L, Hansel, A, Schonherr, Weissbach, H, Brot, N, Hoshi, T, Heinemann, SH. Molecular cloning and functional expression of a human peptide methionine sulfoxide reductase (hMsrA). *FEBS Lett* 1999; 456: 17–21.
27. Kutzbach, C, Stokstad, ELR. Mammalian methylenetetrahydrofolate reductase. Partial purification, properties and inhibition by S-adenosylmethionine. *Biochim Biophys Acta* 1971; 250: 459–77.
27a. Leclerc, D, Wilson, A, Dumas, R, Gafuik, C, Song, D, Watkins, D, Heng, HHQ, Rommens, JM, Scherer, SW, Rosenblatt, DS, Gravel, RA. Cloning and mapping of a cDNA for Methionine synthase reductase, a flavoprotein defective in patients with homocystinuria. *Proc. Natl. Acad. Sci. U. S. A.* 1998; 95: 3059–64.
28. Levine, RL, Berlett, BS, Moskovitz, J, Mosoni, L, Stadtman, ER. Methionine residues may protect proteins from critical oxidative damage. *Mech Ageing Dev* 1999; 107: 323–32.
29. McKeever, MP, Weir, DG, Molloy, A, Scott, JM. Betaine-homocysteine methyltransferase: Organ distribution in man, pig and rat and subcellular distribution in the rat. *Clin Sci* 1991; 81: 551–56.
30. Meister, A. Metabolism and transport of glutathione and other γ-glutamyl compounds. In *Functions of Glutathione: Biochemical, Physiological, Toxicological and Clinical Aspects.* (Larsson, A, Orrenius, S, Holmgren, A, Mannervik, B., eds.). Raven, New York, 1983; 1–21.

methylenetetrahydrofolate reductase content of rat tissues. *Arch Biochem Biophys* 1978; 191: 153–60.

31. Mudd, SH, Ebert, MH, Scriver, CR. Labile methyl group balances in the human: The role of sarcosine. *Metabolism* 1980; 29: 707–20.
32. Mudd, SH, Levy, HL, Tangerman, A, Boujet, C, Buist, N, Davidson-Mundt, A, Hudgins, I, Oyanagi, K, Nagao, M, Wilson, W. Isolated persistent hypermethioninemia. *Am J Hum Genet* 1995; 57: 882–92.
33. Mudd, SH, Poole, JR. Labile methyl balances for normal humans on various dietary regimens. *Metabolism* 1975; 24: 721–35.
34. Rao, PV, Garrow, TA, John, F, Garland, D, Millian, NS, Zigler JS, Jr. Betaine-homocysteine methyltransferase is a developmentally regulated enzyme crystallin in rhesus monkey lens. *J Biol Chem* 1998; 273: 30669–74.
35. Ripp, SL, Itagaki, K, Philpot, RM, Elfarra, AA. Methionine *S*-oxidation in human and rabbit liver microsomes. Evidence for a high-affinity methionine *S*-oxidase activity that is distinct from flavin-containing monooxygenase 3. *Arch Biochem Biophys* 1999; 367: 322–32.
36. Scislowski, PWD, Pickard, K. Methionine transamination—metabolic function and subcellular compartmentation. *Mol Cell Biochem* 1993; 129: 39–45.
37. Surtees, R. Demyelination and inborn errors of the single carbon transfer pathway. *Eur J Pediatr* 1998; 157(Suppl 2): S118–21.
38. Svardal, A, Refsum, H, Ueland, PM. Determination of in vivo protein binding of homocysteine and its relation to free homocysteine in the liver and other tissues of the rat. *J Biol Chem* 1986; 261: 3156–63.
39. Svardal, AM, Ueland, PM. Compartmentalization of *S*-adenosylhomocysteine in rat liver. Determination and characterization of the in vivo protein binding. *J Biol Chem* 1987; 262: 15413–417.
40. Taoka, S, Ohja, S, Shan, X, Kruger, WD, Banerjee, R. Evidence for heme-mediated redox regulation of human cystathionine-β-synthase activity. *J Biol Chem* 1998; 273: 25179–84.
41. Vina, J, Hems, R, Krebs, HA. Maintenance of glutathione content in isolated hepatocytes. *Biochem J* 1978; 170: 627–30.
42. Wagner, C, Briggs, WT, Cook, RJ. Inhibition of glycine *N*-methyltransferase activity by folate derivatives: Implications for regulation of methyl group metabolism. *Biochem Biophys Res Commun* 1985; 127: 746–52.
43. Yeo, E-J, Wagner, C. Tissue distribution of glycine *N*-methyltransferase, a major folate-binding protein of liver. *Proc Natl Acad Sci USA* 1994; 91: 210–14.

10

Microbial Modeling of Human Disease: Homocysteine Metabolism

ROWENA G. MATTHEWS
MARTHA L. LUDWIG

The study of the properties of the purified human enzymes involved in homocysteine metabolism is expected to provide data for estimating the flux through various branches of the pathway and the role of different metabolites in regulating flux through these branches. Furthermore, the molecular phenotypes of clinically significant mutations that affect homocysteine metabolism can be characterized by using purified mutant enzymes. In practice, however, many of the human enzymes have not been fully purified or are available in such limited amounts as to preclude full biochemical and structural characterization. Heterologous expression of human enzymes in bacteria can be problematic, and successful expression in yeast or insect cells often does not provide sufficient amounts of protein for biochemical or structural characterization. Most of the enzymes involved in homocysteine metabolism have homologous counterparts in prokaryotes, and the prokaryotic enzymes are often more amenable to overexpression. Thus some of the information needed to understand human homocysteine metabolism can be obtained by study of judiciously chosen prokaryotic enzymes.

In this chapter, we will illustrate this approach by discussing our studies on prokaryotic methylenetetrahydrofolate reductase (MTHFR; Metabolic Diagram, Enzyme 9) and cobalamin-dependent methionine syn-thase (Metabolic Diagram, Enzyme 4). We have studied the enzymes from *Escherichia coli* because they can be overexpressed readily and purified to homogeneity in amounts sufficient to permit structure determination and detailed biochemical characterization. One caution for such comparative studies is that it is then necessary to ascertain that the human enzymes and their mutant variants really behave the same way as the enzymes from prokaryotes. However, experiments designed to establish similar properties often can be performed with much less material, or with less fully purified material than the initial experiments that established the properties of the enzyme in question.

MTHFR from *Escherichia coli* as a Model for the Role of the Human Enzyme in Hyperhomocysteinemia

Similarities and Differences Between Human and Bacterial Reductases

All MTHFR proteins are flavoproteins. Both the human enzyme and the enzyme from *E. coli* contain 1 equivalent of flavin adenine dinucleotide (FAD) per subunit and catalyze the net transfer of a hydride ion (two electrons and a proton) from reduced pyridine nucleotides (NADH or NADPH) to 5,10-methylenetetrahydrofolate. The FAD cofactor is essential for these transfers, accepting hydride from NADH and donating it to 5,10-methylenetetrahydrofolate.

In *E. coli,* MTHFR is a 33 kDa protein (46) specified by the *metF* gene. It has recently been overexpressed and purified to homogeneity (48), and the x-ray structure has been determined (20). Eukaryotic MTHFRs are much larger proteins, with subunits ranging from 70 to 77 kDa in mass. The enzyme from pig liver has been most extensively characterized, initially by Kutzbach and Stokstad (31) and more recently in the Matthews laboratory (6, 37). Subunits of the larger mammalian enzyme consist of two discrete regions that can be separated after digestion of the native enzyme with trypsin: the N-terminal domain contains bound FAD, and the C-terminal domain contains a binding site for *S*-adenosylmethionine (AdoMet) (50). Proteolytic digestion of the reductase by trypsin is accompanied by loss of allosteric inhibition of the enzyme by AdoMet (39), and catalytic activity is retained, suggesting that the C-terminal region is responsible for the allosteric regulation of the catalytic activity of the N-terminal domain. The DNA sequence of *metF* from *E. coli* aligns with the sequences of the N-terminal regions of the eukaryotic MTHFRs, in agreement with the assumption that this region of the protein is responsible for catalysis (13, 19). Amino acid residues 39 to 343 of the human enzyme, which are specified by bp 46 to 1038 of the MTHFR gene, align with residues 1 to 295 of the bacterial enzyme.

Relative to the enzyme from *E. coli,* the eukaryotic reductases contain N-terminal extensions of varying lengths, and there is little sequence conservation exhibited in this region of the eukaryotic proteins. The 77 kDa subunits of the enzyme from pig liver have the amino acid sequence KQVTSYE at their N-terminus as determined by amino acid sequencing (51). In contrast, the MTHFR gene specifying the human enzyme contains an open reading frame corresponding to a 74.6 kDa protein (13), and no sequence corresponding to the N-terminal sequence of the porcine enzyme has been identified. Western analyses of several human tissues and of porcine liver reveal proteins of 77 and 70 kDa, suggesting that isozymes of MTHFR may exist, but it is also possible that the 5'-end of the open reading frame of the sequenced human cDNA has not yet been recovered.

In addition to the absence of a regulatory domain, the bacterial enzyme differs from the porcine enzyme in its specificity for the reducing substrate; whereas the porcine enzyme uses NADPH as the physiological reductant and has a much lower K_m for NADPH than for NADH (38), the bacterial enzyme preferentially uses NADH (48). The bacterial and porcine enyzmes also differ in quaternary structure. In solution at concentrations between 20 and 60 μmol/L in enzyme-bound flavin, the bacterial enzyme exists as a tetramer, but on dilution the tetramer dissociates into dimers and the flavin is released, with concomitant loss of activity (20, 48). In contrast, the porcine enzyme is a dimer of identical subunits (6), and it is not yet known whether the enzyme dissociates into monomers on dilution.

The Structure of *E. coli* MTHFR

The x-ray structure of bacterial MTHFR provides a prototype for the catalytic domains of the human and other eukaryotic enzymes. The 30% level of sequence identity between the *E. coli* and human enzymes gives assurance that the three-dimensional structure of the catalytic domain of human MTHFR will be mimicked by the bacterial protein. Surveys of known structures show that when sequence identities are 30% or greater, the folds will resemble one another (45). Alignments of MTHFR sequences from many phyla reveal patterns of conserved residues, or fingerprints, that characterize the catalytic region of MTHFR (Figure 10.1). The local structures in which these residues are embedded are also expected to be con-

served so that information about the structural and functional effects of mutations of these conserved residues can be transferred from the model structure to the human enzyme.

The bacterial MTHFR adopts a $\beta_8\alpha_8$ barrel fold (Figure 10.2), a structure that appears rather frequently in nature and is one of the folds known to bind flavins. The structure of MTHFR follows one of the general rules observed for such barrels, the prosthetic group and the substrates are bound near the C-terminal ends of the β-strands that compose the core of the barrel (Figure 10.2A). As in most flavoenzymes, the bound FAD is extended rather than folded back on itself. Many of the conserved residues contribute to the FAD binding site; they are distributed primarily on β-strands 3, 4, and 5, and in helix α5 (Figure 10.1). Mutations of flavin-binding residues that have been characterized in human MTHFR are discussed in Chapter 22. The residues that bind FAD do not match the fingerprints that had been identified in other flavin-dependent enzymes as markers for flavin binding and could not be assigned from the sequence alignments. Thus the structure has been essential to establish which conserved sequences and residues are responsible for FAD binding.

The flavin ring where the redox reactions occur lies near the center of the barrel, exposing the *si* face for hydride transfer. Before the structure was determined, studies of the stereochemistry had shown that the reactions of the folate and pyridine nucleotide substrates occur at this face of the flavin (52). A unique feature of the flavin-binding barrel of MTHFR is the truncation of the final strand and helix, β8 and α8, to produce a groove that adjoins the accessible face of the flavin ring. This groove can be seen best in a side view of the barrel (Figure 10.2B). If a model of 5,10-methylenetetrahydrofolate monoglutamate (the structure is shown in Scheme 1) is built with the folate ring stacked over the open face of the flavin and positioned to allow hydride transfer from the *N*(5) of the flavin, the *p*-aminobenzoic acid and glutamate moieties of the folate extend along the groove, which thus appears to be essential to accommodate the folate substrates of MTHFR. This model of the folate complex has been used to infer roles of conserved residues in folate binding.

Modeling the Ala222Val (677C→T) Polymorphism: The Effect of Folate in Ameliorating Hyperhomocysteinemia

The polymorphism, Ala222Val (bp 677C→T), for which approximately 12% of the Caucasian population is homozygous (13, 30, 56), was initially characterized as a thermolabile mutation (29) (see Chapter 22). It is associated with mildly elevated fasting

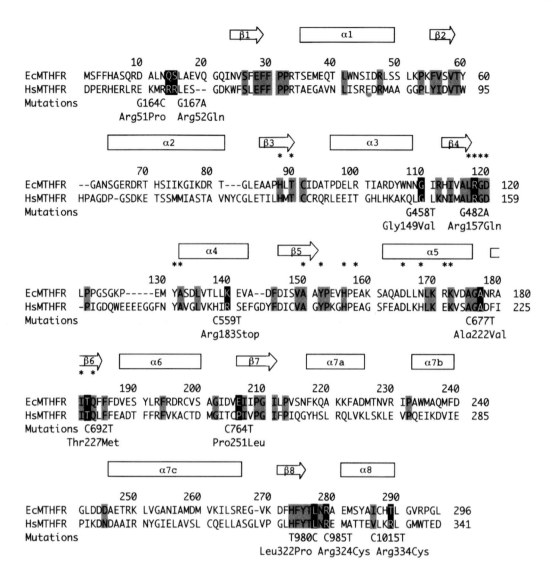

```
                    β1              α1                β2
              10        20        30        40        50        60
EcMTHFR   MSFFHASQRD ALNQSLAEVQ GQINVSFEFF PPRTSEMEQT LWNSIDRLSS LKPKFVSVTY  60
HsMTHFR   DPERHERLRE KMRRRLES-- GDKWFSLEFF PPRTAEGAVN LISREDRMAA GGPLYIDVTW  95
Mutations        G164C   G167A
                 Arg51Pro  Arg52Gln

                     α2           β3           α3              β4
                                  * *                          ****
              70        80        90        100       110       120
EcMTHFR   --GANSGERDRT HSIIKGIKDR T---GLEAAPHLT CIDATPDELR TIARDYWNNG IRHIVALRGD  120
HsMTHFR   HPAGDP-GSDKE TSSMMIASTA VNYCGLETILHMT CCRQRLEEIT GHLHKAKQLG LKNIMALRGD  159
Mutations                                              G458T       G482A
                                                       Gly149Val   Arg157Gln

                  α4          β5                    α5
                  **          * *   * *     *  *  **
              130       140       150       160       170       180
EcMTHFR   LPPGSGKP-----EM YASDLVTLLK EVA--DFDISVA AYPEVHPEAK SAQADLLNLK RKVDAGANRA  180
HsMTHFR   -PIGDQWEEEEGGFN YAVGLVKHIR SEFGDYFDICVA GYPKGHPEAG SFEADLKHLK EKVSAGADFI  225
Mutations                C559T                                          C677T
                         Arg183Stop                                     Ala222Val

            β6        α6          β7          α7a         α7b
            * *
              190       200       210       220       230       240
EcMTHFR   ITQFFFDVES YLRFRDRCVS AGIDVELIPG ILPVSNFKQA KKFADMTNVR IPAWMAQMFD  240
HsMTHFR   ITQLFFEADT FFRFVKACTD MGITCPIVPG IFPIQGYHSL RQLVKLSKLE VPQEIKDVIE  285
Mutations C692T                 C764T
          Thr227Met             Pro251Leu

                    α7c            β8          α8
              250       260       270       280       290
EcMTHFR   GLDDDAETRK LVGANIAMDM VKILSREG-VK DFHFYTLNRA EMSYAICHTL GVRPGL  296
HsMTHFR   PIKDNDAAIR NYGIELAVSL CQELLASGLVP GLHFYTLNRE MATTEVLKRL GMWTED  341
Mutations                                 T980C C985T    C1015T
                                  Leu322Pro Arg324Cys    Arg334Cys
```

Fig. 10.1. An alignment of the sequences of *E. coli* (Ec) and human (Hs) MTHFRs based on the simultaneous alignment of 12 MTHFR sequences and on the positions of secondary structures in the *E. coli* enzyme. Residues highlighted with dark shading indicate the sites of mutations of the human enzyme. Residues highlighted with light shading are strongly conserved fingerprints of MTHFR; residues contacting the FAD cofactor are marked with asterisks. (Reprinted from Guenther et al. [20], with permission.)

plasma total homocysteine levels, especially in patients with low folate levels (23, 25, 36), and with reduced specific activity and thermolability of MTHFR in lymphocyte extracts (13, 25, 53). Homozygosity for the 677C→T mutation is the most common genetic cause of mildly elevated plasma homocysteine. Despite the strong correlation between mild elevations in blood homocysteine and cardiovascular disease, the association of the TT genotype with risk for cardiovascular disease, although plausible (13), remains controversial

(42). One difficulty is that most studies of the risks associated with the TT genotype have not included folate measurements on the patients. The TT genotype in either the mother or the fetus is also suggested to be a risk factor for fetal neural tube defects (54). Folic acid treatment does decrease homocysteine levels in patients homozygous for the 677C→T polymorphism (7). The molecular bases for the dysfunction resulting from the 677C→T mutation and for the protective effects of folate have been analyzed in a recent publication (20) and are discussed later.

The Ala222Val polymorphism in human MTHFR was modeled in the *E. coli* enzyme by introducing the homologous mutation Ala177Val (20, 48). Because the mutant enzyme appeared less stable than wild-type *E. coli* MTHFR and was difficult to isolate in good yields, the coding sequence was modified to include a histidine tag at the C-terminus by insertion into a p*ET*-23b vector (Novagen). This strategy permitted purification of the enzyme to homogeneity in a single step by metal

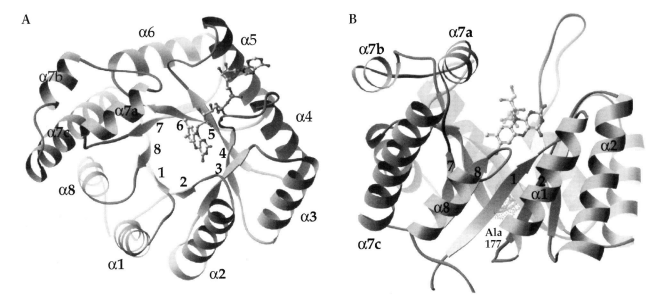

A

B

Fig. 10.2. The structure of *E. coli* MTHFR. (A) A view along the barrel axis looking toward the C-terminal ends of the β strands. (B) A view perpendicular to the barrel axis and toward the *si* face of the flavin ring, showing the groove in which the folate side chain is expected to bind. The side chain of Ala177 is depicted in space-filling mode, and is located at the "bottom of the barrel" in a loop between helix α5 and strand 6. (Reprinted from Guenther et al. [20], with permission.)

chelation chromatography, resulting in isolation of the mutant enzyme in high yield with a full complement of bound FAD. As a control for studies characterizing the mutant, wild-type enzyme was similarly tagged with C-terminal histidines (48).

The Ala177Val mutant of *E. coli* MTHFR exhibits thermolability, the characteristic property of its human counterpart. Differential scanning calorimetry was used to estimate the melting temperatures for the wild-type and mutant *E. coli* enzymes (20). The mutation decreased the melting temperature, relative to wild-type enzyme, by about 37°C at each of a series of protein concentrations. For both mutant and wild-type enzymes melting temperatures also decreased with protein concentration as expected when melting is associated with disaggregation of an oligomer.

The diminished activity of the Ala222Val human enzyme, observed in clinical studies, could arise from changes in the fundamental kinetic properties of MTHFR or from lowered levels of the enzyme resulting from instability. Although impairment of catalysis may seem the most obvious reason for

lowered flux of 5,10-methylenetetrahydrofolate to 5-methyltetrahydrofolate, the kinetic parameters are in fact not altered by introduction of the Ala177Val mutation into the *E. coli* enzyme. When the catalytic properties of the wild-type and Ala177Val mutant enzymes from *E. coli* were compared, the mutation did not affect V_{max} or the K_m values for 5,10-methylenetetrahydrofolate or NADH (20, 48). These determinations were carried out using stopped flow techniques to assay the enzyme at concentrations high enough to avoid inactivation. In retrospect, it is perhaps not sur-

N^5-methyltetrahydrofolate

Hydroxymethylpterin pyrophosphate

Scheme 1

prising that interchange of Ala and Val, residues that cannot serve as catalysts, has no effect on the kinetic properties.

The loss of enzyme activity during purification provided a clue to the molecular phenotype of the Ala177Val mutant. The mutant enzyme was observed to dissociate its essential FAD in a time- and concentration-dependent fashion (20). Dissociation of FAD was examined by following the increase in flavin fluorescence with time, because FAD bound to MTHFR does not fluoresce, but free FAD exhibits strong fluorescence (Figure 10.3A). After dilution of the enzyme from 20 μmol/L to 0.5 μmol/L, flavin was lost from the mutant about 10 times more rapidly than from the wild-type enzyme, and the final fluorescence indicated that all the flavin had been released. In less dilute solutions, only part of the flavin dissociated from the enzyme. The enzyme concentration at which 50% of the flavin dissociated was 1.3 μmol/L for the wild-type enzyme and 5.9 μmol/L for the mutant protein. These data imply that the affinity of the protein for FAD is affected by the Ala177Val mutation. The measurements are not readily converted to dissociation constants because disaggregation of tetramers to dimers accompanies the loss of flavin, as discussed later.

Because FAD is an essential reactant in the enzyme-catalyzed electron transfer from NADH to 5,10-methylenetetrahydrofolate, flavin dissociation is accompanied by loss of enzyme activity. When enzyme activity was monitored under the same conditions as those shown in Figure 10.3A, the loss of activity followed the same time course as the increase in fluorescence. The principal effect of the mutation is thus the impairment of FAD binding.

Because folates act in vivo to maintain the activity of MTHFR, we examined the effects of folate on the properties of the E. coli enzyme in vitro to see whether this model system might offer an explanation for the physiological effects of folic acid therapy. Addition of 5-methyltetrahydrofolate monoglutamate reduced the rate of flavin loss from both the wild-type and mutant enzymes (Figure 10.3B). At any given folate concentration, the mutant enzyme loses flavin faster than the wild-type enzyme; thus more folate must be present to reduce the rate of flavin loss to a level comparable to that of the wild-type enzyme. When activity rather than fluorescence was measured after dilution into solutions containing added folates, the initial activity

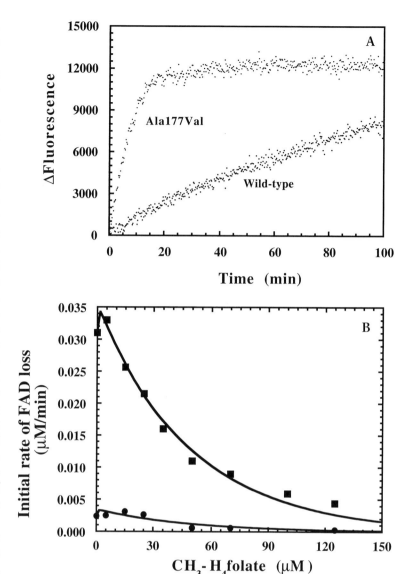

Fig. 10.3. (A) Release of flavin from *E. coli* methylenetetrahydrofolate reductase (MTHFR) on dilution of the enzyme. Concentrated enzyme (20 μmol/L in enzyme-bound FAD) was diluted to 0.5 μmol/L at time zero. Release of flavin is associated with an increase in fluorescence of the cofactor that was monitored in a fluorimeter. The upper curve is observed on dilution of the Ala177Val mutant enzyme, and the lower curve is observed with the wild-type enzyme. The rate of release of flavin is about 11-fold faster for the mutant enzyme. (B) Effect of 5-methyltetrahydrofolate on the rate of release of flavin from wild-type and Ala177Val enzymes. Experiments similar to those performed in (A) were conducted, except that varying amounts of 5-methyltetrahydrofolate (CH_3-H_4 Folate) were present in the buffer into which the enzyme was diluted. The upper curve shows the initial rate of flavin release from diluted Ala177Val enzyme as a function of the concentration of 5-methyltetrahydrofolate in the dilution buffer. The lower curve was obtained for the wild-type enzyme. (Reprinted from Guenther et al. [20], with permission.)

was partially inhibited, but the rate of loss of activity was decreased. For *E. coli*, MTHFR equivalent concentrations of 5-methyltetrahydrofolate triglutamate were more effective than the monoglutamate at reducing the rate of flavin loss. Protection was also observed using the inhibitor dihydrofolate monoglutamate and the folate antagonist 5,10-dideazatetrahydrofolate pentaglutamate. It appears that any folate that binds to the enzyme offers protection against dissociation of the FAD.

The human Ala222Val enzyme is similarly protected from inactivation by folates (20, 48). Addition of folate is effective in preventing the loss of activity that occurs as a result of brief heat treatment. Protection has been demonstrated in experiments with extracts containing human (677C→T) MTHFR expressed in *E. coli* and with mutant enzyme in lymphocyte extracts (see Chapter 22 for details). Higher concentrations of folate are required to maintain activity in Ala222Val (677C→T) than in the wild-type enzyme. Added FAD also protects the wild-type and mutant enzymes against loss of FAD.

The implication of the observed protection by folate and FAD is that the phenotype of the human polymorphism also involves an enhanced tendency to dissociate FAD. One might argue that folic acid therapy, by raising the concentration of folates in the cell, could lead to enzyme inhibition as well as enzyme protection. We assume that supplementation with folic acid increases the concentration of all folate derivatives including the substrate 5,10-methylenetetrahydrofolate.

The structure of the bacterial MTHFR shows that the molecular mechanism for dysfunction in the Ala177Val mutant is more complicated than expected. The mutation occurs at a site near the bottom of the barrel and distant from the FAD (Figure 10.2B). That means that effects of mutation must be mediated through the protein. How this happens is speculation at present, in the absence of a structure for the Ala177Val mutant of *E. coli* MTHFR. We presume that steric overlap is the primary event that triggers the effects of the mutation (i.e., that the larger valine must perturb neighboring residues in the structure). The local displacements may be propagated to the FAD binding site via intervening structures such as helix α5. This propagation mechanism would operate within a single chain and is readily applicable to the homologous human enzyme.

In the wild-type and Ala177Val mutant enzymes from *E. coli*, the dissociation of FAD is accompanied by disaggregation of the MTHFR tetramer to dimeric species. The behavior of these enzymes can be modeled by assuming that FAD is lost primarily from the dimer, and effects of the Ala177Val mutation on the association of the chains to form tetramers can be rationalized from the structure (20). It is not known whether the tetrameric *E. coli* and dimeric human enzymes utilize some of the same interchain interactions so we cannot confidently extrapolate the effects of mutation on subunit interactions to the human enzyme.

In summary, experiments in the *E. coli* model system have demonstrated that the molecular phenotype of the *E. coli* mutant Ala177Val is an enhanced tendency to lose its flavin cofactor. Folates protect against the loss of FAD and stabilize the enzyme by binding directly to the active site. We envision that in the complex with folates, the apparent affinity of MTHFR for FAD is increased because the folate ring lies over the face of the flavin that is solvent accessible in the absence of folates. The basis for the action of folate is a thermodynamic interaction between the binding of folate and flavin; the substrate thereby protects the enzyme against inactivation.

Mutations Causing Severe Hyperhomocysteinemia in Humans

Other mutations that map to the catalytic domain of MTHFR have been identified in patients (17–19). In some cases, the mutations have not been characterized in patients who are homozygous for the mutation, but instead occur in patients heterozygotic for two different mutations. Severe mutations are associated with residual specific activities of 0 to 20% in crude lymphocyte extracts, giving rise to symptoms that include mental retardation, seizures, peripheral neuropathies, and thromboses. The base and amino acid substitutions that define these mutations are compiled in Table 10.1, along with some properties of the mutant MTHFR enzymes. Assignment of the molecular phenotype is sometimes complicated by the simultaneous occurrence of the Ala222Val polymorphism in *cis* and/or *trans* with the more severe mutation (19). As a result, it is not always possible to associate thermolability with the presence of a particular severe mutation.

The positions of the known severe mutations are indicated in the sequences of *E. coli* and human MTHFR in Figure 10.1, which also shows the elements of the three-dimensional structure in which the mutations are embedded. The mutations are mapped onto the structure of the *E. coli* enzyme in Figure 10.4. Some mutations occur at sites near to or in contact with the essential FAD, some modify groups that appear to be critical for substrate binding, and others, like the Ala177Val mutation, are found in more remote parts of the structure. The distribution of observed mutations in the structure suggests that there may be several distinct categories of dysfunction: diminished structural stability, defects in the function of catalytic or substrate-binding residues, or defects in FAD binding. Not all impairments of MTHFR func-

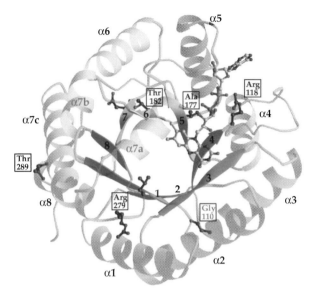

Fig. 10.4. Locations of the known mutations in human MTHFR that map to the catalytic domain. The view is down the axis of the $\beta_8\alpha_8$ barrel as in Figure 10.2A. The residues of *E. coli* MTHFR that occur at the sites of mutations are drawn in ball-and-stick mode.

tion will be amenable to treatment with folates at the level that is effective for the Ala222Val polymorphism. Knowledge of the molecular phenotype associated with a particular mutation might suggest approaches to treatment or contraindicate particular treatments.

The structure leads to hypotheses about the consequences of several of the severe mutations, that can in

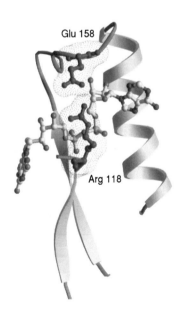

Fig. 10.5. A drawing showing how the belt formed by residues Glu 158 and Arg 118 encircles the side chain of FAD. Dot surfaces represent the volumes occupied by the Arg and Glu residues.

turn be investigated using *E. coli* MTHFR as a model. Here we consider a few of the best studied cases as examples. In the human enzyme, Arg157Gln is a severe mutation, with low activity in heterozygotes. The equivalent residue in *E. coli* MTHFR is Arg 118, part of an intriguing feature of the FAD binding site, a salt bridge between Arg 118 and Glu 158 that encircles the FAD side chain like a belt and appears to secure the FAD to the protein (Figure 10.5). Changes in these belt residues would be expected to have an impact on FAD binding rather than on catalysis. In preliminary experiments, the mutation Arg118Glu has been modeled in the *E. coli* protein (C. Sheppard, H. Campbell, and R. Matthews, unpublished data). FAD is readily lost during the preparation of this mutant enzyme, dissociating even under conditions where FAD remains bound to the Ala177Val mutant. After correction for the amount of apoenzyme, the holoenzyme retains about 20% of its catalytic activity. This is a mutation that should be responsive to riboflavin therapy.

Another intriguing mutation observed in human MTHFR is Thr227Met. The structure of the bacterial protein shows the equivalent Thr 182 on strand β6 close to but not contacting FAD; the succeeding residue is the conserved Gln 183, which is postulated to interact with the pterin of bound 5,10-methylenetetrahydrofolate. Our prediction was that this mutation should affect catalysis and might also alter FAD binding (Table 10.1). The mutation has been emulated in *E. coli* MTHFR, but the resulting enzyme proved too unstable to isolate, even when expressed with a C-terminal histidine tag (P. Althaus, E. Trimmer, and R. Matthews, unpublished data). Changes in packing and interactions in the interior of the protein, resulting from introduction of methionine, had devastating effects on the structure. These observations correlate with the drastic phenotype observed in individuals who are homozygous for the Thr227Met mutation (18). These patients develop severe symptoms within the first year of life.

A final example is the mutation Arg324Cys in the human enzyme. This residue lies in what we have called the folate binding groove and is a good candidate for binding the α-carboxylate group of 5,10-methylenetetrahydrofolate. The enzyme from homozygotes has 20% of normal enzyme activity (19). It will be interesting to construct the homologous bacterial mutation and to examine the kinetic properties of this enzyme form in more detail. One might expect this mutation to result in decreased affinity for 5,10-methylenetetrahydrofolate; folic acid therapy may be indicated for treatment of patients homozygous for this mutation.

The sites of some of the other mutations shown in Figure 10.4 suggest the nature of the defects induced

Table 10.1.   Severe Mutations in Human MTHFR

Mutation Amino Acid (Base)	Activity (%)	E. coli Residue	Location	Proposed Dysfunction	Reference
Arg51Pro (164G→C)	2[a]	Gln 14	Not seen in structure		18
Arg52Gln (167G→A)	10[a]	Ser 15	Not seen in structure		19
Gly149Val (458G→T)	4	Gly 110	"Bottom" of barrel; N-terminus of β4		18
Arg157Gln (482G→A)	6–14[b]	Arg 118	Belt over FAD; C-terminus of β4	FAD binding	20
Thr227Met (692C→T)	0–2	Thr 183	C-terminus of α6	FAD and folate binding	19
Pro251Leu (764C→T)	3	Glu 206	N-terminus of β7		19
Leu322Pro (980T→C)	2[c]	Leu 277	Strand β8	Folate binding	18
Arg324Cys (985C→T)	20	Arg 279	After β8	Folate binding	19
Arg334Cys (1015C→T)	10[a]	Thr 289	C-terminus of α8		19

[a] Patients are heterozygotes with another mutation.
[b] Patients are heterozygous for Arg52Gln and Arg334Cys.
[c] Patients are heterozygotes with Arg376Cys (1141C→T).

in MTHFR. The mutation 458G→T alters a conserved glycine, Gly 110 in *E. coli* MTHFR, at the "bottom" of the barrel and distant from the active site. Glycine residues are often critical in structures because of their ability to adopt conformations that are unfavorable for residues with side chains; this particular glycine seems to be required to allow a tight connection between a helix and a β strand. The 980T→C mutation replaces the conserved Leu 322 in the folate binding groove with proline. Although the wild-type and mutant residues are both hydrophobic, we surmise that leucine plays some specific role in the interaction with folates. In contrast to these examples, it is more difficult to postulate the functional or structural roles of nonconserved surface residues, such as Pro 451, whose mutations affect the human enzyme.

Methionine Synthase from *E. coli* as a Model for Human Methionine Synthase

A complete cDNA sequence for the human methionine synthase (4, 32, 34) is now available. The inferred amino acid sequence of the human enzyme shows 55% identity (34) with the sequence of the enzyme from *E. coli* (2), establishing that the structure of the mammalian enzyme will be homologous to that of the bacterial enzyme (45). As described next, bacterial methionine synthase provides a beautiful example of the assembly of functional and structural modules into a complex enzyme. Mapping polymorphisms and other point mutations of human methionine synthase to one or another module immediately gives some indication of their functional effects.

Methionine Synthase: A Modular Enzyme

The organization, properties, and kinetics of the enzyme from *E. coli* have been intensively studied in the laboratories of Weissbach, Taylor, Huennekens, and Matthews (reviewed in [35]), and crystal structures of two regions making up the C-terminal half of the protein have been determined by Ludwig and colleagues (8, 10). In the conversion of homocysteine to methionine catalyzed by methionine synthase, the cobalamin cofactor is alternately demethylated by homocysteine and remethylated by 5-methyltetrahydrofolate, as shown in Figure 12.1 (see Chapter 12). The intermediate demethylated cofactor is the very reactive cob(I)alamin species, which is occasionally oxidized to cob(II)alamin under aerobic conditions. Return of the inactive cob(II)alamin form of the enzyme to the catalytic cycle requires a reductive methylation in which the methyl group is derived from AdoMet rather than 5-methyltetrahydrofolate. Recent studies of the mechanism of reductive activation, using flavodoxin and methionine synthase from *E. coli* (27), have demonstrated that the first step is reduction of cob(II)alamin to cob(I)alamin. Subsequent transfer of a methyl group from AdoMet to cobalamin drives the overall reaction (3). The reducing equivalents for reactivation are provided by reduced flavodoxin in *E. coli* and in mammalian systems by more complex proteins incorporating flavodoxin-like domains. The proteins responsible for reduction of the human enzyme are discussed in Chapters 12 and 22.

Structural and functional analyses of fragments and constructs, carried out in our laboratories, have established the modular arrangement of methionine synthase. Residues 2 to 353[1] (1 to 368 in the human

---

[1] The N-terminal methionine is removed from the bacterial enzyme in the cell.

enzyme, corresponding to bp 287 to 1390 in the cDNA sequence given by GenBank accession number U75743 [34]) form a region responsible for the binding and activation of homocysteine (16). The homocysteine substrate is coordinated as a thiolate anion to a zinc at the active site of this region; the essential zinc is also coordinated by three thiol residues from the protein (15, 41). In the *E. coli* enzyme, these key residues are Cys 247, Cys 310, and Cys 311; the corresponding residues in the human enzyme are Cys 260, Cys 323, and Cys 324. The homocysteine-binding module of *E. coli* methionine synthase has been independently expressed (16). Although it is unable to catalyze transfer of a methyl group from 5-methyltetrahydrofolate to homocysteine, the homocysteine-binding module can catalyze methyl transfer from exogenous methylcobalamin to homocysteine. This latter assay is useful for assessing the functional effects of mutations in this region of methionine synthase (16). The homocysteine-binding region shows significant sequence homology with betaine-homocysteine methyl transferase (14) (Metabolic Diagram, Enzyme 5). As described in Chapter 13, this protein also contains zinc at its active site (40).

Residues 354 to 649 (369 to 661 in the human enzyme, corresponding to bp 1391 to 2269 in the cDNA sequence) constitute a domain responsible for the binding and activation of 5-methyltetrahydrofolate (16). This region shows significant sequence similarity to the corrinoid iron/sulfur methyltransferase from *Clostridium thermoaceticum* (43), and to dihydropteroate synthases from a variety of organisms (49). X-ray structures of dihydropteroate synthase have been determined (1, 22), including structures with the pterin ligand bound to the enzyme. The synthase are $\beta_8\alpha_8$ barrels, with the pterin bound near the C-terminal ends of the β strands. Because 5-methyltetrahydrofolate and dihydropteroate are structurally similar molecules (Scheme 1), one might expect conservation of the residues that make critical hydrogen bonding interactions with the nitrogen and oxygen atoms of the pterin, or hydrophobic interactions with the pterin ring system. Indeed, residues that are conserved in alignments of methionine synthase with dihydropteroate synthase are primarily involved in binding and activating the pterin cofactor (49). Although the 5-methyltetrahydrofolate-binding domain of methionine synthase has not yet been expressed independently, a construct containing amino acids 1 to 649 has been expressed and characterized. This construct contains both the homocysteine-binding and the 5-methyltetrahydrofolate-binding regions, and catalyzes methyl transfer from exogenous methylcobalamin to homocysteine, and from 5-methyltetrahydrofolate to exogenous cob(I)alamin (16). The latter reaction is particularly useful in assessing the catalytic roles of residues in the methyltetrahydrofolate-binding domain.

Residues 650 to 896 (662 to 922 in the human enzyme corresponding to bp 2270 to 3050 in the cDNA sequence) form domains responsible for binding of the cobalamin cofactor (3, 12). The x-ray structure of this region of the protein (9) is illustrated in Figure 10.6A. The cobalamin is sandwiched between a "cap" domain, which covers the top face of the cobalamin, and a domain that interacts with the dimethylbenzimidazole side chain of the cofactor. This side chain is in an extended conformation and penetrates deeply into the lower domain. The cobalt of cobalamin is coordinated by His 759 from this domain, which is part of a triad of residues linked by hydrogen bonds. The His 759, Asp 757, Ser 810 triad is conserved in all cobalamin-dependent methionine synthases that have been sequenced and forms part of a conserved motif for cobalamin binding (10). The triad is protonated when cob(I)alamin is formed during catalysis and deprotonated when methylcobalamin is formed (26).

Residues 897 to 1227 (923 to 1265 in the human enzyme, corresponding to bp 3051 to 4082 in the cDNA sequence) form a domain that houses the binding site for AdoMet and is required for reactivation of the inactive cob(II)alamin form of methionone synthase (12). Truncated enzymes missing the activation domain are initially active if the cofactor is in the methylcobalamin form, but are gradually converted to the inactive cob(II)alamin form during aerobic turnover. The cob(II)alamin form of the truncated enzyme cannot be reactivated. The x-ray structure of the activation domain (8) is represented in Figure 10.6B. AdoMet is bound to a concave surface of the domain, which is shaped roughly like a kidney, and is positioned with its methyl group exposed to the solvent in the structure of the isolated domain.

The modular arrangement of functional units, connected by linkers, presumably reflects the molecular evolution of the enzyme, but also allows the modules to adopt different arrangements for the alternating reactions of bound homocysteine, 5-methyltetrahydrofolate, and AdoMet at the top face of cobalamin.

Polymorphisms of Methionine Synthase: Asp919Gly

Current working models for the reactions of methionine synthase suggest that the enzyme must undergo conformational changes during turnover to bring the several substrate-binding domains into position for reaction with the cobalamin cofactor (9, 16, 28). The linkers between these domains will play an important role in facilitating such conformational changes. A common polymorphism, Asp919Gly, maps to the linker region

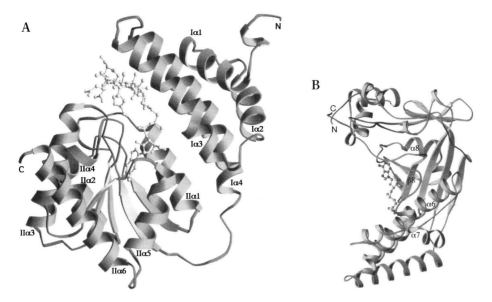

Fig. 10.6. (A) The structure of the cobalamin-binding fragment of methionine synthase from *E. coli*, including residues 649 to 896. α-Helices and sheet strands in the N-terminal "cap" domain (I) and in the cobalamin-binding domain (II) are labeled. Methylcobalamin, with its extended nucleotide tail, is shown in ball-and-stick mode, as is the His 759 that binds cobalt. (B) The structure of the activation domain of methionine synthase from *E. coli*. Bound AdoMet is displayed in ball-and-stick mode. Strands and α helices in the vicinity of bound AdoMet are labeled.

between the cobalamin-binding region and the activation domain and has been modeled using *E. coli* methionine synthase (K. Fluhr and R. G. Matthews, unpublished data). The mutant protein in which the homologous glutamate residue has been changed to glycine, Glu893Gly, exhibits mildly reduced activity, especially when catalysis is initiated with enzyme in the cob(II)alamin form, suggesting that reductive activation is specifically impaired. However, the binding of AdoMet is unaffected by the mutation.

Mutations in Methionine Synthase Associated with Severe Phenotypes

Mutations leading to severe disease in humans have also been identified. One of these is His920Asp, which affects the residue adjacent to Asp 919 in the linker region between the cobalamin-binding and activation domains. This mutation, which results in a change in charge of the linker, is an excellent candidate for modeling in the bacterial enzyme. Another severe mutation is 3804C→T, which results in the substitution of Pro 1173 by Leu (21). The corresponding residue in the enzyme from *E. coli* is Pro 1139, which is located in the C-terminal activation domain in direct contact with the bound AdoMet. This mutation was expected to impair reductive methylation of the cob(II)alamin

form of the enzyme (8). In fact, the enzyme from the mutant cell line shows diminished activity when assayed using the physiological reducing system (21), but is competent in catalysis when assayed using titanium citrate as a reductant. A Pro1135Leu mutant bacterial enzyme has been characterized (K. Fluhr and R. Matthews, unpublished data); the enzyme has very low affinity for AdoMet and is specifically compromised in reductive activation. However, the methylcobalamin form of the mutant enzyme initially exhibits normal catalytic activity.

Proteins that Activate Methionine Synthase: Bacterial Flavodoxin as a Model for the FMN Domain of Methionine Synthase Reductase

Reactivation of the cobalt (II) form of methionine synthase proceeds by a reductive methylation that utilizes AdoMet and requires the C-terminal activation domain of methionine synthase as discussed earlier. Reducing equivalents (electrons) for the reaction are derived from NADPH and supplied via a flavoprotein reductase and an electron carrier. In *E. coli* the carrier is "free-standing" flavodoxin, but human tissues express complex reductases that incorporate flavodoxin-like domains in their sequences. Two methionine synthase reductase systems from human tissues have been described (see Chapter 12). The gene for a methionine synthase reductase (33), the existence of which was first inferred from complementation studies (44), carries mutations that affect the activity of methionine synthase. A partially purified protein with properties resembling cytochrome P450 reductase, but dependent on cytochrome b_5 for reduction of methionine synthase, has been shown to restore the activity of methionine synthase (5). Differences between these systems are not clear at present; the deduced sequence of the first reductase shows that it is also a protein closely resembling P450 reductase.

Because flavodoxin-like domains appear to be the electron donors that interact with methionine synthase in higher organisms, complexes of *E. coli* flavodoxin with *E. coli* methionine synthase furnish models for the activation systems that operate in eukaryotes. For the bacterial system, it is known that binding of flavodoxin to methionine synthase leads to changes in the coordination of the cobalt in cob(II)alamin; His 759 dissociates from the cobalt and the ligand triad becomes protonated (24, 26). Docking experiments using molecular models (11) suggest that in the complex between flavodoxin and methionine synthase, the flavin of flavodoxin, the methyl group of AdoMet, and the cobalt of cobalamin can be positioned close to one another to facilitate electron and methyl transfer to cob(II)alamin. Studies that aim to define the interacting surfaces of flavodoxin and methionine synthase are in progress (D. Mall and R. Matthews, unpublished data). Chemical cross-linking has been used to demonstrate that the primary site of interaction of flavodoxin is the C-terminal activation domain of methionine synthase (21a).

Two structures from cytochrome P450 systems may also be relevant to the interaction of methionine synthase with its reductase. A structure of the P450 and flavodoxin domains from P450BM3 depicts the binding of the electron donor to the P450 acceptor (47), and the structure of human cytochrome P450 reductase (55) reveals the interactions between flavodoxin and FAD domains that presumably are required for reduction of the flavodoxin partner. In both structures, and in the model for flavodoxin binding to methionine synthase, the same surface region of flavodoxin is used for recognition. Comparison of the structures with the hypothetical model of flavodoxin bound to methionine synthase suggests that flavodoxin domains in complex reductases must be able to swing or pivot about linker sequences to act first as electron acceptors from their cognate reductases and then as electron donors to the heme or cobalamin of their target proteins.

Current knowledge of the activation system suggests several plausible mechanisms for functional impairment. Mutations may affect the chemistry of the activation reaction, they may affect conformational changes that are essential to bring the activation domain of methionine synthase in contact with both the cobalamin and activator proteins, or they may disrupt the contacts required for interactions of the activation proteins with methionine synthase.

Some mutations affecting activation map to methionine synthase itself, as already noted for Pro1139Leu, but others affect the accessory proteins of the activation system. Two initial examples of mutations in methionine synthase reductase have been described: the polymorphism Met22Ile in the flavodoxin domain of methionine synthase reductase, and a deletion of Leu 569, a residue that maps to the core of the NADPH-binding domain, according to alignments of methionine synthase reductase with P450 reductase (33). The polymorphism occurs in the region where flavodoxin is proposed to contact methionine synthase and is amenable to functional and structural analysis in *E. coli* model systems.

REFERENCES

1. Achari, A, Somers, DO, Champness, JN, Bryant, PK, Rosemond, J, Stammers, DK. Crystal structure of the anti-bacterial sulfonamide drug target dihydropteroate synthase. *Nature Struct Biol* 1997; 4: 490–97.

2. Banerjee, RV, Johnston, NL, Sobeski, JK, Datta, P, Matthews, RG. Cloning and sequence analysis of the *Escherichia coli metH* gene encoding cobalamin-dependent methionine synthase and isolation of a tryptic fragment containing the cobalamin-binding domain. *J Biol Chem* 1989; 264: 13888–95.

3. Banerjee, RV, Harder, SR, Ragsdale, SW, Matthews, RG. Mechanism of reductive activation of cobalamin-dependent methionine synthase: An electron paramagnetic resonance spectroelectrochemical study. *Biochemistry* 1990; 29: 1129–35.

4. Chen, LH, Liu, M-L, Hwang, H-Y, Chen, L-S, Korenberg, J, Shane, B. Human methionine synthase: cDNA cloning, gene localization and expression. *J Biol Chem* 1997; 272: 3628–34.

5. Chen, Z, Banerjee, R. Purification of soluble cytochrome b_5 as a component of the reductive activation of porcine methionine synthase. *J Biol Chem* 1998; 273: 26248–55.

6. Daubner, SC, Matthews, RG. Purification and properties of methylenetetrahydrofolate reductase from pig liver. *J Biol Chem* 1982; 257: 140–45.

7. Deloughery, TG, Evans, A, Sadeghi, A, McWilliams, J, Henner, WD, Taylor, LH, Jr, Press, RD. Common mutation in methylenetetrahydrofolate reductase. Correlation with homocysteine metabolism and late-onset vascular disease. *Circulation* 1996; 94: 3074–78.

8. Dixon, MM, Huang, S, Matthews, RG, Ludwig, M. The structure of the C-terminal domain of methionine synthase: Presenting *S*-adenosylmethionine for reductive methylation of B_{12}. *Structure* 1996; 4: 1263–75.

9. Drennan, CL, Huang, S, Drummond, JT, Matthews, RG, Ludwig, ML. How a protein binds B_{12}: A 3.0 Å X-ray structure of B_{12}-binding domains of methionine synthase. *Science* 1994; 266: 1669–74.

10. Drennan, CL, Matthews, RG, Ludwig, ML. Cobalamin-dependent methionine synthase: The structure of a methylcobalamin-binding fragment and implications for other B_{12}-dependent enzymes. *Curr Opin Struct Biol* 1994; 4: 919–29.

11. Drennan, CL, Dixon, MM, Hoover, DM. Cobalamin-dependent methionine synthase from *Escherichia coli*: Structure and reactivity. In *Vitamin B_{12} and B_{12} Proteins*.

(Krautler, B, Arigoni, D, Golding, BT, eds). Wiley-VCH, Weinheim, 1998; 131–55.

12. Drummond, JT, Huang, S, Blumenthal, RM, Matthews, RG. Assignment of enzymatic function to specific protein regions of cobalamin-dependent methionine synthase from *Escherichia coli*. *Biochemistry* 1993; 32: 9290–95.

13. Frosst, P, Blom, HJ, Milos, R, Goyette, P, Sheppard, CA, Matthews, RG, Boers, GJH, den Heijer, M, Kluijtmans, LAJ, van den Heuvel, LPWJ, Rozen, R. A candidate genetic risk factor for vascular disease: A common mutation in the methylenetetrahydrofolate reductase gene. *Nat Genet* 1995; 10: 111–13.

14. Garrow, TA. Purification, kinetic properties, and cDNA cloning of mammalian betaine-homocysteine methyltransferase. *J Biol Chem* 1996; 271: 22831–38.

15. Goulding, CW, Matthews, RG. Cobalamin-dependent methionine synthase from *Escherichia coli*: Zinc is required for methyl transfer from methylcobalamin to homocysteine. *Biochemistry* 1997; 36: 15749–57.

16. Goulding, CW, Postigo, D, Matthews, RG. Cobalamin-dependent methionine synthase is a modular protein with distinct regions for binding homocysteine, methyltetrahydrofolate, cobalamin, and adenosylmethionine. *Biochemistry* 1997; 36: 8082–91.

17. Goyette, P, Sumner, JS, Milos, R, Duncan, AMV, Rosenblatt, DS, Matthews, RG, Rozen, R. Human methylenetetrahydrofolate reductase: Isolation of cDNA, mapping and mutation identification. *Nat Genet* 1994; 7: 195–200.

18. Goyette, P, Frosst, P, Rosenblatt, DS, Rozen, R. Seven novel mutations in the methylenetetrahydrofolate reductase gene and genotype/phenotype correlations in severe methylenetetrahydrofolate reductase deficiency. *Am J Hum Genet* 1995; 56: 1052–59.

19. Goyette, P, Christensen, B, Rosenblatt, DS, Rozen, R. Severe and mild mutations in *cis* for the methylenetetrahydrofolate reductase (MTHFR) gene, and description of five novel mutations in MTHFR. *Am J Hum Genet* 1996; 59: 1268–75.

20. Guenther, BD, Sheppard, CA, Tran, P, Rozen, R, Matthews, RG, Ludwig ML. The structure and properties of methylenetetrahydrofolate reductase from *Escherichia coli* suggest how folate ameliorates human hyperhomocysteinemia *Natur Struct Biol* 1999; 6: 359–65.

21. Gulati, S, Baker, P, Li, YN, Fowler, B, Kruger, WD, Brody, LC, Banerjee, R. Defects in human methionine synthase in cb1G patients. *Hum Mol Genet* 1996; 5: 1859–65.

21a. Hall, DA, Jordan-Starck, TC, Loo, RO, Ludwig, ML, Matthews, RG. Interaction of flavodoxin with cobalamin-dependent methionine synthase. *Biochemistry* 2000; 39: 10711–19.

22. Hampele, IC, D'Arcy, A, Dale, GE, Kostrewa, D, Nielsen, J, Oetner, C, Page, MGP, Schoenfeld, M-J, Stoeher, D, Then, RL. Structure and function of the dihydropteroate synthase from *Staphylococcus aureus*. *J Mol Biol* 1997; 268: 21–30.

23. Harmon, DL, Woodside, JV, Yarnell, JW, McMaster, D, Young, IS, McCrum, EE, Gey, KF, Whitehead, AS,

Evans, AE. The common "thermolabile" variant of methylenetetrahydrofolate reductase is a major determinant of mild hyperhomocysteinaemia. *Q J Med* 1996; 89: 515–77.

24. Hoover, DM, Jarrett, JT, Sands, RH, Dunham, WR, Ludwig, ML, Matthews, RG. Interaction of *Escherichia coli* cobalamin-dependent methionine synthase and its physiological partner flavodoxin: Binding of flavodoxin leads to axial ligand dissociation from the cobalamin cofactor. *Biochemistry* 1997; 36: 127–38.

25. Jacques, PF, Bostom, AG, Williams, RR, Ellison, RC, Eckfeldt, JH, Rosenberg, IH, Selhub, J, Rozen, R. Relation between folate status, a common mutation in methylenetetrahydrofolate reductase, and plasma homocysteine concentrations. *Circulation* 1996; 93: 7–9.

26. Jarrett, JT, Choi, CY, Matthews, RG. Changes in protonation associated with substrate binding and cob(I)alamin formation in cobalamin-dependent methionine synthase. *Biochemistry* 1997; 36: 15739–48.

27. Jarrett, JT, Hoover, DM, Ludwig, ML, Matthews, RG. The mechanism of adenosylmethionine-dependent activation of methionine synthase: A rapid kinetic analysis of intermediates in reductive methylation of cob(II)alamin enzyme. *Biochemistry* 1998; 37: 12649–58.

28. Jarrett, JT, Huang, S, Matthews, RG. Methionine synthase exists in two distinct conformations that differ in reactivity toward methyltetrahydrofolate, adenosylmethionine, and flavodoxin. *Biochemistry* 1998; 37: 5372–82.

29. Kang, S-S, Wong, PWK, Zhou, J, Sora, J, Lessick, M, Ruggie, N, Grcevich, G. Thermolabile methylenetetrahydrofolate reductase in patients with coronary artery disease. *Metabolism* 1988; 37: 611–13.

30. Kluijtmans, LAJ, van den Heuvel, LPWJ, Boers, GJH, Frosst, P, Stevens, EM, van Oost, BA, den Heijer, M, Trijbels, FJM, Rozen, R, Blom, HJ. Molecular genetic analysis in mild hyperhomocysteinemia: A common mutation in the methylenetetrahydrofolate reductase gene is a genetic risk factor for cardiovascular disease. *Am J Hum Genet* 1996; 58: 35–41.

31. Kutzbach, C, Stockstad, ELR. Mammalian methylenetetrahydrofolate reductase: Partial purification, properties, and inhibition by S-adenosylmethionine. *Biochim Biophys Acta* 1971; 250: 459–77.

32. Leclerc, D, Campeau, E, Goyette, P, Adjalla, CE, Christensen, B, Ross, M, Eydoux, P, Rosenblatt, DS, Rozen, R, Gravel, RA. Human methionine synthase: cDNA cloning and identification of mutations in patients of the *cblG* complementation group of folate/cobalamin disorders. *Hum Mol Genet* 1996; 5: 1867–74.

33. Leclerc, D, Wilson, A, Dumas, R, Gafuik, C, Song, D, Watkins, D, Heng, HHQ, Rommens, JM, Scherer, SW, Rosenblatt, DS, Gravel, RA. Cloning and mapping of a cDNA for methionine synthase reductase, a flavoprotein defective in patients with homocystinuria. *Proc Natl Acad Sci USA* 1998; 95: 3059–64.

34. Li, YN, Gulati, S, Baker, PJ, Brody, LC, Banerjee, R, Kruger, WD. Cloning, mapping, and RNA analysis of

the human methionine synthase gene. *Hum Mol Genet* 1996; 5: 1851–58.

35. Ludwig, ML, Matthews, RG. Structure-based perspectives on B12-dependent enzymes. *Annu Rev Biochem* 1997; 66: 269–313.

36. Ma, J, Stampfer, MJ, Hennekens, Frosst, P, Selhub, J, Horsford, J, Malinow, MR, Willett, WC, Rozen, R. Methylenetetrahydrofolate reductase polymorphism, plasma folate, homocysteine, and risk of myocardial infarction in US physicians. *Circulation* 1996; 94: 2410–16.

37. Matthews, RG. Methylenetetrahydrofolate reductase from pig liver. *Methods Enzymol* 1986; 122: 372–81.

38. Matthews, RG, Kaufman, S. Characterization of the dihydropterin reductase activity of pig liver methylenetetrahydrofolate reductase. *J Biol Chem* 1980; 255: 6014–17.

39. Matthews, RG, Vanoni, MA, Hainfeld, JF, Wall, J. Methylenetetrahydrofolate reductase. Evidence for spatially distinct subunit domains obtained by scanning transmission electron microscopy and limited proteolysis. *J Biol Chem* 1984; 259: 11647–50.

40. Millian, NS, Garrow, TA. Human betaine-homocysteine methyltransferase is a zinc metalloenzyme. *Arch Biochem Biophys* 1998; 356: 93–98.

41. Peariso, K, Goulding, CW, Matthews, RG, Penner-Hahn, J. The role of zinc in binding of homocysteine to cobalamin-dependent methionine synthase. *J Am Chem Soc* 1998; 120: 8410–16.

42. Refsum, H, Ueland, PM, Nygård, O, Vollset, SE. Homocysteine and cardiovascular disease. *Annu Rev Med* 1998; 49: 31–62.

43. Roberts, DL, Zhao, S, Doukov, T, Ragsdale, SW. The reductive acetyl-CoA pathway: Sequence and heterologous expression of active CH$_3$-H$_4$folate:corrinoid/iron sulfur protein methyltransferase from *Clostridium thermoaceticum*. *J Bacteriol* 1994; 176: 6127–30.

44. Rosenblatt, DS, Cooper, BA, Pottier, A, Lue-Shing, H, Matiaszuk, N, Grauer, K. Altered vitamin B$_{12}$ metabolism in fibroblasts from a patient with megaloblastic anemia and homocystinuria due to a new defect in methionine biosynthesis. *J Clin Invest* 1984; 74: 2149–56.

45. Rost, B. Twilight zone of protein sequence alignments. *Protein Eng* 1999; 12: 85–94.

46. Saint-Girons, I, Duchange, N, Zakin, MM, Park, I, Margarita, D, Ferrara, P, Cohen, GN. Nucleotide sequence of *metF*, the *E. coli* structural gene for 5,10-methylenetetrahydrofolate reductase and of its control region. *Nucleic Acids Res* 1983; 11: 6723–32.

47. Sevrioukova, IF, Li, H, Zhang, H, Peterson, JA, Poulos, TL. Structure of a cytochrome P450-redox partner electron transfer complex. *Proc Natl Acad Sci USA* 1999; 96: 1863–68.

48. Sheppard, CA, Trimmer, EE, Matthews, RG. Purification and properties of NADH-dependent 5,10-methylenetetrahydrofolate reductase (MetF) from *Escherichia coli*. *J Bacteriol* 1999; 181: 718–25.

49. Smith, AE, Matthews, RG. Dihydropteroate synthase as a model for the methyltetrahydrofolate binding region of cobalamin-dependent methionine synthase. *FASEB J* 1999; 13: A1527 (#1121).

50. Sumner, J, Jencks, DA, Khani, S, Matthews, RG. Photoaffinity labeling of methylenetetrahydrofolate reductase with 8-azido-S-adenosylmethionine. *J Biol Chem* 1986; 261: 7697–700.

51. Sumner, JS. Structural and mechanistic properties of methylenetetrahydrofolate reductase and their functional implications. PhD. thesis, University of Michigan, 1992; p. 118.

52. Sumner, JS, Matthews, RG. Stereochemistry and mechanism of hydrogen transfer between NADPH and methylenetetrahydrofolate in the reaction catalyzed by methylenetetrahydrofolate reductase from pig liver. *J Am Chem Soc* 1992; 114: 6949–56.

53. van der Put, N, Steegers-Theunissen, RPM, Frosst, P, Trijbels, FJM, Eskes, TKAB, van den Heuvel, LPWJ, Marinien, ECM, den Heyer, M, Rozen, R, Blom, HJ. Mutated methylenetetrahydrofolate reductase as a risk factor for spina bifida. *Lancet* 1995; 346: 1070–71.

54. van der Put, NM, van der Molen, EF, Kluijtmans, LA, Heil, SG, Trijbels, JM, Eskes, TKAB, Van Oppenraaij-Emmerzaal, D, Banerjee, R, Blom, HJ. Sequence analysis of the coding region of human methionine synthase: Relevance to hyperhomocysteineaemia in neural-tube defects and vascular disease. *Q J Med* 1997; 90: 511–17.

55. Wang, M, Roberts, DL, Paschke, R, Shea, TM, Masters, BSS, Kim, J-JP. Three-dimensional structure of NADPH-cytochrome P450 reductase: Prototype for FMN- and FAD-containing enzymes. *Proc Natl Acad Sci USA* 1997; 94: 8411–16.

56. Wilcken, DE, Wang, XL, Sim, AS, McCredie, RM. Distribution in healthy and coronary populations of the methylenetetrahydrofolate reductase (MTHFR) C677T mutation. *Arterioscler Thromb Vasc Biol* 1996; 16: 878–82.

11

Folate Metabolism

ROBERT J. COOK

Folate is the term used to describe a group of compounds derived from 5,6,7,8-tetrahydropteroyl-glutamate or more commonly referred to as tetrahydrofolate (THF). THF is the central compound to which one-carbon (1-C) units may be added, converted to various oxidation levels, and donated to acceptor molecules or oxidized to CO_2. The biological role of folate is to facilitate the essential cellular metabolism of methionine, serine, glycine, choline,

and histidine, the biosynthesis of purines and 5′-deoxythymidylate (dTMP), and the assimilation or oxidation of formate. When the term folate is used in this chapter it is implied that it is a naturally occurring polyglutamate, unless otherwise stated. Over the past few years several excellent reviews have been published which deal with various aspects of folate metabolism and enzymology (60, 109, 115, 140, 141). For the most part, this chapter provides an overview of mammalian hepatic folate metabolism. Recent efforts have focused on the compartmentalization of folate between the cytosol and mitochondria. This has led to a reappraisal of the roles that some of the folate-dependent enzymes in these two compartments play in the supply and metabolism of 1-C units.

Chemistry

THF is made up of a 2-amino-4-hydroxy pteridine ring system that is linked by a methylene bridge from the C-6 position of the pyrazine ring to *p*-aminobenzoic acid to form tetrahydropteroic acid (Figure 11.1). The pyrazine ring is fully reduced at the 5, 6, 7, and 8 positions in 5,6,7,8-tetrahydropteroyl-γ-glutamate. Reduction of the 7 and 8 positions gives dihydrofolate. In the designation of polyglutamate forms, the use of $H_4PteGlu_n$, where n = 2 to 11, clearly states the number of glutamate residues; however, in this chapter THF is used and when required, the polyglutamate chain length is specified.

Fig. 11.1.   Structure of (6S)-5,6,7,8-tetrahydrofolate (THF).

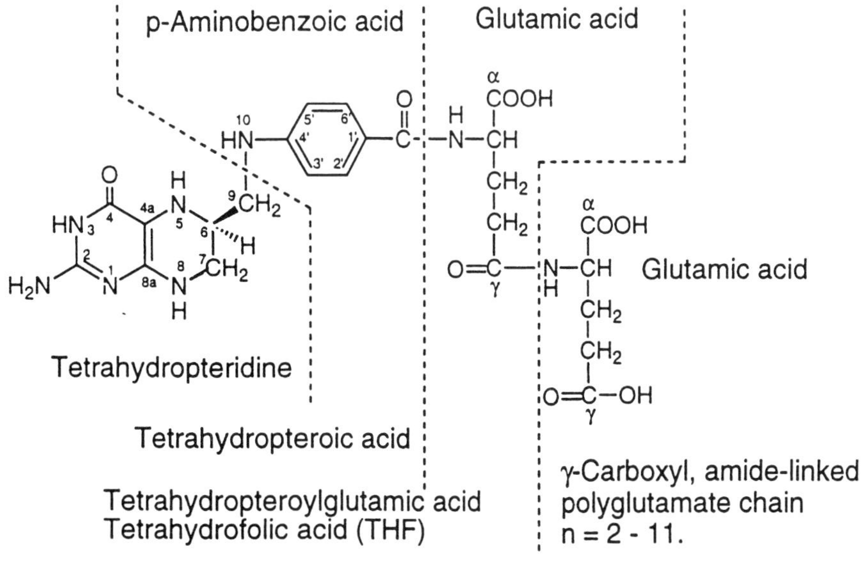

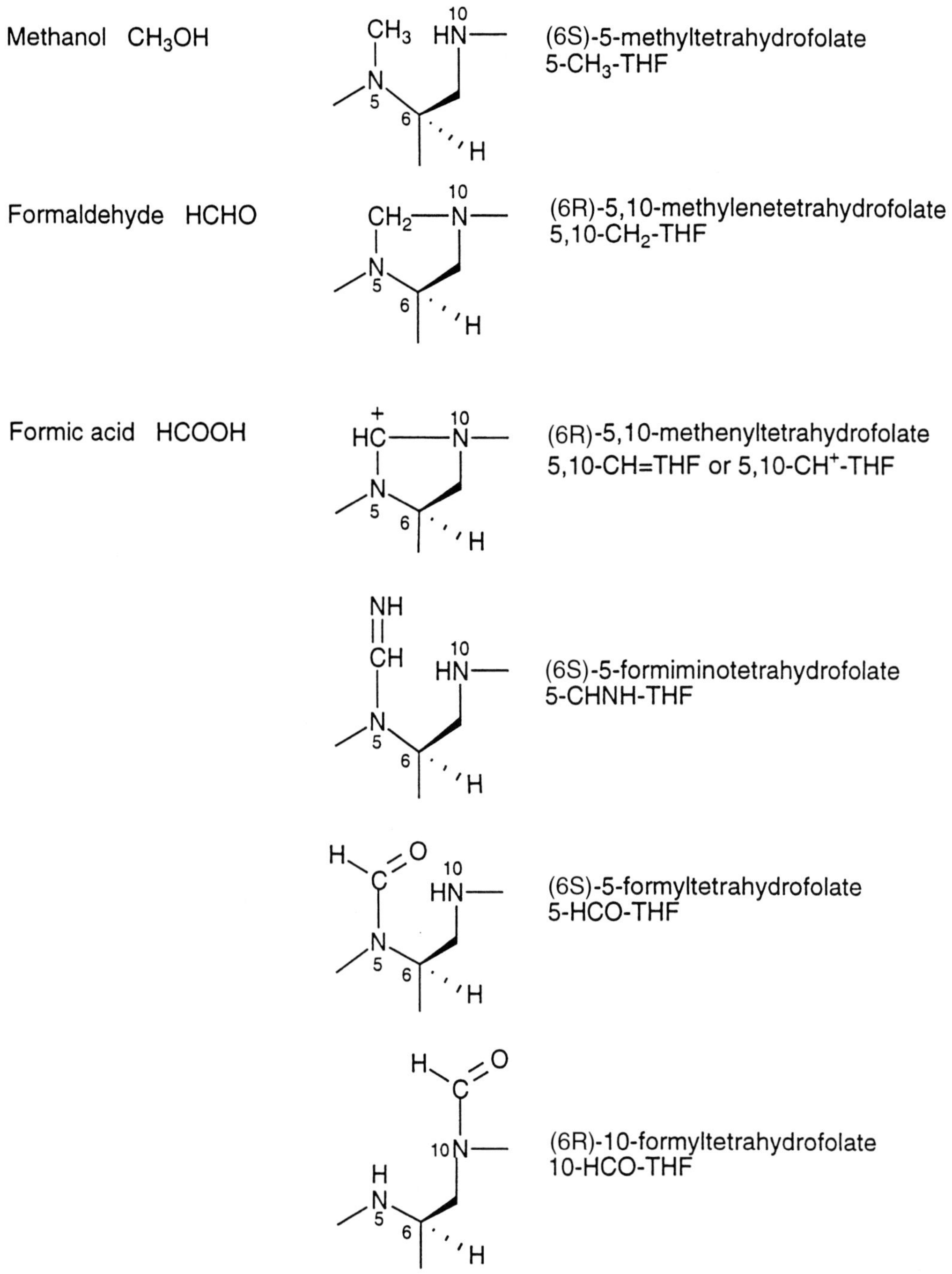

Methanol CH_3OH

(6S)-5-methyltetrahydrofolate
5-CH_3-THF

Formaldehyde HCHO

(6R)-5,10-methylenetetrahydrofolate
5,10-CH_2-THF

Formic acid HCOOH

(6R)-5,10-methenyltetrahydrofolate
5,10-CH=THF or 5,10-CH^+-THF

(6S)-5-formiminotetrahydrofolate
5-CHNH-THF

(6S)-5-formyltetrahydrofolate
5-HCO-THF

(6R)-10-formyltetrahydrofolate
10-HCO-THF

Fig. 11.2. Oxidation states of folate one-carbon substituents.

THF has an asymmetrical center at C-6 of the pyrazine ring. The physiologically active form of THF has the (6S) configuration, as do the forms with adducts at the N-5 position (Figure 11.2). Adducts attached to the N-10 position have a (6R) configuration, even though the absolute configuration has not changed. Thus, (6S)-THF and (6R)-10-HCO-THF have the same configuration at C-6 (109, 139). The

oxidation states of the 1-C adducts range from the most reduced (5-methylTHF) to the intermediate level (methyleneTHF) to the most oxidized methenyl, formimino and formylTHF derivatives. The oxidation levels differ from each other by the addition (reduction) or loss (oxidation) of two electrons for each state. One-carbon units at the fully oxidized formate level or at the formaldehyde level may be added to THF at either the N-5 or N-10 positions or as a bridge between the N-5 and N-10 positions (Figure 11.2). In vivo 5- and 10-formylTHF derivatives can be converted to 5,10-methenylTHF, 5,10-methyleneTHF and, in an irreversible step (48), to 5-methylTHF. 5-MethylTHF is recycled to THF by cobalamin-dependent methionine synthase. 10-FormylTHF can also be converted to CO_2 in an ultimate oxidation step, which recycles THF and eliminates excess 1-C units. The currently known enzymatic interconversions of the various folate forms in liver cytosol and mitochondria are shown in Figure 11.3.

Folates are unstable and require antioxidants such as 2-mercaptoethanol, ascorbate, or dithiothreitol when chemically or enzymatically synthesized, when used in enzyme assays, or when extracted and assayed from tissues. THF and 10-formylTHF are especially unstable, whereas those forms with adducts at the N-5 position are much more stable to air oxidation, although 5-formiminoTHF is readily hydrolyzed by water (139). Fully oxidized folic acid essentially does not exist in nature except under rare circumstances where THF and dihydrofolate oxidize under conditions that do not result in the cleavage of the C-9 – N-10 bridge. Folic acid itself is relatively stable and is used as a dietary supplement (37). Folic acid is assimilated into the reduced folate pool by sequential reduction to dihydrofolate and THF by dihydrofolate reductase (Figure 11.3, Reaction 11).

Polyglutamates

Naturally occurring folates exist as polyglutamate derivatives with an extended γ-amide (γ-carboxyl) linked glutamate side chain. THF in Figure 11.1 has one glutamate residue attached to the p-aminobenzoate; addition of a second γ-linked glutamate yields a diglutamate and this may continue up to 10 or 11 glutamate residues. The length of the polyglutamate side chain varies in mammalian species, with five to eight glutamate residues predominating. Folylpoly-γ-glutamate synthetase (FPGS) catalyzes the adenosine triphosphate (ATP) Mg^{2+} and K^+-dependent γ-amide linkage of glutamate residues to folate (116). The preferred substrates for the enzyme are THF and 10-formylTHF; folic acid, 5-formylTHF, and 5-methylTHF are very poor substrates (3, 116). Folate polyglutamates are the preferred form in 1-C metabolism, and most of the enzymes that use folates show distinctly higher affinities for the polyglutamate forms (116).

Polyglutamates are not transported across cellular membranes, which ensures their cellular retention (66, 116). There also appears to be no transport of polyglutamates from the cytosol into the mitochondrial matrix during short-term studies (58, 65), although there is a specific transport system for reduced folate monoglutamates in rat liver mitochondria (57).

Cytosolic and mitochondrial forms of FPGS are encoded by a single nuclear gene. Exon 1 of the human FPGS gene contains two ATG start sites 126 bp apart, and alternate transcription start sites generate two forms of mRNA. Translation from the first ATG codon generates the mitochondrial isozyme (mFPGS) with a 42 amino acid mitochondrial leader sequence, and translation from the second ATG codon produces the cytosolic isozyme (cFPGS) (3, 24, 41, 65). Accumulation and retention of folates by the mitochondrial and cytosolic compartments are dependent on the activity of FPGS (66).

The Methyl-Trap Hypothesis

The methyl-trap hypothesis was advanced to explain why cobalamin deficiency often results in a functional folate deficiency (51, 86). The hypothesis postulates that in cobalamin deficiency, the cobalamin-dependent enzyme methionine synthase (Figure 11.3, Reaction 4) is inactive and the enzyme that catalyzes the biosynthesis of 5-methylTHF, 5,10-methyleneTHF reductase (MTHFR; Figure 11.3, Reaction 9) is essentially irreversible in vivo (48). Thus 5-methylTHF is "trapped," as it can neither proceed to THF via methionine synthase nor go back to 5,10-methyleneTHF. Eventually the cell folates become trapped as 5-methylTHF. The trap is reinforced because 5-methylTHF is the predominant form supplied to the cell from the circulation and because 5-methylTHF is a very poor substrate for FPGS (116). Thus polyglutamate synthesis ceases, which limits the pool to monoglutamates that are not effectively retained by the cell. Methionine synthase may be rapidly and specifically inactivated by nitrous oxide, which irreversibly oxidizes the enzyme-cobalamin-cobalt complex (22, 38).

Tissue, Cellular, and Subcellular Distribution of Folate

The current methods for analysis of tissue folates include high-performance liquid chromatography (HPLC) coupled to microbiological assays (12, 53, 55, 76), HPLC and spectral analysis (5, 114), enzymatic interconversion (19, 108), and gas chromatography-mass spectrometry (103). A major problem of folate analysis is that one method alone will not determine all the possible folate forms. The most problematic determinations are for 5-formylTHF and 10-formylTHF that interconvert under acidic extraction conditions and THF and 5,10-methyleneTHF, which rapidly interconvert at physiological pH.

A 200 g rat fed a diet containing 1 mg folic acid/kg diet had a whole body folate load of 93 μg (25). Liver

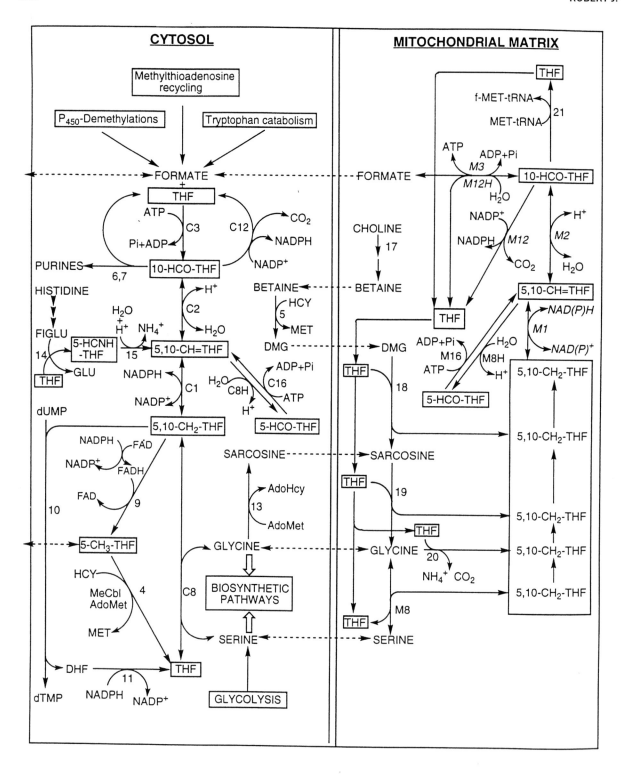

accounted for 36% of total body folate while kidney, gut, red blood cells, and testes contained 6%, 6%, 4%, and 1%, respectively. Rat pancreas contained between 4 and 5 nmol folate/g tissue (56), which is approximately 30% of the level in liver (52, 58) on a per gram basis. Rat brain had approximately 1 nmol/g tissue or 5% compared with liver on a per gram basis (52). In humans the whole body content of folate has been esti-

mated at between 20 and 70 mg (48a, 124), with approximately 50% in the liver (51).

Folates have been extensively studied in liver because the liver contains the highest percentage of body folate, and the levels of the folate-dependent enzymes are high. Studies in mice (18, 134), rats (144), and guinea pigs (34) showed that folate was present primarily in the cytosol and mitochondria, although

Fig. 11.3. Compartmentalization of liver folate-mediated 1-C metabolism. An idealized metabolic scheme that illustrates the interconversion of folates (polyglutamates) and the compartmentalization of folate-dependent enzymes between the cytosol and mitochondrial matrix. The letters C and M refer to cytosolic and mitochondrial isozymes. Italicized numbers refer to mitochondrial enzyme activities that have been identified but are yet to be purified and fully characterized. Included in parentheses is the abbreviation, EC number and coabstrates/coenzymes required for the reaction. The numbers refer to the following enzymatic reactions: C1:*M1*, 5,10-methyleneTHF dehydrogenase (EC 1.5.1.5; NADP); C2:*M2*, 5,10-methenylTHF cyclohydrolase (EC 3.5.4.9); C3:*M3*, 10-formylTHF synthetase (EC 6.3.4.3); 4, methionine synthase (EC 2.1.1.3; MeCbl-AdoMet); 5, betaine:homocysteine methyltransferase (BHMT; E.C. 2.1.1.5); 6, glycinamide ribonucleotide transformylase (EC 2.1.2.2); 7, phosphoribosylamino-imidazole carboxamide transformylase (EC 2.1.2.3); C8:*M8*, serine hydroxymethyltransferase (SHMT; EC 2.1.2.1; PLP); C8H:M8H, the hydrolytic activity of C8:M8; 9, 5,10-methyleneTHF reductase (MTHFR; EC 1.1.99.15; FAD, NADP); 10, thymidylate synthase (EC 2.1.1.45); 11, dihydrofolate reductase (EC1.5.1.3; NADP); C12:*M12*, 10-formylTHF dehydrogenase (FDH; EC 1.5.1.6; NADP); *M12H*, the hydrolytic activity of *M12*, 13, glycine N-methyltransferase (GNMT; EC 2.1.1.20); 14, glutamate formiminotransferase (EC 2.1.2.5); 15, 5-formiminoTHF cyclodeaminase (EC 4.3.1.4); C16:M16, 5,10-methenylTHF synthetase (MTHFS; E.C. 6.3.3.2); 17, choline dehydrogenase (E.C. 1.1.99.1; FAD); 18, dimethylglycine dehydrogenase (EC 1.5.99.2; FAD); 19, sarcosine dehydrogenase (EC 1.5.99.1: FAD); 20, glycine cleavage system (GCS; EC 2.1.2.10; PLP, NAD, FAD); 21, methionyl t-RNA formyltransferase (EC 2.1.2.9). Enzymes 1, 2, and 3 are the three activities associated with the trifunctional C1-THF synthase. Enzymes 14 and 15 form a bifunctional enzyme. Folate abbreviations are as given in Figure 11.2, and are polyglutamates. Other abbreviations are DHF, dihydrofolate; DMG, dimethylglycine; FIGLU, formiminoglutamate; HCY, homocysteine; MET, methionine; f-MET, formyl-methionine; AdoMet, *S*-adenosylmethionine; AdoHcy, *S*-adenosylhomocysteine. The dashed arrows represent transport between the cytosol and the mitochondrion; those to 5-methylTHF and formate represent the transport in and out of the hepatocyte.

some short-term assimilation studies have noted that labeled folate was associated with fractions that contained plasma membrane fragments (26, 156). Time course studies of the assimilation and distribution of [3H]folic acid and [14C]folic acid into the folate pools of rat liver confirmed partition of the label equally between the cytosol and mitochondria (26, 156). Folate in these two pools was bound to high-molecular-weight proteins (156). In the cytosol, they were designated folate binding proteins I and II (FBP-CI and FBP-CII, respectively). Each protein bound reduced polyglutamates, and FBP-CII contained 5-methylTHF. Mitochondria contained a 90 kDa protein that bound an unidentified reduced folate polyglutamate (156). Folate in mitochondria was associated mainly with the inner membrane (28%) and the soluble matrix (52%)

(26). The folates remained bound to these cytosolic and mitochondrial proteins during gel filtration chromatography, indicating very tight binding (26, 156).

Hepatic Cytosolic Folate Binding Proteins

FBP-CI and FBP-CII bind approximately 60% and 25%, respectively, of the rat liver cytosolic folate pool (Cook and Wagner, unpublished results), which leaves approximately 15% of the cytosolic folate unbound. FBP-CI was purified as a dimer with a native mass of 200 kDa. It was composed of two identical subunits of 100 kDa, which contained tightly bound THF-pentaglutamate (33). FBP-CI was identified as $NADP^+$-dependent 10-formylTHF dehydrogenase (83) (Figure 11.3; Reaction C12). THF was a potent inhibitor of 10-formylTHF dehydrogenase (63, 83, 102, 113), and it was suggested that oxidation of 1-C units may be regulated by tight binding of THF to 10-formylTHF dehydrogenase and by the ratio of 10-formylTHF to THF levels in liver cytosol (83). THF was able to bind to a second, noncatalytic tight binding site in 10-formylTHF dehydrogenase and occupation of the second site did not alter catalytic activity (43). This would suggest that the second site is not an allosteric regulatory site but rather a possible storage site for THF (43). In the absence of $NADP^+$, 10-formylTHF dehydrogenase catalyzed the hydrolytic cleavage of 10-formylTHF to formate and THF (63, 83, 102, 113). In pig liver the enzyme's dehydrogenase and hydrolase reactions occurred simultaneously, indicating two reaction sites (102). If the hydrolase activity was coupled to 10-formylTHF synthetase, it could set up a futile cycle of 10-formylTHF synthesis/hydrolysis at the expense of cytosolic ATP. 10-formylTHF dehydrogenase hydrolase activity is strictly dependent on the presence of 2-mercaptoethanol in the assay system, indicating this reaction is probably nonphysiological (30, 106).

Rat liver FBP-CII has a native mass of 150 kDa, is composed of four identical 34 kDa subunits, contains 5-methylTHF pentaglutamate (133), and is abundant in rat liver and pancreas, representing 1% to 2% of the cytosolic protein (14, 32, 151). FBP-CII was identified as glycine N-methyltransferase (Figure 11.3, Reaction 13) and the tightly bound 5-methylTHF-pentaglutamate inhibits the reaction catalyzed by glycine N-methyltransferase (31, 142). The proposed function of glycine N-methyltransferase is to regulate the cytosolic AdoMet pool and to control the AdoMet AdoHcy ratio. Although glycine N-methyltransferase is not a folate-dependent enzyme, it is regulated by folate, and its activity links folate-dependent de novo methyl group synthesis, via MTHFR and methionine synthase, to AdoMet-dependent, methyl group metabolism (140, 142).

Hepatic Mitochondrial Folate Binding Proteins

In rat liver mitochondria, approximately 35% of the folate was bound to two proteins (26) that were identified as dimethylglycine dehydrogenase and sarcosine dehydrogenase (Figure 11.3, Reactions 18 and 19) (27, 28, 148, 149). These proteins represent approximately 1% each of the soluble protein in rat liver mitochondrial matrix (29). Analyses of enzyme activity in the presence or absence of bound THF monoglutamate showed that the folate had no effect on the rate of either reaction (101).

Subcellular Folate Pool Compositions

Horne and co-workers (58) showed that the compositions of the folate pool compositions in rat liver cytosol and mitochondria were distinctly different (Table 11.1A). The cytosol contained most of the 5-methylTHF, whereas the majority of folate in rat liver mitochondria was THF and 10-formylTHF. When rats are exposed to nitrous oxide, which specifically inactivates methionine synthase, the composition of the cytosolic folate pool dramatically shifted to 5-methylTHF (from 44.6% to 84%) at the expense of THF and 5- and 10-formylTHF (Table 11.1B). This was a convincing demonstration of the methyl trap hypothesis, as described previously. Nitrous oxide treatment had no effect on the mitochondrial folates, which strongly suggested that there is little if any transport of free folate polyglutamates between the cytosol and the mitochondria, at least over the 18 hours of the experiment.

Carl et al. (16) reported similar results for rat liver subcellular folate pool distribution, including the polyglutamate chain lengths. Folate pool compositions have also been determined for the cytosol and mitochondria of rat pancreas (56) and rat brain (17) (Table 11.2). 5-MethylTHF was relatively abundant in pancreas cytosol, which might reflect rapid methio-

Table 11.1B. Subcellular Distribution of Folates in Rat Liver After Exposure to Nitrous Oxide (N_2O)[a]

	N_2O Cytosol		N_2O Mitochondria		N_2O Total Pool (Cyto+Mito)	
	nmol/g[b]	%[c]	nmol/g	%	nmol/g	%
10-FTHF[d]	0.87	9.1	2.93	34.7	3.80	21.0
THF	0.45	4.7	4.02	47.6	4.47	24.8
5-FTHF[e]	0.20	2.0	0.92	10.9	1.12	6.2
5-MTHF[f]	8.09	84.2	0.58	6.8	8.67	48.0
Total	9.61	100%	8.45	100%	18.06	100%

[a] Data adapted from Horne et al. (58). Rats were exposed to normal air or an atmosphere containing 80% nitrous oxide/20% oxygen overnight for 18 hours before analyzing the folate pools.
[b] nmol/g liver (wet wt.)
[c] % of the pool.
[d] 10-FTHF is 10-formylTHF
[e] 5-FTHF is 5-formylTHF
[f] 5-MTHF is 5-methylTHF

nine synthesis for the provision of AdoMet-donated methyl groups required for zymogen granule secretion (6, 7). It is also probable that much of the 5-methylTHF is bound to glycine-N-methyltransferase in the pancreas (151). These results illustrate the differences in folate pool compositions in these organs and provide a snapshot of the cytosolic and mitochondrial pools. However, few conclusions can be drawn concerning the 1-C metabolism until there is a catalog of the folate-dependent enzymes present and information about the flux of 1-C units through the various pathways. This problem was clearly demonstrated by Schalinske and Steele (104), who showed that hepatic folate pool sizes and 10-formylTHF dehydrogenase activity (Figure 11.3, Reaction C12) were significantly decreased in hyperthyroidism and by dietary folate restriction. However, the metabolic flux of [2-^{14}C] L-histidine, as measured by oxidation to $^{14}CO_2$ by 10-formylTHF dehydrogenase, was increased threefold in hyperthyroid rats and twofold in folate-restricted rats. Thus, making metabolic predictions based on enzyme activities and folate pools is risky, unless the 1-C flux is also determined.

In summary, the liver is the main organ for the accumulation and interconversion of folates and the main site for folate-dependent enzymes. Folate in rat liver, pancreas, and brain is found almost exclusively in the cytosol and mitochondria. The folate pool compositions of the cytosolic and mitochondrial fractions from various tissues (Tables 11.1 and 11.2) are very different and probably reflect different folate-dependent 1-C metabolic activities.

Table 11.1A. Subcellular Distribution of Folates in Rat Liver[a]

	Cytosol		Mitochondria		Total Pool (Cyto+Mito)	
	nmol/g[b]	%[c]	nmol/g	%	nmol/g	%
10-FTHF[d]	1.99	19.3	2.57	33.1	4.56	25.3
THF	2.82	27.4	3.73	48.1	6.55	36.3
5-FTHF[e]	0.90	8.7	0.89	11.5	1.79	9.9
5-MTHF[f]	4.58	44.6	0.57	7.3	5.15	28.5
Total	10.29	100%	7.76	100%	18.05	100%

Table 11.2. Subcellular Distribution of Folates in Rat Pancreas[a] and Brain[b]

	Pancreas		Brain	
	Cytosol	Mitochondria	Cytosol	Mitochondria
	%[c]	%	%	%
10-FTHF[d]	9	9	9[e]	48
THF	54	60	28	41
DHF	nd[f]	nd	3	2
5-FTHF[g]	6	22	—	—
5-MTHF[h]	31	9	60	9
Total pool[i]	68	32	60	40

[a] Data adapted from Horne et al. (58).
[b] Data adapted from Carl et al. (17).
[c] Data from the two articles have been converted to % of the pools.
[d] 10-FTHF is 10-formylTHF.
[e] The method used does not distinguish between 10-FTHF and 5-FTHF. The value for 10-FTHF includes 5-FTHF.
[f] Not detected.
[g] 5-FTHF is 5-formylTHF.
[h] 5-MTHF is 5-methylTHF.
[i] Represents the % of the total in each compartment.

Serine and Glycine Metabolism

An outline of serine, glycine, and methionine metabolism is given in Figure 11.4. All three amino acids are essential for protein synthesis, but it is their other functions in supplying starting compounds for biosynthetic pathways, 1-C units, and methyl groups that is of interest.

Serine and glycine are both dispensable amino acids. Serine is derived from the diet and from glycolysis via 3-phosphoglycerate and provides much of the glycine requirement via the action of serine hydroxymethyltransferase (71, 107). Serine is also a major contributor to phospholipid, sphingolipid, and cysteine synthesis. In mammals there is a tremendous demand for glycine and thus serine for intermediary metabolism and biosynthetic pathways. Glycine is a major constituent of collagen and is the precursor of several major hepatic biosynthetic pathways, including purines, porphyrins (heme), creatine, glutathione, and bile acids. In the course of supplying glycine from serine via serine hydroxymethyltransferase, a 1-C unit is formed (5,10-methyleneTHF), which is then available for methionine, dTMP, and purine synthesis, or it may be oxidized to CO_2 via 10-formylTHF. The glycine cleavage system, which is found exclusively in mitochondria of certain tissues including liver and kidney (154), cleaves glycine to CO_2, NH_4^+, and 5,10-methyleneTHF. The latter can either be recycled through the 1-C pool or oxidized to CO_2. Thus even in catabolism, glycine conserves 1-C units. Under normal conditions, the supply of glycine must be carefully regulated, probably by the action of the glycine cleavage

system (89). Mutations of the glycine cleavage system in humans result in nonketotic hyperglycinemia, a devastating inherited disease that results in the massive overproduction of glycine (87), suggesting that the glycine cleavage system is the primary regulator of glycine levels.

Mammals are unable to synthesize the carbon–sulfur bond at carbon 4 in methionine, making it an essential amino acid that must be supplied from the diet. Methionine is usually one of the limiting amino acids in the dietary supply of protein and as such has to be efficiently assimilated and recycled. The major role of methionine, apart from protein synthesis, is the supply of methyl groups, via S-adenosylmethionine (AdoMet) to a multitude of substrates ranging from glycine and other small molecules to proteins, RNA, and DNA, in essential cellular methylation reactions (140). The assimilation of methionine into intermediary metabolism proceeds by the synthesis of AdoMet (see Figure 11.4). AdoMet may also be decarboxylated to give adenosylmethylthio-propylamine, which then donates the propylamine moiety, the three-carbon skeleton of methionine without the methylthiol group, to polyamine synthesis. The resulting methylthiol-compound is methylthioadenosine, which is recycled back to methionine (4, 40). Mammals are efficient at recycling the carbon skeleton of methionine, either as homocysteine (105) or methylthioadenosine (40). The contributions of the betaine:homocysteine methyltransferase reaction are discussed in Chapter 13. The contributions of the methylthioadenosine salvage pathway to methionine recycling are not known (40). The betaine:homocysteine methyltransferase reaction is dependent on the degradation of choline and the availability of homocysteine, whereas the methylthioadenosine pathway depends on the production of polyamines from AdoMet. However, both are ultimately dependent on the supply of methionine in the diet for their precursors because there is no net synthesis of methionine, only a recycling of the carbon-sulfur moiety.

Built into this scheme are two reactions that link 1-C metabolism with methyl group metabolism. These two steps provide regulatory points that control the synthesis of de novo methyl groups from the 1-C pool and the use of methionine as AdoMet. AdoMet binds to a specific regulatory domain on MTHFR and

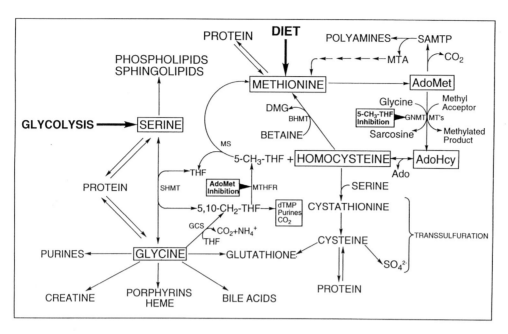

Fig. 11.4. Metabolic interconversions and products of serine, glycine, and methionine. An abbreviated scheme showing the interconversion of serine and glycine and the connection to the methionine cycle. One-carbon units (5,10-CH_2-THF) are generated from the conversion of serine to glycine by serine hydroxymethyltransferase (SHMT) and from the oxidation of glycine by the glycine cleavage system (GCS). These are used for purine and dTMP synthesis or oxidized to CO_2. 5,10-CH_2-THF is reduced by 5,10-methyleneTHF reductase (MTHFR) for the subsequent remethylation of homocysteine by methionine synthase (MS). Homocysteine can also be remethylated to methionine by betaine:homocysteine methyltransferase (BHMT), or it can be directed to the transsulfuration pathway for the production of cysteine and further catabolized to sulfate. Methionine is either used for protein synthesis or converted to AdoMet, which is the primary methyl donor for a multitude of methyltransferase reactions (MTs) and glycine N-methyltransferase (GNMT). AdoHcy is hydrolyzed to homocysteine and adenosine (Ado). AdoMet may also be decarboxylated to S-adenosylmethylthiopropylamine (SAMTP), which donates the propylamine moiety to polyamine biosynthesis and recycles methylthioadenosine (MTA) to methionine.

inhibits enzyme activity (73). Under conditions of adequate dietary methionine supply, AdoMet controls the production of 5-methylTHF by MTHFR and hence the supply of methionine. The level of AdoMet in the liver is regulated by glycine N-methyltransferase (Figure 11.3; Reaction 13), which catalyzes the nonessential, AdoMet-dependent methylation of glycine to sarcosine and AdoHcy (88). Sarcosine is a choline catabolite that has no known metabolic function; it is transported into the mitochondria and converted back to glycine plus 5,10-methyleneTHF by sarcosine dehydrogenase (Figure 11.3, Reaction 19).

These two reactions regulate the cytosolic AdoMet levels while conserving the methyl group as a folate-linked 1-C unit. This reaction was demonstrated in vivo using methionine deuterated in the methyl group and following the production of sarcosine in anesthetized rats (68, 69). The end result is that AdoMet and AdoHcy levels are maintained at a constant ratio, which also regulates all the other biologically important methylation reactions (140). The activity of glycine N-methyltransferase is regulated by 5-methylTHF, which binds tightly to this enzyme and inhibits glycine methylation (142). Under conditions in which dietary methionine is inadequate, AdoMet levels decline and there is decreased inhibition of MTHFR, allowing an increase in the production of 5-methylTHF. Thus homocysteine will be recycled via methionine synthase (Figure 11.3, Reaction 4) to fill the methionine requirement for protein synthesis and methylation. The increased 5-methylTHF pool will also inhibit the activity of glycine N-methyltransferase, thus conserving AdoMet for essential methylation reactions (142). Thus there is a reciprocal regulation of 1-C and methyl group metabolism by AdoMet and 5-methylTHF.

Folate Polyglutamates in the Regulation of 1-C Metabolism

Chinese hamster ovary (CHO) AUXB1 cells have very low folate pools, are auxotrophic for glycine, purines, and thymidine, and have no FPGS activity (90, 135). Shane and co-workers, in a series of elegant studies, showed that CHO-AUXB1 cells, transfected with a mammalian expression vector containing human FPGS cDNA (AUX-*human*), accumulated normal folate pools in both cytosolic and mitochondrial compartments and were no longer dependent on glycine, purines, or thymidine (65). Similar results were obtained for the transfection of *E. coli* FPGS (AUX-*coli*), which was expressed exclusively in the cytosol and only synthesized triglutamates; however, in this instance the glycine auxotrophy was not abolished (65). AUX-*coli* had normal cytosolic folate pools, albeit only at the triglutamate level, but very low folate monoglutamate pools in the mitochondria, indicating that the supply of glycine in CHO cells was dependent on mitochondrial folate polyglutamates. Construction of AUX-*coli* with a mammalian mitochondrial leader sequence resulted in the expression of a mitochondrial form of *E. coli* FPGS in AUX-m*coli* cells, accumulation of mitochondrial folate triglutamates, and glycine independence (67). An interesting observation made for the AUX-m*coli* cells was that despite having expressed *E. coli* FPGS only in the mitochondrial compartment, the cytosol contained triglutamate folate pools. A similar result was reported when AUX-*human* cells expressed only mFPGS (45). In this case the cells were not dependent on glycine, purines, or dTMP, although the cytosolic folate pool was much smaller than that seen in AUX-m*coli* cells, suggesting the longer polyglutamates synthesized by human mFPGS exit the mitochondria more slowly.

These results indicate that although folate polyglutamates are unable to enter the mitochondria from the cytosol, they are able to exit mitochondria. Thus folate polyglutamates in both the cytosolic and mitochondrial compartments are required for CHO cells to grow without exogenous glycine, purines, or dTMP. It should be noted that the glycine auxotrophy was not abolished until a normal mitochondrial folate polyglutamate pool was restored and that purine and dTMP independence were restored with very low cytosolic folate pools (66). It is apparent that polyglutamates are required for folate 1-C metabolism, especially for accumulation in mitochondria and that glycine in CHO cells appears to be supplied primarily from the mitochondrial compartment.

Hepatic Folate–Dependent 1-C Metabolism

Most of the known reactions involving folate mediated 1-C metabolism are shown in Figure 11.3. The exceptions are the reduction of folic acid to dihydrofolate and THF (Figure 11.3, Reaction 11) and folate polyglutamation. All the enzymes in the scheme, with the exception of those italicized in the mitochondria, have been cloned from mammalian sources, and their sequences may be accessed through the National Center for Biotechnology Information (http://www3. ncbi.nlm.nih.gov/Entrez/). Nuclear genes encode all these enzymes.

This complex series of reactions takes place in two subcellular compartments and must be carefully regulated to supply methionine, serine, glycine, purines, and dTMP to the cell and to oxidize excess 1-C units. Perturbations of any of these reactions may result in the restriction or oversupply of any of the products, for example, increased homocysteine.

Cytosolic Folate Metabolism

Folate metabolism in the cytosol is represented as three interconnected cycles shown in Figure 11.3. Two of the cycles start from 5,10-methyleneTHF and produce methionine (Reactions 9 and 4) and dTMP (Reaction 10), and the third uses 10-formylTHF for the biosynthesis of purines (Reactions 6 and 7). All three cycles donate a 1-C unit to a biosynthetic reaction and return THF to the pool for addition of another 1-C unit from three sources: (1) serine via cytosolic serine hydroxymethyltransferase (as 5,10-methyleneTHF (Reaction C8); (2) formate from mitochondria, and cytosolic sources as 10-formylTHF (Reaction C3); and (3) carbon 2 of histidine via formiminoglutamic acid as 5,10-methenylTHF (Reactions 14 and 15).

The bifunctional domain of cytosolic C1-THF synthase (Reactions C2 and C3) catalyzes the reversible oxidation/reduction and cyclohydrolase reactions, which interconvert 10-formylTHF, 5,10-methenylTHF, and 5,10-methyleneTHF. This enzyme links the three biosynthetic cycles and the oxidation reaction that removes excess 1-C units from 10-formylTHF as CO_2 (Reaction C12).

5-MethylTHF monoglutamate is the primary form supplied to the tissues after the absorption of dietary folate. The reduced folate carrier transports 5-methylTHF into the liver (54) where it enters the folate pool by conversion to THF catalyzed by methionine synthase (Reaction 4). This appears to be the obligatory step in the assimilation of exogenous folate. 5-MethylTHF is a very poor substrate for folate polyglutamate synthesis (116), so it must be converted to THF for synthesis of polyglutamate forms, which are retained by cells. THF is the form that accepts 1-C units, which are thought to be generated primarily from serine by cytosolic serine hydroxymethyltransferase (Reaction C8) to produce 5,10-methyleneTHF and glycine (107, 111). 5,10-MethyleneTHF is poised at the mid-point on the oxidation scale of 1-C units and has four possible fates:

1. Reduction to 5-methylTHF in an irreversible reaction catalyzed by MTHFR (Reaction 9), which commits the 1-C unit to methionine biosynthesis and the recycling of homocysteine (48) (see Chapter 12).

2. Transfer and reduction of the methylene group in the addition of a methyl group to deoxyuridylate to produce dTMP, which is catalyzed by thymidylate synthase (Reaction 10). This is an unusual reaction, in that the 1-C unit is initially at the formaldehyde oxidation level and is reduced to the methanol level during the reaction by the reducing power of the tetrahydropyrazine ring. The product of this reaction is dihydrofolate, which is reduced to THF by dihydrofolate reductase (Reaction 11). For efficient folate metabolism, both thymidylate synthase and dihydrofolate reductase must act in a coordinated manner. Adult liver contains very low levels of thymidylate synthase activity; however, higher levels are found in rapidly growing or regenerating tissue (143).

3. Oxidation to 5,10-methenylTHF and then hydrolysis to 10-formylTHF by the sequential actions of 5,10-methylene dehydrogenase and 5,10-methenyl cyclohydrolase (Reactions C1, C2). These two activities reside in the amino terminal domain of C1-THF synthase (71). 10-FormylTHF is used for the synthesis of purines (Reactions 6 and 7) where two reactions, glycinamide ribonucleotide transformylase and phosphoribosylaminoimidazole carboxamide transformylase, add two formyl groups at positions C8 and C2, respectively, during synthesis of the purine ring system.

4. 10-FormylTHF derived from the oxidation of 5,10-methyleneTHF can be oxidized to CO_2 by 10-formylTHF dehydrogenase (Reaction C12), which eliminates excess 1-C units (61). As discussed earlier, this is a curious enzyme that binds the product of the reaction, THF, very tightly and in so doing probably binds most of the liver cytosolic THF (59).

One-carbon units can also arise directly from formate, a product of a number of catabolic pathways including the methylthioadenosine salvage pathway (4), tryptophan degradation (64), and cytochrome P450 demethylation reactions that produce formaldehyde, which is rapidly oxidized to formate (145). Formate is also produced by mitochondria from serine and sarcosine (8). The plasma levels of formate in humans and mice appear to be approximately 0.3 mmol/L (117, 123). Assimilation of formate into the 1-C pool is catalyzed by 10-formylTHF synthetase (Reaction C3) in an ATP-dependent reaction, which is probably irreversible in the cytosol. The synthetase forms the C-terminal domain of C1-THF synthase. The synthetase and dehydrogenase/cyclohydrolase domains do not appear to work in concert; thus it is possible that this enzyme could generate 10-formylTHF from reactions in both domains at the same time (Reactions C1, C2, and C3). It has been shown in vitro that C1-THF synthase plus cytosolic serine hydroxymethyltransferase can convert THF and formate, in the presence of glycine, to serine (131).

As stated previously, cytosolic serine hydroxymethyltransferase has always been assumed to supply the 1-C units for the biosynthetic cycles (107, 111); however, work with CHO-glyA cells indicates this is not the case (23, 84, 100, 128). Most studies on serine and glycine interconversions were done on cell extracts that contained both the cytosolic and mitochondrial forms (128). However, network thermodynamic modeling suggests that cytosolic serine hydroxymethyltransferase has little or no role in the cytosolic supply of 1-C units in murine leukemia L1210 cells (132). The human cytosolic serine hydroxymethyltransferase gene has been localized to chromosome region 17p11.2 (46), a region deleted in the Smith-Magenis syndrome. Analysis of the cytosolic serine hydroxymethyltransferase levels in lymphoblasts from patients with Smith-Magenis syndrome revealed only 50% activity compared with unaffected parent lymphoblasts; however, serine, glycine, and folate levels from three patients were all within the normal clinical ranges (39). This observation also indicates that cytosolic serine hydroxymethyltransferase might not be important in maintaining 1-C metabolite levels and is consistent with the conclusions for this enzyme in L1210 cells (132).

Mitochondrial Folate Metabolism

The choline degradation pathway that converts choline to glycine (42) is strictly mitochondrial (Figure 11.3), except for cytosolic betaine:homocysteine methyltransferase (Reaction 5). The last two enzymes in this pathway are dimethylglycine dehydrogenase and sarcosine dehydrogenase (Reactions 18 and 19), which are major mitochondrial THF binding proteins (101, 148, 149) that catalyze sequential oxidative demethylation reactions, generating 5,10-methyleneTHF and glycine. This pathway conserves all three of the methyl groups of choline. Sarcosine dehydrogenase also serves to recycle sarcosine formed by the action of cytosolic glycine N-methyltransferase (Reaction 13). A lack of sarcosine dehydrogenase results in sarcosinemia, a benign condition in humans (50, 112). Mitochondrial serine hydroxymethyltransferase (Reaction M8) is encoded by its own nuclear gene and is distinct from the cytosolic form (107). The glycine cleavage system (Reaction 20) is exclusive to mitochondria but is tissue specific (e.g., liver and kidney) (153, 155). All four of these mitochondrial folate-dependent enzymes produce 5,10-methyleneTHF and, with the exception of serine hydroxymethyltransferase, are apparently irreversible in vivo (107, 152). Until recently the recycling of 5,10-methyleneTHF to THF in mitochondria had not been specifically addressed (Cook in Wagner [141]), but was considered to be a function of the synthetic reaction of mitochondrial serine hydroxymethyltransferase, which converts glycine and 5,10-methyleneTHF to serine and THF (111).

Initiation of protein synthesis in mitochondria is dependent on formyl-methionine-tRNA, similar to bacterial protein synthesis (122). Formyl-methionine-tRNA is synthesized from methionine-tRNA and 10-formylTHF by methionyl t-RNA formyltransferase (Reaction 21). The flux of 1-C units through this reaction is not known, but it would not be expected to be sufficient to utilize all the 1-C units that arise in mitochondria. 5-FormylTHF and 10-formylTHF are found in mitochondrial folate pools (Tables 11.1 and 11.2) (52, 56), which, coupled with the fact that folate polyglutamates are not transported into mitochondria (52, 65), indicates that there are enzymes present that are capable of oxidizing 5,10-methyleneTHF to 5,10-methenylTHF and 10-formylTHF. 5-FormylTHF is synthesized during the hydrolysis of 5,10-methenylTHF by mitochondrial serine hydroxymethyltransferase. 5,10-MethenylTHF synthetase (Reaction M16) is present in mitochondria (13) and this could account for the recycling of 5-formylTHF. The identity of some of the other mitochondrial folate-dependent enzymes is less certain than their cytosolic counterparts. The inclusion of the various enzymes that oxidize 5,10-methyleneTHF to 10-formylTHF and then either hydrolyze or oxidize 10-formylTHF is controversial and is discussed later.

Extensive work has been reported on folate enzymes and the metabolism of serine and glycine in various species and CHO cells (23, 35, 135–138, 152–154). Investigations have also been reported for *Saccharomyces cerevisiae*, where a number of mutants have been isolated and the effects on folate metabolism have been analyzed (75, 157). Barlowe and Appling (8) investigated the possibility that rat liver mitochondria could supply 1-C units for use by cytosolic folate-dependent pathways. The results demonstrated that the 3-carbon of serine and the *N*-methyl group of sarcosine were converted to formate in mitochondria and could be assimilated in the cytosol by ATP-dependent, 10-formylTHF synthetase (Reaction C1) to give 10-formylTHF for purine synthesis. The study also demonstrated the presence of all three activities of C1-THF synthase and 10-formylTHF dehydrogenase (Reactions *M1, 2, 3* and *M12*) in rat liver mitochondria.

The presence of these enzymes provides a route for recycling 5,10-methyleneTHF, produced by the previously identified mitochondrial folate-dependent enzymes back to THF (Reactions M8, 18, 19, and 20). Further, it details the folate-dependent enzyme complement of mitochondria required to explain the folate pools present in hepatic mitochondria (Table 11.1) (58).

Figure 11.5 depicts this pathway; NADP$^+$-dependent 5,10-methylene dehydrogenase (Reaction M1) oxidizes 5,10-methyleneTHF to 5,10-methenylTHF, which in turn is hydrolyzed to 10-formylTHF by 5,10-methenylTHF cyclohydrolase (Reaction M2). The conversion of 10-formylTHF to THF and formate is possible by a reversal of 10-formylTHF synthetase (Reaction M3) that would require a high concentration of adenosine diphosphate (ADP) which is present only in mitochondria. Alternatively the hydrolytic activity of a mitochondrial form of 10-formylTHF dehydrogenase might also cleave 10-formylTHF to THF and formate (Reaction M12H).

Mitochondrial NADP$^+$-dependent 10-formylTHF dehydrogenase would also be expected to oxidize 10-formylTHF to CO$_2$ and THF in a similar fashion to the cytosolic 10-formylTHF dehydrogenase (Reaction M12). It was reported that formate rapidly exited the mitochondria, which probably protects the electron transport system from formate inhibition (85). Subsequent studies with isolated rat liver mitochondria showed that carbon three of serine (as L-[3-^{14}C]serine) could be oxidized to ^{14}CO$_2$ or converted to [^{14}C]formate via 10-formylTHF (44).

Inspection of the reactions of 10-formylTHF in mitochondria (Figure 11.5) shows a dependence on ADP (Reaction M3) or NADP$^+$ (Reaction M12). The fate of the 1-C unit was not exclusive to one route or the other in intact mitochondria under the different conditions; rather there was a shift toward oxidation to CO$_2$ or a shift to formate production depending on the conditions. Oxidation of carbon three of serine in sonicated, dialyzed mitochondria showed that an adequate supply of NADP$^+$, ADP, and THF-monoglutamate allowed only oxidation to CO$_2$ consistent with the action of a mitochondrial 10-formylTHF dehydrogenase (44). Alternate routes for the oxidation of carbon three of serine were investigated and ruled out (91).

The three publications by Appling and co-workers were the first to point out the *major* importance of formate as a 1-C donor in mammals and provided an explanation for many previous observations concerning the mitochondrial oxidation of serine and sarcosine to formate and CO$_2$, and the composition of the mitochondrial folate pool (1, 8, 44). Subsequent reports have been published on yeast mitochondrial and cytosolic folate enzymes and their role in 1-C metabolism using specific disruption mutants and nuclear magnetic resonance spectroscopy to track metabolites (2, 77–79, 92–95, 146, 147).

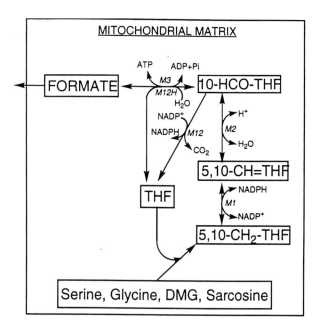

Fig. 11.5. Alternate pathways for the conversion of 1-C units to 10-formylTHF and formate in mitochondria. Conversion of 5,10-methyleneTHF to 10-formylTHF and formate catalyzed by a mitochondrial NADP+-dependent trifunctional C1-THF synthase according to Appling (1). *M1*, 5,10-methyleneTHF dehydrogenase; *M2*, 5,10-methenylTHF cyclohydrolase; *M3*, 10-formylTHF synthetase; *M12*, 10-formylTHF dehydrogenase; *M12H*, the hydrolytic activity of *M12*, 10-formylTHF dehydrogenase. (From Appling [1], with permission).

The original observations that yeast might be a good model for mammalian folate metabolism were complicated because of the apparent lack of certain enzymes in both mammals and yeast, especially in terms of glycine production in mammals compared to yeast (77) and the lack of 10-formylTHF oxidation to CO_2 in yeast. Another problem was that while the mC1-THF synthase and mitochondrial 10-formylTHF dehydrogenase were identified by enzyme activity assays as being present in rat liver mitochondrial matrix, these enzymes have never been purified and characterized from the mitochondria of any mammalian species.

To this end MacKenzie and colleagues have challenged the concept of a specific mammalian mitochondrial NADP+-dependent trifunctional C1-THF synthase, as seen in yeast, and have proposed instead a novel mammalian mitochondrial, bifunctional, NAD-dependent 5,10-methyleneTHF dehydrogenase and 5,10-methenylTHF cyclohydrolase (NMDMC) (80–82). This enzyme has been purified and cloned and is restricted to mitochondria in mammals, whereas the NADP-dependent trifunctional C1-THF synthase is strictly cytosolic (9–11, 98). NAD-dependent 5,10-methyleneTHF is dependent on Mg^{2+} and

inorganic phosphate, which it uses to change the dinucleotide specificity from NADP to NAD.

NMDMC has been proposed as the mammalian homolog of the corresponding yeast mitochondrial C1-THF synthase trifunctional enzyme, encoded by *MIS1* (72, 150). Bifunctional NMDMC was found in fetal tissues, transformed cell lines, and in normal tissues that contain actively differentiating cells (e.g., bone marrow, thymus, and spleen). It does not appear to be present in detectable levels, immunologically or by enzyme activity, in mature adult tissues such as liver, kidney, brain, heart, or skeletal muscle (80). The mRNA for NMDMC was detectable in normal tissues, suggesting it was present (99). NMDMC would generate 10-formylTHF from 5,10-methyleneTHF, via 5,10-methenylTHF using NAD+ (Figure 11.5) exactly as described for the trifunctional enzyme, except that it cannot hydrolyze 10-formylTHF to THF and formate (Reaction M3). Hydrolysis of 10-formylTHF now becomes a requirement of the mitochondrial 10-formylTHF dehydrogenase or another unknown enzyme. It has been known for many years that cytosolic 10-formylTHF dehydrogenase in vitro will hydrolyze 10-formylTHF in the absence of NADP+ (63, 83, 102, 113). However, the cytosolic hydrolytic reaction is dependent on added 2-mercaptoethanol for activity and is considered nonphysiological (30, 106). A similar reaction by a mitochondrial 10-formylTHF dehydrogenase might account for formate production, and it has been reported that rat liver has a mitochondrial 10-formylTHF hydrolase, although this enzyme was never purified from mitochondria (20).

A Model for the Unidirectional Flow of Mitochondrial 1-C Units

There has been a reappraisal of the roles of certain enzymes involved in folate metabolism. This is especially true of mitochondrial enzymes (1, 8) and cytosolic and mitochondrial serine hydroxymethyltransferase (84, 128). A model for adult hepatic 1-C metabolism (Figure 11.6) is based on recent insights into the roles of certain folate-dependent enzymes (1, 8, 84, 128) and updates and expands the model proposed by Appling (1).

Most of the 1-C groups are generated from serine (107) and are primarily produced by mitochondrial serine hydroxymethyltransferase (Figure 11.6; Reaction M8), with contributions from the glycine cleavage system (Figure 11.6; Reaction 20) and the choline catabolite pathway. 5,10-MethyleneTHF is generated in the mitochondria and converted via 10-formylTHF to formate. Formate is delivered to the cytosol and converted by 10-formylTHF synthetase (Figure 11.6; Reaction C3) to 10-formylTHF for

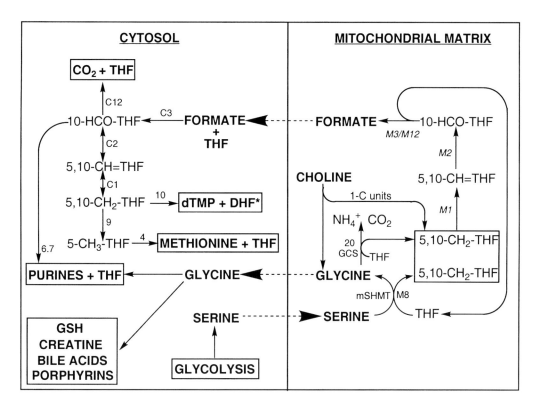

Fig. 11.6. Unidirectional flow of 1-C units from serine, glycine, and choline to methionine, purines, dTMP and CO_2. The figure illustrates the unidirectional flow of 1-C units from serine, glycine and choline through the mitochondrial folate pool to formate that is transferred to the cytosol for conversion to 10-formylTHF. This model does not specify which mitochondrial enzymes *(M1 and M2)* are required to oxidize 5,10-methyleneTHF to 10-formylTHF. Cytosolic 10-formylTHF is the pool of 1-C units that may be used directly for purine synthesis, reduced to 5,10-methyleneTHF for dTMP synthesis, or further reduced to 5-methylTHF for methionine synthesis. Alternatively 10-formylTHF may be oxidized to CO_2 which eliminates excess 1-C units. Each reaction shows the product plus THF, which is recycled to accept another formate from the mitochondria. The enzymes in this scheme are as described in Figure 3. C1, 5,10-methyleneTHF dehydrogenase; C2, 5,10-methenylTHF cyclohydrolase; C3, 10-formylTHF synthetase; *M1, M2, and M3* are not specified but are shown in Figure 11.4A and 11.4B; 4, methionine synthase; 6, glycinamide ribonucleotide transformylase; 7, phosphoribosylaminoimidazole-carboxamide transformylase; 9,5,10-methyleneTHF reductase; C8:M8, serine hydroxymethyltransferase; 10, thymidylate synthase; C12:*M12*, 10-FormylTHF dehydrogenase; *M12H*, the hydrolytic activity of *M12*, 10-FormylTHF dehydrogenase; 20, glycine cleavage system. GSH, glutathione. *DHF produced in the synthesis of dTMP is recycled to THF by dihydrofolate reductase.

purine synthesis, or is reduced to 5,10-methyleneTHF for methionine or dTMP synthesis by the sequential actions of 5,10-methenylTHF cyclohydrolase (Reaction C2) and 5,10-methyleneTHF dehydrogenase (Reaction C1). These three reactions are all catalyzed by the tri-

functional C1-THF synthase (Reactions C1, C2, and C3). Alternatively the 1-C unit as 10-formylTHF can be oxidized to CO_2, which removes excess 1-C groups (Reaction C12). This model separates the synthesis of 1-C units in mitochondria from the biosynthetic reactions that require folate-linked 1-C units in cytosol and provides a unidirectional flow of 1-C units from one compartment to the other. The model relies on the observed rapid transfer of 1-C units as serine and glycine across the inner mitochondrial membrane (35, 36) and the unidirectional transfer of formate out of mitochondria and into the cytosol and does not involve the transport of folate polyglutamates.

If one assumes that cytosolic serine hydroxymethyltransferase does *not* supply the majority of 1-C units, it is appropriate to examine the evidence supporting the model. Both forms of serine hydroxymethyltransferase are differentially expressed and regulated in various tissues during development (119, 120, 128). Mitochondrial serine hydroxymethyltransferase is found in all cell types and is enriched in liver and kidney (128). It has been known for many years that CHO cell mutants of the *glyA* complementation group lack mitochondrial serine hydroxymethyltransferase, have normal levels of cytosolic serine hydroxymethyltransferase, and are auxotrophic for glycine (23). These observations indicate that mitochondrial serine hydroxymethyltransferase is required for the synthesis of glycine in CHO cells. The rates of serine and glycine interconversion have been compared for the *glyA* CHO cell line that has normal cytosolic serine hydroxymethyltransferase, but lacks mitochondrial serine hydroxymethyltransferase (mSHMT$^-$) and a normal CHO cell line with both cytosolic and mitochondrial serine hydroxymethyltransferase (mSHMT$^+$) (84). The relative flux of glycine to serine was similar in both cell lines, suggesting that cytosolic serine hydroxymethyltransferase was responsible for this conversion. Increased serine levels in the media of mSHMT$^+$ cells resulted in the production of more glycine; however, no such increase was seen for mSHMT$^-$ cells. The results clearly demonstrate that the production of glycine was compartmentalized to the mitochondria where mitochondrial serine hydroxymethyltransferase was responsible for approximately all of the synthesis of glycine from serine in CHO cells.

Although these results appear to be clear-cut, it was emphasized that the mutant CHO *glyA* cells were originally obtained by chemical mutagenesis and may be deficient in more than just mitochondrial serine hydroxymethyltransferase (84). Stover and co-workers (128) cloned the human mitochondrial serine hydroxymethyltransferase gene and transfected a modified version of the gene into CHO *glyA* cells. Glycine auxotrophy was eliminated in all of the transfectants, and the intracellular glycine concentrations were restored to levels similar to those of wild-type CHO cells. Additional evidence was presented earlier that showed specific replacement of mitochondrial FPGS in CHO AUXB1 cells restored glycine independence (65). Results from the flux studies and the replacement of mitochondrial serine hydroxymethyltransferase in CHO *GlyA* cells and FPGS in CHO AUXB1 cells strongly support the hypothesis that mitochondrial serine hydroxymethyltransferase supplies most of the cellular glycine and hence 1-C units.

Further support for the model comes from a stable isotope study in a human subject where 1-C units, derived from the hepatic mitochondrial oxidation of infused serine (^{2}H at C-3)serine, were rapidly detected as [C^{2}H$_3$]methionine in plasma apolipoprotein B-100 (48b). Apolipoprotein B-100 is exclusively synthesized in the liver and is used as a marker for hepatic protein synthesis. In this case carbon three of serine, carrying 2 deuterium atoms, was converted to 5,10-[^{2}H]-methyleneTHF by mitochondrial serine hydroxymethyltransferase, oxidized by mC1-THF to 5,10-[^{2}H]-methenylTHF, loosing one deuterium atom, converted to 10-[^{2}H]-formylTHF and released to the cytosol as [^{2}H]-formate. The [^{2}H]-formate was assimilated into the cytosolic 1-C pool and used to remethylate homocysteine to methionine as shown in Figure 11.6.

Consistent with the unidirectional model are the reports describing the kinetics of the 5,10-methylene dehydrogenase/cyclohydrolase bifunctional domains from NADP-dependent C1-THF synthase (Figure 11.6; Reactions C1 and C2) and the mitochondrial NAD-dependent NMDMC enzyme (Reactions M1 and M2) (96, 97). These two articles concluded the following:

1. The cytosolic NADP-dependent 5,10-methylene dehydrogenase/cyclohydrolase activity of C1-THF synthase exists at or near equilibrium and is thus poised to go in either direction, although bound NADP$^+$ stimulates the reverse reaction toward 5,10-methenylTHF.
2. The mitochondrial NAD-dependent NMDMC is far from equilibrium and is poised toward 10-formylTHF synthesis.

Thus in mitochondria the 1-C units are being "pushed" toward 10-formylTHF while the cytosolic enzyme may be "pulled" in the direction of 5,10-methyleneTHF synthesis by the reactions that consume 5,10-methyleneTHF. The second conclusion applies only to the NAD-dependent NMDMC. Predictions about mitochondrial C1-THF synthase will have to await purification and characterization of this enzyme. Another important observation was that the K_m for formate in the synthetic reaction of cytosolic 10-formylTHF synthetase (Reaction C3) was 4 μmol/L when THF pentaglutamate was used in the reaction, which indicates that cytosolic 10-formylTHF synthetase is a very efficient scavenger of formate (130).

For the unidirectional supply of 1-C units to work efficiently cytosolic 5,10-methyleneTHF must be available to thymidylate synthase and MTHFR and methionine synthase for their synthetic reactions. Cytosolic serine hydroxymethyltransferase, which forms 0.5% to 1.0% of the cytosol protein in rabbit liver (110), must be restrained from using cytosolic 5,10-methyleneTHF to synthesize serine from glycine, to prevent the futile cycling of 1-C units. There are two possible mechanisms by which this may be accomplished:

1. 5-FormylTHF is synthesized by cytosolic serine hydroxymethyltransferase and is also a slow tight-binding inhibitor of its activity (125–127). This observation provides a functional role for 5-formylTHF in cellular 1-C metabolism, the presence of which was thought to be an artifact of tissue extraction.
2. 5-MethylTHF is a tight binding inhibitor of serine hydroxymethyltransferase (74). The inhibition of this enzyme by 5-methylTHF is unusual in that the folate binds synergistically in the

presence of glycine, one of the substrate/products of serine hydroxymethyltransferase, to form an inactive ternary complex.

Either one of these options provides a method of regulating the activity of cytosolic serine hydroxymethyltransferase, although inhibition by 5-formylTHF is more attractive in light of recent findings by Stover and co-workers on the effective inhibition of the cytosolic enzyme in neuroblastoma cells (47).

The main advantage of this unidirectional model is that the 1-C units flow in one direction from the mitochondria to the cytosol, unlike previous schemes where 1-C units are generated from serine and formate in the cytosol and then have to compete for interconversion by the NADP-dependent 5,10-methyleneTHF dehydrogenase/cyclohydrolase domain of C1-THF synthase. It allows for the assimilation of the majority of 1-C units as formate from mitochondria or generated in the cytosol from methylthioadenosine, tryptophan and P450 reactions. Histidine contributes 5,10-methenylTHF, which is also incorporated into the 1-C pool. The 1-C units enter the cytosolic pool at the fully oxidized formate level. The 1-C units are then either used directly for purine synthesis, oxidized to CO_2 or distributed by cytosolic NADP-dependent 5,10-methyleneTHF dehydrogenase/cyclohydrolase for methionine or dTMP biosynthesis. The key folate is now 10-formylTHF, which becomes a reservoir of 1-C units in both the cytosol and the mitochondria. In the cytosol, 10-formylTHF is at the branch point where 1-C units are either directed to the biosynthetic folate-dependent cycles or are oxidized to CO_2 by 10-formylTHF dehydrogenase, an enzyme that is considered to be the arbiter in determining the cytosolic THF/10-formylTHF ratio (83). This is supported by work in NEUT2 mice where 10-formylTHF dehydrogenase has been deleted and the 10-formylTHF pools are increased threefold at the expense of THF when compared with normal mice (21). Free formate is toxic to mitochondria (85) and 10-formylTHF provides a convenient way of storing formate before recycling THF and releasing formate to the cytosol.

Production of glycine in mitochondria now consolidates the two major routes of glycine synthesis, mitochondrial serine hydroxymethyltransferase and the choline catabolic pathway. Mitochondrial glycine production now affords close control of glycine levels at the point of synthesis by glycine cleavage system (Figure 11.6; Reaction 20). Mutations in the glycine cleavage system in humans result in nonketotic hyperglycinemia owing to overproduction of glycine (87), indicating that glycine cleavage system may be the major point of control for glycine metabolism. All of these reactions in mitochondria must be tightly cou-

pled to the supply of THF, which accepts the 1-C groups. Unfortunately little is known about the regulation of 1-C supply in mitochondria, although it is likely that mitochondrial serine hydroxymethyltransferase is subject to inhibition by 5-formylTHF in a fashion similar to the cytosol. It should also be noted that small pools of 5-methylTHF present in mitochondria (Tables 11.1 and 11.2) may also influence mitochondrial serine hydroxymethyltransferase activity.

How is the cytosolic use of 1-C units regulated? Krebs, using isolated hepatocytes, made some interesting observations concerning the oxidation of 1-C units by 10-formylTHF dehydrogenase (61). Addition of physiological amounts of methionine accelerated the rate of oxidation of formate and the C2 of histidine to CO_2 via 10-formylTHF dehydrogenase. The explanation for this effect was that methionine was converted to AdoMet, which inhibited MTHFR (outlined in Figure 11.4), and this caused a build-up of 5,10-methyleneTHF, 5,10-methenylTHF and 10-formylTHF. Presumably the increased 1-C folate pool was a signal to oxidize 1-C units via 10-formylTHF dehydrogenase to reequilibrate the THF pool. Neither methionine nor AdoMet has any direct effect on 10-formylTHF dehydrogenase (113), but THF does bind to and inhibit 10-formylTHF dehydrogenase activity (62, 63, 83, 102, 106, 113). Perhaps it is the decreased level of THF bound to 10-formylTHF dehydrogenase that permits the dehydrogenase to oxidize the excess 1-C units and recycle THF. Although this would be a reasonable assumption, Schirch's group has shown that in rabbit 10-formylTHF dehydrogenase, THF was tightly bound to a second, noncatalytic binding site and that it had no effect on the steady-state activity of 10-formylTHF dehydrogenase (43).

Recent work concerning 5-formylTHF and cytosolic serine hydroxymethyltransferase activity has shed some light on the regulation of 1-C assimilation (47). The cytosolic enzyme is inhibited by 5-formylTHF, and this may be responsible for regulating the flow of 1-C units to dTMP and methionine. What happens if the inhibition of cytosolic serine hydroxymethyltransferase by 5-formylTHF is released? Release was accomplished by using a human 5Y neuroblastoma cell line that contained a plasmid expressing high levels of methenylTHF synthetase (*5YMTHFS*), the enzyme that recycles 5-formylTHF to 5,10-methenylTHF (Figure 11.3; Reaction C16:M16). By removing the inhibition of cytosolic serine hydroxymethyltransferase by 5-formylTHF in the presence of glycine, a rapid conversion of available 5,10-methyleneTHF to serine at the expense of dTMP and methionine synthesis occurred. Thus in *5YMTHFS* there was competition between serine synthesis, dTMP synthesis, and remethylation of homocysteine for cytosolic 1-C units. These results support the hypothesis that cytosolic serine hydroxymethyltransferase must be strictly controlled for the efficient use of cytosolic 1-C units.

Hepatic Folate Binding Proteins and the Regulation of 1-C Metabolism

As described earlier, the folate pools in rat liver cytosol and mitochondria appear to be bound to the folate-dependent enzymes 10-formylTHF dehydrogenase, sarcosine dehydrogenase and dimethylglycine dehydrogenase, or glycine N-methyltransferase. Schirch has pointed out that the concentration of folate binding sites on these enzymes in the liver is considerably higher than the concentration of the folate pool (59, 141). The predominant folate bound to 10-formylTHF dehydrogenase, sarcosine dehydrogenase and dimethylglycine dehydrogenase is THF. Thus, how does THF participate in 1-C metabolism if the vast majority is bound to these enzymes?

Schirch and colleagues provided an interesting insight to this problem by investigating the inhibitory effects of THF-pentaglutamate binding to 10-formylTHF dehydrogenase (59). In the presence of excess trifunctional C1-THF synthase or cytosolic serine hydroxymethyltransferase, the product inhibition of 10-formylTHF dehydrogenase by THF-pentaglutamate was relieved and the 10-formylTHF dehydrogenase activity was increased twofold (59). Under these conditions, the THF-pentaglutamate was transferred to C1-THF synthase or cytosolic serine hydroxymethyltransferase. In rabbit liver cytosol, these enzymes are present at approximately equal concentrations (110). They could exist as a core-complex that tightly binds folate and processes 1-C units for assimilation into the synthetic reactions or oxidizes them to CO_2. The other folate-dependent enzymes, which catalyze purine, dTMP, and methionine synthesis, might also be closely associated with the core-complex, resulting in a highly regulated production and distribution of 1-C units.

Evidence for the association of folate-dependent enzymes was provided by showing a functional association of the purine biosynthetic enzyme glycinamide ribonucleotide transformylase and C1-THF synthase in a multiprotein complex consisting of glycinamide ribonucleotide transformylase, phosphoribosylaminoimidazole carboxamide transformylase, cytosolic serine hydroxymethyltransferase and C1-THF synthase in chicken liver (15, 118). The reason that mitochondrial sarcosine dehydrogenase and dimethylglycine dehydrogenase bind THF in rat liver is not known, but they may also form a core-complex that regulates the distribution of THF for 1-C metabolism

in mitochondria. These protein complexes are reminiscent of the "metabolons" proposed by Srere (121).

Glycine N-methyltransferase binds 5-methylTHF and is present in rat liver and pancreas at 1% to 3% of the cytosolic protein (32, 151). Because this enzyme probably binds most of the cytosolic 5-methylTHF, it begs the question how methionine synthase — which is present at much lower levels—accesses the 5-methylTHF pool to recycle homocysteine. There are two possibilities. Methionine synthase may be physically associated with glycine N-methyltransferase and is thus able to acquire 5-methylTHF from it, or MTHFR and methionine synthase may be associated with the core-complex folate enzymes discussed previously and are thus supplied with 1-C units on demand. Alternatively, the 5-methylTHF bound to glycine N-methyltransferase may be a separate pool that equilibrates slowly with the main folate pool.

Folate metabolism in mammalian liver is a complex series of reactions designed to supply 1-C units for the synthesis of purines, dTMP and methionine, and to oxidize excess 1-C units to CO_2. The available evidence indicates that 1-C units are predominantly supplied from the mitochondria to the synthetic reactions in the cytosol as formate. The supply and utilization of 1-C units must be strictly regulated. Perturbations in any of these reactions may lead to an oversupply or undersupply of an essential metabolite.

What causes the perturbations? Primarily it is probably the supply of folate in the diet. This is supported by the observation that hyperhomocysteinemia and 70% of neural tube defects may be treated with folic acid supplements. As Schirch reminds us there are many more enzyme folate-binding sites than there are folate molecules. This sets up a constant battle between the various enzymes that require folate-linked 1-C units for synthetic reactions. The strain on the supply of folate-linked 1-C units, coupled to mutant enzymes that may exhibit less than optimum efficiency, probably results in the observed clinical outcomes. The prime example of this is MTHFR, which has a common $677C{\rightarrow}T$ mutation that leads to decreased enzyme activity and hyperhomocysteinemia (70). The $677C{\rightarrow}T$ mutation results in an accelerated loss of the bound flavin adenine dinucleotide (FAD) cofactor from MTHFR, which leads to decreased enzyme activity (49). Addition of 5-methylTHF greatly retards the loss of FAD and provides a logical explanation of why increased folate intake in the diet lowers plasma homocysteine levels (49).

REFERENCES

1. Appling, DR Compartmentation of folate-mediated one-carbon metabolism in eukaryotes. *FASEB J* 1991; 5: 2645–51.

2. Appling, DR, Kastanos, E, Pasternack, LB, Woldman, YY. Use of 13C nuclear magnetic resonance to evaluate metabolic flux through folate one-carbon pools in *Saccharomyces cerevisiae*. *Methods Enzymol* 1997; 281: 218–31.

3. Atkinson, I, Garrow, T, Brenner, A, Shane, B. Human cytosolic folylpoly-gamma-glutamate synthase. *Methods Enzymol* 1997; 281: 134–40.

4. Backlund, PS, Jr, Smith, RA. Methionine synthesis from 5′-methylthioadenosine in rat liver. *J Biol Chem* 1981; 256: 1533–35.

5. Bagley, PJ, Selhub, J. Analysis of folates using combined affinity and ion-pair chromatography. *Methods Enzymol* 1997; 281: 16–25.

6. Balaghi, M, Horne, DW, Wagner, C. Hepatic one-carbon metabolism in early folate deficiency in rats. *Biochem J* 1993; 291: 145–49.

7. Balaghi, M, Wagner, C. Folate deficiency inhibits pancreatic amylase secretion in rats. *Am J Clin Nutr* 1995; 61: 90–6.

8. Barlowe, CK, Appling, DR. In vitro evidence for the involvement of mitochondrial folate metabolism in the supply of cytoplasmic one-carbon units. *Biofactors* 1: 1988; 171–76.

9. Belanger, C, MacKenzie, RE. Isolation and characterization of cDNA clones encoding the murine NAD-dependent methylenetetrahydrofolate dehydrogenase-methenyltetrahydrofolate cyclohydrolase. *J Biol Chem* 1989; 264: 4837–43.

10. Belanger, C, MacKenzie, RE. Structural organization of the murine gene encoding NAD-dependent methylenetetrahydrofolate dehydrogenase-methenyltetrahydrofolate cyclohydrolase. *Gene* 1991; 97: 283–88.

11. Belanger, C, Peri, KG, MacKenzie, RE. Analysis of the promoter region of the gene encoding NAD-dependent methylenetetrahydrofolate dehydrogenase-methenyltetrahydrofolate cyclohydrolase. *Nucleic Acids Res* 1991; 19: 4341–45.

12. Belz, S, Nau, H. Determination of folate patterns in mouse plasma, erythrocytes, and embryos by HPLC coupled with a microbiological assay. *Anal Biochem* 1998; 265: 157–66.

13. Bertrand, R, Beauchemin, M, Dayan, A, Ouimet, M, Jolivet, J. Identification and characterization of human mitochondrial methenyltetrahydrofolate synthetase activity. *Biochim Biophys Acta* 1995; 1266: 245–49.

14. Capdevila, A, Decha-Umphai, W, Song, KH, Borchardt, RT, Wagner, C. Pancreatic exocrine secretion is blocked by inhibitors of methylation. *Arch Biochem Biophys* 1997; 345: 47–55.

15. Caperelli, CA, Benkovic, PA, Chettur, G, Benkovic, SJ. Purification of a complex catalyzing folate cofactor synthesis and transformylation in de novo purine biosynthesis. *J Biol Chem* 1980; 255: 1885–90.

16. Carl, GF, Hudson, FZ, McGuire, BJ. Rat liver subcellular folate distribution shows association of formyltetrahydropteroylpentaglutamates with mitochondria and methyltetrahydropteroylhexaglutamates with cytoplasm. *J Nutr* 1995; 125: 2096–103.

17. Carl, GF, Hudson, FZ, McGuire, Jr, BS. Formyltetrahydrofolates associated with mitochondria have longer polyglutamate chains than the methyltetrahydrofolates associated with cytoplasm in rat brain. *J Nutr* 1996; 126: 3077–82.

18. Carl, GF, Peterson, JD, McClain, LD, Bridgers, WF. Subcellular localization of folate turnover and folate-dependent enzyme activity in mouse brain. *J Neurochem* 1980; 34: 1442–52.

19. Carl, GF, Smith, ML. Simultaneous measurement of one-carbon and polyglutamate derivatives of folic acid in rat liver using enzymatic interconversions of folates followed by ternary complex formation with thymidylate synthetase and 5-fluorodeoxyuridylic acid: Standardization of the method. *J Nutr* 1995; 125: 1245–57.

20. Case, GL, Kaisaki, PJ, Steele, RD. Resolution of rat liver 10-formyltetrahydrofolate dehydrogenase/hydrolase activities. *J Biol Chem* 1988; 263: 10204–207.

21. Champion, KM, Cook, RJ, Tollaksen, SL, Giometti, CS. Identification of a heritable deficiency of the folate-dependent enzyme 10-formyltetrahydrofolate dehydrogenase in mice. *Proc Natl Acad Sci USA* 1994; 91: 11338–42.

22. Chanarin, I. Cobalamins and nitrous oxide: A review. *J Clin Pathol* 1980; 33: 909–16.

23. Chasin, LA, Feldman, A, Konstam, M, Urlaub, G. Reversion of a Chinese hamster cell auxotrophic mutant. *Proc Natl Acad Sci USA* 1974; 71: 718–22.

24. Chen, L, Qi, H, Korenberg, J, Garrow, TA, Choi, YJ, Shane, B. Purification and properties of human cytosolic folylpoly-gamma-glutamate synthetase and organization, localization, and differential splicing of its gene. *J Biol Chem* 1996; 271: 13077–87.

25. Clifford, AJ, Heid, MK, Muller, HG, Bills, ND. Tissue distribution and prediction of total body folate of rats. *J Nutr* 1990; 120: 1633–39.

26. Cook, RJ, Blair, JA. The distribution and chemical nature of radioactive folates in rat liver cells and rat liver mitochondria. *Biochem J* 1979; 178: 651–59.

27. Cook, RJ, Misono, KS, Wagner, C. The amino acid sequences of the flavin-peptides of dimethylglycine dehydrogenase and sarcosine dehydrogenase from rat liver mitochondria. *J Biol Chem* 1985; 260: 12998–3002.

28. Cook, RJ, Misono, KS, Wagner, C. Identification of the covalently bound flavin of dimethylglycine dehydrogenase and sarcosine dehydrogenase from rat liver mitochondria. *J Biol Chem* 1984; 259: 12475–80.

29. Cook, RJ, and Wagner, C. Dimethylglycine dehydrogenase and sarcosine dehydrogenase: Mitochondrial folate-binding proteins from rat liver. *Methods Enzymol* 1986; 122: 255–60.

30. Cook, RJ, Wagner, C. Enzymatic activities of rat liver cytosol 10-formyltetrahydrofolate dehydrogenase. *Arch Biochem Biophys* 1995; 321: 336–44.

31. Cook, RJ, Wagner, C. Glycine N-methyltransferase is a folate binding protein of rat liver cytosol. *Proc Natl Acad Sci USA* 1984; 81: 3631–34.

32. Cook, RJ, Wagner, C. Measurement of a folate binding protein from rat liver cytosol by radioimmunoassay. *Arch Biochem Biophys* 1981; 208: 358–64.

33. Cook, RJ, Wagner, C. Purification and partial characterization of rat liver folate binding protein: Cytosol I. *Biochemistry* 1982; 21: 4427–34.

34. Corrocher, R, Bhuyan, BK, Hoffbrand, AV. Composition of pteroylpolyglutamates in guinea pig liver and their formation from folic acid. *Clin Sci* 1972; 43: 799–813.

35. Cybulski, RL, Fisher, RR. Intramitochondrial localization and proposed metabolic significance of serine transhydroxymethylase. *Biochemistry* 1976; 15: 3183–87.

36. Cybulski, RL, Fisher, RR. Mitochondrial neutral amino acid transport: Evidence for a carrier mediated mechanism. *Biochemistry* 1977; 16: 5116–20.

37. Czeizel, AE, Dudas, I. Prevention of the first occurrence of neural-tube defects by periconceptional vitamin supplementation. *N Engl J Med* 1992; 327: 1832–35.

38. Drummond, JT, Matthews, RG. Nitrous oxide degradation by cobalamin-dependent methionine synthase: Characterization of the reactants and products in the inactivation reaction. *Biochemistry* 1994; 33: 3732–41.

39. Elsea, SH, Juyal, RC, Jiralerspong, S, Finucane, BM, Pandolfo, M, Greenberg, F, Baldini, A, Stover, P, Patel, PI. Haploinsufficiency of cytosolic serine hydroxymethyltransferase in the Smith-Magenis syndrome. *Am J Hum Genet* 1995; 57: 1342–50.

40. Finkelstein, JD. Methionine metabolism in mammals. *J Nutr Biochem* 1990; 1: 228–37.

41. Freemantle, SJ, Taylor, SM, Krystal, G, Moran, RG. Upstream organization of and multiple transcripts from the human folylpoly-gamma-glutamate synthetase gene. *J Biol Chem* 1995; 270: 9579–84.

42. Frisell, WR, Randolph, VM. N-methyl oxidation in liver mitochondria of triiodothyronine-treated and thyroidectomized rats. *Biochim Biophys Acta* 1974; 347: 145–50.

43. Fu, T-F, Maras, B, Barra, D, Schirch, V. A non-catalytic tetrahydrofolate tight binding site is on the small domain of 10-formyltetrahydrofolate dehydrogenase. *Arch Biochem Biophys* 1999; 367: 161–66.

44. Garcia-Martinez, LF, Appling, DR. Characterization of the folate-dependent mitochondrial oxidation of carbon 3 of serine. *Biochemistry* 1993; 32: 4671–76.

45. Garrow, TA, Admon, A, Shane, B. Expression cloning of a human cDNA encoding folylpoly(gamma-glutamate) synthetase and determination of its primary structure. *Proc Natl Acad Sci USA* 1992; 89: 9151–55.

46. Garrow, TA, Brenner, AA, Whitehead, VM, Chen, XN, Duncan, RG, Korenberg, JR, Shane, B. Cloning of human cDNAs encoding mitochondrial and cytosolic serine hydroxymethyltransferases and chromosomal localization. *J Biol Chem* 1993; 268: 11910–16.

47. Girgis, S, Suh, JR, Jolivet, J, Stover, PJ. 5-Formyltetrahydrofolate regulates homocysteine remethylation in human neuroblastoma. *J Biol Chem* 1997; 272: 4729–34.

48. Green, JM, Ballou, DP, Matthews, RG. Examination of the role of methylenetetrahydrofolate reductase in incorporation of methyltetrahydrofolate into cellular metabolism. *FASEB J* 1988; 2: 42–7.

48a.Gregory, JF, III, Williamson, J, Liao, JF, Bailey, LB, Toth, JP. Kinetic model of folate metabolism in nonpregnant women consuming [^{2}H$_2$] folic acid: isotopic labeling of urinary folate and the catabolite para-acetamidobenzoylglutamate indicates slow, intake-dependent, turnover of folate pools. *J Nutr* 1998; 128: 1896–906.

48b.Gregory, JF, III, Cuskelly, GJ, Shane, B, Toth, JP, Baumgartner, TG, and Stacpoole, PW. Primed-constant infusion of [^{2}H$_3$] serine allows in vivo kinetic measurement of serine turnover, homocysteine remethylation, and transsulfuration processes in human one-carbon metabolism. *Am J Clin Nutr* 2000; 72: 1535–41.

49. Guenther, BD, Sheppard, CA, Tran, P, Rozen, R, Matthews, RG, Ludwig, ML. The structure and properties of methylenetetrahydrofolate reductase from *Escherichia coli* suggest how folate ameliorates human hyperhomocysteinemia. *Nat Struct Biol* 1999; 6: 359–65.

50. Harding, CO, Williams, P, Pflanzer, DM, Colwell, RE, Lyne, PW, Wolff, JA. *sar:* A genetic mouse model for human sarcosinemia generated by ethylnitrosourea mutagenesis. *Proc Natl Acad Sci USA* 1992; 89: 2644–48.

51. Herbert, V, Zalusky, R. Interrelations of vitamin B12 and folic acid metabolism: Folic acid clearance studies. *J Clin Invest* 1962; 41: 1263–76.

52. Horne, DW. Effects of nitrous oxide inactivation of vitamin B12 and of methionine on folate coenzyme metabolism in rat liver, kidney, brain, small intestine and bone marrow. *Biofactors* 1989; 2: 65–8.

53. Horne, DW. Microbiological assay of folates in 96-well microtiter plates. *Methods Enzymol* 1997; 281: 38–43.

54. Horne, DW. Transport of folates and antifolates in liver. *Proc Soc Exp Biol Med* 1993; 202: 385–91.

55. Horne, DW, Briggs, WT, Wagner, C. High-pressure liquid chromatographic separation of the naturally occurring folic acid monoglutamate derivatives. *Anal Biochem* 1981; 116: 393–37.

56. Horne, DW, Holloway, RS. Compartmentation of folate metabolism in rat pancreas: Nitrous oxide inactivation of methionine synthase leads to accumulation of 5-methyltetrahydrofolate in cytosol. *J Nutr* 1997; 127: 1772–75.

57. Horne, DW, Holloway, RS, Said, HM. Uptake of 5-formyltetrahydrofolate in isolated rat liver mitochondria is carrier-mediated. *J Nutr* 1992; 122: 2204–49.

58. Horne, DW, Patterson, D, Cook, RJ. Effect of nitrous oxide inactivation of vitamin B12-dependent methionine synthase on the subcellular distribution of folate coenzymes in rat liver. *Arch Biochem Biophys* 1989; 270: 729–33.

59. Kim, DW, Huang, T, Schirch, D, Schirch, V. Properties of tetrahydropteroylpentaglutamate bound to 10- formyltetrahydrofolate dehydrogenase. *Biochemistry* 1996; 35: 15772–83.

60. Kisliuk, RL. Folate biochemistry in relation to antifolate selectivity. In *Anticancer Drug Development Guide: Antifolate Drugs in Cancer Therapy* (Jackman AL, ed.). Humana Press, Totowa, NJ, 1999; pp. 13–36.

61. Krebs, HA, Hems, R, Tyler, B. The regulation of folate and methionine metabolism. *Biochem J* 1976; 158: 341–53.

62. Kutzbach, C, Stokstad, EL. Partial purification of a 10-formyl-tetrahydrofolate: NADP oxidoreductase from mammalian liver. *Biochem Biophys Res Commun* 1968; 30: 111–17.

63. Kutzbach, C, Stokstad, ELR. 10-Formyl tetrahydrofolate:NADP oxidoreductase. *Methods in Enzymol* 1971; 18B: 793–98.

64. Letter, AA, Zombor, G, Henderson, JF. Tryptophan as a source of one-carbon units for purine biosynthesis de novo. *Can J Biochem* 1973; 51: 486–88.

65. Lin, BF, Huang, RF, Shane, B. Regulation of folate and one-carbon metabolism in mammalian cells. III. Role of mitochondrial folylpoly-gamma-glutamate synthetase. *J Biol Chem* 1993; 268: 21674–79.

66. Lin, BF, Kim, JS, Hsu, JC, Osborne, C, Lowe, K, Garrow, T, Shane, B. Molecular biology in nutrition research: Modeling of folate metabolism. *Adv Food Nutr Res* 1996; 40: 95–106.

67. Lin, BF, and Shane, B. Expression of *Escherichia coli* folylpolyglutamate synthetase in the Chinese hamster ovary cell mitochondrion. *J Biol Chem* 1994; 269: 9705–13.

68. London, RE, and Gabel, SA. A deuterium surface coil NMR study of the metabolism of D-methionine in the liver of the anesthetized rat. *Biochemistry* 1988; 27: 7864–69.

69. London, RE, Gabel, SA, Funk, A. Metabolism of excess methionine in the liver of intact rat: An in vivo 2H NMR study. *Biochemistry* 1987; 26: 7166–72.

70. Ma, J, Stampfer, MJ, Hennekens, CH, Frosst, P, Selhub, J, Horsford, J, Malinow, MR, Willett, WC, Rozen, R. Methylenetetrahydrofolate reductase polymorphism, plasma folate, homocysteine, and risk of myocardial infarction in US physicians. *Circulation* 1996; 94: 2410–16.

71. Mackenzie, RE. Biogenesis and interconversion of substituted tetrahydrofolates. In *Folates and Pterins* (Blakley, RL, Benkovic, SJ, eds.). John Wiley & Sons, New York, 1984; pp. 255–306.

72. MacKenzie, RE, Mejia, N, Yang, XM. Methylenetetrahydrofolate dehydrogenases in normal and transformed mammalian cells. *Adv Enzyme Regul* 1988; 27: 31–9.

73. Matthews, RG, Daubner, SC. Modulation of methylenetetrahydrofolate reductase activity by *S*-adenosylmethionine and by dihydrofolate and its polyglutamate analogues. *Adv Enzyme Regul* 1982; 20: 123–31.

74. Matthews, RG, Ross, J, Baugh, CM, Cook, JD, Davis, L. Interactions of pig liver serine hydroxymethyltransferase with methyltetrahydropteroylpolyglutamate inhibitors and with tetrahydropteroylpolyglutamate substrates. *Biochemistry* 1982; 21: 1230–38.

75. McKenzie, KQ, Jones, EW. Mutants of formyltetrahydrofolate interconversion pathway of *Saccharomyces cerevisiae*. *Genetics* 1977; 86: 85–102.

76. McMartin, KE, Virayotha, V, Tephly, TR. High-pressure liquid chromatography separation and determination of rat liver folates. *Arch Biochem Biophys* 1981; 209: 127–36.

77. McNeil, JB, Bognar, AL, Pearlman, RE. In vivo analysis of folate coenzymes and their compartmentation in *Saccharomyces cerevisiae*. *Genetics* 1996; 142: 371–81.

78. McNeil, JB, McIntosh, EM, Taylor, BV, Zhang, FR, Tang, S, Bognar, AL. Cloning and molecular characterization of three genes, including two genes encoding serine hydroxymethyltransferases, whose inactivation is required to render yeast auxotrophic for glycine. *J Biol Chem* 1994; 269: 9155–65.

79. McNeil, JB, Zhang, F, Taylor, BV, Sinclair, DA, Pearlman, RE, Bognar, AL. Cloning, and molecular characterization of the GCV1 gene encoding the glycine cleavage T-protein from *Saccharomyces cerevisiae*. *Gene* 1997; 186: 13–20.

80. Mejia, NR, MacKenzie, RE. NAD-dependent methylenetetrahydrofolate dehydrogenase is expressed by immortal cells. *J Biol Chem* 1985; 260: 14616–20.

81. Mejia, NR, MacKenzie, RE. NAD-dependent methylenetetrahydrofolate dehydrogenase-methenyltetrahydrofolate cyclohydrolase in transformed cells is a mitochondrial enzyme. *Biochem Biophys Res Commun* 1988; 155: 1–6.

82. Mejia, NR, Rios-Orlandi, EM, MacKenzie, RE. NAD-dependent methylenetetrahydrofolate dehydrogenase-methenyltetrahydrofolate cyclohydrolase from ascites tumor cells. Purification and properties. *J Biol Chem* 1986; 261: 9509–13.

83. Min, H, Shane, B, Stokstad, EL. Identification of 10-formyltetrahydrofolate dehydrogenase-hydrolase as a major folate binding protein in liver cytosol. *Biochim Biophys Acta* 1988; 967: 348–53.

84. Narkewicz, MR, Sauls, SD, Tjoa, SS, Teng, C, Fennessey, PV. Evidence for intracellular partitioning of serine and glycine metabolism in Chinese hamster ovary cells. *Biochem J* 1996; 313: 991–96.

85. Nicholls, P. The effect of formate on cytochrome aa3 and on electron transport in the intact respiratory chain. *Biochim Biophys Acta* 1976; 430: 13–29.

86. Noronha, JM, Silverman, M. On folic acid, vitamin B12, methionine and formiminoglutamic acid metabolism. In *Vitamin B_{12} and Intrinsic Factor* (Heinrich, HC, ed.). Enke, Stuttgart, 1962; pp. 728–36.

87. Nyhan, WL. Nonketotic hyperglycinemia. In *The Metabolic Basis of Inherited Disease* (Scriver, CR, Beaudet, AL, Sly, WS, Valle, D, eds.). McGraw-Hill, New York, 1989, pp. 743–53.

88. Ogawa, H, Gomi, T, Takusagawa, F, Fujioka, M. Structure, function and physiological role of glycine *N*-methyltransferase. *Int J Biochem Cell Biol* 1998; 30: 13–26.

89. Olson, MS, Hampson, RK, Craig, F. Regulation of the hepatic glycine-cleavage system. *Biochem Soc Trans* 1986; 14: 1004–5.

90. Osborne, CB, Lowe, KE, Shane, B. Regulation of folate and one-carbon metabolism in mammalian cells. I. Folate metabolism in Chinese hamster ovary cells expressing *Escherichia coli* or human folylpoly-gamma-glutamate synthetase activity. *J Biol Chem* 1993; 268: 21657–64.

91. Palese, M, Tephly, TR. Metabolism of formate in the rat. *J Toxicol Environ Health* 1975; 1: 13–24.

92. Pasternack, LB, Laude, Jr, DA, Appling, DR. ¹³C NMR analysis of intercompartmental flow of one-carbon units into choline and purines in *Saccharomyces cerevisiae*. *Biochemistry* 1994; 33: 74–82.

93. Pasternack, LB, Laude, Jr, DA, Appling, DR. ¹³C NMR detection of folate-mediated serine and glycine synthesis in vivo in *Saccharomyces cerevisiae*. *Biochemistry* 1992; 31: 8713–39.

94. Pasternack, LB, Laude, Jr, DA, Appling, DR. Whole-cell detection by ¹³C NMR of metabolic flux through the C1-tetrahydrofolate synthase/serine hydroxymethyltransferase enzyme system and effect of antifolate exposure in *Saccharomyces cerevisiae*. *Biochemistry* 1994; 33: 7166–73.

95. Pasternack, LB, Littlepage, LE, Laude, Jr, DA, Appling, DR. 13C NMR analysis of the use of alternative donors to the tetrahydrofolate-dependent one-carbon pools in *Saccharomyces cerevisiae*. *Arch Biochem Biophys* 1996; 326: 158–65.

96. Pawelek, PD, MacKenzie, RE. Methenyltetrahydrofolate cyclohydrolase is rate limiting for the enzymatic conversion of 10-formyltetrahydrofolate to 5,10-methylenetetrahydrofolate in bifunctional dehydrogenase-cyclohydrolase enzymes. *Biochemistry* 1998; 37: 1109–15.

97. Pelletier, JN, MacKenzie, RE. Binding and interconversion of tetrahydrofolates at a single site in the bifunctional methylenetetrahydrofolate dehydrogenase/cyclohydrolase. *Biochemistry* 1995; 34: 12673–80.

98. Peri, KG, Belanger, C, Mackenzie, RE. Nucleotide sequence of the human NAD-dependent methylene tetrahydrofolate dehydrogenase-cyclohydrolase. *Nucleic Acids Res* 1989; 17: 8853.

99. Peri, KG, MacKenzie, RE. NAD(+)-dependent methylenetetrahydrofolate dehydrogenase-cyclohydrolase: detection of the mRNA in normal murine tissues and transcriptional regulation of the gene in cell lines. *Biochim Biophys Acta* 1993; 1171: 281–87.

100. Pfendner, W, Pizer, LI. The metabolism of serine and glycine in mutant lines of Chinese hamster ovary cells. *Arch Biochem Biophys* 1980; 200: 503–12.

101. Porter, DH, Cook, RJ, Wagner, C. Enzymatic properties of dimethylglycine dehydrogenase and sarcosine dehydrogenase from rat liver. *Arch Biochem Biophys* 1985; 243: 396–407.

102. Rios-Orlandi, EM, Zarkadas, CG, MacKenzie, RE. Formyltetrahydrofolate dehydrogenase-hydrolase from pig liver: Simultaneous assay of the activities. *Biochim Biophys Acta* 1986; 871: 24–35.

103. Santhosh-Kumar, CR, Kolhouse, JF. Molar quantitation of folates by gas chromatography-mass spectrometry. *Methods Enzymol* 1997; 281: 26–38.

104. Schalinske, KL, Steele, RD. Quantification of the carbon flow through the folate-dependent one-carbon pool using radiolabeled histidine: effect of altered thyroid and folate status. *Arch Biochem Biophys* 1996; 328: 93–100.

105. Schalinske, KL, and Steele, RD. Quantitation of carbon flow through the hepatic folate-dependent one-carbon pool in rats. *Arch Biochem Biophys* 1989; 271: 49–55.

106. Schirch, D, Villar, E, Maras, B, Barra, D, Schirch, V. Domain structure and function of 10-formyltetrahydrofolate dehydrogenase. *J Biol Chem* 1994; 269: 24728–35.

107. Schirch, L. Folates in serine and glycine metabolism. In *Folates and Pterins* (Blakley, RL, Benkovic, SJ, eds.). John Wiley & Sons, New York, 1984; pp. 399–431.

108. Schirch, V. Enzymatic determination of folylpolyglutamate pools. *Methods Enzymol* 1997; 281: 77–81.

109. Schirch, V. Mechanism of folate-requiring enzymes in one-carbon metabolism. In *Comprehensive Biological Catalysis* (Sinnott, M, ed.). Academic Press, Ltd., New York, 1998; pp. 211–52.

110. Schirch, V. Purification of folate-dependent enzymes from rabbit liver. *Methods Enzymol* 1997; 281: 146–61.

111. Schirch, V, Strong, WB. Interaction of folylpolyglutamates with enzymes in one-carbon metabolism. *Arch Biochem Biophys* 1989; 269: 371–80.

112. Scott, CR. Sarcosinemia. In *The Metabolic Basis of Inherited Disease* (Scriver, CR, Beaudet, AL, Sly, WS, Valle, D, eds.). McGraw-Hill, New York. 1989; pp. 735–41.

113. Scrutton, MC, Beis, I. Inhibitory effects of histidine and their reversal. The roles of pyruvate carboxylase and N10-formyltetrahydrofolate dehydrogenase. *Biochem J* 1979; 177: 833–46.

114. Selhub, J. Determination of tissue folate composition by affinity chromatography followed by high-pressure ion pair liquid chromatography. *Anal Biochem* 1989; 182: 84–93.

115. Shane, B. Folate chemistry and metabolism. In *Folate in Health and Disease* (Bailey, LB, ed.). Marcel Dekker, Inc., New York, 1995; pp. 1–22.

116. Shane, B. Folylpolyglutamate synthesis and role in the regulation of one-carbon metabolism. *Vitam Horm* 1989; 45: 263–335.

117. Smith, EN, Taylor, RT. Acute toxicity of methanol in the folate-deficient acatalasemic mouse. *Toxicology* 1982; 25: 271–87.

118. Smith, GK, Mueller, WT, Wasserman, GF, Taylor, WD, Benkovic, SJ. Characterization of the enzyme complex involving the folate-requiring enzymes of de novo purine biosynthesis. *Biochemistry* 1980; 19: 4313–21.

119. Snell, K. Enzymes of serine metabolism in normal, developing and neoplastic rat tissues. *Adv Enzyme Regul* 1984; 22: 325–400.

120. Snell, K, Fell, DA. Metabolic control analysis of mammalian serine metabolism. *Adv Enzyme Regul* 1990; 30: 13–32.

121. Srere, PA. 17th Fritz Lipmann Lecture. Wanderings (wonderings) in metabolism. *Biol Chem Hoppe Seyler* 1993; 374: 833–42.

122. Staben, C, Rabinowitz, JC. Formation of formylmethionyl-tRNA and initiation of protein synthesis. In *Folates and Pterins* (Blakley, RL, Benkovic, SL, eds.). John Wiley & Sons, New York, 1984; pp. 457–95.

123. Steginjk, LD, Filer, Jr, LJ, Bell, EF, Ziegler, EE, Tephly, TR, Krause, WL. Repeated ingestion of aspartame-sweetened beverages: Further observations in individuals heterozygous for phenylketonuria. *Metabolism* 1990; 39: 1076–81.

124. Stites, TE, Bailey, LB, Scott, KC, Toth, JP, Fisher, WP, Gregory, JF, 3rd. Kinetic modeling of folate metabolism through use of chronic administration of deuterium-labeled folic acid in men. *Am J Clin Nutr* 1997; 65: 53–60.

125. Stover, P, Kruschwitz, H, Schirch, V. Evidence that 5-formyltetrahydropteroylglutamate has a metabolic role in one-carbon metabolism. *Adv Exp Med Biol* 1993; 338: 679–85.

126. Stover, P, Schirch, V. The metabolic role of leucovorin. *Trends Biochem Sci* 1993; 18: 102–26.

127. Stover, P, Schirch, V. Serine hydroxymethyltransferase catalyzes the hydrolysis of 5,10-methenyltetrahydrofolate to 5-formyltetrahydrofolate. *J Biol Chem* 1990; 265: 14227–33.

128. Stover, PJ, Chen, LH, Suh, JR, Stover, DM, Keyomarsi, K, Shane, B. Molecular cloning, characterization, and regulation of the human mitochondrial serine hydroxymethyltransferase gene. *J Biol Chem* 1997; 272: 1842–28.

129. Strong, W, Joshi, G, Lura, R, Muthukumaraswamy, N, Schirch, V. 10-Formyltetrahydrofolate synthetase. Evidence for a conformational change in the enzyme upon binding of tetrahydropteroylpolyglutamates. *J Biol Chem* 1987; 262: 12519–25.

130. Strong, WB, Cook, RJ, Schirch, V. Interaction of tetrahydropteroylpolyglutamates with two enzymes from mitochondria. *Biochemistry* 1989; 28: 106–14.

131. Strong, WB, Schirch, V. In vitro conversion of formate to serine: Effect of tetrahydropteroylpolyglutamates and serine hydroxymethyltransferase on the rate of 10-formyltetrahydrofolate synthetase. *Biochemistry* 1989; 28: 9430–39.

132. Strong, WB, Tendler, SJ, Seither, RL, Goldman, ID, Schirch, V. Purification and properties of serine hydroxymethyltransferase and C1-tetrahydrofolate synthase from L1210 cells. *J Biol Chem* 1990; 265: 12149–55.

133. Suzuki, N, and Wagner, C. Purification and characterization of a folate binding protein from rat liver cytosol. *Arch Biochem Biophys* 1980; 199: 236–48.

134. Swendseid, ME, Bethell, FH, Ackermann, WW. The intracellular disribution of vitamin B12 and folinic acid in mouse liver. *J Biol Chem* 1951; 190: 791–98.

135. Taylor, RT, Hanna, ML. Folate-dependent enzymes in cultured Chinese hamster cells: Folylpolyglutamate synthetase and its absence in mutants auxotrophic for glycine + adenosine + thymidine. *Arch Biochem Biophys* 1977; 181: 331–34.

136. Taylor, RT, and Hanna, ML. Folate-dependent enzymes in cultured Chinese hamster ovary cells: Evidence for mutant forms of folylpolyglutamate synthetase. *Arch Biochem Biophys* 1979; 197: 36–43.

137. Taylor, RT, Hanna, ML. Folate-dependent enzymes in cultured Chinese hamster ovary cells: Impaired mitochondrial serine hydroxymethyltransferase activity in two additional glycine–auxotroph complementation classes. *Arch Biochem Biophys* 1982; 217: 609–23.

138. Taylor, RT, Wu, R, Hanna, ML. Induced reversion of a Chinese hamster ovary triple auxotroph. Validation of the system with several mutagens. *Mutat Res* 1985; 151: 293–308.

139. Temple, C, Montgomery, JA. Chemical and physical properties of folic acid and reduced derivatives. In *Folates and Pterins* (Blakley, RL, Benkovic, SJ, eds.). John Wiley & Sons, New York, 1984; pp. 61–120.

140. Wagner, C. Biochemical role of folate in cellular metabolism. In *Folate in Health and Disease* (Bailey, LB, ed.). Marcel Dekker, Inc., New York; 1995; pp. 23–42.

141. Wagner, C. Symposium on the subcellular compartmentation of folate metabolism. *J Nutr* 1996; 126: 1228S–34S.

142. Wagner, C, Briggs, WT, Cook, RJ. Inhibition of glycine N-methyltransferase activity by folate derivatives: Implications for regulation of methyl group metabolism. *Biochem Biophys Res Commun* 1985; 127: 746–52.

143. Wakabayashi, M, Nakata, R, Tsukamoto, I. Regulation of thymidylate synthase in regenerating rat liver after partial hepatectomy. *Biochem Mol Biol Int* 1994; 34: 345–50.

144. Wang, FK, Koch, J, Stokstad, EL. Folate coenzyme pattern, folate linked enzymes and methionine biosynthesis in rat liver mitochondria. *Biochem Z* 1967; 346: 458–66.

145. Waydhas, C, Weigl, K, Sies, H. The disposition of formaldehyde and formate arising from drug N-demethylations dependent on cytochrome P-450 in hepatocytes and in perfused rat liver. *Eur J Biochem* 1978; 89: 143–50

146. West, MG, Barlowe, CK, Appling, DR. Cloning and characterization of the *Saccharomyces cerevisiae* gene encoding NAD-dependent 5,10-methylenetetrahydrofolate dehydrogenase. *J Biol Chem* 1993; 268: 153–60.

147. West, MG, Horne, DW, Appling, DR. Metabolic role of cytoplasmic isozymes of 5,10-methylenetetrahydrofolate dehydrogenase in *Saccharomyces cerevisiae*. *Biochemistry* 1996; 35: 3122–32.

148. Wittwer, AJ, Wagner, C. Identification of the folate-binding proteins of rat liver mitochondria as dimethylglycine dehydrogenase and sarcosine dehydrogenase. Flavoprotein nature and enzymatic properties of the purified proteins. *J Biol Chem* 1981; 256: 4109–15.

149. Wittwer, AJ, Wagner, C. Identification of the folate-binding proteins of rat liver mitochondria as dimethylglycine dehydrogenase and sarcosine dehydrogenase. Purification and folate-binding characteristics. *J Biol Chem* 1981; 256: 4102–8.

150. Yang, XM, and MacKenzie, RE. NAD-dependent methylenetetrahydrofolate dehydrogenase-methenyltetrahydrofolate cyclohydrolase is the mammalian homolog of the mitochondrial enzyme encoded by the yeast MIS1 gene. *Biochemistry* 1993; 32: 11118–23.

151. Yeo, EJ, Wagner, C. Tissue distribution of glycine N-methyltransferase, a major folate-binding protein of liver. *Proc Natl Acad Sci USA* 1994; 91: 210–14.

152. Yoshida, T, Kikuchi, G. Comparative study on major pathways of glycine and serine catabolism in vertebrate livers. *J Biochem (Tokyo)* 1972; 72: 1503–16.

153. Yoshida, T, Kikuchi, G. Major pathways of glycine and serine catabolism in rat liver. *Arch Biochem Biophys* 1970; 139: 380–92.

154. Yoshida, T, Kikuchi, G. Major pathways of serine and glycine catabolism in various organs of the rat and cock. *J Biochem (Tokyo)* 1973; 73: 1013–22.

155. Yoshida, T, and Kikuchi, G. Significance of the glycine cleavage system in glycine and serine catabolism in avian liver. *Arch Biochem Biophys* 1971; 145: 658–68.

156. Zamierowski, MM, Wagner, C. Identification of folate binding proteins in rat liver. *J Biol Chem* 1977; 252: 933–38.

157. Zelikson, R, Luzzati, M. Mitochondrial and cytoplasmic distribution in *Saccharomyces cerevisiae* of enzymes involved in folate-coenzyme-mediated one-carbon-group transfer. A genetic and biochemical study of the enzyme deficiencies in mutants tmp3 and ade3. *Eur J Biochem* 1977; 79: 285–92.

12

Cobalamin-Dependent Remethylation

HORATIU OLTEANU
RUMA BANERJEE

The two major metabolic avenues for the removal of homocysteine in mammalian cells are remethylation and transsulfuration. Remethylation is catalyzed by methionine synthase and by betaine homocysteine methyltransferase, but the latter enzyme has limited tissue distribution, being confined to the liver and kidney (21). Transsulfuration is catalyzed by cystathionine β-synthase and commits homocysteine to degradation and its ultimate removal as sulfate.

Methionine synthase (Metabolic Diagram, Reaction 4), is an essential housekeeping enzyme found in all three kingdoms of life. In prokaryotes it catalyzes the terminal step in the de novo biosynthesis of methionine, converting homocysteine to methionine. Two classes of methionine synthase have been found in Eubacteria: cobalamin-dependent and cobalamin-independent enzymes. Both catalyze the transfer of a methyl group from 5-methyltetrahydrofolate to homocysteine and represent convergent evolutionary solutions to the same chemical problem (25). In mammals, only the cobalamin-dependent form of methionine synthase has been found.

In mammals, methionine is an essential amino acid and methionine synthase plays an important role in two key metabolic pathways:

1. It functions to conserve homocysteine as methionine, which is a precursor of S-adenosyl-methionine (AdoMet) that supports methylation of RNA, DNA, proteins, and lipids. Aberrations in this pathway may explain the pathogenesis of the neuropathy (subacute combined degeneration) associated with cobalamin deficiency (72).
2. Methionine synthase plays a key role in folate-dependent one-carbon metabolism by releasing 5-methyltetrahydrofolate, the circulating form of the vitamin that is delivered from the blood to the cells, as tetrahydrofolate, which is then available to support DNA and amino acid biosynthetic reactions. Impairments in methionine synthase create a "methyl trap" with a concomitant shift in the intracellular folate pool toward 5-methyltetrahydrofolate (32a, 54).

These changes lead to an effective intracellular folate deficiency and arrested DNA biosynthesis. The metabolic ramifications of impaired methionine synthase activity have led to it being viewed as a choice chemotherapeutic target (48).

Methionine synthase deficiency presents itself with a complex clinical picture including homocystinuria or severe hyperhomocysteinemia, megaloblastic anemia, hypomethioninemia, and neurological disorders with developmental delay and cerebral atrophy (19). Mild hyperhomocysteinemia is related to pregnancy complications (64) and neural tube defects (49) (see Chapter 37). As discussed in the second half of this book, data from numerous clinical and epidemiological studies also point to hyperhomocysteinemia as a strong risk factor for atherosclerotic vascular disease and thromboembolism (28, 56, 63 and references therein). Because of these multiple and intricate pathological connections, the study of methionine synthase is presently enjoying increasing attention.

Characteristics of Methionine Synthase

Physical Properties of the Enzyme

Methionine synthase is a large monomeric protein with a molecular mass of 140 kDa in humans (7, 41, 43) and 139 kDa in rat (77). The mammalian enzyme has been purified to near homogeneity from porcine (9) and rat (76) liver and has a specific activity of 1.6 to 1.7 μmol min^{-1}mg^{-1} protein at 37°C, which corresponds to a turnover number of ~250 min^{-1} (9). The *Escherichia coli* enzyme is highly homologous and only slightly shorter, with a molecular mass of 133 kDa (15) (see also Chapter 10).

Methionine synthase is one of only two known mammalian enzymes that requires a cobalamin cofactor for activity (1, 44). Cobalamin has been appropriately described as "Nature's most beautiful cofactor" (65), and its discovery goes back to the Nobel prize winning work of Whipple (73) and Minot and Murphy (50), which resulted in liver therapy for treatment of pernicious anemia. The role of methylcobalamin in methionine synthase was established in 1962 (29). A single molecule of cobalamin is bound per monomer. In mammalian methionine synthases from pig liver and human placenta, the holoenzyme or cobalamin-bound state represents 90% to 100% of the total enzyme (10). In contrast, only 13% of methionine synthase is in the holoenzyme form in megaloblastic bone marrow cells (67). Fibroblast cells in culture exhibit variable levels of holomethionine synthase (31).

The ultraviolet-visible spectrum of the purified porcine enzyme has absorption maxima at 358 nm, 506 nm, and 536 nm at pH 7.2, consistent with the presence of hydroxocobalamin (10). In free methylcobalamin, the central cobalt atom has a methyl group as the upper axial ligand, and the lower axial coordination site is occupied by a nitrogen atom donated by the intramolecular base, dimethylbenzimidazole (see Figure 24.1). The crystal structure of the cobalamin-binding domain from the *E. coli* methionine synthase therefore was surprising because it showed that a histidine residue from the protein replaces the dimethylbenzimidazole (14). Because the sequences between the *E. coli* and human proteins are highly conserved in the cobalamin-binding domain, including the complete retention of the signature cobalamin-binding sequence (47), a similar conformation for the bound cobalamin is expected in the mammalian enzyme.

Fig. 12.1. Postulated reaction mechanism of methionine synthase. (DTT, dithiothreitol.)

Reductive Activation System

In addition to the cobalamin cofactor, methionine synthase requires a reductive activation system for sustained activity. During catalysis, cobalamin cycles between cob(I)alamin and cob(III)alamin oxidation states (Figure 12.1). In the first transmethylation half reaction, the methyl group from the substrate, 5-methyltetrahydrofolate (methyl-THF), is transferred to the cob(I)alamin form of the cofactor to generate methylcobalamin and tetrahydrofolate (THF) (Equation 1). In the next transmethylation half reaction (Equation 2), the methyl group is transferred to homocysteine to give methionine and cob(I)alamin (5).

$$\text{Methyl-THF} + \text{Cob(I)alamin} \rightarrow \text{THF} + \text{Methylcobalamin} \qquad [1]$$

$$\text{Methylcobalamin} + \text{Homocysteine} \rightarrow \text{Cob(I)alamin} + \text{Methionine} \qquad [2]$$

Cob(I)alamin is a highly reactive species and suffers adventitious oxidation every 200 to 2,000 turnovers, depending on the ambient redox conditions in vitro (15), leading to the inactivation of the enzyme. The oxidative lability of cob(I)alamin renders the activity of methionine synthase dependent on a reductive activation system. The enzyme can be rescued back to the catalytic cycle in a reductive methylation reaction dependent on AdoMet and an electron source. Under in vitro assay conditions, titanium citrate or dithiothreitol and hydroxocobalamin can serve as artificial electron donors (Figure 12.1).

The physiological electron donor to methionine synthase is NADPH in both mammals and in *E. coli*. However, the proteins mediating electron transfer are distinct (Figure 12.2). In *E. coli*, electrons are transferred from NADPH to methionine synthase by the action of two flavoproteins, NADPH-flavodoxin (ferredoxin) reductase and flavodoxin (23, 24) (Figure 12.2). In mammals, two similar solutions to the problem of electron transfer from NADPH to methionine synthase have been described recently using genetic (42) and biochemical approaches (11). A cDNA encoding "methionine synthase reductase" has been cloned by Gravel and co-workers using a genetic-homology-based PCR approach based on the hypothesis that flavodoxin and flavodoxin reductase are fused into a single protein in mammals (42). The cDNA has an open reading frame that encodes a 698-amino acid polypeptide with a predicted molecular mass of 77 kDa. It contains putative

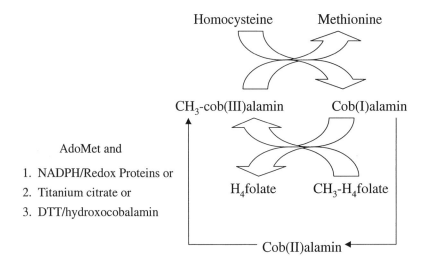

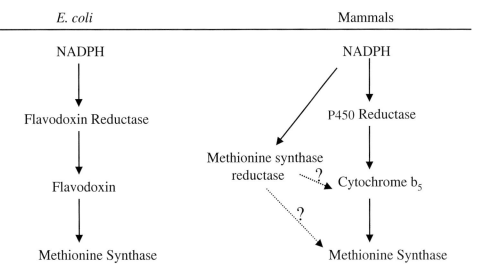

Fig. 12.2. Reductive activation pathway for methionine synthase in *E. coli* and postulated pathways for the mammalian enzyme.

FMN, FAD, and NADPH binding sites. The gene has been mapped to chromosome 5p15.2–15.3 and is 38% identical to human cytochrome P450 reductase. Several mutations have been identified in the methionine synthase reductase gene in *cblE* cell lines from patients and provides compelling evidence that the gene product is involved in the reductive activation of methionine synthase (42). However, the enzyme has not been purified, and its ability to reduce methionine synthase directly has yet to be demonstrated.

Biochemical analysis of the mammalian reductive activation system yielded a similar though not identical solution (11). Based on reconstitution of methionine synthase activity by fractions separated from a porcine liver homogenate, involvement of two protein components was indicated (31). One of the components was purified to homogeneity and identified as soluble cytochrome b_5. The other component is microsomal and could be cytochrome P450 reductase (11). Purified cytochrome b_5 and cytochrome P450 reductase in the presence of NADPH and AdoMet can fully reconstitute methionine synthase activity. The available data suggest that two alternative pathways are capable of electron delivery to mammalian methionine synthase under in vitro conditions: microsomal P450 reductase in the presence of soluble cytochrome b_5 and methionine synthase reductase either singly or in the presence of soluble cytochrome b_5 (Figure 12.2). The physiological relevance of these pathways remains to be established.

Kinetic Properties of the Enzyme

Several methods are available for assaying methionine synthase (3). In the most widely used assay, transfer of the radiolabeled methyl group from the substrate, 5-methyltetrahydrofolate (methyl-THF), to the product, methionine, is monitored (Equation 3).

$$[^{14}C]\text{-Methyl-THF} + \text{Homocysteine} \rightarrow \text{THF} + [^{14}C]\text{-Methionine} \qquad [3]$$

Provision of AdoMet and a source of reducing agents are needed for this assay. Alternative reducing agents can be used under in vitro assay conditions: (1) dithiothreitol and hydroxocobalamin, (2) titanium citrate, or (3) NADPH and redox proteins (3). Whereas the first assay with dithiothreitol and hydoxocobalamin is semianaerobic, the other two assays are conducted under strictly anaerobic conditions (3). A combination of these assays has been used effectively to characterize the nature of the defects in *cblE* and *cblG* cell lines (see Chapter 21). A fixed time assay, which monitors the production of tetrahydrofolate spectrophotometrically following its derivatization to methenyltetrahydrofolate, has been described (16).

Mammalian methionine synthase (9) follows a kinetic pattern similar to the *E. coli* enzyme (2). Kinetic analysis with the purified pig liver enzyme reveals an ordered sequential mechanism, with K_m(Methyl-THF) = 16.8 μmol/L and K_m(Hcy) = 2.2 μmol/L (9). Similar values have been reported for the rat liver enzyme: K_m(Methyl-THF) = 75 μmol/L and K_m(Hcy) = 1.7 μmol/L (76).

Methionine synthase binds polyglutamylated 5-methyltetrahydrofolate more avidly, as has been seen with other folate-dependent enzymes. This preference is reflected in the three-fold lower K_m and two-fold higher V_{max} values for the pentaglutamate and heptaglutamate substrates versus the monoglutamate (12). Polyamines such as putrescine, cadaverine, spermine, and spermidine are reported to stimulate the activity of the rat enzyme. The most prominent effect (up to

400% increase in enzyme activity) was observed with spermine and spermidine (36). The activity of methionine synthase is reported to be inhibited by nitric oxide (NO) (53), ethanol (37), cobalamin analogs (62), and methylmercury (61).

Nitrous oxide (N₂O), or laughing gas, is an anesthetic that can precipitate hematological and neurological abnormalities, including megaloblastic anemia and subacute combined degeneration of the spinal cord (see Chapters 24 and 27). Kondo and co-workers (40) have shown complex deleterious effects of nitrous oxide on cobalamin metabolism in rats, with accompanying inhibition of methionine synthase. The inactivation process has been elucidated mechanistically with the *E. coli* enzyme and results from oxidative damage to the protein, induced by one-electron reduction of nitrous oxide leading to the formation of a reactive hydroxyl radical (17, 18). To increase awareness of nitrous oxide side effects in patients with subclinical cobalamin deficiency, the name *anesthesia paresthetica* has been proposed to describe the associated syndrome (39).

Domain Organization

Characterization of tryptic fragments produced by limited proteolysis of the *E. coli* enzyme (4) has revealed a modular organization for the protein (15, 27) (Figure 12.3). Based on the high degree of primary sequence identity between the *E. coli* and human proteins, the latter is expected to share a similar architecture. The crystal structures of the C-terminal activation domain that binds AdoMet (13) and the central cobalamin-binding domain (14) have been determined (see Chapter 10). These provide a useful structural perspective on the locations and possible consequences of polymorphisms and mutations that have been described in the human gene. The N-terminal domain houses the substrate binding sites and can be further subdivided into a homocysteine binding fragment extending from residues 1-353 (27) and the 5-methyltetrahydrofolate-binding subdomain extending from fragments 354-649 (57) in the *E. coli* sequence. The homocysteine binding site has a tightly bound zinc that plays a role in activation of the substrate thiolate via direct coordination (26, 55). The central cobalamin-binding domain is thus shared between the catalytic and activation functions, and alternative domain conformations appear to control whether the cofactor is accessible for catalysis or reductive methylation (33).

Molecular Cloning and Chromosomal Localization of Human Methionine Synthase

The gene encoding human methionine synthase was cloned and sequenced simultaneously by several groups

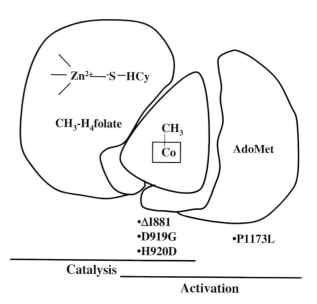

Fig. 12.3. Predicted domain organization of the human methionine synthase showing location of mutations isolated from *cblG* patient cell lines. (Hcy, homocysteine; Co, cobalt.)

(7, 41, 43). This was an important achievement because it opened the door to identification of mutations that specifically affect the human enzyme. The cDNA contains an open reading frame of 3,798 nucleotides encoding a protein of 1,265 amino acids with a predicted molecular mass of 140 kDa. The human gene maps to chromosomal location 1q42.3–43.8 (7). Sequence alignments show 55%, 64%, and 92% identity with the *E. coli*, putative *Caenorhabditis elegans*, and rat liver enzymes, respectively (43, 77). Recently, the cloning of the rat methionine synthase cDNA and overexpression of the recombinant protein in insect cells have been reported (77).

Northern analysis has identified the methionine synthase mRNA in a variety of tissues, including liver, heart, brain, placenta, lung, skeletal muscle, kidney, pancreas, spleen, and thymus (43). Two main mRNA species of ~8 and 10 kb are observed. The 10 kb band appears to be a preprocessed form of the 8 kb species because it hybridizes to a sequence from intron 5 (7). Methionine synthase is expressed early in fetal development (68). The presence of methionine synthase activity during neurulation in the rat embryo may explain the role of altered homocysteine metabolism in the etiology of neural tube defects (68).

Regulation of Mammalian Methionine Synthase

Regulation of mammalian methionine synthase by its cobalamin cofactor was first reported in Hep-2 cells where a 30-fold increase in enzyme activity was observed when the culture medium was supplemented with cyanocobalamin (46). In this study, methionine and choline were replaced by homocysteine and cyanocobalamin in the culture medium. The stimulatory effect was subsequently demonstrated to be independent of the presence or absence of homocysteine, leading to the conclusion that the observed activation of methionine synthase could be attributed solely to the presence of cobalamin. Similar results were later reported with other cell lines in which cyanocobalamin supplementation elicited a 10- to 30-fold activation of the enzyme (45). In contrast, cyanocobalamin supplementation of the culture medium had no effect on the activity of the only other cobalamin-dependent enzyme, methylmalonyl-CoA mutase (38).

An even higher activation (up to fourfold beyond the level induced by cyanocobalamin) was observed when cells were grown in medium containing cyanocobalamin, folic acid, and homocysteine instead of methionine (34). Rats fed a diet deficient in choline and methionine showed a similar pattern of activation on cyanocobalamin supplementation and a further increase in activity resulted after removal of methionine from the cobalamin-containing diet (20).

To gain insight into the nature of the regulation exerted by cobalamin, the effect of the protein inhibitor, puromycin, was studied in hamster kidney cells (34). Puromycin affected activation of methionine synthase induced by low methionine, but not by cobalamin. Based on these results, the effect of cobalamin on methionine synthase activation was ascribed to the conversion of apoenzyme to holoenzyme (34). However, these data are equivocal because the highly efficient import of cyanocobalamin into cells could have surpassed the kinetics of the puromycin effect, accounting for the results. Furthermore, stabilization of the enzyme by cobalamin could not be ruled out.

The availability of the gene sequence and antibodies to the human enzymes, as well as the development of sensitive anaerobic assays, now permit a reexamination of this question by more sensitive techniques. These studies clearly revealed that induction of methionine synthase activity is not correlated with holoenzyme content in cells grown with and without cyanocobalamin supplementation (30). Western blot analysis shows that methionine synthase activation parallels the increase in the methionine synthase protein levels, demonstrating that new protein is synthesized. In contrast, methionine synthase mRNA levels detected by Northern analysis remained unchanged during the same time period. These results preclude both transcriptional regulation and conversion of apoenzyme to holoenzyme as the basis of cobalamin activation of methionine synthase, although the actual mechanism remains to be unraveled. Clinical implications of the cobalamin-dependent increase in methionine synthase activity are many, including consequences of food fortification by cobalamin that is being considered and homocysteine-lowering intervention trials by multivitamin regimens.

Another locus for regulation of methionine synthase is represented by the reductive activation system. Thus, the intracellular NADPH/NADP$^+$ ratio or, more generally, the redox status of the cell might influence methionine synthase activity. In addition, the levels of soluble cytochrome b_5 and/or methionine synthase reductase could represent additional regulatory levers (8). The physiological significance of this level of regulation has yet to be explored. A preliminary report indicated stimulation of methionine synthase activity by protein kinase A under in vitro conditions, leading to the proposal that the enzyme may be regulated by phosphorylation by protein kinase A (35). These studies, however, need to be confirmed.

Remethylation and Hyperhomocysteinemia

Methionine Synthase Mutations Associated with Severe Hyperhomocysteinemia

Intracellular cobalamin metabolism is compartmentalized, complex, and remains incompletely characterized. The final forms of the cofactor derivatives for the cobalamin-containing enzymes, methionine synthase and methylmalonyl-CoA mutase, are synthesized in the cytoplasm (methylcobalamin) and mitochondrion (5′-deoxyadenosylcobalamin), respectively. Genetic complementation analyses have characterized defects at different loci in the cobalamin metabolic pathways (19).

Isolated functional deficiency of methionine synthase is found in *cblE* and *cblG* complementation groups. In *cblC*, *cblD*, and *cblF*, both methylcobalamin and 5′-deoxyadenosylcobalamin-dependent reactions are compromised. Remethylation defects can also result from impairments in 5,10-methylenetetrahydrofolate reductase deficiency, which reduce the availability of 5-methyltetrahydrofolate (see Chapter 21).

The *cblG* phenotype is inherited as an autosomal recessive disorder (71). Initially, two subgroups of *cblG* cell lines were distinguished based on a concentration of [^{57}Co]cobalamin bound to methionine synthase that was either comparable to normal controls or was virtually undetectable (60). In vitro assays using enzyme from fibroblast cells can also detect the heterogeneity in *cblG* patient cell lines (31). In the first subset with normal levels of bound cobalamin, methionine synthase activity is indistinguishable from control cell lines when artificial reductants are used, but the activity is lower when the NADPH-dependent physiological reducing system is used. In the second group (referred to as variants), the catalytic activity is markedly reduced under all assay conditions (31).

The apparently normal methionine synthase activity in one subgroup of *cblG* cells in the presence of artificial but not physiological electron donors strongly implied that the mutations in methionine synthase in these cell lines were likely to be confined to the activation domains. Using single strand conformational polymorphism analysis and nucleotide sequencing approaches, mutations were in fact mapped to the cobalamin- and AdoMet-binding domains (Table 12.1 and Figure 12.3), important in reactivation (32, 41). The crystal structures of these domains available for the *E. coli* enzyme (13, 14), provide a structural framework within which their adverse effects can be rationalized.

In contrast, mutations in the variant cell lines lead to greatly diminished steady-state levels of the methionine synthase mRNA (32, 75). Four mutations have been described in this subgroup (Table 12.1) that are predicted to result in premature termination and are expected to be functionally null (75). However, the biochemical characterization of two of these mutant cell lines, WG1670 and WG1671, contradict the predictions based on the genetic data because measurable, albeit very low, methionine synthase activity was detected in these lines (31). Furthermore, they contradict the results from the mouse knockout experiments discussed later, which reveal that methionine synthase is an essential gene, at least in this organism (66). An explanation for this discrepancy may lie in the nature of the defects. The defect in at least one allele in each of the cell lines carrying functionally null mutations is predicted to unmask a cryptic splice site (75). A low frequency of normal splicing would account for the low level of activity that is measured in these cells (31).

Methionine Synthase Reductase Mutations Associated with Severe Hyperhomocysteinemia

Biochemical and genetic characterization of fibroblast cells provided strong evidence that the defective locus in *cblE* cell lines is in the reductive activation system (31, 58, 59). However, a description of the molecular defects in these cell lines had to await identification of the protein(s) that are involved in reductive activation of mammalian methionine synthases. The solutions that have been discovered to date, methionine synthase reductase (42) and soluble cytochrome b_5 in combination with a P450-type reductase (11), thus represent genetic loci that could be affected by mutations or polymorphisms that are associated with hyperhomocysteinemia. Several mutations in methionine synthase reductase in *cblE* cell lines have been described (42, 74) (see Chapters 21 and 22), but a similar investigation of the cytochrome b_5 gene has yet to be reported. However, in this context it is interesting to note that a third complementation group that is distinct from *cblE* and *cblG* has been reported recently that is associated with an isolated functional deficiency of methionine synthase (22). Because the mutations in *cblE* cell lines are in methionine synthase reductase, this newly described genetic complementation group could have mutations in alternative redox proteins, viz., soluble cytochrome b_5 or the P450-like reductase.

Table 12.1. Polymorphisms and Mutations Identified in Methionine Synthase

Cell Line	Mutation	Phenotype	Reference
Mutations			
1. *cblG* WG1892	2640ΔATC	ΔIle881, single amino acid deletion in cobalamin-binding domain	32, 41
	3517C→T	P1173L, mutation in AdoMet-binding domain	
2. *cblG* WG1505	3517C→T	P1173L, mutation in AdoMet-binding domain	31
3. *cblG* WG2290	2758C→G	H920D, mutation in cobalamin-binding domain	41
4. *cblG* WG1655	3378insA	Frameshift with premature termination	75
	mid IVS-6 G→A substitution	Generation of cryptic 3′-acceptor splice site leading to premature termination	
5. *cblG* WG1670[a]	2112ΔTC	Frameshift with premature termination	75
6. *cblG* WG1671[a]	−166IVS-3 A→G	Generation of cryptic 3′-acceptor splice site leading to premature termination	
Polymorphisms			
1.	2756A→G	D919G, mutation in cobalamin-binding domain	7, 41, 68
2.	2053A→T	K685K, silent polymorphism	69
3.	2127A→G	E709E, silent polymorphism	69
4.	3144A→G	A1048A, silent polymorphism	69

[a] These cell lines were from siblings.

The membrane and soluble forms of cytochrome b_5 are encoded by the same gene that produces two different transcripts by alternative splicing. The presence of a 24 bp insertion into one of the cDNA isoforms brings a stop codon in frame resulting in early termination and leading to the smaller soluble form with a molecular mass of 10,997 Da (70). The small size of the coding sequence and the even smaller size of the unique insertion sequence that distinguishes the soluble from the membrane-bound form predict that mutations in cytochrome b_5 will be statistically rare. The membrane-associated form of cytochrome b_5 serves an essential function in fatty acid desaturation and P450-dependent hydroxylation reactions. Thus, mutations outside the 24-base stretch that is unique to the soluble form could be expected to have multiple detrimental effects.

Polymorphisms in Methionine Synthase

Moderately elevated homocysteine levels have been associated with apparently unrelated pathologies, such as neural tube defects (49) and vascular disease (56 and references cited therein). This has led to an intense effort to identify polymorphisms in the human methionine synthase gene that may be associated with risk for hyperhomocysteinemia. The first study to be reported examined the nucleotide sequence of methionine synthase in cDNA from eight patients with mild hyperhomocysteinemia (69). Four of the patients had neural tube defects, and the other four had experienced pregnancies complicated by spiral (uteroplacental) arterial disease. Of the four polymorphisms detected, three were silent, and the fourth (2756A→G) caused a coding sequence change, D919G, that had been reported previously (7, 41) (Table 12.1). This polymorphism has a fairly high prevalence in the control Dutch population, with the frequency of the AA, AG, and GG genotypes being 71%, 27%, and 3%, respectively. The study, however, revealed no association between this genotype and either neural tube defects or spiral arterial disease, or between the genotype and increased homocysteine levels. A similar study on a British population found no significant association between the 2756A→G genotype and the occurrence of neural tube defects, or between the maternal allele and neural tube defects (52). The 2756A→G polymorphism is also common in the general population in Japan and is not associated with altered homocysteine metabolism or late-onset vascular disease (51). Because the risk for developing colorectal cancer is associated with low-methyl (low folate, low methionine, and high alcohol) diets, the association, if any, between the 667C→T polymorphism in the 5,10-methylenetetrahydrofolate reductase gene, the 2756A→G polymorphism in

methionine synthase and the risk of colorectal adenomas was examined. However, no significant association was found (6). Polymorphisms in the long 3′-untranslated region and in the regulatory sequences have not been reported so far.

Mouse Model for Methionine Synthase Deficiency

Efforts have been directed toward the development of a mouse model for methionine synthase deficiency because of the pathological importance of the enzyme. Using gene targeting technology in embryonic cells, the methionine synthase gene has been knocked out (66). Heterozygous matings indicate that homozygous knockouts are nonviable, as wild-type (+/+), heterozygous (+/−), and homozygous (−/−) progeny are produced in a 1:2:0 ratio. Methionine synthase in heterozygotes displays 65% of the activity found in the wild-type control animals consistent with the genotype. Heterozygotes and controls have similar homocysteine levels (Shane B, personal communication). As expected, there is no difference in the levels of cystathionine-β synthase and methylmalonyl-CoA mutase activities between the wild-type and heterozygous mice.

The study of mammalian methionine synthase is enjoying a resurgence of interest spurred by the associations between hyperhomocysteinemia and cardiovascular diseases and neural tube defects. The introduction of modern biochemical and molecular genetic techniques have resulted in remarkable progress over the last half decade. The important milestones include purification of the mammalian enzyme to homogeneity (9), cloning of the human cDNA (7, 41, 43), description of mutations associated with severe hyperhomocysteinemia (31, 32, 41) and the creation of a mouse knockout model mimicking methionine synthase deficiency (66). Previously unknown components of the mammalian reductive activation system have been described (11, 42). Preliminary results with the common 2756A→G polymorphism in methionine synthase have not found a significant link to vascular disease, neural tube defects (51, 52, 69), or colorectal neoplasia (6). However, the long cDNA encoding methionine synthase must still be fully characterized to complete a comprehensive evaluation of this issue. Besides the basic biochemical importance, the diagnostic and therapeutic implications emerging from these studies may give us a better understanding of the complex pathologies that may involve methionine synthase.

REFERENCES

1. Banerjee, R. The yin-yang of cobalamin biochemistry. *Chem Biol* 1997; 4: 175–186.

2. Banerjee, R, Frasca, V, Ballou, DP, Matthews, RG, Participation of cob(I)alamin in the reaction catalyzed by methionine synthase from *Escherichia coli*: A steady-state and rapid reaction kinetic analysis. *Biochemistry* 1990; 29: 11101–109.

3. Banerjee, R, Gulati, S, Chen, Z: Methionine synthase from pig liver. *Methods Enzymol* 1997; 281: 189–96.

4. Banerjee, RV, Johnston, NL, Sobeski, JK, Datta, P, Matthews, RG. Cloning and sequence analysis of the *Escherichia coli* metH gene encoding cobalamin-dependent methionine synthase and isolation of a tryptic fragment containing the cobalamin-binding domain. *J Biol Chem* 1989; 264: 13888–95.

5. Banerjee, RV, Matthews, RG. Cobalamin-dependent methionine synthase. *FASEB J* 1990; 4: 1450–59.

6. Chen, J, Giovannucci, E, Hankinson, SE, Ma, J, Willett, WC, Spiegelman, D, Kelsey, KT, Hunter, DJ. A prospective study of methylenetetrahydrofolate reductase and methionine synthase gene polymorphisms, and risk of colorectal adenoma. *Carcinogenesis* 1998; 19: 2129–32.

7. Chen, LH, Liu, ML, Hwang, HY, Chen, L-S, Korenberg, J, Shane, B. Human methionine synthase. cDNA cloning, gene localization and expression. *J Biol Chem* 1997; 272: 3628–34.

8. Chen, Z. Purification and characterization of mammalian methionine synthase and its reductive activation proteins. PhD Thesis, University of Nebraska, Lincoln, 1998.

9. Chen, Z, Crippen, K, Gulati, S, Banerjee, R. Purification and kinetic characterization of methionine synthase from pig liver. *J Biol Chem* 1994; 269: 27193–97.

10. Chen, Z, Chakraborty, S, Banerjee, R. Demonstration that the mammalian methionine synthases are predominantly cobalamin-loaded. *J Biol Chem* 1995; 270: 19246–49.

11. Chen, Z, Banerjee, R. Purification of soluble cytochrome b_5 as a component of the reductive activation system of porcine methionine synthase. *J Biol Chem* 1998; 273: 26248–55.

12. Coward, JK, Chello, PL, Cashmore, AR, Parameswaran, KN, DeAngelis, LM, Bertino, JR. 5-Methyl-5,6,7,8-tetrahydropteroyl oligo-γ-L-glutamates: Synthesis and kinetic studies with methionine synthetase from bovine brain. *Biochemistry* 1975; 14: 1548–52.

13. Dixon, MM, Huang, S, Matthews, RG, Ludwig, ML. The activation domain of cobalamin-dependent methionine synthase: A novel fold for AdoMet binding. *Structure* 1996; 4: 1263–75.

14. Drennan, CL, Huang, S, Drummond, JT, Matthews, R, Ludwig, ML. How a protein binds B$_{12}$: A 3A X-ray structure of B$_{12}$-binding domains of methionine synthase. *Science* 1994; 266: 1669–74.

15. Drummond, J, Huang, S, Blumenthal, RM, Matthews, RG. Assignment of enzymatic function to specific protein regions of cobalamin-dependent methionine synthase from *Escherichia coli*. *Biochemistry* 1993; 32: 9290–95.

16. Drummond, JT, Jarrett, J, Gonzalez, JC, Huang, S, Matthews, RG. Characterization of nonradioactive assays for cobalamin-dependent and cobalamin-independent methionine synthase enzymes. *Anal Biochem* 1995; 228: 323–29.

17. Drummond, JT, Matthews, RG. Nitrous oxide degradation by cobalamin-dependent methionine synthase: Characterization of the reactants and products in the inactivation reaction. *Biochemistry* 1994; 33: 3372–41.

18. Drummond, JT, Matthews, RG. Nitrous oxide inactivation of cobalamin-dependent methionine synthase from *Escherichia coli*: Characterization of the damage to the enzyme and prosthetic group. *Biochemistry* 1994; 33: 3742–50.

19. Fenton, WA, Rosenberg, LE. In *The Metabolic and Molecular Bases of Inherited Disease* (Scriver, CR, Beaudet, AL, Sly, WS, Valle, D, eds.). McGraw-Hill, New York, 1995; pp. 3111–28.

20. Finkelstein, JD, Kyle, WE, Harris, BJ. Methionine metabolism in mammals. Regulation of homocysteine methyltransferase in rat tissue. *Arch Biochem Biophys* 1971; 146: 84–92.

21. Finkelstein, JD, Martin, JJ. Methionine metabolism in mammals. Distribution of homocysteine between competing pathways. *J Biol Chem* 1984; 259: 9508–13.

22. Fowler, B, Suormala, T, Gunther, M, Till, J, Wraith, JE. A new patient with functional methionine synthase deficiency: Evidence for a third complementation class. *J Inherit Dis* 1997; 20: 21.

23. Fujii, K, Galivan, JH, Huennekens, FM. Activation of methionine synthase: Further characterization of the flavoprotein system. *Arch Biochem Biophys* 1977; 178: 662–70.

24. Fujii, K, Huennekens, FM. Activation of methionine synthase by a reduced triphosphopyridine nucleotide-dependent flavoprotein system. *J Biol Chem* 1974; 249: 6745–53.

25. Gonzalez, JC, Banerjee, RV, Huang, S, Sumner, JS, Matthews, RG. Comparison of cobalamin-independent and cobalamin-dependent methionine synthases from *Escherichia coli*: Two solutions to the same chemical problem. *Biochemistry* 1992; 31: 6045–56.

26. Goulding, CW, Matthews, RG. Cobalamin-dependent methionine synthase from *Escherichia coli*: Involvement of zinc in homocysteine activation. *Biochemistry* 1997; 36: 15749–57.

27. Goulding, CW, Postigo, D, Matthews, RG. Cobalamin-dependent methionine synthase is a modular protein with distinct regions for binding homocysteine, methyltetrahydrofolate, cobalamin and adenosylmethionine. *Biochemistry* 1997; 36: 8082–91.

28. Graham, IM, Daly, LE, Refsum, HM, Robinson, K, Brattström, LE, Ueland, PM, Palma-Reis, RJ, Boers, GHJ, Sheahan, RG, Israelsson, B, Uiterwaal, CS, Meleady, R, McMaster, D, Verhoef, P, Witteman, J, Rubba, P, Bellet, H, Wautrecht, JC, de Valk, HW, Sales Lúis, AC, Parrot-Rouland, FM, Tan, KS, Higgins, I, Garcon, D, Medrano, MJ, Candito, M, Evans, AE, Andria, G. Plasma homocysteine as a risk factor for vascular disease: The European Concerted Action Project. *JAMA* 1997; 277: 1775–81.

29. Guest, JR, Friedman, S, Woods, DD, Smith, EL. A methyl analog of cobamide coenzyme in relation to methionine synthesis by bacteria. *Nature* 1962; 195: 340–42.

30. Gulati, S, Brody, LC, Banerjee, R. Posttranscriptional regulation of mammalian methionine synthase by B$_{12}$. *Biochem Biophys Res Commun* 1999; 259: 436–42.

31. Gulati, S, Brody, LC, Rosenblatt, DS, Banerjee, R. Defects in auxiliary redox proteins lead to functional methionine synthase deficiency. *J Biol Chem* 1997; 272: 19171–75.

32. Gulati, SG, Baker, P, Fowler, B, Li, Y, Kruger, W, Brody, LC, Banerjee, R. Mutations in human methionine synthase in *cblG* patients. *Hum Mol Genet* 1996; 5: 1859–66.

32a. Herbert, V, Zalusky, R. Interrelations of vitamin B12 and folic acid metabolism: Folic acid clearance studies. *J Clin Invest* 1962; 41: 1263–76.

33. Jarrett, JT, Huang, S, Matthews, RG. Methionine synthase exists in two distinct conformations that differ in the reactivity towards methyltetrahydrofolate, adenosylmethionine and flavodoxin. *Biochemistry* 1998; 37: 5372–82.

34. Kamely, D, Littlefield, JW, Erbe, RW. Regulation of 5-methyltetrahydrofolate:homocysteine methyltransferase activity by methionine, vitamin B$_{12}$, and folate in cultured baby hamster kidney cells. *Proc Natl Acad Sci USA* 1973; 70: 2585–89.

35. Kenyon, SH, Ast, T, Gibbons, WA. In vitro phosphorylation of vitamin B$_{12}$-dependent methionine synthase by protein kinase A. *Biochem Soc Trans* 1995; 2: 335S.

36. Kenyon, SH, Nicolaou, A, Ast, T, Gibbons, WA. Stimulation in vitro of vitamin B$_{12}$-dependent methionine synthase by polyamines. *Biochem J* 1996; 316: 661–65.

37. Kenyon, SH, Nicolaou, A, Gibbons, WA. The effect of ethanol and its metabolites upon methionine synthase activity in vitro. *Alcohol* 1998; 4: 305–9.

38. Kerwar, SS, Spears, C, Brian, M, Weissbach, H. Studies on vitamin B$_{12}$ metabolism in HeLa cells. *Arch Biochem Biophys* 1971; 142: 231–37.

39. Kinsella, LJ, Green, R. "Anesthesia paresthetica": Nitrous oxide-induced cobalamin deficiency. *Neurology* 1995; 45: 1608–10.

40. Kondo, H, Osborne, ML, Kolhouse, JF, Bindier, MJ, Podell, ER, Utley, CS, Abrams, RS, Allen, RH. Nitrous oxide has multiple deleterious effects on cobalamin metabolism and causes decreases in activities of both mammalian cobalamin-dependent enzymes in rats. *J Clin Invest* 1981; 67: 1270–83.

41. Leclerc, D, Campeau, E, Goyette, P, Adjalla, CE, Christensen, B, Ross, M, Eydoux, P, Rosenblatt, DS, Rozen, R, Gravel, RA. Human methionine synthase: cDNA cloning and identification of mutations in patients of the *cblG* complementation group of folate/cobalamin disorders. *Hum Mol Genet* 1996; 5: 1867–74.

42. Leclerc, D, Wilson, A, Dumas, R, Gafuik, C, Song, D, Watkins, D, Heng, HHQ, Rommens, JM, Scherer, SW, Rosenblatt, DS, Gravel, RA. Cloning and mapping of a cDNA for methionine synthase reductase, a flavoprotein defective in patients with homocystinuria. *Proc Natl Acad Sci USA* 1998; 95: 3059–64.

43. Li, YN, Gulati, S, Baker, PJ, Brody, LC, Banerjee, R, Kruger, WD, Cloning, mapping and RNA analysis of the human methionine synthase gene. *Hum Mol Genet* 1996; 5: 1851–58.

44. Ludwig, ML, Matthews, RG. Structure-based perspectives on B$_{12}$-dependent enzymes. *Annu Rev Biochem* 1997; 66: 269–313.

45. Mangum, JH, Murray, BK, North, JA, Vitamin B$_{12}$ dependent methionine biosynthesis in cultured mammalian cells. *Biochemistry* 1969; 8: 3496–99.

46. Mangum, JH, North, JA, Vitamin B$_{12}$-dependent methionine biosynthesis in HEp-2 cells *Biochem Biophys Res Commun* 1968; 32: 105–10.

47. Marsh, ENG, Holloway, DE. Cloning and sequencing of glutamate mutase component S from *Clostridium tetanomorphum FEBS Lett* 1992; 310: 167–70.

48. Matthews, RG, Drummond, JT, Webb, HK. Cobalamin-dependent methionine synthase and serine hydrozymethyltransferase: Targets for chemotherapeutic intervention? *Adv Enzyme Regul* 1998; 38: 377–92.

49. Mills, JL, McPartlin, JM, Kirke, PN, Lee, YJ, Conle, MR, Weir, DG, Scott, JH. Homocysteine metabolism in pregnancies complicated by neural tube defects. *Lancet* 1995; 345: 149–51.

50. Minot, GR, Murphy, WP. Treatment of pernicious anemia by special diet. *JAMA* 1926; 87: 470–76.

51. Morita, H, Kurihara, H, Sugiyama, T, Hamada, C, Kurihara, Y, Shindo, T, Oh-hashi, Y, Yazaki, Y. Polymorphism of the methionine synthase gene: Association with homocysteine metabolism and late-onset vascular diseases in the Japanese population. *Arterioscler Thromb Vasc Biol* 1999; 2: 298–302.

52. Morrison, K, Edwards, YH, Lynch, SA. Methionine synthase and neural tube defects. (1997) *J Med Genet* 1997; 34: 958.

53. Nicolaou, A, Kenyon, SH, Gibbons, JM, Ast, T, Gibbons, WA. In vitro inactivation of mammalian methionine synthase by nitric oxide. *Eur J Clin Invest* 1996; 2: 167–70.

54. Noronha, JM, Silverman, M. On folic acid, vitamin B$_{12}$, methionine and formiminoglutamic acid metabolism. In *Vitamin B$_{12}$ and Intrinsic Factor* (HC Heinrich, ed.), Enke Verlag, Stuttgart, 1962; pp. 728–36.

55. Peariso, K, Goulding, CW, Matthews, RG, Penner-Hahn, J. Characterization of the zinc binding site in methionine synthase enzymes of *Escherichia coli*: The role of zinc in the methylation of homocysteine. *J Am Chem Soc* 1998; 120: 8410–16.

56. Refsum, H, Ueland, PM, Nygård, O, Vollset, SE. Homocysteine and cardiovascular disease. *Annu Rev Med* 1998; 49: 31–62.

57. Roberts, DL, Zhao, S, Doukov, T, Ragsdale, SW. The reductive acetyl coenzyme A pathway: Sequence and heterologous expression of active methyltetrahydrofolate: corrinoid/iron-sulfur protein methyltransferase from *Clostridium thermoaceticum*. *J Bacteriol* 1994; 176: 6127–30.

58. Rosenblatt, DS, Cooper, BA, Pottier, A, Lue-Shing, H, Matiaszuk, N, Grauer, K. Altered vitamin B$_{12}$ metabolism in fibroblasts from patients with megaloblastic anemia and homocystinuria due to a new defect in methionine biosynthesis. *J Clin Invest* 1984; 74: 2149–56.

59. Schuh, W, Rosenblatt, DS, Cooper, BA, Pottier, A, Lue-Shing, H, Matiaszuk, N, Grauer, K. Homocystinuria and megaloblastic anemia responsive to vitamin B$_{12}$ therapy. An inborn error of metabolism due to a single defect in cobalamin metabolism. *N Engl J Med* 1984; 310: 686–90.

60. Sillaots, SL, Hall, CA, Hurteloup, V, Rosenblatt, DS. Heterogeneity in *cblG*: Differential retention of cobalamin on methionine synthase. *Biochem Med Metab Biol* 1992; 47: 242–49.

61. Smith, JR, Smith, JG. Effects of methylmercury in vitro on methionine synthase activity in various rat tissues. *Bull Environ Contam Toxicol* 1990; 45: 649–54.

62. Stabler, SP, Brass, EP, Marcell, PD, Allen, RH. Inhibition of cobalamin-dependent enzymes by cobalamin analogs in rats. *J Clin Invest* 1991; 87: 1422–30.

63. Stampfer, MJ, Malinow, R, Willett, WC. A prospective study of plasma homocysteine and risk of myocardial infaction in United States physicians. *JAMA* 1992; 268: 877–81.

64. Steegers-Theunissen, RPM, Boers, GHJ, Blom, HJ, Trijbels, FJM, Eskes, TKAB. Hyperhomocysteinemia and recurrent spontaneous abortion or abruptio placentae. *Lancet* 1992; 339: 1122–23.

65. Stubbe, J. Binding site revealed of nature's most beautiful cofactor. *Science* 1994; 266: 1663–4.

66. Swanson, DA, Baker, P, Liu, ML, Garrett, L, Stitzel, M, Banerjee, R, Wynshaw-Boris, T, Shane, B, Brody, L. A methionine synthase knock-out mouse. *Am J Hum Genet* 1998; 63: A275.

67. Taylor, RT, Hanna, ML, Hutton, JJ. 5-Methyltetrahydrofolate homocysteine cobalamin methyltransferase in human bone marrow and its relationship to pernicious anemia. *Arch Biochem Biophys* 1974; 165: 787–95.

68. VanAerts, LAGJM, Poirot, CM, Herberts, CA, Blom, HJ, De Abreu, RA, Trijbels, JMF, Eskes, TKAB, Peereboom-Stegeman, JHJC, Noordhoek, J. Development of methionine synthase, cystathionine-β-synthase and *S*-adenosyl-homocysteine hydrolase during gestation in rats. *J Reprod Fertil* 1995; 103: 227–32.

69. van der Put, NMJ, van der Molen, EF, Kluijtmans, LAG, Heil, SG, Trijbels, JMF, Eskes, TKAB, Van Oppenraaij-Emmerzaal, D, Banerjee, R, Blom, HJ. Sequence analysis of the coding region of human methionine synthase: Relevance to hyperhomocysteinemia in neural-tube defects and vascular disease. *Q J Med* 1997; 90: 511–17.

70. VanderMark, PK, Steggles, AW. The isolation and characterization of the soluble membrane-bound porcine cytochrome b$_5$ cDNAs. *Biochem Biophys Res Comm* 1997; 240: 80–3.

71. Watkins, D, Rosenblatt, DS, Genetic heterogeneity among patients with methylcobalamin deficiency. *J Clin Invest* 1988; 81: 1690–94.

72. Weir, DG, Scott, JM. The biochemical basis of the neuropathy in cobalamin deficiency. *Baillieres Clin Haematol* 1995; 3: 479–97.

73. Whipple, GH, Robscheit-Robbins, FS. Blood regeneration in severe anemia: Favorable influence of liver, heart and skeletal muscle in diet. *Am J Physiol* 1926; 72: 408–18.

74. Wilson, A, Leclerc, D, Rosenblatt, DS, Gravel, RA. Molecular basis for methionine synthase reductase deficiency in patients belonging to the *cblE* complementation group of disorders in folate/cobalamin metabolism. *Hum Mol Genet* 1999; 8: 2009–16.

75. Wilson, A, Leclerc, D, Saberi, F, Campeau, E, Hwang, HY, Shane, B, Phillips III, JA, Rosenblatt, DS, Gravel, RA. Functionally null mutations in patients with the *cblG* variant form of methionine synthase deficiency. *Am J Hum Genet* 1998; 63: 409–14.

76. Yamada, K, Tobimatsu, T, Kawata, T, Wada, M, Maekawa, A, Toraya, T. Purification and some properties of cobalamin-dependent methionine synthase from rat liver. *J Nutr Sci Vitaminol* 1997; 43: 177–86.

77. Yamada, K, Tobimatsy, T, Toraya, T. Cloning, sequencing and heterologous expression of rat methionine synthase cDNA. *Biosci Biotechnol Biochem* 1998; 62: 2155–60.

13

Betaine-Dependent Remethylation

TIMOTHY A. GARROW

The betaine-dependent remethylation of homocysteine, catalyzed by betaine:homocysteine methyltransferase (BHMT; Metabolic Diagram, Reaction 5), is an irreversible reaction found in the pathway of choline oxidation. In this pathway, choline is first oxidized to betaine (trimethylglycine) and then demethylated to glycine. BHMT catalyzes the first demethylation step whereby a methyl group of betaine is transferred to homocysteine, producing dimethylglycine and methionine, respectively (Figure 13.1).

Choline Oxidation

Choline, primarily as phosphatidylcholine, is abundant in human diets. In addition, the choline moiety can be synthesized de novo by the S-adenosylmethionine-dependent methylation of phosphatidylethanolamine to form phosphatidylcholine. In animals, as choline-containing phospholipids turn over, the released free choline resides at a metabolic branch-point. Free choline can either be phosphorylated and reincorporated into phospholipids, converted to acetylcholine, or oxidized to glycine. Quantitatively, little choline is converted to acetylcholine. The available data suggest that free choline is first preferentially reincorporated into phospholipids and acetylcholine and that the oxidation of choline provides a way to dispose of excess choline by a pathway that is sensitive to dietary choline intake and subsequent tissue levels.

Five enzymes have traditionally defined the choline oxidation pathway: choline oxidase, betaine aldehyde dehydrogenase, BHMT, dimethylglycine dehydrogenase, and sarcosine dehydrogenase. These reactions are depicted in Figure 13.2. The complete oxidation of choline to glycine takes place primarily in the liver and kidney. Its oxidation begins in mitochondria after transport into this organelle by a specific choline transporter. The first and committed step of the pathway is catalyzed by choline oxidase (Figure 13.2, Reaction 1), an enzyme found in the inner mitochondrial membrane that converts choline to betaine alde-

Fig. 13.1. Betaine:homocysteine methyltransferase catalyzes an ordered Bi Bi reaction (see text later). Structures of substrates and products are shown.

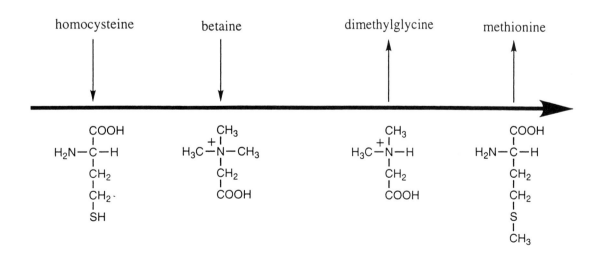

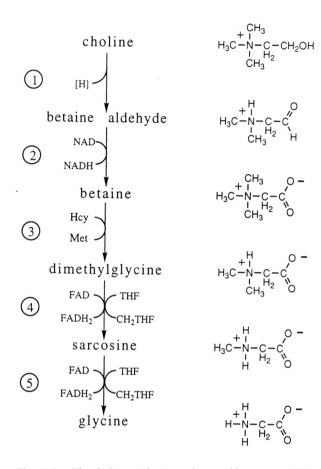

Fig. 13.2. The choline oxidation pathway. Abbreviations: FAD, flavin adenine dinucleotide (oxidized); FADH$_2$, flavin adenine dinucleotide (reduced); NAD, nicotine adenine dinucleotide (oxidized); NADH, nicotine adenine dinucleotide (reduced); THF, tetrahydrofolate; CH$_2$THF, 5,10-methylenetetrahydrofolate. Reactions: 1, choline oxidase; 2, betaine aldehyde dehydrogenase; 3, betaine-homocysteine methyltransferase; 4, dimethylglycine dehydrogenase; and 5, sarcosine dehydrogenase.

hyde. Betaine aldehyde is then rapidly oxidized to betaine by betaine aldehyde dehydrogenase (Figure 13.2, Reaction 2), an activity that is present in both the mitochondria and cytoplasm, although little betaine aldehyde is believed to escape the mitochondria (24).

Betaine leaves the mitochondria to serve as a methyl donor for the cytosolic BHMT-catalyzed reaction (Figure 13.2, Reaction 3). After methyl transfer, the dimethylglycine thus formed is oxidatively demethylated by dimethylglycine dehydrogenase (Figure 13.2, Reaction 4) to form sarcosine, and sarcosine is then oxidized to glycine by sarcosine dehydrogenase (Figure 13.2, Reaction 5). Both dimethylglycine dehydrogenase and sarcosine dehydrogenase are mitochondrial enzymes that require FAD and tetrahydrofolate and produce FADH$_2$ and 5,10-methylenetetrahydrofolate, respectively. In summary, the oxidation of betaine to

glycine results in three carbons entering the one-carbon pool. One of the carbons directly becomes the labile methyl carbon of methionine (Figure 13.2, Reaction 3), and two other carbons enter the folate pool of mitochondria as 5,10-methylenetetrahydrofolate (Figure 13.2, Reactions 4 and 5).

The regulatory features of the choline oxidation pathway are not understood. The enzymes of the pathway are not known to be influenced by any allosteric effectors or covalent modifications. Aside from a report showing that rat liver BHMT was upregulated threefold by hydrocortisone and downregulated threefold by thyroxin (15), in general, the influence of hormones on the concentration of the choline oxidation enzymes or rates of choline oxidation remains to be thoroughly investigated. Although it has not been determined, it is possible that choline transport into mitochondria is coupled to choline oxidase activity, and these initial steps could be rate-limiting for choline oxidation in some species. In previous studies, hepatic choline oxidase activity varied widely across species, with rats and humans on opposite ends of the spectrum. It was reported that rats had 20-fold (23) to 60-fold (42) higher levels of hepatic choline oxidase activity than humans. Another study using isolated rat liver mitochondria indicated that transport into this organelle was the rate-limiting step for the oxidation of choline to betaine and its efflux out of this organelle (24), but this study did not consider the subsequent metabolism of betaine. For example, the BHMT-catalyzed reaction or the transport of dimethylglycine into the mitochondrion are additional factors that could potentially influence the rate of choline oxidation when the pathway is considered in its entirety. It is also possible that substrate availability for BHMT is rate-limiting in the overall oxidation of choline to glycine under some dietary conditions.

In one study, the level of betaine in rat liver increased with the addition of choline to the diet whether dietary methionine was limiting, adequate, or at supplemental levels, and intraperitoneal injection of homocysteine lowered hepatic betaine concentrations (17). This study suggested that the oxidation of betaine, and thus choline, may be limited by the availability of homocysteine under normal dietary conditions. In humans, supplemental dietary choline increases homocysteine remethylation rates (31, 32). This observation indicates that in humans, the production of betaine and the flux through the BHMT reaction are responsive to choline intake. Thus, it appears that BHMT functions below substrate saturation levels in vivo. Although considerable attention has been given to the influence nutrition has on hepatic BHMT expression, which is discussed later, further research on the regulatory features of choline oxidation is warranted.

It is not known whether the choline oxidation pathway, or specifically the BHMT-catalyzed reaction, is metabolically essential. The oxidation of choline to betaine is likely essential because betaine also functions as a renal osmolyte. Other than sarcosinemia, a condition resulting from low sarcosine dehydrogenase activity that appears to be benign (41), no other genetic defect in the choline oxidation pathway has been described.

Characterization of BHMT

Unlike the cobalamin-dependent remethylation of homocysteine catalyzed by methionine synthase, which shows wide tissue distribution, BHMT has a limited tissue distribution in adult animals. In every mammal tested, BHMT activity has been detected in liver (9, 15, 21, 28, 29, 33, 44, 45, 48). In horses (6), rats (19, 27), pigs (10, 20), and humans (30, 43), species in which liver BHMT has been purified to homogeneity, BHMT accounts for up to 1% or more of the total protein in that organ. Some species also have significant levels of BHMT activity in the kidney, including humans (21, 33), rhesus monkeys (44), and pigs (29, 45). The activity in pig kidney was shown to be localized only in the cortex and not the medulla (45). Rat kidney BHMT activity, although measurable, is very low (15, 29, 48). All of the other major organs of pigs (45) and rats (15, 48) either do not express BHMT activity or express low levels of the enzyme compared with levels in liver.

The expression of BHMT primarily in liver and kidney is consistent with the tissue distribution of other choline oxidation enzymes that are highest in liver and kidney, namely, choline oxidase (23), dimethylglycine dehydrogenase (26), and sarcosine dehydrogenase (3). The only known exceptions to this general rule have been the very high levels of BHMT activity in sheep pancreas (48) and a more recent report that BHMT functions as an enzyme, crystallin, in the rhesus monkey lens (39). Whether BHMT is expressed at high levels in the pancreas of other ruminant species or whether other species have recruited BHMT as a lens crystallin remain to be determined.

Several laboratories have studied the physical properties of highly purified samples of liver BHMT. Purified human (30, 43), rat (27), and pig (20) liver BHMT display one band that migrates at about 45 kDa on denaturing polyacrylamide gels. Several liver cDNAs have been cloned, and their deduced amino acid sequences predict a 406 (human) or 407 (rat, mouse) residue protein of about 45 kDa. However, nondenaturing polyacrylamide electrophoresis and gel filtration estimates of the size of BHMT purified from rat (27) and human (43) liver found that it was about 270 kDa, indicating that the native enzyme is a hexamer of 45 kDa subunits. It is unknown whether monomeric, dimeric, or trimeric combinations are catalytically active.

The pH optima of liver BHMT have been determined using enzymes isolated from several species (9). All display a parabolic pH-versus-enzyme activity curve, with the optimum pH between 7 and 8. There is a relatively sharp decrease in activity at lower and higher pH values. Although the BHMT reaction does not result in a net change of proton stoichiometry, the conversion of homocysteine to methionine and betaine to dimethylglycine results in the loss and gain, respectively, of a proton. It is possible that one or more amino acid residues on BHMT facilitate proton movement; if so, these residues remain to be discovered. BHMT has also been shown to be remarkably stable to heat (9), and this property of the enzyme has been exploited in the purification of BHMT from human (30, 43), rat (27), and pig (10, 20) liver. Sucrose gradient and nondenaturing electrophoresis experiments indicated that when BHMT was stored in the absence of a reducing agent, it polymerized into large protein aggregates (7, 43). Adding reducing agents reversed the polymerization, suggesting that the purified enzyme forms intermolecular disulfide linkages when stored in the absence of a reducing agent. It is not known if the polymerized enzyme retains activity, or whether enzyme polymerization occurs in vivo under conditions of oxidative stress.

Several laboratories have studied the kinetic properties of highly purified samples of liver BHMT. Purified rat (27), pig (10, 20), horse (6), and human (30) liver BHMT had specific activities ranging from about 1,000 to 4,000 units per milligram protein (one unit = nmol methionine formed per hour). Most of the assays used saturating levels of homocysteine but subsaturating levels of betaine (near K_m levels). Initial rate analysis of the pig liver enzyme predicted a V_{max} of about 2,000 units/mg protein (20). Assuming that each monomer has one active site, these data indicate that the turnover number for the BHMT hexamer is about 9 per minute. This catalytic rate is remarkably slow, but as indicated previously, liver contains very high levels of BHMT.

BHMT (20) and cobalamin-dependent methionine synthase (5) have both been purified to homogeneity from pig liver. Based on the reported level of purification and specific activities of these two enzymes, it can be calculated that methylation capacity of BHMT in pig liver is similar to the more efficient but less abundant cobalamin-dependent methionine synthase. This calculation is consistent with the results obtained from an in vitro study designed to simulate homocysteine methylation in rat liver (12). The study showed that BHMT and cobalamin-dependent methionine synthase contributed equally to the remethylation of homocysteine when substrates were present at near physiological concentrations. Why BHMT is so abundant in liver and has been selected to retain such low catalytic efficiency is perplexing. Perhaps BHMT has another critical cellular function(s) besides that of a methyltransferase.

The Michaelis constants of recombinant human liver BHMT expressed in *Escherichia coli* and the native enzyme purified from human liver have recently been investigated using highly purified enzyme preparations (30). The K_m for betaine at saturating levels of L-homocysteine was determined to be 2.2 mmol/L. The K_m for L-homocysteine using subsaturating K_m levels of betaine was estimated to be 4 μmol/L. There were no discernible differences between the recombinant human liver enzyme expressed in *E. coli* and the native enzyme purified from human liver. Based on the available metabolite data obtained from rodent liver, which may not reflect the concentrations found in human liver, the data are consistent with BHMT functioning at or below its K_m values and thus increasing concentration of either substrate in liver would be expected to increase flux, as has been observed in whole animals (see previously).

Initial rate studies have also been used to show that the rat liver enzyme catalyzes a sequential reaction (13, 19). Product inhibition studies showed that substrate binding and product release was ordered (Figure 13.1), with homocysteine being the first substrate to bind and methionine being the last product off (13). Dimethylglycine has been shown to be a potent inhibitor of BHMT activity (11, 13), although an affinity constant has never been reported. A putative dual-substrate analog, S-(δ-carboxybutyl)-DL-homocysteine, was shown to be a potent inhibitor of human liver BHMT (2). The Bi Bi (i.e., 2-substrate) kinetic mechanism for BHMT, its high affinity for the dual-substrate analog, S-(δ-carboxybutyl)-DL-homocysteine, and the putative role of zinc in BHMT catalysis (discussed later) thus far support a direct methyl transfer mechanism.

The deduced amino acid sequence of BHMT shares limited homology with the N-terminal region of cobalamin-dependent methionine synthases (20). Two regions of BHMT, GVNC217HRDP and GGC299C300GFEPTHI, are similar to amino acid residues 244–251 and 308–318, respectively, in the cobalamin-dependent methionine synthase of *E. coli*. Specifically, the three cysteine residues in these regions are conserved in all known BHMT and cobalamin-dependent methionine synthase sequences. Both enzymes have been shown to be zinc metalloenzymes (22, 30), and mutating any of these conserved cysteine residues to alanine in BHMT or methionine synthase results in a dramatic loss of activity and a reduced capacity to bind

zinc (4, 22, 30). In the absence of crystal structure, it is presently assumed that these cysteine residues are required for zinc binding in both BHMT and cobalamin-dependent methionine synthase (see Chapters 10 and 12). The mechanism of methyl transfer for cobalamin-dependent methionine synthase and BHMT is believed to proceed through the formation of a zinc tetrathiolate complex by the attack of homocysteine on the zinc to displace a fourth nonthiolate ligand and give a complex with a net charge of –2. The conversion of the thiol of homocysteine to a thiolate activates homocysteine for nucleophilic attack on the methyl group of the methyl donor.

It is unkown whether there is more than one isozyme of BHMT. Evidence exists that there could be two isozymes. Klee et al. (25) showed that two methyltransferase activities could be differentiated in liver extracts by their heat lability and behavior on gel filtration columns. The two proteins separated by gel filtration showed different methyl donor substrate specificities. The larger, more abundant form could use betaine or dimethylacetothetin as methyl donors, whereas the smaller, less abundant form could only use betaine. Thus, whether there is a second BHMT isozyme in liver that can use betaine, its thetin analogs, or both as methyl donors for the methylation of homocysteine, remains to be conclusively determined. The enzyme discussed in this chapter, wherever such a discernment can be made, is a protein that is specifically stable at high temperatures and can use betaine or dimethylacetothetin as a methyl donor.

Structure of the Human BHMT Gene and Its 5′-Flanking Region

The human BHMT gene has recently been shown to be composed of eight exons interrupted by seven introns, and it spans about 20 kilobases of DNA (35) (Figure 13.3). All intron-exon junctions followed the GT-AG rule. The gene was previously shown to reside on chromosome 5q13.1-15 (45). The primary transcriptional start site has been mapped using the 5′ rapid amplification of cDNA ends technique with mRNA isolated from human liver and human hepatoma cells (35). The major transcriptional start site was shown to be an adenine that resides 77 bases upstream from the adenine of the start codon. Centered 26 nucleotides upstream from the transcriptional start site was a consensus TATA binding protein site. The DNA sequence surrounding this TATA box was the only region within the first 3.2 kb of DNA upstream of the transcriptional start site that was recognized as a potential promoter by various DNA analysis programs.

Transcription reporter assays, using human hepatoma cell transfectants expressing various con-

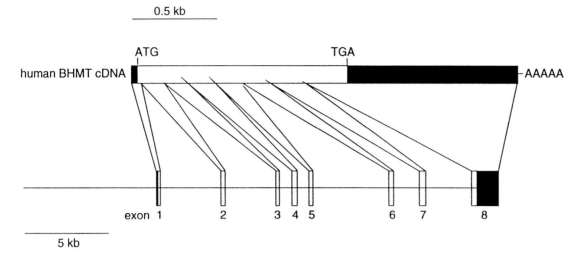

Fig. 13.3. Structure of the human betaine:homocysteine methyltransferase gene. (Adapted from Park and Garrow [35], with permission.)

structs of the 5′-flanking region of the human BHMT gene fused to firefly luciferase, have shown that the region between -254 (*BstX* I site) to -28 (*Sal I* site), relative to the adenine of the start codon, was required for promoter activity (Breksa and Garrow, unpublished data). This region contains the TATA box just described. The location of the transcriptional start site in relation to the TATA box and the luciferase reporter assays suggest that the TATA box region contains the major, if not the sole, promoter in human liver. The genetic determinants specifying the nutritional, hormonal, and tissue-specific expression of BHMT remain unknown. No polymorphisms or mutations have yet been found in the human BHMT gene.

Modulation of BHMT Expression by Diet

Several studies have investigated the effects that nutrition has on hepatic BHMT activity. Some of the earliest studies that involved highly purified diets were conducted by Finkelstein et al. (14, 16, 18). They showed in rats that the specific activity of hepatic BHMT varies with the dietary intake of sulfur amino acids, choline, and betaine. Some of the greatest changes observed were under conditions of methionine deficiency and methionine deficiency in combination with excess dietary choline. However, excess dietary methionine also increased activity. For example, in one study (14), rats that consumed methionine-free diets that contained adequate choline (0.2%) had threefold higher BHMT activity than rats that consumed a diet adequate in methionine (0.3%) but devoid of choline. When dietary choline was adequate (0.2%), rats consuming methionine-supplemented diets (1.0%) had a small increase (30%) in BHMT activity compared with rats fed the diet containing adequate methionine (0.3%).

A study that used chickens reported similar responses of hepatic BHMT-specific activity to varying levels of dietary methionine and choline (8). Although supplemental methionine, either with or without excess methyl donor, slightly increased BHMT activity (10% to 30%), as was observed in rats (14), the study in chickens confirmed that hepatic BHMT activity was most dramatically upregulated (threefold) when the diet was deficient in methionine (0.1%) yet contained adequate choline. Further induction (up to sixfold) was observed when the methionine-deficient diets were supplemented with choline or betaine.

Recent research has elucidated some of the mechanisms involved in the dietary induction of hepatic BHMT expression in rats (35, 36). Figure 13.4 (panel A) shows that restricting methionine in a diet that was adequate in choline and all other essential nutrients caused a fourfold increase in rat liver BHMT activity levels (group 1 vs. group 2). Greater than eightfold increases in BHMT activity were achieved by feeding rats the same methionine-restricted diet containing supplemental betaine (group 1 vs. group 3). As can be seen in Figure 13.4 (panel A), the diet-induced changes in steady-state BHMT mRNA levels mirrored the changes observed for BHMT activity (36). These data suggest that changes in activity reflect changes in message rather than any change in enzyme efficiency. A follow-up study by Park and Garrow (35) confirmed that changes in activity were due to changes in steady-state mRNA levels and showed corresponding changes in immunodetectable protein.

Taken together, these studies indicate that diet-induced changes in BHMT activity are due to changes in BHMT protein secondary to changes in steady-state mRNA levels. It remains to be determined whether diet-induced changes in steady-state mRNA levels are due to changes in transcription, mRNA turnover rates, or a combination of both. The study by Park and Garrow (35) also showed that although high levels of BHMT induction required methionine restriction, methionine restriction alone was not sufficient; there also had to be some choline or a methyl donor substrate for BHMT in the diet. For example, as shown in Figure 13.4 (panel B), BHMT induction levels were directly related to the amount of choline in the methionine-deficient diet (group 4 vs. groups 5 and 6); in addition, the magnitude of induction was inversely related to the severity of methionine deficiency (group 6 vs. group 7). These data support the idea proposed by Finkelstein et al. (14), that BHMT functions to conserve the backbone of homocysteine under conditions of methionine deficiency. The data also indicate that the induction of BHMT occurs only when the diet also contains a source of a methyl donor for the BHMT reaction, namely, choline or betaine.

The requirement for both low dietary methionine and adequate methyl donor levels for the high induc-

Fig. 13.4. Diet-induced changes in BHMT expression. Panel A: weanling rats (*n* = 7) were fed amino acid-defined diets for 14 days as follows: 1, methionine-adequate (3 g/kg); 2, methionine-deficient (1 g/kg); and 3, methionine-deficient (1 g/kg) + betaine (3 g/kg). All diets contained adequate choline (0.5 g/kg). Mean hepatic BHMT activities and mRNA levels are expressed relative to group 1, which was assigned values of 1.0 (Adapted from Park et al. [36], with permission.) Panel B: weanling rats (n = 6) were fed amino acid-defined diets for 14 days as follows: 4, methionine-deficient (1 g/kg) devoid of choline; 5, methionine-deficient (1 g/kg) + adequate choline (0.5 g/kg); 6, methionine-deficient (1 g/kg) + supplemental choline (2 g/kg); and 7, moderately methionine-deficient (1.5 g/kg) + supplemental choline (2 g/kg). Mean hepatic BHMT activities are expressed relative to group 4, which was assigned a relative value of 1.0 (Adapted from Park and Garrow [35], with permission.)

tion of BHMT expression may be a regulatory control to prevent the futile cycling of methyl groups. Because a diet devoid of or low in choline necessitates the synthesis of this compound using *S*-adenosylmethionine, increasing BHMT expression when both dietary methionine and choline are deficient may enhance the oxidation of choline, a compound being synthesized using methyl groups derived from scarce methionine supplies. Synthesizing choline from methyl groups derived from methionine, only to then oxidize it, would be a futile cycle. In contrast, the high induction of BHMT only when dietary methionine levels are low and choline is adequate or high allows the liver to spare the labile methyl carbon of methionine in two ways. First, choline directly spares the methyl group of methionine because the liver cell no longer needs to synthesize as much choline via the methylation of phosphatidylethanolamine to form phosphatidylcholine, as choline can be activated instead by phosphorylation and incorporated into cytidine diphosphocholine and then acylated to phosphatidylcholine. Second, by increasing the expression of BHMT under these nutritional conditions, the liver cell increases the probability of homocysteine being remethylated to methionine, rather than having homocysteine proceed through the transsulfuration pathway.

Dietary Treatment of Homocystinuria

The methylation capacity offered by BHMT has been exploited as an effective treatment for vitamin nonresponsive forms of homocystinuria (1, 38, 40, 46, 47). Individuals with severe deficiencies of cystathionine β-synthase (see Chapter 20), methylenetetrahydrofolate reductase, or one of the *cbl* genes required for the synthesis or maintenance of methylcobalamin (see Chapter 21) respond favorably to gram quantities of betaine taken orally. This treatment generally results in

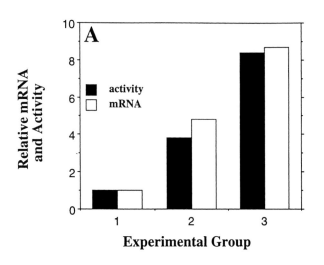
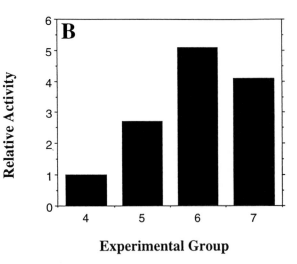

a significant drop in plasma total homocysteine and a greatly improved prognosis. More recently, Yap and Naughten (49) have published data regarding the long-term treatment of cystathionine β-synthase patients using low-methionine cysteine-enriched diets. Their patients experienced significant reductions in plasma homocysteine levels and had significantly improved clinical outcomes compared with untreated cystathionine β-synthase-deficient patients (34).

REFERENCES

1. Allen, RH, Stabler, SP and Lindenbaum, J. Serum betaine, N,N-dimethylglycine and N-methylglycine levels in patients with cobalamin and folate deficiency and related inborn errors of metabolism. *Metabolism* 1993; 42: 1448–60.
2. Awad, WM, Whitney, PL, Skiba, WE, Mangum, JH, Wells, MS. Evidence for a direct methyl transfer in betaine-homocysteine S-methyltransferase. *J Biol Chem* 1983; 258: 12790–792.
3. Bergeron, F, Otto, A, Blache, P, Day, R, Denoroy, L, Brandsch, R, Bataille, D. Molecular cloning and tissue distribution of rat sarcosine dehydrogenase. *Eur J Biochem* 1998; 257: 556–61.
4. Breksa III, AP, Garrow, TA. Recombinant human liver betaine-homocysteine S-methyltransferase: Identification of three cysteine residues critical for zinc binding. *Biochemistry* 1999; 38: 13991–98.
5. Chen, Z, Crippen, K, Gulati, S, Banerjee, R. Purification and kinetic mechanism of a mammalian methionine synthase from pig liver. *J Biol Chem* 1994; 269: 27193–97.
6. Durell, J, Anderson, DG, Cantoni, GL. The synthesis of methionine by enzymic transmethylation: Purification and properties of thetin homocysteine methylpherase. *Biochim Biophys Acta* 1957; 26: 270–82.
7. Durell, J, Cantoni, GL. The synthesis of methionine by transmethylation: Mechanism of the reversible polymerization of thetin-homocysteine methylpherase and its relation to the mechanism of methionine synthesis. *Biochim Biophys Acta* 1959; 35: 515–29.
8. Emmert, JL, Garrow, TA, Baker, DH. Hepatic betaine-homocysteine methyltransferase activity in the chicken is influenced by dietary intake of sulfur amino acids, choline and betaine. *J Nutr* 1996; 126: 2050–58.
9. Ericson, LE. Betaine-homocysteine methyltransferases: Distribution in nature. *Acta Chem. Scand* 1960; 14: 2102–12.
10. Ericson, LE. Betaine-homocysteine methyltransferases: Isolation and properties of the transferase of pig liver. *Acta Chem Scand* 1960; 14: 2113–26.
11. Ericson, LE. Betaine-homocysteine methyltransferases: The methyl donor specificity of the transferase isolated from pig liver. *Acta Chem Scand* 1960; 14: 2127–34.
12. Finkelstein, JD, Martin, JJ. Methionine metabolism in mammals: Distribution of homocysteine between competing pathways. *J Biol Chem* 1984; 259: 9508–13.
13. Finkelstein, JD, Harris, BJ, Kyle, WE. Methionine metabolism in mammals: Kinetic study of betaine-homocysteine

methyltransferase. *Arch Biochem Biophys* 1972; 153: 320–24.
14. Finkelstein, JD, Harris, BJ, Martin, JJ, Kyle, WE. Regulation of hepatic betaine-homocysteine methyltransferase by dietary methionine. *Biochem Biophys Res Commun* 1982; 108: 344–48.
15. Finkelstein, JD, Kyle WE, Harris, BJ. Methionine metabolism in mammals: Regulation of homocysteine methyltransferases in rat tissue. *Arch Biochem Biophys* 1971; 146: 84–92.
16. Finkelstein, JD, Martin, JJ, Harris, BJ. Effect of dietary cystine on methionine metabolism in rat liver. *J Nutr* 1986; 116: 985–90.
17. Finkelstein, JD, Martin, JJ, Harris, BJ, Kyle, WE. Regulation of the betaine content of rat liver. *Arch Biochem Biophys* 1982; 218: 169–73.
18. Finkelstein, JD, Martin, JJ, Harris, BJ, Kyle, WE. Regulation of hepatic betaine-homocysteine methyltransferase by dietary betaine. *J Nutr* 1983; 113: 519–21.
19. Fromm, HJ, Nordlie, RC. On the purification and kinetics of rat liver thetin-homocysteine transmethylase. *Arch Biochem Biophys* 1959; 81: 363–76.
20. Garrow, TA. Purification, kinetic properties, and cDNA cloning of mammalian betaine-homocysteine methyltransferase. *J Biol Chem* 1996; 271: 22831–38.
21. Gaull, GE, von Berg, W, Raiha, NCR, Sturman, JA. Development of methyltransferase activities in human fetal tissues. *Pediatr Res* 1973; 7: 527–33.
22. Goulding, CW, Matthews, RG. Cobalamin-dependent methionine synthase from *Escherichia coli*: Involvement of zinc in homocysteine activation. *Biochemistry* 1997; 36: 15749–57.
23. Haubrich, DR, Gerber, NH. Choline dehydrogenase: Assay, properties and inhibitors. *Biochem Pharmacol* 1981; 30: 2993–3000.
24. Kaplan, CP, Porter, RK, Brand, MD. The choline transporter is the major site of control of choline oxidation in isolated rat liver mitochondria. *FEBS J* 1993; 321: 24–6.
25. Klee, WA, Richards, HH, Cantoni, GL. The synthesis of methionine by enzymatic transmethylation: Existence of two separate homocysteine methylpherases on mammalian liver. *Biochim Biophys Acta* 1961; 54: 157–64.
26. Lang, H, Minaian, K, Freudenberg, N, Hoffmann, R, Brandsch, R. Tissue specificity of rat mitochondrial dimethylglycine dehydrogenase expression. *Biochem J* 1994; 299: 393–98.
27. Lee, K-Y, Cava, M, Amiri, P, Ottoboni, T, Lindquist, RN. Betaine-homocysteine methyltransferase from rat liver: Purification and inhibition by a boronic acid substrate analog. *Arch Biochem Biophys* 1992; 292: 77–86.
28. Maw, GA. Thetin-homocysteine transmethylase: The distribution of the enzyme, studied with the aid of trimethylsulfonium chloride as substrate. *Biochem J* 1959; 72: 602–8.
29. McKeever, MP, Weir, DG, Molloy, A, Scott, JM. Betaine-homocysteine methyltransferase: Organ distribution in man, pig and rat and subcellular localization. *Clin. Sci.* 1991; 81: 551–56.
30. Millian, NS, Garrow, TA. Human betaine-homocysteine methyltransferase is a zinc metalloenzyme. *Arch Biochem Biophys* 1998; 356: 93–8.

31. Mudd, SH, Poole JR. Labile methyl balances for normal humans on various dietary regimens. *Metabolism* 1975; 24: 721–35.

32. Mudd, SH, Ebert, MH, Scriver, CR. Labile methyl group balances in the human: The role of sarcosine. *Metabolism* 1980; 29: 707–20.

33. Mudd, SH, Levy, HL, Abeles RH. A derangement of B_{12} metabolism leading to homocystinemia, cystathionimeia, and methylmalonic aciduria. *Biochem Biophys Res Comm* 1969; 35: 121–26.

34. Mudd, SH, Skovby, F, Levy, HL, Pettigrew, KD, Wilcken, B, Pyeritz, RE, Andria, G, Boers, GH, Bromberg, IL, Cerone, R. The natural history of homocystinuria due to cystathionine β-synthase deficiency. *Am J Hum Genet* 1985; 37: 1–31.

35. Park, EI, Garrow, TA. Interaction between dietary methionine and methyl donor intake on rat liver betaine-homocysteine methyltransferase gene expression and organization of the human gene. *J Biol Chem* 1999; 274: 7816–24.

36. Park, EI, Renduchintala, MS, Garrow, TA. Diet-induced changes in hepatic betaine-homocysteine methyltransferase activity are mediated by changes in steady-state levels of its mRNA. *J Nutr Biochem* 1997; 8: 541–45.

37. Peariso, K, Goulding, CW, Huang, S, Matthews, RG, Pennerhahn, JE. Characterization of the zinc binding site in methionine synthase enzymes of *Escherichia coli*: The role of zinc in the methylation of homocysteine. *J Am Chem Soc* 1998; 120: 8410–16.

38. Pietrzik, K, Bronstrup, A. Causes and consequences of hyperhomocyst(e)inemia. *Int J Vitam Nutr Res* 1997; 67: 389–95.

39. Rao, PV, Garrow, TA, John, F, Garland, D, Millian, NS, Zigler, JS. Betaine-homocysteine methyltransferase is a developmentally regulated enzyme crystallin in Rhesus monkey lens. *J Biol Chem* 1998; 273: 30669–74.

40. Ronge, E, Kjellman, B. Long term treatment with betaine in methylenetetrahydrofolate reductase deficiency. *Arch Dis Child* 1996; 74: 239–41.

41. Scott, R. Sarcosinemia. In *The Metabolic and Molecular Bases of Inherited Disease* (Scriver, CR, ed.). McGraw Hill, Inc., New York, 1995, vol. 1, pp. 1329–35.

42. Sidransky, H, Farber, E. Liver choline oxidase activity in man and in several species of animals. *Arch Biochem Biophys* 1960; 87: 129–33.

43. Skiba, WE, Taylor, MP, Wells, MS, Mangum, JH, Awad, WM. Human hepatic methionine biosynthesis: Purification and characterization of betaine-homocysteine S-methyltransferase. *J Biol Chem* 1982; 257: 14944–48.

44. Sturman, JA, Gaull, GE, Niemann, WH. Activities of some enzymes involved in homocysteine methylation in brain, liver and kidney of the developing rhesus monkey. *J Neurochem* 1976; 27: 425–31.

45. Sunden, LFS, Renduchintala, MS, Park, EI, Miklasz, SD, Garrow, TA. Expression of betaine-homocysteine methyltransferase in porcine and human tissue and chromosomal localization of the human gene. *Arch Biochem Biophys* 1997; 345: 171–74.

46. Walter, JH, Wraith, JE, White, FJ, Bridge, C, Till, J. Strategies for the treatment of cystathionine β-synthase deficiency: The experience of the Willink Biochemical Genetics Unit over the last 30 years. *Eur J Pediatr* 1998; 157: S71–6.

47. Wendel, U, Bremer, HJ. Betaine in the treatment of homocystinuria due to 5,10-methylenetetrahydrofolate reductase deficiency. *Eur J Pediatr* 1984; 142: 147–50.

48. Xue, G-P, Snoswell, AM. Comparative studies on the methionine synthesis in sheep and rat tissues. *Comp Biochem Physiol* 1985; 80B: 489–94.

49. Yap, S, Naughten, E. Homocystinuria due to cystathionine β-synthase deficiency in Ireland: 25 years of experience of a newborn screened and treated population with reference to clinical outcome and biochemical control. *J Inherit Metab Dis* 1998; 21: 738–47.

14

The Transsulfuration Pathway

WARREN D. KRUGER

Sulfur is an essential element in the chemistry of life. It is necessary for the synthesis of the amino acids cysteine and methionine. In humans, all sulfur found in amino acids must be obtained in the diet because humans lack the ability to fix inorganic sulfur, that is, to incorporate inorganic sulfur into amino acids. Transsulfuration is the pathway that allows the transfer of sulfur from methionine to cysteine. The existence of this pathway means that only methionine and not cysteine is essential in the human diet. Transsul-furation also plays a critical role in the removal of homocysteine. Homocysteine is a metabolic intermediary that occupies a critical branch-point in methionine metabolism (see Metabolic Diagram). It can either be recycled to methionine or be acted on by the transsulfuration pathway to form cysteine. Because high levels of homocysteine adversely affect human health, proper functioning of the transsulfuration pathway is essential. This chapter describes the transsulfuration pathway in humans and other organisms, its enzymology and regulation, and the downstream products of the pathway.

Transsulfuration in Evolution

In evolutionary terms, transsulfuration actually consists of two pathways, a forward and a reverse pathway. Some organisms have only one pathway, and others have both (Figure 14.1). The forward pathway, found in mammals (35), archaebacteria (56), and the yeast *Saccharomyces cerevisiae* (10), converts homocysteine to cysteine by first condensing homocysteine with serine to form cystathionine, and then by cleaving cystathionine at the γ-carbon to form cysteine and α-ketobutyrate (Figure 14.2). The reverse pathway, found in bacteria (11) and plants (34), catalyzes the formation of cystathionine by condensing cysteine with O-succinylhomoserine, forming cystathionine and succinate. Cystathionine is then broken down into

Fig. 14.1. Transsulfuration pathways in bacteria *(Escherichia coli)*, yeast *(Saccharomyces cerevisiae)*, and mammals (humans).

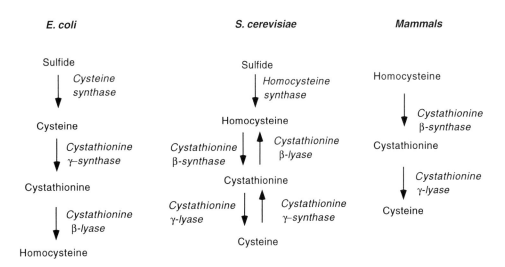

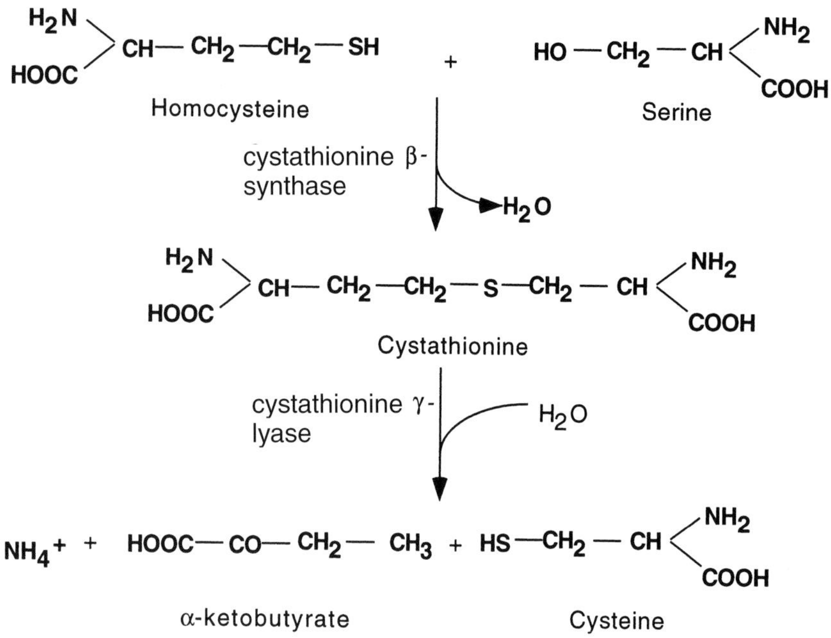

Fig. 14.2. The forward transsulfuration pathway.

homocysteine, ammonia, and pyruvate. Homocysteine can then be methylated to form methionine.

Bacteria and yeast, unlike humans, can fix inorganic sulfate. In bacteria this occurs by reducing sulfate to sulfide and condensing the sulfide to O-acetylserine to form cysteine (11, 29) (Figure 14.1). The reverse transsulfuration pathway must be present to allow the newly produced cysteine to form methionine. Yeast can also fix inorganic sulfur, but the pathway is slightly different. In this case, sulfide is condensed with O-acetylhomoserine to form homocysteine (10). Thus, in yeast a forward transsulfuration pathway is required to allow conversion of homocysteine to cysteine.

The absence of either the forward or the reverse transsulfuration pathways places metabolic constraints on an organism. Bacteria, which lack the forward pathway, cannot use sulfur from methionine to produce cysteine. Because of this, E. coli will not grow in an environment where the sole sulfur source is methionine (29). Humans, who lack the reverse pathway, cannot synthesize methionine from cysteine. This, in combination with the inability to fix inorganic sulfur, means that humans require methionine as an essential amino acid in the diet. Of interest, yeast having both pathways and the ability to fix inorganic sulfur can utilize cysteine, methionine, or inorganic sulfur as its sole sulfur source.

Cystathionine β-Synthase

The first enzyme in the forward transsulfuration pathway is cystathionine β-synthase (CBS) (Metabolic

Diagram, Reaction 6). Because the clinical and genetic aspects of CBS deficiency are covered more fully in Chapter 20, the discussion here focuses on the biochemistry of the enzyme. CBS catalyzes the condensation of homocysteine and serine in a reaction that requires pyridoxal 5′-phosphate, the coenzyme form of vitamin B_6. The human CBS protein is 551 amino acids in length, runs at 63 kDa on sodium dodecyl sulfate-polyacrylamide gel electrophoresis (SDS-PAGE) gels, and is active as a tetramer. Historically, there has been some confusion as to whether the tetramer or a dimer was the active species, as well as the actual size of the monomer. This confusion arose because in early studies the enzyme underwent proteolysis during purification from liver (44). The proteolyzed form runs at about 48 kDa on SDS-PAGE gels and is active as a dimer, and the full length form is a 63 kDa protein and is active as a tetramer. Interestingly, the 48 kDa form appears to have significantly higher specific activity than the full-length form. Recent studies suggest that the 48 kDa form is probably missing the C-terminal portion of the protein. Deletion of the C-terminal 145 amino acids results in the recombinant human protein being active as a dimer and having 10-fold more activity in vitro (43). In addition, treatment of a bacterially produced recombinant human CBS with protease results in a "core" domain missing N- and C-terminal domains. This central domain is also significantly more active in vitro and is active as a dimer (24). These results suggest that the C-terminus of the protein is involved in tetramerization and that it may be involved in regulating enzyme activity.

Kinetic studies on purified recombinant CBS indicate that the K_m for homocysteine is estimated to be 1.5 to 5.0 mmol/L and that of serine is 2.0 to 3.0 mmol/L (24, 52). Methionine synthase, which also uses homocysteine as a substrate, has an estimated K_m of 60 μmol/L (7). Thus, remethylation would be favored, at low concentrations of homocysteine, whereas at high concentrations of homocysteine, the transsulfuration pathway becomes active in removal of the excess homocysteine.

The predicted CBS protein shares significant sequence similarity with several enzymes, including prokaryotic cysteine synthase (which catalyzes the formation of cystathionine from cysteine in bacteria), threonine deaminase, and the β-chain of tryptophan synthase. The region of similarity between all three of these enzymes lies between amino acids 80 and 305 on the protein (28). This similarity in primary amino acid sequence is also reflected in at least some conservation in tertiary structure, as antibodies raised against human CBS strongly cross-react with yeast threonine deaminase (43). All three of the previously mentioned enzymes, such as CBS, utilize pyridoxal 5′-phosphate and catalyze chemical reactions involving serine. Thus, the conserved region probably encompasses the key catalytic regions of CBS, at least with regard to pyridoxal 5′-phosphate and serine. Based on the sequence similarity with tryptophan synthase, whose crystal structure has been determined (20), it was suspected CBS binds pyridoxal 5′-phosphate at lysine 119. Recent biochemical experiments on recombinant human enzyme produced in bacteria have confirmed that pyridoxal 5′-phosphate does indeed bind at this position (25). However, a surprising finding is that within the tetramer, although there are four pyridoxine binding sites, there appear to be two high- and two low-affinity sites (52). This difference in affinity may be related to the stoichiometry of heme binding (see later).

A key role in the biochemistry of human CBS is played by pyridoxal 5′-phosphate. The hypothesized role of pyridoxal 5′-phosphate in the reaction mechanism is to bind serine and help make it more reactive

(57) (Figure 14.3). The pyridoxal 5′-phosphate moiety binds to the ε-amino group of lysine 119 by a Schiff-base linkage. When serine is bound to CBS, this linkage shifts from the lysine to the serine α-amino group. Thus, the aldehyde group of pyridoxal 5′-phosphate attacks the amine group of serine to produce an aldimine intermediate. The pyridoxal ring can act to stabilize electrons, and this allows the β-carbon of serine to be attacked by the sulfur atom of homocysteine. After the reaction is completed, pyridoxal 5′-phosphate is transferred back to lysine again. Therefore, the cofactor is transiently released by CBS during the actual enzyme chemistry.

Another molecule required for human CBS activity is heme (23). In fact the first described mammalian CBS cDNA sequence was initially identified in a search for rat proteins that bound heme (21). Recombinant human CBS enzyme isolated from bacteria shows a linear relationship between increasing heme content and activity (23), and heme ligands, such as carbon monoxide and cyanide, inhibit CBS activity (52). These observations show that heme is required for enzyme activity. The stoichiometry of heme binding is somewhat controversial. Kraus's group has reported that four hemes bind per tetramer (23), whereas Banerjee's group has reported two hemes binding per tetramer (51). The role of heme in CBS chemistry is uncertain because other vitamin B_6-dependent enzymes such as tryptophan synthase and threonine deaminase are not thought to bind heme. One possible model (Figure 14.3) is that the ferric iron in the heme acts to coordinate and activate the homocysteine thiol with its interaction with vitamin B_6-bound serine (51). There are two attractive features of this model. First, the model provides an explanation for the absence of heme in other pyridoxal 5′-phosphate-dependent enzymes because the role of heme is specific to the chemistry of homocysteine and not serine. Second, the model provides a mechanism for the activation of the

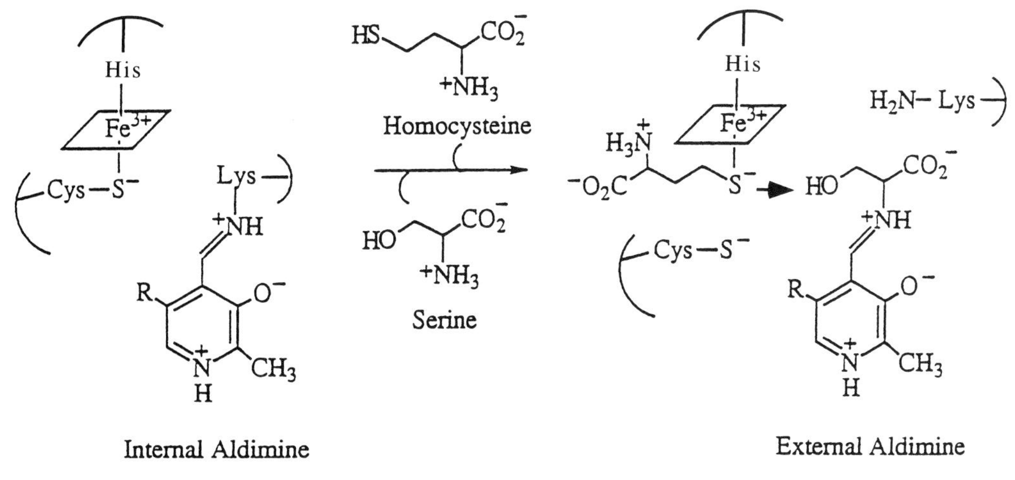

Fig. 14.3. Hypothetical reaction mechanism for cystathionine β-synthase (CBS). On the left is shown the unoccupied active site of the CBS enzyme in the absence of substrate. Pyridoxal 5′-phosphate (PLP) is attached via an aldimine linkage with lysine 119, whereas heme (Fe^{3+}) is attached to CBS via a cysteine-histidine linkage. On the right is shown the reaction of the two substrates, homocysteine and serine, interacting with their respective cofactors (i.e., serine binds to PLP to form an external aldimine), whereas homocysteine interacts with the heme to become activated. The short, thick arrow shows the attack of the activated sulfur on the serine hydroxyl. (Modified from Taoka et al. [51], with permission)

Internal Aldimine   External Aldimine

thiol in lieu of an active site zinc that is used by another homocysteine-utilizing enzyme, cobalamin-independent methionine synthase (18). Interestingly, recent work characterizing the CBS enzyme from *S. cerevisiae* indicates that this enzyme does not bind heme and does not require heme for function (21a).

The activity of CBS is regulated by *S*-adenosylmethionine (16). This regulation helps the cell balance transsulfuration of homocysteine with remethylation of homocysteine. Under conditions of plentiful methionine and *S*-adenosylmethionine, more homocysteine should be shunted down the transsulfuration pathway, whereas under conditions of low methionine and *S*-adenosylmethionine, homocysteine should be remethylated. *S*-adenosylmethionine stimulates CBS activity, increasing the turnover rate of the enzyme twofold to threefold (24, 51). Interestingly, a form of CBS that lacks the C-terminal domain is no longer sensitive to activation by *S*-adenosylmethionine. This has led to the hypothesis that the C-terminal domain of CBS is a negative regulatory domain, and that the binding of *S*-adenosylmethionine to this domain relieves this negative regulation (43). Recent studies indicate that the presence of the C-terminal domain is required for *S*-adenosylmethionine binding to CBS (53).

Sequence similarity analysis has identified a 53-amino acid stretch in CBS C-terminal domain that has been found in proteins in several diverse species ranging from humans to archaebacteria. This domain has been dubbed the "CBS domain" (3). In CBS it is located between amino acids 415 and 468 and thus lies within the C-terminal regulatory region. Other proteins containing the CBS domain include inosine-5'-monophosphate dehydrogenase, 5'-AMP-activated protein kinase, voltage-gated chloride channels, ABC transporters, and several other proteins of undefined function. Interestingly, in all proteins except CBS the motif is found in multiple copies. The functional role of the CBS domain in any of these proteins is not known.

CBS is also sensitive to redox conditions. In vitro the enzyme is 1.7-fold more active under oxidizing than under reducing conditions (51). Because cysteine is required for the production of glutathione, the major intracellular antioxidant, it makes teleological sense that a cell would want to increase cysteine production when under oxidative stress.

CBS enzyme activity is not found in all tissues and cells. It is absent from heart, lung, testes, adrenal, and spleen in rats (15). In humans it has been shown to be absent in heart muscle and primary cultures of human aortic endothelial cells (9). Examination of CBS protein by Western blot suggests that this lack of activity may result from post-translational proteolysis of CBS. The lack of CBS in these tissues implies that these tissues are unable to synthesize cysteine and that cysteine must be supplied extracellularly. It also suggests that these tissues may have increased sensitivity to homocysteine toxicity because they cannot catabolize excess homocysteine via transsulfuration.

Four different CBS RNA isoforms have been described (2, 8). These differ only in their 5' untranslated regions, and all of the isoforms would be expected to encode the same CBS protein. Adult tissues with the highest concentrations of CBS messenger RNA are the liver, pancreas, and kidney. However, some CBS mRNA can be detected by Northern blot analysis in all tissues tested. Certain RNA isoforms are expressed only in specific tissues. For example, isoform 5 is expressed exclusively in the pancreas, and the kidney expresses predominantly isoform 1. The significance of these differences is difficult to assess, as there are no data suggesting that the different mRNA isoforms produce differing levels of CBS protein.

CBS mRNA is also expressed during human fetal development. It is expressed in high levels in fetal human liver and brain (39). In situ hybridization has detected CBS mRNA in the central nervous system from embryos as young as 3 weeks old (39). The gene is expressed in all embryonic tissues that are affected by clinical homocystinuria. Thus, CBS RNA levels are high in the developing neural and vascular systems, and are at somewhat lower levels in the developing skeletal system.

Yeast Assay for Human CBS

The human and the yeast *S. cerevisiae* CBS proteins are 38% identical over 506 amino acids. This high degree of structural conservation has allowed the development of a yeast assay for the human CBS protein (30). Yeast whose endogenous CBS gene *(CYS4)* was deleted require exogenous cysteine for growth because they lack the ability to synthesize cysteine from homocysteine. Expression of the human CBS cDNA can correct the phenotype and allow the yeast to grow on media lacking cysteine. Thus the yeast enzyme is structurally and functionally conserved over 2 billion years of evolution.

The yeast assay has been used to identify and characterize mutations in the human CBS gene found in individuals with homocystinuria (31) (Figure 14.4). One of the major concerns in human mutational analysis is the difficulty of knowing whether a particular point mutation is disease-causing or whether it is a neutral polymorphism. The modeling of mutant forms of CBS in yeast allows the determination of the functional consequences of specific changes. For example, the R266K mutation found in several Norwegian patients with pyridoxine-responsive homocystinuria was shown to give a pyridoxine-responsive phenotype

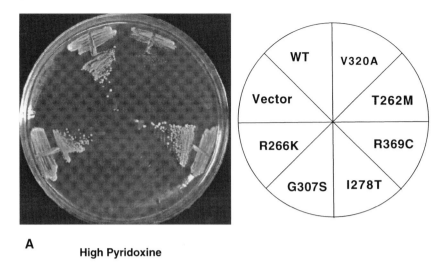

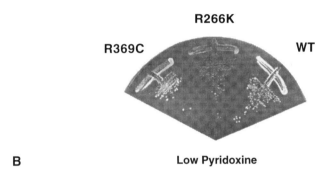

Fig. 14.4.   Yeast assay for functional analysis of cystathionine β-synthase (CBS) mutations. (A) The yeast growing on this plate have a deletion of the endogenous yeast CBS gene, and yeast in each sector express a different human CBS allele identified in a patient with clinical CBS deficiency. The plate lacks cysteine, so the yeast can grow and form colonies only if they have a functional CBS enzyme. Two of the patient-derived mutations, R266K and R369C, do not have any functional effect on yeast grown on standard medium. (B) Yeast expressing R266K, R369C, and wild type (WT) CBS grown on media with only minimal vitamin B_6 supplementation. Note that the R266K allele now shows a phenotypic difference when compared with the other two. R266K is found in several patients who are all highly vitamin B_6-responsive. (Modified from Kim et al. [26], with permission.)

in yeast (26). By using the yeast assay, we have identified and analyzed the functional effects of 12 patient-derived missense mutations and have observed a yeast phenotype for 11 of these mutations. The one mutation that had wild-type behavior in yeast (R369C) now appears to be a rare polymorphism present at about a 1% allele frequency in the population (W.D. Kruger, unpublished observations).

The yeast system can also be used for mutational analysis of the enzyme. The observation that the C-terminus of CBS encoded a regulatory domain that is required for *S*-adenosylmethionine regulation was inferred from a mutation that was originally discovered in the yeast system (43). Recently this laboratory has used PCR-based mutagenesis to identify activating and repression missense mutations located in the C-terminal third of the protein. These sorts of studies should provide insight into the structure/function relations in the enzyme.

Cystathionine γ-Lyase

The second and final enzyme of the forward transsulfuration pathway is cystathionine γ-lyase, which catalyzes the breakdown of cystathionine to cysteine and α-ketobutyrate (Metabolic Diagram, Reaction 7). Like CBS, the enzyme requires pyridoxal 5′-phosphate as a cofactor. Rat cystathionine γ-lyase is a tetramer of four 43 kDa subunits (5). The cDNAs for both the human and the rat cystathionine γ-lyase have been isolated (14, 33). The human protein is predicted to be 405 amino acids long and have a molecular mass of 44.5 kDa. It is 88% similar to the predicted rat protein and shares significant sequence similarities with cystathionine γ-lyases and cystathionine γ-synthases from a variety of species. The rat enzyme has a K_m of 3.5 mmol/L for cystathionine and a V_{max} of 1.3 units/mg (22). No kinetic data exist for the human enzyme.

Propargylglycine is a specific inhibitor of cystathionine γ-lyase. It binds covalently and irreversibly to the active site of the enzyme and is thus a suicide inhibitor (1). Mice treated with propargylglycine show elevated plasma and urinary cystathionine levels (55). Mice given normal diets show minimal weight loss from propargylglycine treatment, but mice on cysteine-free diets show substantial weight loss after 4 days. Thus inhibition of cystathionine γ-lyase will result in cysteine depletion if it is not present in the diet. Mice treated with propargylglycine show no decrease in liver CBS activity, suggesting that high cystathionine levels do not affect CBS activity.

In humans, there have been several documented examples of individuals with cystathionine γ-lyase deficiency leading to cystathioninuria (36). These individuals have elevated cystathionine present in the plasma, as well as other bodily fluids. They also excrete substantial amounts of *N*-acetylcystathionine, presumably after acetylation of cystathionine in the liver and kidney (38). The clinical manifestations of cystathionine γ-lyase deficiency are not entirely clear. Because the initial patient described was mentally retarded, early studies focused exclusively on identifying individuals with low intelligence with cystathioninuria. However, among the 26 patients for whom ascertainment bias was minimal, only five had clinical disorders that could be related to the metabolic disorder (36). Of these five individuals, four had siblings who either had cystathioninuria and were normal, or did not have cystathioninuria and were equally affected clinically. Thus, the current thinking is that there are no clinical implications associated with cystathioninuria. An important point in interpreting these data is that in the normal human diet, cysteine is obtained in abundance, so the absence of a functional transsulfuration pathway would not cause cysteine starvation.

It has also been observed that the livers of fetuses, preterm infants, and term infants have low levels of cystathionine γ-lyase activity. This is consistent with the observation that cysteine is a required amino acid in at least some infants (17, 45, 47).

In rat brain and adipose tissue, cystathionine γ-lyase activity is absent even though CBS activity is present (35). Thus, in these tissues the transsulfuration pathway is "truncated" with the production of cystathionine instead of cysteine. Consistent with this observation is the fact that cystathionine levels are found at very high levels in the human brain (48). Studies on dissected cow brains indicate that the pineal gland has particularly high levels (32). The biological function of cystathionine in neural tissues is not understood. Neural tissue also seems to have relatively high levels of homocysteine (6). Interestingly, homocysteic acid has been shown to act as an excitatory neurotransmitter in cell culture and whole animal models (13, 42, 54). The metabolic pathway by which homocysteine is converted to homocysteic acid is unknown.

The lack of a complete transsulfuration pathway in neurons is probably responsible for the phenomenon of glutamate toxicity in neural cells. High concentrations of extracellular glutamate are known to induce apoptosis by blocking a glutamate/cystine antiporter and thus inhibiting the uptake of cystine from the medium (37). Because these cells lack the ability to synthesize cysteine from methionine, they are starved for cysteine, and this induces cell death by depleting intracellular glutathione levels (49, 50).

Cysteine and Beyond

The sulfur product of the transsulfuration pathway is the amino acid cysteine. Labeling studies in cultured liver hepatocytes reveal that most of the excess cysteine (about 70%) is rapidly converted to glutathione (40). Glutathione is a tripeptide that plays a critical role in maintaining the reducing environment inside the cell. In addition, glutathione is involved in the detoxification of xenobiotics via conjugation by the various glutathione S-transferases.

Most of the remaining cysteine is metabolized to sulfate by the action of the cysteinesulfinate pathway (Figure 14.5). Cysteine is first oxygenated by cysteine dioxygenase to form cysteinesulfinate. Cysteinesulfinate can then have one of two fates. It can be acted on by aspartate aminotransferase to ultimately form pyruvate and sulfate, or it can be decarboxylated to ultimately form taurine. Taurine functions in electrically active tissues such as the brain and heart to help stabilize cell membranes (41). It also has functions in the gallbladder, eyes, and blood vessels and appears to have some antioxidant and detoxifying activity. Taurine aids the movement of potassium, sodium, calcium, and magnesium in and out of cells and thus helps generate nerve impulses. Zinc seems to support this effect of taurine. Taurine is found in the central nervous system, skeletal muscle, and heart; it is con-

Fig. 14.5.   Cysteine metabolism.

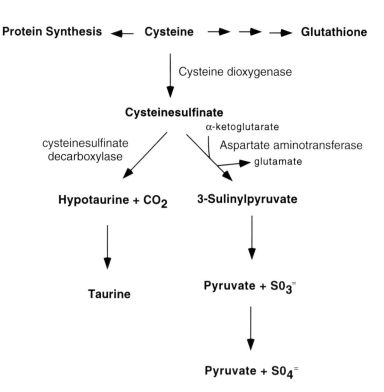

centrated in the brain and heart tissues (41). No human clinical disorders have been ascribed to taurine deficiency.

The sulfate produced by the breakdown of cysteine is thought to be important in the generation of 3′-phosphoadenosine 5′-phosphosulfate (27). In mammals, inorganic sulfate is conjugated to adenine to form 5′-adenylylsulfate, which is then phosphorylated to form 3′-phosphoadenosine 5′-phosphosulfate. This chemistry is catalyzed by a bifunctional enzyme that contains adenosine triphosphate sulfurylase and 5′-adenylyl-sulfate kinase activities. 3′-Phosphoadenosine 5′-phosphosulfate is a sulfate donor in a wide variety of sulfation reactions catalyzed by sulfotransferases. Sulfation has a number of important biological functions such as detoxification of xenobiotics, steroid biosynthesis, and post-translational processing (12). Several drugs and other xenobiotics are directly conjugated with sulfate to inactivate them and increase solubility for excretion. However, in some cases, mutagens and other carcinogens are actually activated by sulfation. Sulfation also is important in steroid biosynthesis. The major circulating steroid and estrogen species (dehydroepiandrosterone sulfate and estrone sulfate) are both conjugated with sulfate. Finally, sulfation of secreted proteoglycans is critical for proper cartilage function (4). Individuals with diastrophic dysplasia and the more severe atelosteogenesis type II have mutations in a gene that encodes a sulfate transporter (19, 46).

In theory, individuals with metabolic blocks in the transsulfuration pathway might be expected to have clinical problems owing to decreased cysteine levels that would result in decreased sulfate levels and taurine levels. However, it should be noted that individuals with both CBS deficiency and cystathionine γ-lyase deficiency would be expected to suffer from this problem and, therefore, to share a set of symptoms in common. However, as there is no solid clinical abnormality associated with cystathionine γ-lyase deficiency, it seems unlikely that cysteine depletion caused by defects in transsulfuration has important clinical consequences.

Why Do We Have Transsulfuration?

Transsulfuration is required for the de novo synthesis of cysteine from methionine. In the human, however, dietary methionine and cysteine are generally found together (i.e., proteins have both of these amino acids). Therefore, it seems unlikely that the purpose of transsulfuration is for biosynthesis of cysteine from methionine. What, then, is the role of transsulfuration? In the absence of transsulfuration, homocysteine levels are tied directly to methionine levels because of the methionine cycle. Thus, high protein diets would result in high methionine and high homocysteine levels. This is, in fact, what is observed in individuals with CBS deficiency. Because most of the clinical features associated with CBS deficiency may be due to homocysteine toxicity, the biological importance of transsulfuration may simply be as a means to reduce homocysteine levels. The real importance of transsulfuration in humans may be as a catabolic pathway in the destruction of homocysteine, rather than an anabolic pathway involved in the formation of cysteine.

REFERENCES

1. Abeles, RH, Walsh, CT. Acetylenic enzyme inactivators. Inactivation of γ-cystathionase, *in vitro* and *in vivo*, by propargylglycine. *J Am Chem Soc* 1973; 95: 6124–25.

2. Bao, L, Vlcek, C, Paces, V, Kraus, JP. Identification and tissue distribution of human cystathionine β-synthase mRNA isoforms. *Arch Biochem Biophys* 1998; 350: 95–103.

3. Bateman, A. The structure of a domain common to archaebacteria and the homocystinuria disease protein. *Trends Biochem Sci* 1997; 22: 12–3.

4. Beaty, NB, Mello, RJ. Extracellular mammalian polysaccharides: Glycosaminoglycans and proteoglycans. *J Chromatogr* 1987; 418: 187–222.

5. Braunstein, AE, Goryachenkova, EV. The β-replacement-specific pyridoxal-P-dependent lyases. *Adv Enzymol Relat Areas Mol Biol* 1984; 56: 1–89.

6. Broch, OJ, Ueland, PM. Regional distribution of homocysteine in the mammalian brain. *J Neurochem* 1984; 43: 1755–57.

7. Burke, GT, Mangum, JH, Brodie, JD. Mechanism of mammalian cobalamin-dependent methionine biosynthesis. *Biochemistry* 1971; 10: 3079–85.

8. Chasse, JF, Paul, V, Escanez, R, Kamoun, P, London, J. Human cystathionine β-synthase: Gene organization and expression of different 5′ alternative splicing. *Mamm Genome* 1997; 8: 917–21.

9. Chen, P, Poddar, R, Tipa, EV, Dibello, PM, Moravec, CD, Robinson, D, Green, R, Kruger, WD, Garrow, TA, Jacobsen, DW. Homocysteine metabolism in the cardiovascular cells and tissues: Implications for hyperhomocysteinemia and cardiovascular disease. *Adv Enzyme Regul* 1999; 39: 93–109.

10. Cherest, H, Surdin-Kerjan, Y. Genetic analysis of a new mutation conferring cysteine auxotrophy in *Saccharomyces cerevisiae:* Updating of the sulfur metabolism pathway. *Genetics* 1992; 130: 51–8.

11. Cohen, GN, Saint-Girons, I. Biosynthesis of threonine, lysine and methionine. In *Escherichia coli and Salmonella typhimurium,* Vol 1 (Neidhart, FC, ed.) American Society for Microbiology, Washington, DC, 1987; 429–44.

12. Coughtrie, MW, Sharp, S, Maxwell, K, Innes, NP. Biology and function of the reversible sulfation pathway catalysed by human sulfotransferases and sulfatases. *Chem Biol Interact* 1998; 109: 3–27.

13. Cuenod, M, Do, KQ, Herrling, PL, Turski, WA, Matute, C, Streit, P. Homocysteic acid, an endogenous agonist of NMDA-receptor: Release, neuroactivity and localization. *Adv Exp Med Biol* 1986; 203: 253–72.

14. Erickson, PF, Maxwell, IH, Su, LJ, Baumann, M, Glode, LM. Sequence of cDNA for rat cystathionine γ-lyase and comparison of deduced amino acid sequence with related *Escherichia coli* enzymes. *Biochem J* 1990; 269: 335–40.

15. Finkelstein, JD. The metabolism of homocysteine: Pathways and regulation. *Eur J Pediatr* 1998; 157: S40–44.

16. Finkelstein, JD, Kyle, WE, Martin, JL, Pick, AM. Activation of cystathionine synthase by adenosylmethionine and adenosylethionine. *Biochem Biophys Res Commun* 1975; 66: 81–7.

17. Gaull, G, Sturman, JA, Raiha, NCR. Development of mammalian sulfur metabolism: Absence of cystathionase in human fetal tissues. *Pediatr Res* 1972; 6: 538–47.

18. Gonzalez, JC, Peariso, K, Penner-Hahn, JE, Matthews, RG. Cobalamin-independent methionine synthase from *Escherichia coli*: A zinc metalloenzyme. *Biochemistry* 1996; 35: 12228–234.

19. Hastbacka, J, Superti-Furga, A, Wilcox, WR, Rimoin, DL, Cohn, DH, Lander, ES. Atelosteogenesis type II is caused by mutations in the diastrophic dysplasia sulfate-transporter gene (DTDST): Evidence for a phenotypic series involving three chondrodysplasias. *Am J Hum Genet* 1996; 58: 255–62.

20. Hyde, CC, Ahmed, SA, Padlan, EA, Miles, EW, Davies, DR. Three-dimensional structure of the tryptophan synthase $\alpha_2\beta_2$ multienzyme complex from *Salmonella typhimurium*. *J Biol Chem* 1988; 263: 17857–71.

21. Ishihara, S, Morohashi, K, Sadano, H, Kawabata, S, Gotoh, O, Omura, T. Molecular cloning and sequence analysis of cDNA coding for rat liver hemoprotein H-450. *J Biochem* 1990; 108: 899–902.

21a. Jhee, KH, McPhie, P, Miles, EW. Yeast cystathionine β-synthase is a pyridoxal phosphate enzyme but, unlike the human enzyme, is not a heme protein. *J Biol Chem* 2000; 275: 11541–44.

22. Kato, A, Ogura, M, Suda, M. Control mechanism in the rat liver enzyme system converting L-methionine to L-cystine. 3. Noncompetitive inhibition of cystathionine synthetase-serine dehydratase by elemental sulfur and competitive inhibition of cystathionase-homoserine dehydratase by L-cysteine and L-cystine. *J Biochem* 1966; 59: 40–8.

23. Kery, V, Bukovska, G, Kraus, JP. Transsulfuration depends on heme in addition to pyridoxal 5′-phosphate. Cystathionine β-synthase is a heme protein. *J Biol Chem* 1994; 269: 25283–88.

24. Kery, V, Poneleit, L, Kraus, JP. Trypsin cleavage of human cystathionine β-synthase into an evolutionarily conserved active core: Structural and functional consequences. *Arch Biochem Biophys* 1998; 355: 222–32.

25. Kery, V, Poneleit, L, Meyer, JD, Manning, MC, Kraus, JP. Binding of pyridoxal 5′-phosphate to the heme protein human cystathionine β-synthase. *Biochemistry* 1999; 38: 2716–24.

26. Kim, CE, Gallagher, PM, Guttormsen, AB, Retsom, H, Veland, PM, Ose, L, Filling, I, Whitehead, AS, Tsai, MY, Kruger, WD. Functional modeling of vitamin responsiveness in yeast: A common pyridoxine-responsive cystathionine β-synthase mutation in homocystinuria. *Hum Mol Genet* 1997; 6: 2213–21.

27. Klaassen, CD, Boles, JW. Sulfation and sulfotransferases 5: The importance of 3′-phosphoadenosine 5′-phosphosulfate (PAPS) in the regulation of sulfation. *FASEB J* 1997; 11: 404–18.

28. Kraus, JP, Le, K, Swaroop M, Ohura, T, Tahara, T, Rosenberg, LE, Roper, MD, Kozich, V. Human cystathionine β-synthase cDNA: Sequence, alternative splicing and expression in cultured cells. *Hum Mol Genet* 1993; 2: 1633–38.

29. Kredich, NM. Biosynthesis of cysteine. In *Escherichia coli and Salmonella typhimurium*, vol. 1 (Neidhardt, FC, ed.). American Society for Microbiology, Washington, DC, 1987; 419–28.

30. Kruger, WD, Cox, DR. A yeast system for expression of human cystathionine β-synthase: Structural and functional conservation of the human and yeast genes. *Proc Natl Acad Sci USA* 1994; 91: 6614–18.

31. Kruger, WD, Cox, DR. A yeast assay for functional detection of mutations in the human cystathionine β-synthase gene. *Hum Mol Genet* 1995; 4: 1155–61.

32. LaBella, F, Vivian, S, Queen, G. Abundance of cystathionine in the pineal body. Free amino acids and related compounds of bovine pineal, anterior and posterior pituitary, and brain. *Biochem Biophys Acta* 1968; 158: 286–88.

33. Lu, Y, O'Dowd, BF, Orrego, H, Israel, Y. Cloning and nucleotide sequence of human liver cDNA encoding for cystathionine γ-lyase. *Biochem Biophys Res Commun* 1992; 189: 749–58.

34. Macnicol, PK, Datko, AH, Giovanelli, J, Mudd, SH. Homocysteine biosynthesis in green plants: Physiological importance of the transsulfuration pathway in *Lemna paucicostata*. *Plant Physiol* 1981; 68: 619–25.

35. Mudd, SH, Finkelstein, JD, Irreverre, F, Laster, L. Transsulfuration in mammals: Microassays and tissue distribution of three enzymes of the pathway. *J Biol Chem* 1965; 240: 4382–92.

36. Mudd, SH, Levy, HL, Skovby, F. Disorders in transsulfuration. In *The Metabolic Basis of Inherited Disease* (Scriver, CR, Beaudet, A, Sly, W, Valle D, eds.). McGraw-Hill, New York, 1995; 693–34.

37. Murphy, TH, Schnaar, RL, Coyle, JT. Immature cortical neurons are uniquely sensitive to glutamate toxicity by inhibition of cystine uptake. *FASEB J* 1990; 4: 1624–33.

38. Perry, TL, Hansen, S, Love, D, Finch, CA. N-acetylcystathionine: A new urinary amino-acid in congenital cystathioninuria. *Nature* 1968; 219: 178–79.

39. Quèrè, I, Paul, V, Rouillac, C, Janbon, C, London, J, Demaille, J, Kamoun, P, Dufier, JL, Abitbol, M, Chassé, J-F. Spatial and temperal expression of the cystathionine β-synthase gene during human development. *Biochem Biophys Res Commun* 1999; 254: 127–37.

40. Rao, AM, Drake, MR, Stipanuk, MH. Role of the transsulfuration pathway and of γ-cystathionase activity

in the formation of cysteine and sulfate from methionine in rat hepatocytes. *J Nutr* 1990; 120: 837–45.

41. Redmond, HP, Stapleton, PP, Neary, P, Bouchier-Hayes, D. Immunonutrition: The role of taurine. *Nutrition* 1998; 14: 599–604.

42. Sawada, S, Takada, S, Yamamoto, C. Excitatory actions of homocysteic acid on hippocampal neurons. *Brain* 1982; 238: 282–85.

43. Shan, X, Kruger, WD. Correction of disease-causing CBS mutations in yeast. *Nat Genet* 1998; 19: 91–3.

44. Skovby, F, Kraus, JP, Rosenberg, LE. Biosynthesis and proteolytic activation of cystathionine β-synthase in rat liver. *J Biol Chem* 1984; 259: 588–93.

45. Sturman, FA, Gaull, G, Raiha, NCR. Absence of cystathionase in human fetal liver: Is cystine essential? *Science* 1970; 169: 74–6.

46. Superti-Furga, A, Hastbacka, J, Wilcox, WR, Cohn, DH, van der Huten, HJ, Rossi, A, Blav, N, Rimoin, DL, Steinmann, B, Lander, ES, GT, Elmann, R. Achondrogenesis type IB is caused by mutations in the diastrophic dysplasia sulphate transporter gene. *Nat Genet* 1996; 12: 100–2.

47. Synderman, SE. The protein and amino acid requirements of the premature infant. In *Metabolic Processes in the Faetus and Newborn Infant* (Ionxix, JHP, Visser, HKA, Troelstra, JD, eds.). HE Stenfert Kroesse NV, Leiden, 1971; pp. 128–41.

48. Tallan, HH, Moore, S, Stein, WH. L-cystathionine in human brain. *J Biol Chem* 1958; 230: 707–16.

49. Tan, S, Sagara, Y, Liu, Y, Maher, P, Schubert, D. The regulation of reactive oxygen species production during programmed cell death. *J Cell Biol* 1998; 141: 1423–32.

50. Tan, S, Wood, M, Maher, P. Oxidative stress induces a form of programmed cell death with characteristics of both apoptosis and necrosis in neuronal cells. *J Neurochem* 1998; 71: 95–105.

51. Taoka, S, Ohja, S, Shan, X, Kruger, WD, Banerjee, R. Evidence of heme-mediated redox regulation of human cystathionine β-synthase activity. *J Biol Chem* 1998; 273: 25179–84.

52. Taoka, S, West, M, Banerjee, R. Characterization of the heme and pyridoxal phosphate cofactors of human cystathionine β-synthase reveals nonequivalent active sites. *Biochemistry* 1999; 38: 2738–44.

53. Taoka, S, Widjata, L, Banerjee, R. Assignment of enzymatic functions to specific regions of the PLP-dependent heme protein cystathionine β-synthase. *Biochemistry* 1999; 38: 13155–61.

54. Turski, WA. Homocysteic acid: Convulsant action of stereoisomers in mice. *Brain* 1989; 479: 371–73.

55. Uren, JR, Ragin, R, Chaykovsky, M. Modulation of cysteine metabolism in mice: Effects of propargylglycine and L-cyst(e)ine-degrading enzymes. *Biochem Pharmacol* 1978; 27: 2807–14.

56. Zhou, D, White, RH. Transsulfuration in archaebacteria. *J Bacteriol* 1991; 173: 3250–51.

57. Zubay, G. *Biochemistry*, Addison-Wesley Publishing Co., Inc., Boston, 1989.

15

Transport and Tissue Distribution of Homocysteine and Related S-Adenosyl Compounds

BRIAN FOWLER

Many factors influence homeostasis of homocysteine and are reflected in its physiological levels. Metabolism of homocysteine depends on correct function of the pertinent enzymes, as well as adequate levels of the many associated amino acids and substrates, other cellular metabolites, and vitamins. The distribution of homocysteine among different tissues, cells, and intracellular compartments is also an important factor affecting physiological concentrations. Distribution is dependent not only on metabolic changes within different tissues and cells but also on transport, cellular uptake and output, and intracellular import and export. Furthermore, the relative distribution of homocysteine in different tissues is an important factor in considering possible disease-causing mechanisms.

Much is known about plasma homocysteine under various physiological conditions and in many disease states, but less information is available on levels in tissues and the processes influencing tissue distribution. An important question is how plasma levels reflect those in the various tissues. It is also necessary to consider how homocysteine crosses cell membranes, whether cellular receptors or membrane channels for homocysteine exist, whether active, specific processes play a role, and whether homocysteine shares systems for other amino acids, such as cysteine, cystine, and glutathione. This chapter addresses these questions for

homocysteine as well as for the important substrates and regulatory compounds, *S*-adenosylmethionine (AdoMet) and *S*-adenosylhomocysteine (AdoHcy).

Source of Homocysteine Production

Because the dietary intake of homocysteine is extremely small, compared with that of methionine, there is no need per se for specific intestinal absorption and cellular uptake of homocysteine. The major determinant of intracellular homocysteine is metabolic production from methionine via AdoMet and AdoHcy.

Finkelstein (29) documented the different homocysteine-metabolizing enzymes in various rat tissues. For example, the activity of cystathionine β-synthase (CBS) is highest in liver, pancreas, kidney, adipose tissue, brain, small intestine, and then spleen; but it is not detectable in adrenal, lung, testes, and heart. In contrast, methionine adenosyltransferase and AdoHcy hydrolase are present in each of these tissues. The highest levels of methionine adenosyltransferase are found in the liver, followed by kidney, pancreas, adrenal, brain, testes, small intestine, lung, adipose tissue, and heart; the activity of AdoHcy hydrolase is highest in the pancreas, then liver, kidney, adrenal, brain, testes, adipose tissue, lung, small intestine, spleen, and heart. Information on the tissue distribution of enzymes that metabolize homocysteine in humans (74), although less comprehensive, supports the idea of variable tissue content of these enzymes.

Thus, the widely differing patterns need to be borne in mind when considering tissue differences of homocysteine concentration (see later). Virtually all tissues contain the enzymes necessary to produce homocysteine from methionine, but differences exist for the remethylation and transsulfuration pathways. For example, erythrocytes produce homocysteine from methionine, but neither the remethylation nor the transsulfuration pathway is present, whereas leukocytes are able to produce labeled cysteine from [^{35}S]methionine (57).

Binding of Homocysteine to Protein

An important factor in the disposition/distribution of homocysteine in physiological fluids, and indeed directly or indirectly in tissues, must be its binding to proteins through the formation of mixed disulfides with protein cysteine residues.

The distribution of the various forms of homocysteine in plasma was determined by Refsum et al. (69),

Ralph Carmel and Donald W. Jacobsen, eds. *Homocysteine in Health and Disease*. © Cambridge University Press 2001. All rights reserved. Printed in the United States of America.

who showed that about 30% was free (cysteine-homo-cysteine disulfide) and 70% was protein-bound. Only 0.1 to 0.35 μmol/L free, reduced homocysteine was reported by Araki and Sako (4), who found a mean total free homocysteine level of 1.94 μmol/L and a mean plasma total homocysteine (protein-bound plus free) level of 6.18 μmol/L in healthy subjects. Gel filtration studies suggested that albumin was the plasma protein binding homocysteine (69).

The degree of protein binding of homocysteine seems to be less in tissues. For example in the rat, liver total homocysteine was 7.6 μmol/kg, with 60% free and 40% bound, and in spleen 2.15 μmol/kg, with 75% free and 25% bound. The highest ratio of free to bound homocysteine was found in cerebellum, where total homocysteine was 5.44 μmol/kg, with 95% free and 5% bound (77).

A critical question remains whether both free and bound homocysteine are available for metabolism and able to evoke toxic effects in humans. For example, assuming that tissue levels in animals can be extrapolated to humans, there is a gradient of free homocysteine from intracellular to extracellular fluids and

export will predominate, but this gradient may not be apparent if free plus bound homocysteine are considered together. However, this consideration may be of limited importance because of rapid turnover of homocysteine bound to protein in liver cells, suggesting that the protein-bound fraction may indeed be metabolically available (77). This turnover is probably related to enzymatic reduction of disulfide bonds and may not necessarily apply to protein-bound homocysteine in plasma.

Homocysteine Concentrations in Different Tissues

An enormous body of information exists on plasma or serum levels of total homocysteine in various healthy and disease groups, but data in other tissues are more limited. Some information exists on human erythrocyte, cerebrospinal fluid, and urine levels. For other tissues, however, we must rely on data from animals or cultured cells, both of which have limitations in extrapolation to human subjects. Table 15.1 summarizes homocysteine levels in humans, both in control subjects and in some pathological states. Table 15.2

Table 15.1.   Homocysteine Levels in Humans

Tissue	Free[a]	Protein-bound[a]	Total[a]	Reference
Plasma				
Normal	1.94 ± 0.46		6.18 ± 1.19	4
Normal	(M) 2.27 ± 0.48	(M) 6.5 ± 1.35		69
Normal	(F) 1.95 ± 0.56	(F) 7.3 ± 2.26		69
Normal	2.06 ± 0.33		9.0 ± 1.1	3
Normal			11 ± 2	75
Uremic patients			39 ± 10	75
CSF				
Normal			0.46 ± 0.13	46
Normal			< 0.1	76
Normal			0.02–0.08 (n = 7)	91
CBS deficiency			1.18 (0.7–1.99)[b]	76
NKH			0.10 – 0.28 (n = 4)	91
Erythrocytes				
Normal			8.2 ± 1.2 (n = 11)	61
Normal			0.8 ± 1.05	86
Normal			3.9 ± 0.6	75
Uremic patients			32.0 ± 6	61
Uremic patients			5.6 ± 1.9	75
Urine				
Normal			3.5 – 9.5	69
Normal			7.2(1.4–24.7)	73
			(0.2–3.67)[c]	73

[a]All values are expressed in μmol/L.
[b] 95% confidence limits
[c] μmol/mmol creatinine
CSF, cerebrospinal fluid; CBS, cystathionine β-synthase; NKH, nonketotic hyperglycinemia; M, male; F, female

Table 15.2. Brain Homocysteine Levels in Various Species

Species	Area of Brain	Total Free Hcy[a]
Mouse	Cerebrum	0.34 ± 0.012
	Cerebellum	0.91 ± 0.099
Rat	Hypothalamus	1.09 ± 0.11
	Thalamus	0.67 ± 0.10
	Hippocampus	0.90 ± 0.18
	Corpus striatum	1.12 ± 0.13
	Cerebellum	6.40 ± 0.65
Guinea pig	Hypothalamus	0.48 ± 0.14
	Thalamus	0.25 ± 0.06
	Hippocampus	0.25 ± 0.10
	Corpus striatum	0.54 ± 0.17
	Cerebellum	1.07 ± 0.25
Rabbit	Hypothalamus	5.17 ± 0.56
	Hippocampus	3.83 ± 0.13
	Corpus striatum	6.61 ± 1.17

[a] Total free Hcy = total free homocysteine (reduced + oxidized; nmol/g wet weight (± SEM).
Adapted from Broch and Ueland (12).

and 15.3 show values obtained in various tissues from animals, in particular the mouse and rat. (77, 87).

The presence of low tissue levels compared with those in plasma has been suggested as evidence that homocysteine is exported from cells, but levels are higher in some tissues (e.g., liver) in the rat and mouse. The concentration of free homocysteine in samples frozen in vivo ranged from 5.1 μmol/kg in rat cerebellum to about 4 μmol/kg in liver, with lower levels in other tissues.

It is important to note that levels of homocysteine in the mouse do vary in different tissues, possibly reflecting the degree of metabolic activity. They are similar to plasma levels of 1.17 μmol/L (87) and 3 μmol/L (94) for free and total homocysteine, respectively, in the mouse. However, this variation is much

less than might be expected, considering the variability of homocysteine metabolism in specific tissues.

Little information is available on tissue levels of homocysteine in humans and, in particular, on tissue level changes as a result of pathological concentrations of plasma total homocysteine seen in the homocystinurias. Early investigations, performed soon after the discovery of CBS deficiency, used classical ion-exchange chromatography, which had low sensitivity. Homocystine and homocysteine-cysteine disulfide were undetectable in the postmortem brains of two patients (11). However, increased homocystine (7.5 μmol/L) was found in the cerebrospinal fluid of one patient with CBS deficiency (14). Homocystine levels of 13 to 61.8 μmol/100 g liver were reported (82, 83) (although the methodological details were not given), but none was detected in a later study of four liver samples (66). A comparison of erythrocyte and plasma levels in four untreated patients revealed much lower intracellular homocysteine levels than in plasma, in contrast to the comparable levels of tissue and plasma methionine that were observed (6). Taken together, these anecdotal observations in CBS deficiency reinforce rather than negate the idea that accumulating homocysteine is exported from tissues into the extracellular compartment.

Transport of Homocysteine and Homocystine

Transport of either homocysteine or its disulfide form homocystine, as well as homocysteine-cysteine mixed disulfide, may be important in tissue disposition, bearing in mind that there may be ready interconversion of these two forms. L-[35S]Homocystine uptake has been studied in isolated renal cortical tubules from the rat (30). Uptake in these cells reached a plateau after 60 minutes, and the compound was mainly converted to transsulfuration metabolites, predominantly cystathionine. Evidence was obtained for two transport systems

Table 15.3. Free and Protein-bound Homocysteine Concentrations in Mouse and Rat Tissue[a]

	Liver	Kidney	Brain	Heart	Lung
Mouse					
Free	3.63 ± 0.89	1.29 ± 0.11	0.89 ± 0.09	1.12 ± 0.1	1.02 ± 0.12
Rat					
Free	3.79 ± 0.55	1.21 ± 0.12	0.76 ± 0.07	0.97 ± 0.08	1.13 ± 0.08
Rat					
Free	4.57 (2.22–7.4)	2.10 (1.40–2.88)	0.78[b] (0.31–1.46)	1.70 (1.13–2.34)	1.87 (1.40–2.39)
Bound	3.04 (2.35–3.8)	1.73 (0.75–2.88)	0.34[b] (0.23–0.46)	1.10 (0.76–1.49)	1.40 (1.07–1.77)

[a] Results are shown in nmol/g, wet weight.
[b] Cerebrum
Data from Svardal, Refsam, and Ueland (77) and from Ueland et al. (87).

with K_m values of 0.17 and 7.65 mmol/L. The low K_m system is responsible for cystine and dibasic amino acid transport. The two systems resemble those described for cysteine. Homocysteine uptake has also been investigated in cultured human umbilical vein endothelial cells (26). Uptake at a concentration of 50 μmol/L achieved a steady state after 10 to 20 minutes. Inhibition studies suggest that homocysteine shares sodium-independent (system L) and sodium-dependent (system ASC) transport mechanisms already described for cysteine. The physiological role of these transport systems remains unclear. However, interactions between cysteine and homocysteine redox couples may be relevant in CBS deficiency where cells are dependent on uptake of extracellular cysteine (26).

The many studies investigating homocysteine damage in vitro provide indirect evidence of uptake of this amino acid. For example, Wang et al. (93) showed inhibition of DNA synthesis in vascular endothelial cells with specific alterations of the level of carboxymethylation of $p21^{ras}$. The concentration of homocysteine used was 10 to 50 μmol/L, implying an uptake into cells at levels seen in patients with vascular disease. Further evidence of active transport is afforded by the observation that added DL-homocysteine (100 μmol/L) increased intracellular levels from 0.3 to 2.4 nmol/mg protein in a human endothelial cell line (45). Finally, injection of homocysteine in rats resulted in changes in neutrophil-endothelial interactions in vivo (24).

More recently the idea of a "homocysteine receptor" has been reported (85). In studies on the effect of homocysteine on the growth of human vascular smooth muscle cells, homocystine bound to membranes and appeared in the cytosol. Binding was disrupted by N-acetylcysteine but not homocysteine, so the exact physiological transport role of this receptor remains to be established. A study on the uptake of different sulfur-containing compounds and their conversion to glutathione in astroglia-rich cultures derived from neonatal rat brain reported that homocysteine did not substitute for cysteine. This may reflect lack of cellular uptake or lack of conversion of homocysteine to cysteine in this particular tissue (48). In contrast, homocysteine was able to increase glutathione in mouse embryo fibroblasts by an unidentified, probably nonspecific mechanism (21).

Further evidence that homocysteine must be taken up into cells is provided by observations of neurological changes in response to homocysteine administration. These changes include seizures in rats (50), inhibition of taurine and γ-aminobutyrate uptake into cultured brain cells (2), inhibition of muscinol binding to calf synaptic membranes (38), and increased hippocampal electrical activity in mouse brain (20). These effects imply uptake of homocysteine, although measurements of homocysteine in the target tissue were not reported.

There is also considerable evidence that homocysteine and other related sulfur-containing amino acids, which occur naturally in the mammalian central nervous system, can interact with N-methyl-D-aspartate receptors (glutamate-gated calcium ion channel receptors), which play a crucial role in neurotransmission. Such interaction may explain neurological changes observed after homocysteine administration. Evidence supporting the role of L-homocysteine-sulfinate and L-homocysteic acid as endogenous ligands of the N-methyl-D-aspartate receptors was reported (60, 65). Subsequently it was shown that high concentrations of homocysteine, possibly after conversion to homocysteic acid, caused neuronal damage in rat cerebellar granule cells (47). Further studies showed that homocysteine shows dual action, both as an agonist at the glutamate-binding site and as a partial antagonist of the glycine coagonist site at the N-methyl-D-aspartate type glutamate receptor. It was suggested that high levels of homocysteine cause neurotoxicity by overstimulation of these receptors (51).

Recent findings confirmed the interaction of homocysteine with N-methyl-D-aspartate receptors in vascular smooth muscle cells and related this action to a signal cascade involving phospholipids and protein kinase C (19). They also found evidence that homocysteine may affect neural crest and neural tube development in chicken embryos by inhibition of such receptors (71). Whether interactions with N-methyl-D-aspartate receptors indicate that homocysteine plays a specific role in a signal transduction mechanism remains to be established.

Homocysteine Loading and Clearance

Oral administration of L-homocysteine, freshly prepared from the thiolactone, to 13 healthy subjects established that this compound is well absorbed, with an estimated bioavailability of 0.53 (39, 68). The elimination of L-homocysteine from plasma followed first-order kinetics for at least 6 hours with an average half-life of 225 minutes. Administration of 67 μmol/kg body weight (18 mg/kg) resulted in a transient hyperhomocysteinemia, with peak levels higher than those seen after oral administration of 10 times higher concentrations (on a molar basis) of methionine. Homocysteine administration resulted in clear increases of plasma methionine concentrations, implying that there was cellular uptake and remethylation of homocysteine. Less than 2% of the administered dose of homocysteine was excreted in the urine, providing further evidence for intracellular metabolism. Furthermore, in cobalamin-

or folate-deficient patients, only 6.5% of the administered homocysteine was found in the urine (40).

Urine Levels of Homocysteine

Urinary excretion of homocysteine may also help maintain plasma and tissue levels. Although marked increases of homocystine are found in patients with homocystinuria as a consequence of high plasma levels (31), the relation of urine to plasma levels in health and moderate hyperhomocysteinemia is less well known. Only low levels of homocysteine are detected in healthy subjects (Table 15.1).

The role of the kidney in disposition of homocysteine has been addressed by a few investigators (see Chapter 16). A study of free and total homocysteine in arterial versus renal venous blood in 20 fasting humans with normal renal function (mean total homocysteine, 10.8 µmol/L) allowed calculation of renal extraction (90). It was concluded that no net renal uptake of homocysteine occurs. In contrast, a study in rats revealed that in vivo, 20% of plasma homocysteine was removed by the kidney in one pass (8). A follow-up study reported the loss of about 15% of arterial plasma homocysteine at physiological concentrations, with 85% renal reabsorption but less than 2% urinary excretion (44). Infusion of homocysteine to increase plasma levels of homocysteine led to renal extraction of about 50% of the infused dose, with essentially no urinary excretion. Therefore, the rat kidney appears to play a major role in removing homocysteine from plasma by a metabolic mechanism rather than by loss to the urine.

Whether differences in enzyme activities are responsible for differences between the rat and humans is not clear. As one example, human but not rat kidney, contains betaine methyltransferase activity (29).

Tissue Disposition and Export of Homocysteine

The concept of cellular export or egress of homocysteine from cells has been established by Ueland and colleagues (87), although the molecular mechanism of the process in not fully known. They first observed that homocysteine is present at relatively low levels in the tissues of mice and rats. The free but not protein-bound form was measured. Some release of bound homocysteine could have occurred during processing, with values ranging from 0.5 to 6 nmol/g compared with 1.17 µmol/L in mouse plasma. Subsequently, it was shown that the bound homocysteine fraction is lower than free homocysteine in rat tissues (77) (see previous discussion). Rat hepatocytes in culture revealed an intracellular ratio of free to bound homocysteine of

0.6, similar to that in liver, and much higher levels were found in medium than intracellularly, indicating export (77).

These studies established that the protein-bound homocysteine fraction in tissues is lower than the approximately 80% fraction found in plasma. The observations corrected the previously held view that nearly all intracellular homocysteine is protein-bound. The free fraction of homocysteine was located in the cytosol, whereas the bound fraction was microsomal and cytosolic (77). It was concluded that, although a substantial fraction of intracellular homocysteine is associated with proteins in various rat tissues, at least in liver cells there is a rapid turnover rate of homocysteine in the bound form, in equilibrium with free homocysteine, so that it is metabolically available. In cultured human lymphoid cells, homocysteine accumulated in the growth medium, reaching a level of 12.4 µmol/L at maximum cell density, with a concomitant decline in methionine, indicating export in this cell type (32).

Further studies have helped to characterize the nature of the export process. In particular, factors that increased homocysteine production or inhibited its metabolism (16, 67, 70, 78, 81, 88) led to marked increases of homocysteine export. Furthermore, a lower degree of export was observed during pharmacological inhibition of homocysteine production (22, 79), suggesting that homocysteine export reflects the balance between its production and catabolism. A study of various cell types indicated that homocysteine export was dependent on cell density in proliferating cells or on time in quiescent cells (16). Different response patterns of homocysteine export to methionine loading (15 to 1,000 µmol/L) were observed: 1) Little or no increase was seen in quiescent fibroblasts, growing murine lymphoma cells and human lymphocytes; 2) a threefold to eightfold increase occurred in proliferating hepatoma cells and benign and transformed fibroblasts; and 3) a 15-fold increase was found in nontransformed primary hepatocytes in stationary culture. Furthermore, the kinetic properties of the rate of export and its method of calculation were defined (16). This study concluded that the export of homocysteine is likely to be a function of intracellular homocysteine concentration, although a direct enhancement of export by methionine could not be ruled out.

Increased endogenous formation of homocysteine by methotrexate treatment led to a marked export of homocysteine to the medium, but only small amounts were found intracellularly in both nonmalignant and transformed mouse fibroblasts. Export from malignant cells was not associated with increases of intracellular AdoHcy, suggesting that homocysteine concentrations were kept below the level needed for inhibition of AdoHcy hydrolase (88).

In addition, in cultured human fibroblasts with specific enzyme deficiencies (CBS, methionine synthase) (17) or in normal cells exposed to nitrous oxide to inactivate methionine synthase (17, 18), homocysteine increases in the medium were linked to loss of function of these enzymes. The level of export of homocysteine was lowered when its production was reduced by inhibition of AdoHcy hydrolase in rat hepatocytes and transformed and nontransformed mouse embryo fibroblasts (78). The egress of homocysteine was reduced in a manner that mirrored the inhibition of AdoHcy hydrolysis, which led to an increase of both free and protein-bound homocysteine in liver cells but reduced levels of homocysteine in fibroblasts. The differences between liver cells and mouse fibroblasts were explained by the existence of a different pool of homocysteine for export and a greater nonexportable pool in liver cells (78). An additional finding in this study was that inhibition of AdoHcy hydrolase by 3-deazaaristeromycin greatly reduced intracellular and extracellular homocysteine and increased both intracellular and extracellular levels of AdoHcy, indicating export of the latter also, which reached levels of 15 nmol/10^6 cells after 96 hours. This work suggests a close link between homocysteine egress and AdoHcy accumulation. The appearance of AdoHcy in the medium is also an important finding.

Ueland and co-workers postulated that an export mechanism for L-homocysteine exists that ensures low intracellular homocysteine levels, and this may be critical for maintaining vital cellular functions (16–18, 67, 78, 79, 88). Extracellular homocysteine is thus likely to be a measure of the balance between homocysteine formation and utilization (89) (Figure 15.1).

The mechanism of homocysteine export has also been investigated in endothelial, HeLa and hepatoma cells (45). An increase of export was demonstrated in the presence of copper ions, but intracellular levels were unaffected by copper. A correlation was also shown between the concentration of fetal calf serum and total homocysteine in the medium.

In summary, there is convincing evidence that cells in culture export homocysteine against a concentration gradient of high extracellular homocysteine in the medium. Extrapolation of this in vitro process to the in vivo situation in humans should be made with caution because the intracellular levels of homocysteine in relation to plasma levels in healthy subjects and in patients with disturbances of homocysteine metabolism are not known. Moreover, the driving force for this process needs to be established. Possibilities include the binding of homocysteine with plasma protein cysteine residues, binding with free cysteine (or homocys-

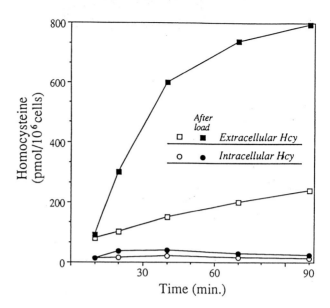

Fig. 15.1. Homocysteine (Hcy) export showing much larger increases of extracellular than intracellular homocysteine concentrations in isolated rat hepatocytes. Methionine concentrations in the medium are 1 µmol/L and, after loading, 200 µmol/L. (Reproduced from Ueland and Refsum [89], with permission.)

teine itself), and some exchange mechanism in the transport of glutathione (23).

Homocysteine Levels in Erythrocytes and Cerebrospinal Fluid

Erythrocyte total homocysteine levels have been reported in healthy subjects and in uremic patients (61, 75, 86, see Table 15.1). Although reported levels vary considerably in healthy subjects, the values are consistently lower in erythrocytes than in plasma in each study. Suliman et al. (75) reported much higher plasma (mean, 39 µmol/L) than erythrocyte values (mean, 5.6 µmol/L) in uremic patients; this difference was much less marked in the report by Perna et al. (61) (plasma mean level, 40.6 µmol/L; erythrocyte mean level, 32 µmol/L). Thus, there is general support for the idea of lower erythrocyte than plasma levels, but there is no obvious explanation for the apparent discrepancy in reported concentrations.

The limited information available on cerebrospinal fluid levels of homocysteine shows much lower levels than in plasma, possibly reflecting both the much lower protein content of cerebrospinal fluid and relatively low brain levels of homocysteine. Increased cerebrospinal fluid levels of total homocysteine have been reported in the homocystinurias (76), as well as slight increases in nonketotic hyperglycinemia in which folate metabolism is disturbed (91).

Table 15.4. *S*-Adenosylmethionine and *S*-Adenosylhomocysteine in Different Tissues

	AdoMet		AdoHcy		Reference
Human CSF control	0.214 μmol/L[a] (n=27)				76
	0.161 ± 0.03[b] μmol/L				9
Human plasma	60 ± 3 nmol/L		24.4 ± 1.1 nmol/L		52
	103 ± 9.9 nmol/L		22.7 ± 3.1 nmol/L		13
Human RBC[c]	3.5 ± 0.5		1.3 ± 0.5		59
Human whole blood	0.68 ± 0.03 μmol/L		0.48 μmol/L		15
	1.8 ± 0.3 μmol/L				54
Cultured lymphoblast	98 nmol/10⁹ cells		—		32
Rat cult. hepatocytes					27
Nucleus (mean)	3.2 nmol/2×10⁸ cells		—		
Mitochondrion (mean)	2.44 nmol/2×10⁸ cells		—		
Human Brain	Control	AD[d]	Control	AD[d]	58
Frontal cortex[e]	0.95	0.25	0.45	0.2	
Occipital cortex[e]	1.15	0.3	0.65	0.3	
Temporal cortex[e]	1.2	0.25	0.7	0.15	
Putamen[e]	0.75	0.15	0.6	0.25	
Hyppocampus[e]	1.5	0.6	0.65	0.2	
Rat brain (19–22 months)	nmol/g wet wt		nmol/g wet wt		36
Cortex	23.0 ± 1.9		2.67 ± 0.11		
Striatum	18.9 ± 1.2		4.10 ± 0.23		
Midbrain	26.5 ± 2.2		2.53 ± 0.2		
Hypothalamus	21.6 ± 0.9		2.58 ± 0.28		
Brainstem	20.5 ± 1.6		2.10 ± 0.02		
Cerebellum	21.6 ± 1.0		2.28 ± 0.17		
Rat perfused liver	45 ± 13 nmol/g		8 ± 6 nmol/g		42
Rat tissues					
Liver					
(standard diet)[f]	141		20		29
(excess methionine)[f]	673		427		29
Liver[f]	60–90		10–15 (adult)		41
	67.5 ± 1.1		43.8 ± 3.2		25
	83.6 ± 11.4		12.9 ± 7.0		28
	139.6 ± 16.3		17.5 ± 2.9		81
	95.6 ± 11.4		46.7 ± 2.4		72
	63.4 ± 7.3		25.3 ± 2.6		10
Adrenals[f]	51.5		16.1		25
Brain[f]	25.4 ± 0.9		3.4 ± 1.2		25
	26.7 ± 3.4		3.7 ± 0.7		28
Brain cortex[f]	18.9 ± 1.74		2.4 ± 0.32		10
Heart[f]	38.5		3.9		25
Kidney[f]	47.2		22.5 ± 3.4		25
	53.5 ± 8.1		9.9 ± 1.4		28
	81.0 ± 12.0		11.3 ± 3.4		81
Pancreas[f]	39.8		11.4		25
Skeletal muscle[f]	22.7 ± 2.1		4.7 ± 0.7		25
Spleen[f]	42.2		6.4		25
	76.5 ± 14.9		1.0 ± 0.4		81

[a] 95% confidence limit; 0.19 to 0.24 μmol/L.

[b] Bottiglieri (9) summarizes CSF values in control subjects and in patients with psychiatric and neurological disorders

[c] RBC, red blood cells concentration given in μmol/L packed RBC

[d] AD, Alzheimer's disease

[e] Original values are nmol/mg protein. These have been converted to nmol/g based on reported brain protein concentrations. (From Gomes-Trolin et al., 37.)

[f] nmol/g.

Tissue Distribution of AdoMet and AdoHcy

The levels of AdoMet and AdoHcy have been determined in many tissues from various species, as summarized in Table 15.4. Rat tissues, particularly regions of the brain, have been studied extensively. In the rat AdoMet and AdoHcy occur in all tissues studied with reasonably comparable results in different studies; the highest levels are seen in the liver. Of importance, hepatic levels increased dramatically when rats were fed excessive amounts of methionine (3.0% dietary methionine vs. 0.3% as normal intake) (29).

Considerable variation exists in the AdoMet/AdoHcy ratio, ranging from 6 to 10 in the liver and brain to approximately 3 in erythrocytes. A very high ratio of 87 was reported in the spleen (81), although other workers found a value of 6.6 in this tissue (25). Similar levels were found in the various areas of adult rat brain and human brain (36), and the ratio of AdoMet/AdoHcy decreased as a function of maturation in the rat (33).

Two pools of AdoMet have been identified in rat hepatocytes using short and long labeling periods with [14C]methionine. Subcellular fractionation localized the stable metabolic pool to the mitochondria and the labile pool to the cytosol (27). Methionine adenosyltransferase is not present in mitochondria; this infers a carrier-mediated system for AdoMet, which has been characterized in isolated rat liver mitochondria (43). Uptake characteristics included incorporation of the methyl group into phospholipids and mitochondrial uptake via a specific carrier-mediated system.

Similarly, two pools of AdoHcy have been described in the rat liver and isolated rat hepatocytes whereby 30% to 50% of AdoHcy is protein-bound and is associated with the microsomal fraction, whereas the free fraction is found in the cytosol (80). Thus, tissue levels of AdoMet and AdoHcy reflect the ubiquitous presence of the methionine to AdoHcy pathway.

Erythrocyte and Plasma Levels

AdoMet and AdoHcy are both readily detectable in isolated erythrocytes or whole blood (Table 15.4). The levels probably reflect intracellular methyltransferase activity, such as in the methylation of erythrocyte membrane proteins (61).

Reduced levels of AdoMet have been reported in whole blood from patients with coronary artery disease (53). The authors speculated that low AdoMet levels may be an independent risk factor for vascular disease, but this finding needs to be examined in other patients. In a subsequent study, lower levels were found in erythrocytes of 61 patients with peripheral vascular disease than in control subjects (mean AdoMet levels, 3.35 vs. 3.73 μmol/L in the control group, $p < 0.01$) (56).

Human plasma levels of AdoMet and AdoHcy are in the nanomolar range and are much lower than those in tissues. Nevertheless, with newer methods levels of these two compounds can be clearly determined in plasma (13, 54) (see Table 15.4 for control values). Clear increases also can be demonstrated in normal subjects, both after methionine loading (54) and after administration of AdoMet (55) (Figure 15.2). The importance of such low concentrations (8 to 409 nmol/L) is not yet established, but much higher levels ranging from 531 to 1,587 nmol/L AdoHcy and 223 to 841 nmol/L AdoMet were found in patients with renal disease (52) in whom the elevated levels and disturbed ratio of AdoMet/AdoHcy are likely to be linked to intracellular changes. Furthermore, AdoHcy and AdoMet levels as high as 614 and 831 nmol/L, respectively, were found in patients with peripheral vascular disease (56). It is likely that a disturbance of intracellular levels of AdoMet and AdoHcy, whether or not directly related to homocysteine, may result in the export of these compounds into plasma, which ties in with the finding of export of AdoHcy by rat liver cells described above (79).

Transport and Uptake of AdoMet and AdoHcy

Transport of AdoMet has been well studied in various microorganisms such as trypanosomes (35), *crithidia* (1), *leishmania* (5), and *saccharomyces* (62). Indeed the ability of parasites to take up AdoMet selectively has been exploited in the design of antiparasitic drugs. In contrast, specific transport into mammalian cells is not fully established. Goldberg et al. (35), describing the AdoMet transporter in trypanosomes, stated that only small quantities of AdoMet enter mammalian cells. However, an early article on transport of AdoMet presented evidence that AdoMet crosses the cell membrane and described a biphasic uptake of AdoMet in the range of 0.5 to 90 μmol/L in isolated rat hepatocytes (63). Those authors also found that differentially labeled AdoMet, administered intravenously to rats, was metabolized efficiently to creatine, for example; and the label was distributed comparably between decarboxylation, transmethylation and catabolism to homoserine and methylthioadenosine (34, 95). It is claimed that these results indicate unambiguously that AdoMet is taken up and metabolized by the liver. In other studies, [14C]methyl AdoMet was shown to cross the placental barrier, albeit slowly, and to accumulate in various fetal tissues, including intestine, liver, lung, and kidney (64).

In contrast, no uptake of [14C]methyl AdoMet was found in perfused rat liver (42), and isolated rat hepatocytes did not take up AdoMet at concentrations of 50 μmol/L (92). In light of these conflicting results, the

a)

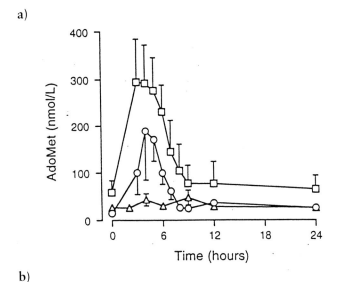

b)

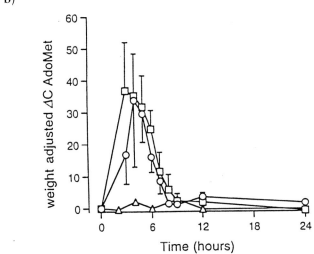

Fig. 15.2. Increase of plasma S-adenosylmethionine (AdoMet) after oral administration of 400 mg AdoMet in 14 subjects and 3 control subjects (Δ) without AdoMet intake. Values shown in panel A are mean concentrations and in panel B means of the weight-adjusted increase above baseline (ΔC) of AdoMet [(nmol/L*BW(kg)] in male (O) and female subjects (□) over a 24-hour period. (Reproduced from Loehrer et al. [55], with permission.)

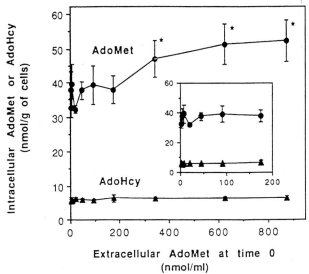

Fig. 15.3. The effect of extracellular S-adenosylmethionine (AdoMet) on the intracellular concentrations of AdoMet and S-adenosylhomocysteine (AdoHcy) in isolated hepatocytes incubated for 15 minutes with various concentrations of [methyl-^{14}C]AdoMet. Inset shows an enlargement of the lower end of the x-axis. Asterisks denote significant increases of intracellular AdoMet ($p \leq 0.05$). (Reproduced from Bontemps and Van den Berghe [7], with permission.)

mechanism of action for the favorable effects of AdoMet on liver disorders has been investigated in rat hepatocyte cultures (7) (Figure 15.3). Administration of [^{14}C]methyl AdoMet at lower concentrations (2 and 50 μmol/L) resulted in the appearance of less than 0.2% intracellularly. Only with concentrations greater than 200 μmol/L was a slight increase of intracellular AdoMet detected. These and other extensive findings led the authors to propose that, in liver cell suspensions, AdoMet provided exogenously is used mostly for the methylation of plasma membrane phospholipids. This suggests that the beneficial effects of AdoMet are modulated through a direct effect on membrane structure and function, although the link between membrane and hepatic function remains to be found. Such a link may be indicated by the finding that AdoMet induced an increased uptake of ^{45}Ca^{2+} into those liposomes containing integral membrane proteins but not into those without membrane proteins (84). Interestingly calcium uptake was inhibited by AdoHcy. Little is known about transport of AdoHcy, although the link between its intracellular levels and the transport of adenosine and homocysteine has been addressed in a novel mathematical model (49) based on findings in guinea pig heart.

A mechanism whereby the methyl group of AdoMet is used to methylate outer cell membrane phospholipids or other components and the possibility that methyl groups can be further transferred across the inner membranes need to be considered. Furthermore, possible differences between the various in vivo and in vitro systems that were investigated may be responsible for the different conclusions reached about the ability of AdoMet to cross membranes.

Summary

The tissue distribution and transport of homocysteine and its closely related S-adenosyl derivatives are important to the understanding of physiological and pathological mechanisms of homocysteine homeostasis. Current concepts point to homocysteine as a predominantly extracellular compound that is mainly protein-bound at physiological levels. Many in vitro studies show that disturbed intracellular homocysteine metabolism leads to its accumulation in the extracellular medium. Although the exact mechanism of export of homocysteine into the extracellular compartment is unclear, it may share transport systems with other sulfhydryl amino acids. In contrast, *S*-adenosyl derivatives occur mainly intracellularly. Transport mechanisms in humans are not fully understood. There is conflicting evidence that AdoMet can cross cell membranes, although pathological disturbance of membrane structure may lead to substantially increased levels in plasma.

REFERENCES

1. Allemann, MM, Mann, VH, Bacchi, CJ, Yarlett, N, Gottlieb, M, Dwyer, DM. *Crithidia luciliae:* Effect of purine starvation on *S*-adenosyl-L-methionine uptake and protein methylation. *Exp Parasitol* 1986; 81: 519–28.
2. Allen, IC, Schousboe, A, Griffiths, R. Effect of L-homocysteine and derivatives on the high-affinity uptake of taurine and gaba into synaptosomes and cultured neurons and astrocytes. *Neurochem Res* 1986; 11: 1487–96.
3. Andersson, A, Isaksson, A, Hultberg, B. Homocysteine export from erythrocytes and its implication for plasma sampling. *Clin Chem* 1992; 38: 1311–15.
4. Araki, A, Sako, Y. Determination of free and total homocysteine in human plasma by high-performance liquid chromatography with fluorescence detection. *J Chromatogr Biomed Sci App* 1987; 422: 43–52.
5. Avila, JL, Polegre, MA. Uptake and metabolism of *S*-adenosyl-L-methionine by *Leishmania mexicana* and *Leishmania braziliensis* promastigotes. *Mol Biochem Parasitol* 1993; 58: 123–34.
6. Barber, GW, Spaeth, GL. The successful treatment of homocystinuria with pyridoxine. *J Pediatr* 1969; 75: 463–78.
7. Bontemps, F, Van den Berghe, G. Metabolism of exogenous *S*-adenosylmethionine in isolated rat hepatocyte suspensions: Methylation of plasma-membrane phospholipids without intracellular uptake. *Biochem J* 1997; 327: 383–89.
8. Bostom, A, Brosnan, JT, Hall, B, Nadeau, M, Selhub, J. Net uptake of plasma homocysteine by the rat kidney in vivo. *Atherosclerosis* 1995; 116: 59–62.
9. Bottiglieri, T. Isocratic high performance liquid chromatographic analysis of *S*-adenosylmethionine and *S*-adenosylhomocysteine in animal tissues: The effect of exposure to nitrous oxide. *Biomed Chromatogr* 1990; 4: 239–41.
10. Bottiglieri, T, Hyland, K. *S*-adenosylmethionine levels in psychiatric and neurological disorders: A review. *Acta Neurol Scand Suppl* 1994; 154: 19–26.
11. Brenton, DP, Cusworth, DC, Gaull, GE. Homocystinuria. Biochemical studies of tissues including a comparison with cystathinuria. *Science* 1964; 145: 50–6.
12. Broch, OJ, Ueland, PM. Regional distribution of homocysteine in the mammalian brain *J Neurochem* 1984; 43: 1755–57.
13. Capdevila, A, Wagner, C. Measurement of plasma *S*-adenosylmethionine and *S*-adenosylhomocysteine as their fluorescent isoindoles. *Analy Biochem* 1998; 264: 180–84.
14. Carson, NAJ, Dent, CE, Field, CMB, Gaull, GE. Homocystinuria. *J Pediatr* 1965; 66: 565–83.
15. Cheng, H, Gomes-Trolin, C, Aquilonius, S-M, Steinberg, A, Löfberg, C, Ekblom, J, Oereland, L. Levels of L-methionine *S*-adenosyltransferase activity in erythrocytes and concentrations of *S*-adenosylmethionine and *S*-adenosylhomocysteine in whole blood of patients with Parkinson's disease. *Exp Neurol* 1997; 145: 580–85.
16. Christensen, B, Refsum, H, Vintermyr, O, Ueland, PM. Homocysteine export from cells cultured in the presence of physiological or superfluous levels of methionine—methionine loading of non-transformed, transformed, proliferating, and quiescent cells in culture. *J Cell Physiol* 1991; 146: 52–62.
17. Christensen, B, Rosenblatt, DS, Chu, RC, Ueland, PM. Effect of methionine and nitrous oxide on homocysteine export and remethylation in fibroblasts from cystathionine synthase-deficient, *cblG*, and *cblE* patients. *Pediatr Res* 1994; 35: 3–9.
18. Christensen, B, Ueland, PM. Methionine synthase inactivation by nitrous oxide during methionine loading of normal human fibroblasts—homocysteine remethylation as determinant of enzyme inactivation and homocysteine export. *J Pharmacol Exp Ther* 1993; 267: 1298–1303.
19. Dalton, ML, Gadson, PF Jr, Wrenn, RW, Rosenquist, TH. Homocysteine signal cascade: Production of phospholipids, activation of protein kinase C, and the induction of c-*fos* and c-*myb* in smooth muscle cells. *FASEB J* 1997; 11: 703–11.
20. Dewhurst, IC, Hagan, JJ, Morris, RGM, Griffiths, R. Hippocampal electrical activity and γ-aminobutyrate metabolism in brain tissue following administration of homocysteine. *J Neurochem* 1983; 40: 752–57.
21. Djurhuus, R, Svardal, AM, Ueland, PM. Cysteamine increases homocysteine export and glutathione content by independent mechanisms in C3H/10T1/2 cells. *Mol Pharmacol* 1990; 38: 327–32.
22. Djurhuus, R, Svardal, AM, Ueland, PM. Differential effects on growth, homocysteine, and related compounds of two inhibitors of *S*-adenosylhomocysteine catabolism, 3-deazaadenosine, and 3-deazaaristeromycin, in C3H/10T1/2 cells. *Cancer Res* 1989; 49: 324–30.
23. Djurhuus, R, Svardal, AM, Ueland, PM. Growth state dependent increase of glutathione by homocysteine and other thiols, and homocysteine formation in glutathione depleted mouse cell lines. *Biochem Pharmacol* 1990; 39: 421–29.
24. Dudman, NPB, Temple, SE, Guo, XW, Fu, W, Perry, MA. Homocysteine enhances neutrophil-endothelial interactions in both cultured human cells and rats in vivo. *Circ Res* 1999; 84: 409–16.
25. Eloranta, TO. Tissue distribution of *S*-adenosylmethionine and *S*-adenosylhomocysteine in the rat. Effect of age, sex and methionine administration on the metabolism of *S*-adenosylmethionine, *S*-adenosylhomocysteine and polyamines. *Biochem J* 1977; 166: 521–29.

26. Ewadh, MJA, Tudball, N, Rose, FA. Homocysteine uptake by human umbilical vein endothelial cells in culture. *Biochem Biophys Acta* 1990; 1054: 263–66.

27. Farooqui, JZ, Lee, HW, Kim, S, Ki Paik, W. Studies on compartmentation of S-adenosyl-L-methionine in *Saccharomyces cerevisiae* and isolated rat hepatocytes. *Biochim Biophys Acta* 1983; 757: 342–51.

28. Finkelstein, JD, Kyle, WE, Harris, BJ, Martin, JJ. Methionine metabolism in mammals: Concentration of metabolites in rat tissue. *J Nutr* 1982; 112: 1011–18.

29. Finkelstein, JD. Methionine metabolism in mammals. *J Nutr Biochem* 1990; 1: 228–37.

30. Foreman, JW, Wald, H, Blumberg, G, Pepe, LM, Segal, S. Homocystine uptake in isolated rat renal cortical tubules. *Metabolism* 1982; 31: 613–19.

31. Fowler, B, Jakobs, C. Post- and Prenatal diagnostic methods for the homocystinurias. *Eur J Pediatr* 1998; 157: S88–93.

32. German, DC, Bloch, CA, Kredich, NM. Measurements of S-adenosylmethionine and L-homocysteine metabolism in cultured human lymphoid cells. *J Biol Chem* 1983; 258: 10997–11003.

33. Gharib, A, Rey, C, Fonlupt, P, Sarda, N, Pacheco, H. Phospholipid methylase activity, 3[H]S-adenosyl-L-homocysteine binding, and S-adenosyl-L-methionine and S-adenosyl-L-homocysteine levels in rat brain during maturation. *J Neurochem* 1985; 45: 33–6.

34. Giulidori, P, Galli-Kienle, M, Catto, E, Stramentinoli, G. Transmethylation, transsulfuration and aminopropylation reactions of S-adenosyl-L-methionine in vivo. *J Biol Chem* 1984; 359: 4205–11.

35. Goldberg, B, Yarlett, N, Sufrin, J, Lloyd, D, Bacchi, CJ. A unique transporter of S-adenosylmethionine in African trypanosomes. *FASEB J* 1997; 11: 256–60.

36. Gomes Trolin, C, Löfberg, C, Trolin, G, Oreland, L. Brain ATP:L-methionine S-adenosyltransferase (MAT), S-adenosylmethionine (SAM) and S-adenosylhomocysteine (SAH): Regional distribution and age-related changes. *Eur Neuropsychopharmacol* 1994; 4: 469–77.

37. Gomes-Trolin, C, Gottfries, CG, Regland, B, Oreland, L. Influence of vitamin B_{12} on brain methionine adenosyltransferase activity in senile dementia of the Alzheimer's type. *J Neural Tansm* 1996; 103: 861–72.

38. Griffiths, R, Williams, DC, O'Neill, C, Dewhurst, IC, Ekuwem, CE, Sinclair, CD. Synergistic inhibition of [3H]muscimol binding to calf-brain synaptic membranes in the presence of L-homocysteine and pyridoxal 5′-phosphate. *Eur J Biochem* 1983; 137: 4467–78.

39. Guttormsen, A, Mansoor, AM, Fiskerstrand, T, Ueland, PM, Refsum, H. Kinetics of plasma homocysteine in healthy subjects after peroral homocysteine loading. *Clin Chem* 1993; 39: 1390–97.

40. Guttormsen, AB, Schneede, J, Ueland, PM, Refsum, H. Kinetics of total plasma homocysteine in subjects with hyperhomocysteinemia due to folate or cobalamin deficiency. *Am J Clin Nutr* 1996; 63: 194–202.

41. Hoffman, DR, Cornatzer, WE, Duerre, JA. Relationship between tissue levels of S-adenosylmethionine, S-adenosylhomocysteine, and transmethylation reactions. *Can J Biochem* 1979; 57: 56–65.

42. Hoffman, DR, Marion, DW, Cornatzer, WE, Duerre, J. S-Adenosylmethionine and S-adenosylhomocysteine metabolism in isolated rat liver. *J Biol Chem* 1980; 255: 10822–27.

43. Horne, DW, Holloway, RS, Wagner, C. Transport of S-adenosylmethionine in isolated rat liver mitochondria. *Arch Biochem Biophys* 1997; 2: 201–6.

44. House, JD, Brosnan, ME, Brosnan, JT. Renal uptake and excretion of homocysteine in rats with acute hyperhomocysteinemia. *Kidney Int* 1998; 54: 1601–7.

45. Hultberg, B, Andersson, A, Isaksson, A. Higher export rate of homocysteine in a human endothelial cell line than in other human cell lines. *Biochim Biophys Acta* 1998; 1448: 61–9.

46. Hyland, K, Bottiglieri, T. Measurement of total plasma and cerebrospinal fluid homocysteine by fluorescence following high-performance liquid chromatography and precolumn derivatization with o-phthaldialdehyde. *J Chromatogr* 1992; 579: 55–62.

47. Kim, WK, Pae, YS. Involvement of N-methyl-D-aspartate receptor and free radical in homocysteine-mediated toxicity on rat cerebellar granule cells in culture. *Neurosci Lett* 1996; 216: 117–20.

48. Kranich, O, Dringen, R, Sandberg, M, Hamprecht, B. Utilization of cysteine and cysteine precursors for the synthesis of glutathione in astroglial cultures: Preference for cystine. *Glia* 1998; 22: 11–8.

49. Kroll, K, Deussen, A, Sweet, IR. Comprehensive model of transport and metabolism of adenosine and S-adenosylhomocysteine in the Guinea pig heart. *Circ Res* 1992; 71: 590–604.

50. Kubová, H, Folbergrová, J, Mares, P. Seizures induced by homocysteine in rats during ontogenesis. *Epilepsia* 1995; 36: 750–56.

51. Lipton, SA, Kim, WK, Choi, YB, Kumar, S, D'Emilia, DM, Rayudu, PV, Arnelle, DR, Stamler, JS. Neurotoxicity associated with dual actions of homocysteine at the N-methyl-D-aspartate receptor. *Proc Natl Acad Sci* 1997; 94: 5923–28.

52. Loehrer, FMT, Angst, CP, Brunner, FP, Haefeli, WE, Fowler, B. Evidence for disturbed S-adenosylhomocysteine ratio in patients with end-stage renal failure: A cause for disturbed methylation reactions? *Nephrol Dial Transplant* 1998; 13: 656–61.

53. Loehrer, FMT, Angst, CP, Haefeli, WE, Jordan, PP, Ritz, R, Fowler, B. Low whole-blood S-adenosylmethionine and correlation between 5-methyltetrahydrofolate and homocysteine in coronary artery disease. *Arterioscler Thromb Vasc Biol* 1996; 16: 727–33.

54. Loehrer, FMT, Haefeli, WE, Angst, CP, Browne, G, Frick, G, Fowler, B. Effect of methionine loading on 5-methyltetrahydrofolate, S-adenosylmethionine and S-adenosylhomocysteine in plasma of healthy humans. *Clin Sci* 1996; 91: 79–86.

55. Loehrer, FMT, Schwab, R, Angst, CP, Haefeli, WE, Fowler, B. Influence of oral S-adenosylmethionine on plasma 5-methyltetrahydrofolate, S-adenosylhomocysteine, homocysteine and methionine in healthy humans. *J Pharmacol Exp Ther* 1997; 282: 845–50.

56. Loehrer, FMT, Tschöpl, M, Angst, CP, Litynski, P, Jäger, K, Fowler, B, Haefeli, WE. Disturbed ratio of erythrocyte and

plasma *S*-adenosylmethionine/*S*-adenosylhomocysteine in peripheral arterial occlusive disease. *Atherosclerosis,* in press.

57. Malinow, MR, Axthelm, MK, Meredith, MJ, MacDonald, NA, Upson, BM. Synthesis and transulfuration of homocysteine in blood. *J Lab Clin Med* 1994; 123: 421–29.

58. Morrison, LD, Smith, DD, Kish, SJ. Brain *S*-adenosylmethionine levels are severely decreased in Alzheimer's disease. *J Neurochem* 1996; 67: 1328–31.

59. Oden, KL, Clarke, S. *S*-adenosyl-L-methionine synthetase from human erythrocytes: Role in the regulation of cellular *S*-adenosylmethionine levels. *Biochemistry* 1983; 22: 2978–86.

60. Olney, JW, Price, MT, Salles, KS, Labruyere, J, Ryerson, R, Mahan, K, Frierdich, G, Samson, L. L-homocysteic acid: An endogenous excitotoxic ligand of the NMDA receptor. *Brain Res Bull* 1987; 19: 595–602.

61. Perna, AF, Ingrosso, D, De Sandto, NG, Galletti, P, Zappia, V. Mechanism of erythrocyte accumulation of methylation inhibitor *S*-adenosylhomocysteine in uremia. *Kidney Int* 1995; 47: 247–53.

62. Petrotta-Simpson, TF, Talmadge, JE, Spence, KD. Specificity and genetics of *S*-adenosylmethionine transport in *Saccharomyces cerevisiae. J Bacteriol* 1975; 123: 2516–22.

63. Pezzoli, C, Stramentinoli, G, Galli-Kienle, M, Pfaff, E. Uptake and metabolism of *S*-adenosyl-L-methionine by isolated rat hepatocytes. *Biochem Biophys Res Commun* 1978; 85: 1031–38.

64. Placidi, GF, Fornaro, P, Guarneri, M, Stramentinoli, G. Localization of *S*-[methyl-^{14}C]adenosyl-L-methionine in pregnant mice and fetuses as determined by autoradiography. *Eur J Drug Metab Pharmacokine* 1979; 4: 157–61.

65. Pullan, LM, Olney, JW, Price, MT, Compton, RP, Hood, WF, Michel, J, Monahan, JB. Excitatory amino acid receptor potency and subclass specificity of sulfur-containing amino acids. *J Neurochem* 1987; 49: 1301–7.

66. Rassin, DK, Longhi, RC, Gaull, GE. Free amino acids in liver of patients with homocystinuria due to cystathionine synthase deficiency: Effects of vitamin B$_6$. *J Pediatr* 1977; 91: 574–77.

67. Refsum, H, Christensen, B, Djurhuus, R, Ueland, PM. Interaction between methotrexate, rescue agents and cell proliferation as modulators of homocysteine export from cells in culture. *J Pharmacol Exp Ther* 1991; 258: 559–566.

68. Refsum, H, Guttormsen, AB, Fiskerstrand, T, Ueland, PM. Hyperhomocysteinemia in terms of steady-state kinetics. *Eur J Pediatr* 1998; 157: S45–9.

69. Refsum, H, Helland, S, Ueland, PM. Radioenzymic determination of homocysteine in plasma and urine. *Clin Chem* 1985; 31: 624–28.

70. Refsum, H, Ueland, PM, Kvinnsland, S. Acute and long-term effects of high-dose methotrexate treatment on homocysteine in plasma and urine. *Cancer Res* 1986; 46: 5385–91.

71. Rosenquist, TH, Schneider, AM, Monogham, DT. *N*-methyl-D-aspartate receptor agonists modulate homocysteine-induced developmental abnormalities. *FASEB J* 1999; 13: 1523–31.

72. She, QB, Nagao, I, Hayakawa, T, Tsuge, H. A simple HPLC method for the determination of *S*-adenosylmethionine and *S*-adenosylhomocysteine in rat tissues: The effect of vitamin B$_6$ deficiency on these concentrations in rat liver. *Biochem Biophys Res Commun* 1994; 205: 1748–54.

73. Stabler, SP, Marcell, PD, Podel, ER, Allen, RH. Quantitation of total homocysteine, total cysteine, and methionine in normal serum and urine using capillary gas chromatography—mass spectrometry. *Anal Biochem* 1987; 162: 185–96.

74. Sturman, JA, Rassin, DK, Gaull, GE. Distribution of transulphuration enzymes in various organs and species. *Int J Biochem* 1970; 1: 251–53.

75. Suliman, ME, Divino, Filho, JC, Barany, P, Anderstam, B, Lindholm, B, Bergstrom, J. Effects of high dose folic acid and pyridoxine on plasma and erythrocyte sulfur amino acids in hemodialysis patients. *J Am Soc Nephrol* 1999; 10: 1287–96.

76. Surtees, R, Bowron, A, Leonard, J. Cerebrospinal fluid and plasma total homocysteine and related metabolites in children with cystathionine β-synthase deficiency: The effect of treatment. *Pediatr Res* 1997; 5: 577–82.

77. Svardal, A, Refsum, H, Ueland, PM. Determination of in vivo protein binding of homocysteine and its relation to free homocysteine in the liver and other tissues of the rat. *J Biol Chem* 1986; 261: 3156–63.

78. Svardal, AM, Djurhuus, R, Refsum, H, Ueland, PM. Disposition of homocysteine in rat hepatocytes and in nontransformed and malignant mouse embryo fibroblasts following exposure to inhibitors of *S*-adenosylhomocysteine catabolism. *Cancer Res* 1986; 46: 5095–5100.

79. Svardal, AM, Djurhuus, R, Ueland, PM. Disposition of homocysteine and *S*-3-deazaadenosylhomocysteine in cells exposed to 3-deazaadenosine. *Mol Pharmacol* 1986; 30: 154–58.

80. Svardal, AM, Ueland, PM. Compartmentalization of *S*-adenosylhomocysteine in rat liver. Determination and characterization of the in vivo protein binding. *J Biol Chem* 1987; 262: 15413–17.

81. Svardal, AM, Ueland, PM, Berge, RK, Aarsland, A, Aarsaether, N, Lonning, PE, Refsum, H. Effect of methotrexate on homocysteine and other sulfur compounds in tissues of rats fed a normal or a defined, choline-deficient diet. *Cancer Chemother Pharmacol* 1988; 21: 313–18.

82. Tada, K, Yoshida, T, Arakawa, T. Free amino acid pattern in the liver from the patients with amino acid disorders: Post-mortem diagnosis of inborn errors of amino acid metabolism. *Tohoku J Exp Med* 1970; 101: 223–26.

83. Tada, K, Yoshida, T, Hirono, H, Arakawa, T. Homocystinuria: Amino acid pattern of the liver. *Tohoku J Exp Med* 1967; 92: 325–32.

84. Toyoshima, S, Saido, T, Makishima, F, Osawa, T. Induction of increased calcium uptake in liposomes having membrane proteins of chicken erythrocytes by *S*-adenosylmethionine. *Biochem Biophys Res Commun* 1983; 114: 1126–31.

85. Tyagi, SC. Homocysteine redox receptor and regulation of extracellular matrix components in vascular cells. *Am J Physiol Cell Physiol* 1998; 43: C396–C405.

86. Ubbink, JB, Hayward Vermaak, WJ, van der Merwe, A, Becker, PJ. The effect of blood sample aging and food consumption on plasma total homocysteine levels. *Clin Chim Acta* 1992; 207: 119–28.

87. Ueland, PM, Helland, S, Broch, O-J, Schanche, J-S. Homocysteine in tissues of the mouse and rat. *J Biol Chem* 1984; 259: 2360–64.

88. Ueland, PM, Refsum, H, Male, R, Lillehaug, JR. Disposition of endogenous homocysteine by mouse fibroblast C3H/10T1/2 CL8 and the chemically transformed C3H/10T1/2 MCA CL 16 cells following methotrexate exposure. *J Natl Cancer Inst* 1986; 77: 283–89.

89. Ueland, PM, Refsum, H. Plasma homocysteine, a risk factor for vascular disease: Plasma levels in health, disease, and drug therapy. *J Lab Clin Med* 1989; 114: 473–501.

90. Van Guldener, C, Donker, AJM, Jakobs, C, Teerlink, T, De Meer, K, Stehouwer, CDA. No net renal extraction of homocysteine in fasting humans. *Kindney Int* 1998; 54: 166–69.

91. Van Hove, JLK, Lazeyras, F, Zeisel, SH, Bottiglieri, T, Hyland, K, Charles, HC, Gray, L, Jaeken, J, Kahler, SG. One-methyl group metabolism in non-ketotic hyperglycinaemia: Mildly elevated cerebrospinal fluid homocysteine levels. *J Inherit Metab Dis* 1998; 21: 799–811.

92. Van Phi, L, Soling, HD. Methyl group transfer from exogenous *S*-adenosylmethionine on to plasma-membrane phospholipids without cellular uptake in isolated hepatocytes. *Biochem J* 1982; 206: 481–87.

93. Wang, H, Yoshizumi, M, Lai, K, Tsai, JC, Perrella, MA, Haber, E, Lee, ME. Inhibition of growth and p21ras methylation in vascular endothelial cells by homocysteine but not cysteine. *J Biol Chem* 1997; 272: 25380–85.

94. Watanabe, M, Osada, J, Aratani, Y, Kluckman, K, Reddick, R, Malinow, MR, Maeda, N. Mice deficient in cystathionine β-synthase: Animal models for mild and severe homocyst(e)inemia. *Proc Natl Acad Sci USA* 1995; 92: 1585–89.

95. Zappia, V, Galletti, P, Porcelli, M, Ruggiero, G, Andrena, A. Uptake of adenosylmethionine and related sulfur compounds by isolated rat liver. *FEBS Lett* 1978; 90: 331–35.

16

Homocysteine and the Kidney

JOHN T. BROSNAN

The major interest in homocysteine and the kidney arises from the well-established increase in plasma total homocysteine that occurs in end-stage renal disease (see Chapter 26). Of direct relevance to this phenomenon is the renal handling of homocysteine, including the possibility that homocysteine metabolism by renal tissue may play a role in the hyperhomocysteinemia of renal disease.

Plasma Total Homocysteine and Renal Function

Plasma total homocysteine is elevated in renal disease (5, 22, 42). Typical increases in patients with advanced renal failure are more than 100%, from about 10 μmol/L to above 20 μmol/L. In such patients, the increase in plasma total homocysteine is inversely correlated with the glomerular filtration rate and is already appreciably increased in patients with moderate renal failure (1). There are also some differences in the relative amounts of the different components of plasma total homocysteine in renal disease; a decrease in reduced homocysteine has been reported (23). Increased plasma total homocysteine concentrations that occur with increasing age also correlate with decreased glomerular filtration rate (23). Of course, a decreased glomerular filtration rate is not the only

determinant of elevated plasma total homocysteine in these situations. As in other populations, decreased folate and vitamin B_6 status can contribute to the phenomenon (6, 35). However, aggressive B-vitamin therapy, in particular with folic acid, only partly corrects the elevated plasma total homocysteine of renal failure (2, 7). Bostom et al. (5) have shown elevated plasma total homocysteine in renal patients, despite normal to supernormal B-vitamin status. Elevated plasma total homocysteine levels (both fasting and postmethionine load) are also found in renal transplant recipients (2, 7), and it is clear that treatment with the immunosuppressive drug, cyclosporine, contributes significantly to these elevations (2).

In summary, an impressive body of evidence links elevated plasma total homocysteine to the loss of renal function, in particular to the decrease in glomerular filtration rate. A key question, therefore, concerns the basis for this. In theory, an increase in the plasma level of any metabolite can be brought about by an increased rate of its production, a decreased rate of its removal, or both.

In the case of patients with chronic renal failure, it is clear that a decreased rate of removal is a key event. An elegant study by Guttormsen et al. (19) showed that high-dose folic acid therapy in such patients can reduce the fasting plasma total homocysteine by about 25%. However, folate therapy did not affect the elimination of homocysteine from plasma after oral homocysteine loading. Patients' ability remained highly impaired (only about 30% that of control subjects). These results point to two defects in homocysteine metabolism in patients with renal disease: a defect in homocysteine remethylation, which contributes to the fasting hyperhomocysteinemia and which can be corrected by folate, and a massive decrease in total homocysteine clearance from plasma which is not corrected by folate (19).

A recent study by van Guldener et al. (44) applied stable isotope methodology to methionine and homocysteine metabolism in fasting patients with end-stage renal disease. They were also able to show a decrease in whole body remethylation reactions in these patients with renal failure. A key, unresolved question concerns the basis for these decreases in homocysteine metabolism and how they relate to renal function.

Renal Amino Acid Metabolism

The kidney plays a major role in amino acid metabolism. Amino acid reabsorption by renal tubules recovers about 70 g of filtered amino acids per day in a 70 kg man. The principal site of amino acid reabsorption is the proximal tubule. The kidney is rich in peptidases and is a major site for the catabolism of circulating peptides. Even in healthy individuals there is some loss of plasma proteins through the glomerulus; these proteins are taken into the proximal cells where they undergo proteolysis, with the component amino acids released into the venous outflow (8).

The kidney also plays a specific role in the removal of certain amino acids from the circulation and the addition of others (8). In particular, the kidney plays major roles in the metabolism of glycine, serine, citrulline, arginine, and glutamine. The kidney removes glycine from the circulation and converts it to serine, which is released into the renal vein. This occurs in the cells of the proximal tubule, which are well endowed with both the glycine cleavage enzyme and serine hydroxymethyltransferase. Thus, the cells of the proximal tubule have an abundant supply of one-carbon units from the glycine cleavage enzyme. In fact, the kidney produces more serine than can be accounted for by the uptake of glycine, and it is apparent that serine is also produced from glycolytic intermediates. The kidney of a 70-kg man produces about 4 g of serine per day, which is approximately equivalent to the daily dietary intake of serine from a typical Western diet (8). Renal serine output decreases in patients with chronic renal insufficiency and is accompanied by a decreased plasma serine concentration (41). This could, conceivably, have implications for the decreased rate of disposal of homocysteine in such patients because serine depletion could limit the transsulfuration pathway. In addition, because serine is the ultimate supplier of the one-carbon groups that produce 5-methyltetrahydrofolate, it is possible that serine depletion could also limit remethylation. However, Bostom et al. (5) showed that oral serine supplementation in patients with renal disease did not affect their hyperhomocysteinemia.

Kidneys of various species, including rat and human, remove citrulline from the circulation, convert it to arginine and release this arginine into the renal vein (8, 41). This is part of a metabolic pathway that is shared between the intestine (which produces the citrulline), and the kidney and is responsible for the endogenous synthesis of arginine (8). Again, the proximal tubules are the cellular sites of this renal amino

Table 16.1. Arterial Plasma Levels and Renal Arteriovenous Differences for Plasma Total Homocysteine and Other Amino Acids in Humans and Rats

	Rat			Human		
	Artery	A-V	Reference	Artery	A-V	Reference
Plasma total homocysteine	7.9	+ 1.1[a]	4	10.8	+ 0.1	43
Glycine	231	+ 12[a]	9	274	+ 3	41
Serine	208	− 31[a]	9	127	− 20[a]	41
Citrulline	50	+ 7[a]	9	29	+ 7[a]	41
Arginine	260	− 9[a]	9	69	− 6[a]	41
Glutamine	547	+10	9	530	+ 32[a]	41

All units are μmol/L.
A-V = arteriovenous difference.
[a] Significant A-V difference. A positive sign indicates an uptake and a negative sign indicates an output.

acid metabolism (12). Citrulline does provide us with an example of an amino acid that is normally removed by the kidney and whose plasma level increases markedly in renal insufficiency. This occurs both in the rat and in humans (25, 41). Table 16.1 shows arteriovenous differences across kidneys of human and rat for homocysteine and a number of other amino acids. It should be emphasized that, in general, except for homocysteine, both human and rat kidneys display the same pattern of renal amino acid metabolism.

Finally, mention should be made of the role of the kidney in creatine synthesis. This is particularly relevant because creatine synthesis, which must proceed at the same rate as creatinine excretion to maintain creatine status, is by far the major sink for labile methyl groups. Indeed, Mudd and Poole (30) have estimated that as much as 80% of labile methyl groups are required for creatine synthesis in humans. Creatine synthesis involves two enzyme-catalyzed steps:

Glycine + Arginine → Guanidinoacetate + Ornithine (1)

Guanidinoacetate + S-adenosylmethionine → Creatine + S-adenosylhomocysteine   (2)

Reaction 1 is catalyzed by L-arginine:glycine amidinotransferase and Reaction 2 by guanidinoacetate methyltransferase. These enzymes have a limited tissue distribution: The guanidinoacetate methyltransferase is restricted to the liver (32), thus implying that the dominant endogenous origin of homocysteine is hepatic. Glycine transamidinase is essentially restricted to the kidney and the pancreas (26), and the kidney is considered to be the source of guanidinoacetate for creatine synthesis, which occurs as an interorgan metabolic pathway — renal synthesis of guanidinoac-etate and the hepatic methylation of this compound. Thus the kidney, by producing guanidinoacetate, plays an essential role in the pathway that produces the greater part of S-adenosylhomocysteine and hence of homocysteine in the body.

Renal Homocysteine Metabolism

Reabsorption of Total Homocysteine

Plasma total homocysteine is not a homogenous chemical species. In normal humans, protein-S-S-homocysteine accounts for about 80% of total homocysteine, with homocystine, the homocysteine-cysteine mixed disulfide, and free reduced homocysteine accounting for the remainder (17). In the rat, however, only about 30% of plasma total homocysteine is protein-bound (21, 38). The important point is that protein-bound homocysteine will not be filtered by the glomerulus; but homocysteine, homocystine, and the homocysteine-cysteine mixed disulfide will. A comparison of the filtered load of these species with their urinary excretion reveals substantial renal reabsorption (Table 16.2). In both rats and humans, urinary excretion is only about 1% of the filtered load. Renal homocysteine excretion in humans is so small, approximately 6 μmol per day (25) compared with the approximately 24 mmol of methionine ingested per day on a normal Western diet (24), that loss of this homocysteine excretion can, in no way, account for the hyperhomocysteinemia of renal disease.

The renal handling of total homocysteine in the rat has been examined in detail (24). These kidneys have a substantial reserve capacity for reabsorption of filtered total homocysteine. After increasing the plasma concentration and the filtered load of total homocysteine by up to sixfold (either by homocysteine infusion or by exposure to nitrous oxide) the percentage of total homocysteine lost to the urine (about 1%) remained unchanged. However, the kidney's ability to reabsorb homocysteine/homocystine is clearly limited and when excessive amounts are presented to the renal tubules, a pronounced homocystinuria is evident as, for example, the 300 μmol per day of homocystine and of the homocysteine-cysteine mixed disulfide found in the urine of patients with cystathionine β-synthase deficiency (10). Homocystinuria of a similar magnitude is also found in patients with 5,10-methylenetetrahydrofolate reductase deficiency (36).

Renal reabsorption is a transepithelial process. This involves transport of a substance from the renal tubular fluid via a transporter on the luminal membrane of the epithelial cell as well as its transport out of the cell via a transporter on the basolateral membrane. Generally, these two transporters are different. It is very likely that separate mechanisms may apply to reduced homocysteine compared with either of the oxidized forms, homocystine or the homocysteine-cysteine mixed disulfide. There is some information about the renal transport of the oxidized forms. Cusworth and Gattereau (11) speculated that homocystine reabsorption may occur via the transporter responsible for cystine reabsorption. This transporter is also involved in the reabsorption of arginine, ornithine, and lysine; and those investigators showed that injection of either lysine or arginine into rats led to a substantial increase in homocystine excretion. Infusion of arginine into a homocystinuric patient also markedly increased (20-fold) urinary homocystine excretion in the absence of any change in its plasma concentration (11).

Foreman et al. (14) examined ^{35}S-labeled homocystine uptake and metabolism in isolated rat renal tubules. Their results provided evidence for two saturable transport systems. A high affinity system ($K_m = 0.17$ mmol/L) was inhibited by cystine and the dibasic amino acids, whereas a low affinity system ($K_m = 7.7$ mmol/L) was not affected by the dibasic amino acids but also appeared to transport cystine. These transporters appear to correspond to two systems previously described for cystine uptake. If homocystine (or the homocysteine-cysteine mixed disulfide) is taken up from the glomerular filtrate by a transporter that also transports cystine, then one would expect increased urinary excretion of these compounds if this transporter is defective. This prediction is borne out in cystinuria, an autosomal recessive disorder with impaired renal transport of cystine and the dibasic amino acids. In

---

Table 16.2. Renal Reabsorption of Homocysteine/Homocystine in Rats and Humans

	Rat[a]	Human[b]
Arterial plasma total homocysteine	7.9 μmol/L	10.8 μmol/L
Filterable total homocysteine	5.85 μmol/L	3.2 μmol/L
Glomerular filtration rate	0.85 ml/min/100g	125 ml/min
Filtered total homocysteine load	5.4 nmol/min/100g	400 nmol/min
Urinary total homocysteine excretion	0.07 nmol/min/100g	3.5 nmol/min

[a] Rat data from Bostom et al. (4).
[b] Human data from van Guldener (43) (plasma total homocysteine and filterable total homocysteine) and Refsum et al. (34) (urinary total homocysteine excretion). 125 ml/min is a standard value for the glomerular filtration rate in healthy adult humans.

such patients, there is a substantial excretion of the homocysteine-cysteine mixed disulfide in amounts up to about 900 μmol/day (37).

It is clear, therefore, that reabsorption of the oxidized forms (homocystine and the homocysteine-cysteine mixed disulfide) from the filtrate occurs via the cystine/dibasic amino acid transporter located on the luminal, brush-border membrane. In view of the multiplicity of amino acid transporters and their overlapping specificity, it is probably not safe to assume that all of the transport of these species occurs via this single transporter. The role of the low affinity system is not clear, nor is it evident which transporter(s) on the basolateral membrane may complete the reabsorptive process. In some cystinuric patients, there is good evidence that urinary cystine excretion is greater than the filtered load, indicating cystine secretion (37). However, there are no data on this point for homocystine.

Homocysteine Metabolism

Homocysteine arises in the kidney endogenously, from the multiplicity of methyltransferase reactions that occur within the organ, and exogenously, from the plasma. Although the focus of this chapter is on exogenous homocysteine, one particular renal methylation reaction should be noted. It is now clear that a critical protein methylation is crucial for the regulation of aldosterone-induced Na^+ transport, a key renal function (39).

With regard to exogenous total homocysteine, the crucial issue is whether renal metabolism provides an important route for the removal of plasma total homocysteine. If such is the case, then we have a satisfactory explanation for the hyperhomocysteinemia of renal disease, as the loss of a major route of homocysteine disposal would lead to an elevation in its plasma concentration. A consideration of this question will focus on the rat and humans, the two species for which direct evidence (in terms of measurements of arteriovenous differences across the kidney) is available (Table 16.1). The evidence is contradictory; there is a clear renal uptake in rats (4) but not in humans (43). We have been able to reproduce our original observation of uptake by the rat kidney (21), but we have also measured arteriovenous differences across nine human kidneys (unpublished data) and have been able to confirm van Guldener's finding (43) of no net renal extraction in humans. In attempting to understand these quite different results, there are two possibilities: Either there is a fundamental difference between rat and human kidneys, in that the human kidney really does not significantly remove plasma homocysteine, or there is some experimental or methodological difference between the two situations. Two such differences

are evident. One difference is that the human studies, both published (43) and unpublished, were carried out on fasting humans and, conceivably, an uptake might be evident in the fed state when methionine (and, therefore, homocysteine) catabolism is more pronounced. It would be interesting to know whether there is a renal uptake of total homocysteine in the fed human.

Perhaps a more important difference relates to the relative amounts of the different forms of plasma total homocysteine in these two species — about 80% protein-bound (protein-S-S-homocysteine) in humans but only about 30% in rats. Because protein-bound homocysteine is not filterable, only 20% of plasma total homocysteine in humans, but 70% in rats is available for glomerular filtration. When one considers that the filtration fraction (percentage of plasma filtered by the glomeruli) is about 20% in humans and 35% in rats, one can calculate that only about 6% of plasma total homocysteine would be filtered in humans but about 24% in rats. Thus, if filtration is the exclusive means of delivering homocysteine to the kidney, then the maximum arteriovenous difference that could be expected in humans would be about 6%; differences of this magnitude should be detectable. The maximum arteriovenous difference for the rat would be about 24%, which is about 50% more than that observed in vivo (4, 21). It is conceivable that the human kidney removes plasma homocysteine, but to a much lesser degree than does the rat kidney. For example, if the human kidney removed about two thirds of the filtered total homocysteine (as does the rat), the arteriovenous difference would be 4% and might be difficult to detect.

It is possible to calculate what the renal arteriovenous difference should be if the kidneys were the principal sites of disposal of plasma total homocysteine. On the basis of clearance studies in healthy humans, Guttormsen et al. (18) have calculated that about 1.2 mmol of total homocysteine are added by cells to the plasma in 24 hours. Given that renal plasma flow to the kidneys is about 600 ml/min, one can calculate that a renal arteriovenous difference of 1.4 nmol/ml would be required if the kidneys disposed of all of this plasma flux. Such an arteriovenous difference would be about 13%, given an arterial concentration of 10.8 nmol/ml, and would be readily detected. Even if the kidneys removed only half the plasma flux, we would have an arteriovenous difference of 6.5%, which would be detected. Smaller arteriovenous differences, however, would be difficult to detect.

Strong evidence, however, against a role for the human kidney in homocysteine metabolism comes from studies of its enzyme complement, compared with that of the rat (Table 16.3). Rat renal homocysteine metabolism has been studied extensively.

Homocysteine is metabolized almost exclusively via the transsulfuration pathway (20). Foreman et al. (14) came to a similar conclusion. The rat kidney does have methionine synthase activity (13), but it does not seem to play a role in the removal of exogenous homocysteine. The transsulfuration enzymes are primarily found in the cells of the proximal tubule (20), which is consistent with a role in metabolizing filtered homocysteine, as the proximal tubule is the primary site of amino acid reabsorption. Curiously, the two transsulfuration enzymes do not exactly colocalize. Both cystathionine β-synthase and cystathionine γ-lyase occur in the cells of the proximal convoluted tubule, but there is also a substantial enrichment of the lyase in cells of the proximal straight tubule (20). This points to a possible independent function for this enzyme. Rat kidney contains no detectable betaine:homocysteine methyltransferase (27).

The complement of enzymes that can remove homocysteine in human kidney shows two striking differences from that in the rat. First, human kidney contains the betaine:homocysteine methyltransferase (27). However, more important for the present discussion, human kidney has been reported to contain only very low activities of cystathionine β-synthase (40). It does, however, express mRNA for this gene (3, 33). Because flux through the transsulfuration pathway is the metabolic fate of exogenous homocysteine in the rat, it is clear that a very low activity of the cystathionine β-synthase could account for the fact that human kidneys do not appear to metabolize plasma total homocysteine.

Sturman's assays of transsulfuration enzymes in human tissues did find appreciable renal activities of cystathionine γ-lyase (40). Such activities of the lyase in the virtual absence of the synthase recalls rat kidney

data where the synthase occurred primarily in cells of the proximal convoluted tubule and the lyase occurred primarily in cells of the proximal straight tubule (20). Such enzyme distributions argue for a separate function for the cystathionase, independent of the synthase. House et al. (20) argued that this may lie in catabolism of cysteine because the lyase can also catabolize this amino acid. There is also the possibility that it may play a role in the catabolism of circulating cystathionine. Filtered cystathionine is partly reabsorbed (15), and it is possible that it may be catabolized by the lyase after it enters the renal cells.

Further Outlook

Filtered homocystine and the homocysteine–cysteine mixed disulfide are reabsorbed by the kidney via the lumenal cystine/basic amino acid transporter. Increased urinary homocysteine and mixed disulfide excretion occur when the capacity of this transporter is exceeded owing to a massively increased filtered load of homocysteine (as in cystathionine β-synthase or methylenetetrahydrofolate reductase deficiency) or when the transporter is defective (as in cystinuria). The pattern of amino acid metabolism across the kidney is generally similar among different species. Total plasma homocysteine presents an important exception, however, in that there is a substantial uptake and metabolism by the rat kidney, but no such renal uptake and metabolism can be found in the human. This may be due to the fact that human kidneys filter much less plasma total homocysteine than do rat kidneys. Alternatively, it may be due to a very low activity of cystathionine β-synthase in the human kidney. There seems to be only one report on the activity of this

Table 16.3. Enzymes of Homocysteine Metabolism in Kidneys and Livers from Rats and Humans

	Rat			Human		
	Liver	Kidney	Reference	Liver	Kidney	Reference
Methionine synthase	—	7	21	1.3	0.8	16
	4	16	13	1.1	2.3	29
Betaine:homocysteine	81	ND	27	32	14	27
methyltransferase	69	ND	13	8	23	16
				8	14	29
Cystathionine β-synthase	184	83	28	98	1	40
	—	52	21	120	—	28
Cystathionine γ-lyase	108	40	28	126	45	40
				—	32	16
				32	—	28

All activities are given as nmol/mg protein/hour.
ND = not detected.

enzyme in human kidney, and it will be important to see whether this result can be replicated. It will also be of importance to measure arteriovenous differences for plasma total homocysteine across the kidneys of fed humans so as to determine whether an uptake can be found in this state. The balance of evidence currently available, however, is that the human kidney, unlike the rat, does not appreciably remove plasma total homocysteine from the circulation.

REFERENCES

1. Arnadottir, M, Hultberg, B, Nilsson-Ehle, P, Thysell, H. The effect of reduced glomerular filtration rate on plasma total homocysteine concentration. *Scand J Clin Lab Invest* 1996; 56: 41–46.

2. Arnadottir, M, Hultberg, B, Wahlberg, J, Fellstrom, B, Dimeny, E. Serum total homocysteine concentration before and after renal transplantation. *Kidney Int* 1998; 54: 1380–84.

3. Bao, L, Vlcek, C, Paces, V, Kraus, JP. Identification and tissue distribution of human cystathionine β-synthase mRNA isoforms. *Arch Biochem Biophys* 1998; 350: 95–103.

4. Bostom, AG, Brosnan, JT, Hall, B, Nadeau, MR, Selhub, J. Net uptake of plasma homocysteine by the rat kidney in vivo. *Atherosclerosis* 1995; 116: 59–62.

5. Bostom, AG, Shemin, D, Lapane, KL, Miller, JW, Sutherland, P, Nadeau, M, Seyoum, E, Hartman, W, Prior, R, Wilson, PWF, Selhub, J. Hyperhomocysteinemia and traditional cardiovascular risk factors in end-stage renal disease patients on dialysis: A case control study. *Atherosclerosis* 1995; 114: 93–103.

6. Bostom, AG, Shemin, D, Lapane, KL, Nadeau, MR, Sutherland, P, Chan, J, Rozen, R, Yobum, D, Jacques, PF, Selhub, J, Rosenberg, IH. Folate status is the major determinant of fasting total plasma homocysteine levels in maintenance dialysis patients. *Atherosclerosis* 1996; 123: 193–202.

7. Bostom, AG, Gohh, RY, Tsai, MY, Hopkins-Garcia, BJ, Nadeau, MR, Bianchi, LA, Jacques, PF, Rosenberg, IH, Selhub, J. Excess prevalence of fasting and postmethionine-loading hyperhomocysteinemia in stable renal transplant recipients. *Arterioscler Thromb Vasc Biol* 1997; 17: 1894–900.

8. Brosnan, JT. The 1986 Borden Award Lecture. The role of the kidney in amino acid metabolism and nutrition. *Can J Physiol Pharmacol* 1987; 65: 2355–62.

9. Brosnan, JT, Man, K-C, Hall, DE, Colbourne, SA, Brosnan, ME. Interorgan metabolism of amino acids in the streptozotocin-diabetic ketoacidotic rat. *Am J Physiol* 1983; 244: E151–58.

10. Carson, NAJ, Cusworth, DC, Dent, CE, Field, CMB, Neill, DW, Westal, RG. Homocystinuria: A new inborn error of metabolism associated with mental deficiency. *Arch Dis Child.* 1963; 38: 425–35.

11. Cusworth, DW, Gattereau, A. Inhibition of renal tubular reabsorption of homocystine by lysine and arginine. *Lancet* 1968; 2: 916–17.

12. Dhanakoti, SN, Brosnan, ME, Herzberg, GR, Brosnan, JT. Cellular and subcellular localization of enzymes of arginine metabolism in rat kidney. *Biochem J* 1992; 282: 369–75.

13. Finkelstein, JD, Kyle, WE, Harris, BJ. Methionine metabolism in mammals. Regulation of homocysteine methyltransferases in rat tissue. *Arch Biochem Biophys* 1971; 146: 84–92.

14. Foreman, JW, Wald, H, Blumberg, G, Pepe, LM, Segal, S. Homocystine uptake in isolated rat renal tubules. *Metabolism* 1982; 31: 613–19.

15. Frimpter, GW, Greenberg, AJ. Renal clearance of cystathionine in homozygous and hetereozygous cystathionuria, cystinuria and in the normal state. *J Clin Invest* 1967; 46: 975–82.

16. Gaull, GE, von Berg, W, Raiha, NCR, Sturman, JA. Development of methyltransferase activities of human fetal tissues. *Pediatr Res* 1973; 7: 527–33.

17. Green, R, Jacobsen, DW. Clinical implications of hyperhomocysteinemia. In *Folate in Health and Disease* (Bailey, LB, ed.). M. Dekker, New York, 1995; pp. 75–122.

18. Guttormsen, AB, Mansoor, MA, Fiskerstrand, T, Ueland, PM, Refsum, H. Kinetics of plasma homocysteine in healthy subjects after peroral homocysteine loading. *Clin Chem* 1993; 39: 1390–97.

19. Guttormsen, AB, Ueland, PM, Svarstad, E, Refsum, H. Kinetic basis of hyperhomocysteinemia in patients with chronic renal failure. *Kidney Int* 1997; 52: 495–502.

20. House, JD, Brosnan, ME, Brosnan, JT. Characterization of homocysteine metabolism in the rat kidney. *Biochem J* 1997; 328: 287–92.

21. House, JD, Brosnan, ME, Brosnan, JT. Renal uptake and excretion of homocysteine in rats with acute hyperhomocysteinemia. *Kidney Int* 1998; 54: 1601–7.

22. Hultberg, B, Andersson, A, Sterner, G. Plasma homocysteine in renal failure. *Clin Nephrol* 1993; 40: 230–35.

23. Hultberg, B, Andersson, A, Arnadottir, M. Reduced, free and total fractions of homocysteine and other thiol compounds in plasma from patients with renal failure. *Nephron* 1995; 70: 62–7.

24. Jungas, RL, Halperin, ML, Brosnan, JT. Quantitative analysis of amino acid oxidation and related gluconeogenesis in humans. *Physiol Rev* 1992; 72: 419–48.

25. Levillain, O, Parvy, P, Hassler, C. Amino acid handling in uremic rats: Citrulline, a reliable marker of renal insufficiency and proximal tubular dysfunction. *Metabolism* 1997; 46: 611–18.

26. McGuire, DM, Tormanen, CD, Segal, IS, Van Pilsum, JF. The effect of growth hormone and thyroxine on the amount of L-arginine: Glycine amidinotransferase in kidneys of hypophysectomized rats. Purification and some properties of rat kidney transamidinase. *J Biol Chem* 1980; 255: 1152–59.

27. McKeever, MP, Weir, DG, Molloy, A, Scott, JM. Betaine-homocysteine methyltransferase: Organ distribution in man, pig and rat and subcellular distribution in the rat. *Clin Sci* 1991; 81: 551–56.

28. Mudd, SH, Finkelstein, JD, Irreverre, F, Laster, L. Transsulfuration in mammals. Microassays and tissue distributions of three enzymes of the pathway. *J Biol Chem* 1965; 240: 4382–91.

29. Mudd, SH, Levy, HL, Abeles, RH. A derangement in B_{12} metabolism leading to homocystinemia, cystathioninemia and methylmalonic aciduria. *Biochem Biophys Res Commun* 1969; 35: 121–26.

30. Mudd, SH, Poole, JR. Labile methyl balances for normal humans on various dietary regimens. *Metabolism* 1975; 24: 721–35.

31. Norlund, L, Grubb, A, Fex, G, Leskell, H, Nilsson, JE, Schenck, H, Hultberg, B. The increase of plasma homocysteine concentration with age is partly due to the deterioration of renal function as determined by plasma cystatin C. *Clin Chem Lab Med* 1998; 36: 175–78.

32. Ogawa, H, Ishiguro, Y, Fujioka, M. Guanidinoacetate methyltransferase from rat liver: Purification, properties, and evidence for the involvement of sulfhydryl groups for activity. *Arch Biochem Biophys* 1983; 226: 265–75.

33. Quere, I, Paul, V, Rouillac, C, Janbon, C, London, J, Kamoun, P, Dufier, J-L, Abitbol, M, Chasse, J-F. Spatial and temporal expression of the cystathionine β-synthase gene during early human development. *Biochem Biophys Res Commun* 1999; 254: 127–37.

34. Refsum, H, Helland, S, Ueland, PM. Radioenzymic determination of homocysteine in plasma and urine. *Clin Chem* 1985; 31: 624–28.

35. Robinson, K, Gupta, A, Dennis, V, Arheart, K, Chaudary, D, Green, R, Vigo, P, Mayer, EL, Selhub, J, Kutner, M, Jacobsen, DW. Hyperhomocysteinemia confers an independent risk of atherosclerosis in end-stage renal disease and is closely linked to plasma folate and pyridoxine concentrations. *Circulation* 1996; 94: 2743–48.

36. Rosenblatt, DS. Inherited disorders of folate transport and metabolism In *The Metabolic and Molecular Bases of Inherited Disease*, Vol. III. (Scriver, CR, Beaudet, AL, Sly, WS, Valle, D, eds.). McGraw-Hill Inc, New York, 1995; pp. 3111–18.

37. Segal, S, Thier SO. Cystinuria, In *The Metabolic and Molecular Bases of Inherited Disease*, Vol. III. (Scriver, CR, Beaudet, AL, Sly, WS, Valle, D, eds.). McGraw-Hill Inc, New York, 1995; pp. 3581–3601.

38. Smolin, LA, Benevenga, NJ. Accumulation of homocysteine in vitamin B_6 deficiency: A model for the study of cystathione β-synthase deficiency. *J Nutr* 1982; 112: 1264–72.

39. Stockand, JD, A1-Baldawi, NF, Al-Khalili, OK, Wonell, R, Eaton, DC. S-adenosyl-L-homocysteine hydrolase regulates aldosterone-induced Na⁺ transport. *J Biol Chem* 1999; 274: 3842–50.

40. Sturman, JA, Rassin, DK, Gaull, GE. Distribution of transsulfuration enzymes in various organs and species. *Int J Biochem* 1970; 1: 251–53.

41. Tizianello, A, Deferrari, G, Garibotto, G, Gurreri, G, Robaudo, C. Renal metabolism of amino acids and ammonia in subjects with normal renal function and in patients with chronic renal insufficiency. *J Clin Invest* 1980; 65: 1162–72.

42. Wilcken, DEL, Gupta, VJ, Reddy, SG. Accumulation of sulphur-containing amino acids including cysteine-homocysteine mixed disulfide in patients on maintenance haemodialysis. *Clin Sci* 1980; 58: 426–330.

43. van Guldener, C, Donker, AJM, Jakobs, C, Tearlink, T, de Meer, K, Stenouwer, CDA. No net renal extraction of homocysteine in fasting humans. *Kidney Int* 1998; 54: 166–69.

44. van Guldener, C, Kulik, W, Berger, R, Dijkstra, DA, Jacobs, C, Reijngoud, D-J, Donker, AJM, Stehouwer, CDA, deMeer, K. Homocysteine and methionine metabolism in ESRD: A stable isotope study. *Kidney Int* 1999; 56: 1064–71.

17

Homocysteine and the Nervous System

ANNE M. MOLLOY
DONALD G. WEIR

Over the last decade a clear picture has emerged of the risks to cardiovascular health associated with elevated blood levels of homocysteine. This picture has been built up by linking disorders affecting homocysteine metabolism with morbidity and mortality caused by a variety of forms of cardiovascular disease. There is a parallel and equally rich literature linking disorders affecting homocysteine metabolism and disturbances of the nervous system. This chapter reviews these latter links and discusses the evidence that exists to implicate 1) a direct effect of homocysteine on the nervous system through its interactions with cellular components such as cell membranes or through its excitotoxic action on neural receptors and 2) the indirect effects on essential brain methylation reactions resulting from disturbances in the neural cell's ability to recycle homocysteine.

Homocysteine Metabolism in Brain

The Metabolic Diagram describes a generalized version of homocysteine metabolism that probably occurs in its entirety only in a few tissues such as the liver or kidney (25). In the brain, there is a limited capacity for homocysteine metabolism. In addition, it is important to highlight certain aspects of folate metabolism within the brain that play critical roles in the metabolism of homocysteine.

Brain Folate Metabolism

The level of 5-methyltetrahydrofolate in cerebrospinal fluid is at least three times that found in plasma (39) and an active transport process exists at the blood-brain barrier (111, 112). This suggests an important role for folates in the brain and the necessity for protection against the effects of deficiency. As in other tissues, the requirements for one-carbon units in the brain change over the period from early development to adulthood. The folate-related enzymes involved in purine and pyrimidine synthesis decline almost 10-fold in adulthood indicating that the provision of methyl groups for S-adenosylmethionine (AdoMet) and methylation reactions coupled with the recycling of homocysteine through methionine synthase may be the dominant function of adult brain folate metabolism (18, 98). Brain serine metabolism through serine hydroxymethyltransferase and 5,10-methylenetetrahydrofolate reductase (MTHFR) (Metabolic Diagram, Reactions 8 and 9) probably supplies most of the one-carbon units destined for folate-related pathways (35, 55, 57). This pathway, operating through the remethylation of homocysteine to methionine and formation of AdoMet, ultimately provides the majority of methyl groups for the wide variety of methyltransferase reactions that take place in the nervous system.

Cobalamin and Methionine Synthase

The brain has an absolute requirement for cobalamin to function as a cofactor for methionine synthase (Metabolic Diagram, Reaction 4). This requirement is necessary because methionine synthase is the only enzyme in the brain capable of remethylating homocysteine to methionine (96, 98). The other remethylation enzyme, betaine homocysteine methyltransferase (Metabolic Diagram, Reaction 5), is not expressed in neural tissue (23, 58, 99). About 50% of homocysteine produced by the liver is remethylated (24); however, because liver is also a catabolic organ and has two remethylating enzymes, this may have little bearing on the flux of homocysteine in the brain. Remethylation of homocysteine through methionine synthase in the brain has not been quantified directly. However, it must be substantial, as evidence from animal studies shows 10-fold increases in the levels of S-adenosylhomocysteine (AdoHcy) in the brain and spinal cord when methionine synthase is inactivated through nitrous oxide treatment (67).

Control of AdoMet in the Brain (see also Chapter 6)

Animal studies show that the brain expresses isoform II of methionine adenosyltransferase, which has a K_m for methionine of approximately 10 µmol/L (66) and is, therefore, probably saturated with methionine in vivo. The methionine adenosyltransferase II isoform is sensitive to tissue levels of AdoMet (46), which act as a feedback inhibitor of its activity. Thus, the rate of AdoMet synthesis in brain is dependent on the rate of its utilization. This prevents wide fluctuations in the levels of AdoMet and probably maintains a steady-state flow of folate substrates through the mini-folate cycle (Metabolic Diagram, Reactions 4, 8, and 9). Studies in pigs and rats report concentrations of AdoMet between 50 and 90 µmol/L (31, 67). The K_m values of AdoMet for the vast majority of methyltransferase enzymes are considerably lower, on the order of 5 to 15 µmol/L (77). Thus, under normal conditions, the brain concentration of AdoMet is not a limiting factor for enzymatic methylation in vivo.

AdoHcy Inhibition of Methyltransferase Enzymes

As described in Chapters 7 and 8, AdoHcy is a powerful competitive inhibitor of methyltransferase enzymes, often having a greater affinity for these enzymes than the substrate AdoMet. Protein methylase II (AdoMet:protein-carboxyl O-methyltransferase) has a K_m for AdoMet of about 9 µmol/L and a K_i for AdoHcy of about 1 µmol/L (48), the highest activity being in brain, which suggests a role in neurological or secretory processes. The enzyme catalyzes the transfer of methyl groups from AdoMet to the terminal carboxyl group of farnesylated cysteine residues. Recent work indicates that this methylation is involved in the regulation of tumor necrosis factor and that elevated AdoHcy potentiates and AdoMet administration protects against its cytotoxicity (7, 15).

Protein methylase I (AdoMet:protein-arginine N-methyltransferase) is similarly sensitive to AdoHcy. This enzyme is also elevated in the brain and plays a pivotal role in the methylation of arginine residue 107 of myelin basic protein (32, 45). The increased hydrophobicity caused by this methylation may facilitate the interaction of myelin basic protein with the phospholipid membrane and may function in the long-term maintenance of myelin (45).

In brain, as in other tissues, AdoHcy is rapidly converted to adenosine and L-homocysteine such that the intracellular concentration is maintained between 1 and 5 µmol/L (31, 67). However, because the AdoHcy hydrolase reaction (Metabolic Diagram, Reaction 3) is reversible and favors the synthesis of AdoHcy, any rise in the level of homocysteine in neural tissue will alter the AdoHcy concentration and disturb the AdoMet/AdoHcy ratio, potentially affecting the activity of methyltransferase enzymes and leading to cellular hypomethylation. It is likely therefore that elevated intracellular AdoHcy levels have an important role to play in the development of diseases associated with elevated plasma (or cerebrospinal fluid) homocysteine.

Homocysteine Catabolism

A final important consideration regarding brain homocysteine metabolism is the apparent absence of a complete transsulfuration pathway. Whereas cystathionine β-synthase (CBS) (Metabolic Diagram, Reaction 6) is present in brain at about 20% of the proportion in liver, cystathionine γ-lyase (Metabolic Diagram, Reaction 7) occurs at very low activity or possibly not at all (24). This is supported by the finding that astroglial cells in culture could not substitute methionine or homocysteine for cysteine (47). In addition, relatively high cystathionine concentrations are found in mammalian brain (97), the highest levels being in humans (105). There is also a dramatic increase in brain cystathionine levels after nitrous oxide inactivation of methionine synthase in pigs, suggesting that homocysteine catabolism is substantially blocked beyond this point (92).

In summary, the brain tissues utilize three mechanisms for maintaining low steady-state concentrations of homocysteine: 1) efficient recycling through cobalamin-dependent methionine synthase, given an adequate supply of cobalamin and folate; 2) catabolism through CBS to cystathionine, a reportedly nontoxic product; and 3) export into the circulation.

Links Between Disorders Affecting Homocysteine Metabolism and Disturbances of Brain Function

In brain, as elsewhere, disruption of homocysteine metabolism can arise from nutritional imbalances, genetic defects, or drug therapy. In recent years, much progress has been made in understanding the mechanisms involved in some of the pathologies that result from this disruption, largely owing to the development of highly sensitive methods to measure plasma and cerebrospinal fluid homocysteine concentrations and other metabolic indices of folate and cobalamin deficiency.

Cobalamin Deficiency

Neurological disabilities associated with cobalamin deficiency have been described for more than a century. Long-term severe cobalamin deficiency can cause a classic vacuolar demyelination of the spinal cord and brain, the primary pathological change being a swelling and subsequent degeneration of the myelin sheath. This spinal cord lesion has sometimes been termed subacute combined degeneration, but cobalamin deficiency affects all parts of the central nervous system, including the brain and peripheral nerves (see Chapter 24). Up to 30% of subjects with cobalamin deficiency present with neurological symptoms only (36, 53). Although cobalamin therapy leads to an arrest of the degenerative process, a reversal of existing symptoms appears to be related to the severity of involvement and they can be irreversible (53, 110).

Present knowledge suggests that there are only two enzymes in mammalian systems requiring cobalamin, methionine synthase and methylmalonyl CoA mutase. The plasma concentrations of homocysteine and methylmalonic acid, being substrates of these enzymes, are sensitive biological indices of cobalamin status. Nevertheless, biochemical studies of patients with cobalamin deficiency have been unhelpful in identifying which of these two enzymes is responsible for the neurological defects. Both plasma total homocysteine and methylmalonic acid can be elevated to varying extents and are not predictive of patients with and without neurological symptoms (1, 53). However, estimations of homocysteine levels in cerebrospinal fluid are rarely performed, and it is possible that these would be more informative.

Folate Deficiency

Patients with megaloblastic anemia caused by cobalamin or folate deficiency have a comparable prevalence of symptoms such as dementia and cognitive impairment, but peripheral neuropathy occurs frequently in cobalamin deficiency, whereas psychiatric disorders such as depression may be more common in folate deficiency (94) (see also Chapter 23). Herbert (38) reported a range of neuropsychiatric symptoms including irritability, fatigue, and depression after 4 months on a folate-deficient diet. There have been occasional reports of myelopathy in cases of severe folate deficiency (52, 62, 84) and methotrexate therapy (30). In addition, severe congenital deficiency of MTHFR, which supplies folate substrate for the methionine synthase reaction, also results in the classic myelopathic lesion (40), possibly linking the enzyme methionine synthase with the development of the neuropathy. Occasional reports have described cases of "folate responsive" schizophrenia (29) or psychoses (72) where homocystinuria was a common feature. MTHFR deficiency was implicated as the underlying mechanism.

Genetic Defects of Homocysteine Metabolism

Acquired deficiencies of folate, cobalamin, and vitamin B_6 have such a broad range of effects that the underlying mechanisms of the neurological disorders are difficult to unravel. By contrast, the biochemical, clinical and neuropathological sequelae of a small number of genetic defects have been pivotal in establishing the importance of homocysteine metabolism in the brain. These include mutations in MTHFR, methionine synthase, the putative cobalamin processing enzymes (see Chapter 21), which result in functional deficiency of methionine synthase, AdoMet synthetase, and CBS (40, 70, 88, 104). These defects can be broadly grouped into two classes: those that affect the remethylation of homocysteine and those that affect the catabolism of homocysteine.

Inborn Errors Affecting the Remethylation of Homocysteine

Congenital mutations in MTHFR limit the supply of the folate remethylation substrate 5-methyltetrahydrofolate, whereas defects in methionine synthase or the *Cbl* mutations mentioned previously limit the remethylation process itself (see Chapter 21). The major clinical problems arising from these defects include hypotonia, lethargy, seizures, mental retardation, and ataxia. Demyelination has been demonstrated both pathologically and radiologically in children with MTHFR deficiency and with functional methionine synthase deficiency (40, 104). Biochemically, these defects were associated with abnormally high cerebrospinal fluid homocysteine and low methionine and AdoMet. Myelin abnormalities were also demonstrated in patients with defects in AdoMet synthetase in the face of normal cerebrospinal fluid homocysteine plus a 200-fold elevation of methionine, the common factor being AdoMet deficiency (104). When patients having one or another of these three enzyme defects were treated with AdoMet, the demyelination was reversed to some extent (40, 104).

Inborn Errors Affecting the Catabolism of Homocysteine

The principal neurological complications of CBS deficiency are mental retardation and epileptic seizures (see Chapter 20). Although these symptoms have been attributed to episodes of intracranial or venous thromboses, clinical observations are not always consistent with this theory (26). Cerebrospinal fluid and plasma levels of total homocysteine, as well as AdoMet were measured in 10 children with CBS deficiency before and after the children were treated with betaine (102).

Plasma and cerebrospinal fluid total homocysteine levels were elevated before treatment and were significantly reduced after betaine treatment, but were not normalized. Levels of AdoMet in cerebrospinal fluid were normal before treatment and rose after treatment, suggesting that the neurological complications associated with this deficiency may be secondary to an accumulation of homocysteine in the central nervous system.

Other Disorders Affecting Brain Function

All of the preceding disorders may cause severe hyperhomocysteinemia and homocystinuria; thus it is not surprising that pathological effects have been attributed either directly or indirectly to the toxicity of homocysteine. However, in the last decade, there has been a surge of interest in the role of moderate elevations of plasma total homocysteine in a variety of neurodegenerative conditions, particularly where there is impairment of cognitive processing. These conditions include vascular and nonvascular dementia in elderly patients, schizophrenia, and depression.

There is mounting evidence that deficiencies of cobalamin, folate, and vitamin B_6 increase with age (5, 41, 79). As described in Chapter 24, up to 15% of elderly people were reported to be cobalamin deficient, based on elevated serum homocysteine or methylmalonic acid and low or low-normal serum cobalamin (5, 79). The clinical and biochemical manifestations associated with cobalamin and folate deficiency in the elderly are discussed in Chapters 23 and 24. The point to emphasize here is that elevated homocysteine is a common finding in older persons, substantially as a result of reduced vitamin status. It is possible that hyperhomocysteinemia may be the fundamental link between the observed associations of reduced vitamin status and severity of cognitive dysfunction. Plasma total homocysteine may be a stronger predictor of some cognitive skills than either plasma folate or cobalamin levels (86).

Vascular and Nonvascular Dementia

Current evidence that hyperhomocysteinemia may be a risk factor for stroke is discussed in Chapter 31. The prevalence of hyperhomocysteinemia in stroke victims is reported to range from 19% to 42% (20). Furthermore, in patients with a history of stroke, those with hyperhomocysteinemia had a more pronounced impairment of cognitive function (20). Low serum and cerebrospinal fluid cobalamin concentrations have been reported in both vascular dementia and Alzheimer's disease (4, 13, 16, 74), although these parameters could not be correlated with cognitive

function (4). Similarly, low folate status was reported to occur predominantly in demented subjects (73), which is consistent with the generally high prevalence of folate deficiency in geriatric patients with depression and dementia. Overall, estimations of vitamin levels in these subjects have not been of great diagnostic value (5), because different populations, cut-off points, and assay methods have resulted in large variations in study outcomes. However, hyperhomocysteinemia was reported to be an early and sensitive marker for cognitive impairment in Alzheimer's disease and other dementias (6, 16, 56). In a study of 741 psychogeriatric patients, plasma total homocysteine was elevated in both demented and nondemented patients compared with control subjects (73). Furthermore, patients with both vascular disease and dementia tended to have higher plasma total homocysteine levels than those without vascular disease (6, 73).

An emerging hypothesis suggests that homocysteine-associated damage may impact more on the small penetrating cerebral arteries and arterioles than on the brain macrovasculature (16). In support of this hypothesis, a recent study showed that elderly patients with a characteristic form of microangiopathic vascular dementia known as subcortical vascular encephalopathy had higher plasma total homocysteine levels than either healthy control subjects or patients with cerebral macroangiopathy (21).

Overall, there seems to be little doubt that vitamin deficiencies causing hyperhomocysteinemia are associated with the evolution of certain brain diseases that lead to cognitive decline in elderly persons. Nevertheless, further work is required to definitively establish whether elevated homocysteine levels occur before or after the disease develops and to determine the mechanism by which elevated homocysteine is related to cognitive dysfunction. (74a, 93a)

Depression

There appear to be strong links between folate status and mood regulation. Plasma folate levels less than 5.7 nmol/L (2.5 μg/L) or red cell folate levels less than 453 nmol/L (200 μg/L) may occur in 15% to 38% of patients with depression and lower folate levels seem to correlate with severity of depression (2, 8). In addition, treatment with antidepressant drugs is less effective in subjects with major depression who are also folate deficient than in those who have normal folate levels (2). It is not clear which folate-dependent mechanism may be involved in mood regulation, although it has been suggested that deficient methylation of monoamine neurotransmitters is involved and that AdoMet has effective antidepressant properties (8).

Cobalamin status is equally important in the metabolism of AdoMet, and one might expect similar links between cobalamin deficiency and depression, but this is not the case. Neither cobalamin status nor plasma total homocysteine seems to correlate with degree or subtype of depression in psychiatric patients (22). On the other hand, dramatic changes in the levels of the monoamine metabolites, hydroxyindoleacetic acid, and homovanillic acid have been associated with severe folate deficiency (101). The mechanism is unknown, but it appears to be independent of changes in the AdoMet concentration.

Schizophrenia

For many years a folate-related mechanism or a methylation deficiency has been proposed in schizophrenia. Several groups have found low folate status in schizophrenics and folate-responsive schizophrenic-like behavior have been reported in subjects with deficiency of MTHFR (29). In one study, high plasma total homocysteine was a common finding (83). Homozygosity for the TT genotype of the MTHFR 677C→T variant was also found to be a risk factor for this disorder (3). However, it is not known whether treatment with cobalamin or folate to lower the plasma total homocysteine would have any effect on the psychosis.

Direct Effects of Homocysteine on the Nervous System

It is clear that hyperhomocysteinemia represents a metabolic link among a multitude of neurological disorders. However, the role that homocysteine plays has not been established. It could vary from a direct action, by exerting a toxic effect either on glutamate neurotransmitter receptors in neural cells or on vascular endothelial cells in the cerebral blood vessels, to an indirect action by disruption of methylation systems via its conversion to AdoHcy, to a combination of these two mechanisms. The evidence that one or the other of these mechanisms may be involved is discussed next.

Evidence that Homocysteine May Act as a Transmitter

It is considered that epileptic seizures result from a marked predominance of neuronal excitation over inhibition. There is now substantial evidence that homocysteine, cysteine, and other sulfur-containing metabolites including homocysteine thiolactone, homocysteic acid, and homocysteine sulfinic acid can cause convulsions and act as excitatory agonists on the N-methyl-D-aspartate (NMDA) subtype of the glutamate receptor (34, 113).

Broch and Ueland (10) found homocysteine in all regions of the brain of several animal species, with a marked abundance in cerebellum. Both homocysteic acid and homocysteine sulfinic acid have been detected in rat brain slices and shown to be released from nerve terminals in a Ca^{2+}-dependent manner (17). Although its exact physiological function is unclear, homocysteic acid appears to be exclusively localized to glial cells (17, 34) where it has recently been hypothesized to function as a "gliotransmitter" that is released on stimulation by noradrenaline (17). There is considerable evidence that excitatory amino acids play a role in a wide variety of neurodegenerative diseases as a consequence of excessive activation of the excitatory amino acid receptors (64). Parsons et al. (78) showed that homocysteine was selectively toxic to medulloblastoma cells at relatively low concentrations (5 to 15 μmol/L), emphasizing that cell-specific and toxin-specific patterns might vary according to the number and subunit isoforms of NMDA receptors found on the cell surface. This finding has relevance in elucidating the possible mechanisms of homocysteine neurotoxicity in clinical conditions.

Although it has been suggested that the neurotoxic action of homocysteine may be through its conversion to homocysteic acid or homocysteine sulfinic acid (26), it is not clear how this could occur because homocysteine and homocysteic acid caused different types of seizures in immature rats (63). However, it is known that the excitatory neurotransmitter system undergoes marked changes during postnatal development and that younger animals are more sensitive to the convulsant action of these compounds. Recent evidence suggests that homocysteine may not be an effective agonist for conventional ionotropic glutamate receptors but that it may be active at some of the NMDA modulatory sites (27). In addition, free radical formation may be involved in homocysteine induced neuronal death (27). Lipton et al. (54) showed that homocysteine is a partial agonist at the glutamate site but a partial antagonist of the glycine coagonist site, and under normal conditions, with physiological levels of glycine, homocysteine does not become toxic until it reaches millimolar concentrations. Under pathological conditions (such as stroke or head trauma), however, when glycine levels are elevated, the neurotoxic (agonist) effect of homocysteine, even at 10 to 100 μmol/L concentrations, far outweighs its neuroprotective (antagonist) activity. Under these conditions, neuronal damage could be caused by excessive Ca^{2+} influx and reactive oxygen generation (54).

Contribution of Homocysteine Toxicity to the Pathogenesis of Diseases of the Nervous System

Epileptic seizures, mental retardation, dystonia, and other degenerative effects within the nervous system are among the classic symptoms of genetic and acquired disorders that cause severe hyperhomocysteinemia, irrespective of whether the disturbance is in the remethylation or the catabolism of homocysteine. Therefore, it is attractive to hypothesize that some of these symptoms are precipitated through the neurotoxic effect of homocysteine, although no direct evidence exists to verify this possibility. Both homocysteic acid and homocysteine sulfinic acid are elevated in the urine of patients with homocystinuria (75), and homocysteic acid was identified in human neurosurgical samples (28). Very high levels of protein-bound homocysteine were found in postmortem brain tissue from a subject with MTHFR deficiency (42). Children who received methotrexate for treatment of cancer had elevated cerebrospinal fluid homocysteine and a marked accumulation of homocysteic acid and cysteinsulfinic acid in the fluid (82). Thus, it is likely that the elevated cerebrospinal fluid homocysteine seen in children with homocysteine-related inborn errors (70, 104) reflects sufficiently high concentrations in the cells of the nervous system to potentially cause convulsive seizures and neuronal degeneration.

It is less clear how moderately elevated brain homocysteine levels might exert a neurotoxic effect. In vitro studies show that both homocysteine and AdoHcy can significantly alter vascular endothelial cell function, acting through entirely separate pathways (19). Thus, both metabolites can contribute to the development of vascular disease. A possible mechanism suggested by Clarke et al. (16) in relation to Alzheimer's dementia is that homocysteine-associated microvascular disease in a critical region of the brain, such as the hippocampus, may trigger neuronal degeneration and the deposition of β-amyloid plaques. Alternatively, the combination of elevated homocysteine with microvascular disease or repeated ischemic episodes may provide sufficiently adverse conditions within the neural cell to promote the neurotoxic effect of homocysteine on the NMDA receptors as shown in vitro by Lipton et al. (54).

Indirect Effects of Homocysteine on the Nervous System

As discussed, studies of patients with inborn errors of enzymes associated with the remethylation of homocysteine demonstrate that abnormal AdoMet and AdoHcy metabolism is associated with neurological lesions. The underlying process has not been elucidated, but experimental evidence suggests that it is probably triggered by inhibition of essential methylation processes. Alteration of AdoMet and AdoHcy levels may also cause and prevent mood disturbances via the methylation of neurotransmitters.

Experimental Evidence for the Role of AdoMet and AdoHcy Remethylation Disorders

There is accumulating evidence that many of the neurological manifestations of cobalamin deficiency (and perhaps folate deficiency) result from alterations of AdoMet and AdoHcy within the nervous system. Much of this evidence has been derived experimentally, by inactivating methionine synthase with nitrous oxide (110) or by inhibiting the synthesis of AdoMet with cycloleucine (50), both of which produce abnormalities indistinguishable from those seen in clinical subacute combined degeneration.

Nitrous oxide inactivates methionine synthase (110). Recovery of enzyme activity requires synthesis of new enzyme and can take from several days in liver, kidney, and brain to more than 2 weeks in spinal cord (68). In humans, chronic exposure to nitrous oxide also produces myelopathy (49). Nitrous oxide has been successfully used in monkeys (93), fruit bats (107), and pigs (108) to produce a myelopathy that could be prevented by methionine supplementation.

Biochemically, nitrous oxide causes dramatic increases in the level of AdoHcy in brain and spinal cord along with a moderate reduction in AdoMet levels (67, 108) (Figure 17.1). Methionine supplementation greatly increases the level of methionine within the brain and spinal cord (92), thereby helping to normalize the AdoMet level, but AdoHcy remains abnormally high because the betaine-dependent pathway of homocysteine remethylation is not present in brain. The change in methionine synthase activity during periods of inactivation and resynthesis closely correlates with changes in the AdoMet/AdoHcy ratio in brain and spinal cord but not in liver, emphasizing the importance of that enzyme to AdoMet and AdoHcy homeostasis in neural tissues (68).

Using the pig model, O- and N-hypomethylation was demonstrated in vitro (59) and in vivo (60) in the brains of nitrous oxide-treated animals. Methionine supplementation reduced the level of hypomethylation in vitro (59), which is consistent with the apparent protection by methionine against demyelination in vivo (108).

An attractive hypothesis for the mechanism of this demyelination implicates hypomethylation of arginine 107 in myelin basic protein, leading to changes in the protein structure and breakdown of the myelin sheath. However, this model does not provide a good correlation between the period of maximal myelin deposition and the clinical observations of when demyelination has been noted in children with inborn errors involving homocysteine remethylation (104).

Recently, Scalabrino et al. (89, 90) proposed a new experimental model for neurological abnormality, the totally gastrectomized rat. This model developed a widespread spongiform vacuolation of the brain, and only cobalamin administration was capable of decreasing the severity of the neurological dysfunction. The spongy vacuolation did not correlate either with early impairment of methylmalonyl CoA mutase or with the more delayed impairment of methionine synthase (91), but

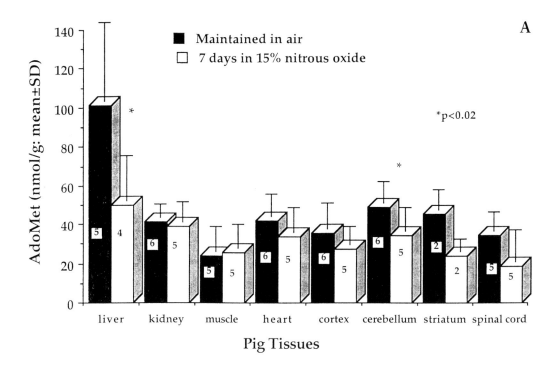

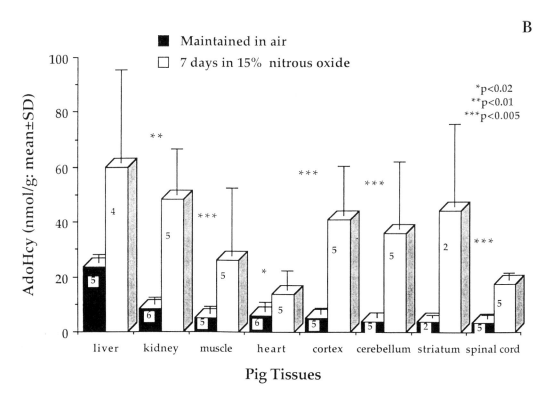

Fig. 17.1. Concentrations of (A) S-adenosylmethionine (AdoMet) and (B) S-adenosylhomocysteine (AdoHcy) in tissues of pigs maintained in air (shaded boxes) or an atmosphere of 15% nitrous oxide (white boxes) for 7 days. Air and nitrous oxide treatment were compared using a Mann-Whitney test. The numbers in the boxes represent the numbers of animals in each group.

tumor necrosis factor was overexpressed in the spinal cord and treatment with cobalamin substantially reduced its levels. (11). Treatment with tumor necrosis factor was capable of producing the same lesions in normal rats, suggesting a pathological role in the neurological disorders. The mechanism of these effects is not understood, nor is it known what causes the abnormalities in cytokine levels. However, reports have linked elevated AdoHcy with tumor necrosis factor cytotoxicity through the inhibition of carboxyl-O-methyltransferase (7, 15, 19, 51). These new observations, therefore, are not inconsistent with other experimental models showing abnormal AdoMet and AdoHcy concentrations in brain before the development of the lesion.

Clinical Evidence of AdoMet and AdoHcy Abnormalities in Homocysteine Related Disorders

Using the nitrous oxide model, it can be demonstrated that the plasma total homocysteine concentration is closely correlated with brain AdoHcy levels (Figure 17.2). Furthermore, the concentration of AdoHcy in cerebrospinal fluid is strongly associated with the concentrations in cortex, cerebellum, or spinal cord (109), confirming that methods to measure the levels of AdoMet and AdoHcy in cerebrospinal fluid would be important tools. Because of methodological problems, AdoHcy levels in cerebrospinal fluid are rarely reported but low concentrations of AdoMet have been observed in disease processes featuring demyelination or other neurological abnormalities. In some instances, a disruption of specific methylation processes can be hypothesized, whereas in others, the relevance of the measurement to the disease process is unclear.

Cobalamin or Folate Deficiency Concentrations of AdoMet are significantly reduced in the cerebrospinal fluid of patients with neurological abnormalities owing to folate deficiency or cobalamin deficiency (8) and in patients receiving methotrexate for the treatment of acute lymphoblastic leukemia (103). In the latter study, the reduction in AdoMet closely mirrored a rise in cerebrospinal fluid myelin basic protein levels. Concentrations of AdoHcy in cerebrospinal fluid have not yet been measured in humans with cobalamin or folate deficiency but would be expected to be elevated given the dramatic elevation in homocysteine concentrations.

Depression Disturbances in the metabolism of monoamine neurotransmitters have been implicated in a variety of neurological and psychiatric diseases. AdoMet is required by catechol-O-methyltransferase to catalyze the breakdown of catechols such as dopamine, serotonin, and noradrenaline. Tyrosine hydroxylase, a rate-limiting enzyme catalyzing catecholamine synthesis, is activated by AdoMet and inhibited by AdoHcy in vitro (61). AdoMet administration increases the levels of noradrenaline, dopamine, serotonin, and 5-hydroxyindole-3-acetic acid in rat brain (76). AdoMet also participates in the biosynthesis of melatonin, being a substrate for hydroxyindole-O-methyltransferase. Sitaram et al. (95) found that AdoMet undergoes a marked circadian rhythm in rat pineal gland, and there was a relationship between AdoMet levels and the degree of melatonin biosynthesis that could be altered either by changing the light-dark cycle or by administration of a β-adrenergic agonist or antagonist. These results suggest that abnormal concentrations of AdoMet in the central nervous system may contribute to mood disturbances by altering the pattern of melatonin biosynthesis in the pineal gland.

In some studies, severely depressed patients had significantly reduced cerebrospinal fluid levels of AdoMet, which could be increased by either intravenous or oral administration of AdoMet (8). A meta-analysis of clinical trials using AdoMet and other tricyclic antidepressants concluded that AdoMet was as effective in treating depression as standard tricyclic antidepressants, and it had relatively few side effects (9).

Parkinson's Disease One of the side effects of L-dopa (3-hydroxy-L-tyrosine) in the rat is a reduction of brain AdoMet levels and an increase in brain AdoHcy and homocysteine, which could be prevented with a catechol-O-methyltransferase inhibitor (65). This side effect appears to occur in human therapy because patients with Parkinson's disease who were treated with L-dopa had significantly higher plasma total homocysteine than untreated patients or healthy controls (71). Apart from this, abnormalities of homocysteine metabolism have not been noted. One study found no change in the AdoMet and AdoHcy levels of postmortem brain tissue from Parkinson's disease sufferers compared with control subjects (69). Conversely, an excitotoxic mechanism involving cysteine or cysteine sulfinic acid may occur.

Human Immunodeficiency Virus Encephalitis and Vacuolar Myelopathy Human immunodeficiency virus (HIV) infection commonly results in the development of neurological complications, most frequently subacute encephalitis (81). The resultant neuropsychiatric condition is known as acquired immune deficiency syndrome (AIDS) dementia complex. The other neurological manifestation of HIV infection, vacuolar myelopathy of the spinal cord, bears a striking resemblance to the myelopathy associated with cobalamin deficiency (37, 80), suggesting either deficiency or altered metabolism of cobalamin.

An increased incidence of low serum cobalamin levels occurs in HIV-positive patients (12, 44). However, Robertson et al. (87) found no relationship between a range of neurological symptoms in AIDS patients and their cobalamin status. Trimble et al. (106) found no

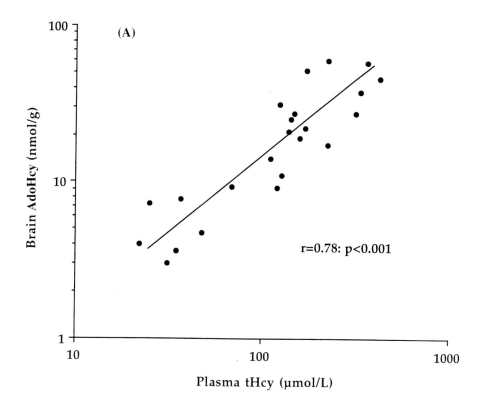

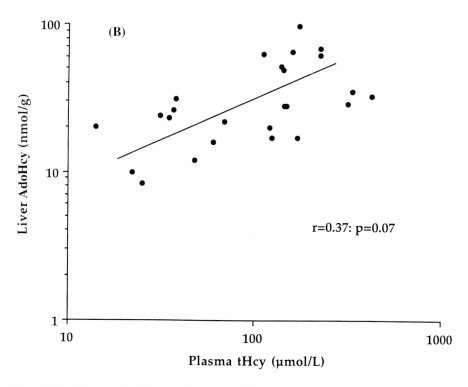

Fig. 17.2. The relationship of plasma total homocysteine (tHcy) to S-adenosylhomocysteine (AdoHcy) in brain (A) and liver (B).

evidence of subtle, localized cobalamin deficiency, based on measurement of cerebrospinal fluid levels of methylmalonic acid. Surtees et al. (100) reported significantly reduced levels of 5-methyltetrahydrofolate and AdoMet in the cerebrospinal fluid of children with neurological complications associated with HIV infection. Keating et al. (43) also showed reduced cerebrospinal fluid AdoMet and elevated levels of AdoHcy in the cerebrospinal fluid in 20 HIV-positive patients compared with control subjects, suggesting that there may be inhibition of methylation reactions in the central nervous system. However, these HIV-positive patients had normal cobalamin and folate status. Furthermore, Goggins et al. (33) found no evidence of hypomethylation in postmortem brain tissue from AIDS patients.

Although it seems unlikely that the alteration in the AdoMet/AdoHcy ratio in HIV infection could be due to inhibition of methionine synthase, the association of altered methylation capacity with the disease remains unexplained. Other workers have reported low cerebrospinal fluid levels of AdoMet and glutathione in HIV-positive patients, but cerebrospinal fluid homocysteine levels were not elevated (14). Administration of AdoMet as the butanedisulfonate

salt (800 mg/day) led to significant increases of AdoMet and glutathione concentrations in cerebrospinal fluid (14); the effect, if any, on their clinical condition is not known.

Dementia It is not known whether methylation reactions are involved in the dementia process. Lower than normal AdoMet concentrations in cerebrospinal fluid have been reported in patients with Alzheimer's dementia (8), as well as a significant reduction in the levels of AdoMet and AdoHcy in postmortem brain (69). On the other hand, Goggins et al. (33) found evidence of protein hypermethylation in postmortem brain tissue from patients with Alzheimer's dementia.

Multiple Sclerosis The clinical and pathological manifestations of multiple sclerosis are usually clearly distinguishable from those of cobalamin deficiency. Although most patients with multiple sclerosis do not have cobalamin deficiency, there have been reports of low serum and cerebrospinal fluid cobalamin levels (74, 85) and some evidence of an overlap between the two conditions (85). No consistent associations

Table 17.1. Association of Homocysteine Metabolism with Neurological Disorders that Have Been Linked to Elevated Plasma Or Cerebrospinal Fluid Homocysteine Levels

Condition	Direct Effect Owing to Homocysteine Toxicity	Indirect Effect Owing to Abnormalities of AdoMet or AdoHcy	Biomarker for Other Folate or Cobalamin-Related Abnormalities	References
Severe elevation of homocysteine				
Folate deficiency	Possibly	Occasional myelopathy	Yes	8, 38, 52, 62, 84, 94
Cobalamin deficiency	Possibly	Strong evidence	Yes	8, 36, 53, 110
Remethylation defects	Possibly	Strong evidence	Probably	40, 42, 49, 104,
CBS deficiency	Probably	Unlikely	Unlikely	70, 75, 102
Mild to moderate elevation of homocysteine				
Depression	No evidence	AdoMet ↓ in CSF; AdoMet therapeutic	Strong link with low folate	2, 8, 22, 73, 101
Schizophrenia	No evidence	Speculation of a methylation defect	No evidence	3, 29, 72, 83
Parkinson's disease	No evidence	Drug related	No evidence	69, 71
AIDS dementia complex	No evidence	AdoMet ↓ in CSF	Low cobalamin noted but not linked to dementia	12, 14, 33, 43, 44, 87, 100, 106
Multiple sclerosis	No evidence	No evidence	Low cobalamin often noted	74, 85
Vascular dementia and Alzheimer's disease	Speculation of a toxic mechanism	AdoMet ↓ in CSF	Low folate and cobalamin often noted	4, 6, 8, 13, 16, 20, 21, 33, 56, 69, 73, 74

CSF, Cerebrospinal fluid.

between homocysteine and AdoMet concentrations have been reported.

Concluding Remarks

The role of homocysteine in the nervous system is a new and rapidly developing area of research, and our present understanding is, at best, superficial even though the metabolic pathways controlling the remethylation and catabolism of homocysteine in the brain are largely known. Attempting to link specific aspects of homocysteine metabolism with some of the classic neurological and neuropsychiatric symptoms of diseases featuring elevated homocysteine yields a complex picture (Table 17.1). In some cases, there is an argument for a direct neurotoxic effect of homocysteine, whereas in others, an indirect effect seems more likely by contributing to abnormalities of AdoMet and AdoHcy metabolism. There are many puzzles. A variety of degenerative disorders as disparate as AIDS dementia complex and Alzheimer's disease have been linked either to reduced cerebrospinal fluid concentrations of AdoMet, elevated plasma or cerebrospinal fluid homocysteine, or reduced folate or cobalamin status. What, if any, is the link between these observations and the disease processes?

On a separate point, what is the function of AdoMet therapy in mood regulation? AdoMet appears to have antidepressant properties, which are speculated to act through enhanced activity of methylation steps in the synthesis and catabolism of neurotransmitters. However, depression is associated with folate deficiency much more than with cobalamin deficiency. Could the therapy be functioning at a different locus to the metabolic disorder causing the depression in many cases? Finally, what is the significance of elevated homocysteine in cognitive dysfunction? Is it a forerunner or a consequence of the disease process? Does it have an intrinsic pathogenic action, does it act by exacerbating an existing disease process, or is it merely functioning as a biological marker for an impaired folate, cobalamin, or vitamin B_6-related event?

REFERENCES

1. Allen, RH, Stabler, SP, Lindenbaum, J. Relevance of vitamins, homocysteine and other metabolites in neuropsychiatric disorders. *Eur J Pediatr* 1998; 157: S122–26.
2. Alpert, JE, Fava, M. Nutrition and depression: The role of folate. *Nutr Rev* 1997; 55: 145–49.
3. Arinami, T, Yamada, N, Yamakawa-Kobayashi, K, Hamaguchi, H, Toru, M. Methylenetetrahydrofolate reductase variant and schizophrenia/depression. *Am J Med Genet* 1997; 74: 526–28.
4. Basun, H, Forsell, LG, Bendz, R, Wahlund, L-O, Wetterberg, L, Winblad, B. Cobalamin in blood and cerebrospinal fluid in Alzheimer's disease and related disorders. *Dementia* 1991; 2: 324–32.
5. Basun, H, Fratiglioni, L, Winblad, B. Cobalamin levels are not reduced in Alzheimer's disease: Results from a population-based study. *J Am Geriatr Soc* 1994; 42: 132–36.
6. Bell, IR, Edman, JS, Selhub, J, Morrow, FD, Marby, DW, Kayne, HL, Cole, JO. Plasma homocysteine in vascular disease and in nonvascular dementia of depressed elderly people. *Acta Psychiatr Scand* 1992; 86: 386–90.
7. Bergmann, S, Shatrov, V, Ratter, F, Schiemann, S, Schulze-Osthoff, K, Lehmann, V, Adenosine and homocysteine together enhance TNF-mediated cytotoxicity but do not alter activation of nuclear factor-κB in L929 cells. *J Immunol* 1994; 153: 1736–43.
8. Bottiglieri, T. Folate, vitamin B_{12} and neuropsychiatric disorders. In *Homocysteine Metabolism: From Basic Science to Clinical Medicine*. (Graham, I, Refsum, H, Rosenberg, IH, Ueland, PM, eds.). Kluwer Boston, Academic Publishers, 1997; pp. 117–26.
9. Bressa, GM. S-Adenosyl-L-methionine (SAMe) as antidepressant: Meta-analysis of clinical studies. *Acta Neurol Scand Suppl* 1994; 154: 7–14.
10. Broch, OJ, Ueland, PM. Regional distribution of homocysteine in the mammalian brain. *J. Neurochem* 1984; 43: 1755–57.
11. Buccellato, FR, Miloso, M, Braga, M, Nicolini, G, Morabito, A, Pravettoni, G, Tredici, G, Scalabrino, G. Myelinolytic lesions in spinal cord of cobalamin-deficient rats are TNFα-mediated. *FASEB J* 1999; 13: 297–304.
12. Burkes, RL, Cohen, H, Krailo, M, Sinow, RM, Carmel, R. Low serum cobalamin levels occur frequently in the acquired immune deficiency syndrome and related disorders. *Eur J Haematol* 1987; 38: 141–47.
13. Carmel, R, Gott, PS, Waters, CH, Cairo, K, Green, R, Bondareff, W, DeGiorgio, CM, Cummings, JL. The frequently low cobalamin levels in dementia usually signify treatable metabolic, neurologic and electrophysiologic abnormalities. *Eur J Haematol* 1995; 54: 245–53.
14. Castagna, A, LeGrazie, C, Accordini, A, Giuilidori, P, Cavalli, G, Bottiglieri, T, Lazzarin, A. Cerebrospinal fluid S-adenosylmethionine (SAMe) and glutathione concentrations in HIV infection: Effect of parenteral treatment with SAMe. *Neurology* 1995; 45: 1678–83.
15. Chawla, RK, Watson, WH, Eastin, CE, Lee, EY, Schmidt, J, McClain, CJ. S-Adenosylmethionine deficiency and TNFα in lipopolysaccharide-induced hepatic injury. *Am J Physiol* 1998; 275: G125–29.
16. Clarke, R, Smith, D, Jobst, KA, Refsum, H, Sutton, L, Ueland, PM. Folate, vitamin B_{12}, and serum total homocysteine levels in confirmed Alzheimer disease. *Arch Neurol* 1998; 55: 1449–55.
17. Do, KQ, Benz, B, Sorg, O, Pellerin, L, Magistretti, PJ. β-adrenergic stimulation promotes homocysteic acid release from astrocyte cultures: Evidence for a role of astrocytes in the modulation of synaptic transmission. *J Neurochem* 1997; 68: 2386–94.
18. Dominguez, J, Ordonez, LA. Developmental changes in the folate-dependent enzymes of de novo purine biosynthesis in rat brain. *J Neurochem* 1982; 38: 625–30.
19. Dudman, NPB, Hale, SET. Endothelial and leucocyte-mediated mechanisms in homocysteine-associated occlu-

sive vascular disease. In *Homocysteine Metabolism: From Basic Science to Clinical Medicine.* (Graham, I, Refsum, H, Rosenberg, IH, Ueland, PM, eds.). Boston, Kluwer Academic Publishers, 1997; pp. 267–71.

20. Evers, S, Koch, HG, Grotemeyer, KH, Lange, B, Deufel, T, Ringelstein, EB. Features, symptoms, and neurophysiological findings in stroke associated with hyperhomocysteinemia. *Arch Neurol* 1997; 54: 1276–82.

21. Fassbender, K, Mielke, O, Bertsch, T, Nafe, B, Froschen, S, Hennerici, M. Homocysteine in cerebral macroangiography and microangiopathy. *Lancet* 1999; 353: 1586–87.

22. Fava, M, Borus, JS, Alpert, JE, Nierenberg, AA, Rosenbaum, JF, Bottiglieri, T. Folate, vitamin B$_{12}$, and homocysteine in major depressive disorder. *Am J Psychiatry* 1997; 154: 426–28.

23. Finkelstein, JD, Kyle, WE, Harris, BJ. Methionine metabolism in mammals: Regulation of homocysteine methyltransferase in rat tissue. *Arch Biochim Biophys* 1971; 146: 84–92.

24. Finkelstein, JD. Methionine metabolism in mammals. *J Nutr Biochem* 1990; 1: 228–37.

25. Finkelstein, JD. The regulation of homocysteine metabolism. In *Homocysteine Metabolism: From Basic Science to Clinical Medicine.* (Graham, I, Refsum, H, Rosenberg, IH, Ueland, PM, eds.). Boston Kluwer Academic Publishers, 1997; pp. 3–9.

26. Flott-Rahmel, B, Schurmann, M, Schluff, P, Fingerhut, R, Musshoff, U, Fowler, B, Ullrich, K. Homocysteic and homocysteine sulphinic acid exhibit excitotoxicity in organotypic cultures from rat brain. *Eur J Pediatr* 1998; 157: S112–17.

27. Folbergrova, J, Lisy, V, Haugvicova, R, Stastny, F. Specific [^{3}H]glutamate binding in the cerebral cortex and hippocampus of rats during development: Effect of homocysteine-induced seizures. *Neurochem Res* 1997; 22: 637–46.

28. Francis, PT, Poynton, A, Lowe, SL, Najlerahim, A, Bridges, PK, Bartlett, JR, Procter, AW, Bruton, CJ, Bowen, DM. Brain amino acid concentrations and Ca^{2+}-dependent release in intractable depression assessed antemortem. *Brain Res* 1989; 494: 315–24.

29. Freeman, JM, Finkelstein, JD, Mudd, SH. Folate-responsive homocystinuria and "schizophrenia". A defect in methylation due to deficient 5, 10-methylenetetrahydrofolate reductase activity. *N Engl J Med* 1975; 292: 491–96.

30. Gagliano, RG, Costanzi, JJ. Paraplegia following intrathecal methotrexate: Report of a case and review of the literature. *Cancer* 1976; 37: 1663–68.

31. Gharib, A, Sarda, N, Chabannes, B, Cronenberger, L, Pacheco, H. The regional concentrations of S-adenosyl-L-methionine, S-adenosyl-L-homocysteine and adenosine in rat brain. *J Neurochem* 1982; 38: 810–15.

32. Ghosh, SK, Paik, WK, Kim, S. Purification and molecular identification of two protein methylase I from calf brain. *J Biol Chem* 1988; 263: 19024–33.

33. Goggins, M, Scott, JM, Weir, DG. Methylation of cortical brain proteins from patients with HIV infection. *Acta Neurol Scand* 1999; 100: 326–31.

34. Grandes, P, Do, KQ, Morino, P, Cuenod, M, Streit, P. Homocysteate, an excitatory transmitter candidate localised in glia. *Eur J Neurosci* 1991; 3: 1370–73.

35. Grange, E, Gharib, A, Lepetit, P, Guillaud, J, Sarda, N, Bobillier, P. Brain protein synthesis in the conscious rat using L[^{35}S]methionine: Relationship of methionine specific activity between plasma and precursor compartment and evaluation of methionine metabolic pathways. *J Neurochem* 1992; 59: 1437–43.

36. Healton, EB, Savage, DG, Brust, JC, Garrett, TJ, Lindenbaum, J. Neurologic aspects of cobalamin deficiency. *Medicine* 1991; 70: 229–45.

37. Henin, D, Smith, TW, DeGirolami, U, Sughayer, M, Hauw, JJ. Neuropathology of the spinal cord in acquired immune deficiency syndrome. *Hum Pathol* 1992; 23: 1106–14.

38. Herbert, V. Experimental nutritional folate deficiency in man. *Trans Assoc Am Physicians* 1961; 75: 307–20.

39. Herbert, V, Zalusky, R. Selective concentration of folic acid activity in cerebrospinal fluid. *Fed Proc* 1961; 20: 453.

40. Hyland, K, Smith, I, Bottiglieri, T, Perry, J, Wendel, U, Clayton, PT, Leonard, JV. Demyelination and decreased S-adenosylmethionine in 5,10-methylenetetrahydrofolate reductase deficiency. *Neurology* 1988; 38: 459–62.

41. Joosten, E, van den Berg, A, Riezler, R, Naurath, HJ, Lindenbaum, J, Stabler, SP, Allen, RH. Metabolic evidence that deficiencies of vitamin B$_{12}$ (cobalamin), folate, and vitamin B$_6$ occur commonly in elderly people. *Am J Clin Nutr* 1993; 58: 468–76.

42. Kang, SS, Wong, PW, Becker, N. Protein-bound homocyst(e)ine in normal subjects and in patients with homocystinuria. *Pediatr Res* 1979; 13: 1141–43.

43. Keating, JN, Trimble, KC, Mulcahy, F, Scott, JM, Weir, DG. Evidence of brain methyltransferase inhibition and early brain involvement in HIV positive patients. *Lancet* 1991; 337: 935–39.

44. Kieburtz, KD, Giang, DW, Schiffer, RB, Vakil, N. Abnormal vitamin B$_{12}$ metabolism in human immunodeficiency virus infection: Association with neurological dysfunction. *Arch Neurol* 1991; 48: 312–14.

45. Kim, S, Lim, IK, Park, G-H, Paik, WK. Biological methylation of myelin basic protein: Enzymology and biological significance. *Int J Biochem Cell Biol* 1997; 29: 743–51.

46. Kotb, M, Geller, AM, Markham, GD, Kredich, NM, De La Rosa, J, Beachey, EH. Antigenic conservation of primary structural regions of S-adenosylmethionine synthetase. *Biochim Biophys Acta* 1990; 1040: 137–44.

47. Kranich, O, Dringen, R, Sandberg, M, Hamprecht, B. Utilization of cysteine and cysteine precursors for the synthesis of glutathione in astroglial cultures: Preference for cystine. *Glia* 1998; 22: 11–8.

48. Lawrence, F, Robert-Gero, M. Natural and synthetic analogs of S-adenosylhomocysteine and protein methylation. In *Protein Methylation*, 2nd ed. (Paik, WK, Kim, S, eds.). CRC Press, Boca Raton, Fla, 1990; pp. 305–40.

49. Layzer, RB, Fishman, RA, Schafer, JA. Neuropathy following abuse of nitrous oxide. *Neurology* 1978; 28: 504–6.

50. Lee, CC, Surtees, R, Duchen, LW. Distal motor axonopathy and central nervous system myelin vacuolation caused by cycloleucine, an inhibitor of methionine adenosyltransferase. *Brain* 1992; 115: 935–55.

51. Lehmann, V, Ratter, F. S-Adenosylhomocysteine as a modulator of tumor necrosis factor (TNF)-mediated cytotoxicity: Mode of action. In *III Workshop on Methionine Metabolism: Molecular Mechanisms and Clinical Implications.* (Mato, JM, Caballero, A, eds.). Madrid, Instituto de Investigaciones Biomedicas, 1996; pp. 85–94.

52. Lever, EG, Elwes, RD, Williams, A, Reynolds, EH. Subacute combined degeneration of the cord due to folate deficiency: Response to methyl folate treatment. *J Neurol Neurosurg Psychiatry* 1986; 49: 1203–7.

53. Lindenbaum, J, Healton, EB, Savage, DG, Brust, JC, Garrett, TJ, Podell, ER, Marcell, PD, Stabler, SP, Allen, RH. Neuropsychiatric disorders caused by cobalamin deficiency in the absence of anemia or macrocytosis. *N Engl J Med* 1988; 318: 1720–28.

54. Lipton, SA, Kim, WK, Choi, YB, Kumar, S, D'Emilia, DM, Rayudu, PV, Arnelle, DR, Stamler, JS. Neurotoxicity associated with dual actions of homocysteine at the *N*-methyl-D-aspartate receptor. *Proc Natl Acad Sci USA* 1997; 94: 5923–28.

55. Long, M, Weir, D, Scott, J. Source of methyl groups in brain and nerve tissue in the rat. *J Neurochem* 1989; 52: 377–80.

56. McCaddon, A, Davies, G, Hudson, P, Tandy, S, Cattell, H. Total serum homocysteine in senile dementia of Alzheimer type. *Int J Geriatr Psychiatry* 1998; 13: 235–39.

57. McClain, LD, Carl, GF, Bridgers, WF. Distribution of folic acid coenzymes and folate dependent enzymes in mouse brain. *J Neurochem* 1975; 24: 719–22.

58. McKeever, MP, Weir, DG, Molloy, AM, Scott, JM. Betaine-homocysteine methyltransferase: Organ distribution in man, pig and rat and subcellular distribution in the rat. *Clin Sci* 1991; 81: 551–56.

59. McKeever, MP, Molloy, AM, Weir, DG, Young, PB, Kennedy, DG, Kennedy, S, Scott, JM. An abnormal methylation ratio induces hypomethylation *in vitro* in the brain of pig and man, but not in rat. *Clin Sci* 1995; 88: 73–9.

60. McKeever, MP, Molloy, AM, Young, PB, Kennedy, S, Kennedy, DG, Scott, JM, Weir, DG. Demonstration of hypomethylation of proteins in the brain of pigs (but not in rats) associated with chronic B$_{12}$ inactivation. *Clin Sci* 1995; 88: 471–77.

61. Mann, S, Hill, MW. Activation and inactivation of striatal tyrosine hydroxylase: The effect of pH, ATP, cyclic AMP, S-adenosylmethionine and S-adenosylhomocysteine. *Biochem Pharmacol* 1983; 32: 3369–74.

62. Manzoor, M, Runzie, J. Folate responsive neuropathy: Reports of ten cases. *Br Med J* 1976; i: 1176–78.

63. Mares, P, Folbergrova, J, Langmeier, M, Haugvicova, R, Kubova, H. Convulsant action of D,L-homocysteic acid and its stereoisomers in immature rats. *Epilepsia* 1997; 38: 767–76.

64. Meldrum, B, Garthwaite, J. Excitatory amino acid neurotoxicity and neurodegenerative disease. *Trends Pharmacol Sci* 1990; 11: 379–87.

65. Miller, JW, Shukitt-Hale, B, Villalobos-Molina, R, Nadeau, MR, Selhub, J, Joseph, JA. Effect of L-dopa and the catechol-O-methyltransferase inhibitor Ro 41-0960 on sulfur amino acid metabolites in rats. *Clin Neuropharmacol* 1997; 20: 55–66.

66. Mitsui, K, Teraoka, H, Tsukada, K. Complete purification and immunochemical analysis of S-adenosylmethionine synthetase from bovine brain. *J Biol Chem* 1988; 263: 11211–16.

67. Molloy, AM, Weir, DG, Kennedy, DG, Kennedy, S, Scott, JM. A new high performance liquid chromatography method for the simultaneous measurement of S-adenosylmethionine and S-adenosylhomocysteine: Concentrations in pig tissue after inactivation of methionine synthase by nitrous oxide. *Biomed Chromatogr* 1990; 4: 257–60.

68. Molloy, AM, Orsi, B, Kennedy, DG, Kennedy, S, Weir, DG, Scott, JM. The relationship between the activity of methionine synthase and the ratio of S-adenosylmethionine to S-adenosylhomocysteine in the brain and other tissues of the pig. *Biochem Pharmacol* 1992; 44: 1349–55.

69. Morrison, LD, Smith, DD, Kish, SJ. Brain S-adenosylmethionine levels are severely decreased in Alzheimer's disease. *J Neurochem* 1996; 67: 1328–31.

70. Mudd, SH, Skovby, F, Levy, HL, Pettigrew, KD, Wilken, B, Pyeritz, RE, Andria, G, Boers, GHJ, Bromberg, IL, Cerone, R, Fowler, B, Gröbe, H, Schmidt, H, and Schweitzer, L. The natural history of homocystinuria due to cystathionine β-synthase deficiency. *Am J Hum Genet* 1985; 37: 1–31.

71. Muller, T, Werne, B, Fowler, B, Kuhn, W. Nigral endothelial dysfunction, homocysteine, and Parkinson's disease. *Lancet* 1999; 354: 126–27.

72. Murphy, JV, Thome, LM, Michals, K, Matalon, RJ. Folic acid responsive rages, seizures and homocystinuria. *Inherit Metab Dis* 1985; 8 Suppl 2: 109–10.

73. Nilsson, K, Gustafson, L, Faldt, R, Andersson, A, Brattstrom, L, Lindgren, A, Israelsson, B, Hultberg, B. Hyperhomocysteinaemia—a common finding in a psychogeriatric population. *Eur J Clin Invest* 1996; 26: 853–59.

74. Nijst, TQ, Wevers, RA, Schoonderwaldt, HC, Hommes, OR, de Haan, AF. Vitamin B$_{12}$ and folate concentrations in serum and cerebrospinal fluid of neurological patients with special reference to multiple sclerosis and dementia. *J Neurol Neurosurg Psychiatry* 1990; 53: 951–54.

74a. Nourhashemi, F, Gillette-Guyonnet, S, Andrieu, S, Ghisolfi, A, Ousset, PJ, Grandjean, H, Grand, A, Pous, J, Vellas, B, Albarede, J-L. Alzheimer disease: Protective factors. *Am J Clin Nutr* 2000; 71 (Suppl): 643S–49S.

75. Ohmori, S, Kodama, H, Ikegami, T, Mizuhara, S, Oura, T, Isshiki, G, Uemura, I. Unusual sulfur-containing amino acids in the urine of homocystinuric patients. III. Homocysteic acid, homocysteine sulfinic acid, S-(carboxymethylthio)homocysteine and S-(3-hydroxy-3-carboxy-n-propyl)homocysteine. *Physiol Chem Phys Med NMR* 1972; 4: 286–94.

76. Otero-Losada, ME, Rubio, MC. Acute effects of S-adenosylmethionine on cholaminergic central function. *Eur. J. Pharmacol* 1990; 163: 353–56.

77. Paik, WK, Kim, S. Protein methylation. In *Enzymology of Protein Methylation* (Meister, A, ed.). John Wiley & Sons, New York, 1980; pp. 112–141.

78. Parsons, RB, Waring, RH, Ramsden, DB, Williams, AC. In vitro effect of the cysteine metabolites homocysteic

acid, homocysteine and cysteic acid upon human neuronal cell lines. *Neurotoxicology* 1998; 19: 599–603.

79. Pennypacker, LC, Allen, RH, Kelly, JP, Mathews, LM, Grigsby, J, Kaye, K, Lindenbaum, J. High prevalence of cobalamin deficiency in elderly outpatients. *J Am Geriatr Soc* 1992; 40: 1197–204.

80. Petito, CK, Navia, BA, Cho, E-S, Jordan, BD, George, DC, Price, RW. Vacuolar myelopathy pathologically resembling subacute combined degeneration in patients with the acquired immunodeficiency syndrome. *N Engl J Med* 1985; 312: 874–79.

81. Price, RW, Brew, BJ, Sidtis, J, Rosenblum, M, Scheck, AC, Cleary, P. The brain in AIDS: Central nervous system HIV-1 infection and AIDS dementia complex. *Science* 1988; 239: 586–92.

82. Quinn, CT, Griener, JC, Bottiglieri, T, Hyland, K, Farrow, A, Kamen, BA. Elevation of homocysteine and excitatory amino acid neurotransmitters in the CSF of children who receive methotrexate for the treatment of cancer. *J Clin Oncol* 1997; 15: 2800–6.

83. Regland, B, Johansson, BV, Grenfeldt, B, Hjelmgren, LT, Medhus, M. Homocysteinemia is a common feature of schizophrenia. *J Neural Transm Gen Sect* 1995; 100: 165–69.

84. Reynolds, EH, Rothfeld, P, Pincus, JH. Neurological disease associated with folate deficiency. *Br Med J* 1973; 2: 398–400.

85. Reynolds, EH. Multiple sclerosis and vitamin B$_{12}$ metabolism. *J Neurol Neurosurg Psychiatry* 1992; 55: 339–40.

86. Riggs, KM, Spiro, A 3rd, Tucker, K, Rush, D. Relations of vitamin B$_{12}$, vitamin B$_6$, folate, and homocysteine to cognitive performance in the Normative Aging Study. *Am J Clin Nutr* 1996; 63: 306–14.

87. Robertson, KR, Stern, RA, Hall, CD, Perkins, DO, Wilkins, JW, Gortner, DT, Donovan, MK, Messenheimer, JA, Whaley, R, Evans, DL. Vitamin B$_{12}$ deficiency and nervous system disease in HIV infection. *Arch Neurol* 1993; 50: 807–11.

88. Rosenblatt, DS, Whitehead, VM. Cobalamin and folate deficiency: Acquired and hereditary disorders in children. *Semin Hematol* 1999; 36: 19–34.

89. Scalabrino, G, Monzio-Compagnoni, B, Feroli, ME, Lorenzini, EC, Chiodini, E, Candiani, R. Subacute combined degeneration and induction of ornithine decarboxylase in spinal cord of total gastrectomized rats. *Lab Invest* 1990; 62: 297–304.

90. Scalabrino, G, Lorenzini, EC, Monzio-Campagnoni, B, Colombi, RP, Chiodini, E, Buccellato, FR. Subacute combined degeneration of the spinal cords of totally gastrectomized rats. Ornithine decarboxylase induction, cobalamin status and astroglial reaction. *Lab Invest* 1995; 72: 114–21.

91. Scalabrino, G, Buccellato, FR, Tredici, G, Morabito, A, Lorenzini, EC, Allen, RH, Lindenbaum, J. Enhanced levels of biochemical markers for cobalamin deficiency in totally gastrectomized rats: Uncoupling of the enhancement from the severity of spongy vacuolation in spinal cord. *Exp Neurol* 1997; 144: 258–65.

92. Scott, JM, Molloy, AM, Kennedy, DG, Kennedy, S, Weir, DG. Effects of the disruption of transmethylation in the central nervous system: An animal model. *Acta Neurol Scand* 1994; 89 (Suppl 154): 27–31.

93. Scott, JM, Dinn, JJ, Wilson, P, Weir, DG. Pathogenesis of subacute combined degeneration: A result of methyl group deficiency. *Lancet* 1981; ii: 334–37.

93a. Selhub, J, Bagley, LC, Miller, J, Rosenberg, IH. B vitamins, homocysteine and neurocognitive function in the elderly. *Am J Clin Nutr* 2000; 71 (suppl): 614S–20S.

94. Shorvon, SD, Carney, MW, Chanarin, I, Reynolds, EH. The neuropsychiatry of megaloblastic anaemia. *Br Med J* 1980; 281: 1036–38.

95. Sitaram, BR, Sitaram, M, Traut, M, Chapman, CB. Nyctohemeral rhythm in the levels of S-adenosylmethionine in the rat pineal gland and its relationship to melatonin biosynthesis. *J Neurochem* 1995; 65: 1887–94.

96. Spector, R, Coakley, G, Blakely, R. Methionine recycling in brain: A role for folates and vitamin B$_{12}$. *J Neurochem* 1980; 34: 132–37.

97. Sturman, JA, Gaull, GE, Niemann, WH. Cystathionine synthesis and degradation in brain, liver and kidney of the developing monkey. *J Neurochem* 1976; 26: 457–63.

98. Suleiman, SA, Spector, R. Methionine synthetase in mammalian brain: Function, development and distribution. *Life Sci* 1980; 27: 2427–32.

99. Sunden, SLF, Renduchintala, MS, Park, EI, Miklasz, SD, Garrow, TA. Betaine-homocysteine methyltransferase expression in porcine and human tissues and chromosomal localization of the human gene. *Arch Biochem Biophys* 1997; 345: 171–74.

100. Surtees, R, Hyland, K, Smith, I. Central nervous system methyl group metabolism in children with neurological complication of HIV infection. *Lancet* 1990; 335: 619–21.

101. Surtees, R, Heales, S, Bowron, A. Association of cerebrospinal fluid deficiency of 5-methyltetrahydrofolate, but not S-adenosylmethionine, with reduced concentrations of the acid metabolites of 5-hydroxytryptamine and dopamine. *Clin Sci* 1994; 86: 697–702.

102. Surtees, R, Bowron, A, Leonard, J. Cerebrospinal fluid and plasma total homocysteine and related metabolites in children with cystathionine β-synthase deficiency: Effect of treatment. *Pediatr Res* 1997; 42: 577–82.

103. Surtees, R, Clelland, J, Hann, I. Demyelination and single-carbon transfer pathway metabolites during the treatment of acute lymphoblastic leukemia. *J Clin Oncol* 1998; 16: 1505–11.

104. Surtees, R. Demyelination and inborn errors of the single carbon transfer pathway. *Eur J Pediatr* 1998; 157: S118–21.

105. Tallan, HH, Moore, S, Stein, WH. L-Cystathionine in human brain. *J Biol Chem* 1958; 230: 707–16.

106. Trimble, KC, Goggins, MG, Molloy, AM, Mulcahy, F, Scott, JM, Weir, DG. Vitamin B$_{12}$ deficiency is not the cause of HIV-associated neuropathy. *AIDS* 1993; 7: 1132–33.

107. Van der Westhuyzen, J, Fernandez-Costa, F, Metz, J. Cobalamin inactivation by nitrous oxide produces severe neurological impairment in fruit bats: Protection by methionine and aggravation by folates. *Life Sci* 1982; 31: 2001–10.

108. Weir, DG, Keating, JN, Molloy, AM, McPartlin, J, Kennedy, S, Blanchflower, J, Kennedy, DG, Rice, D, Scott, JM. Methylation deficiency causes B₁₂-associated neuropathy in the pig. *J Neurochem* 1988; 51: 1949–52.

109. Weir, DG, Molloy, AM, Keating, JN, Young, PB, Kennedy, S, Kennedy, DG, Scott, JM. Correlation of the ratio of *S*-adenosylmethionine to *S*-adenosylhomocysteine in the brain and cerebrospinal fluid of the pig: Implications for the determination of this methylation ratio in human brain. *Clin Sci* 1992; 82: 93–7.

110. Weir, DG, Scott, JM. The biochemical basis of the neuropathy in cobalamin deficiency. *Clin Haematol* 1995; 8: 479–97.

111. Weitman, SD, Weinberg, AG, Coney, LR, Zurawski, VR, Jennings, DS, Kamen, BA. Cellular localization of the folate receptor: Potential role in drug toxicity and folate homeostasis. *Cancer Res* 1992; 52: 6708–11.

112. Wu, D, Pardridge, WM. Blood-brain barrier transport of reduced folic acid. *Pharm Res* 1999; 16: 415–19.

113. Wuerthele, SE, Yasuda, RP, Freed, WJ, Hoffer, BJ. The effect of local application of homocysteine on neuronal activity in the central nervous system of the rat. *Life Sci* 1982; 31: 2683–91.

18

Methodologies of Testing

KARSTEN RASMUSSEN
JAN MØLLER

The increasing clinical interest in measuring homocysteine has called for rapid, automated, and reliable methods with high sample capacity, suitable for routine use, which could meet the stringent requirements of a clinical assay. This chapter discusses the current analytical methods for measuring plasma total homocysteine, which were developed in the mid to late 1980s. Equally important issues are the role of controlled blood collection, stability of samples, analytical performance based on current quality goals and laboratory requirements, and quality assurance and interpretation of results.

Historical Aspects

In the late 1960s, the disulfide homocysteine was detected in plasma of patients with homocystinuria, whereas it was not detectable at all in normal human plasma. Sometimes, if homocystinuric plasma was chromatographed on an ion-exchange amino acid analyzer promptly after blood was drawn, free homocysteine could be detected as a shoulder on the leading edge of the methionine peak (42). In the mid-1970s, when the second-generation amino acid analyzers became available, the reduced form, free homocysteine, was detected in the acid-soluble fraction of plasma or serum from healthy subjects. However, the level of analytical sensitivity necessary for the clinical application of measuring homocysteine in plasma as a marker of vitamin deficiency states, and in studies of homocysteine and occlusive vascular disease, was first achieved in the mid-1980s with the introduction of measurement of total homocysteine in plasma after addition of a reducing agent.

In 1993, Ueland et al. (70) reviewed the subject of techniques for the determination of homocysteine in plasma. Since then, new methods have been developed and old techniques have been refined. This chapter focuses mainly on the more recent literature and developments in this area.

Biochemical Aspects

Homocysteine in plasma probably derives from cellular homocysteine. The site of formation is uncertain, but in vitro experiments point to the liver and proliferating cells as important sources (55). The reactive sulfhydryl group in free homocysteine readily forms disulfide bonds with another molecule of homocysteine, cysteine, or a protein sulfhydryl group to form the circulating oxidized species of homocysteine: homocystine, homocysteine-cysteine mixed disulfide, or protein bound homocysteine. Therefore, the concentration of free homocysteine in plasma is very low and accounts for less than 2% of total homocysteine in normal subjects (5, 34, 35); homocystine and homocysteine-cysteine mixed disulfide represent approximately 10% to 15%, and protein-bound homocysteine accounts for more than 80% of the total measured homocysteine in normal plasma (23, 25, 27, 52). Binding of homocysteine to plasma proteins seems to be saturable, with a maximal capacity of about 140 μmol/L (70, 74).

Measurement of Free Homocysteine in Plasma

Determination of free homocysteine has largely been abandoned because reliable measurement requires immediate acid treatment and centrifugation of plasma. This procedure is inconvenient and, indeed, impossible in most clinical settings (70). There is also no documentation that it provides more useful clinical information than measurement of total homocysteine in plasma.

Measurement of Total Homocysteine in Plasma

The term *total homocysteine,* as applied to biological samples such as plasma, refers to the sum of the concentrations of all the aforementioned homocysteine species in plasma (see also Chapter 2). Total homocysteine is measured after chemical reduction of the disulfides. Early studies used ion-exchange amino acid analyzers (3) or radioenzymatic determination (52), but newer methods include capillary gas chromatography, stable-isotope dilution combined with capillary gas chromatography-mass spectrometry (GC-MS) or with liquid chromatography electrospray tandem mass spectrometry, capillary electrophoresis, and high-performance liquid chromatography (HPLC). Today, total homocysteine is usually measured by an HPLC assay, which has become the preferred approach because it is easily automated (73). However, an easily performed immunoassay (60), which may simplify measurement of total homocysteine in the future, has been found useful in a multicenter evaluation (40a).

Preanalytical Variables

Because homocysteine is bound to plasma albumin to a large extent (52), the position of the person during venipuncture and the amount of venous stasis may affect the measured value.

Effect of Posture during Sample Collection

Only two studies have been published on the effect of posture on homocysteine, both in 1999. Thirup and Ekelund (65) found that homocysteine declined up to 29.9% (3.5 μmol/L), with a mean of 19% (2.1 μmol/L) in nine healthy adults after 30 minutes at supine rest; the changes correlated only weakly with the albumin change. Rasmussen et al. (49) observed a decline in homocysteine of up to 15.3% (1.7 μmol/L), with a mean of 6.3% (0.54 μmol/L) in 24 healthy subjects after 30 minutes in the horizontal posture. The decrease correlated significantly with the decrease in albumin, and the homocysteine/albumin ratio did not change with posture. Because homocysteine is predominantly bound to albumin, the change in homocysteine with posture is explained by orthostatic changes. The total analytical imprecision was 3.0%, so the position of the subject during venipuncture may have a greater effect on the laboratory result than the analysis itself. Thus, blood should not be collected with the patient at supine rest.

Effect of Venous Stasis

Few data concerning a possible effect of tourniquet application are available. The effect of a 3-minute tourniquet application — the duration of tourniquet time that is often required when blood is drawn from a patient whose veins are difficult to see or palpate, or when several blood specimens are taken at one venipuncture — was evaluated (49). An observed 2.8% increase (range of increases, –7.4% to 13.6%) was relatively small compared with the 8.1% intraindividual variation and does not add an appreciable variation to measurement of homocysteine. The increase correlated significantly, as expected, with the increase in albumin, and the homocysteine/albumin ratio did not change with application of the tourniquet.

Stability of Homocysteine in Whole Blood

After sampling, the blood cells continue to produce and release homocysteine, resulting in an artificial increase of homocysteine in plasma at ~10%/hour at room temperature (6, 72). For this reason, homocysteine should never be measured in serum, because the homocysteine concentration will increase by 5% to 10% during the time required for completion of coagulation before centrifugation of the blood specimen. Cooling stabilized blood on ice and separating the plasma from the cells as soon as possible, or at least within 1 hour, inhibits the cellular release of homocysteine (6, 72). However, this procedure will be impractical in many clinical settings.

Alternatively, inhibitors of cell metabolism have been used. Ubbink et al. (69) demonstrated that sodium fluoride inhibits the release of homocysteine from the cells. Investigation of the dose-response effect found that adding 2 g/L (48 mmol/L) or 4 g/L (95 mmol/L) of sodium fluoride to the blood minimized the increase of homocysteine for the first 2 hours at room temperature (Figure 18.1). Sodium fluoride inhibits cell metabolism but also results in hyperosmosis, drawing intracellular water into the plasma and reducing the concentrations of all plasma constituents including homocysteine (24). Tubes with sodium fluoride and heparin as an anticoagulant are readily available, making their use more practical than collecting ethylenediaminetetraacetic acid (EDTA) plasma on ice.

Several other procedures have been suggested. However, addition of acidic citrate (75) does not seem to be more efficient than sodium fluoride, and even though the proposed blood collection tubes are available commercially, they are not easily accessible everywhere. Lysing EDTA-anticoagulated blood and measuring homocysteine in the lysate has been suggested (48). The concentration of homocysteine in the lysate seems to be stable, but because the homocysteine concentration within the erythrocytes is very low, the resulting concentration in the hemolysate, depending on the hematocrit, will be less than half the concentration in the plasma, necessitating the use of special reference and decision limits.

A promising alternative is 3-deazaadenosine, a specific inhibitor of S-adenosylhomocysteine hydrolase

Increase in Homocysteine

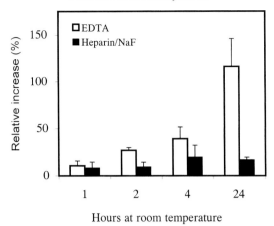

Fig. 18.1. The effect of incubation at room temperature (22 to 24°C) on the concentration of homocysteine in blood. Two blood samples, collected with EDTA and heparin with sodium fluoride, 4 g/L blood, respectively, were drawn from five volunteers and left to incubate at room temperature. Aliquots of blood were centrifuged immediately, and after 1, 2, 4, and 24 hours. Homocysteine was measured in all samples within the same run. The mean relative increases as a function of time is depicted. The error bars represent the 95% confidence interval. In EDTA plasma, the homocysteine concentration rises at the rate of 10% per hour in the first few hours (39).

(Metabolic Diagram, Reaction 3) (1). However, 3-deazaadenosine is contraindicated for current immunoassays, which are based on the conversion of homocysteine to S-adenosylhomocysteine by the hydrolase (30). Vacuum tubes for blood collection containing an appropriate amount of 3-deazaadenosine in addition to EDTA or heparin will have to be made available.

The production of homocysteine by the cells after blood sampling is a major, if not the major, source of error when measuring homocysteine. If possible, collecting blood on ice and then separating the plasma from the cells as soon as possible and at least within 1 hour is still the best procedure. However, if that is impossible in the clinical setting, collecting blood in a heparin tube with 2 or 4 g of sodium fluoride/L blood can be a practical alternative and prevents a significant increase in homocysteine for 2 hours.

Stability of Homocysteine in Plasma and Appropiate Anticoagulants

After plasma is separated from the cells, homocysteine is stable for at least 2 days at ambient temperature, 3 to 4 days at 4°C and more than 1 year at −20°C. The choice of anticoagulant depends on the subsequent analytical procedure, but most methods are compatible with standard concentrations of EDTA or heparin.

General Considerations of Methodology

Reduction

Because less than 2% of the total homocysteine in plasma is in the reduced form, any analytical method must include a reduction step before separation and detection. The use of the sulfhydryl-containing reagents dithiothreitol, dithioerythritol and mercaptoethanol, sodium or potassium borohydride, and tri-*n*-butylphosphine (referred to as TBP in the literature) has been described (70); more recently the use of tris(2-carboxylethyl)phosphine (referred to as TCEP) has been documented (22, 43, 44). Most of the reagents are unstable in solution and have additional specific drawbacks; thus the choice of reagent or combination of reagents depends on the subsequent analytical procedures. The sulfhydryl-containing reagents may compete with homocysteine in derivatization; the borohydride reduction results in gas development, which might be impractical in automated procedures; tri-*n*-butylphosphine and other tri-alkylphosphine reagents are almost insoluble in water and must be dissolved in dimethylformamide. However, tris(2-carboxylethyl)phosphine is more soluble in water and is reported to be quite stable as well (22).

Reoxidation

After removal of the reducing agent, homocysteine can undergo reoxidization to form disulfides. One way to correct for this occurrence is to use internal standards. However, only homocysteine labeled with stable isotopes (i.e., deuterium) corrects accurately for reoxidation. Stable-isotope internal standards, quantitated by mass spectrometry, have the additional advantage of correcting for varying efficiency of the initial reduction step (63). Alternatively, reoxidation can be limited by speeding up the subsequent analytical steps, or it can be inhibited by the use of EDTA (70).

Current Analytical Methods

A variety of methods for measuring total homocysteine, comprehensively reviewed in 1993 (70), was introduced during the 1980s. These include the most widely applied HPLC separation and subsequent fluorescent detection methods, radioenzymatic assay, gas chromatography combined with mass spectrometry, and determination by optimized amino acid analyzers.

Generally, these methods were laborious, and their analytical precision was inadequate for investigating the slight increases in homocysteine concentration (e.g., <3 μmol/L) that constitute a risk factor for vascular disease. The growing clinical interest in measuring homocysteine called for rapid, automated, and reliable methods with high sample capacity that were suitable for routine use and that could meet the stringent requirements of a clinical assay.

Capillary Gas Chromatography

Kataoka et al. (28) described a method for determining sulfhydryl-containing amino acids by gas chromatography with flame detection. Plasma samples were chemically reduced with sodium borohydride; and homocysteine and related aminothiols, such as cysteine and cysteinylglycine in plasma together with added S-2-aminoethyl-L-cysteine (as an internal standard), were analyzed as their N,S-diisopropoxycarbonyl methyl ester derivatives. The sample preparation included three extractions with diethyl ether. The sensitivity of the assay was 2 μmol/L for total homocysteine. Recoveries of 10 μmol/L homocysteine added to plasma samples containing 4.3 and 10.5 μmol homocysteine/L were 95% and 103%, respectively (n = 4). The interassay coefficient of variation (CV) for the aminothiols was 5.5% to 14.5% (n = 4). However, the imprecision for homocysteine was not specified explicitly and sample capacity of the method was not stated.

Capillary Gas Chromatography–Mass Spectrometry

The first gas chromatography–mass spectrometry (GC-MS) method for quantifying total homocysteine in blood from normal humans was developed by Stabler et al. (63). It involved laborious sample preparation. In 1990 to 1993, the authors simplified the method and made it more robust (2, 62). The method is based on the stable-isotope dilution principle. The steps before GC-MS are: 1) addition of homocystine, which contains eight deuterium atoms (internal standard) to the sample before reduction of disulfides, including the deuterated internal standard; 2) reduction with dithiothreitol; 3) solid-phase extraction of homocysteine from plasma, together with the reduced internal standard, onto an anion-exchange column; and then, 4) elution with acetic acid in methanol. The eluate is taken to dryness by vacuum centrifugation and the residue is then derivatized in silylating reagents. The resulting *tert*-butyldimethylsilyl derivatives are separated and quantified by capillary GC-MS with the mass spectrometer in the selected-ion monitoring mode. After correcting for the 1.7% natural iso-

tope abundance contributing to the internal standard peak, the ratio of unlabeled homocysteine to labeled homocysteine is measured. The variable recovery through sample preparation steps and reoxidation of homocysteine are corrected for by the inclusion of deuterated homocystine as an internal standard, which results in an accurate assay.

When assayed 11 times over 6-months, a normal control sample (8.0 μmol/L) gave a CV of 5.3% (62). Allen et al. (2) reported that the within-run CV is approximately 2% and the between-run CV is approximately 6%, which gives a total analytical imprecision of about 6.3%. An attractive feature is that with some modifications, codetermination of cysteine, methionine, cystathionine, N,N-dimethylglycine, N-methylglycine, methylmalonic acid, 2-methylcitric acid, and betaine is possible. Ueland et al. (70) reported that with semiautomated pipetting equipment, a technician can process 320 samples in 8 hours. Using a benchtop GC-MS equipped with an autosampler, the capacity is about 160 derivatized samples per 24 hours.

Møller and Rasmussen (39) modified the GC-MS assay by reducing the amount of d_8-homocystine added to plasma, resulting in smaller imprecision and analytical inaccuracy at borderline homocysteine concentrations (12 to 14 μmol/L). The method provides the most useful clinical information in this range, namely from high-normal to moderately above normal. Furthermore, the rate of temperature increase during gas chromatography was decreased to obtain a good separation. The method proved to be linear over the concentration range examined (0.5 to 300 μmol/L) (51). The internal 4-month quality-control system (n = 82) yielded total analytical imprecisions of 0.36 and 1.28 μmol/L standard deviations at mean concentrations of 7.1 and 23.2 μmol/L, respectively, which corresponds to CVs of 5.1% and 5.5% (51). A technician using manual pipetting equipment can process about 90 samples a day, and a GC-MS equipped with an autosampler has a capacity of 90 derivatized samples per 24 hours.

Pietzsch et al. (46) described an assay for total homocysteine using tri-n-butylphosphine as reductant and d_8-homocystine as internal standard. After precipitation of protein with sulfosalicylic acid, total homocysteine and the internal standard are isolated by cation exchange, dried by lyophilization, and derivatized to $N(O,S)$-ethoxycarbonyl ethyl esters, which are extracted with chloroform and injected into a capillary GC-MS. The method proved to be linear over the concentration range examined (0.5 to 280 μmol/L). The authors reported good precision (within-day CV < 3.2%, between-day CV < 3.5%, equivalent to a total analytical imprecision < 4.7%); however, the number of measurements and the length of the study period were not stated. The method is said to be less laborious and time consuming and requires cheaper reagents than the GC-MS methods most widely used. With a benchtop GC-MS equipped with an autosampler, the capacity is about 100 samples per 24 hours, but apparently it takes 3 days to work up a batch of about 100 samples. Another drawback is that the derivatized samples have sufficient stability for "at least 3 days", making reruns impractical.

Sass and Endres (58) described an assay using dithiothreitol as reductant and unlabeled aminoethylcystine as internal standard. These thiols are derivatized to N(O,S)-propoxycarbonyl propyl esters. The within- and between-assay CVs in 3 "normal plasma samples" were 5.3% and 11.1%, respectively, adding up to a total analytical imprecision of about 12.3%. The method requires only inexpensive and easy to obtain chemicals, but this hardly justifies the use of GC-MS instrumentation in an imprecise assay not using isotope dilution.

Liquid Chromatography Electrospray Tandem Mass Spectrometry

Magera et al. (31a) developed a liquid chromatography electrospray tandem mass spectrometry method based on the analysis of 100 µl of plasma with d_8-homocystine (2 nmol) added as internal standard. The method proved to be linear over the concentration range examined (2.5 to 60 µmol/L). Interassay and intraassay CVs were 2.9% to 5.9% and 3.6% to 5.6%, respectively, at mean concentrations of 3.9, 22.7, and 52.8 µmol/L. Preparation of a batch of 40 specimens is completed in less than 1 hour, and the analysis of 200 samples requires no more than 10 hours of instrument time, which could be conveniently set up overnight. The assay awaits further evaluation.

HPLC Assays

Fluorescence Detection Ubbink et al. (68) improved the method of Araki and Sato (8) who reduced plasma with tri-n-butylphosphine and derivatized with ammonium 7-fluoro-2,1,3-benzoxadiazole-4-sulfonate (SBD-F). By modifying the chromatographic conditions, they separated and quantified the homocysteine derivatives by gradient elution of a reversed-phase column. Their system is able to resolve the homocysteine, cysteine, glutathione, and cysteinylglycine adducts within 6 minutes. The authors reported within- and between-run CVs of 4.5 and 6.6%, respectively (mean concentration = 8.2 µmol/L; n = 12), with a total analytical imprecision of about 8.1%.

Vester and Rasmussen (72) also improved the method of Araki and Sato (8) and made it more suit-able for routine clinical use. The most important changes were the use of a plasma pool for calibration instead of the buffer and the addition of an internal standard, mercaptopropionylglycine, that corrects for inaccuracy and ensures precision. The total imprecision is 3.0% (mean concentration = 8.92 µmol/L; n = 11 assays done over 4 weeks). The method is sensitive, with a limit of detection at 0.3 µmol/L, and linear over the range of 0 to 500 µmol/L. The capacity of the automated assay is 70 tubes (calibrators + 60 samples) per 24 hours. The assay remains a widely used HPLC method.

Pfeiffer et al. (43) modified the method of Vester and Rasmussen (72) by using the newer, stable, water-soluble phosphine derivative, tris(2-carboxyethyl)-phosphine, as the reducing agent, cystamine as the internal standard, and isocratic separation of the thiols within 6 minutes. When analyzed over 20 days, quality-control plasma pools showed a total imprecision of 6.7% (low pool, 6.5 µmol/L), 5.0% (medium pool, 12.4 µmol/L), and 4.4% (high pool, 29.9 µmol/L). The method is sensitive, with a limit of detection at 0.16 µmol/L, and linear up to 200 µmol/L. It is a rapid and user-friendly assay, using a less hazardous reducing agent.

Fiskerstrand et al. (18) substantially improved the first fully automated HPLC assay they had described 4 years earlier (54). This modified version, which omits column switching, is based on a single-solvent delivery system using simultaneous reduction with dithioerythritol and sodium borohydride and derivatization with monobromobimane. The new method measures cysteine and cysteinylglycine in addition to homocysteine. The method proved to be linear over the concentration range examined (approximately 2 to 65 µmol/L). The within- and between-day CVs at 9.2 µmol/L were 2.6% and 2.2% (n = 10), respectively, a total analytical imprecision of about 3.4%. The sample output is about 70 samples in 24 hours.

Jacobsen et al. (26) extensively modified their earlier procedure (25), allowing rapid determination of plasma total homocysteine, cysteine, and cysteinylglycine by using simultaneous sodium borohydride reduction and derivatization with monobromobimane and eliminating steps such as solid-phase extraction of samples before HPLC. The method is sensitive, with a limit of detection <1 µmol/L and is linear over the range of 0 to 200 µmol/L. The total analytical imprecision is 5.9% (mean concentration = 10.80 µmol/L; n = 7 assays done over 4 weeks). The capacity of the automated assay is high. More than 80 samples plus appropriate calibrators and quality-control samples can be analyzed within 24 hours.

Feussner et al. (17) reported an isocratic HPLC assay with manual derivatization as described by

Araki and Sako (8) with slight modifications. Insufficient data were provided for assay validation and assessment of imprecision.

Pastore et al. (41) improved the Fiskerstrand method (18) to measure, in a 6-minute run (plus 5 minutes column equilibration time), the total concentrations of the most important thiols in plasma, as well as the concentrations of cysteamine and mercaptopropionylglycine, two compounds used to treat disorders of cysteine metabolism. The method was linear for homocysteine in an aqueous matrix over a range of 0.625 to 100 µmol/L; however, linearity data for plasma were not shown. The intraassay imprecision (2.4%) was obtained by analyzing a sample (12.6 µmol/L) 10 times in the same day. The interassay imprecision (4.9%) was determined by analyzing the same sample on 10 different days over 1 month. Thus, the total analytical imprecision is at least 5.5%.

Recently, an HPLC kit was introduced by Bio-Rad, which uses 4-(aminosulfonyl)-7-fluoro-2,1,3-benzoxadiazole (ABD-F) as the derivatizing agent. The kit assay was evaluated and compared with another HPLC fluorescence assay that uses ammonium 7-fluoro-2,1,3-benzoxadiazole-4-sulfonate and to the enzyme immunoassay produced by Axis-Shields ASA, Oslo, Norway (14). The assay proved to be linear over a concentration range of 0.5 to 100 µmol/L. When control samples (7.6 and 23.1 µmol/L) were assayed daily in duplicate for 21 days, the within- and between-run CVs were 3.5% and 6.2%, respectively, with a total analytical imprecision of about 7.1%. The capacity of the assay was not stated, but the assay is rapid.

Electrochemical Detection The presence of a sulfhydryl group in homocysteine makes it potentially suited for detection based on oxidation-reduction reactions. The method of Smolin and Schneider (61) was optimized by Malinow et al. (32). Sample processing is simple, the reductant is sodium borohydride, and no derivatization of the sample is required. Autoinjection and a short run time at about 11 to 12 minutes allow the processing of a large sample throughput. The authors reported that the total variance of 16 paired, external quality control samples was 10.9% (33). The stability (and, more than likely, the precision) of the assay depends on careful maintenance to avoid contamination of the flow cell and deterioration of the gold-mercury electrode (16, 70). Evrovski et al. (15) offered a possible solution to avoid contamination of the flow cell and electrode fouling by using pulsed integrated amperometry and a solid gold electrode. The total imprecision, however, was above 11% (n = 11).

D'Eramo et al. (13) reported an assay using a glassy-carbon electrode that is not specific for thiol groups. The assay proved to be linear from 1.8 µmol/L up to 100 µmol/L. Interassay and intraassay CVs were 5.6% and 3.9%, respectively (mean concentration = 9.4 µmol/L; n = 6), a total analytical imprecision of about 7%.

Martin et al. (36) improved their previously reported method by using penicillamine as an internal standard. A guard cell was installed between the pump and the autosampler to clean the mobile phase electrochemically before addition of sample and to reduce the background current at the detector. The intraassay CV at 7 µmol/L was 2.2% (n = 20), and the interassay CV at 8.5 µmol/L is 8.6% (n = 8), a total analytical imprecision of about 9%.

Melnyk et al. (37) reported a new HPLC method for the simultaneous determination of oxidized and reduced plasma aminothiols using coulometric electrochemical detection. The method was linear over the concentration range examined (0.5–100 µmol/L). Inter- and intraassay CVs were 4.0% and 3.9%, respectively (mean concentration = 7.6 µmol/L; n = 10), a total analytical imprecision of about 5.6%. This method was not intended for routine analysis, but is best suited for refinement of diagnoses, for interpretation of nutritional intervention, and for mechanistically based research studies.

Colorimetric Detection Andersson et al. (5) described a HPLC method in which homocysteine is directly chromatographed. The assay involves reduction of sample with dithiothreitol, postcolumn derivatization with 4,4'-dithiodipyridine, and colorimetric detection at 324 nm. Using three different procedures for preparation of plasma, the assay can determine total, non-protein-bound disulfides and the reduced forms of homocysteine and other thiols. The method is highly precise, with a total imprecision at 2.9%. The sample capacity was not stated, but homocysteine elutes after 15.9 minutes.

Candito et al. (9) modified an amino acid analyzer, using ninhydrin for postcolumn derivatization to improve separation of homocysteine and methionine. It is not clear whether the reported imprecision of 7.8% is total or between-day imprecision. A run time of 52 minutes limits sample capacity, which is low compared with other HPLC assays.

Capillary Electrophoresis

Caussé et al. (10) described an assay with laser-induced fluorescence detection. Plasma samples and an internal standard (D-penicillamine) are reduced with tris(2-carboxyethyl)phosphine, deproteinized with 5-sulfosalicylic acid, and incubated overnight with 6-iodoacetamidofluorescein. The sample capacity is not stated, but the migration time for the homocysteine derivative is 7.2 minutes. The authors reported a limit of detection at 0.25 µmol/L and linearity over the concentration range 2 to 200 µmol/L. When aliquots were assayed in triplicate, the within- and between-assay CVs were 4.9% and 7.8% (n = 10), respectively, a total analytical imprecision of 9.2%. The average recovery of homocysteine added to six plasma samples was 101.1% ± 6.99% (n = 18). However, compared with ion-exchange chromatography, one of the methods appeared to be highly inaccurate (mean control values: 11.73 ± 4.45 µmol/L [capillary electrophoresis] vs. 8.89 ± 2.85 µmol/L, respectively, n = 27).

Vecchione et al. (71) also described an assay with laser-induced fluorescence detection. Plasma samples (200 µl) and internal standard (n-(2-mercaptopropionyl)-glycine) are reduced with tri-n-butylphosphine, deproteinized with trichloroacetic acid, and incubated for 15 minutes at 60°C with 5-bromomethylfluoresceine in dimethylformamide. The migration time for the homocysteine derivative is 7.4 minutes, and the whole procedure is done within 15 minutes. The authors reported a limit of detection at 0.01 µmol/L and linearity over the concentration range 5 to 100 µmol/L. Insufficient data were provided for assay validation and assessment of imprecision. However, when results were compared with results obtained by a HPLC-based method, a satisfactory correlation was observed.

Immunoassays

The first method for measuring total homocysteine in plasma was a radioenzymatic assay based on the conversion of homocysteine to S-adenosylhomocysteine using S-adenosylhomocysteine hydrolase (52). Shipchandler at al. (60) described an immunoassay based on the same conversion, using a monoclonal antibody against S-adenosylhomocysteine. The assay is a fluorescence polarization immunoassay based on the IMx instrument (Abbott Laboratories, Chicago, IL). The initial reduction is performed by dithiothreitol, and in the same reaction mixture, conversion to S-adenosylhomocysteine is accomplished during 30 minutes of incubation at 34°C, using S-adenosylhomocysteine hydrolase and an excess of adenosine. Subsequently, the S-adenosylhomocysteine reacts with the antibody in competition with a fluoresceinated analog. The capacity of the instrument is about 20 samples an hour. The total imprecision was reported to be 10.2% at 5.0 µmol/L, and 5.7% to 6.8% at 8.6 to 33.2 µmol/L (3 determinations on different instruments in 5 days, n = 15).

The manufacturer has collected data from trials of the fluorescence polarization immunoassay. In 21 European laboratories, the total imprecision was 3.3% at 7.3 µmol/L, 2.3% at 12.8 µmol/L, and 2.3% at 25.8 µmol/L, ranging from 1.4% to 6.0% for the different laboratories. Independent evaluations have also been published. Pfeiffer et al. (45) reported a total imprecision of 3.2% at 6.0 µmol/L, 4.9% at 11.4 µmol/L, and 2.5% at 28.8 µmol/L (n = 21); Leino (29) using guidelines from the National Committee for Clinical Laboratory Standards for evaluation of precision performance (7) reported 1.9% at 7.0 µmol/L, 1.8% at 12.5 µmol/L, and 1.4% at 25.0 µmol/L.

The same analytical principles and reagents are also adapted to an enzyme immunoassay using coated microtiter wells (19). The capacity of the assay varies. A technician should be able to process 80 to 100 samples in a working day. The intraassay CV was 5.0% at 8.1 µmol/L, 4.3% at 13.6 µmol/L, and 5.5% at 27.3 µmol/L (n = 21). The interassay imprecision was 5.4% at 8.1 µmol/L, 6.2% at 13.6 µmol/L, and 8.2% at 27.3 µmol/L (n = 21). A further evaluation reported an intraassay CV of <6.2% and a interassay CV of <8.0% (47).

Ubbink et al. (67) compared both immunoassays to a GC-MS method (62) and a HPLC method (68) with tris(2-carboxyethyl)phosphine for reduction and ammonium 7-fluoro-2,1,3-benzoxadiazole-4-sulfonate for derivatization. They found a interassay CV of 6.9% for the enzyme immunoassay method and 4.5% for the fluorescence polarization immunoassay method, respectively. However, when the GC-MS method was used as a reference, the three other methods showed negative bias for fasting samples, emphasizing the need for standardization of the assays, in particular of the calibrators.

An independent European multicenter project (76) reported good linearity and correlation to reference methods for both methods and imprecisions of 3.1% to 5.0% for the fluorescence polarization immunoassay method and 6.6% to 11.7% for the enzyme immunoassay method. The authors concluded that the fluorescence method shows excellent performance and that the enzyme immunoassay method is suitable for screening purposes.

The analytical principle has several advantages. Performing reduction and derivatization in the same reaction mixture prevents reoxidation, and the enzymatic conversion to S-adenosylhomocysteine, as well as the reaction with the monoclonal antibody, ensures specificity. However, S-adenosylhomocysteine interferes in the assays, but concentrations in plasma (20 to 40 nmol/L [31]) are usually too low to give a significant contribution. S-adenosylmethionine may interfere as well. According to Frantzen et al. (19), a concentration above 10 µmol/L will show an effect. Basal concentrations of S-adenosylmethionine are about 10 to

70 nmol/L (31), so this should not be a problem. Caution should be exercised when patients are being treated with *S*-adenosylmethionine for depression, liver disease, pancreatitis, and osteoarthritis, among other diseases. After an oral load of 400 mg, the maximum concentration in plasma is 362 ± 66 nmol/L and the half-life is only 1.7 ± 0.3 hours (31).

Interpretation of Results

Frequently, the result of only a single plasma total homocysteine test is used to assess risk for cardiovascular disease. A prerequisite for the interpretation of a single homocysteine test, however, is knowledge of the magnitude of preanalytical variables, analytical variation, and intraindividual and interindividual variations. The influence of preanalytical variables and the analytical variations of the different analytical methods was described earlier in this chapter.

Intraindividual Variation

All studies but one agree that the intraindividual variation of homocysteine in healthy subjects is relatively small and have reported CVs < 10% (11, 12, 21, 49, 56, 65). The explanation for the one discrepant report, describing a threefold higher variation (57), is not clear, but the 8% imprecision of that method was high. Other factors could also contribute to the variation (e.g., the sampling procedure using serum instead of plasma or a higher prevalance of folate deficiency in the study population).

Interindividual Variation and Reference Intervals

The interindividual variation of homocysteine in healthy subjects is 21% to 34%, depending on the age and gender of the participants (11, 12, 21, 49, 56, 65).

For several years, concentrations of total homocysteine in plasma ranging from 5 to 15 μmol/L have been considered the so-called "normal range" in adults (53, 70). Nonetheless, upper reference limits (mean + 2 SD) differ greatly between laboratories. The variability may be related not only to different methodologies or differences in sample collection but also, and perhaps more importantly, to the selection of reference individuals (50). Studies from the United States, South Africa, and Denmark suggest that a large proportion of the population, perhaps 40%, is not consuming enough folate to keep the concentrations of homocysteine in plasma low (50, 59, 64, 66). Furthermore, plasma homocysteine depends on age and gender; homocysteine increases with age, and until menopause, women have lower homocysteine levels than men (4, 50). Studies on targeted segments of populations indicate

that the formerly accepted upper limit of 15 μmol/L is far too high in well-nourished populations without vitamin deficiency (50, 56, 66). In our laboratory, the upper limits are 8.1 to 11.9 μmol/L, depending on age and gender (50). These limits are based on results, obtained *before* supplementation with folic acid, in apparently healthy individuals who were weak responders to reduction of plasma homocysteine through subsequent supplementation. However, instead of defining reference intervals for healthy individuals, investigators are currently faced with the far more important task of defining desirable low homocysteine levels in populations at risk for vascular disease (see Chapter 40).

Evaluation of Methods

Quality Goals

As mentioned previously, the difference in plasma homocysteine associated with the absence and presence of risk for vascular disease is about 3 μmol/L or less. The analytical quality required must be seen in this context and in the context of biological variability. Fraser et al. (20) have suggested a way of calculating analytical quality goals based on biological variations. The quality goal for the precision of analysis should be calculated as a fraction of the intraindividual variation, $CV_{within\ subject}$, and the analytical bias as a fraction of the group variation, calculated as $(CV^2_{within\ subject} + CV^2_{between\ subject})^{1/2}$. Briefly, the argument for the analytical goal for precision is that the analytical contribution to the variability of the test result is a function of the fraction of the analytical variation of the biological variation (i.e., an analytical variation of $0.5*CV_{within\ subject}$ will add 12% to the total variability of the test result).

To be able to use identical reference intervals and decision limits, the bias of the methods should be less than a fraction of the group variation, because the percentage of individuals outside the limits is a function of the fraction of the analytical bias of the group variation. Fraser et al. (20) proposed empirically that, for precision, the fraction recommended for optimum performance is 0.25, and for desirable and minimum performance 0.50 and 0.75, respectively. For the bias, the recommended fractions for optimum performance are suggested to be 0.125, for desirable performance 0.25, and for minimum performance 0.375.

The $CV_{within\ subject}$ for homocysteine is between 7.0% and 9.4% (see section on intraindividual variation). Using 8% as an average, the analytical goals for optimum, desirable, and minimum performance for analytical imprecision are 2%, 4% and 6%, respectively, as described by Møller et al. (40). The $CV_{between\ subject}$ is reported to be between 21% and 34% (see section on interindividual variation), depending on the age and gender of the study subjects. Assuming a value of about 29% for the $CV_{between\ subject}$, the total group variation, calculated as $(CV^2_{within\ subject} + CV^2_{between\ subject})^{1/2}$, is 30%, and the analytical goals for optimum, desirable, and minimum performance for analytical bias is 4%, 8%, and 11%, respectively (40).

Quality Assessment

Internal Quality Assessment The purpose of internal quality assessment is documentation of performance in accordance with the quality goals just calculated. For the assessment of precision, choice of material must depend on the method of analysis. Because plasma is the preferred sample material, an unmodified plasma pool with identical anticoagulant is preferred. Interest should center on the upper reference limit, 10 to 12 µmol/L, possibly supplemented with material having a higher concentration. For the documentation of bias, several materials with a certified concentration of homocysteine are commercially available. Alternatively, recovery of the disulfide, homocystine, added to a plasma pool can be used. However, for the immunoassays, the homocystine should be the L-homocystine, because the *S*-adenosylhomocysteine hydrolase does not react as efficiently with D-homocystine. There will be a theoretical difference, however, between the bias and the recovery of homocystine, because a plasma

pool supplemented with the disulfide homocystine has a distribution of homocysteine quite different from the physiological sample, in which most of the homocysteine is protein bound.

External Quality Assessment Programs Several programs for the external quality control of homocysteine are available. The results of a Scandinavian-based program were classified into three groups: 12 sets of results from various HPLC methods, 6 sets of results from mass-spectrometric methods, and 16 sets of results from the two immunoassays (40). The average intralaboratory CV was 7.5%, with a range of 6.3% to 12.5%; the interlaboratory CV was 5.5%. The intra-

Fig. 18.2. Results from an external quality assessment program (40). The 28 laboratories submitted 34 sets of results, with several laboratories submitting results from more than one method. The imprecision is calculated from the results of an unmodified pool of EDTA plasma sent to each laboratory four times with different codes in four of six different rounds. One laboratory achieved "desirable" performance and nine achieved "minimum" performance, corresponding to imprecisions better than 4% and 6%, respectively. To obtain a measure of the bias, the same plasma pool was supplemented with increasing amounts of L-homocystine to produce three sets of samples with increased concentrations of homocysteine. These samples were sent out twice to each laboratory in different rounds, and the recovery of homocysteine was calculated for each laboratory. Ten laboratories had recoveries within the range for "optimum" performance (bias less than 4%), 22 achieved "desirable" performance (bias less than 8%), and 26 "minimum" performance (bias less than 11%).

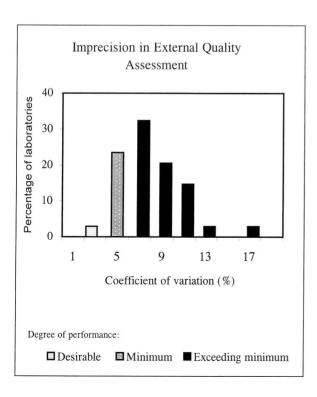

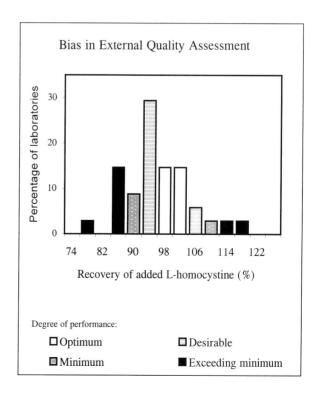

laboratory variation was highest for the HPLC methods, 8.4%; and the HPLC group was the only group with a significant interlaboratory variation, probably because the group of HPLC methods is the least homogenous. Only one set of results achieved desirable performance, and nine achieved only minimum performance as calculated previously (Figure 18.2).

The average recovery of the added L-homocystine was 96%, with a range of 76% to 117%. Using the recovery as the best approximation of bias, 22 and 26 participants of the 34 achieved desirable and minimum performance, respectively (Figure 18.2).

A round robin between 14 selected laboratories reporting results from 17 analytical methods found a mean interlaboratory variation of 7.6% and an intramethod variation of 4.2%, respectively (44). Two of the HPLC methods (electrochemical detection and fluorescence detection with sodiumborohydride reduction and monobrobimane derivatization) and the enzyme immunoassay showed a positive bias compared with the GC-MS results, and a large negative bias (16%) was found for a HPLC method with trialkylphosphine reduction and derivatization with ABD-F. The fluorescence polarization immunoassay method and HPLC with ammonium 7-fluoro-2,1,3-benzoxadiazole-4-sulfonate derivatization were in good agreement with the GC-MS method. There is an urgent need to improve analytical imprecision and, for some methods, to decrease analytical bias.

Selecting the Method That Best Fits Laboratory Requirements

The choice of method depends on different factors such as personnel and instrument resources, training, the number of samples to be analyzed, special interests concerning codetermination of other metabolites, and cost (16). Use of hazardous chemicals for derivatization or use of potentially toxic solvents for extractions and chromatography should be limited.

An important determinant will always be the analytical quality. Thorough testing demands many resources, making it cost-effective to adapt a method whose performance is documented and published. Many reports, including several cited in this chapter, are quite unsatisfactory, mainly because of very limited data for control samples in the evaluations. Only 26% of the methods in an external quality assessment (40) had an imprecision within the minimum limits calculated on the basis of biological variation (20), whereas in most methods (76%), recoveries of added homocystine in spiked samples corresponded to a bias within the minimum limits. Because the quality goals for allowable precision correspond to a minimum performance at an imprecision of 6%, the candidate method

should be able to meet this standard. Apparently, bias is not that great a problem, but the chosen assay must conform to the quality goals to use and compare international reference and decision limits.

The stable-isotope-dilution technique is the candidate definitive method for accurate determination of homocysteine in plasma. The GC-MS assay combines the speed, simplicity, and reproducibility of solid-phase extraction with the sensitivity, specificity, and accuracy of the stable-isotope-dilution GC-MS. Other major advantages include the capacity for codetermination, using the appropriate internal standards, of other metabolites. The disadvantages have been the expense of the equipment and the need for highly experienced staff, but with the introduction of benchtop GC-MS instruments, the stable-isotope-dilution method has become more attractive.

Several HPLC methods have sufficient sensitivity, specificity, and accuracy for the routine determination of homocysteine. Major advantages are the relatively low cost of chemicals and solvents, the routine availability of HPLC equipment as part of the hospital laboratory instrumentation, and the existence of a fully automated assay. Approaches using the less hazardous reducing agent, tris(2-carboxyethyl)phosphine (TCEP), (22, 43) are gaining acceptance.

The most attractive feature of the fluorescence polarization immunoassay method based on the IMx instrument is its complete automation. The instrument is also often part of the hospital laboratory instrumentation. The analytical quality and feasibility as a routine method look promising.

Costs of supplies, reagents, equipment, and labor vary among the methods. Generally, the final cost of a measurement depends on the number of samples to be processed. Prices of reagents and disposables also vary geographically. In contrast, GC-MS assays are more labor intensive. Many laboratories have found the HPLC methods a reasonable compromise because the prices of reagents and consumables are comparable to the GC-MS assays, and more laboratories have experience with HPLC.

REFERENCES

1. Al-Khafaji, F, Bowron, A, Day, AP, Scott, J, Stansbie, D. Stabilization of blood homocysteine by 3-deazaadenosine. *Ann Clin Biochem* 1998; 35: 780–82.
2. Allen, RH, Stabler, SP, Savage, DG, Lindenbaum, J. Diagnosis of cobalamin deficiency I: Usefulness of serum methylmalonic acid and total homocysteine concentrations [see comments]. *Am J Hematol* 1990; 34: 90–8.
3. Andersson, A, Brattstrom, L, Isaksson, A, Israelsson, B, Hultberg, B. Determination of homocysteine in plasma by ion-exchange chromatography. *Scand J Clin Lab Invest* 1989; 49: 445–49.

4. Andersson, A, Brattstrom, L, Israelsson, B, Isaksson, A, Hamfelt, A, Hultberg, B. Plasma homocysteine before and after methionine loading with regard to age, gender, and menopausal status. *Eur J Clin Invest* 1992; 22: 79–87.

5. Andersson, A, Isaksson, A, Brattstrom, L, Hultberg, B. Homocysteine and other thiols determined in plasma by HPLC and thiol-specific postcolumn derivatization. *Clin Chem* 1993; 39: 1590–97.

6. Andersson, A, Isaksson, A, Hultberg, B. Homocysteine export from erythrocytes and its implication for plasma sampling. *Clin Chem* 1992; 38: 1311–15.

7. Anonymous. *National Committee for Clinical Laboratory Standards. Evaluation of Precision Performance of Clinical Chemistry Devices; Tentative Guideline EP5-T2,* 2nd ed. NCCLS, Villanova, Pa, 1992; pp. 1–43.

8. Araki, A, Sako, Y. Determination of free and total homocysteine in human plasma by high-performance liquid chromatography with fluorescence detection. *J Chromatogr* 1987; 422: 43–52.

9. Candito, M, Bedoucha, P, Mahagne, MH, Scavini, G, Chatel, M. Total plasma homocysteine determination by liquid chromatography before and after methionine loading. Results in cerebrovascular disease. *J Chromatogr B Biomed Sci Appl* 1997; 692: 213–16.

10. Caussé, E, Siri, N, Bellet, H, Champagne, S, Bayle, C, Valdiguié, P, Salvayre, R, Couderc, F. Plasma homocysteine determined by capillary electrophoresis with Lascr-induced fluorescence detection. *Clin Chem* 1999; 45: 412–14.

11. Clarke, R, Woodhouse, P, Ulvik, A, Frost, C, Sherliker, P, Refsum, H, Ueland, PM, Khaw, KT. Variability and determinants of total homocysteine concentrations in plasma in an elderly population. *Clin Chem* 1998; 44: 102–7.

12. Cobbaert, C, Arentsen, JC, Mulder, P, Hoogerbrugge, N, Lindemans, J. Significance of various parameters derived from biological variability of lipoprotein(a), homocysteine, cysteine, and total antioxidant status. *Clin Chem* 1997; 43: 1958–64.

13. D'Eramo, JL, Finkelstein, AE, Boccazzi, FO, Fridman, O. Total homocysteine in plasma: High-performance liquid chromatographic determination with electrochemical detection and glassy carbon electrode. *J Chromatogr B* 1998; 720: 205–10.

14. Dias, VC, Bamforth, FJ, Tesanovic, M, Hyndman, ME, Parsons, HG, Cembrowski, GS. Evaluation and intermethod comparison of the Bio-Rad high-performance liquid chromatographic method for plasma total homocysteine. *Clin Chem* 1998; 44: 2199–201.

15. Evrovski, J, Callaghan, M, Cole, DE. Determination of homocysteine by HPLC with pulsed integrated amperometry. *Clin Chem* 1995; 41: 757–58.

16. Fermo, I, De Vecchi, E, Arcelloni, C, D'Angelo, A, Paroni, R. Methodological aspects of total plasma homocysteine measurement *Haematologica* 1997; 82: 246–50.

17. Feussner, A, Rolinski, B, Weiss, N, Deufel, T, Wolfram, G, Roscher, AA. Determination of total homocysteine in human plasma by isocratic high-performance liquid chromatography. *Eur J Clin Chem Clin Biochem* 1997; 35: 687–91.

18. Fiskerstrand, T, Refsum, H, Kvalheim, G, Ueland, PM. Homocysteine and other thiols in plasma and urine: Automated determination and sample stability. *Clin Chem* 1993; 39: 263–71.

19. Frantzen, F, Faaren, AL, Alfheim, I, Nordhei, AK. Enzyme conversion immunoassay for determining total homocysteine in plasma or serum. *Clin Chem* 1998; 44: 311–16.

20. Fraser, CG, Hyltoft Petersen, P, Libeer, JC, Ricos, C. Proposals for setting generally applicable quality goals solely based on biology. *Ann Clin Biochem* 1997; 34: 8–12.

21. Garg, UC, Zheng, ZJ, Folsom, AR, Moyer, YS, Tsai, MY, McGovern, P, Eckfeldt, JH. Short-term and long-term variability of plasma homocysteine measurement. *Clin Chem* 1997; 43: 141–45.

22. Gilfix, BM, Blank, DW, Rosenblatt, DS. Novel reductant for determination of total plasma homocysteine. *Clin Chem* 1997; 43: 687–88.

23. Green, R, Jacobsen, DW. Clinical implications of hyperhomocysteineamia. In: Baily, LB., ed. *Folate in health and disease.* Marcel Dekker, Inc., New York 1995; pp: 75–122.

24. Hughes, MP, Carlson, TH, McLaughlin, MK, Bankson, DD. Addition of sodium fluoride to whole blood does not stabilize plasma homocysteine but produces dilution effects on plasma constituents and hematocrit. *Clin Chem* 1998; 44: 2204–6.

25. Jacobsen, DW, Gatautis, VJ, Green, R. Determination of plasma homocysteine by high-performance liquid chromatography with fluorescence detection. *Anal Biochem* 1989; 178: 208–14.

26. Jacobsen, DW, Gatautis, VJ, Green, R, Robinson, K, Savon, SR, Secic, M, Ji, J, Otto, JM, Taylor, LM. Rapid HPLC determination of total homocysteine and other thiols in serum and plasma: Sex differences and correlation with cobalamin and folate concentrations in healthy subjects. *Clin Chem* 1994; 40: 873–81.

27. Kang, SS, Wong, PW, Becker, N. Protein-bound homocyst(e)ine in normal subjects and in patients with homocystinuria. *Pediatr Res* 1979; 13: 1141–43.

28. Kataoka, H, Takagi, K, Makita, M. Determination of total plasma homocysteine and related aminothiols by gas chromatography with flame photometric detection. *J Chromatogr B Biomed Appl* 1995; 664: 421–25.

29. Leino, A. Fully automated measurement of total homocysteine in plasma and serum on the Abbott IMx analyzer. *Clin Chem* 1999; 45: 569–71.

30. Loehrer, FM, Angst, CP, Brunner, FP, Haefeli, WE, Fowler, B. Evidence for disturbed S-adenosylmethionine. S-adenosylhomocysteine ratio in patients with end-stage renal failure: A cause for disturbed methylation reactions? *Nephrol Dial Transplant* 1998; 13: 656–61.

31. Loehrer, FM, Schwab, R, Angst, CP, Haefeli, WE, Fowler, B. Influence of oral S-adenosylmethionine on plasma 5-methyltetrahydrofolate, S-adenosylhomocysteine, homocysteine and methionine in healthy humans. *J Pharmacol Exp Ther* 1997; 282: 845–50.

31a. Magera, MJ, Lacey, JM, Casetta, B, Rinaldo, P. Method for the determination of total homocysteine in plasma and urine by stable isotope dilution and electrospray tandem mass spectrometry. *Clin Chem* 1999; 45: 1517–22.

32. Malinow, MR, Kang, SS, Taylor, LM, Wong, PW, Coull, B, Inahara, T, Mukerjee, D, Sexton, G, Upson, B. Prevalence of hyperhomocyst(e)inemia in patients with peripheral arterial occlusive disease. *Circulation* 1989; 79: 1180–88.

33. Malinow, MR, Nieto, FJ, Szklo, M, Chambless, LE, Bond, G. Carotid artery intimal-medial wall thickening and plasma homocyst(e)ine in asymptomatic adults. The Atherosclerosis Risk in Communities Study. *Circulation* 1993; 87: 1107–13.

34. Mansoor, MA, Bergmark, C, Svardal, AM, Lonning, PE, Ueland, PM. Redox status and protein binding of plasma homocysteine and other aminothiols in patients with early-onset peripheral vascular disease. Homocysteine and peripheral vascular disease. *Arterioscler Thromb Vasc Biol* 1995; 15: 232–40.

35. Mansoor, MA, Svardal, AM, Schneede, J, Ueland, PM. Dynamic relation between reduced, oxidized, and protein-bound homocysteine and other thiol components in plasma during methionine loading in healthy men. *Clin Chem* 1992; 38: 1316–21.

36. Martin, SC, Tsakas-Ampatzis, I, Bartlett, WA, Jones, AF. Measurement of plasma total homocysteine by HPLC with coulometric detection. *Clin Chem* 1999; 45: 150–52.

37. Melnyk, S, Pogribna, M, Pogribny, I, Hine, RJ, James, SJ. A new HPLC method for the simultaneous determination of oxidized and reduced plasma aminothiols using coulometric electrochemical detection. *J Nutr Biochem* 1999; 10: 490–97.

38. Moat, SJ, Bonham, JR, Tanner, MS, Allen, JC, Powers, HJ. Recommended approaches for the laboratory measurement of homocysteine in the diagnosis and monitoring of patients with hyperhomocysteinaemia. *Ann Clin Biochem* 1999; 36: 372–79.

39. Møller, J, Rasmussen, K. Homocysteine in plasma: Stabilization of blood samples with fluoride. *Clin Chem* 1995; 41: 758–59.

40. Møller, J, Rasmussen, K, Christensen, L. External quality assessment of methylmalonic acid and total homocysteine. *Clin Chem* 1999; 45: 1536–42.

40a. Nexø, E, Engbaek, F, Ueland, PM, Westby, C, O'Gorman, P, Johnston, C, Kase, BF, Guttormsen, AB, Alfheim, I, McPartlin, J, Smith, D, Møller, J, Rasmussen, K, Clarke, R, Scott, JM, Refsum, H. Evaluation of novel assays in clinical chemistry: Quantification of plasma total homocysteine. *Clin Chem* 2000; 46: 1150–56.

41. Pastore, A, Massoud, R, Motti, C, Lo Russo, A, Fucci, G, Cortese, C, Federici, G. Fully automated assay for total homocysteine, cysteine, cysteinylglycine, glutathione, cysteamine, and 2-mercaptopropionylglycine in plasma and urine. *Clin Chem* 1998; 44: 825–32.

42. Perry, TL. Unsolved problems in homocytiuria. In: Nyhan, WL., ed. *Amino Acid Metabolism and Genetic Variation.* McGraw-Hill Book Company, New York 1967; pp: 279–96.

43. Pfeiffer, CM, Huff, DL, Gunter, EW. Rapid and accurate HPLC assay for plasma total homocysteine and cysteine in a clinical laboratory setting. *Clin Chem* 1999; 45: 290–92.

44. Pfeiffer, CM, Huff, DL, Smith, SJ, Miller, DT, Gunter, EW. Comparison of plasma total homocysteine measurements in 14 laboratories: An international study. *Clin Chem* 1999; 45: 1261–68.

45. Pfeiffer, CM, Twite, D, Shih, J, Holets-McCormack, SR, Gunter, EW. Method comparison for total plasma homocysteine between the Abbott IMx analyzer and an HPLC assay with internal standardization. *Clin Chem* 1999; 45: 152–53.

46. Pietzsch, J, Julius, U, Hanefeld, M. Rapid determination of total homocysteine in human plasma by using N(O,S)-ethoxycarbonyl ethyl ester derivatives and gas chromatography-mass spectrometry. *Clin Chem* 1997; 43: 2001–4.

47. Pietzsch, J, Pixa, A. Determination of total homocysteine [letter]. *Clin Chem* 1998; 44: 1781–82.

48. Probst, R, Brandl, R, Blumke, M, Neumeier, D. Stabilization of homocysteine concentration in whole blood. *Clin Chem* 1998; 44: 1567–69.

49. Rasmussen, K, Møller, J, Lyngbak, M. Within-person variation of plasma homocysteine and effects of posture and tourniquet application. *Clin Chem* 1999; 45: 1850–55.

50. Rasmussen, K, Møller, J, Lyngbak, M, Pedersen, AM, Dybkjaer, L. Age- and gender-specific reference intervals for total homocysteine and methylmalonic acid in plasma before and after vitamin supplementation. *Clin Chem* 1996; 42: 630–36.

51. Rasmussen, K, Møller, J. Measurement of homocysteine in plasma: Experience with the GC-MS method. [abstract]. *Irish J Med Sci* 1995; 164 (Suppl 15): 16.

52. Refsum, H, Helland, S, Ueland, PM. Radioenzymic determination of homocysteine in plasma and urine. *Clin Chem* 1985; 31: 624–28.

53. Refsum, H, Ueland, PM, Nygard, O, Vollset, SE. Homocysteine and cardiovascular disease. *Annu Rev Med* 1998; 49: 31–62.

54. Refsum, H, Ueland, PM, Svardal, AM. Fully automated fluorescence assay for determining total homocysteine in plasma. *Clin Chem* 1989; 35: 1921–27.

55. Refsum, H, Guttormsen, AB, Fiskerstrand, T, Ueland, PM. On the formation and fate of total homocysteine. In: Graham, I, Refsum, H, Rosenberg, IH, Ueland, PM, eds. *Homocysteine Metabolism: From Basic Science to Clinical Medicine.* Kluwer Academic Publishers, Boston 1997; pp: 23–29.

56. Rossi, E, Beilby, JP, McQuillan, BM, Hung, J. Biological variability and reference intervals for total plasma homocysteine. *Ann Clin Biochem* 1999; 36: 56–61.

57. Santhosh Kumar, CR, Deutsch, JC, Ryder, JW, Kolhouse, JF. Unpredictable intra-individual variations in serum homocysteine levels on folic acid supplementation. *Eur J Clin Nutr* 1997; 51: 188–92.

58. Sass, JO, Endres, W. Quantitation of total homocysteine in human plasma by derivatization to its N(O,S)-propoxycarbonyl propyl ester and gas chromatography-mass spectrometry analysis. *J Chromatogr A* 1997; 776: 342–47.

59. Selhub, J, Jacques, PF, Wilson, PW, Rush, D, Rosenberg, IH. Vitamin status and intake as primary determinants of homocysteinemia in an elderly population [see comments]. *JAMA* 1993; 270: 2693–98.

60. Shipchandler, MT, Moore, EG. Rapid, fully automated measurement of plasma homocyst(e)ine with the Abbott IMx analyzer. *Clin Chem* 1995; 41: 991–94.

61. Smolin, LA, Schneider, JA. Measurement of total plasma cysteamine using high-performance liquid chromatography with electrochemical detection. *Anal Biochem* 1988; 168: 374–79.

62. Stabler, SP, Lindenbaum, J, Savage, DG, Allen, RH. Elevation of serum cystathionine levels in patients with cobalamin and folate deficiency. *Blood* 1993; 81: 3404–13.

63. Stabler, SP, Marcell, PD, Podell, ER, Allen, RH. Quantitation of total homocysteine, total cysteine, and methionine in normal serum and urine using capillary gas chromatography-mass spectrometry. *Anal Biochem* 1987; 162: 185–96.

64. Stampfer, MJ, Willett, WC. Homocysteine and marginal vitamin deficiency. The importance of adequate vitamin intake [editorial]. *JAMA* 1993; 270: 2726–27.

65. Thirup, P, Ekelund, S. Day-to-day, postprandial, and orthostatic variation of total plasma homocysteine [technical brief]. *Clin Chem* 1999; 45: 1280–83.

66. Ubbink, JB, Becker, PJ, Vermaak, WJ, Delport, R. Results of B-vitamin supplementation study used in a prediction model to define a reference range for plasma homocysteine. *Clin Chem* 1995; 41: 1033–37.

67. Ubbink, JB, Delport, R, Riezler, R, Vermaak, WJH. Comparison of three different plasma homocysteine assays with gas chromatography-mass spectrometry. *Clin Chem* 1999; 45: 670–75.

68. Ubbink, JB, Hayward Vermaak, WJ, Bissbort, S. Rapid high-performance liquid chromatographic assay for total homocysteine levels in human serum. *J Chromatogr* 1991; 565: 441–46.

69. Ubbink, JB, Vermaak, WJ, van der Merwe, A, Becker, PJ. The effect of blood sample aging and food consumption on plasma total homocysteine levels. *Clin Chim Acta* 1992; 207: 119–28.

70. Ueland, PM, Refsum, H, Stabler, SP, Malinow, MR, Andersson, A, Allen, RH. Total homocysteine in plasma or serum: Methods and clinical applications. *Clin Chem* 1993; 39: 1764–79.

71. Vecchione, G, Margaglione, M, Grandone, E, Colaizzo, E, Cappucci, G, Fermo, I, D'Angelo, A, Di Minno, G. Determining sulfur-containing amino acids by capillary electrophoresis: A fast novel method for total homocyst(e)ine human plasma. *Electrophoresis* 1999; 20: 569–74.

72. Vester, B, Rasmussen, K. High performance liquid chromatography method for rapid and accurate determination of homocysteine in plasma and serum. *Eur J Clin Chem Clin Biochem* 1991; 29: 549–54.

73. Wilcken, DEL. Novel risk for vascular disease: The homocysteine hypothesis of cardiovascular disease. *J Cardiovas Risk* 1998; 5: 217–21.

74. Wiley, VC, Dudman, NP, Wilcken, DE. Interrelations between plasma free and protein-bound homocysteine and cysteine in homocystinuria. *Metabolism* 1988; 37: 191–95.

75. Willems, HP, Bos, GM, Gerrits, WB, den Heijer, M, Vloet, S, Blom, HJ. Acidic citrate stabilizes blood samples for assay of total homocysteine. *Clin Chem* 1998; 44: 342–45.

76. Woltersdorf, WW, Bowron, A, Day, AP, Scott, J, Stansbie, D. Abbott IMx homocysteine assay: Significant interference by 3-deazaadenosine [letter]. *Ann Clin Biochem* 1999; 36: 533.

19

Methionine Loading

JONATHAN SILBERBERG
NICHOLAS DUDMAN*

Methionine loading has been used as a clinical diagnostic tool to study the efficiency of homocysteine metabolism, primarily through the transsulfuration pathway. The technique has been used since the condition known as homocystinuria was first described in the early 1960s (10, 23). Initially, methionine was administered orally (10) or intravenously (8) at a dose of 0.10 g/kg. This dose is still used today. In the early tests, a methionine load was followed by blood and urine analysis for changes in the concentrations of homocystine and the homocysteine-cysteine mixed disulfide.

Methionine loading and other analytical techniques were used to establish the diagnosis of homocystinuria and to help identify the impaired metabolic pathway(s) responsible for elevated homocysteine levels. Later, the methionine loading test was used to identify individuals who were suspected of being heterozygous for mutations in the genes that code for the enzymes involved in homocysteine metabolism, particularly cystathionine β-synthase (CBS) (Metabolic Diagram, Reaction 6). A belief developed that heterozygosity for a mutant CBS gene would alter the enzyme's activity and cause moderately elevated postmethionine plasma homocysteine levels (4, 16). However, the application of molecular genetic techniques in the mid 1990s cast doubt on the use of this test for identifying heterozygotes (20). After publication of the work by Wilcken and Wilcken (41), researchers began using the oral methionine load test to assess homocysteine metabolism empirically in selected patients. Oral methionine load testing is still used extensively for that purpose.

During the first 25 years of the study of homocystinuria, the methods used to accurately measure the concentrations of the various homocysteine-containing compounds in body fluids, particularly homocystine, were insensitive and often inadequate. One of the important early reasons for using the methionine loading test was to increase the plasma concentrations of homocystine and homocysteine-cysteine mixed disulfide, whereby these augmented levels could be determined with precision by the amino acid analyzers of the time. In the late 1980s, much more sensitive and precise techniques were developed that could accurately measure low levels of plasma total homocysteine and other sulfhydryl-containing amino acids after chemical reduction (39). Thereafter, precise, accurate, and reliable measurement of fasting plasma total homocysteine became available in many laboratories; and the methionine loading test became less relevant as the tool for assessing abnormal plasma homocysteine levels in most patients. This chapter describes the current methionine loading practice and the various influences on its outcomes, as well as applications and limitations of the technique.

Loading Protocols

Timing and Dose

In subjects with normal renal function given oral L-methionine, plasma total homocysteine peaks at 6 to 8 hours postmethionine administration, and levels remain above baseline for more than 24 hours (Figure 19.1) (38). It is customary for the postload homocysteine measurement to be done 4 hours after dosing, although alternative techniques have been used.

Oral methionine is given as the L-isomer, most commonly in water or orange juice, after an overnight fast. Side effects are common, with nausea in about one third of the subjects and vomiting in up to 5%. Some investigators allow a standardized meal of known protein content, typically containing no more than 100 mg methionine, at 0, 2 or 4 hours. This reduces nausea and allows for measurements at later time periods without the need for prolonged fasting.

* Deceased

Ralph Carmel and Donald W. Jacobsen, eds. *Homocysteine in Health and Disease.* © Cambridge University Press 2001. All rights reserved. Printed in the United States of America.

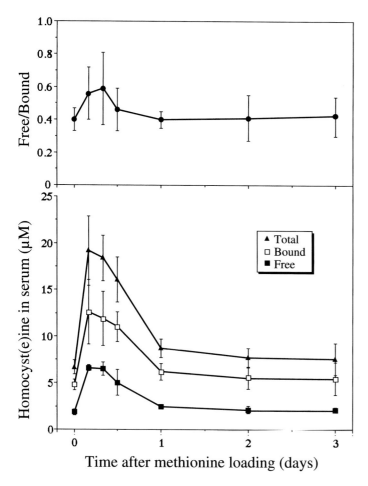

Fig. 19.1. Time course of change in homocysteine levels after methionine loading in normal subjects. Healthy premenopausal women were given 0.1 g methionine/kg orally. Top panel, postload ratio of free/bound homocysteine over time. Bottom panel, postload total, protein-bound, and free homocysteine levels. (Reproduced from Ueland and Refsum [38], with permission.)

The usual dose is 0.10 g/kg body weight or 3.8 to 4.0 g/m² body surface area. In view of the differences in body fat between men and women, weight-adjusted dosing leads to higher increments in homocysteine in women (see later). Protocols based on lean body mass would correct this problem, but these protocols have not yet been developed.

For population testing, an alternative 2-hour collection protocol may be more convenient (5). Two- and 4-hour plasma total homocysteine levels are highly correlated, but the predictive value of the 2-hour level has not been independently established. In renal failure, testing is often deferred to 6 or 24 hours after dosing because levels remain high for several days.

Food and Dietary Methionine

Humans on diets with differing methionine contents might be expected to display different responses to loading. In healthy volunteers exposed to either a threefold increase in methionine intake or a fivefold reduction in protein intake for several weeks, neither methionine clearance nor the postload homocysteine levels were affected (1, 18). This result does not comment on effects of longer term dietary patterns, but it does indicate that small variations in daily intake are unlikely to affect the test results. In contrast, substantial protein intake during the test is likely to affect interpretation (25).

Defining an Abnormal Result

In early studies the absolute postload homocysteine level was compared with the 95th percentile for control subjects in defining postload hyperhomocysteinemia. However, subjects with high basal values commonly have high postload levels, so the absolute value does not clearly identify those with an exaggerated response to oral methionine loading.

Two parameters of the loading test describe the *increment* in homocysteine: the absolute rise (ΔHcy; equation 1) and percent or relative rise (%ΔHcy; equation 2) in homocysteine level. Of these, the percent rise is preferred, but is unfortunately rarely used.

$$\Delta Hcy = postload\ Hcy - preload\ Hcy \qquad (1)$$

$$\%\Delta Hcy = (postload\ Hcy - \\ preload\ Hcy)*100/preload\ Hcy \qquad (2)$$

The ΔHcy is the arithmetic difference between postload and fasting plasma total homocysteine values; the latter is the difference relative to the fasting values, with the result expressed on a log scale. Plots depicting the relationship between the absolute difference in the preload and postload homocysteine values (ΔHcy) and the relative or percent differences (%ΔHcy) are shown in Figure 19.2 (32). The absolute rise in levels is directly proportional to the mean of two measurements, but the percent rise is not.

The absolute rise in homocysteine is commonly used to describe the increment in plasma total homocysteine after loading, but it tends to be higher when fasting homocysteine is high. Unless the baseline value is known, the significance of the absolute rise in levels is unclear. Most studies examining determinants of the postload response have used the absolute rise and therefore actually describe determinants of both the basal level and postload response. If the percent rise in homocysteine is used instead, the changes in postload response relative to basal values are far more

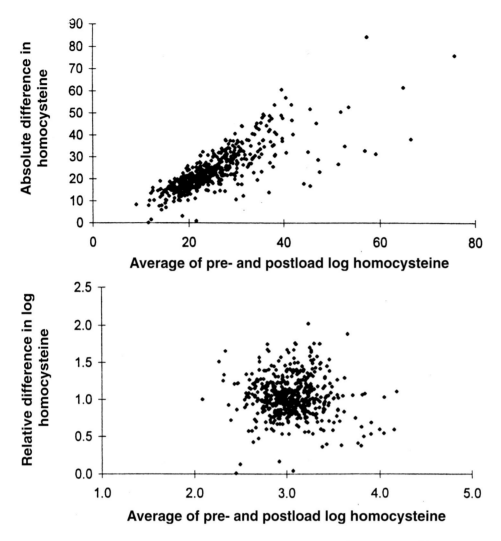

Fig. 19.2. Plots comparing the absolute and relative (%) rise in homocysteine levels after methionine loading. Top panel, the absolute, arithmetic difference in total homocysteine levels before and after methionine loading (ΔHcy) is compared with the mean of the two values. Bottom panel, the relative or percent difference in homocysteine levels before and after loading (%ΔHcy) is compared with the mean of the two values (log-log plot). The absolute change in homocysteine levels is directly proportional to the mean of the two measurements, but the relative difference is not. (Reproduced from Silberberg et al. [32], with permission.)

significant than the absolute difference between the two values.

Normal Variation: Age, Sex, and Race

Age

The increase in plasma total homocysteine that follows methionine loading declines with age (Figure 19.3) (32). The relation between the percent rise in homocysteine and age is quadratic and negative such

that many subjects over 75 years of age have only a very slight rise in plasma total homocysteine. It is likely that methionine absorption is impaired in some older persons, but this has not yet been explicitly tested.

Sex

Women have greater increases in plasma total homocysteine after loading than do men, approximately 25% overall. This probably represents excess dosing based on body weight or body surface area rather than lean body mass. If sex-specific reference ranges are not used, women are particularly apt to be labeled as suffering from postload hyperhomocysteinemia.

Race

Few studies have adequately assessed the effect of race or ethnicity on the methionine loading test, as opposed to effects on fasting plasma total homocysteine levels. South African blacks were reported to have lower fast-

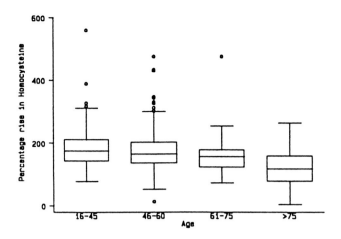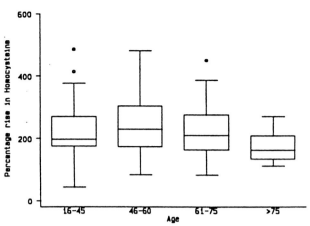

Fig. 19.3. Effect of age on percentage rise in homocysteine levels (%ΔHcy) after methionine loading. Box plots of percent rise in homocysteine levels (%ΔHcy) in four age strata. Left: males. Right: females. The percent rise is higher in females at all ages ($p < 0.0001$). The effect of age is nonlinear, being less over the age of 75 years. (Reproduced from Silberberg et al. [32], with permission.)

ing plasma total homocysteine levels and a lower response to load, measured as either the absolute rise in homocysteine or the percent rise, than South African whites (35). The difference in fasting levels was more marked between urban and traditional-living black populations, but persisted when blacks and whites with similar lifestyles were compared. In a small study, young black males had lower levels of plasma pyridoxal-5'-phosphate, yet had lower fasting plasma total homocysteine, absolute rise, and percent rise in homocysteine. After vitamin supplementation, their absolute rise in homocysteine was similar to whites, but the percent rise was higher (34). Other than differences resulting from differing basal levels, there is no evidence yet that race specifically affects the methionine load test.

Clearance of Homocysteine after Oral Methionine Load

Insights from Animal Studies

After in vivo homocysteine loading in the rat, there is net uptake of homocysteine by the kidney, indicating that the kidney is the major site of clearance. Miller et al. (29) formulated a hypothesis of coordinate regulation of remethylation and transsulfuration based on methionine loading studies in vitamin B_6- and folate-deficient rats (see Chapter 9). In rats with vitamin B_6 deficiency, marked increases in plasma total homocysteine were seen after loading with 0.10 g/kg, but folate-deficient rats displayed no increase. Miller et al. (29) suggested that this could be explained by S-adenosylmethionine inhibiting 5,10-methylenetetrahy-

drofolate reductase (MTHFR) and activating CBS. In vitamin B_6-deficiency, increased hepatic S-adenosylmethionine suppresses homocysteine remethylation and leads to increases in plasma homocysteine after methionine loading. In folate deficiency, increased S-adenosylmethionine activates the transsulfuration pathway and allows rapid clearance of excess homocysteine. However, the role of folate in the cellular production of methionine and thus S-adenosylmethionine has yet to be accounted for by this hypothesis.

Human Studies

Numerous studies have examined the relation between folate, cobalamin, or vitamin B_6 status and the response to methionine loading. Because most studies have used absolute postload homocysteine change, the effect of vitamins on the load response as distinct from the baseline level is difficult to disentangle. Because basal homocysteine is negatively related to levels of folate and cobalamin, these vitamins are similarly correlated with the absolute rise in homocysteine (lower folate, higher increment). When examined as the percent rise in homocysteine, the correlation is positive (lower folate, lower increment), in keeping with the Miller-Selhub hypothesis. A useful implementation of the response to methionine loading has been to define a normal (i.e., physiological) range for folate, below which neither fasting nor postload homocysteine levels exceed a population percentile (9).

Renal metabolism contributes significantly to clearance of homocysteine in normal subjects, and fasting plasma total homocysteine levels increase in renal failure. As in subjects with normal renal function, folate status affects plasma total homocysteine levels by its effect on remethylation in tissues (26). In renal failure the loading test is particularly difficult to interpret.

Homocysteine increases after methionine loading in dialysis patients; the magnitude of the rise is proportional to basal levels. Here the kinetics of homocysteine elimination after oral methionine loading are uncertain, with some methodological problems preventing accurate kinetic modeling. Accordingly, no single model fits all patients. In about one fifth of the patients, homocysteine levels continue to rise between 6 and 24 hours after loading, but in others there is a 20% decrease in homocysteine levels (compared with 40% to 50% in healthy subjects), demonstrating first-order kinetics and a half-life estimated at 27 hours (40). Although these clearances are similar to the clearance of homocysteine after oral homocysteine loading (which approximates first-order kinetics with a half-time of 13 hours) (26), many assumptions must hold for kinetic models to be meaningful. In 23 stable transplant patients, fasting plasma total homocysteine was increased compared with control subjects (18.0 vs. 9.8 µmol/L) (7). After loading, the absolute rise in homocysteine levels was higher (22 vs. 15 µmol/L), but not the percent rise (approximately 122% vs. 155%).

Effects of Vitamin Supplementation

In mild hyperhomocysteinemia, vitamin levels influence the response to load predominantly through effects on basal homocysteine levels. No report has used the percent rise in homocysteine levels in the primary analysis, so the effect of supplementation with folic acid or vitamin B_6 on the load parameter itself is unclear.

In a physiological model of vitamin B_6 deficiency (humans treated with theophylline for asthma), vitamin B_6 supplements reduced the absolute rise in homocysteine levels after methionine loading (36). In another study, three vitamin supplements had no effect on the methionine load test results when measured as the absolute rise in levels (34). However, calculated as the percent rise in homocysteine levels, the response to load with supplementation may have been greater, but the sample was small (34).

Among women with recurrent miscarriage, folic acid supplementation lowered fasting plasma total homocysteine. The effect was greatest in those homozygous for the MTHFR 677C→T mutation, who consequently had lower absolute rises in homocysteine levels (30).

In patients with homozygous homocystinuria, treatment with vitamin B_6 lowered fasting plasma total homocysteine levels but had little effect on postload levels (3). Both fasting and postload levels are lowered by folic acid supplementation in dialysis patients, as in those with normal renal function. There appear to be no additional effects of betaine (40).

Influence of Genotype

Several studies have confirmed that fasting plasma total homocysteine levels are higher in relatives of

hyperhomocysteinemic patients (22). The same has been shown for postload homocysteine levels (22). Considerations of the absolute and percent rises in homocysteine levels similarly compound interpretation of the effect of genotypic markers on the methionine load test. When homocysteine levels are measured as the absolute rise, most studies show a greater response to load in those homozygous for the 677C→T variant at the gene for MTHFR (14). Likewise the 133T→C mutation in the gene for CBS has been associated with elevated fasting and postload homocysteine levels. In contrast, the 2756A→G variation in the gene for methionine synthase affects neither the basal nor postload homocysteine levels (33).

Methionine Loading in Diagnosis

Hyperhomocysteinemia

In early studies, the term *hyperhomocysteinemia* was defined with reference to the population 95th percentile for either basal or postload homocysteine levels. Not surprisingly, the methionine loading test identifies 5% of individuals as having the hyperhomocysteinemia phenotype. If the comparison uses inappropriate reference ranges, the diagnosis of postload hyperhomocysteinemia is more readily made, a problem that often develops when investigators use a published reference range from another laboratory. Similarly, as many as 50% of patients with renal failure have levels above the 95th percentile for healthy persons (7).

Because females have a greater response to load doses based on body weight, the use of overall rather than age- and gender-specific ranges is prone to identify a high proportion of females as having the hyperhomocysteinemia trait (5, 24). With gender-specific ranges, the proportion of males and females with hyperhomocysteinemia is similar.

Vascular Disease

Coronary Atherosclerosis Numerous case-control studies have reported differences in fasting plasma total homocysteine between patients with coronary heart disease and control subjects and similarly higher postload homocysteine levels and absolute rises in homocysteine in patients with heart disease compared with controls subjects (reviewed in [31]). Although the diagnosis of hyperhomocysteinemia in patients with arterial disease is enhanced by the methionine loading test, this is largely due to the use of absolute postload homocysteine rises rather than the percent rise. The only study examining the percent rise found no association with coronary disease, but also found no association for fasting homocysteine levels (J. Silberberg, unpublished data).

Thrombotic Disorders In patients with recurrent venous thrombosis, both fasting and 6-hour postmethionine homocysteine levels were higher than in control subjects (17). The proportion above the 90th percentile was 25% for fasting and 24% for postload homocysteine, suggesting that the diagnosis was not particularly enhanced by the loading protocol. Neither the absolute not the percent rises in homocysteine levels were reported. It has been suggested that in venous thrombosis, synergism exists between fasting plasma total homocysteine and other markers of a procoagulant state such as resistance to activated protein C, an abnormal clotting factor V, or prothrombin levels (11, 13). These studies have not been extended to include the methionine loading test.

A study of eight families with homocystinuria found venous thrombosis to be more common in patients with activated protein C resistance because of the factor V Leiden mutation (27). In these families, postload homocysteine levels were markedly increased, and cell culture studies confirmed a deficiency of CBS (27). It seems likely that in a few individuals with normal fasting plasma total homocysteine levels and a coexistent thrombotic disorder, the methionine loading test will identify clinically significant hyperhomocysteinemia postload that is not evident from basal levels.

Inborn Errors of Metabolism

In an early case study, several patients were identified with premature coronary disease and high postload homocysteine values. They were shown by cell culture to have a deficiency in CBS activity (19). Because most had very large increments in homocysteine, both the absolute and percent rises in homocysteine levels were clearly abnormal. However, when some of these patients were later studied by mRNA sequencing techniques, no relevant CBS mutations were found (20). Studies of obligate heterozygotes for CBS deficiency have shown that not all affected individuals have an abnormal methionine loading test or even abnormal activity in enzyme assays (28).

Neural Tube Defects

Although both elevated fasting homocysteine levels and folate deficiency have been associated with neural tube defects, no relation has been shown with the absolute or percent rises in homocysteine levels. Ubbink et al. (37) found paradoxically low absolute rises in homocysteine in women with affected pregnancies but also failed to confirm the common finding of lower folate or elevated fasting homocysteine levels.

Methionine Loading in Clinical Research

The acute rise in plasma total homocysteine that follows an oral methionine load has been used to examine the physiological effects of mild homocysteinemia in vivo. Because these studies induce a rapid rise in homocysteine level, their relevance to chronic increases in homocysteine remains uncertain.

Clotting Factors

Neither the absolute level of activated protein C nor its ratio to total protein C is altered in methionine loading tests by the postload increases in plasma total homocysteine levels. Conversely, the postload homocysteine level is not influenced by the activated protein C level (12).

Vasodilator Reserve

The increase in homocysteine after methionine loading was associated with abnormal vasodilator reserve as measured by the brachial artery occlusion technique (2). Pretreatment with vitamin C prevented reduction in flow-mediated dilatation but did not affect the absolute rise in homocysteine levels, suggesting that the redox state of plasma total homocysteine is relevant to this response (15).

Summary: Not an Oral Glucose Tolerance Test

Long considered a cornerstone of diagnosis in diabetes mellitus, the oral glucose tolerance test may offer an analogy to the methionine loading test. Apparently similar, there are in fact important differences between the two. Foremost, the oral glucose tolerance test is never suggested when the fasting level is high. The glucose load is intended as a stress test for latent disease; at follow-up evaluation, those with an abnormal load response are more likely to have a raised fasting glucose. This, in turn, defines the diabetic condition and future risk of end-organ damage.

In contrast, the methionine loading test does not identify those who will later have high fasting levels. It was developed to augment basal levels to overcome problems with measuring small amounts of free homocysteine in the laboratory. The significance of high postload values with respect to a causal role in cardiovascular disease remains uncertain.

Despite established credentials, even the oral glucose tolerance test has recently come under question. Those who would do without the test reason that lowering the level of fasting blood sugar adequately identifies those with latent diabetes. The current recommendation of the American Diabetes Association taskforce is that the oral glucose tolerance test need rarely be used for diagnosis (21).

In the assessment of homocysteine metabolism, the oral methionine loading test continues to have a limited place. For the present, the test may be of value in the diagnosis of heterozygotes for CBS deficiency, particularly in known affected families. We think it unlikely that the oral methionine loading test will have a lasting role in the assessment of common forms of mild homocysteinemia.

REFERENCES

1. Andersson, A, Brattstrom, L, Israelsson, B, Hultberg, B. The effect of excess daily methionine intake on plasma homocysteine after a methionine loading test in humans. *Clin Chim Acta* 1990; 192: 69–76.

2. Bellamy, MF, McDowell, IFW, Ramsey, MW, Brownlee, M, Bones, C, Newcombe, RG, Lewis, MJ. Hyperhomocysteinemia after an oral methionine load acutely impairs endothelial function in healthy adults. *Circulation* 1998; 98: 1848–52.

3. Boers, GHJ, Smals, AGH, Drayer, JIM, Trijbels, FJM, Leermakers, AI, Kloppenborg, PW. Pyridoxine treatment does not prevent homocysteinemia after methionine loading in adult homocystinuria patients. *Metabolism* 1983; 32: 390–97.

4. Boers, GHJ, Smals, AGH, Trijbels, FJM, Fowler, B, Bakkeren, JAJM, Schoonderwald, HC, Kleijer, WJ, Kloppenborg, PWC. Heterozygosity for homocystinuria in premature peripheral and cerebral occlusive arterial disease. *N Engl J Med* 1985; 313: 709–15.

5. Bostom, AG, Jacques, PF, Nadeau, MR, Williams, RR, Ellison, RC, Selhub, J. Post-methionine load hyperhomocysteinemia in persons with normal fasting total plasma homocysteine: Initial results from the NHLBI Family Heart Study. *Atherosclerosis* 1995; 116: 147–51.

6. Bostom, AG, Roubenoff, R, Dellaripa, P, Nadeau, MR, Sutherland, P, Wilson, PWF, Jacques, PF, Selhub, J, Rosenberg, F.H. Validation of an abbreviated oral methionine-load test (letter). *Clin Chem* 1995; 41: 948–49.

7. Bostom, AG, Gohh, RY, Tsai, MY, Hopkins-Garcia, BJ, Nadeau, MR, Bianchi, LA, Jacques, PF, Rosenberg, IH, Selhub, J. Excess prevalence of fasting and postmethionine-loading hyperhomocysteinemia in stable renal transplant recipients. *Arterioscl Thromb Vasc Biol* 1997; 17: 1894–900.

8. Brenton, DP, Cusworth, DC, Gaull, GE. Homocystinuria: Metabolic studies on 3 patients. *J Pediatr* 1965; 67: 58–68.

9. Brouwer, DAJ, Welten, HTME, Reijngoud, DJ, Van Doormaal, JJ, Muskiet, FAJ. Plasma folic acid cutoff value, derived from its relationship with homocyst(e)ine. *Clin Chem* 1998; 44: 1545–50.

10. Carson, NAJ, Cusworth, DC, Dent, CE, Field, CMB, Neill, DW, Westall, RG. Homocystinuria: A new inborn error of metabolism associated with mental deficiency. *Arch Dis Child* 1963; 38: 425–36.

11. Cattaneo, M, Tsai, MY, Bucciarelli, P, Taioli, E, Zighetti, ML, Bignell, M, Mannucci, PM. A common mutation in the methylenetetrahydrofolate reductase gene (C677T) increases the risk for deep vein thrombosis in patients with mutant factor V (Factor V:Q^{506}). *Arterioscl Thromb Vasc Biol* 1997; 17: 1662–66.

12. Cattaneo, M, Franchi, F, Zighetti, ML, Martinelli, I, Asti, D, Mannucci, PM. Plasma levels of activated protein C in healthy subjects and patients with previous venous thromboembolism: Relationships with plasma homocysteine levels. *Arterioscl Thromb Vasc Biol* 1998; 18: 1371–75.

13. Cattaneo, M, Chantarangkul, V, Taioli, E, Samtos, JH, Tagliabue, L. The G20210A mutation of the prothrombin gene in patients with previous first episodes of deep vein thrombosis: Prevalence and association with factor V G1691A, methylenetetrahydrofolate reductase C677T and plasma prothrombin levels. *Thromb Res* 1999; 93: 1–8.

14. Cattaneo, M, Lombardi, R, Lecchi, A, Zighetti, ML. Is the oral methionine loading test insensitive to the remethylation of homocysteine? (letter). *Blood* 1999; 93: 1118–20.

15. Chambers, JC, McGregor, A, Jean-Marie, J, Obeid, OA, Kooner, JS. Demonstration of rapid onset vascular endothelial dysfunction after hyperhomocysteinemia: An effect reversible with vitamin C therapy. *Circulation* 1999; 99: 1156–60.

16. Clarke, R, Daly, L, Robinson, K, Naughten, E, Cahalane, S, Fowler, B, Graham, I. Hyperhomocysteinemia: An independent risk factor for vascular disease. *N Engl J Med* 1991; 325: 967–60.

17. den Heijer, M, Blom, HJ, Gerrits, WBJ, Rosendaal, FR, Haak, HL, Wijermans, PW, Bos, GM. Is hyperhomocysteinaemia a risk factor for recurrent venous thrombosis? *Lancet* 1995; 345: 882–85.

18. den Heijer, M, Bos, GJM, Brouwer, IA, Gerrits, WB, Blom, HJ. Variability of the methionine loading test: No effect of a low protein diet. *Ann Clin Biochem* 1996; 33: 551–54.

19. Dudman NPB, Guo XW, Gordon RB, Dawson PA, Wilcken DEL. Human homocysteine catabolism: Three major pathways and their relevance ot development of arterial occlusive disease. *J. Nutr.* 1996;126 Suppl.: 1295S–1300S.

20. Dudman NPB, Wilcken DEL, Wang J, Lynch JF, Macey D, Lundberg P. Disordered methionine/homocysteine metabolism in premature vascular disease: Its occurrence, cofactor therapy, and enzymology. *Arterioscler. Thromb.* 1993;13: 1253–1260.

21. Expert Committee on the Diagnosis and Classification of Diabetes Mellitus. Report of the Expert Committee on the Diagnosis and Classification of Diabetes Mellitus. *Diabetes Care* 1997; 20: 1183–97.

22. Franken, DG, Boers, GHJ, Blom, HJ, Cruysberg, JRM, Trijbels, FJM, Hamel, BCJ. Prevalence of familial mild hyperhomocysteinemia. *Atherosclerosis* 1996; 125: 71–80.

23. Gerritsen, T, Waisman, HA. Homocystinuria, an error in the metabolism of methionine. *Pediatrics* 1964; 33: 413–20.

24. Graham, IM, Daly, LE, Refsum, HM, Robinson, K, Brattström, L, Ueland, PM, Palma-Reis, RJ, Boers, GHJ, Sheahan, RG, Israelsson, B, Uiterwaal, CS, Meleady, R, McMaster, D, Verhoef, P, Witteman, J, Rubba, P, Bellet,

H, Wautrecht, JC, De Valk, HW, Sales Lúis, AC, Parrot-Roulaud, FM, Tan, KS, Higgins, I, Garcon, D, Medrano, MJ, Candito, M, Evans, AE, Andria G. Plasma homocysteine as a risk factor for vascular disease. The European Concerted Action Project. *J Am Med Assoc* 1997; 277: 1775–81.

25. Guttormsen, AB, Schneede, J, Fiskerstrand, T, Ueland, PM, Refsum, HM. Plasma concentrations of homocysteine and other aminothiol compounds are related to food intake in healthy human subjects. *J Nutr* 1994; 124: 1934–41.

26. Guttormsen, AB, Ueland, PM, Svarstad, E, Refsum, H. Kinetic basis of hyperhomocysteinemia in patients with chronic renal failure. *Kidney Int* 1997; 52: 495–502.

27. Mandel, H, Brenner, B, Berant, M, Rosenberg, N, Lanir, N, Jakobs, C, Fowler, B, Seligsohn, U. Coexistence of hereditary homocystinuria and factor V Leiden—effect on thrombosis. *N Engl J Med* 1996; 334: 763–68.

28. McGill, JJ, Mettler, G, Rosenblatt, DS, Scriver, CR. Detection of heterozygotes for recessive alleles. Homocysteinemia: Paradigm of pitfalls in phenotypes. *Am J Med Genet* 1990; 36: 45–52.

29. Miller, JW, Nadeau, MR, Smith, D, Selhub, J. Vitamin B$_6$ deficiency vs folate deficiency: Comparison of responses to methionine loading in rats. *Am J Clin Nutr* 1994; 59: 1033–39.

30. Nelen, WLDM, Blom, HJ, Thomas, CMG, Steegers, EAP, Boers, GHJ, Eskes, TKAB. Methylenetetrahydrofolate reductase polymorphism affects the change in homocysteine and folate concentrations resulting from low dose folic acid supplementation in women with unexplained recurrent miscarriages. *J Nutr* 1998; 128: 1336–41.

31. Refsum, H, Ueland, PM, Nygard, O, Vollset, SE. Homocysteine and cardiovascular disease. *Annu Rev Med* 1998; 49: 31–62.

32. Silberberg, JS, Crooks, R, Fryer, J, Wlodarczyk, J, Nair, B, Guo, XW, Xie, LJ, Dudman, N. Gender differences and other determinants of the rise in plasma homocysteine after L-methionine loading. *Atherosclerosis* 1997; 133: 105–10.

33. Tsai, MY, Welge, BG, Hanson, NQ, Bignell, MK, Vessey, J, Schwichtenberg, K, Yang, F, Bullemer, FE, Rasmussen, R, Graham, KJ. Genetic causes of mild hyperhomocysteinemia in patients with premature occlusive coronary artery diseases. *Atherosclerosis* 1999; 143: 163–70.

34. Ubbink, JB, Vermaak, H, Delport, R, van der Merwe, A, Becker, PJ, Potgieter, H. Effective homocysteine metabolism may protect South African blacks against coronary heart disease. *Am J Clin Nutr* 1995; 62: 802–8.

35. Ubbink, JB, Delport, R, Vermaak, WJ. Plasma homocysteine concentrations in a population with a low coronary heart disease prevalence. *J Nutr* 1996; 126: 1254S–7S.

36. Ubbink, JB, vd Merwe, A, Delport, R, Allen, RH, Stabler, SP, Riezler, R, Vermaak, WJH. The effect of a subnormal vitamin B$_6$ status on homocysteine metabolism. *J Clin Invest* 1996; 98: 177–84.

37. Ubbink, JB, Christianson, A, Bester, MJ, Van Allen, MI, Venter, PA, Delport, R, Blom, HJ, van der Merwe, A, Potgieter, H, Vermaak, WJH. Folate status, homocysteine metabolism, and methylene tetrahydrofolate reductase genotype in rural South African blacks with a history of pregnancy complicated by neural tube defects. *Metabolism* 1999; 48: 269–74.

38. Ueland, PM, Refsum, H. Plasma homocysteine, a risk factor for vascular disease: Plasma levels in health, disease, and drug therapy. *J Lab Clin Med* 1989; 114: 473–501.

39. Ueland, PM, Refsum, H, Stabler, SP, Malinow, MR, Andersson, A, Allen, RH. Total homocysteine in plasma or serum: Methods and clinical applications. *Clin Chem* 1993; 39: 1764–79.

40. Van Guldener, C, Janssen, MJFM, de Meer, K, Donker, AJM, Stehouwer, CDA. Effect of folic acid and betaine on fasting and postmethionine-loading plasma homocysteine and methionine levels in chronic haemodialysis patients. *J Intern Med* 1999; 245: 175–83.

41. Wilcken, DEL, Wilcken, B. The pathogenesis of coronary artery disease. A possible role for methionine metabolism. *J Clin Invest* 1976; 57: 1079–82.

PART TWO

CLINICAL DYSFUNCTION AND
HYPERHOMOCYSTEINEMIA

20

Cystathionine β-Synthase and Its Deficiency

JAN P. KRAUS
VIKTOR KOŽICH

Homocysteine occupies a branch point in methionine, cysteine, and S-adenosylmethionine metabolism. About half the homocysteine formed is conserved by remethylation to methionine in the "methionine cycle" (31). The other half is irreversibly converted by cystathionine β-synthase (CBS) [L-serine hydrolyase] and cystathionine γ-lyase to cysteine (Metabolic Diagram, Reactions 6 and 7). Thus, CBS is involved directly in the removal of homocysteine from the cycle and in the biosynthesis of cysteine, a precursor of glutathione, the major redox regulating metabolite of the cell.

In vitro studies have indicated that S-adenosylmethionine functions as a switch between the methionine cycle and the transsulfuration pathway (32) (see Chapter 9). At low S-adenosylmethionine concentrations its resynthesis is unimpaired. High concentrations of S-adenosylmethionine, however, limit homocysteine remethylation by inhibiting 5,10-methylenetetrahydrofolate reductase (26) and betaine methyltransferase (32). Transsulfuration, by contrast, is enhanced by the stimulatory effect of S-adenosylmethionine on CBS activity (30, 56).

Deficient CBS activity was recognized as a cause of homocystinuria in 1964 (80). CBS deficiency (MIM 236200 [76a]) is now considered to be the major cause of inherited homocystinuria.

The Human Cystathionine β-Synthase Gene

The locus for human CBS was mapped to chromosome 21 (65, 101). The gene has subsequently been localized more precisely to the subtelomeric region of band 21q22.3 (87) where the gene for α-A-crystallin, a major structural protein of the ocular lens, is also found. Synteny of these two loci is conserved in the mouse on chromosome 17 (106), in the rat on chromosome 20 (69), and in the cow in the syntenic group U10 (58). The entire human CBS gene was cloned and sequenced in 1998 (62). A total of 28,046 nucleotides were reported spanning the entire CBS gene and an additional 5 kbp of 5′-flanking sequence (Figure 20.1).

Alternative Splicing of Cystathionine β-synthase Pre-mRNA

The human CBS gene contains 23 exons; the CBS polypeptide of 551 amino acids is encoded by exons 1 to 14 and 16. Exon 15 is alternatively spliced. It encodes 14 amino acids and is incorporated in relatively few mature human CBS mRNA molecules. The CBS polypeptide containing exon 15 has not yet been detected in any human tissues. Consequently, the biological significance, if any, of exon 15 remains obscure (62). The 5′-untranslated region of human CBS mRNA is formed by one of five alternatively used exons, designated -1a to -1e, and one invariably present, exon 0, whereas the 3′-untranslated region is encoded by exons 16 and 17 (5, 21, 22). Interestingly, intron 16 appears to be retained in the 3′- untranslated region of most of the fibroblast and liver mRNA of every individual tested (61). While the exon-intron organization of the human CBS gene in the protein-coding region is perfectly conserved with the rat and mouse CBS genes, the genomic organization of the untranslated regions is quite different (5, 62, 92, 108).

Cystathionine β-Synthase Promoters

The human gene has at least two alternatively used promoters. These are located upstream of exons -1a and -1b. They are GC-rich (~80%) and contain numerous putative binding sites for Sp1, Ap1, Ap2, and c-myb, but lack the classic TATA box. Evaluation of the relative levels of the -1a and -1b promoter activities by transfection of the reporter constructs into COS 7, and HepG cells indicated that both of these regions contain all of the sequences essential for promoter activity. Under the conditions tested, the -1b

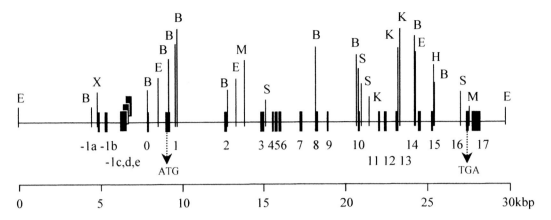

Fig. 20.1. Genomic organization of the human cystathionine β-synthase (CBS) gene. All exons, including the alternatively used exons -1a, b, c, d, e, and 15 are represented by solid boxes. The beginning and the end of the coding region are indicated by the codons ATG and TGA, respectively. The restriction sites are B, *Bam*H I; E, *Eco*R I; H, *Hin*d III; K, *Kpn* I; M, *Mlu* I; S, *Sfi* I; X, *Xba* I (reproduced from Kraus [62], with permission).

promoter activity was approximately 7- to 10-fold stronger than that of -1a (62).

Polymorphisms

The CBS locus contains DNA sequence repeats and single base variations that are polymorphic in Caucasians (60, 62) (Table 20.1). One variation deserves special mention because of its relatively high incidence in the normal population. Sebastio et al. (97) described an insertion of 68 base pairs (bp) in exon 8 (844ins68) in an allele from a CBS-deficient patient that also con-

tained the frequent I278T mutation. The 844ins68 was shown to be a frequent polymorphism occurring in about 5–13% of Caucasian and up to 40% of sub-Saharan African alleles (54, 90a, 105, 112). The insertion duplicates the intron 7 acceptor splice site and may lead to two alternatively spliced transcripts. The most abundant transcript, and the only one that has been detected in the cytosol of patient-derived fibroblasts, contains the wild-type mRNA sequence. The other transcript carrying the I278T mutation and a premature termination codon may be unstable and was detected in very low amounts only in the nucleus (105).

The Cystathionine β-Synthase Enzyme

The primary translational product of the CBS gene is a polypeptide with a molecular weight of 63 kDa (103). In fresh liver extracts, the enzyme is found as a tetramer of this subunit, whereas after a procedure in which the enzyme is first "aged" at 4°C and then puri-

---

Table 20.1. Polymorphisms and Repeats in the CBS Gene

Position gDNA	cDNA	Polymorphism	Repeat Unit	Tested Alleles	Allele 1	Allele 2	Allele 3	Allele 4	Allele 5
−6,921		STR	TTTC	30	5 × TTTC 0.667	6×TTTC 0.333			
−5,697		STR	GT	120	14 × GT 0.075	15 × GT 0.016	16 × GT 0.557	17 × GT 0.27	18 × GT 0.016
6,955	699	SNP	C/T	116	C 0.65	T 0.35			
9,132	844	Ins/Del	68 bp	880	Del 0.945	Ins 0.055			
11,686	1,080	SNP	C/T	111	C 0.55	T 0.45			
14,048		VNTR	31 bp	142	16 × 31 bp 0.098	17 × 31 bp 0.797	18 × 31 bp 0.07	19×31 bp 0	20 × 31 bp 0.035
18,854	1,985	SNP	C/T	78	T 0.63	C 0.37			

STR, short tandem repeats; VNTR, variable number of tandem repeats; SNP, single nucleotide polymorphism; ins/del, presence or absence of 844ins68; bp, base pairs.
Polymorphisms and repeats were tested in genomic DNA and cDNA samples derived from North American and Czech Caucasians. The A in the initiator Met codon has been designated as number 1 in both genomic DNA (gDNA) and cDNA sequences. (Reproduced from Kraus et al. [60], with permission.)

fied, CBS is isolated as a dimer of a 48 kDa subunit (64, 103). The reduction in size, caused by limited proteolysis, is accompanied by a significant increase in the specific activity of the enzyme. The purified hepatic enzyme contains firmly bound pyridoxal 5'-phosphate, on which it depends for activity (13, 51, 63).

Expression of Recombinant Human Cystathionine β-Synthase

The CBS cDNA has been used in various vectors to express the human recombinant enzyme in *Escherichia coli* (14), in yeast (66), and in Chinese hamster ovary cells (61). Significant amounts of the recombinant human CBS were purified from *E. coli* and characterized (14, 46, 109). Each hepatic or recombinant CBS subunit of 551 amino acid residues binds, in addition to the two substrates, three additional ligands: pyridoxal 5'-phosphate, *S*-adenosylmethionine (an allosteric activator), and, surprisingly, heme.

The Pyridoxal 5'-Phosphate-Binding Site of Cystathionine β-Synthase

Each mole of CBS subunit binds one mole of pyridoxal 5'-phosphate (46, 110). Kery et al. (49) demonstrated that the treatment of CBS with sodium borohydride selectively reduces the enzyme-pyridoxal 5'-phosphate Schiff base without affecting the heme. Sequencing of the pyridoxal 5'-phosphate-cross-linked peptide from a trypsin digest of the reduced enzyme identified the evolutionarily conserved Lys119 to be the pyridoxal 5'-phosphate-binding residue in human CBS. Serine and hydroxylamine form an α-aminoacrylate and an oxime with pyridoxal 5'-phosphate in CBS, respec-

tively. Homocysteine disturbs the heme environment but does not interact with pyridoxal 5'-phosphate.

S-Adenosylmethionine Activation of Cystathionine β-Synthase

The homocysteine branch point in the methyl cycle appears to be controlled by *S*-adenosylmethionine (32, 98). CBS in crude extracts is activated by *S*-adenosylmethionine two- to fourfold with an apparent K_{act} of 15 μmol/L (57). A human mutation, D444N, appears to interfere with the activation process (53). In addition, *S*-adenosylmethionine does not activate CBS that has been truncated at W409 or R413, and does not contain ~140 residues from the COOH terminus but exhibits increased activity (48, 99).

The Role of Heme in Cystathionine β-Synthase

Heme binding was first assigned to protein "H-450" (44, 89). Later comparison of the cDNA sequences revealed that H-450 and CBS were identical. The visible spectrum of CBS is due mostly to heme rather than pyridoxal 5'-phosphate. CBS exhibits the characteristic features of a heme protein: a sharp Soret peak at 428 nm with a shoulder at 363 nm and a broad band at 550 nm (Figure 20.2). The presence of heme in CBS is striking because the mechanism of the β-replacement reactions catalyzed by the enzyme can be

Fig. 20.2. Ultraviolet-visible spectra of the full-length cystathionine β-synthase (CBS) and the 45 kDa active core. The spectra were measured in Tris-buffered saline, pH 8.6. Full-length enzyme (thick line); the active core (thin line).

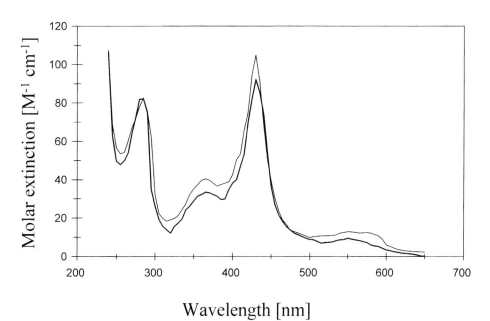

Wavelength [nm]

explained solely by pyridoxal 5′-phosphate-mediated catalysis (10, 11). The role of heme in this pyridoxal 5′-phosphate enzyme is unclear at present. Taoka et al. (109) proposed a catalytic role for the heme by activating homocysteine, similar to the action of zinc in the enzymes involved in the remethylation of homocysteine (42, 78). These workers also suggested that there are only 2 hemes per tetramer and that the hemes are nonequivalent (109, 110). However, Kery et al. (46) found that the specific activity of CBS increases with its heme saturation and that at full saturation 1 mol of the 63 kDa subunit binds 1 mol of heme. Heme incorporation into CBS is a prerequisite for pyridoxal 5′-phosphate binding and the amount of pyridoxal 5′-phosphate bound to the enzyme is limited by its heme saturation. Thus, the issues of heme stoichiometry and function in CBS await further clarification. Recently, two groups (45a, 70a) characterized purified CBS from *Saccharomyces cerevisiae*. They found that the yeast enzyme does not contain heme and is not activated by *S*-adenosylmethionine. Given the degree of sequence and mechanistic similarity between yeast and human CBS, this result indicates that heme is unlikely to play a direct catalytic role in the human CBS reaction mechanism. In support of this conclusion, another group found that the heme could be removed from a CBS crystal without affecting the ability of the crystal to condense homocysteine and serine (13a). Very recently, the two axial ligands of the heme were identified as Cys 52 and His 65 in the x-ray structure of human CBS (Kraus, unpublished observation).

Active Core of Cystathionine β-Synthase

Activation of human and rat CBS by proteolysis in crude liver extracts has been described previously (104). The cleaved dimeric enzyme of 48 kDa subunits was purified from human liver extracts and its properties were described (64). It was also shown that trypsin cleaves and activates the enzyme similarly to the hepatic protease (56, 79, 104). Recently, the active core of the enzyme was generated by limited digestion of the full-length CBS enzyme with trypsin and was subsequently characterized. The active core, extending from Glu 37 to Arg 413, forms a dimer of 45 kDa subunits, which is about twice as active as the tetramer. It binds both pyridoxal 5′-phosphate and heme cofactors, but is no longer activated by *S*-adenosylmethionine (48). This 45 kDa active core is the portion of CBS most homologous with the evolutionarily related enzymes isolated from plants or bacteria. Similar results were observed when human CBS cDNA containing a premature stop codon at position 409 was expressed in CBS-deficient yeast. The enzyme lacking the carboxy-terminal 143 amino acids was twice as active as the wild-type enzyme. Surprisingly, when any

one of several human inactivating pathogenic mutations were expressed in yeast in *cis* with this truncation, CBS activity was restored sufficiently to permit growth of the yeast on medium lacking cysteine. Of interest, activities of some of the mutant CBS approached wild-type levels (99).

Other β-Replacement Reactions and Evolutionary Conservation of Cystathionine β-Synthase

CBS can catalyze alternative β-replacement reactions in which sulfide is a substrate or a product (11) according to the general scheme:

$$XCH_2CH(NH_2)COOH + YH \rightarrow XH + YCH_2CH(NH_2)COOH$$

where, X = OH or SH and Y = SH or S-alkyl

The alternative reactions catalyzed by CBS may turn out to be of significance because the putative neuromodulator, hydrogen sulfide, is produced in rat brain by the activity of CBS (2).

The amino acid sequence of the active core of human CBS shares a high degree of structural similarity (52% if conservative replacements are counted) with the related *O*-acetylserine sulfhydrases (cysteine synthases) from plants and bacteria (59, 108) (Figure 20.3). This enzyme catalyzes the synthesis of cysteine from sulfide and acetylserine (15). It has been suggested that during evolution, the capacity to synthesize cystathionine was acquired by broadening the substrate specificity of such enzymes to include homocysteine as well as inorganic sulfide (108). Exon 3 is the most highly conserved region with about 50% identity to the bacterial enzymes. This highly conserved region contains lysine 119, the pyridoxal 5′-phosphate binding residue (49).

A more detailed discussion of the evolutionary conservation of CBS can be found in Chapter 14.

Cystathionine β-Synthase Deficiency

Clinical Picture of Cystathionine β-Synthase–Deficiency

Vitamin B₆ Responsiveness   The clinical and biochemical consequences of CBS deficiency are profoundly influenced by vitamin B₆ responsiveness. Responsiveness was originally defined as elimination of homocystine from plasma and urine and decrease of plasma methionine into the normal range after vitamin B₆ administration (12, 83). Various doses ranging between 25 and 1,200 mg/day have been shown to elicit the biochemical response, although occasionally a response was reported after a 2-mg dose of vitamin B₆ (83). In the original definition of responsiveness as "virtual elimination of

```
                →1                                    Q  →2
                ▼         R       R   S              PN  ▼              V R
CBS   HS 68 TAPAKSPKILPDILKKIGDTPMVRINKIGKKFGLKCELLAKCEFFNAGGS         117
CBS   RN 65 TVPTKSPKILPDILRKIGNTPMVRINRISKNAGLKCELLAKCEFFNAGGS         114
CYSK  EC  1 ---SKIFED-NSLT--IGHTPLVRLNRIGNG---R--ILAKVESRNPSFS          39
CYSK  ST  1 ---SKIYED-NSLT--IGHTPLVRLNRIGNG---R--ILAKVESRNPSFS          39
CSYN  SO  1 MVEEKAFIA-KDVTELIGKTPLVYLNTVADGCVAR--VAAKLEGMEPCSS          47
              .*         ..    **.**.* .*  ...  .   . ** *   .. .  *
                L
                H       W
                C       QV  D     D         R         KL  R   RM   T           Y
CBS   HS    VKDRISLRMIEDAERDGTLKPGDT-IIEPTSGNTGIGLA-LAAAVRGYRCI        166
CBS   RN    VKDRISLRMIEDAERAGTLKPGDT-IIEPTSGNTGIGLA-LAAAVKGYRCI        163
CYSK  EC    VKCRIGANMIWDAEKRGVLKPGVE-LVEPTSGNTGIALAYVAAA-RGYKLT         88
CYSK  ST    VKCRIGANMIWDAEKRGVLKPGVE-LVEPTNGNTGIALAYVAAA-RGYKLT         88
CSYN  SO    VKDRIGFSMITDAEKSGLITPGESVLIEPTSGNTGIGLAFIAAA-KGYKLI         97
            ** **. .** ***. * ..** .  .***.*****.** *** ..**. .
                    →4
                M       K▼  A            M       V
CBS   HS    IVMPEKMSSEKVDVLRALGAEIVRTPTNARFDSPESHVGVAWRLKNEIPN        216
CBS   RN    IVMPEKMSMEKVDVLRALGAEIVRTPTNARFDSPESHVGVAWRLKNEIPN        213
CYSK  EC    LTMPETMSIERRKLLKALGANLVLTEGAKGMKGA-IQKAEE-IVASNPEK        136
CYSK  ST    LTMPETMSIERRKLLKALGANLVLTEGAKGMKGA-IQKAEE-IVASDPQK        136
CSYN  SO    ITMPASMSLERRTILRAFGAELILTDPAKGMKGA-VQKAEE-IRDKTPNS        145
            ..**..** *.  ..*.*.** ...  *     . .... .      .. .
                →5                 →6                        G
                ▼ H T K      N     K     ▼              M S M     K
CBS   HS    SHILDQYRNASNPLAHYDTTADEILQQCDGKLDMLVASVGTGGTITGIAR        266
CBS   RN    SHILDQYRNASNPLAHYDDTAEEILQQCDGKVDMLVASAGTGGTITGIAR        263
CYSK  EC    YLLLQQFSNPANPEIHEKTTGPEIWEDTDGQVDVFIAGVGTGGTLTGVSR        186
CYSK  ST    YLLLQQFSNPANPEIHEKTTGPEIWEDTDGQVDVFISGVGTGGTLTGVTR        186
CSYN  SO    YIL-QQFENPANPKVHYETTGPEIWKGTGGKIDIFVSGIGTGGTITGAGR        194
             .  .*. .*..** *  ..*. ** ...*..*...  *****.** .*
                →7
                ΔQ      ▼ T               L              K  R S
CBS   HS    KLKEKCPGCRIIGV--DP-EGSILAEPEELNQTEQTTYEVEGIGYDFIPT        313
CBS   RN    KLKEKCPGCKIIGV--DP-EGSILAEPEELNQTEQTAYEVEGIGYDFIPT        310
CYSK  EC    YIKGTKGKTDLISVAVEPTDSPVIAQALAGEEIKPGPHKIQGIGAGFIPA        236
CYSK  ST    YIKGTKGKTDLITVAVEPTDSPVIAQALAGEEIKPGPHKIQGIGAGFIPG        236
CSYN  SO    YLKEQNPDVKLIGL--EPVESAV----LSGG--KPGPHKIQGLGAGFIPG        236
            .*.      .*...  .*  .... .    ..   *.* .***.
                →8             E     H        →9
                ▼ A            V     C        ▼       NMMP
CBS   HS    VLDRTVVDKWFKSNDEEAFTFARMLIAQEGLLCGGSAGSTVAVAVKAAQE        363
CBS   RN    VLDRAVVDRWFKSNDDDSFAFARMLISQEGLLCGGSSGSAMAVAVKAAQE        360
CYSK  EC    NLDLKLVDKVIGITNEEAISTARRLMEEEGILAGISSGAAVAAALKLQED        286
CYSK  ST    NLDLKLIDKVVGITNEEAISTARRLMEEEVFLAGISSGAAVAAALKLQED        286
CSYN  SO    VLDVNIIDEVVQISSEESIEMAKLLALKEGLLVGISSGAAAAAAIKVAKR        286
            **   ..*  .......  *. *  .* .* *.* *.*.*.*.* ..
                C              →10N                      →11
                HY    M        ▼ E     XI                ▼X
CBS   HS    LQEGQRC---VVILPDSVRNYMTKFLSDRWMLQKGFLKEEDLTEKKPWWW        410
CBS   RN    LKEGQRC---VVILPDSVRNYMSKFLSDKWMLQKGFMKEE-LSVKRPWWW        406
CYSK  EC    --ESFTNKNIVVILPSSGE-----------------------------        303
CYSK  ST    --ESFTNKNIVVILPSSGE-----------------------------        303
CSYN  SO    -PE-NAGKLIVAVFPSFGE-----------------------------        303
                *       *...*
```

Fig. 20.3. Evolutionary conservation of the active core of cystathionine β-synthase (CBS) and mutations. CBS HS, human CBS; CBS RN, rat CBS; CYSK EC, *E. coli* O-acetylserine lyase; CYSK ST, *Salmonella typhimurium* O-acetylserine lyase; CSYN SO, spinach cysteine synthase. Asterisks (*) signify absolute conservation of amino acid residues; dots (•) show conservative replacements. Approximate positions of the introns are indicated by solid, numbered triangles (∗). The human CBS mutations are noted above the sequences by bold letters. (Reproduced from Mudd et al. [83], with permission.)

homocystine from plasma and urine," the limit for detecting any plasma homocystine corresponded to a plasma total homocysteine concentration of ≈50 to 60 μmol/L. Because free homocystine determination has been universally replaced by the total homocysteine analysis, we propose to classify vitamin B_6 responsiveness as a decrease of total homocysteine below 50 μmol/L, and nonresponsiveness as no change in plasma total homocysteine after a dose of up to 10 mg/kg of vitamin B_6 per day administered for at least 2 weeks. Intermediate response should be reserved for those cases with some decrease in total homocysteine, although with levels remaining above 50 μmol/L. Because no general consensus on the classification exists, other definitions of vitamin B_6 responsiveness may be acceptable.

Age of Manifestation First reviews suggested that CBS deficiency was a severe disorder of childhood associated with profound mental retardation and seizures, connective tissue involvement, and thromboembolic episodes resulting in early death (76). In the last 30 years, however, evidence has accumulated showing that the manifestation of CBS deficiency may be much broader and may include adults with a very mild phenotype. Such adult patients may lack some of the typical features of the disease and may be diagnosed as late as 61 years of age (25). The development of a generally available immunoassay for total homocysteine determination (37, 91) and increasing clinical awareness of this disease may lead to the detection of numerous mildly affected adult patients.

Organ Involvement The most complete clinical description of CBS deficiency in patients with a proven or presumed enzymatic defect analyzed the spectrum and onset of symptoms and signs in 629 homocystinuric patients (86). The frequent symptoms and signs are summarized in Table 20.2. Further details are available in references 40, 83, and 85.

EYE Lens dislocation is the most common sign leading to diagnosis. The finding has been instrumental in the diagnosis in more than 80% of symptomatic, unrelated patients (25, 86). Although lens ectopia was detected in one patient by 4 weeks of age (84), it is rarely seen before 2 years of age. In untreated patients, the likelihood of developing ectopia lentis increases with age and correlates positively with vitamin B_6 nonresponsiveness. The probability of having dislocated lenses at 10 years of age is 55% and 92% in vitamin B_6 responders and nonresponders, respectively; at 20 years of age, it is 80% and 100% in responders and nonresponders, respectively (86). Lens dislocation may lead to an acute pupillary block with glaucoma, other ocular complications including retinal detachment and degeneration, and optic atrophy. It was

shown that myopia, as an important sign suggestive of homocystinuria, preceded lens dislocation in all patients who presented with ectopic lenses (25).

SKELETAL ABNORMALITIES Numerous skeletal abnormalities may be observed (84) (Table 20.2) by both clinical and x-ray examinations. The most remarkable abnormalities resembling the Marfan syndrome include scoliosis/kyphosis, dolichostenomelia (long and thin extremities), decreased upper/lower body segment ratio, and arachnodactyly (100). Osteoporosis was present in lateral radiographs of the spine in many CBS-deficient patients. Patients nonresponsive to vitamin B_6 were more likely to exhibit osteoporosis; by 20 years of age it was present in 50% and 72% of vitamin B_6 responders and nonresponders, respectively (86).

VASCULATURE Vascular disorders are another peculiar feature of this disease. Generally, they can be characterized as a thrombotic diathesis that may manifest in the venous or arterial system and/or as accelerated atherosclerosis.

A survey reported 253 thromboembolic events in 158 patients (86). About half of all events were thromboses of peripheral veins, with embolism in about one fourth of them. The second most common event was a cerebrovascular accident, which accounted for about one-third of cases. Occlusions of peripheral, coronary, or other arteries were much less common. Patients responsive to vitamin B_6 had an almost identical probability of developing thromboembolic episodes as nonresponders (by 20 years of age, 28% and 32% of responders and nonresponders, respectively, suffered from thromboembolism).

Signs of early atherosclerosis were originally reported in autopsies of CBS deficient patients (71). In contrast, other reports did not find changes typical for atherosclerosis and the observed pathology was suggestive of an arterial wall repair response to repeated mural thromboses (summarized in reference 10a). Improved diagnostic methods have now made it possible to detect subclinical vascular changes. These changes include impaired nitric oxide-related relaxation (18) and decreased ankle/arm systolic pressure index with early, non-flow-reducing lesions of iliac arteries (94). However, the early signs of carotid atherosclerosis were not detected in nine CBS-deficient patients (95), and the extent of atherosclerosis in CBS deficiency remains to be critically evaluated.

CENTRAL NERVOUS SYSTEM Mental retardation is common. Data from 284 patients showed a median IQ of 78 and 56 for the vitamin B_6 responders and nonresponders, respectively (86). Average or above average IQ (defined as IQ > 90), as one of the determinants of social performance, was present in only 4% of nonresponders, but in 22% of vitamin B_6 respon-

Table 20.2. Symptoms and Signs in CBS Deficiency[a]

System/Organ	Frequent	Less Frequent
Connective Tissue		
Eye	Progressive spherophakia with lenticular myopia, resulting in lens dislocation	Retinal microcystoid degeneration, retinal detachment, acute glaucoma due to pupillary block, optic atrophy, cataracts with zonular appearance
Skeletal system	Changes in vertebrae and ribs: biconcave vertebrae, osteoporosis, scoliosis	Kyphosis, pectus carinatum, pectus excavatum,
	Abnormalities of long bones: dolichostenomelia, growth arrest lines, widened metaphyses, metaphyseal spicules	Arachnodactyly, genua valga, short fourth metacarpal
	High arched palate, pes cavus	Enlarged carpal bones, abnormal bone age
Skin	Fair, brittle and thin skin	Hypopigmented hair
		Inguinal hernia
Vasculature		
Venous system	Crural thrombosis resulting in embolism	
Arterial system	Arterial occlusion (especially cerebral and peripheral arteries), livedo reticularis, and malar flush	Myocardial infarction
Central nervous system		
Brain development	Mental retardation	
CNS functions	Psychiatric disturbances (personality and behavior disorder, episodic depression, obsessive-compulsive disorder)	Schizophrenia
	Abnormal electroencephalogram	Seizures, focal signs due to vascular occlusion, extrapyramidal signs
Other		Fatty liver
		Pancreatitis, hyperinsulinism
		Asthma

[a] Data adapted from Gerding (40), Mudd et al. (83), and Skovby and Kraus (100).

ders. About one-fifth of the patients exhibited seizures, approximately 70% of which were of grand mal type. Psychiatric disturbances are also common; clinically important psychiatric disorders were reported in about half of 63 CBS-deficient patients (1). Personality/behavioral disorders were more common than depression or obsessive-compulsive disorder (approximately 70%, 20%, and 10%, respectively).

Determinants of Disease Severity In untreated patients, vitamin B_6 responsiveness was shown to be the major determinant of the clinical outcome (86). At any age, vitamin B_6-responsive patients are less likely to die of the disease and are less likely to develop lens dislocation, osteoporosis, or thromboembolism than their nonresponsive counterparts. In addition, mental development is better in vitamin B_6 responders.

In treated patients, two major determinants seem to influence the clinical course of the disease. They are the age at which the treatment is started and the degree of patient compliance with the difficult regimen. Outcomes in treated patients are summarized in Table 20.3. This table demonstrates that in nonresponders, the outcome is much better in patients detected by neonatal screening and treated since the newborn period than in their counterparts who were detected late. However, the generally beneficial outcome in patients treated early may be hampered by a lack of compliance (114, 118).

Mortality Untreated CBS deficiency was originally considered a very severe disease, with 75% mortality by the age of 30 years (76). However, a large international study found that mortality by that age was only 15% (86). A significant difference in mortality was observed between vitamin B_6 responders (4%) and nonresponders (23%). A further decrease in mortality was apparent in treated patients (Table 20.3).

Table 20.3. Outcome in Treated Patients

Clinical End-Point / Origin of patients	Patients Treated Early				Patients Treated Late							
	Vitamin B_6 Nonresponders				Vitamin B_6 Responders				Vitamin B_6 Nonresponders			
	Number	Patient Years	Events Observed	Events Expected	Number	Patient Years	Events Observed	Events Expected	Number	Patient Years	Events Observed	Events Expected
Lens dislocation												
Worldwide	39	N/A	6	16.2	26	N/A	5	10.8	23	N/A	9	6.9
English	11	166	0	8.8								
Irish	18	249	0	14.2								
Thromboembolism												
Worldwide	41	N/A	1	2.9	135	169	4	19.9	68	69	8	6.2
Australian					17	281	2	11	15	258	0	10
English	11	166	0	2.7								
Irish	18	249	0	4.8								
Mental development												
Worldwide	16	N/A	94[a]	56[b]	N/A	N/A	N/A	N/A	N/A	N/A	58[a]	56[b]
English	11	166	100[a]	56[b]								
Irish	18	249	Normal[a]	56[b]								

Treatment varied in different studies; in general vitamin B_6 nonresponders were on a methionine-restricted diet, supplemented with cystine and betaine; vitamin B_6-responsive patients received high doses of vitamin B_6, and some were also given a methionine-restricted diet and betaine. Combined mortality in English and Irish patients treated early (29 vitamin B_6 non-responders; total of 415 patient years): 0 death observed vs. 5.7 deaths expected. The other data for the worldwide population were taken from Mudd et al. (86) and for Australians from Wilcken and Wilcken (116). The number of events was calculated using the method described in Mudd et al. (86) for patients of English (114) and Irish (118) ancestry. N/A, data not available.

[a] Mean IQ values in treated patients.
[b] Mean IQ values in untreated patients.

Thromboembolism was the major cause or a contributing factor in 47 of 59 deaths (86). The remaining deaths were attributable to pneumonia, sepsis, or other causes.

Reproduction in Cystathionine β-Synthase Deficiency

Two clinical issues relate to pregnancies in women with CBS deficiency: an increased maternal risk of thromboembolism and the potential of a teratogenic effect of homocysteine on the offspring. In a recent study, four pregnancies were complicated by preeclampsia, one with thrombophlebitis in the third trimester, and four women suffered from venous or arterial occlusions postpartum. Although these reports suggest the possibility of increased vascular complications during pregnancy in CBS-deficient women, other pregnancies proceeded without complication (83).

Both men and women with CBS deficiency have had offspring. Normal offspring were reported in all but one of 38 recognized conceptions involving CBS-deficient men. Mudd et al. (83) summarized data from 141 pregnancies in CBS-deficient women, approximately 75% of whom were vitamin B_6 responders. Fetal loss was observed in 30% of pregnancies (of which 70% were due to spontaneous abortion, 21% stillbirth, and 9% ectopic pregnancy). Of 98 live births, 5% were born preterm and 88% were apparently normal at birth and at follow-up evaluation. In addition, 7% of the newborns exhibited various congenital malformations, such as coloboma iridis, congenital heart disease, microcephaly, neural tube defect, and psychomotor retardation. These findings suggest that elevated homocysteine concentrations during pregnancy may exhibit some teratogenic effect. However, the teratogenic effect does not seem as great as in maternal phenylketonuria (96).

Molecular Mechanisms

Cystathionine β-Synthase Mutations THE NATURE OF CYSTATHIONINE β-SYNTHASE MUTATIONS A recent review of CBS mutations identified 92 disease-associated CBS-gene mutations in 310 examined homocystinuric alleles (60). An updated list of mutant CBS alleles is maintained on the CBS website (http://www.uchsc.edu/sm/cbs). By October 1999, the number of CBS mutations had reached 100 (Figure 20.4). Most of the mutations are missense mutations, and the vast majority of them are private mutations. There are only four known nonsense mutations; the remainder are deletions, insertions, and splicing mutations. About half of all point substitutions in the coding region of the gene originate from deaminations of methylcytosines in CpG dinucleotides (60).

A total of 71 missense mutations have been identified. Nearly one-third of these have been expressed in

E. coli, and all of them significantly decrease the level of CBS activity (60). As can be seen on the left in Figure 20.4, many of the missense mutations are found in exon 3, the most evolutionarily conserved part of the CBS polypeptide (Figure 20.3). The two most frequent mutations, I278T and G307S, are in exon 8. They change absolutely conserved isoleucine and glycine residues, respectively.

The I278T mutation is panethnic and accounts for nearly one-fourth of all homocystinuric alleles. However, in some countries (e.g., the Netherlands) (52), it accounts for more than half of the affected alleles. A DNA-based screening of newborns in Denmark showed 1.4% of them to be heterozygous for the I278T mutation (39). This value corresponds to a homozygote frequency of about 1: 20,000, which is significantly higher than the often quoted incidence of 1:335,000 (85).

The G307S mutation is undoubtedly the leading cause of homocystinuria in Ireland (71% of affected alleles) (38). It has also been detected frequently in North American and Australian patients of Celtic origin, including families with Irish, Scottish, English, French, and Portuguese ancestry. In contrast, the G307S mutation has not been detected in Italy, the Netherlands, Germany, and the Czech Republic. A recent finding of this mutation in Norway (50), however, may indicate that this allele originated in Scandinavia.

The third most frequent alteration is a splice mutation in intron 11, 1224-2 A→C (IVS 11-2 A→C), which results in the deletion of exon 12. Surprisingly, although it was found in Germany in about 20% of affected chromosomes of German and Turkish origin (55), it has never been detected in Italy and the Netherlands in nearly 70 alleles studied. Together with the I278T mutation, it is the most prevalent mutation in patients of Czech and Slovak origin.

In nine isolated cases, a mutation was linked to another mutation on the same allele. Most of these mutations have been reproduced separately by in vitro mutagenesis, and each was found to be deleterious to CBS activity (60). The origin of double mutant alleles in the CBS gene is not clear, as there is no evidence of a CBS pseudogene in the human genome. Homologous recombination between the numerous *Alu* sequences or other repetitive elements within the CBS gene is a possible alternative explanation for some of the double mutations found *in cis* (62).

THE MOLECULAR MECHANISMS OF VITAMIN B_6 RESPONSIVENESS Vitamin B_6 responsiveness in vivo is not due to a correction of vitamin B_6 deficiency but originates from the properties of the mutant CBS enzyme (83). In vivo responsiveness to vitamin B_6, and the in vitro changes in enzyme activity after the addition of pyridoxal 5′-phosphate to cell extracts do not always correlate. Lipson et al. (67) suggested that

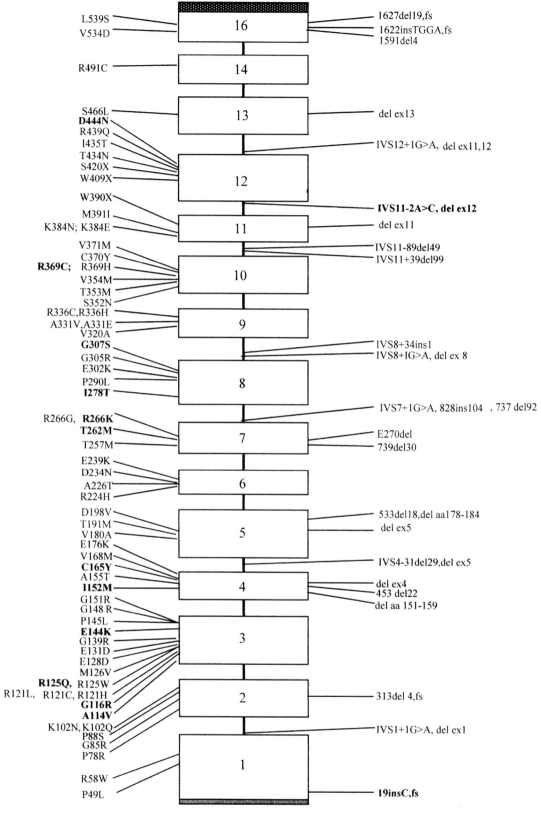

Fig. 20.4. Location of human cystathionine β-synthase (CBS) mutations. The exons in the coding region are drawn as boxes to scale; the introns are not. The shaded areas are parts of the 5′- and 3′-untranslated regions of CBS mRNA found in exon 1 and exon 16, respectively. The mutations shown on the left are missense and nonsense; the mutations on the right are deletions, insertions, and splicing errors. The mutations shown in bold type have been detected in three or more alleles. (Reproduced from Skovby and Kraus [100], with permission.)

mutant enzymes, with a twofold to fivefold reduced affinity for pyridoxal 5'-phosphate, can be activated in vivo by vitamin B_6 administration. However, mutant enzymes with a 20- to 70-fold reduced affinity for pyridoxal 5'-phosphate cannot be so modulated in vivo because of limits on the capacity of cells to accumulate and retain pyridoxal 5'-phosphate. It should be noted that residual CBS activity can be stimulated under in vitro conditions even in those mutant enzymes with severely reduced affinity. The lack of residual CBS activity in a fibroblast extract or the absence of detectable cross-reacting material does not preclude an in vivo response to vitamin B_6 (27, 102).

Most homocystinuric patients other than I278T/I278T and G307S/G307S homozygotes are compound heterozygotes. The I278T mutation usually confers vitamin B_6 responsiveness, whether in the homozygote or the compound heterozygote state (Table 20.4). With the exception of a group of Dutch patients (52), the clinical phenotype usually appears to be mild (43). Although the genotype by itself does not always predict the phenotype, several general statements can be drawn from Table 20.4. In addition to the I278T mutation, the A114V, R266K, R336H, K384E, and L539S mutations also appear to correlate with vitamin B_6 responsiveness in vivo. By contrast, the R121L, R125Q, C165Y, E176K, T191M, T257M, and T262M mutations, as well as the G307S mutation in one or two copies, appear to be incompatible with vitamin B_6 responsiveness. Accordingly, patients carrying the frequent G307S mutation seem to have moderate to severe phenotypes (83), except for those who have been treated since birth (118). Taken together, it seems that the patient genotype is the major determinant of vitamin B_6 responsiveness, as demonstrated by the absolute correlation of responsiveness within sibships (86).

The molecular mechanisms that determine vitamin B_6 responsiveness have not been elucidated. It is unclear how mutations alter the binding or function of pyridoxal 5'-phosphate. In addition, it is unknown whether mutant polypeptides may be less saturated with heme, which in turn may limit the binding of pyridoxal 5'-phosphate (47).

Metabolic Sequelae (Table 20.5)

Homocysteine Marked elevation of plasma total homocysteine and free homocystine has been reported in patients with CBS deficiency, as summarized by Mudd et al. (83). The plasma concentrations of total homocysteine in untreated patients are typically 100 to 500 μmol/L, but much lower concentrations such as 45 μmol/L have also been observed (27). In earlier reports, free homocystine was routinely analyzed and reported. Free homocystine levels of 0, 1 to 20 and

Table 20.4. Correlation Between Genotype and Vitamin B_6 Responsiveness in CBS Deficiency

Cell Line	Genotype		B_6[b]
419	19insC (fs,K36X)	19insC (fs,K36X)	–
LT	A114V	A114V	+
R600	R121L	R121L	–
SGo	R125Q	R125Q	–
AP	C165Y	C165Y	–
428	E176K	E176K	–
S	T191M	T191M	–
NO	T257M	T257M	–
N2	T262M	T262M	–
N1,N4a[a], N4b,N9	R266K	R266K	+
RB,C110, MP,426,PA, CG,M	I278T	I278T	+
AB, B-H, H.B/G, JU,GE,W.S/J	I278T	I278T	+
L209, L188	I278T	I278T	+
NM, MW	I278T	I278T	+
NM	I278T	I278T	+
426	I278T	I278T	+
RS[a],SS	I278T	P88S	+
LM[a],AM	I278T	G116R	+
L264	I278T	G139R	+
L265	I278T	E144K	+
JC[a], MC	I278T	I152M	+
403	I278T	A155T	+
HvE(RD55)	I278T	C165Y	+
GC	I278T	G305R	+
IWa	I278T	T353M	–
N6a[a], N6b	I278T	R369C	+
AC	I278T	C370Y	+
JM, JR	I278T	V371M	+
DS	I278T	R439Q	+
366	I278T	IVS11-2A>C, del ex12	+
427	I278T	IVS11-2A>C, del ex12	+/–
TD	I278T	IVS11-2A>C, del ex12	+
ST,FH	G307S	G307S	–
N10	G307S	G307S	–
MGL166, MGL246	G307S	G307S	–
AP,DA	G307S	G307S	–
7215	R336H	R336H	+
P465	K384E	K384E	+
P325	L539S	L539S	+

[a] Sibling pairs
[b] Positive or negative response to vitamin B_6 treatment.
(Reproduced from Skovby and Kraus [100], with permission.)

Table 20.5.   Pathophysiology of Cystathionine β-Synthase (CBS) Deficiency

Metabolite	Typical Change	Putative Consequences	Possible Clinical Relevance
Accumulation of metabolites proximal to the CBS step			
Homocysteine and homocysteine thiolactone	$\uparrow \approx 10-30 \times$ in plasma	Numerous consequences in vascular system	Thromboembolism and atherosclerosis
		Inhibition of lysyloxidase/ homocysteinylation of proteins resulting in impaired crosslinking and/or disruption of disulfide bridges in connective tissue fibers	Connective tissue disorder
		NMDA receptor activation	CNS involvement and congenital anomalies in pregnancies of CBS-deficient women
Homocysteic acid		Inhibition of tyrosinase due to copper chelation by Hcy	Hypopigmentation
		NMDA receptor activation	Seizures
		Excess of phosphoadenosine-phosphosulfate and sulfation	Connective tissue disorder, atherosclerosis
Homocysteine sulfinic acid		Non-NMDA receptor activation	Seizures
Methionine	$\uparrow \approx 1-50\times$ in plasma	Unknown, probably harmless	Unknown
S-adenosylhomocysteine	$\uparrow$ in liver, urine	Alteration of AdoMet/AdoHcy ratio resulting in changes of protein and nucleic acid methylations, impaired neuro-transmitter synthesis	CNS involvement and atherosclerosis
S-adenosylmethionine	no change in CSF		
Deficiency of metabolites distal to the CBS block			
Cystathionine	$\downarrow$ up to 2×	Cystathionine may be a neuromodulator	CNS involvement
Cysteine	$\downarrow$ up to 2×	Lack of cross-linking in connective tissue proteins (e.g., collagen VI)	Connective tissue disorder
Hydrogen sulfide		Hydrogen sulfide may be a neuromodulator	CNS involvement, atherosclerosis
Taurine		Impaired conjugation of xenobiotics and bile acids, altered cholesterol metabolism	Atherosclerosis and liver disease (in animal model of CBS deficiency)
Other mechanisms			
Stimulation of the remethylation pathway		Increased demand for methyltetrahydrofolate-dependent remethylation	Folate deficiency with megaloblastic anemia
Unexplained metabolic sequelae		Ornithine accumulation ($\uparrow \approx 2-3x$), ceruloplasmin increase ($\uparrow \approx 1.4\times$), pyroglutamic aciduria	Unknown

NMDA, N-methyl-D-aspartate; AdoMet, S-adenosylmethionine; Hcy, homocysteine; AdoHcy, S-adenosylhomocysteine; CNS, central nervous system; CSF, cerebrospinal fluid; $\uparrow$, increased; $\downarrow$, decreased.

>20 μmol/L correspond to total homocysteine concentrations of <60, 60 to 150, and >150 μmol/L, respectively (9).

Accumulation of homocysteine in cells and plasma leads to additional biochemical changes such as an increase of homocysteine-cysteine and homocysteine-cysteinylglycine disulfides in plasma and to the production and excretion of other metabolites, such as homocysteic acid, homocysteine sulfinic acid, homo-lanthionine, 5-amino-4-imidazolecarboxamide-5'-Shomocysteinylriboside and homocysteine thiolactone (45, 81, 84).

The pleiotropic effects of homocysteine and related metabolites on cellular systems are discussed in other chapters.

Methionine   An elevation of plasma methionine is a typical biochemical hallmark of CBS deficiency. Hypermethioninemia has been absent in only 1% of vitamin B_6 nonresponders but in 10% of patients responsive to vitamin B_6 (86). In CBS-deficient patients, elevation of plasma methionine usually reaches several hundreds of μmol/L but may be as high as 2,000 μmol/L, whereas reference values are usually 40 μmol/L or less (83). In a cohort of Czech and Slovak patients, the median plasma methionine concentration at the time of diagnosis was 116 and 600 μmol/L in responders and nonresponders, respectively (Janosik et al, unpublished observation). The absence of hypermethioninemia is an important issue for neonatal screening of CBS deficiency. Most programs are based on detecting hypermethioninemia with cutoff levels ranging between 67 and 270 μmol/L (88). The lack of hypermethioninemia or too high a cut-off level may have led to some patients, particularly the vitamin B_6-responsive ones, being missed during neonatal screening.

High methionine levels lead to an enhanced rate of S-adenosylmethionine synthesis while part of the methionine undergoes transamination in an alternative pathway. There is no evidence that hypermethioninemia directly causes any deleterious clinical consequences except for a malodor that has been observed in some patients with CBS deficiency (83).

S-Adenosylmethionine and S-Adenosylhomocysteine
Accumulation of homocysteine has far-reaching consequences for the steady-state levels of S-adenosylmethionine and S-adenosylhomocysteine, as discussed in Chapters 6, 9, and 17. Early studies showed that S-adenosylhomocysteine was increased in liver and urine and normal in erythrocytes of CBS-deficient patients compared with control subjects, as summarized by Mudd and Levy (82). In contrast, a recent study showed that the S-adenosylhomocysteine concentration in whole blood was increased about five-fold in CBS-deficient patients compared with controls (Kožich V, unpublished observation). Because activity of many methyltransferases is inhibited by a decreased S-adenosylmethionine/S-adenosylhomocysteine ratio (16), a depressed ratio has profound effect on methylation reactions in all cells. Recently, evidence of altered tissue concentrations of these two metabolites was shown in a CBS-deficient mouse (23). The S-adenosylmethionine concentration in the liver increased

twofold, and S-adenosylhomocysteine increased 10-fold resulting in an abnormal ratio. Even more profound changes in the ratio were found in the brain, with approximately 200-fold increases in S-adenosylhomocysteine concentration and no change in S-adenosylmethionine levels.

Metabolites Distal to the Cystathionine β-Synthase Block (see also Chapter 14)   Cystathionine and cysteine deficiencies are well-known biochemical consequences of CBS deficiency. Lack of cysteine may also impair the synthesis of cysteine-rich peptides and proteins. One of these compounds, the antioxidant tripeptide glutathione (γ-glutamylcysteinylglycine) is present within cells in millimolar concentrations (77). Preliminary data show that the reduced glutathione concentration in whole blood is not depressed in homocystinuric patients (Kožich et al, unpublished observation). It is unclear whether the normal blood concentration reflects the situation in tissues and whether a supposed decrease in glutathione plays any role in the pathogenesis of CBS deficiency. Other molecules that may be affected by the lack of cysteine are the cysteine-rich proteins of connective tissue. It is conceivable that a decreased availability of cysteine alters their synthesis and leads to the characteristic connective tissue disorders associated with CBS deficiency (100). Direct evidence to support this hypothesis in CBS-deficient patients has not yet been obtained.

Pathophysiology

Connective Tissue Abnormalities   Skovby and Kraus (100) summarized several hypotheses for mechanisms of lens dislocation and skeletal abnormalities in patients with CBS deficiency. In lens ectopy, zonular fibers attached to either the ciliary body or the lens itself are disrupted. Normal human zonules contain microfilaments, which have a high cysteine content with almost no hydroxylysine or hydroxyproline. These findings suggest that disulfide bonds play a greater role in maintaining the structure of zonular fibers than the cross-linking ensured by hydroxylysines. Although there is no direct proof of altered amino acid composition of zonular fibers in CBS-deficient patients, other evidence suggests that cysteine deficiency may play a role in the pathogenesis of lens dislocation. Lens dislocation has never been reported in patients with various homocysteine remethylation defects (29, 93; Surtees R, personal communication; Rosenblatt DS, personal communication), who exhibit severe hyperhomocysteinemia but synthesize normal amounts of cysteine. This suggests that the lack of cysteine rather than the accumulation of homocysteine or related compounds leads to zonular fiber disruption.

No evidence exists that fiber damage results from the disruption of disulfide bonds caused by homocysteine or other compounds or from a lack of collagen cross-linking by inhibited lysyloxidase.

Excessive growth of long bones resulting in dolichostenomelia was hypothesized to result from either homocysteic acid or homocysteine accumulation because both of these metabolites promote proliferation of cells. Other putative mechanisms for skeletal changes, especially for osteoporosis, include impaired cross-linking of collagen. This may be caused by direct interaction of homocysteine with lysine and hydroxylysine residues in collagen, or by inhibition of lysyloxidase. Experimental evidence suggests that cross-linking of collagen in patients with CBS deficiency is indeed impaired (70). However, the true role of these mechanisms is unclear in the development of skeletal changes in CBS-deficient patients, as accumulation of homocysteine and other metabolites also occurs in patients with remethylation defects in whom no skeletal changes have been reported (29, 93; Surtees R, personal communication; Rosenblatt DS, personal communication).

Vascular Abnormalities Thromboembolic disease and premature atherosclerosis are frequent in CBS-deficient patients. Typically, fibrous plaques with smooth muscle hyperplasia, deposition of extracellular matrix and collagen, and degeneration and destruction of elastic fibers have been found in arteries of patients with CBS deficiency (72). In addition, venous thromboemboli have been reported at both clinical and postmortem examinations in CBS deficiency. Because the vascular changes were also found in patients with remethylation defects, homocysteine or its derivatives have been proposed as a possible cause for the atherosclerosis present in all homocystinuric patients (72). However, no widely accepted unifying theory of vascular changes currently exists.

Central Nervous System Impairment Mudd et al. (83) suggested that mental retardation, seizures, and psychoses in patients with CBS deficiency may be caused by chemical abnormalities in the brain and/or repeated and perhaps subclinical thromboemboli. Although the thromboembolic hypothesis has not been verified, it is plausible and may account for some of the neurological dysfunction. The chemical abnormalities, however, seem to be better candidates for explaining nervous system abnormalities.

Several compounds accumulating or lacking in CBS deficiency have been implicated as neurotransmitters in brain. Homocysteine interacts with the N-methyl-D-aspartate receptor (68) and may have a direct toxic effect on neural cells (90). In addition, homocysteine may decrease adenosine concentrations by forming S-

adenosylhomocysteine (75). Depletion of adenosine may alter functions associated with the adenosine receptor such as vasodilatation, sedation, inhibition of neutrotransmitter release, and inhibition of nerve cell firing (28). By-products of homocysteine accumulation, homocysteic acid and homocysteine sulfinic acid have excitotoxic properties and interact with various subtypes of the glutamate family of receptors (33, 34, 90). Lack of cystathionine, a putative neurotransmitter, was proposed as a cause of mental retardation (83).

Recent reports have indicated that hydrogen sulfide is produced by CBS in rat brains and may function as a neuromodulator, possibly by selectively enhancing the N-methyl-D-aspartate receptor–mediated responses in the hippocampus (2). It is unclear whether CBS-deficient patients exhibit any disturbances in hydrogen sulfide metabolism and whether hydrogen sulfide plays any role in organ damage.

CBS-deficient patients accumulate S-adenosylhomocysteine, which may result in the abnormal methylation of nucleic acids and proteins and in the impaired synthesis of phospholipids and neurotransmitters. However, S-adenosylmethionine does not accumulate in the cerebrospinal fluid of CBS-deficient patients (107). A disturbed ratio of S-adenosylmethionine/S-adenosylhomocysteine was clearly demonstrated in the brain of CBS-deficient mice (23). The role of the S-adenosylmethionine to S-adenosylhomocysteine ratio in the development of brain dysfunction requires further study.

Animal Models Animal models of hyperhomocysteinemia were generated by manipulating dietary intake of homocysteine (73) or vitamins (24) and by administration of nitrous oxide (119). None of these models, however, mimicked both the homocysteine accumulation and the deficiency of the metabolites beyond the CBS step.

A CBS knockout mouse was generated by excising exons 3 and 4 of the CBS gene by homologous recombination (115). The resulting biochemical phenotype resembled that of the human disease. The homozygous animals exhibited average plasma total homocysteine concentrations of ≈200 μmol/L, which is approximately 40 times the normal value. Nevertheless, these mice did not exhibit any of the typical clinical features of the human disease. Instead, they failed to thrive and developed liver disease with microvesicular steatosis; 77% of them died by 4 weeks of age. The reasons for the differing clinical outcomes are unknown.

Diagnosis

Neonatal Screening Screening newborns for CBS deficiency has involved determining hypermethioninemia in blood samples using a bacterial inhibition method or paper chromatography or by screening for homocystine excretion in urine samples (88). For the last 30 years, this approach has identified many patients, most of who have been vitamin B_6 nonresponders (83, 114, 118).

Debate persists about whether neonates should be screened for CBS deficiency (20, 88, 111). The favorable effects of early treatment demonstrated in Table 20.3 are clear. By contrast, a problematic screening method that misses many of the vitamin B_6 responders and the reported low incidence led to the termination of newborn screening in many countries. Novel techniques such as tandem mass spectrometry (19) and reports of a much higher incidence of mutant alleles than expected (39) suggest that CBS deficiency should be reconsidered as a disease suitable for newborn screening.

Selective Screening Most patients with the CBS deficiency have been identified by selective screening of clinically affected individuals (86). Older methods have been almost universally replaced by more precise methods that measure total plasma homocysteine by high performance liquid chromatography or immuno-assay methods.

For selective screening, the most important signs that should alert the clinician to the possibility of CBS deficiency are summarized in Table 20.6. Clinicians should be encouraged to think of CBS deficiency not only in terms of typical cases manifesting in childhood but also in adult patients with a very mild phenotype. Some practical considerations for establishing the diagnosis are also given in Table 20.6. The most important issue concerns vitamin B_6 withdrawal before homocysteine levels are determined.

Differential Diagnosis Several inherited and acquired conditions cause hyperhomocysteinemia, with plasma homocysteine exceeding 50 μmol/L. The minimum set of analyses that needs to be performed for patients with such a finding should include plasma and erythrocyte folate, cobalamin and vitamin B_6, plasma and urinary amino acids, and urinary organic acids. Typically, patients with CBS deficiency exhibit severe hyperhomocysteinemia with massive urinary excretion of homocystine, decreased plasma cysteine, absent urinary cystathionine, and highly elevated plasma methionine levels. In addition, they will rarely show methylmalonic aciduria or a vitamin deficiency other than occasional secondary folate deficiency.

Confirmation of Diagnosis Although CBS activity has been measured in liver, phytohemagglutinin-stimulated lymphocytes, and brain, the most practical tissue

---

Table 20.6. A Practical Approach to the Diagnosis of CBS Deficiency

Age: First signs mostly in childhood; occasionally as late as the seventh decade

Alerting signs (only one of the signs may be present):

- **Dislocation of ocular lenses**
- **Lenticular myopia** preceding lens dislocation (correction: > −1 diopter in children,
- > −5 diopters in adults, especially if progressive and if signs of axial myopia are absent; non-corneal astigmatism)
- **Marfan-like appearance** (dolichostenomelia with arachnodactyly)
- **Thrombosis or thromboembolism**
- **Early-onset atherosclerosis** below age 40 years (after excluding more common causes of atherosclerosis)
- **Mental retardation** and/or **psychosis or seizures,** especially if combined with the above signs

Important consideration before performing metabolite assays

The patient **should not be taking any vitamin B_6** supplements for at least 1 to 2 weeks before the sample collection (even 2 mg of vitamin B_6 per day may decrease plasma homocysteine).

Metabolite assays

Plasma total homocysteine: Expected values of fasting total homocysteine in CBS deficiency are usually > 50 μmol/L (typically in the range of 100 to 500μmol/L).

Plasma amino acids: Hypermethioninemia >> 40μmol/L is present in most untreated patients (typically several hundreds of μmol/L).

---

for confirming diagnosis is cultured skin fibroblasts (83). Molecular genetic diagnosis is not practical at this time because the number of private mutations is large (60), and analysis of the entire gene or mRNA is laborious and expensive. Furthermore, the newly observed mutations still require expression analyses to characterize the relative pathogenicity of their phenotypic effect. However, new approaches such as the use of nucleic acid microarrays may soon become more prominent in the diagnostic process.

Prenatal Diagnosis Prenatal diagnosis is possible by measuring CBS activity in cultured amniocytes (36). The activity in control amniocytes (8 to 33 nmol/hr/mg protein) was clearly distinguishable from amniocytes obtained from two affected fetuses (0.04 and 0.18 nmol/hr/mg protein) (36). Uncultured chorionic villi exhibit very low activity (35), but cultured villi were used to measure the CBS activity in at least three pregnancies at risk (Kraus J, unpublished observation).

Management

Compounds in the Treatment of Cystathionine β-Synthase Deficiency VITAMIN B_6 Vitamin B_6 is the key agent for the treatment of patients with CBS deficiency. Approximately 44% of patients can be expected to respond to vitamin B_6 administration, and another 13% will exhibit some response (86). Most reports used about 200 to 500 mg/day given in two to four doses; however, the range was wide, between 25 and 1,200 mg/day (83). It is generally agreed that vitamin B_6 has beneficial clinical effects in vitamin B_6-responsive patients (83). Several reports have been published on the toxicity of vitamin B_6. Acute toxicity resulting in apnea in infants receiving 500 mg/day was reported by Mudd et al. (83); they concluded that in infants "prudence suggests limiting the oral dose of vitamin B_6 to considerably less than 500 mg daily." Another review concluded that doses of up to 500 mg/day for 2 years or total doses of less than 1,000 g appear to be safe in adults as far as the side effects of sensory neuropathy and ataxia are concerned (6).

Several practical issues should be considered when treating patients with vitamin B_6. First, the individual dose exhibiting the maximal biochemical response, as indicated by the total homocysteine, cysteine, and methionine levels, should be optimized for each patient by gradually increasing the dose up to 10 mg/kg. Second, folate or cobalamin deficiency should be corrected before vitamin B_6 responsiveness is assessed. Third, we propose that the maximum dose should be kept below ≈100 mg/day in infants, ≈150 to 400 mg/day in children, and ≈700 mg/day in adults to prevent neurological complications. It has been suggested that a cutoff value of 50 μmol/L of plasma total homocysteine be used to determine vitamin B_6 responsiveness.

METHIONINE RESTRICTION AND CYSTEINE SUPPLEMENTATION Dietary manipulation of methionine and cysteine intake is an option for treating patients who are partially or fully nonresponsive to vitamin B_6. This approach decreases the load of the affected pathway and replaces the deficient product in the transsulfuration pathway. Its efficiency has been unequivocally demonstrated in patients nonresponsive to vitamin B_6 who are treated early (Table 20.3). Methionine restriction is achieved by limiting protein intake in food, but some methionine must be provided to ensure positive nitrogen balance. For patients with no residual CBS

activity, cysteine must also be provided to maintain a positive nitrogen balance (81). In CBS-deficient patients, the recommended daily intakes of methionine and cysteine, respectively, is 10 to 30 and 200 to 300 mg/kg in infants, 6 to 20 and 100 to 200 mg/kg in children, and 5 to 15 and 25 to 100 mg/kg in adults (3). Because the low-methionine diet does not provide enough protein, supplemental amino acid mixtures should be given. These mixtures contain two to three times more L-cysteine or L-cystine than formulas used in treating patients with other inborn errors of amino acid metabolism (3).

BETAINE Betaine stimulates remethylation of homocysteine to methionine by serving as a methyl donor for betaine-homocysteine methyltransferase (Metabolic Diagram, Reaction 5; see Chapter 13). Betaine was advocated as a safe drug without adverse effects (117), although occasional patients have complained of a fishy odor (83). Wilcken and Wilcken (116) showed that betaine administration of 6 to 9 g/day decreased the probability of developing thromboembolic disease. Homocysteine levels in the cerebrospinal fluid of 10 patients with CBS deficiency decreased from 1.2 μmol/L to 0.32 μmol/L during betaine treatment (107). Other reports suggest that betaine may not be as efficient as originally thought. Walter et al. (114) administered 250 mg/kg of betaine to CBS-deficient patients and did not observe a significant change in free homocystine levels (35 vs. 33 μmol/L). Moreover, large doses of betaine lead to an increase of plasma N,N-dimethylglycine, an inhibitor of betaine-homocysteine methyltransferase (4). However, betaine in doses of 100 to 200 mg/kg may be considered a safe drug in nonresponsive patients in whom biochemical control cannot be achieved by dietary treatment.

FOLIC ACID AND CYANO/HYDROXOCOBALAMIN The increased flux of homocysteine through the remethylation pathway in patients with CBS deficiency may result in secondary disturbances of folate metabolism (17). Nutritionally deprived CBS-deficient patients might develop severe folate deficiency and pancytopenia (113). Monitoring of folate and cobalamin status is a common practice (116, 118), and some have even used preventive supplementation (116).

Management of Responsive and Partially Responsive Patients Vitamin B_6 administration is the primary therapeutic measure in responsive and partially responsive patients. The goal is to maintain plasma homocysteine levels as low as possible, usually below 30 to 40 μmol/L. In full responders this might be achieved solely by vitamin B_6 administration, but in partially responsive patients some methionine restriction, occasionally combined with betaine administration, may be necessary.

Management of Patients Unresponsive to Vitamin B₆
In these patients, the primary measure is methionine restriction with cysteine supplementation and betaine administration, if needed, to maintain homocysteine levels as low as possible. In some vitamin B₆-nonresponders, total homocysteine levels as low as 20–50 μmol/L may be achieved. In other patients, despite all measures and strict dietary control, levels may stay in the range of 50 to 100 μmol/L.

Treatment in Patients Undergoing Surgery A high rate of postoperative thromboembolic disease and death was originally reported in CBS-deficient patients (76). However, a study of 451 surgical procedures reported only 18 nonfatal and 9 fatal thromboembolic events (86), probably due to improved preoperative and postoperative management.

Several practical issues should be considered when planning surgical intervention in CBS-deficient patients (83; Wilcken DL, personal communication). Nitrous oxide should be avoided in anesthesia to prevent the inhibition it causes of methionine synthase. Patients should be hydrated adequately, and other general antithrombotic measures, including miniheparinization, should be observed. Vitamin B₆ should be added to the continuous infusion preoperatively and postoperatively in a daily dose of 100 to 200 mg. Oral vitamin B₆ and betaine should be started as early as possible after surgery. In the catabolic postoperative period, methionine intake should be reduced by about 20%, and the methionine-free, cysteine-enriched amino acid mixture should be increased appropriately. Monitoring of plasma metabolite levels and adjustment of therapy are needed to manage CBS-deficient patients undergoing surgery.

Maternal Cystathionine β-Synthase Deficiency There are few reports on the management of pregnancy in patients with CBS deficiency (83). In an analogy to maternal phenylketonuria, it appears sensible to treat maternal CBS deficiency before conception. Homocysteine levels during pregnancy should be kept as low as possible to minimize any possible teratogenic effect on the embryo/fetus and to prevent thromboembolism in the mother. Patients responsive to vitamin B₆ have been treated with vitamin B₆ and nonresponsive patients with a methionine-restricted diet, folate, aspirin, and dipyridamole. More recently, three patients were given betaine during pregnancy (83). Additional studies are needed to establish a consensus on safe and efficacious treatment.

Genetic Counseling

The estimated prevalence of heterozygotes, which is of great importance in genetic counseling, varies with the ethnic background of the population. The worldwide estimate of homozygote frequency (or more precisely, the rate of detection of homozygotes by neonatal screening) is 1:344,000 (85). This number suggests that the prevalence of heterozygotes is about 1:300. Neonatal screening in countries such as Ireland yielded a much higher prevalence of heterozygotes of about 1:120 (118). These estimates, however, include only the nonresponsive patients with severe biochemical phenotype in the neonatal period, and they represent only a fraction of all CBS-deficient patients. Recent data showed that the prevalence of heterozygotes for the relatively mild, common I278T mutation is about 1:70 in Denmark (39).

The detection of heterozygotes has been extensively reviewed by Mudd et al. (83). Despite reports on detection of heterozygotes by methionine loading (8), homocysteine/cysteine ratio measurement (7), and CBS activity measurement in fibroblasts (74) or phytohemagglutinin-stimulated lymphocytes (41), no universal method can be advised. Currently, the best approach for detecting heterozygosity is to directly analyze mutations in the CBS gene.

REFERENCES

1. Abbott, MH, Folstein, SE, Abbey, H, Pyeritz, RE. Psychiatric manifestations of homocystinuria due to cystathionine β-synthase deficiency. *Am J Med Genet* 1987; 26: 959–69.

2. Abe, K, Kimura, H. The possible role of hydrogen sulfide as an endogenous neuromodulator. *J Neurosci* 1996; 16: 1066–71.

3. Acosta, P, Yannicelli, S. *The Ross Metabolic Formula System: Nutrition Support Protocols*, 3rd ed. Ross Products Division, Columbus, Ohio, 1997.

4. Allen, RH, Stabler, SP, Lindenbaum, J. Serum betaine, N,N-dimethylglycine and N-methylglycine levels in patients with cobalamin and folate deficiency and related inborn errors of metabolism. *Metabolism* 1993; 42: 1448–60.

5. Bao, L, Vlcek, C, Paces, V, Kraus, JP. Identification and tissue distribution of human cystathionine β-synthase messenger-RNA isoforms. *Arch Biochem Biophys* 1998; 350: 95–103.

6. Bendich, A, Cohen, M. Vitamin B₆ safety issues. *Ann NY Acad Sci* 1990; 585: 321–30.

7. Boddie, AM, Steen, MT, Sullivan, KM, Pasquali, M, Dembure, PP, Coates, RJ, Elsas, LJ, II. Cystathionine-β-synthase deficiency: Detection of heterozygotes by ratios of homocysteine to cysteine and folate. *Metabolism* 1997; 47: 207–11.

8. Boers, GHJ, Fowler, B, Smals, AGH, Trijbels, FJM, Leermakers, AI, Kleijer, WJ, Kloppenborg, PWC. Improved identification of heterozygotes for homocystinuria due to cystathionine synthase deficiency by the combination of methionine loading and enzyme determi-

nation in cultured fibroblasts. *Hum Genet* 1985; 69: 164–69.

9. Bonham, JR, Moat, SJ, Allen, JC, Powers, HJ, Tanner, MS, McDowell, I, Bellamy, MF. Free homocystine may be a poor measure of control in homocystinuria. *J Inherit Metab Dis* 1997; 20 (Suppl 1): P2.9.

10. Borcsok, E, Abeles, RH. Mechanism of action of cystathionine synthase. *Arch Biochem Biophys* 1982; 213: 695–707.

10a. Brattstrom, L, Wilcken, DE. Homocysteine and cardiovascular disease: cause or effect? *Am J Clin Nutr* 2000; 72: 315–23.

11. Braunstein, AE, Goryachenkova, EV. The β-replacement-specific pyridoxal-*P*-dependent lyases. *Adv Enzymol* 1984; 56: 1–89.

12. Brenton, DP, Cusworth, DC. The response of patients with cystathionine synthase deficiency to pyridoxine. In *Inherited Disorders of Sulphur Metabolism*. (Carson, NAJ, Raine, DN, eds.) Churchill Livingstone, Ltd, London, 1971; pp. 264–74.

13. Brown, FC, Gordon, PH. Cystathionine synthase from rat liver: Partial purification and properties. *Can J Biochem* 1971; 49: 484–91.

13a. Bruno, S, Schiaretti, F, Burkhard, P, Kraus, JP, Janošik, M, Mozzarelli, A. Functional properties of the active core of human cystathionine β-synthase crystals. *J Biol Chem* 2001; 276: 16–19.

14. Bukovska, G, Kery, V, Kraus, JP. Expression of human cystathionine β-synthase in *Escherichia coli*: Purification and characterization. *Protein Expr Purif* 1994; 5: 442–48.

15. Burkhard, P, Rao, GS, Hohenester, E, Schnackerz, KD, Cook, PF, Jansonius, JN. Three-dimensional structure of *O*-acetylserine sulfhydrylase from *Salmonella typhimurium*. *J Mol Biol* 1998; 283: 121–33.

16. Cantoni, GL, Richards, HH, Chiang, PK. Inhibitors of *S*-adenosylhomocysteine hydrolase and their role in the regulation of biological methylation. In *Transmethylation* (Usdin, E, Borchardt, RT, Creveling, CR, eds.). Elsevier/North-Holland, New York, 1979: pp. 155–72.

17. Carey, MC, Fennelly, JJ, Fitzgerald, O. Homocystinuria. II. Subnormal serum folate levels, increased folate clearance and effects of folic acid therapy. *Am J Med* 1968; 45: 26–31.

18. Celermajer, DS, Sorensen, K, Ryalls, M, Robinson, J, Thomas, O, Leonard, JV, Deanfield, JE. Impaired endothelial function occurs in the systemic arteries of children with homozygous homocystinuria but not in their heterozygous parents. *J Am Coll Cardiol* 1993; 22: 854–58.

19. Chace, DH, Hillman, SL, Millington, DS, Kahler, SG, Adam, BW, Levy, HL. Rapid diagnosis of homocystinuria and other hypermethioninemias from newborns' blood spots by tandem mass spectrometry. *Clin Chem* 1996; 42: 349–55.

20. Champion, MP, Turner, C, Bird, S, Dalton, RN. Delay in diagnosis of homocystinuria. Neonatal screening avoids complications of delayed treatment. *Br Med J* 1997; 314: 369–70.

21. Chassé, JF, Paly, E, Paris, D, Paul, V, Sinet, PM, Kamoun, P, London, J. Genomic organization of the human cystathionine β-synthase gene: Evidence for various cDNAs. *Biochem Biophys Res Commun* 1995; 211: 826–32.

22. Chassé, JF, Paul, V, Escañez, R, Kamoun, P, London, J. Human cystathionine β-synthase: Gene organization and expression of different 5' alternative splicing. *Mamm Genome* 1997; 8: 917–21.

23. Choumenkovitch, SF, Bagley, P, Maeda, N, Nadeau, M, Smith, D, Selhub, J. *S*-adenosylmethionine (SAM) and *S*-adenosylhomocysteine (SAH) in mice deficient in cystathionine β-synthase (CBS). *FASEB J* 1998; 12: A550.

24. Cravo, M, Mason, J, Salomon, RN, Ordovas, J, Osada, J, Selhub, J, Rosenberg, IH. Folate deficiency in rats causes hypomethylation of DNA. *FASEB J* 1991; 5: A914.

25. Cruysberg, JRM, Boers, GHJ, Trijbels, JMF, Deutman, AF. Delay in diagnosis of homocystinuria: Retrospective study of consecutive patients. *Br Med J* 1996; 313: 1037–40.

26. Daubner, SC, Matthews, RG. Purification and properties of methylenetetrahydrofolate reductase from pig liver. *J Biol Chem* 1982; 257: 140–45.

27. de Franchis, R, Kozich, V, McInnes, RR, Kraus, JP. Identical genotypes in siblings with different homocystinuric phenotypes: Identification of three mutations in cystathionine β-synthase using an improved bacterial expression system. *Hum Mol Genet* 1994; 3: 1103–8.

28. Dunwiddie, T. The physiological role of adenosine in the central nervous system. *Int Rev Neurobiol* 1985; 27: 63–139.

29. Fenton, WA, Rosenberg, LE. Inherited disorders of cobalamin transport and metabolism. In *The Metabolic and Molecular Bases of Inherited Disease*. 7th ed. (Scriver, CR, Beaudet, AL, Sly, WS, Valle, D, eds.). McGraw-Hill, Inc, New York, 1995; pp. 3129–49.

30. Finkelstein, JD, Kyle, WE, Martin, JJ, Pick, A-M. Activation of cystathionine synthase by adenosylmethionine and adenosylethionine. *Biochem Biophys Res Commun* 1975; 66: 81–7.

31. Finkelstein, JD, Martin, JJ. Methionine metabolism in mammals. Distribution of homocysteine between competing pathways. *J Biol Chem* 1984; 259: 9508–13.

32. Finkelstein, JD, Martin, JJ. Inactivation of betaine-homocysteine methyltransferase by adenosylmethionine and adenosylethionine. *Biochem Biophys Res Commun* 1984; 118: 14–9.

33. Flott-Rahmel, B, Schürmann, M, Mushoff, U, Ullrich, K. Neurotoxic potency of metabolites accumulating in homocystinuria. *J Inherit Metab Dis* 1996; 19(Suppl.1): 55.

34. Flott-Rahmel, B, Schürmann, M, Schluff, P, Fingerhut, R, Musshoff, U, Fowler, B, Ullrich, K. Homocysteic and homocysteine sulphinic acid exhibit excitotoxicity in organotypic cultures from rat brain. *Eur J Pediatr* 1998; 157(Suppl 2): S112–17.

35. Fowler, B, Giles, L, Cooper, A, Sardharwalla, IB. Chorionic villus sampling: Diagnostic uses and limitations of enzyme assays. *J Inherit Metab Dis* 1989; 12(Suppl 1): 105–17.

36. Fowler, B, Jakobs, C. Post- and prenatal diagnostic methods for the homocystinurias. *Eur J Pediatr* 1998; 157(Suppl 2): S88–S93.

37. Frantzen, F, Faaren, AL, Alfheim, I, Nordhei, AK. Enzyme conversion immunoassay for determining total homocysteine in plasma or serum. *Clin Chem* 1998; 44: 311–16.

38. Gallagher, PM, Ward, P, Tan, S, Naughten, E, Kraus, JP, Sellar, GC, McConnell, DJ, Graham, I, Whitehead, AS. High frequency (71%) of cystathionine β-synthase mutation G307S in Irish homocystinuria patients. *Hum Mutat* 1995; 6: 177–80.

39. Gaustadnes, MIJ, Rüdiger, N. Prevalence of congenital homocystinuria in Denmark. *N Engl J Med* 1999; 340: 1513.

40. Gerding, H. Ocular complications and a new surgical approach to lens dislocation in homocystinuria due to cystathionine-β-synthetase deficiency. *Eur J Pediatr* 1998; 157(Suppl 2): S94–S101.

41. Goldstein, JL, Campbell, BK, Gartler, SM. Homocystinuria: Heterozygote detection using phytohemagglutinin-stimulated lymphocytes. *J Clin Invest* 1973; 52: 218–21.

42. Goulding, CW, Matthews, RG. Cobalamin-dependent methionine synthase from *Escherichia coli*: Involvement of zinc in homocysteine activation. *Biochemistry* 1997; 36: 15749–57.

43. Hu, FL, Gu, Z, Kozich, V, Kraus, JP, Ramesh, V, Shih, VE. Molecular basis of cystathionine β-synthase deficiency in pyridoxine responsive and nonresponsive homocystinuria. *Hum Mol Genet* 1993; 2: 1857–60.

44. Ishihara, S, Morohashi, K, Sadano, H, Kawabata, S, Gotoh, O, Omura, T. Molecular cloning and sequence analysis of cDNA coding for rat liver hemoprotein H-450. *J Biochem (Tokyo)* 1990; 108: 899–902.

45. Jakubowski, H. Metabolism of homocysteine thiolactone in human cell cultures: Possible mechanism for pathological consequences of elevated homocysteine levels. *J Biol Chem* 1997; 272: 1935–42.

45a. Jhee, KH, McPhie, P, Miles, EW. Yeast cystathionine β-synthase is a pyridoxal phosphate enzyme but, unlike the human enzyme, is not a heme protien. *J Biol Chem* 2000; 275: 11541–4.

46. Kery, V, Bukovska, G, Kraus, JP. Transsulfuration depends on heme in addition to pyridoxal 5′-phosphate. Cystathionine β-synthase is a heme protein. *J Biol Chem* 1994; 269: 25283–88.

47. Kery, V, Elleder, D, Kraus, JP. δ-Aminolevulinate increases heme saturation and yield of human cystathionine β-synthase expressed in *Escherichia coli*. *Arch Biochem Biophys* 1995; 316: 24–9.

48. Kery, V, Poneleit, L, Kraus, JP. Trypsin cleavage of human cystathionine β-synthase into an evolutionary conserved active core: Structural and functional consequences. *Arch Biochem Biophys* 1998; 355: 222–32.

49. Kery, V, Poneleit, L, Meyer, J, Manning, M, Kraus, JP. Binding of pyridoxal 5′-phosphate to a hemeprotein—human cystathionine β-synthase. *Biochemistry* 1999; 38: 2716–24.

50. Kim, CE, Gallagher, PM, Guttormsen, AB, Refsum, H, Ueland, PM, Ose, L, Folling, I, Whitehead, AS, Tsai, MY, Kruger, WD. Functional modeling of vitamin responsiveness in yeast: A common pyridoxine-responsive cystathionine β-synthase mutation in homocystinuria. *Hum Mol Genet* 1997; 6: 2213–21.

51. Kimura, H, Nakagawa, H. Studies on cystathionine synthetase: Characteristics of purified rat liver enzyme. *J Biochem (Tokyo)* 1971; 69: 711–23.

52. Kluijtmans, LA, Boers, GH, Kraus, JP, van den Heuvel, LP, Cruysberg, JR, Trijbels, FJ, Blom, HJ. The molecular basis of cystathionine beta-synthase deficiency in Dutch patients with homocystinuria: Effect of CBS genotype on biochemical and clinical phenotype and on response to treatment. *Am J Hum Genet* 1999; 65: 59–67.

53. Kluijtmans, LAJ, Boers, GHJ, Stevens, EMB, Renier, WO, Kraus, JP, Trijbels, FJM, van den Heuvel, LPWJ, Blom, HJ. Defective cystathionine β-synthase regulation by *S*-adenosylmethionine in a partially pyridoxine responsive homocystinuria patient. *J Clin Invest* 1996; 98: 285–89.

54. Kluijtmans, LAJ, Boers, GHJ, Trijbels, FJM, van Lith-Zanders, HMA, van den Heuvel, LPWJ, Blom, HJ. A common 844INS68 insertion variant in the cystathionine β-synthase gene. *Biochem Mol Med* 1997; 62: 23–5.

55. Koch, HG, Ullrich, K, Deufel, T, Harms, E. High prevalence of a splice site mutation in the cystathionine β-synthase gene causing pyridoxine nonresponsive homocystinuria. Sixth International Congress, Inborn Errors of Metabolism, Milan, May 27–31, 1994; abstr. W11.3.

56. Koracevic, D, Djordjevic, V. Effect of trypsin, *S*-adenosylmethionine and ethionine on serine sulfhydrase activity. *Experientia* 1977; 33: 1010–11.

57. Kožich, V, Kraus, JP. Screening for mutations by expressing patient cDNA segments in *E. coli*—homocystinuria due to cystathionine β-synthase deficiency. *Hum Mutat* 1992; 1: 113–23.

58. Kraus, JP. Molecular analysis of cystathionine β-synthase—a gene on chromosome 21. *Prog Clin Biol Res* 1990; 360: 201–14.

59. Kraus, JP. Molecular basis of phenotype expression in homocystinuria. *J Inherit Metab Dis* 1994; 17: 383–90.

60. Kraus, JP, Janosik, M, Kozich, V, Mandell, R, Shih, V, Sperandeo, MP, Sebastio, G, de Franchis, R, Andria, G, Kluijtmans, LAJ, Blom, H, Boers, GHJ, Gordon, RB, Kamoun, P, Tsai, MY, Kruger, WD, Koch, HG, Ohura, T, Gaustadnes, M. Cystathionine β-synthase mutations in homocystinuria. *Hum Mutat* 1999; 13: 362–75.

61. Kraus, JP, Le, K, Swaroop, M, Ohura, T, Tahara, T, Rosenberg, LE, Roper, MD, Kozich, V. Human cystathionine β-synthase cDNA: Sequence, alternative splicing and expression in cultured cells. *Hum Mol Genet* 1993; 2: 1633–38.

62. Kraus, JP, Oliveriusova, J, Sokolova, J, Kraus, E, Vlcek, C, de Franchis, R, Maclean, KN, Bao, L, Bukovska, G, Patterson, D, Paces, V, Ansorge, W, Kozich, V. The human cystathionine β-synthase (CBS) gene: Complete sequence, alternative splicing and polymorphisms. *Genomics* 1998; 52: 312–24.

63. Kraus, JP, Packman, S, Fowler, B, Rosenberg, LE. Purification and properties of cystathionine β-synthase from human liver. *J Biol Chem* 1978; 253: 6523–28.

64. Kraus, JP, Rosenberg, LE. Cystathionine β-synthase from human liver: Improved purification scheme and additional characterization of the enzyme in crude and pure form. *Arch Biochem Biophys* 1983; 222: 44–52.

65. Kraus, JP, Williamson, CL, Firgaira, FA, Yang-Feng, TL, Münke, M, Francke, U, Rosenberg, LE. Cloning and screening with nanogram amounts of immunopurified mRNAs: cDNA cloning and chromosomal mapping of

cystathionine β-synthase and the β subunit of propionyl-CoA carboxylase. *Proc Natl Acad Sci USA* 1986; 83: 2047–51.

66. Kruger, WD, Cox, DR. A yeast system for expression of human cystathionine β-synthase: Structural and functional conservation of the human and yeast genes. *Proc Natl Acad Sci USA* 1994; 91: 6614–18.

67. Lipson, MH, Kraus, J, Rosenberg, LE. Affinity of cystathionine β-synthase for pyridoxal 5′-phosphate in cultured cells. A mechanism for pyridoxine-responsive homocystinuria. *J Clin Invest* 1980; 66: 188–93.

68. Lipton, SA, Kim, W-K, Choi, Y-B, Kumar, S, D'Emilia, DM, Rayudu, PV, Arnelle, DR, Stamler, JS. Neurotoxicity associated with dual actions of homocysteine at the *N*-methyl-D-aspartate receptor. *Proc Natl Acad Sci USA* 1997; 94: 5923–28.

69. Locker, J, Gill, TJ III, Kraus, JP, Ohura, T, Swarop, M, Rivière, M, Islam, MQ, Levan, G, Szpirer, J, Szpirer, C. The rat MHC and cystathionine β-synthase gene are syntenic on chromosome 20. *Immunogenetics* 1990; 31: 271–74.

70. Lubec, B, Fang-Kircher, S, Lubec, T, Blom, HJ, Boers, GHJ. Evidence for McKusick's hypothesis of deficient collagen cross-linking in patients with homocystinuria. *Biochim Biophys Acta* 1996; 1315: 159–62.

70a. Maclean, KN, Janošik, M, Oliveriusová, J, Kery, V, Kraus, JP. Transsulfuration in *Saccharomyces cerevisiae* is not dependent on heme: Purification and characterization of recombinant yeast cystathionine β-synthase. *J Inorg Chem*; 81: 161–71.

71. McCully, KS. Vascular pathology of homocysteinemia: Implications for the pathogenesis of arteriosclerosis. *Am J Pathol* 1969; 56: 111–28.

72. McCully, KS. Homocysteine theory of arteriosclerosis: Development and current status. *Arterioscler Rev* 1983; 11: 157–246.

73. McCully, KS, Ragsdale, BD. Production of arteriosclerosis by homocysteinemia. *Am J Pathol* 1970; 61: 1–8.

74. McGill, JJ, Mettler, G, Rosenblatt, DS, Scriver, CR. Detection of heterozygotes for recessive alleles. Homocyst(e)inemia: Paradigm of pitfalls in phenotypes. *Am J Med Genet* 1990; 36: 45–52.

75. McIlwain, H, Poll, JD. Interaction between adenosine generated endogenously in neocortical tissues, and homocysteine and its thiolactone. *Neurochem Int* 1985; 7: 103–10.

76. McKusick, VA, Hall, JG, Char, F. The clinical and genetic characteristics of homocystinuria. In *Inherited Disorders of Sulphur Metabolism*. (Carson, NAJ, Raine, DN, eds.). Churchill Livingstone Ltd, London, 1971; pp. 179–203.

76a. McKusick, VA. *Mendelian Inheritance in Man. A Catalog of Human Genes and Genetic Disorders*. 12th ed. Johns Hopkins University Press, Baltimore, 1998.

77. Meister, A, Larsson, A. Glutathione synthetase deficiency and other disorders of the γ-glutamyl cycle. In *The Metabolic and Molecular Bases of Inherited Disease*, 7th ed (Scriver, CR, Beaudet, AL, Sly, WS, Valle, D, eds.). McGraw-Hill, Inc, New York, 1995, pp. 1461–77.

78. Millian, NS, Garrow, TA. Human betaine-homocysteine methyltransferase is a zinc metalloenzyme. *Arch Biochem Biophys* 1998; 356: 93–8.

79. Mudd, SH, Edwards, WA, Loeb, PM, Brown, MS, Laster, L. Homocystinuria due to cystathionine synthase deficiency: The effect of pyridoxine. *J Clin Invest* 1970; 49: 1762–73.

80. Mudd, SH, Finkelstein, JD, Irreverre, F, Laster, L. Homocystinuria: An enzymatic defect. *Science* 1964; 143: 1443–45.

81. Mudd, SH, Levy, HL. Disorders of transsulfuration. In *The Metabolic Basis of Inherited Disease*, 4th ed. (Stanbury, JB, Wyngaarden, JB, Frederickson, DS, eds.). McGraw-Hill Book Co, New York, 1978; pp. 458–503.

82. Mudd, SH, Levy, HL. Disorders of transsulfuration. In *The Metabolic Basis of Inherited Disease*, 5th ed. (Stanbury, JB, Wyngaarden, JB, Frederickson, DS, Goldstein, JL, Brown, MS, eds). McGraw-Hill Book Co, New York, 1983; pp. 522–59.

83. Mudd, SH, Levy, HL, Kraus, JP. Disorders of transsulfuration. In *The Metabolic and Molecular Bases of Inherited Disease*, 8th ed. (Scriver, CR, Beaudet, AL, Sly, WS, Valle, D, Childs, B, Vogelstein, B, eds.). McGraw-Hill, New York, 2001; pp 2007–56.

84. Mudd, SH, Levy, HL, Skovby, F. Disorders of transsulfuration. In *The Metabolic Basis of Inherited Disease*, 6th ed. (Scriver, CR, Beaudet, AL, Sly, WS, Valle, D, eds.). McGraw-Hill, Inc, New York, 1989; pp. 693–734.

85. Mudd, SH, Levy, HL, Skovby, F. Disorders of transsulfuration. In *The Metabolic and Molecular Bases of Inherited Disease*, 7th ed. Scriver, CR, Beaudet, AL, Sly, WS, Valle, D, eds.). McGraw-Hill, Inc, New York, 1995; pp. 1279–1327.

86. Mudd, SH, Skovby, F, Levy, HL, Pettigrew, KD, Wilcken, B, Pyeritz, RE, Andria, G, Boers, GHJ, Bromberg, IL, Cerone, R, Fowler, B, Grobe, H, Schmidt, H, Schweitzer, L. The natural history of homocystinuria due to cystathionine β-synthase deficiency. *Am J Hum Genet* 1985; 37: 1–31.

87. Münke, M, Kraus, JP, Ohura, T, Francke, U. The gene for cystathionine β-synthase (CBS) maps to the sub-telomeric region on human chromosome 21q and to proximal mouse chromosome 17. *Am J Hum Genet* 1988; 42: 550–59.

88. Naughten, ER, Yap, S, Mayne, PD. Newborn screening for homocystinuria: Irish and world experience. *Eur J Pediatr* 1998; 157 (Suppl 2): S84–7.

89. Omura, T, Sadano, H, Hasegawa, T, Yoshida, Y, Kominami, S. Hemoprotein H-450 identified as a form of cytochrome P-450 having an endogenous ligand at the 6th coordination position of the heme. *J Biochem (Tokyo)* 1984; 96: 1491–1500.

90. Parsons, RB, Waring, RH, Ramsden, DB, Williams, AC. *In vitro* effect of the cysteine metabolites homocysteic acid, homocysteine and cysteic acid upon human neuronal cell lines. *Neurotoxicology* 1998; 19: 599–604.

90a. Pepe, G, Vanegas, OC, Rickards, O, Giusti, B, Comeglio, P, Brunelli, T, Marcucci, R, Prisco, D, Gensini, GF, Abbate, R. World distribution of the T833C/844INS68 CBS in cis double mutation: a reliable anthropological marker. *Hum Genet* 1999; 104: 126–9.

91. Pietzsch, J, Pixa, A. Determination of total homocysteine. *Clin Chem* 1998; 44: 1781–82.

92. Roper, MD, Straubhaar, JR, Kraus, E, Sokolová, J, Hrebicek, M, Kraus, JP. Comparison of the 5′ end of the

rat and mouse cystathionine β-synthase genes. *Mamm Genome* 1996; 7: 754–57.

93. Rosenblatt, DS. Inherited disorders of folate transport and metabolism. In *The Metabolic and Molecular Bases of Inherited Disease.* 7th ed. (Scriver, CR, Beaudet, AL, Sly, WS, Valle, D, eds.). McGraw-Hill, Inc, New York, 1995; pp. 3111–28.

94. Rubba, P, Faccenda, F, Pauciullo, P, Carbone, L, Mancini, M, Strisciuglio, P, Carrozzo, R, Sartorio, R, Del Giudice, E, Andria, G. Early signs of vascular disease in homocystinuria: A noninvasive study by ultrasound methods in eight families with cystathionine-β-synthase deficiency. *Metabolism* 1990; 39: 1191–95.

95. Rubba, P, Mercuri, M, Faccenda, F, Iannuzzi, A, Irace, C, Strisciuglio, P, Gnasso, A, Tang, R, Andria, G, Bond, MG, Mancini, M. Premature carotid artery atherosclerosis: Does it occur in both familial hypercholesterolemia and homocystinuria? Ultrasound assessment of arterial intima-media thickness and blood flow velocity. *Stroke* 1994; 25: 943–50.

96. Scriver, CR, Kaufman, S, Eisensmith, RC, Woo, SLC. The hyperphenylalaninemias. In *The Metabolic and Molecular Bases of Inherited Disease.* 7th ed. (Scriver, CR, Beaudet, AL, Sly, WS, Valle, D, eds.). McGraw-Hill, Inc, New York, 1995; pp. 1015–75.

97. Sebastio, G, Sperandeo, MP, Panico, M, de Franchis, R, Kraus, J, Andria, G. The molecular basis of homocystinuria due to cystathionine β-synthase deficiency in Italian families, and report of four novel mutations. *Am J Hum Genet* 1995; 56: 1324–33.

98. Selhub, J, Miller, JW. The pathogenesis of homocysteinemia: Interruption of the coordinate regulation by *S*-adenosylmethionine of the remethylation and transsulfuration of homocysteine. *Am J Clin Nutr* 1992; 55: 131–38.

99. Shan, X, Kruger, WD. Correction of disease-causing *CBS* mutations in yeast. *Nat Genet* 1998; 19: 91–3.

100. Skovby, F, Kraus, JP. The homocystinurias. In *Connective Tissue and its Heritable Disorders: Molecular, Genetic, and Medical Aspects.* (Royce, PM, Steinmann, B, eds.). Wiley-Liss, New York, in press.

101. Skovby, F, Krassikoff, N, Francke, U. Assignment of the gene for cystathionine β-synthase to human chromosome 21 in somatic cell hybrids. *Hum Genet* 1984; 65: 291–94.

102. Skovby, F, Kraus, JP, Rosenberg, LE. Homocystinuria: Biogenesis of cystathionine β-synthase subunits in cultured fibroblasts and in an in vitro translation system programmed with fibroblast messenger RNA. *Am J Hum Genet* 1984; 36: 452–59.

103. Skovby, F, Kraus, JP, Rosenberg, LE. Biosynthesis of human cystathionine β-synthase in cultured fibroblasts. *J Biol Chem* 1984; 259: 583–87.

104. Skovby, F, Kraus, JP, Rosenberg, LE. Biosynthesis and proteolytic activation of cystathionine β-synthase in rat liver. *J Biol Chem* 1984; 259: 588–93.

105. Sperandeo, MP, de Franchis, R, Andria, G, Sebastio, G. A 68-bp insertion found in a homocystinuric patient is a common variant and is skipped by alternative splicing of the cystathionine β-synthase mRNA. *Am J Hum Genet* 1996; 59: 1391–93.

106. Stubbs, L, Kraus, J, Lehrach, H. The α-A-crystallin and cystathionine β-synthase genes are physically very closely linked in proximal mouse chromosome 17. *Genomics* 1990; 7: 284–88.

107. Surtees, R, Bowron, A, Leonard, J. Cerebrospinal fluid and plasma total homocysteine and related metabolites in children with cystathionine β-synthase deficiency: The effect of treatment. *Pediatr Res* 1997; 42: 577–82.

108. Swaroop, M, Bradley, K, Ohura, T, Tahara, T, Roper, MD, Rosenberg, LE, Kraus, JP. Rat cystathionine β-synthase. Gene organization and alternative splicing. *J Biol Chem* 1992; 267: 11455–61.

109. Taoka, S, Ohja, S, Shan, X, Kruger, WD, Banerjee, R. Evidence for heme-mediated redox regulation of human cystathionine β-synthase activity. *J Biol Chem* 1998; 273: 25179–84.

110. Taoka, S, West, M, Banerjee, R. Characterization of the heme and pyridoxal phosphate cofactors of human cystathionine β-synthase reveals nonequivalent active sites. *Biochemistry* 1999; 38: 2738–44.

111. Thomason, MJ, Lord, J, Bain, MD, Chalmers, RA, Littlejohns, P, Addison, GM, Wilcox, AH, Seymour, CA. A systematic review of evidence for the appropriateness of neonatal screening programmes for inborn errors of metabolism. *J Public Health Med* 1998; 20: 331–43.

112. Tsai, MY, Bignell, M, Schwichtenberg, K, Hanson, NQ. High prevalence of a mutation in the cystathionine β-synthase gene. *Am J Hum Genet* 1996; 59: 1262–67.

113. Wagstaff, J, Korson, M, Kraus, JP, Levy, HL. Severe folate deficiency and pancytopenia in a nutritionally deprived infant with homocystinuria caused by cystathionine β-synthase deficiency. *J Pediatr* 1991; 118: 569–72.

114. Walter, JH, Wraith, JE, White, FJ, Bridge, C, Till, J. Strategies for the treatment of cystathionine β-synthase deficiency: The experience of the Willink Biochemical Genetics Unit over the past 30 years. *Eur J Pediatr* 1998; 157 (Suppl 2): S71–6.

115. Watanabe, M, Osada, J, Aratani, Y, Kluckman, K, Reddick, R, Malinow, MR, Maeda, N. Mice deficient in cystathionine β-synthase: Animal models for mild and severe homocyst(e)inemia. *Proc Natl Acad Sci USA* 1995; 92: 1585–89.

116. Wilcken, DEL, Wilcken, B. The natural history of vascular disease in homocystinuria and the effects of treatment. *J Inherit Metab Dis* 1997; 20: 295–300.

117. Wilcken, DEL, Wilcken, B, Dudman, NPB, Tyrrell, PA. Homocystinuria: The effects of betaine in the treatment of patients not responsive to pyridoxine. *N Engl J Med* 1983; 309: 448–53.

118. Yap, S, Naughten, E. Homocystinuria due to cystathionine beta-synthase deficiency in Ireland: 25 years experience of a newborn screened and treated population with reference to clinical outcome and biochemical control. *J Inherit Metab Dis* 1998; 21: 738–47.

119. Young, PB, Kennedy, S, Molloy, AM, Scott, JM, Weir, DG, Kennedy, DG. Lipid peroxidation induced by hyperhomocysteinaemia in pigs. *Atherosclerosis* 1997; 129: 67–71.

21

Inborn Errors of Folate and Cobalamin Metabolism

DAVID S. ROSENBLATT

Although hyperhomocysteinemia is not a prominent feature of all of the inherited disorders of folate and cobalamin metabolism, these disorders have played a major role in our understanding of the spectrum of clinical phenotypes that can be associated with hyperhomocysteinemia. The enzyme methionine synthase (Metabolic Diagram, Reaction 4) plays the critical role in determining whether an elevation of homocysteine will be associated with a particular disease. Because this enzyme requires three methyl donors (5-methyltetrahydrofolate, *S*-adenosylmethionine, methylcobalamin), a functional deficiency of either folate or cobalamin can result in a buildup of homocysteine and a lack of methionine. In addition, the conversion of homocysteine to methionine by methionine synthase is associated with the regeneration of tetrahydrofolate from 5-methyltetrahydrofolate. Tetrahydrofolate is needed as a precursor for both 5,10-methylenetetrahydrofolate, which is required for thymidylate synthesis (Metabolic Diagram, Reaction 10) and for 10-formyltetrahydrofolate, which is required for the synthesis of the purine ring. Thus, patients who are blocked in the methionine synthase reaction, either on the basis of a genetic disorder or on the basis of a nutritional deficiency of folate or cobalamin, will also have abnormalities in purine and pyrimidine biosynthesis.

This is the reason that megaloblastic anemia is a frequent finding in patients with a functional block in methionine synthase. However, megaloblastic anemia is not expected and not usually found in patients with a defect in methylenetetrahydrofolate reductase (MTHFR) (Metabolic Diagram, Reaction 9) because this reaction is thought to run physiologically in the direction of 5-methyltetrahydrofolate formation. Even with a block in the reaction, there are adequate levels of reduced folates in the form of 5,10-methylenetetrahydrofolate and its derivatives and thus no impairment of endogenous purine and pyrimidine synthesis. However, there is a deficiency of 5-methyltetrahydrofolate and a consequent hyperhomocysteinemia and hypomethioninemia.

Inborn Errors of Folate Absorption and Transport

There are only three well-defined inherited disorders of folate transport or metabolism: hereditary folate malabsorption, MTHFR deficiency, and glutamate formiminotransferase deficiency. Hyperhomocysteinemia is a major manifestation of MTHFR deficiency.

Hereditary Folate Malabsorption

This disorder is associated with severe megaloblastic anemia, usually in the first few months of life. Other clinical features include failure to thrive, stomatitis, diarrhea, and developmental delay. Less than 20 patients have been described, and they have been mostly female (41, 90, 94, 95, 105–107, 118, 133, 134, 157, 158, 171, 172, 175, 200). There is clinical heterogeneity among patients. Most showed progressive neurological deterioration; a peripheral neuropathy that responded to folinic acid has been seen (171, 172). In some, seizures were ameliorated by folate therapy, whereas in others they were exacerbated. One of the affected boys had a partial deficiency in both humoral and cellular immunity (175). In contrast to other cases, he did not have mental retardation, and correction of the serum folate levels did result in normalization of folate levels in the cerebrospinal fluid. The occurrence of siblings with hereditary folate malabsorption and the documented cases of consanguinity all suggest inheritance as autosomal recessive (94, 107, 118, 158, 175, 200). In one of the families, there is the suggestion of another possibly affected male (41), and all but four of the documented cases have been female (171, 175, 200). One patient's father had intermediate absorption of oral folate, consistent with autosomal recessive inheritance (158).

All patients were severely restricted in their ability to absorb oral folic acid or reduced folates, which was reflected in low folate levels in serum as well as cerebrospinal fluid. There may be urinary excretion of formiminoglutamic acid and orotic acid (41, 46). The levels of homocysteine in most patients have not been reported; two unpublished cases had either normal or mildly elevated homocysteine levels. Large doses of oral folates did lead to a hematological response in some patients (41, 94, 107). Parenteral therapy with folates has been effective in correcting anemia, but has been of limited effectiveness in correcting the levels of folate in the cerebrospinal fluid. There is evidence that folinic acid (133, 134) or 5-methyltetrahydrofolic acid is effective in increasing cerebrospinal fluid folate. Treatment is aimed at maintaining blood and cerebrospinal folate levels in the normal range by the use of high dose oral folates or of oral or parenteral reduced folates. There has also been the suggestion that intrathecal folate therapy may be necessary.

Patients with hereditary folate malabsorption provide the best evidence for the existence of a specific folate carrier in the intestine and in the choroid plexus. All folates appear to share this system because the absorption of both oxidized and reduced folates is effectively blocked. A single gene mediates both intestinal and choroid plexus transport because, except in the two affected males (171, 175), cerebrospinal fluid folate levels remained low when blood folate levels were raised sufficiently to correct the anemia. A cDNA for the putative intestinal transporter has been cloned that is identical to that for the reduced folate carrier (122). Uptake of folates into other cells of the body appears to be normal in patients with hereditary folate malabsorption, because the anemia is reversed in the presence of relatively low blood folate levels. Also, the content and distribution of folates were normal in cultured fibroblasts from the one patient studied (41). It remains to be seen whether mutations in the putative gene for intestinal transport will be found in patients with hereditary folate malabsorption.

Methylenetetrahydrofolate Reductase Deficiency

MTHFR catalyzes the reduction of 5,10-methylenetetrahydrofolate to 5-methyltetrahydrofolate (Metabolic Diagram, Reaction 9). This activity is thought to be essentially irreversible under physiological conditions, and the enzyme activity is regulated by levels of S-adenosylmethionine, which is an inhibitor (82, 92, 151). Nearly 50 patients with autosomal recessive, severe MTHFR deficiency are known, and the age of diagnosis has ranged from before birth to adult life (1,

2, 14–16, 19, 20, 22, 23, 31, 35, 36, 39, 51, 54–56, 72, 74, 75, 77, 81, 85, 117, 119–121, 126, 127, 141, 148, 152, 163, 164, 166, 170, 178, 186, 191, 192). The major biochemical findings are moderate hyperhomocysteinemia with low or relatively normal levels of plasma methionine. The clinical severity of this disorder varies greatly; clinical features include developmental delay, microcephaly, motor and gait abnormalities, seizures, and psychiatric manifestations (47, 87, 127, 128). Because there is no deficiency of tetrahydrofolate, megaloblastic anemia is not a usual feature. Many, but not all, patients have low serum folate levels on at least one determination, but serum cobalamin levels are almost always normal. Neurotransmitter levels in the cerebrospinal fluid have usually been low (47, 87).

The enzyme deficiency has been confirmed in the liver, leukocytes, and cultured fibroblasts and lymphoblasts of severely affected patients. The specific activity of MTHFR depends on the stage of the culture cycle of fibroblasts, with the specific activity in control cells being highest in confluent cultures (151). The residual specific activity in fibroblasts and clinical severity correlate roughly, but both the measurement of the proportion of folate present as 5-methyltetrahydrofolate (141) and the synthesis of methionine from formate (22, 53) provide a better correlation. Fibroblasts from patients cannot grow when homocysteine is substituted for methionine in the culture medium (117, 152). This inability to grow on homocysteine is shared by fibroblasts from patients who are functionally deficient in methionine synthase (cblC, cblD, cblE, cblF, and cblG) (60).

MTHFR deficiency has been diagnosed or excluded prenatally by enzyme assay or by measurement of the incorporation of labeled formate into methionine by cultured amniotic fluid cells (23, 35, 54, 111, 166, 185). Enzyme activity is detectable in normal chorionic villi (35, 166). If both MTHFR mutations segregating in a family are known, molecular analysis allows for early prenatal diagnosis.

The gene is on chromosome 1p36.3 and has 11 exons (66). Although nonsense and splice site mutations have been reported, most mutations have been missense, and each has been reported in only one or two families with severe deficiency (63–65, 88). More than 20 different mutations that cause severe disease are known in addition to the polymorphisms that may contribute to disease in the general population.

Biochemical heterogeneity in severe MTHFR deficiency was noted in the original families; fibroblast extracts from different patients had different levels of residual specific activity after preincubation at 55°C (152). Although several of the later-onset patients also had a thermolabile reductase under these conditions, thermolability was found in patients with early-onset disease as well (146). In some patients, this condition was due to the presence of severe mutations in combination with the common 677C→T mutation that is responsible for most enzyme thermolability in the general population (57, 65). The subject of common polymorphisms in the reductase gene is covered in detail in Chapter 22.

The pathological changes have included dilated cerebral ventricles, internal hydrocephalus, microgyria, perivascular changes, demyelination, macrophage infiltration, gliosis, and astrocytosis (14, 15, 19, 36, 47, 72, 81, 85, 192). Thrombosis of arteries and cerebral veins appears to have been a major factor in the death of these patients. These thromboses were the major pathological findings shared with cystathionine β-synthase deficiency. The combination of MTHFR deficiency and factor V Leiden may contribute to the vascular pathology in some patients (67, 110). Demyelination, astrogliosis, and lipid-filled macrophages are associated in many MTHFR-deficient patients with a progressive course of seizures, microcephaly, and severe psychomotor retardation. At least two patients had subacute combined degeneration of the cord similar to that in patients with untreated cobalamin deficiency (19, 36). It has been proposed that methionine deficiency causes demyelination by interfering with methylation.

MTHFR deficiency has been resistant to treatment (37, 47, 51, 200). Rationales for therapy include folates to maximize residual enzyme activity, 5-methyltetrahydrofolate to replace the missing product, methionine to correct the cellular methionine deficiency, pyridoxine to lower homocysteine levels because of its role as a cofactor for cystathionine β-synthase, cobalamin because of its role as a cofactor for methionine synthase, carnitine because of its requirement for S-adenosylmethionine, riboflavin because of the enzyme's flavin requirement, and betaine because it is a substrate for betaine methyltransferase (51, 61). Betaine has the advantage of both lowering homocysteine levels and raising methionine levels.

The best therapeutic results have included a patient who was treated with a combination of methionine, 5-formyltetrahydrofolic acid and vitamin B_6, and cobalamin (74, 75) and several patients in whom betaine was included in the regimen (23, 35, 47, 186). Betaine (23, 80, 139, 186) is the most promising agent for therapy. Many authors have stressed the importance of early diagnosis and therapy because of the poor prognosis in this disorder once there is evidence of neurological involvement (1, 46, 47, 139). Even with early diagnosis, none of the therapeutic regimens is universally successful, and it is possible that genetic heterogeneity in the disease itself is responsible for some of the variability in clinical response to therapy.

Glutamate Formiminotransferase Deficiency

In histidine catabolism, a formimino group is transferred to tetrahydrofolate, followed by the release of ammonia and the formation of 5,10-methenyltetrahydrofolate. The two enzyme activities involved in these steps, glutamate formiminotransferase and formiminotetrahydrofolate cyclodeaminase, share a single octameric enzyme (17, 109) that channels folylpolyglutamates from one reaction to the next. This pathway, which is thought to be present only in the liver and kidney, represents a minor source of single-carbon units. Defects in this pathway result in the excretion of formiminoglutamate. Formiminoglutamate excretion is also seen in patients deficient in folate or cobalamin. Hyperhomocysteinemia is not a feature of glutamate formiminotransferase deficiency.

Fewer than 20 patients with glutamate formiminotransferase deficiency are known. Patients have come to medical attention from 3 months to 42 years of age (7–12, 18, 43, 44, 47, 78, 123, 124, 129, 155, 156). It is unclear whether the enzyme deficiency is associated with a disease state or whether the association of clinical findings with formiminoglutamate excretion is a result of bias of ascertainment (47, 51, 176, 200). Two distinct phenotypes have been described. In one there is mental and physical retardation, cortical atrophy with dilatation of cerebral ventricles, and abnormal electroencephalograms. In the other there is no mental retardation but massive excretion of formiminoglutamate. Although it has been proposed that the severe form is associated with a block in the cyclodeaminase enzyme and the mild form with a block in the formiminotransferase enzyme (154), no direct enzyme measurements have been presented to support this hypothesis. Glutamate formiminotransferase deficiency has been found in both male and female offspring of unaffected parents, but there has not been any consanguinity. The deficiency is presumed to be inherited as an autosomal recessive disorder.

Inborn Errors of Cobalamin Absorption and Transport

In the inborn errors of cobalamin absorption and transport, cobalamin is not delivered to its target cells. Although hyperhomocysteinemia has been reported, it is not as prominent a feature as in the inborn errors of cobalamin metabolism that affect the synthesis of methylcobalamin, the cofactor for methionine synthase. Disorders of cobalamin absorption and transport should be considered in the differential diagnosis of patients with anemia, infection, or myelopathy because they are much more readily treated than the inborn errors of intracellular metabolism. The defect may be at the level of transport across the intestine (intrinsic factor deficiency or defective cobalamin transport by enterocytes), or at the level of a circulating cobalamin binding protein (transcobalamin I, transcobalamin II). When searched for, methylmalonic acid and homocystine have been found in the urine of some patients. The cobalamin absorption test (Schilling test) will be abnormal in all except transcobalamin I deficiency.

Transcobalamin I (Haptocorrin, R Binder) Deficiency

R binders are glycoproteins containing variable polysaccharide complexes and are secreted in exocrine secretions and by granulocytes (see Chapter 24). R binders carry the major quantitative pool of bound cobalamin in serum but do not deliver their cobalamin to cells for utilization.

A deficiency or complete absence of R binder has been reported in plasma, saliva, and leukocytes in six adults and one child; but it is not clear that this was the cause of the clinical findings in any of them (27, 28, 30, 38, 82, 201). However, the entity is not homogenous; two brothers had coexisting deficiency of lactoferrin (103). The younger of these two brothers had optic atrophy, ataxia, long tract signs, and dementia in his 40s (30). Another man, whose R binder deficiency was limited to plasma and who had normal levels in secretions, had findings resembling those seen in subacute combined degeneration of the spinal cord in his 40s and 50s (168). Although serum cobalamin levels were low, transcobalamin II-cobalamin levels were normal, and the patients were not clinically cobalamin deficient.

Intrinsic Factor Deficiency

Intrinsic factor carries cobalamin to its site of intestinal absorption in the distal ileum. At least 45 patients have been found to have absent or defective intrinsic factor as a result of an autosomal recessive disorder. The patients have otherwise normal stomachs with adequate acid secretion. Megaloblastic anemia, developmental delay, and myelopathy usually appear after the first year of life but may be delayed until adolescence or adulthood (29, 86, 137). Mixing the vitamin with a source of normal intrinsic factor corrects the abnormal absorption of cobalamin. Whereas some patients have no detectable intrinsic factor, others have intrinsic factor that lacks function but can be detected immunologically. In one patient, the intrinsic factor had a low affinity for cobalamin and was labile to destruction by acid and pepsin (195). There has been a report of a patient with a combined deficiency of intrinsic factor and R binder (201). Human intrinsic factor is coded by a gene on chromosome 11 (79). The mutations responsible for inherited intrinsic factor deficiency have not yet been described. Most patients are treated with parenteral cobalamin, and if treatment is started before neurological deterioration has occurred, outcomes are excellent.

Defective Cobalamin Transport by Enterocytes (Imerslund-Gräsbeck Syndrome, Megaloblastic Anemia 1)

Both intestinal and renal proximal tubule cells produce a receptor for the intrinsic factor–cobalamin complex (161). This receptor is a peripheral membrane protein with a clear membrane-spanning domain. The sequence has eight epidermal growth factor repeats followed by 27 contiguous, 110-amino acid *CUB* domains (21). Thus, the receptor has been named cubilin. Cubilin has been copurified with megalin, an even larger receptor, and colocalization of these two receptors suggests that both may be needed for cobalamin transport (21, 160).

Defective cobalamin transport by enterocytes (Imerslund-Gräsbeck syndrome) is an autosomal recessive disorder. Patients have symptoms and signs of cobalamin deficiency, anorexia, failure to thrive, recurrent infections, and gastrointestinal symptoms, usually within the first 2 years of life (3, 33, 68, 193). Of the approximately 180 known patients, most are found in Finland, in Norway, among Sephardic Jews in Israel, and in Saudi Arabia (3). They have normal intrinsic factor and normal intestinal morphology. They have a selective defect in cobalamin absorption that is not corrected by treatment with an external source of intrinsic factor. Many patients also have proteinuria of the tubular type that does not correct with cobalamin therapy.

The defect resides in the ileal intrinsic factor–cobalamin receptor (24). The locus was mapped to a 6 cM region on chromosome 10p12.1, based on data from linkage studies of multiplex families from Finland and Norway, and cubilin was mapped to the same interval (3, 91). Two independent, disease-specific mutations have been found in the cubilin gene in 17 Finnish families (4). A canine model has been described in which the receptor protein is not transported to the apical surface of ileal mucosal cells (58, 59). The canine defect is in a gene other than that coding for cubilin (195).

A decrease in the number of new cases diagnosed in Finland and Norway in recent years has been reported (3). The authors suggested that changing dietary factors may influence the expression of this disease or that there might be a drop in the birth rate in subpopulations showing enrichment of the responsible mutations.

Transcobalamin II Deficiency

Transcobalamin II is the physiologically important carrier of newly absorbed cobalamin and is encoded by a gene on chromosome 22 (132). It is recognized by a 62 kDa surface receptor, and the receptor-transcobalamin II-cobalamin complex is taken up by receptor-mediated endocytosis (45, 136; see Chapter 24 and Figure 24.2). Transcobalamin II deficiency is an autosomal recessive disease and about 30 patients are known (73, 84, 101, 104, 153). Because the majority of cobalamin in serum is bound to transcobalamin I and not transcobalamin II, most but not all patients have serum cobalamin levels within the control range. Infants with undetectable transcobalamin II in their blood are born healthy and do not demonstrate cobalamin deficiency until several days after birth, even though the transcobalamin II in cord blood is of fetal origin (135). Clinical findings include failure to thrive, infections, weakness, and diarrhea, as well as severe megaloblastic anemia in the first few months of life, pancytopenia, or even isolated erythroid hypoplasia (125). Neurological disease is not present at diagnosis and occurs much later; it is associated with suboptimal treatment with cobalamin or with treatment of the anemia with folate instead of cobalamin (24, 73, 115, 173, 199). Immunological deficiency with defective cellular and humoral immunity as well as defective granulocyte function have been seen. Both homocystinuria and methylmalonic aciduria may be present (38).

In most patients, transcobalamin II is undetectable, although some have immunologically reactive protein with abnormal cobalamin-binding properties or the inability to bind to the receptor (76, 162, 196). It appears that transcobalamin II also has a role in the transport of cobalamin across the ileal cell (see Figure 24.2). Most patients with transcobalamin II deficiency show intestinal cobalamin malabsorption by Schilling test; some patients with normal Schilling test results have immunoreactive transcobalamin II.

Successful treatment requires maintaining high serum cobalamin levels in the range of 750 to 7,500 pmol/L. These serum levels have been achieved with twice weekly doses of hydroxocobalamin or cyanocobalamin orally (500 to 1,000 μg) or of parenteral cyanocobalamin or hydroxocobalamin (1,000 μg) weekly or more often. Although folic or folinic acid in milligram doses has been successful in reversing the hematological findings in most patients, they should not be given as the only therapy. Hematological relapse and neurological damage can occur when folate supplementation is given without cobalamin (38).

The first mutant alleles in transcobalamin II deficiency have included deletions (100) and nonsense mutations (101). The protein is synthesized by amnio-cytes, which allows for prenatal diagnosis even when the causal mutations are not known (113, 145).

Inborn Errors of Cobalamin Metabolism (Figure 21.1)

After endocytosis of the transcobalamin II-cobalamin complex, transcobalamin II must be cleaved from cobalamin, and the cobalamin must exit the lysosome and undergo a series of reductions of its central cobalt from trivalent (cob(III)alamin) to the monovalent state (cob(I)alamin). Cobalamin is then converted to methylcobalamin in the cytoplasm and adenosylcobalamin in the mitochondrion. The prominent biochemical features of patients with inborn errors of cobalamin metabolism are hyperhomocysteinemia and methylmalonic acidemia, either alone or in combination. Hyperhomocysteinemia occurs as a result of a functional defect in the cytoplasmic methionine synthase (Metabolic Diagram, Reaction 4) for which methylcobalamin is a cofactor. A functional test for the integrity of methionine synthase is the ability of cultured fibroblasts to incorporate label from [^{14}C]methyltetrahydrofolate into high-molecular-weight products. Methylmalonic acidemia occurs as a result of a functional defect in the mitochondrial methylmalonyl CoA mutase for which adenosylcobalamin is a cofactor. A functional test for the integrity of methylmalonyl CoA mutase is the ability of cells to incorporate label from [^{14}C]propionate into high-molecular-weight products. The disorders of cobalamin metabolism have been grouped into eight complementation classes *cblA*, *cblB*, *cblC*, *cblD*, *cblE*, *cblF*, *cblG*, and *mut* on the basis of somatic cell complementation analysis (69, 181, 183, 187). Defects in methylmalonyl CoA mutase responsible for the *mut* complementation class will not be discussed, as they are not primary defects in cobalamin metabolism, and they do not result in hyperhomocysteinemia. The defects in adenosylcobalamin synthesis are reviewed even though they also result only in methylmalonic acidemia and not hyperhomocysteinemia.

Adenosylcobalamin Deficiency—*cblA*, *cblB*

Newborn screening gave an incidence of 1:61,000 and of 1:48,000 in Quebec and Massachusetts, respectively, for all forms of methylmalonic aciduria (42, 99). Mutations in the mutase gene on chromosome 6p21 are responsible for methylmalonic aciduria in those patients who do not respond to cobalamin therapy (98). Defects in the synthesis of adenosylcobalamin are responsible for the cobalamin-responsive forms of methylmalonic aciduria. There are at least 45 *cblA* and 33 *cblB* patients known and both are inher-

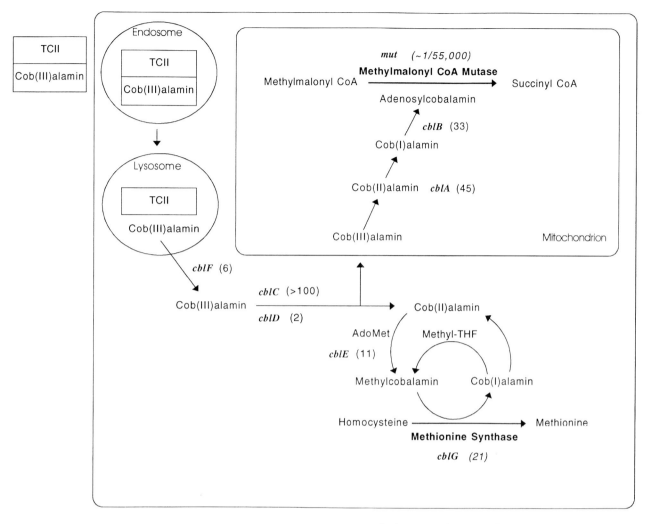

Fig. 21.1. Inborn errors of cobalamin metabolism. The number of patients with each disease are given in parentheses. AdoMet, *S*-adenosylmethionine; TC II, transcobalamin II; Cob(III)alamin, Cob(II)alamin, Cob(I)alamin represent cobalamin with its cobalt in the trivalent, divalent, or monovalent oxidation state; methyl-THF, 5-methyltetrahydrofolate.

ited as autosomal recessive diseases. Most patients are ill within the first year of life, and although patients in both groups respond to cobalamin treatment, prognosis is usually better in the *cblA* group (112). Symptoms including vomiting, failure to thrive, lethargy, hypotonia, and severe acidosis are induced by infection or protein consumption. In addition to the accumulation of large amounts of methylmalonic acid in both blood and urine, elevated levels of ammonia, glycine, glucose, and ketones may be seen, as well as low levels of leukocytes and platelets. Although prenatal therapy with cobalamin has been beneficial in some patients, it is possible that treatment started at birth would have been equally effective (5, 198).

Intact fibroblasts from both *cblA* and *cblB* patients fail to synthesize adenosylcobalamin from labeled cyanocobalamin. Whereas cell extracts of *cblA* fibroblasts can synthesize adenosylcobalamin when provided with an appropriate reducing system, those of *cblB* cannot. Fibroblasts from both disorders have decreased incorporation of label from propionate, and the two disorders are best distinguished by complementation analysis. The defect in *cblA* has been reported to be related to deficiency of a mitochondrial NADPH-linked aquacobalamin reductase (180). The defect in *cblB* is in an adenosyltransferase, which is the final step in adenosylcobalamin synthesis (48). Obligate heterozygotes of *cblB* patients show decreased activity of this adenosyltransferase (49, 152a). There is evidence for interallelic complementation with the *cblA* complementation class (40).

Combined Adenosylcobalamin and Methylcobalamin Deficiencies—*cblC, cblD, cblF*

These three disorders involve early steps in intracellular cobalamin metabolism leading to a failure of synthesis of both methylcobalamin—resulting in hyperhomocysteinemia, homocystinuria and hypomethioninemia—and adenosylcobalamin, resulting in methylmalonic aciduria (93). The levels of homocysteine and methylmalonic acid are lower than those found in cystathionine β-synthase and methylmalonyl CoA mutase deficiency, respectively. In all three disorders, incorporation of label from propionate and 5-methyltetrahydrofolate is decreased. When control fibroblasts are incubated with labeled cyanocobalamin, virtually all of the label is ultimately found as adenosylcobalamin bound to methylmalonyl CoA mutase or as methylcobalamin bound to methionine synthase. In contrast, fibroblasts from *cblC* and *cblD* patients accumulate almost no labeled cobalamin derivatives when incubated with labeled cyanocobalamin, and fibroblasts from *cblF* patients accumulate excess cobalamin, but it remains as unmetabolized, nonprotein-bound cyanocobalamin in lysosomes (149, 177). In *cblC* and *cblD*, the defect is thought to involve the reduction of cob(III)alamin, and partial deficiencies of cyanocobalamin β-ligand transferase and microsomal cob(III)alamin reductase have been described in fibroblasts as well (114, 130, 131). In *cblF*, the defect involves the exit of cobalamin within lysosomes after it has been released from transcobalamin II following endocytosis.

There is considerable heterogeneity among the more than 100 known patients with *cblC* disease. Most come to medical attention in the first year of life with poor feeding, failure to thrive, and megaloblastic anemia; some also have thrombocytopenia (116, 147). Other patients have onsets later in childhood, adolescence, or even adult life with spasticity, delirium, and psychosis (167). Hydrocephalus, cor pulmonale, and hepatic failure have been described, as well as a pigmentary retinopathy with perimacular degeneration (26, 38, 116, 138, 140, 174, 184). The *cblD* group consists of a single sibship of two brothers who had mild mental retardation and behavioral problems (62). One of them developed a pulmonary embolism and recurrent deep vein thromboses (49, 152a). Of the six *cblF* patients, four were ill in the first year of life and the fifth at age 4 years (108, 144, 166, 190). One patient died suddenly in infancy, two had minor malformations, and the oldest patient had arthritis and a pigmentary skin abnormality. One patient, treated from early infancy, had normal development and no adverse neurological findings at age 20 months (179). The *cblF* patients have also shown abnormal intestinal cobalamin absorption, suggesting that cobalamin passes through a lysosomal stage in the enterocyte (93, 190). The patients with *cblF* disease have responded to systemic hydroxocobalamin therapy (108, 144, 166, 190); the first patient also responded to oral hydroxocobalamin.

Treatment of *cblC* disease is difficult, and about one third of patients with symptom onset in the first month of life have died (49, 147, 152a). Patients with a later age of onset have a better prognosis. Parenteral therapy with hydroxocobalamin is better than therapy with oral hydroxocobalamin, and cyanocobalamin is not effective (6). Betaine is helpful in combination with hydroxocobalamin, but neither folinic acid nor carnitine is beneficial (13). Most patients respond to hydroxocobalamin therapy by reducing homocystine and methylmalonic acid excretion, although there are not many reported measurements of total plasma homocysteine in patients with *cblC* disease. In some patients, daily therapy with oral betaine and twice weekly injections of hydroxocobalamin improve the lethargy, irritability, and failure to thrive. There is usually incomplete reversal of the neurological and retinal findings. Surviving patients usually have moderate to severe developmental delay, even with good metabolic control (38, 49, 147, 152a).

All three disorders are thought to be inherited as autosomal recessive conditions, although none of the responsible genes have yet been cloned. There are roughly equal numbers of male and female patients with *cblC,* and both males and females have been reported with *cblF.* Both siblings with *cblD* disease are males, and the possibility of X linkage cannot be excluded. Prenatal diagnosis has been successful in *cblC* disease with the use of amniocytes, and the diagnosis has been excluded using chorionic villus biopsy material and cultured chorionic villus cells (32, 197).

Methylcobalamin Deficiency—Methionine Synthase Reductase Deficiency (cblE) and Methionine Synthase Deficiency (cblG)

In the methylation of homocysteine to methionine by methionine synthase (Metabolic Diagram, Reaction 4), the methyl group of 5-methyltetrahydrofolate is transferred to enzyme-bound cob(I)alamin to form methylcobalamin, and then it is transferred to homocysteine with the regeneration of cob(I)alamin. Over many cycles, cob(I)alamin oxidizes to cob(II)alamin and regeneration of a functional methionine synthase requires a reductive methylation of cob(II)alamin. A better understanding of the roles of these activities in human cells has been provided by the two complementation classes *cblE* and *cblG* with deficiencies of methylcobalamin and functional deficiencies in methionine synthase activity.

Hyperhomocysteinemia, homocystinuria, and hypomethioninemia without methylmalonic aciduria characterize functional methionine synthase deficiency *(cblE, cblG).* Most patients become ill within the first 2 years of life, although some are first diagnosed in adulthood. There are at least 11 *cblE* and 21 *cblG* patients known. In contrast to MTHFR deficiency, megaloblastic anemia is a prominent clinical feature because the block in methionine synthase results in a deficiency of the tetrahydrofolate needed for purine and pyrimidine synthesis. Other clinical findings have included developmental delay, cerebral atrophy, electroencephalogram abnormalities, nystagmus, hypotonia, hypertonia, seizures, blindness, and ataxia (183). Therapy with systemic hydroxocobalamin daily at first, then once or twice weekly, usually has corrected the anemia and the metabolic abnormalities. Once established, the neurological defects have been difficult to reverse, particularly in *cblG* disease. A mother carrying a *cblE* fetus was treated from the second trimester, and the infant was treated from birth (143). His development has been much better into the second decade than his older brother, who had metabolic decompensation during the first few months of life.

Relative to control fibroblasts, those from *cblE* and *cblG* patients show decreased accumulation of methylcobalamin with normal accumulation of adenosylcobalamin after incubation with labeled cyanocobalamin, as well as decreased incorporation of labeled 5-methyltetrahydrofolate (182). Cyanocobalamin uptake and binding to both cobalamin-dependent enzymes is normal in *cblE* fibroblasts and in most *cblG* fibroblasts, but in fibroblasts from a few *cblG* patients (*cblG* variants), there is no binding of labeled cyanocobalamin to methionine synthase (169). Most *cblG* extracts have low methionine synthase activity in the standard assay system. The standard assay for methionine synthase gives activities within the control range in *cblE* fibroblast extracts, but a deficiency in methionine synthase activity can be detected when the assay is performed using specific reducing conditions (71, 142, 150).

A cDNA for methionine synthase has been cloned, and the gene has been localized to chromosome 1q43. The first missense and nonsense mutations in methionine synthase have been described in *cblG* patients (70, 71, 96, 102, 188) (see Table 12.1 in chapter 12). The *cblG* variant patients all have functionally null mutations in methionine synthase (70, 188).

A cDNA for methionine synthase reductase has been cloned and localized to chromosome 5p15.2-15.3 by using consensus sequences to the predicted binding sites for flavin mononucleotide, flavin adenine dinucleotide, and NADPH (97). This novel deduced protein has a predicted molecular mass of 77 kDa and contains 698 amino acids. It is a member of the ferridoxin (flavodoxin) $NADP^+$ reductase family and shares 38% identity with human cytochrome P450 reductase. It also shows homology to nitric oxide synthase, sulfite reductase, flavodoxin reductase, and flavodoxin. It has been suggested that there has been a convergent evolution of the two genes specifying for flavodoxin and flavodoxin reductase to a single human gene encoding a fused ver-

sion of the two proteins. However, a two-component system for human cells has been proposed based on fractionation of the reducing system by DEAE chromatography (34). To date, 13 mutations, of which 4 have been nonsense and the remainder have been missense or in-frame disruptions of the coding sequence in methionine synthase reductase, have been identified in 11 patients (97, 189). A preliminary report described a patient whose cells complemented both *cblE* and *cblG* cells (52). It remains to be seen whether this patient has a defect in the postulated second reducing protein (34). The findings to date confirm that the defect in *cblE* is in the regeneration of active methionine synthase (71, 142).

REFERENCES

1. Abeling, NGGM, van Gennip, AH, Blom, H, Wevers, RA, Vreken, P, van Tinteren, HLG, Bakker, HD. Rapid diagnosis and methionine administration: Basis for a favourable outcome in a patient with methylenetetrahydrofolate reductase deficiency. *J Inherit Metab Dis* 1999; 22: 240–42.
2. Allen, RJ, Wong, PWK, Rothenberg, SP, Dimauro, S, Headington, JT. Progressive neonatal leukoencephalomyopathy due to absent methylenetetrahydrofolate reductase, responsive to treatment. *Ann Neurol* 1980; 8: 211.
3. Aminoff, M, Tahvanainen, E, Gräsbeck, R, Weissenbach, J, Broch, H, de la Chapelle, A. Selective intestinal malabsorption of vitamin B12 displays recessive mendelian inheritance: Assignment of a locus to chromosome 10 by linkage. *Am J Hum Genet* 1995; 57: 824–31.
4. Aminoff, M, Carter, JE, Chadwick, RB, Johnson, C, Gräsbeck, R, Abdelaal, MA, Broch, H, Jenner, LB, Verroust, PJ, Moestrup, SK, de la Chapelle, A, Krahe, R. Mutations in CUBN, encoding the intrinsic factor-vitamin B12 receptor, cubilin, cause hereditary megaloblastic anaemia 1. *Nat Genet* 1999; 21: 309–13.
5. Ampola, M, Mahoney, MJ, Nakamura, E, Tanaka, K. Prenatal therapy of a patient with vitamin B12 responsive methylmalonic acidemia. *N Engl J Med* 1975; 293: 313–17.
6. Anderson, HC, Shapira, E. Biochemical and clinical response to hydroxocobalamin versus cyanocobalamin treatment in patients with methylmalonic acidemia and homocystinuria (*cblC*). *J Pediatr* 1998; 132: 121–24.
7. Arakawa, T, Ohara, K, Kudo, Z, Tada, K, Hayashi, T, Mizuno, T. Hyperfolic-acidemia with formiminoglutamic-aciduria following histidine loading: Suggested for a case of congenital deficiency in formiminotransferase. *Tohoku J Exp Med* 1963; 80: 370–82.
8. Arakawa, T, Ohara, K, Takahashi, Y, Ogasawara, J, Hayashi, T, Chiba, R, Wada, Y, Tada, K, Mizuno, T, Ohamura, T, Yoshida, T. Formiminotransferase-deficiency syndrome: A new inborn error of folic acid metabolism. *Ann Pediatr* 1965; 205: 1–11.
9. Arakawa, T, Fujii, M, Hirono, H. Tetrahydrofolate-dependent enzyme activity in formiminotransferase

deficiency syndrome. *Tohoku J Exp Med* 1966; 88: 305–10.

10. Arakawa, T, Fujii, M, Ohara, K. Erythrocyte formiminotransferase activity in formiminotransferase deficiency syndrome. *Tohoku J Exp Med* 1966; 88: 195–202.

11. Arakawa, T, Tamura, T, Ohara, K, Narisawa, K, Tanno, K, Honda, Y, Higashi, O. Familial occurrence of formiminotransferase deficiency syndrome. *Tohoku J Exp Med* 1968; 96: 211–17.

12. Arakawa, T, Yoshida, T, Konna, T, Honda, Y. Defect of incorporation of glycine-1-14C into urinary uric acid in formiminotransferase deficiency syndrome. *Tohoku J Exp Med* 1972; 106: 213–18.

13. Bartholomew, DW, Batshaw, ML, Allen, RH, Roe, CR, Rosenblatt, D, Valle, DL, Francomano, CA. Therapeutic approaches to cobalamin-C methylmalonic acidemia and homocystinuria. *J Pediatr* 1988; 112: 32–9.

14. Baumgartner, ER, Schweizer, K, Wick, H. Different congenital forms of defective remethylation in homocystinuria. Clinical, biochemical, and morphological studies. *Pediatr Res* 1977; 11: 1015.

15. Baumgartner, ER, Stokstad, ELR, Wick, H, Watson, JE, Kusano, G. Comparison of folic acid coenzyme distribution patterns in patients with methylenetetrahydrofolate reductase and methionine synthetase deficiencies. *Pediatr Res* 1985; 19: 1288–92.

16. Baumgartner, R, Wick, H, Ohnacker, H, Probst, A, Maurer, R. Vascular lesions in two patients with congenital homocystinuria due to different defects of remethylation. *J Inherit Metab Dis* 1980; 3: 101–3.

17. Beaudet, R, Mackenzie, RE. Formiminotransferase-cyclohydrolase from porcine liver. An octameric enzyme containing bifunctional polypeptide. *Biochim Biophys Acta* 1976; 453: 151–61.

18. Beck, B, Christensen, E, Brandt, NJ, Pederson, M. Formiminoglutamic aciduria in a slightly retarded boy with chronic obstructive lung disease. *J Inherit Metab Dis* 1981; 14: 225–28.

19. Beckman, DR, Hoganson, G, Berlow, S, Gilbert, EF. Pathological findings in 5,10-methylenetetrahydrofolate reductase deficiency. *Birth Defects: Original Article Series* 1987; 23: 47–64.

20. Berlow, S. Critical review of cobalamin-folate interrelations. *Blood* 1986; 67: 1526.

21. Birn, H, Verroust, PJ, Nexo, E, Hager, H, Jacobsen, C, Christensen, EI, Moestrup, SK. Characterization of an epithelial ~460-kDa protein that facilitates endocytosis of intrinsic factor-vitamin B_{12} and binds receptor-associated protein. *J Biol Chem* 1997; 272: 26497–504.

22. Boss, G, Erbe, RW. Decreased rates of methionine synthesis by methylenetetrahydrofolate reductase-deficient fibroblasts and lymphoblasts. *J Clin Invest* 1981; 67: 1659–64.

23. Brandt, NJ, Christensen, E, Skovby, F, Djernes, B. Treatment of methylenetetrahydrofolate reductase deficiency from the neonatal period. *The Society for the Study of Inborn Errors of Metabolism* (abstract) Amersfoort, The Netherlands 1986.

24. Burman, JF, Mollin, DL, Sourial, NA, Sladden, RA. Inherited lack of transcobalamin II in serum and megaloblastic anemia: A further patient. *Br J Haematol* 1979; 43: 27–38.

25. Burman, JF, Jenkins, KJ, Walker-Smith, JA, Philips, AD, Sourial, NA, Williams, CB, Mollin, DL. Absent ileal uptake of IF-bound-vitamin B_{12} in the Imerslund-Gräsbeck syndrome (familial vitamin B_{12} malabsorption with proteinuria). *Gut* 1985; 26: 311–14.

26. Caouette, G, Rosenblatt, D, Laframboise, R. Hepatic dysfunction in a neonate with combined methylmalonic aciduria and homocystinuria (abstract). *Clin Invest Med* 1992; 15: A112.

27. Carmel, R. A new case of deficiency of the R binder for cobalamin, with observations on minor cobalamin binding proteins in serum and saliva. *Blood* 1982; 59: 152–56.

28. Carmel, R. R-binder deficiency. A clinically benign cause of cobalamin pseudodeficiency. *JAMA* 1983; 250: 1886–90.

29. Carmel, R. Gastric juice in congenital pernicious anaemia contains no immunoreactive intrinsic factor molecule: Studies of three kindreds with variable ages of presentation including a patient in adulthood. *Am J Hum Genet* 1983; 35: 67–77.

30. Carmel, R, Herbert, V. Deficiency of vitamin B_{12} alpha globulin in two brothers. *Blood* 1969; 33: 1–12.

31. Cederbaum, SD, Shaw, KNF, Cox, DR, Erbe, RW, Boss, GR, Carrel, RE. Homocystinuria due to methylenetetrahydrofolate reductase (MTHFR) deficiency: Response to a high protein diet. *Pediatr Res* 1981; 15: 560.

32. Chadefaux-Vekemans, B, Rolland, MO, Lyonet, S, Rabier, D, Divry, P, Kamoun, P. Prenatal diagnosis of combined methylmalonic aciduria and homocystinuria (cobalamin *CblC* or *CblD* mutant). *Prenat Diagn* 1994; 14: 417–18.

33. Chanarin, I. *The Megaloblastic Anaemias*. Blackwell Scientific Publications, London, 1979.

34. Chen, Z, Banerjee, R. Purification of soluble cytochrome b5 as a component of the reductive activation of porcine methionine synthase. *J Biol Chem* 1998; 273: 26248–55.

35. Christensen, E, Brandt, NJ. Prenatal diagnosis of 5,10-methylenetetrahydrofolate reductase deficiency. *N Engl J Med* 1985; 313: 50–1.

36. Clayton, PT, Smith, I, Harding, B, Hyland, KI, Leonard, JV, Leeming, RJ. Subacute combined degeneration of the cord, dementia and Parkinsonian due to an inborn error of folate metabolism. *J Neurol Neurosurg Psychiatry* 1986; 49: 920–27.

37. Cooper, BA. Anomalies congenitales du metabolisme des folates. In *Folates et Cobalamines*. (Zittoun, J, Cooper, BA, eds.). Doin, Paris, 1987, p. 193–208.

38. Cooper, BA, Rosenblatt, DS. Inherited defects of vitamin B_{12} metabolism. *Annu Rev Nutr* 1987; 7: 291–320.

39. Cooper, BA, Rosenblatt, DS. Folate coenzyme forms in fibroblasts from patients deficient in 5,10-methylenetetrahydrofolate reductase. *Biochem Soc Trans* 1976; 4: 921–22.

40. Cooper, BA, Rosenblatt, DS, Watkins, D. Methylmalonic aciduria due to a new defect in adenosylcobalamin accumulation by cells. *Am J Hematol* 1990; 34: 115–20.

41. Corbeel, L, Van Den Berghe, G, Jaeken, J, Vantornout, J, Eeckels, R. Congenital folate malabsorption. *Eur J Pediatr* 1985; 143: 284–90.

42. Coulombe, JT, Shih, VE, Levy, HL. Massachusetts Metabolic Disorders Screening Program. II Methylmalonic aciduria. *Pediatrics* 1981; 67: 26–31.

43. Duran, M, Ketting, D, deBree, PK, van Sprang, FJ, Wadman, SK, Penders, TJ, Wilms, RHH: A case of formiminoglutamic aciduria and biochemical studies. *Eur J Pediatr* 1981; 136: 319–23.

44. Duran, M, Bruinvis, L, Wadman, SK. Quantitative gas chromatographic determination of urinary hydantion-5-propionic acid in patients with disorders of folate/vitamin B_{12} metabolism. *J Chromatogr* 1986; 381: 401–5.

45. Eiberg, H, Moller, N, Mohr, J, Nielsen, LS. Linkage of transcobalamin II (TC2) to the P blood group system and assignment to chromosome 22. *Clin Genet* 1986; 29: 354–59.

46. Erbe, RW. Genetic aspects of folate metabolism. *Adv Hum Genet* 1979; 9: 293–354.

47. Erbe, RW. Inborn errors of folate metabolism. In *Nutritional, Pharmacological and Physiological Aspects,* vol. 3. (Blakley, RL, Whitehead, VM, eds.). Wiley, New York, 1986; pp. 413–66.

48. Fenton, WA, Rosenberg, LE. The defect in the cbl B class of human methylmalonic acidemia: Deficiency of cob(I)alamin adenosyltransferase activity in extracts of cultured fibroblasts. *Biochem Biophys Res Commun* 1981; 98: 283–89.

49. Fenton, W, Rosenberg, LE. Inherited disorders of cobalamin transport and metabolism. In *The Metabolic and Molecular Bases of Inherited Disease.* (Scriver, CR, Beaudet, AL, Sly, WS, Valle, D, eds.). McGraw-Hill, New York, 1995; pp. 3129–49.

50. Fowler, B. Homocystinuria, remethylation defects. Methionine synthesis and cofactor response in cultured fibroblasts. Society for the Study of Inborn Errors of Metabolism, 24th Annual Symposium, Amersfoort, the Netherlands, Sept 9–12, 1986.

51. Fowler, B. Genetic defects of folate and cobalamin metabolism. *Eur J Pediatr* 1998; 157: S60–6.

52. Fowler, B, Suormala, T, Gunther, M, Till, J, Wraith, JE. A new patient with methionine synthase deficiency: Evidence for a third complementation class (abstract). *J Inherit Metab Dis* 1997; 20: 21.

53. Fowler, B, Whitehouse, C, Wenzel, F, Wraith, JE. Methionine and serine formation in control and mutant human cultured fibroblasts: Evidence for methyl trapping and characterization of remethylation defects. *Pediatr Res* 1997; 41: 145–51.

54. Fowler, B, Jakobs, C. Post- and prenatal diagnostic methods for the homocystinurias. *Eur J Pediatr* 1998; 157: S88–S93.

55. Freeman, JM, Finkelstein, JD, Mudd, SH, Uhlendorf, BW. Homocystinuria presenting as reversible "schizophrenia:" A new defect in methionine metabolism with reduced 5,10-methylenetetrahydrofolate reductase activity. *Pediatr Res* 1972; 6: 423.

56. Freeman, JM, Finkelstein, JD, Mudd, SH. Folate-responsive homocystinuria and "schizophrenia:" A defect in methylation due to deficient 5,10-methylenetetrahydrofolate reductase activity. *N Engl J Med* 1975; 292: 491–96.

57. Frosst, P, Blom, HJ, Milos, R, Goyette, P, Sheppard, CA, Matthews, RG, Boers, GJH, den Heijer, M, Kluijtmans, LAJ, van den Heuvel, LP, Rozen, R. A candidate genetic risk factor for vascular disease: A common methylenetetrahydrofolate reductase mutation causes thermoinstability. *Nat Genet* 1995; 10: 111–13.

58. Fyfe, JC, Giger, U, Hall, CA, Jezyk, PF, Klumpp, SA, Levine, JS, Patterson, DF. Inherited selective intestinal cobalamin malabsorption and cobalamin deficiency in dogs. *Pediatr Res* 1991; 29: 24–31.

59. Fyfe, JC, Ramanujam, KS, Ramaswamy, K, Patterson, DF, Seetharam, B. Defective brush-border expression of intrinsic factor-cobalamin receptor in canine inherited intestinal cobalamin malabsorption. *J Biol Chem* 1991; 266: 4489–94.

60. Garovic-Kocic, V, Rosenblatt, DS. Methionine auxotrophy in inborn errors of cobalamin metabolism. *Clin Invest Med* 1992; 15: 395–400.

61. Gaull, GE, Von Berg, W, Raiha, NCR, Sturman, JA. Development of methyltransferase activities of human fetal tissues. *Pediatr Res* 1973; 7: 527–33.

62. Goodman, SI, Moe, PG, Hammond, KB, Mudd, SH, Uhlendorff, BW. Homocystinuria with methylmalonic aciduria: Two cases in a sibship. *Biochem Med* 1970; 4: 500–15.

63. Goyette, P, Sumner, JS, Milos, R, Duncan, AM, Rosenblatt, DS, Matthews, RG, Rozen, R. Human methylenetetrahydrofolate reductase: Isolation of cDNA, mapping and mutation identification. *Nat Genet* 1994; 7: 195–200.

64. Goyette, P, Frosst, P, Rosenblatt, DS, Rozen, R. Seven novel mutations in the methylenetetrahydrofolate reductase gene and genotype/phenotype correlations in severe methylenetetrahydrofolate reductase deficiency. *Am J Hum Genet* 1995; 56: 1052–59.

65. Goyette, P, Christensen, B, Rosenblatt, DS, Rozen, R. Severe and mild mutations in *cis* for the methylenetrahydrofolate (MTHFR) gene, and description of 5 novel mutations in MTHFR. *Am J Hum Genet* 1996; 59: 1268–75.

66. Goyette, P, Pai, A, Milos, R, Frosst, P, Tran, P, Chen, ZT, Chan, M, Rozen, R. Gene structure of human and mouse methylenetetrahydrofolate reductase (MTHFR). *Mamm Genome* 1998; 9: 652–56.

67. Goyette, P, Rosenblatt, D, Rozen, R. Homocystinuria (Methylenetetrahydrofolate reductase deficiency) and mutation of Factor V gene. *J Inherit Metab Dis* 1998; 21: 690–91.

68. Gräsbeck, R. Familial selective vitamin B_{12} malabsorption (letter). *N Engl J Med* 1972; 287: 358.

69. Gravel, RA, Mahoney, MJ, Ruddle, FH, Rosenberg, LE. Genetic complementation in heterokaryons of human fibroblasts defective in cobalamin metabolism. *Proc Natl Acad Sci USA* 1975; 72: 3181–85.

70. Gulati, S, Baker, P, Li, YN, Fowler, B, Kruger, WD, Brody, LC, Banerjee, R. Defects in human methionine synthase in *cblG* patients. *Hum Mol Genet* 1996; 5: 1859–65.

71. Gulati, S, Chen, Z, Brody, LC, Rosenblatt, DS, Banerjee, R. Defects in auxillary redox proteins lead to functional methionine synthase deficiency. *J Biol Chem* 1997; 272: 19171–75.

72. Haan, E, Rogers, J, Lewis, G, Rowe, P. 5,10-Methylenetetrahydrofolate reductase deficiency: Clinical and biochemical features of a further case. *J Inherit Metab Dis* 1985; 8: 53–7.

73. Hall, CA. The neurologic aspects of transcobalamin II deficiency. *Br J Haematol* 1992; 80: 117–20.

74. Harpey, JP, Rosenblatt, DS, Cooper, BA, Le Moel, G, Roy, C, Lafourcade, J. Homocystinuria caused by 5,10-methylenetetrahydrofolate reductase deficiency: A case in an infant responding to methionine, folinic acid, pyridoxine, and vitamin therapy. *J Pediatr* 1981; 98: 275–78.

75. Harpey, JP, Lemoel, G, Zittoun, J. Follow-up in a child with 5,10-methylenetetrahydrofolate reductase deficiency (letter). *J Pediatr* 1983; 103: 1007.

76. Haurani, FI, Hall, CA, Rubin, R. Megaloblastic anemia as a result of an abnormal transcobalamin II. *J Clin Invest* 1979; 64: 1253–59.

77. Haworth, JC, Dilling, LA, Surtees, RAH, Seargeant, LE, Lue-Shing, H, Cooper, BA, Rosenblatt, DS. Symptomatic and asymptomatic methylenetetrahydrofolate reductase deficiency in two adult brothers. *Am J Med Genet* 1993; 45: 572–76.

78. Herman, RH, Rosenweig, NS, Stifel, FB, Herman, YF. Adult formiminotransferase deficiency: A new entity (abstract). *Clin Res* 1969; 17: 304.

79. Hewitt, JE, Gordon, MM, Taggart, RT, Mohandas, TK, Alpers, DH. Human gastric intrinsic factor: Characterization of cDNA and genomic clones and localization to human chromosome 11. *Genomics* 1991; 10: 432–40.

80. Holme, E, Kjellman, B, Ronge, E. Betaine for treatment of homocystinuria caused by methylenetetrahydrofolate reductase deficiency. *Arch Dis Child* 1989; 64: 1061–64.

81. Hyland, K, Smith, I, Howell, DW, Clayton, PT, Leonard, JV. The determination of pterins, biogenic amino metabolites, and aromatic amino acids in cerebrospinal fluid using isocratic reverse phase liquid chromatography within series dual cell coulometric electrochemical and fluorescence determinations. Use in the study of inborn errors of dihydropteridine reductase and 5,10-methylenetetrahydrofolate reductase. In *Biochemical and Clinical Aspects of Pteridines*, vol. 4. (Wachter, H, Curtius, H, Pfleiderer, W, eds.). Walter de Gruyter, Berlin, 1985; pp. 85–99.

82. Jencks, DA, Matthews, RG. Allosteric inhibition of methylenetetrahydrofolate reductase by adenosylmethionine. *J Biol Chem* 1987; 262: 2485–93.

83. Jenks, J, Begley, J, Howard, L. Cobalamin-R binder deficiency in a woman with thalassemia. *Nutr Rev* 1983; 41: 277–80.

84. Kaikov, Y, Wadsworth, LD, Hall, CA, Rogers, PC. Transcobalamin II deficiency: Case report and review of the literature. *Eur J Pediatr* 1991; 150: 841–43.

85. Kanwar, YS, Manaligod, JR, Wong, PWK. Morphologic studies in a patient with homocystinuria due to 5,10-methylenetetrahydrofolate reductase deficiency. *Pediatr Res* 1976; 10: 598–609.

86. Katz, M, Lee, SK, Cooper, BA. Vitamin malabsorption due to a biologically inert intrinsic factor. *N Engl J Med* 1972; 287: 425–29.

87. Kishi, T, Kawamura, I, Harada, Y, Eguchi, T, Sakura, N, Ueda, K, Narisawa, K, Rosenblatt, DS. Effect of betaine on S-adenosylmethionine levels in the cerebrospinal fluid in a patient with methylenetetrahydrofolate reductase deficiency and peripheral neuropathy. *J Inherit Metab Dis* 1994; 17: 560–65.

88. Kluijtmans, LAJ, Wendel, U, Stevens, EMB, van den Heuvel, LPWJ, Trijbels, FJM, Blom, HJ. Identification of four novel mutations in severe methylenetetrahydrofolate reductase deficiency. *Eur J Hum Genet* 1998; 6: 257–65.

89. Kolhouse, JF, Allen, RH. Recognition of two intracellular cobalamin binding proteins and their identification as methylmalonyl-CoA mutase and methionine synthase. *Proc Natl Acad Sci USA* 1977; 74: 3: 921–25.

90. Konomi, H, Kuwajima, K, Yanagisawa, M, Kamoshita, S, Narisawa, K. A case of congenital folic acid malabsorption with infantile spasms. *Brain Dev* 1978; 3: 234.

91. Kozyraki, R, Kristiansen, M, Silahtaroglu, A, Hansen, C, Jacobsen, C, Tommerup, N, Verroust, PJ, Moestrup, SK. The human intrinsic factor-vitamin receptor, *cubilin*: Molecular characterization and chromosomal mapping of the gene to 10p within the autosomal recessive megaloblastic anemia (MGA1) region. *Blood* 1998; 91: 3593–600.

92. Kutzbach, C, Stokstad, ELR. Feedback inhibition of methylene tetrahydrofolate reductase in rat liver by S-adenosylmethionine. *Biochim Biophys Acta* 1967; 139: 217–20.

93. Laframboise, R, Cooper, BA, Rosenblatt, DS. Malabsorption of vitamin from the intestine in a child with cblF disease: Evidence for lysosomal-mediated absorption. *Blood* 1992; 80: 291–92.

94. Lanzkowsky, P, Erlandson, ME, Bezan, AI. Isolated defect of folic acid absorption associated with mental retardation and cerebral calcification. *Blood* 1969; 34: 452–65.

95. Lanzkowsky, P. Congenital malabsorption of folate. *Am J Med* 1970; 48: 580–83.

96. Leclerc, D, Campeau, E, Goyette, P, Adjalla, CE, Christensen, B, Ross, M, Eydoux, P, Rosenblatt, DS, Rozen, R, Gravel, RA. Human methionine synthase: cDNA cloning and identification of mutations in patients of the cblG complementation group of folate/cobalamin disorders. *Hum Mol Genet* 1996; 5: 1867–74.

97. Leclerc, D, Wilson, A, Dumas, R, Gafuik, C, Song, D, Watkins, D, Heng, HHQ, Rommens, JM, Scherer, SW, Rosenblatt, DS, Gravel, RA: Cloning and mapping of a cDNA for methionine synthase reductase, a flavoprotein defective in patients with homocystinuria. *Proc Natl Acad Sci USA* 1998; 95: 3059–64.

98. Ledley, FD, Lumetta, MR, Zoghbi, HY, VanTuinen, P, Ledbetter, DH. Mapping of human methylmalonyl CoA mutase (MUT) locus on chromosome 6. *Am J Hum Genet* 1988; 42: 839–46.

99. Lemieux, B, Auray-Bay, C, Guiguere, R, Shapeon, D, Scriver, CR. Newborn urine screening experience with over one million infants in Quebec network of genetic medicine. *J Inherit Met Dis* 1988; 11: 45–55.

100. Li, N, Rosenblatt, DS, Kamen, BA, Seetharam, S, Seetharam, B. Identification of two mutant alleles of transcobalamin II in an affected family. *Hum Mol Genet* 1994; 3: 1835–40.

101. Li, N, Rosenblatt, DS, Seetharam, B. Nonsense mutations in human transcobalamin II deficiency. *Biochem Biophys Res Comm* 1994; 204: 1111–18.

102. Li, YN, Gulati, S, Baker, PJ, Brody, LC, Banerjee, R, Kruger, WD. Cloning, mapping and RNA analysis of the human methionine synthase gene. *Hum Mol Genet* 1996; 5: 1851–58.

103. Lin, JC, Borregaard, N, Liebman, HA, Carmel, R. Deficiency of the specific granule proteins, transcobalamin I and lactoferrin, in plasma and saliva: A new disorder. *Am J Med Genet* 2001; in press.

104. Linnell, JC, Bhatt, HR. Inherited errors of cobalamin metabolism and their management. *Baillieres Clin Haematol* 1995; 8: 567–601.

105. Luhby, AL, Eagle, FJ, Roth, E, Cooperman, JM. Relapsing megaloblastic anemia in an infant due to a specific defect in gastrointestinal absorption of folic acid. *Am J Dis Child* 1961; 102: 482–83.

106. Luhby, AL, Cooperman, JM. Folic acid deficiency in man and its interrelationship with vitamin metabolism. *Adv Metab Disord* 1964; 1: 263–334.

107. Luhby, AL, Cooperman, JM. Congenital megaloblastic anemia and progressive central nervous system degeneration. Further clinical and physiological characterization and therapy of syndrome due to inborn error of folate transport. Proceedings of the American Pediatric Society, Philadelphia, Atlantic City, April 26–29, 1967.

108. MacDonald, MR, Wiltse, HE, Bever, JL, Rosenblatt, DS. Clinical heterogeneity in two patients with *cblF* disease (abstract). *Am J Hum Genet* 1992; 15: A353.

109. Mackenzie, RE. Formiminotransferase-cyclodeaminase, a bifunctional protein from pig liver. In *Chemistry and Biology of Pteridines*. (Kisliuk, RL, Brown, GM, eds.). Elsevier, New York, 1979; p. 443.

110. Mandel, H, Brenner, B, Berant, M, Rosenberg, N, Lanir, N, Jakobs, C, Fowler, B, Seligsohn, U. Coexistence of hereditary homocystinuria and factor V Leiden-Effect on thrombosis. *N Eng J Med* 1996; 334: 763–68.

111. Marquet, J, Chadefaux, B, Bonnefont, JP, Saudubray, JM, Zittoun, J. Methylenetetrahydrofolate reductase deficiency: Prenatal diagnosis and family studies. *Prenat Diagn* 1994; 14: 29–33.

112. Matsui, SM, Mahoney, MJ, Rosenberg, LE. The natural history of the inherited methylmalonic acidemias. *N Engl J Med* 1983; 308: 857–61.

113. Mayes, JS, Say, B, Marcus, DL. Prenatal diagnosis in a family with transcobalamin II deficiency. *Am J Hum Genet* 1987; 41: 686–87.

114. Mellman, I, Willard, HF, Youngdahl-Turner, P, Rosenberg, LE. Cobalamin coenzyme synthesis in normal and mutant fibroblasts: Evidence for a processing

enzyme activity deficient in *cblC* cells. *J Biol Chem* 1979; 254: 11847–53.

115. Meyers, PA, Carmel, R. Hereditary transcobalamin II deficiency with subnormal serum cobalamin levels. *Pediatrics* 1984; 74: 866–71.

116. Mitchell, GA, Watkins, D, Melancon, SB, Rosenblatt, DS, Geoffroy, G, Orquin, J, Homsy, MB, Dallaire, L. Clinical heterogeneity in cobalamin C variant of combined homocystinuria and methylmalonic aciduria. *J Pediatr* 1986; 108: 410–15.

117. Mudd, SH, Uhlendorf, BW, Freeman, JM, Finkelstein, JD, Shih, VE. Homocystinuria associated with decreased methylenetetrahydrofolate reductase activity. *Biochem Biophys Res Commun* 1972; 46: 905–12.

118. Narisawa, K. Personal communication describing siblings reported in the Japanese literature: Kobayashi K and Hoshino M: Japan. *J Pediatr* 1976; 29: 1788.

119. Narisawa, K, Wada, Y, Saito, T, Suzuki, K, Kudo, M, Arakawa, TS, Katsushima, NA, Tsuboi, R. Infantile type of homocystinuria with N5,10-methylenetetrahydrofolate reductase defect. *Tohoku J Exp Med* 1977; 121: 185–94.

120. Narisawa, K. Brain damage in the infantile type of 5,10-methylenetetrahydrofolate reductase deficiency. In *Folic Acid in Neurology, Psychiatry, and Internal Medicine*. (Botez, MI, Reynolds, EH, eds.). Raven, New York, 1979; pp. 391–400.

121. Narisawa, K. Folate metabolism in infantile type of 5,10-methylenetetrahydrofolate reductase deficiency. *Acta Paediatr Jpn* 1981; 23: 82.

122. Nguyen, TT, Dyer, DL, Dunning, DD, Rubin, SA, Grant, KE, Said, HM. Human intestinal folate transport: Cloning, expression, and distribution of complementary RNA. *Gastroenterology* 1997; 112: 783–91.

123. Niederwieser, A, Giliberti, P, Matasovic, A, Pluznik, S, Steinmann, B, Baerlocher, K. Folic acid non-dependent formiminoglutamic aciduria in two siblings. *Clin Chim Acta* 1974; 54: 293–316.

124. Niederwieser, A, Matasovic, A, Steinmann, B, Baerlocher, K, Kempen, B. Hydantoin-5-propionic aciduria in folic acid non-dependent formiminoglutamic aciduria observed in two siblings. *Pediatr Res* 1976; 10: 215–19.

125. Nierbrugge, DJ, Benjamin, DR, Christie, D, Scott, CR. Hereditary transcobalamin II deficiency presenting as red cell hypoplasia. *J Pediatr* 1982; 101: 732–35.

126. Nishimura, M, Yoshino, K, Tomita, Y, Takashina, S, Tanaka, J, Narisawa, K, Kurobane, I. Central and peripheral nervous system pathology of homocystinuria due to 5,10-methylenetetrahydrofolate reductase deficiency. *Pediatr Neurol* 1985; 1: 375–78.

127. Ogier de Baulny, H, Gerard, M, Saudubray, JM, Zittoun, J. Remethylation defects: Guidelines for clinical diagnosis and treatment. *Eur J Pediatr* 1998; 157: S77–S83.

128. Pasquier, F, Lebert, F, Petit, H, Zittoun, J, Marquet, J. Methylenetetrahydrofolate reductase deficiency revealed by a neuropathy in a psychotic adult. *J Neurol Neurosurg Psychiatry* 1994; 57: 765–66.

129. Perry, TL, Applegarth, DA, Evans, ME, Hansen, S. Metabolic studies of a family with massive formiminoglutamic aciduria. *Pediatr Res* 1975; 9: 117–22.

130. Pezacka, EH. Identification and characterization of two enzymes involved in the intracellular metabolism of cobalamin. Cyanocobalamin beta-ligand transferase and microsomal cob(III)alamin reductase. *Biochim Biophys Acta* 1993; 1157: 167–77.

131. Pezacka, EH, Rosenblatt, DS. Intracellular metabolism of cobalamin. Altered activities of β-axial-ligand transferase and microsomal cob(III)alamin reductase in cblC and cblD fibroblasts. In *Advances in Thomas Addison's Diseases.* (Bhatt, HR, James, VHT, Besser, GM, Bottazzo, GF, Keen, H, eds.). J Endocrinol: Bristol, UK 1994; pp. 315–23.

132. Platica, O, Janeczko, R, Quadros, EV, Regec, A, Romain, R, Rothenberg, SP. The cDNA sequence and the deduced amino acid sequence of human transcobalamin II show homology with rat intrinsic factor and human transcobalamin I. *J Biol Chem* 1991; 66: 7860–63.

133. Poncz, M, Colman, N, Herbert, V, Schwartz, E, Cohen, AR. Therapy of congenital folate malabsorption. *J Pediatr* 1981; 98: 76–9.

134. Poncz, M, Colman, N, Herbert, V, Schwartz, E, Cohen, AR. Congenital folate malabsorption. *J Pediatr* 1981; 99: 828–29.

135. Porck, HJ, Frater-Schroder, M, Frants, KI, Kierat L, Eriksson, AW. Genetic evidence for fetal origin of transcobalamin II in human cord blood. *Blood* 1983; 62: 234–37.

136. Quadros, EV, Sai, P, Rothenberg, SP. Characterization of the human placental membrane receptor for transcobalamin II-cobalamin. *Arch Biochem Biophys* 1994; 308: 192–99.

137. Remacha, AF, Sambeat, MA, Barcelo, MJ, Mones, J, Garcia-Die, J, Gimferrer, E. Congenital intrinsic factor deficiency in a Spanish patient. *Ann Hematol* 1992; 64: 202–4.

138. Robb, RM, Dowton, SB, Fulton, AB, Levy, HL. Retinal degeneration in vitamin disorder associated with methylmalonic aciduria and sulfur amino acid abnormalities. *Am J Ophthalmol* 1984; 97: 691–96.

139. Ronge, E, Kjellman, B. Long-term treatment with betaine in methylenetetrahydrofolate reductase deficiency. *Arch Dis Child* 1996; 74: 239–41.

140. Rosenblatt, DS. Inherited errors of cobalamin metabolism: An overview. In *Advances in Thomas Addison's Diseases.* (Bhatt, HR, James, VHT, Besser, GM, Bottazzo, GF, Keen, H, eds.). Bristol, UK. J Endocrinol 1994; Volume 1, pp. 303–13.

141. Rosenblatt, DS, Cooper, BA, Lue-Shing, S, Wong, PW, Berlow, S, Narisawa, K, Baumgartner, R. Folate distribution in cultured human cells. Studies on 5,10-CH2-H4PteGlu reductase deficiency. *J Clin Invest* 1979; 63: 1019–25.

142. Rosenblatt, DS, Cooper, BA, Pottier, A, Lue-Shing, H, Matiaszuk, N, Grauer, K. Altered vitamin metabolism in fibroblasts from a patient with megaloblastic anemia and homocystinuria due to a new defect in methionine biosynthesis. *J Clin Invest* 1984; 74: 2149–56.

143. Rosenblatt, DS, Cooper, BA, Schmutz, SM, Zaleski, WA, Casey, RE. Prenatal vitamin therapy of a fetus with methylcobalamin deficiency (cobalamin E disease). *Lancet* 1985; 1: 1127–29.

144. Rosenblatt, DS, Laframboise, R, Pichette, J, Langevin, P, Cooper, BA, Costa, T. New disorder of vitamin metabolism (cobalamin F) presenting as methylmalonic aciduria. *Pediatrics* 1986; 78: 51–4.

145. Rosenblatt, DS, Hosack, A, Matiaszuk, N. Expression of transcobalamin II by amniocytes. *Prenat Diagn* 1987; 7: 35–9.

146. Rosenblatt, DS, Lue-Shing, H, Arzoumanian, A, Low-Nang, L, Matiaszuk, N. Methylenetetrahydrofolate reductase (MR) deficiency: Thermolability of residual MR activity, methionine synthase activity, and methylcobalamin levels in cultured fibroblasts. *Biochem Med Metab Biol* 1992; 47: 221–25.

147. Rosenblatt, DS, Aspler, AL, Shevell, MI, Pletcher, BA, Fenton, WA, Seashore, MR. Clinical heterogeneity and prognosis in combined methylmalonic aciduria and homocystinuria *(cblC). J Inherit Metab Dis* 1997; 20: 528–38.

148. Rosenblatt, DS, Cooper, BA. Methylenetetrahydrofolate reductase deficiency: Clinical and biochemical correlations. In *Folic Acid in Neurology, Psychiatry, and Internal Medicine.* Botez, MI and Reynolds, EH, ed. Raven Press, New York, 1979; pp. 385–90.

149. Rosenblatt, DS, Cooper, BA. Inherited disorders of vitamin metabolism. *Blood Rev* 1987; 1: 177–82.

150. Rosenblatt, DS, Cooper, BA. Selective deficiencies of methyl *(cblE* and *cblG). Clin Invest Med* 1989; 12: 270–71.

151. Rosenblatt, DS, Erbe, RW. Methylenetetrahydrofolate reductase in cultured human cells. Growth and metabolic studies. *Pediatr Res* 1977; 11: 1137–41.

152. Rosenblatt, DS, Erbe, RW. Methylenetetrahydrofolate reductase in cultured human cells. II. Studies of methylenetetrahydrofolate reductase deficiency. *Pediatr Res* 1977; 11: 1141–43.

152a. Rosenblatt, DS, Fenton, WA. Inherited disorders of folate and cobalamin transport and metabolism. In *The Metabolic and Molecular Bases of Inherited Metabolic Disease.* (Scriver, CR, Beaudet, AL, Sly, WS, Valle, D, eds.) McGraw-Hill, New York, 2001; pp. 3897–933.

153. Rothenberg, SP, Quadros, EV. Transcobalamin II and the membrane receptor for the transcobalamin II-cobalamin complex. In *Megaloblastic Anaemia.* (Wickramasinghe, SN, ed.). Baillière Tindall, London, 1995; pp. 499–514.

154. Rowe, PB. Inherited disorders of folate metabolism. In *The Metabolic Basis of Inherited Diseases.* (Stanbury, JB, Wyngaarden, JB, Frederickson, DS, Goldstein, JL, Brown, MS, eds.) McGraw-Hill, New York, 1983; p. 498.

155. Russell, A, Statter, M, Abzug-Horowitz, S. Methionine-dependent formiminoglutamic acid transferase deficiency: Human and experimental studies in its therapy. *Monogr Hum Genet* 1978; 9: 65–74.

156. Russell, A, Statter, M, Abzug-Horowitz, S. Methionine-dependent glutamic acid formiminotransferase deficiency. In *Inborn Errors of Metabolism. in Man.* (Sperling, O, de Vries, H, eds.). S. Karger, Basel, 1978; p. 65.

157. Sakiyama, T, Tsuda, M, Nakabayashi, H, Shimizu, H, Owaka, M, Kitagawa, T. Clinical and biochemical observations in a case with congenital defect of folate absorption. Annual Meeting of the SSIEM: Newcastle upon Tyne, 5–8 Sept., 1984.

158. Santiago-Borrera, PJ, Santini, R, Jr, Perez-Santiago, E, Maldonado, N, Millan, S, Coll-Camalez, G. Congenital isolated defect of folic acid absorption. *J Pediatr* 1973; 82: 450–55.

159. Sass, JO, Endres, W. Quantitation of total homocysteine in human plasma by derivatization to its N(O,S)-propoxycarbonyl propyl ester and gas chromatography-mass spectrometry analysis. *J Chromatogr* 1997; 776: 342–47.

160. Seetharam, B, Presti, M, Frank, B, Tiruppathi, C, Alpers, DH. Intestinal uptake and release of cobalamin complexed with rat intrinsic factor. *Am J Physiol* 1985; 248: G326–G31.

161. Seetharam, B, Levine, JS, Ramasamy, M, Alpers, DH. Purification, properties, and immunochemical localization of a receptor for inrinsic factor-cobalamin complex in the rat kidney. *J Biol Chem* 1988; 263: 4443–49.

162. Seligman, PA, Steiner, LL, Allen, RH. Studies of a patient with megaloblastic anemia and an abnormal transcobalamin II. *N Engl J Med* 1980; 303: 1209–12.

163. Sewell, AC, Neirich, U, Fowler, B. Early infantile methylenetetrahydrofolate reductase deficiency: A rare cause of progressive brain atrophy (abstract). *J Inherit Metab Dis* 1998; 21: 22.

164. Shih, VE, Salam, MZ, Mudd, SH, Uhlendorf, BV, Adams, RD. A new form of homocystinuria due to N5,N10-methylenetetrahydrofolate reductase deficiency. *Pediatr Res* 1972; 6: 395.

165. Shih, VE, Axel, SM, Tewksbury, JC, Watkins, D, Cooper, BA, Rosenblatt, DS. Defective lysosomal release of vitamin (*cblF*): A hereditary cobalamin metabolic disorder associated with sudden death. *Am J Med Genet* 1989; 33: 555–63.

166. Shin, YS, Pilz, G, Enders, W. Methylenetetrahydrofolate reductase and methylenetetrahydrofolate methyltransferase in human fetal tissues and chorionic villi. *J Inherit Med Dis* 1986; 9: 275–76.

167. Shinnar, S, Singer, HS. Cobalamin C mutation (methylmalonic aciduria and homocystinuria) in adolescence. A treatable cause of dementia and myelopathy. *N Engl J Med* 1984; 311: 451–54.

168. Sigal, SH, Hall, CA, Antel, JP. Plasma R binder deficiency and neurologic disease. *N Engl J Med* 1988; 317: 1330–32.

169. Sillaots, SL, Hall, CA, Hurteloup, V, Rosenblatt, DS. Heterogeneity in cblG: Differential retention of cobalamin on methionine synthase. *Biochem Med Metab Biol* 1992; 47: 242–49.

170. Singer, HS, Butler, I, Rothenberg, S, Valle, D, Freeman, J. Interrelationships among serum folate, CSF folate, neurotransmitters, and neuropsychiatric symptoms. *Neurology* 1980; 30: 419.

171. Steinschneider, M, Sherbany, A, Pavlakis, S, Emerson, R, Lovelace, R, DeVivo, DC. Congenital folate malabsorption: Reversible clinical and neurophysiologic abnormalities. *Neurology* 1990; 40: 1315.

172. Su, PC. Congenital folate deficiency. *N Engl J Med* 1976; 294: 1128.

173. Thomas, PK, Hoffbrand, AV, Smith, IS. Neurological involvement in hereditary transcobalamin II deficiency. *J Neurol Neurosurg Psychiatry* 1982; 45: 74–7.

174. Traboulsi, EI, Silva, JC, Geraghty, MT, Maumenes, IH, Valle, D, Green, WR. Ocular histopathologic characteristics of cobalamin C complementation type vitamin defect with methylmalonic aciduria and homocystinuria. *Am J Ophthalmol* 1992; 113: 269–80.

175. Urbach, J, Abrahamov, A, Grossowicz, N. Congenital isolated folic acid malabsorption. *Arch Dis Child* 1987; 62: 78–80.

176. van Gennip, AH, Abeling, NGGM, Nijenhuis, AA, Voute, PA, Bakker, HD. Formiminoglutamic/hydantoinpropionic aciduria in three patients with different tumors. *J Inherit Metab Dis* 1994; 17: 642–43.

177. Vassiliadis, A, Rosenblatt, DS, Cooper, BA, Bergeron, JJ. Lysosomal cobalamin accumulation in fibroblasts from a patient with an inborn error of cobalamin metabolism (*cblF* complementation group): Visualization by electron microscope radioautography. *Exp Cell Res* 1991; 195: 295–302.

178. Visy, JM, Le Coz, P, Chadefaux, B, Fressinaud, C, Woimant, F, Marquet, J, Zittoun, J, Visy, J, Vallat, JM, Haguenau, M. Homocystinuria due to 5,10-methylenetetrahydrofolate reductase deficiency revealed by stroke in adult siblings. *Neurology* 1991; 41: 1313–15.

179. Waggoner, DJ, Ueda, K, Mantia, C, Dowton, SB. Methylmalonic aciduria (*cblF*): Case report and response to therapy. *Am J Med Genet* 1998; 79: 373–75.

180. Watanabe, F, Saido, H, Yamaji, R, Miyatake, K, Isegawa, Y, Ito, A, Yubisui, T, Rosenblatt, DS, Nakano, Y. Mitochondrial NADH- or NADP-linked aquacobalamin reductase activity is low in human skin fibroblasts with defects in synthesis of cobalamin coenzymes. *J Nutr* 1996; 126: 2947–51.

181. Watkins, D, Rosenblatt, DS. Complementation studies in functional methionine synthase deficiency: Evidence for heterogeneity in CblE (abstract). *Am J Hum Genet* 1986; 39: 22a.

182. Watkins, D, Rosenblatt, DS. Genetic heterogeneity among patients with methylcobalamin deficiency: Definition of two complementation groups, *cblE* and *cblG*. *J Clin Invest* 1988; 81: 1690–94.

183. Watkins, D, Rosenblatt, DS. Functional methionine synthase deficiency (*cblE* and *cblG*): Clinical and biochemical heterogeneity. *Am J Med Genet* 1989; 34: 427–34.

184. Weintraub, L, Tardo, C, Rosenblatt, DS, Shapira, E. Hydrocephalus as a possible complication of the *cblC* type of methylmalonic aciduria (abstract). *Am J Hum Genet* 1991; 49: 108.

185. Wendel, U, Claussen, U, Dickmann, E. Prenatal diagnosis for methylenetetrahydrofolate reductase deficiency. *J Pediatr* 1983; 102: 938–40.

186. Wendel, U, Bremer, HJ. Betaine in the treatment of homocystinuria due to 5,10-methylenetetrahydrofolate reductase deficiency. *Eur J Pediatr* 1984; 142: 147–50.

187. Willard, HF, Mellman, IS, Rosenberg, LE. Genetic complementation among inherited deficiencies of methyl-

malonyl-CoA mutase activity: Evidence for a new class of human cobalamin mutant. *Am J Hum Genet* 1978; 30: 1–13.

188. Wilson, A, Leclerc, D, Saberi, F, Phillips, JA III, Rosenblatt, DS, Gravel, RA. Functionally null mutations in patients with the *cblG* variant form of methionine synthase deficiency. *Am J Hum Genet* 1998; 63: 409–14.

189. Wilson, A, Leclerc, D, Rosenblatt, DS, Gravel, RA. Molecular basis for methionine synthase reductase deficiency in patients belonging to the *cblE* complementation group of disorders in folate/cobalamin metabolism. *Hum Mol Genet* 1999; 8: 2009–16.

190. Wong, LTK, Rosenblatt, DS, Applegarth, DA, Davidson, AGF. Diagnosis and treatment of a child with *cblF* disease (abstract). *Clin Invest Med* 1992; 15: A111.

191. Wong, PWK, Justice, P, Berlow, S. Detection of homozygotes and heterozygotes with methylenetetrahydrofolate reductase deficiency. *J Lab Clin Med* 1977; 90: 283–88.

192. Wong, PWK, Justice, P, Hruby, M, Weiss, EB, Diamond, E. Folic acid non-responsive homocystinuria due to methylenetetrahydrofolate reductase deficiency. *Pediatrics* 1977; 59: 749–56.

193. Wulffraat, NM, De Schryver, J, Bruin, M, Pinxteren-Nagler, E, Van Dijken, PJ. Failure to thrive is an early symptom of the Imerslund Gräsbeck syndrome. *Am J Hematol Oncol* 1994; 16: 177–80.

194. Xu, D, Kozyraki, R, Newman, TC, Fyfe, JC. Genetic evidence of an accessory activity required specifically for cubilin brush-border expression and intrinsic factor-cobalamin absorption. *Blood* 1999; 94: 3604–6.

195. Yang, Y-M, Ducos, R, Rosenberg, AJ, Catrou, PG, Levine, JS, Podell, ER, Allen, RH. Cobalamin malabsorption in three siblings due to an abnormal intrinsic factor that is markedly susceptible to acid and proteolysis. *J Clin Invest* 1985; 76: 2057–65.

196. Youngdahl-Turner, P, Mellman, IS, Allen, RH, Rosenberg, LE. Protein mediated vitamin uptake: Adsorptive endocytosis of the transcobalamin II-cobalamin complex by cultured human fibroblasts. *Exp Cell Res* 1979; 118: 127–34.

197. Zammarchi, E, Lippi, A, Falorni, S, Pasquini, E, Cooper, BA, Rosenblatt, DS: *cblC* Disease: Case report and monitoring of a pregnancy at risk by chorionic villus sampling. *Clin Invest Med* 1990; 13: 139–42.

198. Zass, R, Leupold, MA, Fernandez, MA, Wendel, U. Evaluation of prenatal treatment in newborns with cobalamin-responsive methylmalonic acidaemia. *J Inherit Metab Dis* 1995; 18: 100–1.

199. Zeitlin, HC, Sheppard, K, Bolton, FG, Hall, CA. Homozygous transcobalamin II deficiency maintained on oral hydroxocobalamin. *Blood* 1985; 66: 1022–27.

200. Zittoun, J. Congenital errors of folate metabolism. In *Megaloblastic Anaemias*. (Wickringamasinghe, S, ed.). Baillière Tindall, London, 1995; pp. 603–16.

201. Zittoun, J, Leger, J, Marquet, J, Carmel, R. Combined congenital deficiencies of intrinsic factor and R binder. *Blood* 1988; 72: 940–43.

22

Polymorphisms of Folate and Cobalamin Metabolism

RIMA ROZEN

Substantial genetic variation exists in the human genome. A mutation, or DNA sequence alteration, can result in a protein variant with altered properties and a disease phenotype. Although disease is the most obvious manifestation of genetic change, it merely represents one extreme in the spectrum of normal genetic diversity. Not all mutations or irregularities in nucleotide sequence have phenotypic consequences. Silent mutations that conserve the amino acid residue and mutations in intronic regions may have no impact on the gene product. Furthermore, many sequence changes can result in amino acid substitutions (missense mutations) that have no clinical consequences. By definition, a mutation is simply a sequence variant; it can be benign or deleterious.

When a mutation is present in a population at a frequency ≥ 1.0% of alleles, it is called a polymorphism (79). Although it is often assumed that mutations are deleterious and polymorphisms are benign, the term *polymorphism* simply refers to the prevalence and not to the functional consequence of the mutation.

Other chapters in this book focus on the relatively rare mutations in genes encoding enzymes of homocysteine metabolism. These rare changes result in homocystinuria, an inborn error of metabolism with serious clinical consequences. This chapter concentrates on the common mutations, or polymorphisms, in some of the same genes/enzymes in the homocysteine remethylation pathway. Because polymorphisms are quite prevalent in the general population, their clinical impact is often less dramatic than the rare variants that cause homocystinuria; they may require an interaction with other factors (e.g., nutritional deficiencies, other genetic variants) to display an abnormal phenotype.

Methylenetetrahydrofolate Reductase

Methylenetetrahydrofolate reductase (MTHFR) (Metabolic Diagram, Reaction 9) catalyzes the conversion of 5, 10-methylenetetrahydrofolate to 5-methyltetrahydrofolate, the primary circulating form of folate and a carbon donor for homocysteine remethylation to methionine. The human cDNA was isolated in 1994, and the human gene was mapped to 1p36.3 (21). The isolation of the cDNA enabled the identification of rare and common sequence variants in the MTHFR gene. The rare mutations in MTHFR that cause homocystinuria are discussed in Chapter 21. Five common sequence changes in MTHFR are listed in Table 22.1. The sequence variants are designated by the nucleotide rather than by codon numbers. Analysis of the 5′ region of human MTHFR has resulted in identification of additional exons, with alternative splicing (8). Until this complex genetic structure is solved, the initiator ATG codon of the existing cDNA should not necessarily be considered as the only translation start site.

Table 22.1. Polymorphic Mutations in 5,10-Methylenetetrahydrofolate Reductase

Mutation	Change in Amino Acid or Splice Site	Exon or Intron	Reference
677 C/T	Alanine/valine	Exon 4	18
1068 T/C	Serine/serine	Exon 6	22
1178 + 31 T/C	5′ Splice site	Intron 6	23
1298 A/C	Glutamate/alanine	Exon 7	84, 86, 87
1317 T/C	Phenylalanine/ phenylalanine	Exon 7	87

Sequence numbering is based on the cDNA sequence reported in Goyette et al. (21), GenBank accession number U09806. Exon designations are based on Goyette et al. (24).

The first common variant, the 677C→T substitution (an alanine to valine change), has been studied extensively. It is an interesting model for multifactorial diseases that are characterized by an interplay between genetic and environmental factors. The frequency of this variant in the homozygous state for several different populations is listed in Table 22.2. The second missense mutation, 1298A→C (a glutamate to alanine change), is a more recent finding and has been studied less often. The two sequence variants that do not alter the amino acid (bp 1068 and bp 1317) and the polymorphism that is quite far into intron 6 (bp 1178 +31) are not likely to have clinical consequences and are not discussed here.

677C→T Mutation

Functional Aspects Kang et al. (34) identified a common biochemically distinct form of MTHFR in patients with coronary artery disease by enzymatic assays of lymphocyte extracts. This variant had decreased specific activity at 37°C and increased thermolability at 46°C. A common C→T substitution at

Table 22.2. Frequency of Methylenetetrahydrofolate Reductase 677C→T Variant in Control Populations

	Percent Homozygous	Reference
North America		
Canada and United States	11%–15%	18, 32, 44
Hispanic Americans	25%	72
African Americans	0–1%	60, 77
South America		
Brazil	4%	5
Colombia	24%	85
Europe		
Austria	10%	17
Finland	5%	60
France	10%	58
Ireland	8%	74
Italy	18%–23%	7, 49
Netherlands	8%	82
Norway	10%	28
Russia	8%	78
Turkey	6%	2
United Kingdom	13%	50
Asia		
Israel	15%	71
Japan	10%–12%	31, 55
Korea	16%	66
Australia	11%	91

bp 677 that converted an alanine to a valine codon was identified by Frosst et al. (18). Expression studies with the mutagenized cDNA in vitro demonstrated that this variant encodes a thermolabile enzyme (18) and that specific activity at 37°C is approximately 45% of wild type (88). The values obtained in vitro correlate well with those obtained in lymphocyte extracts (11, 18, 81). Lymphocyte extracts of homozygous mutant individuals have approximately 35% of control activity at 37°C, whereas those of heterozygotes have values that are intermediate between control and homozygous mutant. Residual activities after heating of lymphocytes at 46°C are approximately 30% of control values for homozygous mutants, with heterozygotes having intermediate values.

The alanine residue at bp 677 in the human enzyme is conserved in the MTHFRs of several species. The recent structural determination of bacterial MTHFR has led to the prediction that this residue may indirectly affect the binding of cofactor flavin adenine dinucleotide to the enzyme (27). The decrease in binding of flavin adenine dinucleotide results in dissociation of the bacterial tetramer with loss of activity. Mammalian MTHFR is a dimer, with approximately 30% identity to the bacterial enzyme (21) in the catalytic region; the mammalian enzyme has an additional regulatory domain that is absent in bacterial MTHFR (52). Although human MTHFR has not been purified to homogeneity, studies of the recombinant wild-type and mutagenized human enzyme have shown that the residual activity after heating is increased for wild-type and mutant proteins in the presence of folate and flavin adenine dinucleotide (Figure 22.1) (27). These data support the hypothesis that the mutant enzyme is unstable and that the instability may be overcome by folate or its cofactor; the clinical implications for this observation are discussed later.

Association with Hyperhomocysteinemia Numerous studies have identified an association between the 677C→T sequence change and increased plasma homocysteine (11, 18, 28, 29, 32, 44, 81). Because the product of the MTHFR reaction is utilized for homocysteine remethylation, a disruption of MTHFR activity would be expected to increase homocysteine levels. A study of 625 men in the general population of Northern Ireland reported that the risks for hyperhomocysteinemia conferred by the mutant genotype were 9.7, 5.7, 2.6 and 1.7 (odds ratios) for being in the top 5%, 10%, 20%, and 50% of individuals, respectively, ranked by homocysteine levels (29). In a Norwegian study where individuals were selected on the basis of having high homocysteine levels (>40 µmol/L), 73% of individuals in this group were homozygous for the valine allele (28).

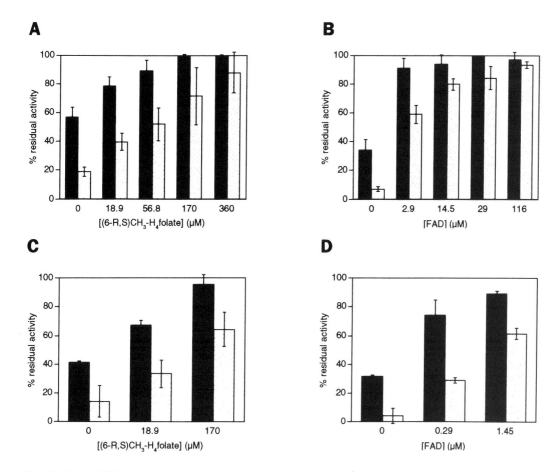

Fig. 22.1. Stabilization of normal and mutant (677C→T) human MTHFR by 5-methyltetrahydrofolate (CH$_3$-H$_4$ folate) and flavin adenine dinucleotide (FAD) against heat inactivation. In each panel, the dark columns represent data obtained for normal (Ala) MTHFR, and the light columns represent data obtained for mutant (Val) MTHFR. Panels A,B: Stabilization of recombinant wild-type and mutant MTHFR expressed in *Escherichia coli*. Aliquots of crude-sonicate supernatants containing 100 μg protein were preincubated at 46°C in the presence of the indicated concentrations of (6-RS)CH$_3$-H$_4$ folate (A) or FAD (B). After cooling to 37°C, additional (6-RS)CH$_3$-H$_4$ folate and/or FAD was added to the reaction mixtures, and the samples were assayed in duplicate using the CH$_3$-H$_4$ folate-menadione oxidoreductase assay. Values reported have been corrected for the activity in a control JM105 strain. The bars represent the mean ± standard deviation of data obtained from three experiments. Panels C,D: Stabilization of normal (Ala/Ala) and mutant (Val/Val) MTHFR in human lymphocyte extracts (90 μg of protein) by CH$_3$-H$_4$ folate (C) and FAD (D). The bars represent the mean ± standard deviation of data obtained from duplicate assays of the enzyme extracts of three individuals. (Reproduced from Guenther et al. [27], with permission.)

This association between mutant genotype and hyperhomocysteinemia is observed predominantly in individuals with lower plasma folate levels. In the original description of this genetic-nutrient interactive effect, Jacques et al. (32) demonstrated that the homozygous mutant genotype was not associated with mild hyperhomocysteinemia when plasma folate was above the median value; homozygous mutant individuals had higher homocysteine levels only when their folate was below the median. The folate levels that are associated with hyperhomocysteinemia in these individuals are not in the deficient range; they appear to be in the lower end of the normal range.

Individuals with the mutant genotype have been reported to have decreased plasma folate levels (29, 81) and an altered distribution of folates in red blood cells (6), reflecting their decreased ability to synthesize methylated folates. Maintenance of adequate plasma folate by diet or by vitamin supplementation could conceivably ameliorate hyperhomocysteinemia in mutant individuals in two ways: by stabilizing the mutant enzyme and allowing it to function normally (Figure 22.1 and above discussion) or by providing exogenous 5-methyltetrahydrofolate for the remethylation pathway. Individuals with the mutant genotype are quite responsive to exogenous folate with respect to homocysteine lowering (14, 28, 47).

Association with Cardiovascular Disease   Because mild hyperhomocysteinemia is a risk factor for cardiovascular disease, the MTHFR variant has been extensively investigated for its role in many forms of cardiovascular disease. The subject is discussed in greater detail in Chapter 30. Homozygosity for the valine allele has been associated with increased risk for premature coronary artery disease (19, 30, 31, 36, 55), cerebral infarction (56), and venous thrombosis (5, 7, 49, 71). In a large Japanese study of 362 patients with coronary artery disease, the genotype showed a stronger association in those with the greater degree of stenosis and in those with triple-vessel disease compared with single-vessel or double-vessel disease (55). Several studies, however, have not observed an association of the MTHFR genotype with risk for cardiovascular disease (37, 38, 44, 50). Nonetheless, a meta-analysis of eight early studies concluded that the polymorphism was a modest but significant risk factor (37). A recent review of this literature discussed some of the factors that may have contributed to the controversy in this field (16).

As indicated, the MTHFR mutation is highly dependent on folate status for manifestation of hyperhomocysteinemia and, presumably, disease risk. Very few of the disease-association studies have examined folate status in conjuction with the genotype. It is likely that the genotype may be a risk factor only in groups with lower nutritional status. A second concern with association studies is the variable frequency of this polymorphism between populations, as indicated in Table 22.2. Study subjects and control subjects must be closely matched for ethnic background, particularly in heterogeneous populations such as those in the United States.

The presence of other cardiovascular disease risk factors in the study groups can affect outcome. When patients with conventional risk factors (such as hypertension or hyperlipidemia) are excluded from the analysis, the risk conferred by the MTHFR genotype can be more significant (5, 36). Because cardiovascular disease is a multifactorial disorder, the influence of a single polymorphism may be small, but it could have a greater impact when combined with other risk factors (genetic and nongenetic). The Factor V Leiden mutation has been suggested to increase the risk for thrombosis in homocystinuric patients with severe MTHFR deficiency (25, 48). Similarly, the combination of Factor V Leiden and the homozygous V/V genotype has significantly increased the risk of thrombosis in some studies (7, 49). The MTHFR genotype has been reported to increase risk for cardiovascular disease in individuals with non-insulin-dependent diabetes (3), with apolipoprotein variants (30), as well as those with multiple risks (20). It is evident that the combination of genetic and nongenetic factors in ethnically distinct populations has contributed to the variable outcomes in the assessment of this polymorphism. It is also likely that the effect of MTHFR on the cardiovascular system is through an elevation of homocysteine,

although the exact mechanism by which hyperhomocysteinemia increases cardiovascular disease risk is still under discussion, as mentioned in other chapters.

Association with Other Disorders The MTHFR polymorphism is the first genetic risk factor reported to increase risk for neural tube defects such as spina bifida (81, 90). Several studies have confirmed a positive association with risk for neural tube defects, although some studies have not reached the same conclusion. A meta-analysis by van der Put et al. (82) supports this polymorphism as a risk factor, as does a recent Irish study containing the largest number of cases examined thus far (74). The association is consistent with earlier reports of mild hyperhomocysteinemia in families with neural tube defects (53, 76), as well as with the dramatic response to folate supplementation in reducing risk (13, 61). The risk is clearly dependent on folate status, particularly in individuals with the mutant genotype (12, 54). The benefit of additional folate is presumably due to the same factors discussed for cardiovascular disease (i.e., stabilization of a mutant enzyme and/or dietary supply of the 5-methyltetrahydrofolate required for homocysteine remethylation).

Although elevated homocysteine levels could affect the developing nervous system and increase the risk of neural tube defects (69), another important pathogenetic mechanism could involve the decreased synthesis of methionine and S-adenosylmethionine, with subsequent effects on methylation reactions. As discussed in Chapter 7, S-adenosylmethionine is utilized for over 100 methylation reactions, including lipid, DNA, and protein methylation. The reported association between MTHFR and psychiatric disturbances (4, 68) could also be due to altered methylation reactions in the nervous system. A recent preliminary report suggests that the MTHFR variant may also increase the risk for Down syndrome, through DNA hypomethylation and maternal meiotic nondysjunction (33).

Other disorders in which disease risk is increased by the 677 MTHFR polymorphism are likely to be related through homocysteine-induced vascular damage. Several studies have reported that this polymorphism increases the risk for preeclampsia and other complications of pregnancy, such as abruptio placentae and recurrent early pregnancy loss (26, 39, 63, 75); these effects may be mediated through damage to the placental vasculature. The increased risk in homozygous mutant individuals for retinal vein occlusion (43, 71) and for diabetic retinopathy (64) presumably stems from damage to the retinal vasculature.

It is interesting to speculate why a deleterious polymorphism should be maintained at high frequency in many different populations. Selective advantage has been proposed for common mutations in other genes, including those for hemoglobin and for cystic fibrosis. The only advantage demonstrated thus far for the MTHFR polymorphism is a twofold reduction in risk for colorectal cancer in homozygous mutant individuals (9, 45). Again, this effect is modulated by environmental factors, because the protective effect is not seen when individuals are folate-deficient or when alcohol intake is high. Proposed mechanisms for the protective effect include altered DNA methylation or an increased conversion of deoxyuridine monophosphate to thymidine monophosphate in the presence of an increased amount of the MTHFR substrate, 5,10-methylenetetrahydrofolate (Metabolic Diagram, Reaction 10). Because colorectal cancer, a late adult-onset disorder, is not likely to alter reproductive fitness, studies of other neoplasias might be instructive. On the other hand, the enhanced thymidine and DNA synthesis may offer a selective advantage during fetal development, for example.

The role of MTHFR in neoplasia requires additional investigation. Using the common 677 variant, it has been reported that loss of heterozygosity of MTHFR in tumor cells occurs at a frequency of approximately 40% to 50% in ovarian carcinomas (86) and 15% to 20% in colorectal carcinomas (67). Although the study numbers were small, the valine allele appeared to be preferentially lost in colorectal tumors, consistent with the protective role of this variant (67).

Many of the aforementioned clinical studies are still preliminary and require confirmation. All the caveats expressed for associations with cardiovascular disease risk are equally applicable for the other disorders in which the 677 variant has been implicated. Of additional interest is the implication that the homozygous mutant genotype is associated with decreased viability at both ends of the age spectrum. The increased complications of pregnancy (26, 39, 63, 75), reports on genetic selection based on MTHFR genotype (62, 89), and the decreased numbers of control female newborns with the mutant genotype are consistent with early losses (70). At the other end of the age spectrum, some reports have suggested that the mutant genotype is decreased in frequency in older individuals owing to increased mortality (15, 51).

1298A→C Mutation

Functional Aspects In a loss of heterozygosity study in ovarian carcinoma cell lines, Viel et al. (86) identified a novel sequence change at the MTHFR locus that converted a glutamate residue to an alanine codon in the C-terminal regulatory domain. The original published human MTHFR cDNA sequence (21) contained the C allele at bp 1298; therefore this muta-

tion was initially reported as a 1298C→A base change. However, after investigating its frequency in several studies, it became clear that the more prevalent base at this position was the A nucleotide. Accordingly, the 1298A→C nomenclature has been adopted for this MTHFR variant.

In vitro bacterial expression data suggest that the 1298A→C mutation reduces overall MTHFR specific activity, although to a lesser degree than the 677C→T polymorphism (88). Four cDNA constructs, containing all possible combinations of the two MTHFR polymorphisms (designated by their amino acid codes: AE, AA, VE, VA), were created by site-directed mutagenesis and assayed for MTHFR activity in bacterial extracts. The specific activity of the wild-type construct (AE, alanine for the 677 polymorphism and glutamate for the 1298 polymorphism) was designated as 100% activity, and all other constructs were evaluated in relation to this control value. The recombinant enzyme mutant for the 1298A→C polymorphism alone (AA) showed 65% of wild-type activity, whereas the presence of the 677C→T (VE) mutation alone was associated with a much greater reduction in overall activity (≈ 45% of wild-type activity).

Because the 677C→T mutation encodes a thermolabile MTHFR variant, these constructs were assayed for MTHFR activity following heat inactivation. Irrespective of the 1298A→C genotype, when the enzyme was wild-type for the 677C→T mutation (AE or AA), residual activity remained approximately 40% to 50% after heating. However, when the enzyme was mutant for the 677C→T change (VE or VA), activity fell to 10% to 12% residual activity. These data suggest that the 1298A→C mutation, unlike the 677C→T polymorphism, does not render the enzyme thermolabile.

There appears to be good correlation between the enzyme activity observed in the in vitro expression system and the activity seen in lymphocyte extracts. Individuals who are homozygous mutant for the 1298 variant have approximately 60% of control activity (84, 87), and the enzyme in these extracts does not appear to be thermolabile (84).

Although the bacterial enzyme has recently been crystallized, it does not include the C-terminal regulatory domain, which contains the binding site for the allosteric inhibitor, S-adenosylmethionine. Consequently, the mechanism by which the 1298 bp mutation affects MTHFR activity remains speculative at this time. Because allosteric inhibition does not appear to be compromised (MTHFR activity is reduced rather than enhanced in the presence of the C allele), the 1298A→C base change is not likely to disrupt binding of S-adenosylmethionine. The mutation could influence protein stability or alter the conformation such that catalytic activity (in the N-terminal region) would be affected.

However, the glutamate residue is not conserved in yeast MTHFR, for example, and, based on main chain folding angles, the substitution is highly conservative (65).

Association with Homocysteine and Disease The potential association of this polymorphism with hyperhomocysteinemia has been examined (84, 87). Both reports concluded that individuals with one or two copies of this polymorphism did not have elevated plasma homocysteine. Similar frequencies for this mutation were observed in the two studies; approximately 10% of Canadian and Dutch individuals were homozygous mutant. Of interest, the mutant allele of this polymorphism (alanine) has not been seen *in cis* with the mutant allele of the 677 polymorphism (valine), suggesting that the two mutations occurred independently.

Although there are no data thus far to suggest that the 1298 polymorphism alone influences homocysteine levels, combined heterozygosity for the 1298 and 677 polymorphism might be associated with increased plasma homocysteine (84, 88).

Two studies have examined the 1298 polymorphism for risk for neural tube defects. Consistent with the lack of association with plasma homocysteine, the 1298 polymorphism alone is not associated with increased risk for this birth defect (84, 87). However, individuals heterozygous for both polymorphisms were reported to be at increased risk in one study (84), although the odds ratios were not statistically significant. Additional studies are required to evaluate the clinical significance of combined heterozygosity for both MTHFR polymorphisms; the influence of folate status as well as the aforementioned caveats for the 677 polymorphism need to be considered.

Methionine Synthase

Methionine synthase (Metabolic Diagram, Reaction 4) catalyzes homocysteine remethylation to methionine, using 5-methyltetrahydrofolate (the product of the MTHFR reaction) as the carbon donor. The cDNA for human methionine synthase has been isolated and the human gene has been mapped to 1q43 (10, 40, 42). Rare mutations in the gene for methionine synthase that cause homocystinuria are discussed in Chapters 12 and 21. Other nonsilent sequence variants have been reported (10, 40, 42), but the only change that has been extensively studied and shown to be polymorphic is the 2756A→G (D919G) substitution (Table 22.3).

2756A→G Mutation

Functional Aspects The 2756A→G mutation results in the substitution of an aspartic acid with a glycine

Table 22.3. Polymorphic Mutations in Methionine Synthase and Methionine Synthase Reductase

Mutation	Change in Amino Acid	Reference
Methionine synthase		
2756A→G	D919G	10, 40
Methionine synthase reductase		
66A→G	I22M	92

residue (D919G). Functional studies of this polymorphism have not been performed because human methionine synthase has not been expressed in vitro. However, the corresponding amino acid (glutamine) in the bacterial enzyme (Q893) lies in a linker region connecting the cobalamin binding domain to the activation domain. As discussed in Chapter 12, the functional consequence of the 2756A→G mutation was recently tested by converting the bacterial Q893 residue into glycine. The mutated enzyme displayed a slight decrease in activity, with impaired reductive activation.

Association with Homocysteine and Disease Several groups have assessed the 2756A→G (D919G) polymorphism for an association with neural tube defects (12, 59, 73, 83) or with vascular disease (57, 80). The substitution is less prevalent than the aforementioned variants in MTHFR, with homozygosity frequencies of less than 5%; these relatively lower frequencies may have limited the statistical power of the above studies. Nonetheless, the polymorphism thus far does not appear to be associated with hyperhomocysteinemia or with an increased risk of neural tube defects or vascular disease.

In contrast, a possible association with homozygosity for this polymorphism and decreased risk for colorectal cancer has been observed, particularly among men with low alcohol intake (46). These findings are similar to the aforementioned results for MTHFR.

Methionine Synthase Reductase

Methionine synthase reductase catalyzes the reductive activation of methionine synthase. The human cDNA was recently cloned, and the human gene was mapped to 5p15.2–15.3 (41). Rare mutations causing homocystinuria are discussed in Chapter 12. One common variant (Table 22.3) has been recently investigated (92).

66A→G Mutation

Functional Aspects The 66A→G mutation results in the conversion of an isoleucine residue into a methionine at codon 22, in the putative binding domain for flavin mononucleotide, within the N-terminal region. The functional significance of this change remains to be determined. The human enzyme has not been expressed in vitro. However, this gene has significant homology to related proteins with binding sites for flavin mononucleotide, including a putative methionine synthase reductase from *Caenorhabditis elegans,* as well as sulfite reductases, nitric oxide synthases, cytochrome P450 reductases, and flavodoxins. In 123 of 130 entries in GenBank, the equivalent codon was isoleucine, leucine, or valine; none of the entries contained a methionine in this position. These findings allude to a functional role for this residue, possibly in the binding of flavin mononucleotide.

Association with Homocysteine and Disease In the only report for this mutation thus far, the homozygosity frequency (for the methionine allele) in Canadians was approximately 25% to 30%, but an association with plasma homocysteine levels was not observed (92). However, this polymorphism was proposed as a second genetic risk factor for neural tube defects, in the presence of low cobalamin levels. Children with spina bifida and their mothers were nearly twice as likely as control populations to have the homozygous mutant genotype, although this result was not statistically significant. When the mutant genotype was assessed in combination with low cobalamin levels, the odds ratio for mothers increased to 4.8 (95% confidence interval, 1.5 to 15.8), and the odds ratio for the children was 2.5 (95% confidence interval, 0.63 to 9.7). These results are consistent with earlier suggestions that cobalamin and methionine synthase might be involved in the risk for neural tube defects (1, 35).

Because the MTHFR 677C→T polymorphism had already been implicated as a risk factor for neural tube defects, the interaction between these two mutant genotypes was also investigated. Mothers and children who were homozygous for both the methionine synthase reductase and MTHFR mutations had threefold and fourfold increase in risk, respectively. If the results from this first report are confirmed, they substantiate the notion of multifactorial inheritance for this common birth defect, by adding cobalamin deficiency and a common polymorphism in methionine synthase reductase to the growing list of risk factors for neural tube defects (folate deficiency, MTHFR polymorphism). Studies of this polymorphism in cardiovascular disease are required; if a disease association is identified, without significant hyperhomocysteinemia as seen in the aforementioned report, other pathogenetic mechanisms would have to be considered.

Several polymorphisms have now been identified in folate- and cobalamin-dependent enzymes, but the 677C→T substitution in MTHFR has been studied most extensively and serves as a prototype for polymorphisms in homocysteine metabolic pathways, as well as for associations with complex traits. Although clinical studies for all these polymorphisms will continue to appear in the literature, a critical piece of information that is still missing for methionine synthase and methionine synthase reductase is the confirmation that the common variant affects enzyme function.

The identification of genetic predisposing factors could offer a means of disease prevention, particularly if treatment is simple. It is clear that folate supplementation ameliorates the effects of the 677 variant in MTHFR. The data for the polymorphism in methionine synthase reductase and cobalamin status are still preliminary. Nonetheless, an understanding of common variants and of the genetic/nongenetic factors with which they interact can improve public health by focusing on genetic individuality in the diagnosis and treatment of disease.

REFERENCES

1. Adams, MJ Jr, Khoury, MJ, Scanlon, KS, Stevenson, RE, Knight, GJ, Haddow, JE, Syvester, GC, Cheek, JE, Henry, JP, Stabler, SP, Allen, RH. Elevated midtrimester serum methymalonic acid levels as a risk factor for neural tube defects. *Teratology* 1995; 51: 311–17.
2. Akar, N, Akar, E, Misirhoglu, M, Avcu, F, Yalcin, A, Cin, S. Search for genetic factors favoring thrombosis in Turkish population. *Thromb Res* 1998; 92: 79–82.
3. Arai, K, Yamasaki, Y, Kajimoto, Y, Watada, H, Umayahara, Y, Kodama, M, Sakamoto, K, Hori, M. Association of methylenetetrahydrofolate reductase gene polymorphism with carotid arterial wall thickening and myocardial infarction risk in NIDDM. *Diabetes* 1997; 46: 2102–4.
4. Arinami, T, Yamada, N, Yamakawa-Kobayashi, K, Hamaguchi, H, Toru, M. Methylenetetrahydrofolate reductase variant and schizophrenia/depression. *Am J Med Genet* 1997; 74: 526–28.
5. Arruda, VR, von Zuben, PM, Chiaparini, LC, Annichino-Bizzacchi, JM, Costa, FF. The mutation Ala677→Val in the methylenetetrahydrofolate reductase gene: A risk factor for arterial disease and venous thrombosis. *Thromb Haemost* 1997; 77: 818–21.
6. Bagley, PJ, Selhub, J. A common mutation in the methylenetetrahydrofolate reductase gene is associated with an accumulation of formylated tetrahydrofolates in red bood cells. *Proc Natl Acad Sci USA* 1998; 95: 13217–20.
7. Cattaneo, M, Tsai, MY, Bucciarelli, P, Taioli, E, Zighetti, ML, Bignell, M, Mannucci, PM. A common mutation in the methylenetetrahydrofolate reductase gene (C677T) increases the risk for deep-vein thrombosis in patients with mutant factor V (factor V:Q506). *Arterioscler Thromb Vasc Biol* 1997; 17: 1662–66.

8. Chan, M, Tran, P, Goyette, P, Chen, Z, Milos, R, Artigas, C, Rozen, R. Analysis of the 5' region of the methylenetetrahydrofolate reductase (MTHFR) gene reveals multiple exons with alternative splicing and an overlapping gene. *FASEB J* 1999; 13: A1375.

9. Chen, J, Giovannucci, E, Kelsey, K, Rimm, EB, Stampfer, MJ, Colditz, GA, Spiegelman, D, Willett, WC, Hunter, DJ. A methylenetetrahydrofolate reductase polymorphism and the risk of colorectal cancer. *Cancer Res* 1996; 56: 4862–64.

10. Chen, LH, Liu, M-L, Hwang, H-Y, Chen, L-S, Korenberg, J, Shane, B. Human methionine synthase. cDNA cloning, gene localization and expression. *J Biol Chem* 1997; 272: 3628–34.

11. Christensen, B, Frosst, P, Lussier-Cacan, S, Selhub, J, Goyette, P, Rosenblatt, DS, Genest, J Jr, J, Rozen, R. Correlation of a common mutation in the methylenetetrahydrofolate reductase (MTHFR) gene with plasma homocysteine in patients with premature coronary artery disease. *Arterioscler Thromb Vasc Biol* 1997; 17: 569–73.

12. Christensen, B, Arbour, L, Tran, P, Leclerc, D, Sabbaghian, N, Platt, R, Gilfix, BM, Rosenblatt, DS, Gravel, RA, Forbes, P, Rozen, R. Genetic polymorphisms in methylenetetrahydrofolate reductase and methionine synthase, folate levels in red blood cells, and risk of neural tube defects, *Am J Med Genet* 1999; 84: 151–57.

13. Czeizel, AE, Dudas, I. Prevention of the first occurrence of neural-tube defects by periconceptional vitamin supplementation. *N Engl J Med* 1992; 327: 1832–35.

14. Deloughery, TG, Evans, A, Sadeghi, A, McWilliams, J, Henner, WD, Taylor, LM, Press, RD. Common mutation in methylenetetrahydrofolate reductase. Correlation with homocysteine metabolism and late-onset vascular disease. *Circulation* 1996; 94: 3074–78.

15. Faure-Delanef, L, Quéré, I, Chassé, JF, Guerassimenko, O, Lesaulnier, M, Bellet, H, Zittoun, J, Kamoun, P, Cohen, D. Methylenetetrahydrofolate reductase thermolabile variant and human longevity. *Am J Hum Genet* 1997; 60: 999–1001.

16. Fletcher, O, Kessling, AM. MTHFR association with arteriosclerotic vascular disease? *Hum Genet* 1998; 103: 11–21.

17. Födinger, M, Mannhalter, C, Wölfli, G, Pabinger, I, Müller, E, Schmid, R, Hörl, WH, Sunder-Plassman, G. Mutation (677 C to T) in the methylenetetrahydrofolate reductase gene aggravates hyperhomocysteinemia in hemodialysis patients. *Kidney Int* 1997; 52: 517–23.

18. Frosst, P, Blom, HJ, Milos, R, Goyette, P, Sheppard, CA, Matthews, RG, Boers, GJH, den Heijer, M, Kluijtmans, LAJ, van den Heuvel, LP, Rozen, R. A candidate genetic risk factor for vascular disease: A common mutation in methylenetetrahydrofolate reductase. *Nature Genet* 1995; 10: 111–13.

19. Gallagher, P, Meleady, R, Shields, D, Tan, KS, McMaster, D, Rozen, R, Evans, A, Graham, I, Whitehead, AS. Homocysteine and risk of coronary heart disease: Evidence for a common gene mutation. *Circulation* 1996; 94: 2154–58.

20. Gardemann, A, Weidemann, H, Philipp, M, Katz, N, Tillmanns, H, Hehrlein, FW, Haberbosch, W. The TT genotype of the methylenetetrahydrofolate reductase C677T gene polymorphism is associated with the extent of coronary atherosclerosis in patients at high risk for coronary artery disease. *Eur Heart J* 1999; 20: 584–92.

21. Goyette, P, Sumner, JS, Milos, R, Duncan, AMV, Rosenblatt, DS, Matthews, RG, Rozen, R. Human methylenetetrahydrofolate reductase: Isolation of cDNA, mapping and mutation identification. *Nat Genet* 1994; 7: 195–200.

22. Goyette, P, Frosst, P, Rosenblatt, DS, Rozen, R. Seven novel mutations in the methylenetetrahydrofolate reductase gene and genotype/phenotype correlations in severe MTHFR deficiency. *Am J Hum Genet* 1995; 56: 1052–59.

23. Goyette, P, Christensen, B, Rosenblatt, DS, Rozen, R. Severe and mild mutations in *cis* for the methylenetetrahydrofolate reductase (MTHFR) gene, and description of 5 novel mutations in MTHFR. *Am J Hum Genet* 1996; 59: 1268–75.

24. Goyette, P, Pai, A, Milos, R, Frosst, P, Tran, P, Chen, Z, Chan, M, Rozen, R. Gene structure of human and mouse methylenetetrahydrofolate reductase (MTHFR). *Mamm Genome* 1998; 9: 652–56.

25. Goyette, P, Rosenblatt, D, Rozen, R. Homocystinuria (methylenetetrahydrofolate reductase deficiency) and mutation of factor V gene. *J Inherit Metab Dis* 1998; 21: 690–91.

26. Grandone, E, Margaglione, M, Colaizzo, D, Cappucci, G, Paladini, D, Martinelli, P, Montanaro, S, Pavone, G, Di Minno, G. Factor V Leiden, C→T MTHFR polymorphism and genetic susceptibility to preeclampsia. *Thromb Haemost* 1997; 77: 1052–54.

27. Guenther, BG, Sheppard, CA, Tran, P, Rozen, R, Matthews, RG, Ludwig, ML. The structure and properties of methylenetetrahydrofolate reductase from *Escherichia coli*: A model for the role of folate in ameliorating hyperhomocysteinemia in humans. *Nat Struct Biol* 1999; 6: 359–65.

28. Guttormsen, AB, Ueland, PM, Nesthus, I, Nygard, O, Schneede, J, Vollset, SE, Refsum, H. Determinants and vitamin responsiveness of intermediate hyperhomocysteinemia (≥ 40 µmol/liter) *J Clin Invest* 1996; 98: 2174–83.

29. Harmon, DL, Woodside, JV, Yarnell, JWG, McMaster, D, Young, IS, McCrum, EE, Gey, KF, Whitehead, AS, Evans, AE. The common "thermolabile" variant of methylene tetrahydrofolate reductase is a major determinant of mild hyperhomocysteinaemia. *Q J Med* 1996; 89: 571–77.

30. Inbal, A, Freimark, D, Modan, B, Chetrit, A, Matetzky, S, Rosenberg, N, Dardik, R, Baron, Z, Seligsohn, U. Synergistic effects of prothrombotic polymorphisms and atherogenic factors on the risk of myocardial infarction in young males. *Blood* 1999; 93: 2186–90.

31. Izumi, M, Iwai, N, Ohmichi, N, Nakamura, Y, Shimoike, H, Kinoshita, M. Molecular variant of 5,10-methylenetetrahydrofolate reductase is a risk factor of ischemic heart disease in the Japanese population. *Atherosclerosis* 1996; 121: 293–94.

32. Jacques, PF, Bostom, AG, Williams, RR, Ellison, RC, Eckfeldt, JH, Rosenberg, IH, Selhub, J, Rozen, R. Relation between folate status, a common mutation in

methylenetetrahydrofolate reductase, and plasma homocysteine concentrations. *Circulation* 1996; 93: 7–9.

33. James, SJ, Pogribna, M, Pogribny, II, Melnyk, S, Hine, RJ,
    Gibson, JB, Yi, P, Tafoya, DL, Swenson, DH, Wilson, VL,
    Gaylor, DW. Abnormal folate metabolism and mutation
    in the methylenetetrahydrofolate reductase gene may be
    maternal risk factors for Down syndrome. *Am J Clin Nutr*
    1999; 70: 495–501.

34. Kang, S-S, Wong, PWK, Susmano, A, Sora, J, Norusis, M,
    Ruggie, N. Thermolabile methylenetetrahydrofolate
    reductase: An inherited risk factor for coronary disease.
    Am J Hum Genet 1991; 48: 536–45.

35. Kirke, PN, Molloy, AM, Daly, LE, Burke, H, Weir, DG,
    Scott, JM. Maternal plasma folate and vitamin B$_{12}$ are
    independent risk factors for neural tube defects. *Q J Med*
    1993; 86: 703–8.

36. Kluijtmans, LAJ, van den Heuvel, LP, Boers, GHJ, Frosst,
    P, Stevens, EMB, van Oost, BA, den Heijer, M, Trijbels,
    FJM, Rozen, R, Blom, HJ. Molecular genetic analysis in
    mild hyperhomocysteinemia: A common mutation in the
    methylenetetrahydrofolate reductase gene is a genetic risk
    factor for cardiovascular disease. *Am J Hum Genet* 1996;
    58: 35–41.

37. Kluijtmans, LAJ, Kastelein, JJ, Lindemans, J, Boers, GHJ,
    Heil, SG, Bruschke, AVG, Jukema, JW, van den Heuvel,
    LPWJ, Trijbels, FJM, Boerma, GJM, Verheugt, FWA,
    Willems, F, Blom, HJ. Thermolabile methylenetetrahydro-
    folate reductase in coronary artery disease. *Circulation*
    1997; 96: 2573–77.

38. Kluijtmans, LA, den Heijer, M, Reitsma, PH, Heil, SG,
    Blom, HJ, Rosendaal, FR. Thermolabile methylenetetrahy-
    drofolate reductase and factor V Leiden in the risk of deep-
    vein thrombosis. *Thromb Haemost* 1998; 79: 254–58.

39. Kupferminc, MJ, Eldor, A, Steinman, N, Many, A, Bar-
    Am, A, Jaffa, A, Fait, G, Lessing, JB. Increased frequency
    of genetic thrombophilia in women with complications of
    pregnancy. *N Engl J Med* 1999; 340: 9–13.

40. Leclerc, D, Campeau, E, Goyette, P, Adjalla, CE,
    Christensen, B, Ross, M, Eydoux, P, Rosenblatt, DS,
    Rozen, R, Gravel, RA. Human methionine synthase:
    cDNA cloning, chromosomal localization, and identifica-
    tion of mutations in patients of the *cblG* complementa-
    tion group of folate/cobalamin disorders. *Hum Mol
    Genet* 1996; 5: 1867–74.

41. Leclerc, D, Wilson, A, Dumas, R, Gafuik, C, Song, D,
    Watkins, D, Heng, HHQ, Rommens, JM, Scherer, SW,
    Rosenblatt, DS, Gravel, RA. Cloning and mapping of a
    cDNA for methionine synthase reductase, a flavoprotein
    defective in patients with homocystinuria. *Proc Natl Acad
    Sci USA* 1998; 95: 3059–64.

42. Li, YN, Gulati, S, Baker, PJ, Brody, LC, Banerjee, R,
    Kruger, WD. Cloning, mapping and RNA analysis of the
    human methionine synthase gene. *Hum Mol Genet* 1996;
    5: 1851–58.

43. Loewenstein, A, Winder, A, Goldstein, M, Lazar, M,
    Eldor, A. Bilateral retinal vein occlusion associated with
    5,10-methylenetetrahydrofolate reductase mutation. *Am J
    Ophthalmol* 1997; 124: 840–41.

44. Ma, J, Stampfer, MJ, Hennekens, CH, Frosst, P, Selhub, J,
    Horsford, J, Malinow, MR, Willett, WC, Rozen, R.

Methylenetetrahydrofolate reductase polymorphism,
plasma folate, homocysteine, and risk of myocardial
infarction in U.S. physicians. *Circulation* 1996; 94:
2410–16.

45. Ma, J, Stampfer, MJ, Giovannucci, E, Artigas, C, Hunter,
    D, Fuchs, C, Willett, W, Selhub, J, Hennekens, CH,
    Rozen, R. Methylenetetrahydrofolate reductase polymor-
    phism, reduced risk of colorectal cancer and dietary inter-
    actions. *Cancer Res* 1997; 57: 1098–102.

46. Ma, J, Stampfer, MJ, Christensen, B, Giovannucci, E,
    Hunter, DJ, Chen, J, Willett, WC, Selhub, J, Hennekens,
    CH, Gravel, R, Rozen, R. A polymorphism of the methio-
    nine synthase gene: Association with plasma folate, vita-
    min B12, homocysteine, and colorectal cancer risk.
    Cancer Epidemiol Biomarkers Prev 1999; 8: 825–29.

47. Malinow, MR, Nieto, FJ, Kruger, WD, Duell, PB, Hess,
    DL, Gluckman, RA, Block, PC, Holzgang, CR, Anderson,
    PH, Seltzer, D, Upson, B, Lin, QR. The effects of folic acid
    supplementation on plasma total homocysteine are modu-
    lated by multivitamin use and methylenetetrahydrofolate
    reductase genotypes. *Arterioscler Thromb Vasc Biol*
    1997; 17: 1157–62.

48. Mandel, H, Brenner, B, Berant, M, Rosenberg, N, Lanir,
    N, Jakobs, C, Fowler, B, Seligsohn, U. Coexistence of
    hereditary homocystinuria and factor V Leiden: Effect on
    thrombosis. *N Engl J Med* 1996; 334: 763–68.

49. Margaglione, M, D'Andrea, G, d'Addedda, M, Giuliani,
    N, Cappucci, G, Iannaccone, L, Veccione, G, Grandone,
    E, Brancaccio, V, Di Minno, G. The methylenetetrahydro-
    folate reductase TT677 genotype is associated with
    venous thrombosis independently of the coexistence of
    the FV Leiden and the prothrombin A20210 mutation.
    Thromb Haemost 1998; 79: 907–11.

50. Markus, HS, Ali, N, Swaminathan, R, Sankaralingam, A,
    Molloy, J, Powell, J. A common polymorphism in the
    methylenetetrahydrofolate reductase gene, homocysteine,
    and ischemic cerebrovascular disease. *Stroke* 1997; 28:
    1739–43.

51. Matsushita, S, Muramatsu, T, Arai, H, Matsui, T,
    Higuchi, S. The frequency of the methylenetetrahydrofo-
    late reductase-gene mutation varies with age in the nor-
    mal population. *Am J Hum Genet* 1997; 61: 1459–60.

52. Matthews, RG, Vanoni, MA, Hainfeld, JF, Wall, J.
    Methylenetetrahydrofolate reductase. Evidence for spa-
    tially distinct subunit domains obtained by scanning
    transmission electron microscopy and limited proteolysis.
    J Biol Chem 1984; 259: 11647–40.

53. Mills, JL, McPartlin, JM, Kirke, PN, Lee, YJ, Conley,
    MR, Weir, DG, Scott, JH. Homocysteine metabolism in
    pregnancies complicated by neural-tube defects. *Lancet*
    1995; 345: 149–51.

54. Molloy, AM, Daly, S, Mills, JL, Kirke, PN, Whitehead,
    AS, Ramsbottom, D, Conley, MR, Weir, DG, Scott, JM.
    Thermolabile variant of 5,10-methylenetetrahydrofolate
    reductase associated with low red-cell folates:
    Implications for folate intake recommendations. *Lancet*
    1997; 349: 1591–93.

55. Morita, H, Taguchi, J-I, Kurihara, H, Kitaoka, M,
    Kaneda, H, Kurihara, Y, Maemura, K, Shindo, T,
    Minamino, T, Ohno, M, Yamaoki, K, Ogasawara, K,

Aizawa, T, Suzuki, S, Yazaki, Y. Genetic polymorphism of 5,10-methylenetetrahydrofolate reductase (MTHFR) as a risk factor for coronary artery disease. *Circulation* 1997; 95: 2032–36.

56. Morita, H, Kurihara, H, Tsubaki, S, Sugiyama, T, Hamada, C, Kurihara, Y, Shindo, T, Oh-hashi, Y, Kitamura, K, Yazaki, Y. Methylenetetrahydrofolate reductase gene polymorphism and ischemic stroke in Japanese. *Arterioscler Thromb Vasc Biol* 1998; 18: 1465–69.

57. Morita, H, Kurihara, H, Sugiyama, T, Hamada, C, Kurihara, Y, Shindo, T, Oh-hashi, Y, Yazaki, Y. Polymorphism of the methionine synthase gene: Association with homocysteine metabolism and late-onset vascular diseases in the Japanese population. *Arterioscler Thromb Vasc Biol* 1999; 19: 298–302.

58. Mornet, E, Muller, F, Lenvoisé-Furet, A, Delezoide, A-L, Col, J-Y, Simon-Bouy, B, Serre, J-L. Screening of the C677T mutation on the methylenetetrahydrofolate reductase gene in French patients with neural tube defects. *Hum Genet* 1997; 100: 512–14.

59. Morrison, K, Edwards, YH, Lynch, SA, Burn, J, Hol, F, Mariman, E. Methionine synthase and neural tube defects. *J Med Genet* 1997; 34: 958–60.

60. Motulsky, AG. Nutritional ecogenetics: Homocysteine-related arteriosclerotic vascular disease, neural tube defects, and folic acid. *Am J Hum Genet* 1996; 58: 17–20.

61. MRC Vitamin Study Research Group. Prevention of neural-tube defects: Results of the Medical Research Council vitamin study. *Lancet* 1991; 352: 1120–21.

62. Muñoz-Moran, E, Dieguez–Lucena, JL, Fernandez-Arcas, N, Peran-Mesa, S, Reyes-Engel, A. Genetic selection and folate intake during pregnancy. *Lancet* 1998; 352–53.

63. Nelen, WLDM, Steegers, EAP, Eskes, TKAB, Blom, HJ. Genetic risk factor for unexplained recurrent early pregnancy loss. *Lancet* 1997; 350: 861.

64. Neugebauer, S, Baba, T, Kurokawa, K, Watanabe, T. Defective homocysteine metabolism as a risk factor for diabetic retinopathy. *Lancet* 1997; 349: 473–74.

65. Niefind, K, Schomburg, D. Amino acid similarity coefficients for protein modeling and sequence alignment derived from main-chain folding angles. *J Mol Biol* 1991; 219: 481–97.

66. Park, KS, Podskarbi, T, Yoo, EA, Shin, YS. The C677T mutation in the methylenetetrahydrofolate reductase gene in Koreans. *Korean J Genet* 1998; 20: 23–8.

67. Pereira, P, Stanton, V, Jothy, S, Tomlinson, IPM, Foulkes, WD, Rozen, R. Loss of heterozygosity of methylenetetrahydrofolate reductase in colon carcinomas. *Oncol Reports* 1999; 6: 597–99.

68. Regland, B, Germgard, T, Gottfries, CG, Grenfeldt, B, Koch-Schmidt, AC. Homozygous thermolabile methylenetetrahydrofolate reductase in schizophrenia-like psychosis. *J Neural Transm* 1997; 104: 931–41.

69. Rosenquist, TH, Ratashak, SA, Selhub, J. Homocysteine induces congenital defects of the heart and neural tube: Effect of folic acid. *Proc Natl Acad Sci USA* 1996; 93: 15227–32.

70. Rozen, R, Fraser, FC, Shaw, GM. Decreased proportion of female newborn infants homozygous for the 677C→T mutation in methylenetetrahydrofolate reductase. *Am J Med Genet* 1999; 83: 142–43.

71. Salomon, O, Moisseiev, J, Rosenberg, N, Vidne, O, Yassur, I, Zivelin, A, Treister, G, Steinberg, DM, Seligsohn, U. Analysis of genetic polymorphisms related to thrombosis and other risk factors in patients with retinal vein occlusion. *Blood Coagul Fibrinolysis* 1998; 9: 617–22.

72. Shaw, GM, Rozen, R, Finnell, RH, Wasserman, CR, Lammer, EJ. Maternal vitamin use: Genetic variation of infant methylenetetrahydrofolate reductase and risk for spina bifida. *Am J Epidemiol* 1998; 148: 30–7.

73. Shaw, GM, Todoroff, K, Finnell, RH, Lammer, EJ, Leclerc, D, Gravel, RA, Rozen, R. Infant methionine synthase variants and risk for spina bifida, *J Med Genet* 1999; 36: 86–7.

74. Shields, DC, Kirke, PN, Mills, JL, Ramsbottom, D, Molloy, AM, Burke, H, Weir, DG, Scott, JM, Whitehead, AS. The thermolabile variant of methylenetetrahydrofolate reductase and neural tube defects: An evaluation of genetic risk and the relative importance of the genotypes of the embryo and the mother. *Am J Hum Genet* 1999; 64: 1045–55.

75. Sohda, S, Arinami, T, Hamada, H, Yamada, N, Hamaguchi, H, Kubo, T. Methylenetetrahydrofolate reductase polymorphism and pre-eclampsia. *J Med Genet* 1997; 34: 525–26.

76. Steegers-Theunissen, RPM, Boers, GHJ, Trijbels, FJM, Finkelstein, JD, Blom, HJ, Thomas, CMG, Borm, GF, Wouters, MGAJ, Eskes, TKAB. Maternal hyperhomocysteinemia: A risk factor for neural-tube defects? *Metabolism* 1994; 43: 1475–80.

77. Stevenson, RE, Schwartz, CE, Du, YZ, Adams, MJ. Differences in methylenetetrahydrofolate reductase genotype frequencies between whites and blacks. *Am J Hum Genet* 1997; 60: 230–33.

78. Sverdlova, AM, Bubnova, NA, Baranovskaya, SS. Vasina, VI, Avitisjan, AO, Schwartz, EI. Prevalence of the methylenetetrahydrofolate reductase (MTHFR) C677T mutation in patients with varicose veins of lower limbs. *Mol Genet Metab* 1998; 63: 35–6.

79. Thompson, MW, McInnes, RR, Willard, HF. *Genetics in Medicine,* 5th ed. WB, Saunders, Philadelphia, 1991.

80. Tsai, MY, Welge, BG, Hanson, NQ, Bignell, MK, Vessey, J, Schwichtenberg, K, Yang, F, Bullemer, FE, Rasmussen, R, Graham, KJ. Genetic causes of mild hyperhomocysteinemia in patients with premature occlusive coronary artery diseases. *Atherosclerosis* 1999; 143: 163–70.

81. van der Put, NMJ, Steegers-Theunissen, RPM, Frosst, P, Trijbels, FJM, Eskes, TKAB, ven den Heuvel, LP, Mariman, ECM, den Heyer, M, Rozen, R, Blom, HJ. Mutated methylenetetrahydrofolate reductase as a risk factor for spina bifida. *Lancet* 1995; 346: 1070–71.

82. van der Put, NMJ, Eskes, TKAB, Blom, HJ. Is the common 677C→T mutation in the methylenetetrahydrofolate reductase gene a risk factor for neural tube defects? A meta-analysis. *Q J Med* 1997; 90: 111–15.

83. van der Put, NMJ, van der Molen, EF, Kluijtmans, LAJ, Heil, SG, Trijbels, JMF, Eskes, TKAB, van Oppenraaij-Emmerzaal, D, Banerjee, R, Blom, HJ. Sequence analysis

of the coding region of human methionine synthase: Relevance to hyperhomocysteinaemia in neural-tube defects and vascular disease. *Q J Med* 1997; 90: 511–17.

84. van der Put, NMJ, Gabreels, F, Stevens, EMB, Smeitink, JAM, Trijbels, FJM, Eskes, TKAB, van den Heuvel, LP, Blom, HJ. A second common mutation in the methylenetetrahydrofolate reductase gene: An additional risk factor for neural-tube defects? *Am J Hum Genet* 1998; 62: 1044–51.

85. Vanegas, OC, Giusti, B, Fernandez, CMR, Abbate, R, Pepe, G. Frequency of Factor V (FV) Leiden and C677T methylenetetrahydrofolate reductase (MTHFR) mutations in Colombians. *Thromb Haemost* 1998; 79: 883–84.

86. Viel, A, Dall'Agnese, L, Simone, F, Canzonieri, V, Capozzi, E, Visentin, MC, Valle, R, Boiocchi, M. Loss of heterozygosity at the 5,10-methylenetetrahdyrofolate reductase locus in human ovarian carcinomas. *Br J Cancer* 1997; 75: 1105–10.

87. Weisberg, I, Tran, P, Christensen, B, Sibani, S, Rozen, R. A second genetic polymorphism in methylenetetrahydrofolate reductase (MTHFR) associated with decreased enzyme activity. *Mol Genet Metab* 1998; 64: 169–72.

88. Weisberg, IS, Jacques, PF, Selhub, J, Bostom, AG, Chen, Z, Ellison, RC, Eckfeldt, JH, Rozen, R. The 1298A→C polymorphism in methylenetetrahydrofolate reductase (MTHFR): In vitro expression and association with homocysteine. *Atherosclerosis*, 2001; in press.

89. Weitkamp, LR, Tackels, DC, Hunter, AGW, Holmes, LB, Schwartz, CE. Heterozygote advantage of the MTHFR gene in patients with neural-tube defect and their relatives. *Lancet* 1998; 351: 1554–55.

90. Whitehead, AS, Gallagher, P, Mills, JL, Kirke, PN, Burke, H, Molloy, AM, Weir, DG, Shields, DC, Scott, JM. A genetic defect in 5,10 methylenetetrahydrofolate reductase in neural tube defects. *Q J Med* 1995; 88: 763–66.

91. Wilcken, DEL, Wang, XL, Sim, AS, McCredie, RM. Distribution in healthy and coronary populations of the methylenetetrahydrofolate reductase (MTHFR) C_{677} T mutation. *Arterioscler Thromb Vasc Biol* 1996; 16: 878–82.

92. Wilson, A, Platt, R, Wu, Q, Leclerc, D, Christensen, B, Yang, H, Gravel, R, Rozen, R. A common variant in methionine synthase reductase combined with low cobalamin (vitamin B12) increases risk for spina bifida. *Mol Genet Metab* 1999; 67: 317–23.

23

Folate Deficiency

RALPH CARMEL

Folate Metabolism and Physiology

Reduced, polyglutamated folates play many roles in one-carbon metabolism involving amino acids, purines, and pyrimidines. The biochemistry is discussed in detail in Chapter 11. From the clinical perspective of the discussion here, two reactions are particularly important. 5,10-Methylenetetrahydrofolate is necessary for the de novo synthesis of thymidylate from deoxyuridylate (Metabolic Diagram, Reaction 10). The failure of this reaction ultimately leads to the characteristic megaloblastic changes in folate-deficient cells. The second reaction, the remethylation of homocysteine in which 5-methyltetrahydrofolate is a cosubstrate and methylcobalamin a cofactor (Metabolic Diagram, Reaction 4), has a critical role in homocysteine metabolism and sits at the crossroad of folate and cobalamin metabolism.

Folate and Diet

Many foods contain folate. Rich sources include beans, nuts, meat (especially organ meats), dairy products, fruits, grains, and cereals. Yeast is the single richest source of folate available. Dietary analysis of 24-hour food collections varied from 69 to 601 μg of folate in studies of Western diets (32).

Despite folate's widespread distribution in foods, nutrition can be problematic, in part because folates are labile. Many cooking and preservation processes can destroy much of the folate in food (32). Reducing substances such as ascorbic acid provide some degree of protection.

The liver stores 7.5 to 22.5 mg of folate, which declines to about 1.5 mg when megaloblastic anemia appears (32). A minimum intake of 50 μg of folate is needed daily to prevent signs of deficiency, although it may not maintain folate stores. The Recommended Daily Allowance, based on an intake from all sources that is sufficient to maintain red cell folate levels, has been revised upward recently (5, 76) and is shown in Table 23.1. It is expressed in Dietary Folate Equivalents to take into account the different availabilities of folates from food, supplements, and fortification. Synthetic folic acid taken in supplements appears to be twice as bioavailable as most food folate (132), and the folic acid that fortifies cereal grain foods has been estimated to have 1.7 times the bioavailability of most natural food folate (122).

Folate Absorption and Excretion

Absorption occurs throughout the small intestine, especially in the jejunum. The process is poorly understood and may consist of several discrete mechanisms. The polyglutamated forms that predominate in the diet are less well absorbed than monoglutamated folic

Table 23.1. Recommended Daily Allowance (RDA)[a] of Folate Proposed by the Institute of Medicine, National Academy of Sciences (76).

Subgroup	DFE[b] (μg/day)
Infants	—
1–3 years old	150
4–8 years old	200
9–13 years old	300
14–18 years old	400
Adults	400[c]
Pregnant women	600
Lactating women	500

[a] The RDA is expressed in dietary folate equivalents (DFE).
[b] 1 μg DFE = 1 μg of food folate = 0.6 μg of synthetic folic acid fortifying food = 0.5 μg of synthetic folic acid supplement.
[c] For women of reproductive age, the RDA is expanded with a recommended additional intake of 400 μg of folic acid supplement or folic acid-fortified food.

acid in supplements. Especially when present in high concentrations, the latter is absorbed by nonsaturable mechanisms and appears unchanged in the portal circulation. The γ-linked glutamate side chains of the polyglutamated folates are hydrolyzed by pteroylpolyglutamate hydrolases that are found on small intestinal cell brush borders and in lysosomes. Two folate-binding activities have been identified at the intestinal cell membrane. The more important of the two may reside in the reduced folate carrier, which is discussed in the next section.

Folate Transport, Cellular Uptake, and Excretion

Absorbed folate is cleared from the circulation within minutes and is taken up by liver and other tissues. About 90 μg of folate is recycled daily via the enterohepatic cycle (151). Much of the folate circulating in plasma is in equilibrium with freshly absorbed dietary folate and reabsorbed biliary folate. Unlike cobalamin, circulating folate is attached only weakly and nonspecifically to serum proteins and approximately one third is unattached. A tiny fraction is bound to a specific folate-binding protein, which appears to be derived from folate receptors from cell membranes (86). This circulating protein's function is uncertain (3).

Cell membranes have two folate binders. One is a glycosyl-phosphatidylinositol-anchored receptor (100) found in hematopoietic cells, kidney tubular cells, placenta, and other tissues. This receptor is active at physiological folate concentrations, has a high affinity for 5-methyltetrahydrofolate, and mediates its endocytosis via clathrin-coated pits. The second protein, reduced folate carrier, binds only reduced folates and has a wide tissue distribution, including the brain (130). It is a low-affinity carrier but has a much greater capacity than the previously mentioned receptor and thus may promote uptake in settings where folate concentrations are great, such as in the intestine. The roles of these two proteins are still unclear and vary considerably among different cell types (3, 144). Some cellular folate uptake also occurs by diffusion.

Once internalized by the cell, folate tends to be retained well if polyglutamated but poorly if in the monoglutamate form (139). Retention of folate in red blood cells is also enhanced by association with hemoglobin (12).

Folate is filtered by the kidney, but much of it is reabsorbed in the proximal tubule after binding by the tubular cells' folate receptors (136).

Folate Deficiency

The definition of folate deficiency is surprisingly elusive and susceptible to subjective interpretation. The definition was long based on clinical signs and symptoms, especially the presence of megaloblastic changes in hematopoiesis. Reliance on serum folate levels alone or even on red cell folate levels was somewhat suspect, in part because of technical variations in both the assay results and their interpretations. At the same time, it was also abundantly clear that low folate values, even conservatively defined, were much more common than megaloblastic anemia.

As metabolic information—especially homocysteine data—accumulated in the last decade, it has become clear that even low-normal and sometimes mid-normal folate levels coexist with hyperhomocysteinemia that responds to folate therapy. As a result, the pendulum shifted greatly and people are often labeled automatically as folate deficient on that basis. However, it remains unclear how often that is justified. For example, an independent, inverse correlation between homocysteine and riboflavin status was described recently (72a). If confirmed, this vitamin, which is a cofactor in Reaction 9 (Metabolic Diagram), may be yet another vitamin with a role in hyperhomocysteinemia.

Table 23.2 lists the usual ways used to diagnose folate deficiency. The table also includes the major confounders of each of those criteria, above and beyond such problems as vagaries in cut-off point selection and assay problems. It is important to remember, too, that folate deficiency is rarely an isolated deficiency. Because of the multitude of confounders, reliable identification of deficiency in both clinical and study settings should be based on abnormality in more than one of the diagnostic criteria in Table 23.2. However, care must be taken not to rely on criteria that share confounders.

Low Serum and Red Blood Cell Folate Levels

Serum folate, which is predominantly 5-methyltetrahydrofolate, is influenced by absorbed dietary folate and enterohepatically recycled folate and is therefore sensitive to even transient disruptions in either of those two equilibria. Serum folate levels sometimes reflect a relatively brief disruption of supply to the bloodstream rather than a state of depletion with dwindling folate stores. Reversal of the disruption rapidly restores the serum level to normal. The sometimes high frequency of low serum folate levels in hospitalized patients may reflect this transitory fluctuation to some degree. Serum folate is also unstable on storage unless protective measures are taken.

There is limited consensus on the normal reference range for serum folate levels (32). The ranges vary among assays, as methods have changed from microbiological to radioisotopic to chemiluminescent ones, as well as among laboratories. Most laboratories have

Table 23.2. Findings Used to Diagnose Folate Deficiency, and Confounders of Abnormal Results[a]

Diagnostic Finding	Major Confounders of Abnormal Results
Biochemical	
1. Low serum folate level	Transiently negative folate balance
2. Low red blood cell folate level	Cobalamin deficiency
3. High total homocysteine level	Cobalamin deficiency Renal insufficiency Enzyme defects
4. Abnormal deoxyuridine suppression	Cobalamin deficiency (if vitamin additive controls not used)
Hematological	
5. Anemia and/or macrocytosis[b]	Other causes of either or both are more common than folate deficiency
6. Megaloblastic changes[b]	Cobalamin deficiency
Clinical	
7. Presence of disorders known to cause folate deficiency[b]	Folate deficiency does not invariably follow Such disorders often cause multiple deficiencies
8. Response of any of # 1–7 to folic acid therapy[c]	Some abnormalities "improve" whether or not deficiency was present (e.g., #1 and 2) Some abnormalities respond to folate even though due to other causes (e.g., hematologic abnormalities of cobalamin deficiency; hyperhomocysteinemia of enzyme defects)

[a] Many confounders of negative or normal findings also exist but are not listed here.
[b] Often not seen in mild or subclinical folate deficiency
[c] Response to folic acid taken with other vitamins in a supplement cannot be interpreted diagnostically.

used 4.8 to 5.7 nmol/L (or 1.8 to 2.5 µg/L; 2.266 nmol = 1 µg) as the defining cutoff points between subnormal and normal levels. The validity of a cut-off within that range was supported by homocysteine data in elderly community dwellers (137). A rise in homocysteine levels was seen in the lowest two deciles of folate levels, with folate levels <4.8 nmol/L (Figure 23.1). However, after adjusting for age, sex, and status of other vitamins, that study found increased odds ratios

for high homocysteine levels for folate levels <9.2 nmol/L and recommended that folate supplementation be considered for such persons even though the folate levels were well within the accepted normal range. In a later study, these investigators used 11 nmol/L as the cutoff point for folate deficiency (138). The lack of a consensus on the "gold standard" to define folate deficiency has left this issue unresolved. Abnormal folate status by the deoxyuridine suppression test has also been described in occasional patients with a normal serum folate level (162).

The folate content is fixed in red blood cells before the cells emerge from the bone marrow. As a result,

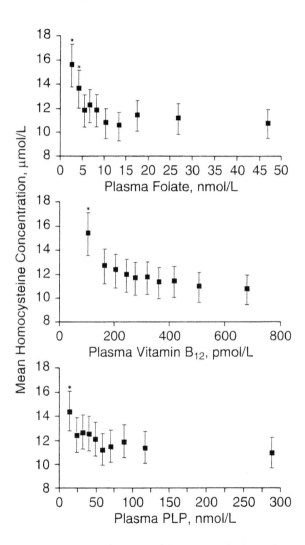

Fig. 23.1. Mean (and 95% confidence interval) plasma homocysteine levels by deciles of vitamin status in 1,160 elderly subjects from the Framingham Heart Study (137). Panels from top to bottom show homocysteine levels by deciles of folate, vitamin B_{12} (cobalamin) and pyridoxal 5′-phosphate (PLP; vitamin B_6) levels. The homocysteine values were adjusted for age, sex, and other vitamins; the asterisks indicate significantly different values from the highest decile of vitamin status. (Reproduced from Selhub et al. [137], with permission.)

red cell folate levels, which are about 30 times higher than in serum, are not subject to the frequent fluctuations seen in serum. Although more reflective of body stores (169), the red cell folate level is also a slightly less sensitive indicator of early developing deficiency than serum folate because the red cell's life span in the circulation is 120 days. Only 14% of patients with low serum folate also had low red cell folate levels (32). A limitation in interpreting the folate level in red cells is that it is low in cobalamin deficiency as well as in folate deficiency. This low level occurs because 5-methyltetrahydrofolate, which accumulates when cobalamin deficiency impairs the methionine synthase reaction, is monoglutamated and readily diffuses out of cells. As a result, the folate content of red blood cells decreases while the level in serum increases.

The red cell folate assay is also subject to many technical influences, including the adequacy of preparing the hemolysate. Assay problems are common, both with specific commercial kits and with variability among laboratories. In one survey, the interlaboratory coefficient of variation was 20.8% to 64.7% for red cell folate and 17.9% to 34.5% for serum folate (22). As with serum folate, little consensus exists about the normal reference range; most cutoff points between deficiency and normality have been set between 220 and 390 nmol/L. Some authors have advocated deemphasis of the red cell assay (83), but others find that its usefulness outweighs its disadvantages.

Consequences of Deficiency

Like the biochemical consequences, the megaloblastic changes that come after them affect all dividing cells. The traditional clinical picture has revolved around megaloblastic anemia, with limited expression in other organ systems. Nonhematological complications are being increasingly described, many of which tend to appear in more chronic folate deficiency states that are low grade and thus not severe enough to produce megaloblastic anemia.

Hematological Consequences The chief clinical expression of folate deficiency is megaloblastic anemia. Figure 23.2 illustrates the characteristic changes in the appearance of the hematopoietic precursors in the bone marrow and their progeny in the bloodstream. Most of the precursors become arrested or retarded at various stages in interphase (161). These cells do not divide further. Their appearance suggests appropriate cytoplasmic maturation but abnormal nuclear maturation. The chromatin appears abnormal and the nuclei are large.

The cells themselves are enlarged too, although red cell macrocytosis, easily identified by an elevated

mean corpuscular volume, is also found in many other conditions (Table 23.3). Indeed, megaloblastic anemia is not even the most common cause of macrocytosis. The diagnostic usefulness of a high mean corpuscular volume, although substantial, is further limited by the fact that macrocytosis may be masked when iron deficiency or thalassemia, both of which induce microcytosis, coexist. A normal mean corpuscular volume was found in 25% of folate-deficient patients (133), although seemingly normal mean corpuscular volumes sometimes decline after folate or cobalamin therapy (27, 107), indicating a hidden macrocytosis. In general, however, macrocytosis precedes anemia, as has been shown in cobalamin-deficient patients (25).

The functional end result of the megaloblastic process is ineffective hematopoiesis. This hematopoiesis is intense, but the precursors do not mature normally, and as many as 90% of them are destroyed by phagocytes within the bone marrow. Apoptosis has been identified in folate-deficient leukemic cell lines (92), but not in patients (75). Red cell death is marked clinically by rising serum bilirubin levels, as large amounts of hemoglobin are broken down.

White blood cell and platelet precursors undergo ineffective production as well. Neutropenia and thrombocytopenia usually are not noticeable, however, until the anemia has become quite marked, at which point pancytopenia can become severe. A morphological change, hypersegmentation of neutrophil

Table 23.3. Causes of Macrocytic Red Blood Cells	
Megaloblastic Processes	Nonmegaloblastic Processes
Acquired and hereditary cobalamin disorders	Hematological disorders
Acquired and hereditary folate disorders	myelodysplastic syndrome[a]
Thiamine-reponsive megaloblastic anemia	aplastic anemia
Chemotherapeutic drugs	pure red cell aplasia
Orotic aciduria	sideroblastic anemia
	hemolytic anemia/intense reticulocytosis
	Nonhematological disorders
	liver disease
	hypothyroidism
	Alcohol abuse
	Physiological
	infancy
	pregnancy
	Technical artifacts

[a] Nuclear changes resembling megaloblastic changes are sometimes seen.

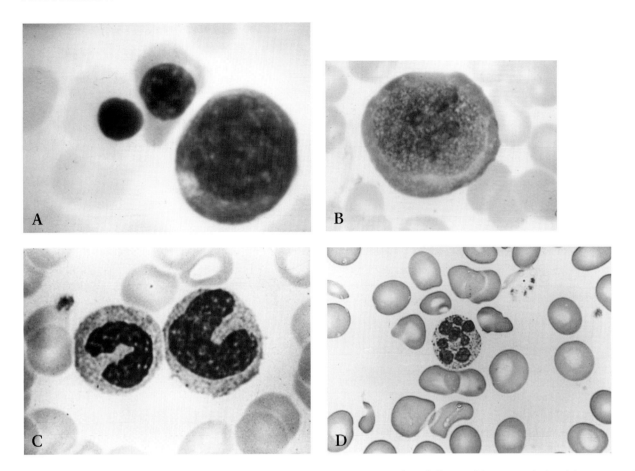

Fig. 23.2. Megaloblastic changes in blood cells. (A) Normal bone marrow aspirate: three red blood cell precursors of increasing maturation from large to progressively smaller cells with more compact nuclei. (B) Megaloblastic bone marrow aspirate: a megaloblastic early red blood cell precursor comparable in maturation stage to the largest cell in panel A. Note the abnormal nuclear chromatin compared with the compact chromatin in panel A. (C) Megaloblastic peripheral blood: a megaloblastic, "giant" band cell (late precursor of segmented neutrophil) on the right can be compared with its smaller, normal neighbor. (D) Megaloblastic peripheral blood: a hypersegmented neutrophil with seven or eight nuclear lobes (most normal neutrophils have two to four nuclear lobes); most of the mature (non-nucleated) red blood cells, such as the cell to 4 o'clock of the neutrophil, are larger than normal.

nuclei (Figure 23.2D), however, precedes macrocytic anemia (69) and is considered an even more sensitive marker of deficiency than is macrocytosis (97). Nevertheless, as shown in cobalamin deficiency, it does not appear in the preclinical stages (28).

The megaloblastic changes occur because an inadequate 5,10-methylenetetrahydrofolate supply compromises de novo synthesis of thymidylate (Metabolic Diagram, Reaction 10) (14, 160, 161). The decreased deoxythymidylate availability combined with the accumulation of deoxyuridylate leads to extensive misincorporation of uracil in place of thymine into DNA (15, 58). The greatly expanded excision repair process that follows this expanded misincorporation may result in critical DNA strand breaks (14).

Neurological Consequences The traditional view has held that folate deficiency does not cause neurological dysfunction, in clear contradistinction to cobalamin deficiency, which does. Indeed, folate deficiency rarely causes the striking myelopathy found in many cobalamin-deficient patients. However, reports have accumulated of mild or even moderate neurological impairment in some folate-deficient patients—just as it occurs in only some cobalamin-deficient patients. Those reports are compelling, but careful studies coupled with metabolic data are needed, given the many other deficiencies that often accompany folate deficiency.

The severe mental changes, seizures, and even occasional myelopathy of children with hereditary folate disorders such as 5,10-methylenetetrahydrofolate reductase (MTHFR) deficiency and congenital folate malabsorption provide incontrovertible examples of neurological sequelae of folate deficiency (see Chapter 21). Chronic methotrexate toxicity, too, produces severe cerebral and spinal cord abnormalities (140).

The most commonly reported neurological association with folate deficiency has been with mood and other mental changes (74, 143). Indeed, the experimental nutritional induction of relatively pure folate deficiency described forgetfulness and irritability in the test subject (69). The review by Hutto (74) detailed the mixed results of studies on folate deficiency and psychiatric manifestations. Neuropathy and myelopathy have also been described (143).

Botez et al. (16) described cerebral dysfunction and atrophy in 16 older folate-deficient adults. With the spread of metabolic testing, additional reports have suggested significant and independent associations of cognitive dysfunction and dementia in older adults with low folate levels (37, 126, 147). The association was often stronger with folate levels than with cobalamin levels (37, 147). However, others have not found an association with vitamin status (85, 94, 95). Moreover, whether low vitamin levels represent an effect rather than the cause of such changes is unresolved, especially for folate, which is more readily affected by poor diet than is cobalamin. Also unknown is whether putative hyperhomocysteinemic cerebrovascular mechanisms contribute to the cognitive dysfunction in folate deficiency (47).

The mechanism for the more obvious neurological damage in cobalamin deficiency is unknown but is suspected to involve cobalamin interaction with methionine metabolism, especially with *S*-adenosylmethionine and *S*-adenosylhomocysteine (see Chapter 17). If this suspicion is true, it is difficult to understand why folate deficiency would not produce comparable neurological dysfunction, given its equally intimate involvement with methionine metabolism. There may be still unknown metabolic explanations for the difference between cobalamin and folate in this respect. The difference may also turn out to be one of degree only. One factor could be the usually greater chronicity of cobalamin deficiency. Until the mechanism of the neurological pathology is clearly identified, however, these questions will be difficult to resolve.

Other Consequences Occasional folate-deficient patients may have oral symptoms and glossitis. However, few other overt symptoms have been noted, which is surprising because folate deficiency affects all cells and tissues.

Gastrointestinal symptoms have been described, but they tend to be nonspecific. It is not always clear whether they are due to the deficiency or to the underlying causes of the deficiency. Mucosal morphological and absorptive changes that reverse with folate therapy have been noted in folate-deficient adults (13, 43), and severe changes were reported in infants with goat's milk anemia (42). However, others have described only minor mucosal changes (166). For unknown reasons, serum cholesterol levels are low in folate deficiency and tend to rise with folic acid therapy.

Possible Consequences of Folate Deficiency One of the general difficulties in interpreting reported associations is that folate deficiency usually exists as part of a wider dietary insufficiency. Whereas cobalamin deficiency tends to be caused by a cobalamin-specific disruption of absorption, folate deficiency is most often part of general malnutrition, alcohol abuse, or multinutrient malabsorption syndromes. Moreover, response to folate supplementation does not always prove that folate deficiency was causative. Folate, especially in higher doses, may ameliorate metabolic defects not caused by folate deficiency, best illustrated by the response of the anemia of cobalamin deficiency to high doses of folic acid (see Chapter 24).

Greater attention is being paid now to the less acute, "low grade" aspects of folate deficiency, which may be viewed in many respects as subclinical. Because hyperhomocysteinemia arises even in mild folate deficiency, potential patients and phenomena that previously escaped attention now can be identified and studied. Particular interest has focused on the possibility of homocysteine-related vascular complications. Little evidence exists for increased prevalences of vascular disease or thrombosis in clinically overt folate deficiency. Nevertheless, as discussed in other chapters, epidemiological surveys suggest that the risk for vasoocclusive disease is associated with lower, although not necessarily subnormal, folate levels (48, 156).

Various adverse outcomes of pregnancy have been associated with poor folate status. For example, folate supplementation of African and Indian mothers during pregnancy has increased their infants' birth weight significantly compared with unsupplemented control subjects (10, 78). However, a causative relationship for most complications remains unproven (134). This includes neural tube defects, as discussed in Chapter 37, in which folate's preventive role often may be a partially pharmacological modulation of unknown metabolic defects. Immune dysfunction has been reported in folate-deficient animals but evidence of immune hypofunction in folate-deficient humans is not yet convincing.

Considerable epidemiologic and animal data suggest that folate insufficiency, or perhaps conditions for which it is a marker, may contribute to carcinogenesis. Kim (89) has provided an extensive and careful assessment of the data on the subject. Cervical dysplasia served as an early model for epithelial cell atypia in folate deficiency. An increased risk of cervical epithelial dysplasia was described in women with low red cell folate levels who were also infected with papilloma virus (24). Compelling linkage with colon neoplasia has developed. A possible protective effect of high folate intake has been shown in prospective surveys and case-control studies (55-57, 159). The

Nurses' Health Study showed a greater protective effect on colon cancer rates with folic acid supplements than with increased food folate intake (55), but found no protective effect against breast cancer (170). To illustrate the complexities of analysis, a protective effect was found in nurses who ingested >15 gm of alcohol daily.

While intriguing, none of the reports on neoplasia are conclusive. Nearly all are observational analyses. Because folate supplementation is rarely taken alone and because dietary patterns reflect many things, it may be that folate status is a confounder for still unidentified factors despite the great care taken in many studies to exclude such factors. As reviewed elsewhere (59, 89), putative folate-related mechanisms for predisposition to cell transformation include changes in DNA methylation, effects on DNA damage and repair processes, and interactions with carcinogens.

Metabolic Consequences. The most sensitive and specific test for cellular folate deficiency, which antedated sensitive and accurate homocysteine assays, was the deoxyuridine suppression test. This test was conceived by Killmann (88) and adapted for clinical testing by Metz et al. (110). It is directed at the de novo thymidine synthesis pathway and 5,10-methylenetetrahydrofolate adequacy.

The cells most often tested have been bone marrow cells. The measured baseline incorporation of [³H]thymidine into their DNA is assigned the value of 100% incorporation. Other aliquots of the cells are preincubated with deoxyuridine, which "suppresses" the incorporation of the subsequently added [³H]thymidine. The suppression is >90% effective; normal cells incorporate <8.5% of the expected amount of [³H]thymidine. Cells from folate-deficient patients (or, as discussed in Chapter 24, cobalamin-deficient patients) demonstrate substandard suppression by deoxyuridine. In patients with mild, often preclinical deficiency, 8.5% to 20% of the expected [³H]thymidine is usually incorporated. Patients with clinically obvious deficiency have incorporation rates sometimes exceeding 50%. The test is made diagnostically vitamin-specific by preincubating additional cell aliquots with folate or cobalamin before measuring suppression (26, 109, 110, 162, 171). All forms of folate correct the abnormal suppression due to folate deficiency, but cobalamin does not. In cobalamin deficiency, addition of cobalamin or most folates corrects the abnormality, with the critical distinction that addition of 5-methyltetrahydrofolate does not; in fact, the latter sometimes worsens the suppression abnormality in mildly cobalamin-deficient cells (26, 27).

Although the mechanism of the deoxyuridine effect is more complex than originally assumed (121), the test has proven reliable when combined with proper controls (26, 109, 110, 162, 171). It has correlated well with clinical data (162) and with methylmalonic acid and homocysteine levels (29). Indeed, the test is slightly more sensitive than either of those metabolite assays in patients with preclinical cobalamin deficiency (29).

The homocysteine issues related to folate are discussed later in this chapter. Older metabolite tests, such as the measurement of formiminoglutamic acid, which depends on folate for its metabolism, have proven nonspecific and have largely been abandoned.

Causes of Folate Deficiency

It is not unusual for folate deficiency to arise from a combination of several causes in a single individual.

Dietary Inadequacy A classic self-experiment produced folate deficiency in an adult male given a diet restricted to 5 µg folic acid daily (69). The study demonstrated how rapidly nutritional folate deficiency can be induced. The serum folate level fell below 6.8 nmol/L after 3 weeks, and neutrophil hypersegmentation appeared in the seventh week. The experiment was complicated by iron deficiency, which may have delayed the onset of macrocytosis, and by potassium deficiency. These complications, even in the experimental setting, help illustrate how infrequently folate deficiency occurs alone.

Dietary folate insufficiency in Western societies tends to predominate in certain groups at high risk, such as alcoholics, the poor, and premature infants. Special diets, such as the one used for phenylketonuria, also place people at risk, as does unsupplemented parenteral nutrition.

Nutritional folate deficiency is more common in developing parts of the world, where it affects broader segments of the population. Women are at special risk in many of these countries, perhaps largely owing to the extra demands put on them by pregnancy and lactation. However, Indian and Pakistani women even in the United Kingdom had significantly lower red cell folate levels than non-Asian women (112). High rates of hyperhomocysteinemia and low serum folate levels were noted in Bangladeshi men and women in London (117). In the United States, too, higher prevalences of low serum and red cell folate levels have been noted in blacks and Latin Americans than in whites or Asian Americans (30, 51, 131, 150). The causes are still uncertain. Studies have not always confirmed a socioeconomic explanation (51), and dietary intake analyses have been inconclusive.

Malabsorption Because folate can be absorbed without involving specific, saturable transport and uptake processes, folate malabsorption is usually part of a generalized malabsorptive disorder involving several nutrients. With the exception of congenital folate malabsorption, malabsorption specific to folate alone is rare.

Folate deficiency has been noted in >80% of patients with celiac disease, a common and underdiagnosed disorder (65). However, coexisting iron deficiency anemia sometimes makes megaloblastic anemia hard to recognize in these patients. Folate deficiency is also common in tropical sprue (11). Folate deficiency tends to predominate early in the course because of the relatively low ratio of body stores to daily turnover of folate, whereas cobalamin deficiency with its much higher ratio tends to appear several years later. Folate deficiency also occurs in inflammatory bowel disease, but is less frequent than in the foregoing disorders. Rarer disorders, such as the small bowel dysfunction in dermatitis herpetiformis, also cause folate deficiency. Some drugs, such as sulfasalazine, reportedly interfere with folate absorption (52). However, the evidence for many drugs that have been implicated as causes of folate malabsorption has been questioned. Treatment of pancreatic insufficiency with pancreatic extracts and alkalinization interferes with folate absorption (129).

Metabolic Disorders, Including Alcohol and Drugs

Alcohol is a very important and common contributor to folate deficiency, and it affects folate metabolism in many ways. People who abuse wine and spirits are more prone to deficiency than beer drinkers, presumably because beer itself contains about 100 µg of folate/L. Serum folate levels decline within hours of alcohol ingestion. Several mechanisms have been implicated, primarily from animal studies. These include interference with enterohepatic recycling of folates and increased breakdown and urinary excretion of folate (141, 158). Interference with folate absorption has also been described (7, 66). Acetaldehyde, a major breakdown product of ethanol, may also form adducts with tetrahydrofolates (63). Finally, of course, alcoholics often have diminished nutritional intake.

Alcohol also partially inhibits methionine synthase and increases betaine:homocysteine methyltransferase (101). Elevated homocysteine levels that reverse in 1 or 2 weeks have been described in alcohol abusers (39, 73), who had lower serum vitamin B_6 and red cell folate (but not serum folate) levels than control subjects (39). The homocysteine levels did not correlate with the vitamin levels.

In addition to its many effects on folate status, alcohol causes red cell macrocytosis directly by a still unknown mechanism (168). Indeed, alcohol abuse may be the most common cause of macrocytosis in general. The macrocytosis is usually mild, and the patient may not even be anemic.

Other drugs also interfere with folate metabolism (see Chapter 27). Several, such as methotrexate, which binds and inhibits dihydrofolate reductase (Metabolic Diagram, Reaction 11), were designed specifically as antifolates for use in antineoplastic or immunosuppressive therapy. Several antibiotics, such as trimethoprim-sulfamethoxazole, are directed against microbial dihydrofolate reductase. Because these antibiotics bind the human enzyme 30,000-fold less avidly (71), patients rarely develop clinical signs unless additional factors compromise folate status. Cytopenias have been described in occasional folate-deficient or cobalamin-deficient patients who took the antibiotics (33, 34). Despite the general infrequency of clinical manifestations, 27% to 333% increases in homocysteine levels were seen in seven healthy subjects given the antibiotics (146). Similar considerations to those mentioned for the antibiotics apply to other weak inhibitors of dihydrofolate reductase, such as pyrimethamine and the antidiuretic triamterene.

Anticonvulsants of several types have been associated with folate deficiency. Patients taking anticonvulsants that inhibit cytochrome P450 had lower folate levels and higher homocysteine levels than control subjects (4). A proposed effect of hydantoins on folate absorption is still uncertain. Increased folate catabolism appears to occur (125).

Sulfasalazine may inhibit several folate-related enzymes, such as dihydrofolate reductase and MTHFR (135), in addition to interfering with folate absorption (52). The effects of oral contraceptives on folate metabolism are uncertain, but, as reviewed by Shojania (142), low folate levels have been described in some studies. A folate deficiency state specific to the cervical epithelium has been proposed.

The hereditary metabolic disorders are discussed in Chapter 21. In addition, homozygotes for the thermolabile 677C→T variant of the MTHFR enzyme (see Chapter 22) tend to have slightly lower folate levels and higher homocysteine levels than unaffected persons (19, 81, 114).

Increased Requirements and Increased Losses

The most common example of increased folate demand is in pregnancy. Both serum and red cell folate levels decline as pregnancy progresses. The published data summarized by Chanarin in 1979 (32) are instructive even though the prevalences are surely lower today in Western societies. Low serum folate levels were found in 15% to 54% of pregnant women and low red cell folate levels in 24% to 32%. Some megaloblastic changes in the bone marrow were described in about one fourth of all women in late pregnancy, while actual anemia was found in only 0 to 12%, with the lower prevalences in Western countries. A negative folate balance has also been found in lactating women unless supplementation was given (103).

Another example of increased folate demand is chronic hemolytic anemia such as sickle cell anemia. As in pregnant women, a negative folate balance can be demonstrated in most patients. There is disagreement whether hyperhomocysteinemia is common in children with sickle cell anemia (127, 155). In occasional cases, the negative folate balance produces clinical signs such as megaloblastic anemia. Most often, however, such developments occur when other causes of folate deficiency are superimposed, such as poor diet, alcohol abuse, or a malabsorptive disorder. The routine provision of folic acid to pregnant women has largely eliminated folate deficiency as a clinical issue in pregnancy. Routine folic acid supplementation is also given to patients with sickle cell anemia. However, controlled, prospective studies have shown no clinical benefits to folic acid supplementation in sickle cell anemia, although better indices of folate status were seen (123).

Folate is lost during hemodialysis. It is now standard to give supplements to all patients who undergo dialysis.

Demographic Factors and Folate

Age The demographic groups thought to be at greatest risk for most nutritional deficiencies are infants, women—especially pregnant women—the elderly, and the poor. This demographic susceptibility is thought to apply to folate deficiency as well. However, surveys of healthy populations do not always bear this out, especially in industrialized countries, and more so in the last decade or two as folic acid supplement use has increased. Thus, full-term infants in Illinois, especially when formula-fed, tended to have higher serum folate levels than did adults (145). Adolescents, however, have had high prevalences of low folate levels. Two studies in the United States described serum folate levels of <6.8 nmol/L in 11.7% to 15% and red cell folate levels of <316 nmol/L in 42% to 47.6% of adolescents (6, 36). Moreover, in both studies the folate status was worst in the older adolescents, presumably reflecting unmet needs for their growth spurt.

Until the mid-1980s, surveys in the elderly population reported often quite high frequencies of low serum folate levels. The frequencies sometimes exceeded 20% (49, 104, 108, 113). Low red cell folate levels were less common. For example, 8% of 229 community-dwelling elderly subjects in Wales had low red cell folate compared with a 30% prevalence of low serum levels (49), and a study of 216 nursing home residents in Norway

showed the respective prevalences of low red cell and serum levels to be 17.6% and 27.8% (104).

Certain patterns were consistent, as summarized by a panel of experts who reviewed the literature on folate and aging in 1982 (128). First, elderly subjects living in their own homes generally had fewer low folate levels than nursing home residents or hospitalized patients (8, 84). Second, even with low folate levels, megaloblastic anemia was distinctly uncommon (60). Third, dietary folate intake by elderly persons was only marginally lower than in younger persons. Finally, little evidence existed for diminished folate absorption, diminished hepatic stores of folate, or increased folate requirements in the elderly. The panel concluded that elderly persons were not disproportionately susceptible to folate deficiency unless they were institutionalized, of low income, or alcoholic (128).

On the contrary, higher folate levels are increasingly being shown in the elderly population than in younger persons. Thus, data from a subset of the Third National Health and Nutrition Examination Survey in the United States in 1991 to 1994 reported a 50th percentile serum folate level of 14.3 nmol/L for men above the age of 60 years compared with 9.5 to 11.1 nmol/L for the various age groups below 60 years (138); the comparable folate levels in women were 15.9 and 10.7 to 11.3 nmol/L, respectively. Four other surveys of 200 to 548 healthy elderly subjects, although using different cutoff points for folate levels, found low serum folate levels in only 1% to 8% and low red cell folate levels in only 1.5% to 3.3% of subjects (53, 67, 68, 98).

This better folate status stands in sharp contrast to cobalamin deficiency, whose prevalence remains high in elderly persons. Studies in the 1970s and early 1980s usually showed prevalences of low folate levels that were greater than (49, 53, 104) or similar to (113) prevalences of low cobalamin levels in the elderly. Since then, with rare exceptions (118), low folate levels have been less common than low cobalamin levels in the elderly population (30, 44, 67, 68, 70, 84, 90, 98, 150). This dichotomy is even more pronounced in persons >85 years old (70).

Ethnic and Racial Background Blacks and Latin Americans living in the United States have lower folate levels than do whites (30, 51, 138). The ethnic differences tend to be more significant among women than among men (30, 51). The Third National Health and Nutrition Examination Survey data from 8,457 adults from 1988 to 1991 found mean folate levels in black men and women of 15.6 and 16.3 nmol/L, respectively, and in Mexican-American men and women of 16.0 and 15.9 nmol/L, respectively, compared with 16.9 and 18.4 nmol/L in white men and women, respectively (51). Although these values needed adjustment because of assay kit calibration problems, the ethnic differences were closely matched by another study in part of the same survey (138). It is also instructive to compare the results with those of the First National Health and Nutrition Examination Survey from 1971 to 1975, in which folate levels were only 7.5 nmol/L in blacks and 8.0 nmol/L in whites.

The ethnic differences are evident at all ages. They were reported in the elderly, both among healthy community dwellers, including Asian-Americans whose folate levels were comparable to those in whites (30), and among disabled elderly women (150). A study of premenopausal women also showed that folate levels were lower in blacks than in whites (54). The difference in folate levels remained significant even after adjustment for the greater use of folate supplements and intake of ready-to-eat cereal by white women. Similar ethnic differences in folate levels were seen in schoolchildren, although levels in Mexican-American schoolchildren were not significantly lower than those in white schoolchildren (119).

Sex   Although intake is generally higher in men than in women and despite past attributions of higher risk for folate deficiency and anemia in women of reproductive age, population-wide surveys do not show lower serum or red cell folate levels in women. In fact, several recent studies, including the National Health and Nutrition Examination Survey, reported higher levels in women than in men (51, 102, 138), especially white women and especially among the elderly population. Evidence indicates that elderly white women use supplements more frequently than men.

Treatment of Folate Deficiency

Oral therapy is usually effective because most folate deficiencies are not malabsorptive in origin. Moreover, even in the presence of malabsorption, crystalline folic acid (pteroyl monoglutamate) is adequately absorbed. Although large doses have been given in the past, especially when malabsorption was suspected, 1 mg doses are now used. Parenteral therapy is rarely necessary, but it can be given safely if desired.

In cases involving any metabolic block, especially when dihydrofolate reductase is impaired (e.g., in methotrexate therapy), bypassing the block by giving a tetrahydrofolate form is effective. Folinic acid (5-formyltetrahydrofolate) is stable and is commonly used. 5-Methyltetrahydrofolate, although unstable, has been used in some studies.

Response to folic acid is rapid. If megaloblastic anemia was present, reticulocytosis appears within 2 days and reaches a peak at 7 to 10 days. Serum lactate dehydrogenase and bilirubin levels decline within a few days, as ineffective hematopoiesis is replaced by effective hematopoiesis.

Folic acid is not toxic over a wide dosage range. Exacerbation of seizures has been described in exceptional cases when large intravenous doses were given to epileptic children with anticonvulsant-associated folate deficiency. Animal studies produced renal damage only when massive doses of folic acid were infused.

Folate Supplementation and Food Fortification

A sharp rise has been noted in folate levels in the United States. A review of 98,351 physician-requested folate assay results in the Kaiser Permanente system in California showed that median serum folate levels had risen from 28.5 nmol/L in 1994 to 42.3 nmol/L in 1998, with a parallel decline in the frequency of subnormal levels < 6.1 nmol/L (93). Both food fortification and increased use of supplements were thought to have contributed to this change. The use of supplements has become increasingly common in industrialized countries, especially in the United States. Use is particularly high among whites and is higher in women than in men. For example, 29.8% of white women used supplements, compared with 19.7% of white men, 18.1% of black women, and 11.9% of black men in a national survey (51).

As mentioned earlier, folate bioavailability is greatest from folic acid supplements. Studies of pregnant women with megaloblastic anemia in South Africa showed a 30% to 60% bioavailability of folic acid from fortified staple foods (38). A controlled trial of 41 healthy women showed that 400 μg folic acid taken daily in fortified food raised red cell folate levels (52.8% increase) as effectively as 400 μg folic acid supplements (40.6% increase) and more effectively than increasing general food folate intake by 400 μg (7.7% increase) (41).

Fortification of cereal grain foods with 1.4 μg folic acid/g was mandated for the United States by the Food and Drug Administration in 1998 to reduce neural tube defect births (50), but this practice began earlier on a voluntary basis. The bioavailability of this fortification was estimated to be 85% (122). Some have criticized the level of fortification as inadequate, whereas others focus on the risk fortification may pose to people with unrecognized cobalamin deficiency. Malinow et al. (105) concluded that fortification must exceed the projected 127 μg/day level to affect homocysteine levels (see Table 30.1 in Chapter 30). Nevertheless, a follow-up study of 248 middle-aged and elderly subjects from Framingham showed that median folate levels rose from 10.4 to 22.5 nmol/L after fortification was instituted, and the prevalence of low levels declined from

22% to 7% (82). It appears that homocysteine levels declined during approximately the same time or with a slight delay (91). However, widespread use of folic acid (and cobalamin) supplements may have played an even greater role than fortification in these changes.

Preliminary reports have not yet found evidence for a decline in neural tube defect incidence despite the improved folate and homocysteine status (111). If this finding is true, it is not clear whether that is because the fortification dose is too low, because other factors have intervened, or because folate fortification is not the optimal remedy. A readjusted analysis of data from the Third National Health and Nutrition Examination Survey done to take into account fortification and supplementation estimated that 67% to 95% of the population now met or exceeded the recommended daily intake, yet 68% to 87% of women of reproductive age still did not exceed daily intakes of 400 µg/day (96).

Folate and Homocysteine

The biochemical explanation for homocysteine elevation in folate deficiency is clear from the impairment of remethylation. Kinetic studies in folate-deficient patients indicate an increased influx of homocysteine into plasma from tissues (61) Plasma clearance of homocysteine is normal in folate deficiency and appears to involve alternate metabolic pathways, although wide individual variation exists.

Total Homocysteine Levels in Patients with Folate Deficiency

Kang et al. (87) provided the first demonstration of an association between folate status and homocysteine. Subjects with serum folate levels <4.5 nmol/L had strikingly increased serum protein-bound homocysteine levels. Indeed, homocysteine levels were also significantly higher in subjects with low-normal folate levels of 4.5 to 8.8 nmol/L than in those with folate levels > 8.8 nmol/L (87). This finding, combined with earlier demonstrations by Wilcken et al. (163–165) and Brattström et al. (17) that high-dose folic acid consistently lowered homocysteine or mixed disulfide levels in renal transplant recipients, patients with heart disease, and postmenopausal women with normal folate levels, set the stage for the many subsequent studies that established the strong connection between folate status and homocysteine levels.

Studies in patients with unequivocal clinical evidence of deficiency, usually diagnosed by the presence of megaloblastic anemia, confirmed the association in 1988 by showing hyperhomocysteinemia in 2 of 2 (35) and 18 of 19 folate-deficient patients (148). The largest study of clinically overt folate deficiency to date reported hyper-

homocysteinemia in 112 of 123 patients, a diagnostic sensitivity of 91.1% (133). The homocysteine levels (median = 67 µmol/L; range 17 to 185 µmol/L) tended to be not as high as in cobalamin-deficient patients (median = 113 µmol/L; range 11 to 476 µmol/L).

A study using a cross-over, low-folate diet design to induce folate insufficiency demonstrated that homocysteine levels rose even before serum folate levels fell below the normal range (79). This finding supports the concept that traditional serum folate reference ranges may not capture early or mild folate deficiency. However, it was equally noteworthy that individual subjects varied greatly in their responses.

Homocysteine levels increase regardless of how the folate deficiency arose. For example, methotrexate therapy in children with leukemia raised their homocysteine levels by 55.6% to 61.7% (23).

Homocysteine Levels and Folate Status in the Population

Not surprisingly, the prevalence of hyperhomocysteinemia in persons found to have low folate levels in the course of surveys of the general population is smaller than in patients identified during clinical encounters. As noted in Table 23.2, not all low folate levels, especially in serum, represent folate deficiency. Interpretation of prevalence rates must also take into account great variations among surveys in cutoff points for both low folate and high homocysteine levels, in methods, in taking creatinine values into consideration, and in subject recruitment.

One of the earliest studies reported homocysteine levels >13.6 µmol/L in 27 of 48 (56.3%) selected patients with serum folate levels <4.5 nmol/L (64). Homocysteine levels >13.7 µmol/L were found in 35 of 130 (26.9%) inpatients with red cell folate levels <362 nmol/L (40). A recent survey reported homocysteine levels > 16.8 µmol/L for women or >17.1 nmol/L for men in 12 of 22 (54.5%) presumably healthy elderly persons who had folate levels <5.7 nmol/L (30).

Folate Levels in Relation to Homocysteine

Serum folate levels correlate inversely with total homocysteine levels in virtually all surveys, whether national surveys of presumably healthy persons (9, 51, 137, 138) or surveys of patients with cardiovascular (31, 77, 120, 156) or psychogeriatric disorders (37, 115). The correlation exists in children (45, 119, 152) as well as elderly persons (30, 90, 126, 137), including the very old who have little folate deficiency (70). Exceptions are rare (99).

The inverse correlation with homocysteine levels is stronger with folate than with cobalamin levels (2, 45,

51, 126, 137, 138, 156) or as strong (9, 37, 54, 80, 90, 98, 102, 115, 119, 150). Indeed, some studies found a correlation with folate levels but not with cobalamin levels (40, 70, 152, 153). Only a few studies have noted a stronger correlation of homocysteine with cobalamin than with folate levels (20, 30, 31). In general, folate seems a stronger determinant of homocysteine levels than does cobalamin (62, 138). This is especially true in younger individuals, the effect of cobalamin becoming stronger with age (40, 138, 150, 167).

An inverse correlation has also been described between homocysteine levels and folate intake (9, 116, 156). Elderly subjects with folate intakes <253 µg/day had significantly higher homocysteine levels than subjects with the highest folate intakes (137). That survey found similar homocysteine associations with vitamin B_6 intake but not with cobalamin intake. Given the much greater role of malabsorption as a cause of cobalamin deficiency than of folate deficiency, the disparity in associations with intake between the two vitamins is not surprising.

Response of Total Homocysteine Levels to Folic Acid (see also Chapter 38)

Homocysteine levels decline within a day (1) to a few days (148) of beginning folic acid therapy of folate deficiency. The hyperhomocysteinemia of cobalamin deficiency does not respond to folic acid (1).

However, homocysteine responses to folic acid also often occur in persons without clear evidence of folate deficiency. This finding has been reported in many large studies of presumably healthy subjects (72) but tends to occur primarily in those with low or low-normal folate levels and high or high-normal homocysteine levels (157). In the latter study, the homocysteine levels returned to their original levels 10 weeks after folate supplementation was discontinued (157).

The response of seemingly normal subjects to folic acid has led to questions concerning the validity of existing reference ranges for both folate and homocysteine (85, 124). An unsettled question is whether the previously mentioned responses indicate widespread subclinical folate deficiency, heretofore unrecognized because of an undue reliance on folate reference ranges built to detect florid folate deficiency, or represent a pharmacological effect of folic acid on genetic or other phenomena not representing folate deficiency. It is also important to keep in mind the phenomenon of regression to the mean, wherein abnormal values spontaneously tend to become more normal on retesting. Equally instructive is the importance of control subjects, illustrated by the incidental finding that homocysteine levels declined in 7 of 30 placebo control subjects (46).

Many broad population and subgroup studies have been conducted on the effect of folic acid on homocysteine levels. The double-blind, crossover trial in 75 patients with coronary artery disease of different levels of folic acid fortification (105) has already been mentioned. Whereas 127 µg/day increased folate levels by 30.8% but lowered homocysteine levels by only 3.7%, fortification with 499 and 655 µg raised folate levels by 64.8% and 105.7%, respectively, and lowered homocysteine more effectively, 11.0% and 14.0%, respectively.

A meta-analysis of 12 controlled trials testing 1,112 subjects for 3 weeks or longer established the effectiveness of folate supplementation (72). Daily amounts of 0.5 to 5.0 mg folic acid were all equally effective, reducing homocysteine levels by 25%. As mentioned earlier, the best effects occurred in persons with lower folate and higher homocysteine levels. A later trial in 114 healthy women showed a similar effect with 0.5 mg folic acid daily but only an 11.4% lowering of homocysteine when the folic acid was given every other day (21). The meta-analysis noted that adding cobalamin to the regimen lowered homocysteine by an additional 7%, but adding vitamin B_6 had no further effect (72). Other studies showed similar results (154); in one report, adding cobalamin increased the homocysteine lowering effect from 11% to 18% (20).

The lowest effective dose of folic acid supplement (not fortification) appears to be <400 µg/day. In a trial of progressively increasing supplement doses in 30 normal men, homocysteine levels responded significantly to 100 µg folic acid and fell further again when 200 µg doses were used (157). However, no further effect was seen when the dose was increased from 200 to 400 µg daily.

Homocysteine-Related Metabolites and Folate

Changes in methionine levels are variable in folate deficiency. Low serum methionine levels were found in only 54% of folate-deficient patients (106), whereas another survey reported no low levels in 20 patients (149). However, methionine levels, although unremarkable before treatment, increased after folic acid therapy in four of six folate-deficient patients (61). By contrast, methionine levels did not rise when folate therapy reduced homocysteine levels in patients with renal failure who were not obviously folate deficient (163, 165).

Serum cystathionine levels were elevated in 19 of 20 folate-deficient patients, although the levels did not correlate with homocysteine levels (149). Cysteine levels were low in 5 of 19 folate-deficient patients (148) and did not correlate with vitamin levels (18).

Although not related to homocysteine metabolism, methylmalonic acid is of interest because of its relationship with cobalamin deficiency (see Chapter 24). The few cases in which elevated methylmalonic acid levels were reported in folate deficiency seem to reflect renal insufficiency or "volume contraction" (133, 148).

REFERENCES

1. Allen, RH, Stabler, SP, Savage, DG, Lindenbaum, J. Diagnosis of cobalamin deficiency. I. Usefulness of serum methylmalonic acid and total homocysteine concentrations. *Am J Hematol* 1990; 34: 90–8.

2. Andersson, A, Brattström, L, Israelsson, B, Isaksson, A, Hamfelt, A, Hultberg, B. Plasma homocysteine before and after methionine loading with regard to age, gender, and menopausal status. *Eur J Clin Invest* 1992; 22: 79–87.

3. Antony, AC. Folate receptors. *Annu Rev Nutr* 1996; 16: 501–21.

4. Apeland, T, Mansoor, MA, Strandjord, RE, Kristensen, O. Homocysteine concentrations and methionine loading in patients on antiepileptic drugs. *Acta Neurol Scand* 2000; 101: 217–23.

5. Bailey, LB. Dietary reference intakes for folate: The debut of dietary folate equivalents. *Nutr Rev* 1998; 56: 294–99.

6. Bailey, LB, Wagner, PA, Christakis, GJ, Davis, CG, Appledorf, H, Araujo, PE, Dorsey, E, Dinning, JS. Folacin and iron status and hematological findings in black and Spanish-American adolescents from urban low-income households. *Am J Clin Nutr* 1982; 35: 1023–32.

7. Baker, H, Frank, O, Zetterman, RK, Rajan, KS, ten Hove, W, Leevy, CM. Inability of chronic alcoholics with liver disease to use food as a source of folates, thiamine, and vitamin B6. *Am J Clin Nutr* 1975; 28: 1377–80.

8. Baker, H, Frank, O, Thind, IS, Jaslow, SP, Louria, DB. Vitamin profiles in elderly persons living at home or in nursing homes, versus profiles in healthy young subjects. *J Am Geriatr Soc* 1979; 27: 444–50.

9. Bates, CJ, Mansoor, MA, van der Pols, J, Prentice, A, Cole, TJ, Finch, S. Plasma total homocysteine in a representative sample of 972 British men and women aged 65 and over. *Eur J Clin Nutr* 1997; 51: 691–97.

10. Baumslag, N, Edelstein, T, Metz, J. Reduction of incidence of prematurity by folic acid supplements in pregnancy. *Br Med J* 1970; 1: 16–7.

11. Bayless TM, Wheby, MS, Swanson, VL. Tropical sprue in Puerto Rico. *Am J Clin Nutr* 1968; 21: 1030–41.

12. Benesch, RE, Kwong, S, Benesch, R, Baugh, CM. The binding of folyl- and antifolylpolyglutamates to hemoglobin. *J Biol Chem* 1985; 260: 14653–58.

13. Bianchi, A, Chipman, DW, Dreskin, A, Rosenzweig, NS. Nutritional folate deficiency with megaloblastic changes in the small-bowel epithelium. *N Engl J Med* 1970; 282: 859–61.

14. Blount, BC, Ames, BN. DNA damage in folate deficiency. *Baillieres Clin Haematol* 1995; 8: 461–78.

15. Blount, BC, Mack, MM, Wehr, CM, MacGregor, JT, Hiatt, RA, Wang, G, Wickramasinghe, SN, Everson, RB, Ames, BN. Folate deficiency causes uracil misincorporation into human DNA and chromosome breakage: Implications for cancer and neuronal damage. *Proc Natl Acad Sci USA* 1997; 94: 3290–95.

16. Botez, MI, Fontaine, F, Botez, T, Bachevalier, J. Folate-responsive neurological and mental disorders: Report of 16 cases. Neuropsychological correlates of computerized transaxial tomography and radionuclide cisternography in folic acid deficiencies. *Eur Neurol* 1977; 16: 230–46.

17. Brattström, LE, Hultberg, BL, Hardebo, JE. Folic acid responsive postmenopausal homocysteinemia. *Metabolism* 1985; 34: 1073–77.

18. Brattström, L, Lindgren, A, Israelsson, B, Andersson, A, Hultberg, B. Homocysteine and cysteine: Determinants of plasma levels in middle-aged and elderly subjects. *J Intern Med* 1994; 236: 633–41.

19. Brattström, L, Wilcken, DE, Ohrvik, J, Brudin, L. Common methylene tetrahydrofolate reductase gene mutation leads to hyperhomocysteinemia but not to vascular disease: The result of a meta-analysis. *Circulation* 1998; 98: 2520–26.

20. Brönstrup, A, Hages, M, Prinz-Langenohl, R, Pietrzik, K. Effects of folic acid and combinations of folic acid and vitamin B-12 on plasma homocysteine concentrations in healthy young women. *Am J Clin Nutr* 1998; 68: 1104–10.

21. Brouwer, IA, van Dusseldorp, M, Thomas, CMG, Duran, M, Hautvast, JGAJ, Eskes, TKAB, Steegers-Theunissen, RPM. Low-dose folic acid supplementation decreases plasma homocysteine concentrations: A randomization trial. *Am J Clin Nutr* 1999; 69: 99–104.

22. Brown, RD, Jun, R, Hughes, W, Watman, R, Arnold, B, Kronenberg, H. Red cell folate assays: Some answers to current problems with radioassay variability. *Pathology* 1990; 22: 82–7.

23. Broxson, EH Jr, Stork, LC, Allen, RH, Stabler, SP, Kolhouse, JF. Changes in plasma methionine and total homocysteine levels in patients receiving methotrexate infusions. *Cancer Res* 1989; 49: 5879–83.

24. Butterworth, CE Jr, Hatch, KD, Macaluso, M, Cole, P, Sauberlich, HE, Soong, SJ, Borst, M, Baker, VV. Folate deficiency and cervical dysplasia. *JAMA* 1992; 267: 528–33.

25. Carmel, R. Macrocytosis, mild anemia and delay in the diagnosis of pernicious anemia. *Arch Intern Med* 1979; 139: 47–50.

26. Carmel, R, Goodman, SI. Abnormal deoxyuridine suppression test in congenital methylmalonic aciduria-homocystinuria without megaloblastic anemia: Divergent biochemical and morphological bone marrow manifestations of disordered cobalamin metabolism in man. *Blood* 1982; 59: 306–11.

27. Carmel, R, Sinow, RM, Karnaze, DS. Atypical cobalamin deficiency: Subtle biochemical evidence of deficiency is commonly demonstrable in patients without megaloblastic anemia and is often associated with protein-bound cobalamin malabsorption. *J Lab Clin Med* 1987; 109: 454–63.

28. Carmel, R, Green, R, Jacobsen, DW, Qian, GD. Neutrophil nuclear segmentation in mild cobalamin deficiency: Relation to metabolic tests of cobalamin status

and observations on ethnic differences in neutrophil segmentation. *Am J Clin Pathol* 1996; 106: 57–63.

29. Carmel, R, Rasmussen, K, Jacobsen, DW, Green, R. Comparison of deoxyuridine suppression test with serum levels of methylmalonic acid and homocysteine in mild cobalamin deficiency. *Br J Haematol* 1996; 93: 311–18.

30. Carmel, R, Green, R, Jacobsen, DW, Rasmussen, K, Florea, M, Azen, C. Serum cobalamin, homocysteine, and methylmalonic acid concentrations in a multiethnic elderly population: Ethnic and sex differences in cobalamin and metabolite abnormalities. *Am J Clin Nutr* 1999; 70: 904–10.

31. Chambers, JC, Obeid, OA, Refsum, H, Ueland, P, Hackett, D, Hooper, J, Turner, RM, Thompson, SG, Kooner, JS. Plasma homocysteine concentrations and risk of coronary heart disease in UK Indian Asian and European men. *Lancet* 2000; 355: 523–27.

32. Chanarin, I. *The Megaloblastic Anaemias,* 2nd ed. Blackwell Scientific, Oxford, 1979.

33. Chanarin, I. Folate deficiency. In *Folates and Pterins* vol 3. *Nutritional, Pharmacological and Physiological Aspects.* (Blakley, RL, Whitehead, VM, eds.). John Wiley & Sons, New York, 1986; pp. 75–146.

34. Chanarin, I, England, JM. Toxicity of trimethoprim-sulphamethoxazole in patients with megaloblastic haemopoiesis. *Br Med J* 1972; 1: 651–53.

35. Chu, RC, Hall, CA. The total serum homocysteine as an indicator of vitamin B12 and folate status. *Am J Clin Pathol* 1988; 90: 446–49.

36. Clark, AJ, Mossholder, S, Gates, R. Folacin status in adolescent females. *Am J Clin Nutr* 1987; 46: 302–6.

37. Clarke, R, Smith, AD, Jobst, KA, Refsum, H, Sutton, L, Ueland, PM. Folate, vitamin B12, and serum total homocysteine levels in confirmed Alzheimer disease. *Arch Neurol* 1998; 55: 1449–55.

38. Colman, N, Green, R, Metz, J. Prevention of folate deficiency by food fortification. II. Absorption of folic acid from fortified staple foods. *Am J Clin Nutr* 1975; 28: 459–64.

39. Cravo, ML, Glória, LM, Selhub, J, Nadeau, MR, Camilo, ME, Resende, MP, Cardoso, JN, Leitao, CN, Mira, FC. Hyperhomocysteinemia in chronic alcoholism: Correlation with folate, vitamin B-12, and vitamin B-6 status. *Am J Clin Nutr* 1996; 63: 220–24.

40. Curtis, D, Sparrow, E, Brennan, L, van der Weyden, MB. Elevated serum homocysteine as a predictor for vitamin B12 or folate deficiency. *Eur J Haematol* 1994; 52: 227–32.

41. Cuskelly, GJ, McNulty, H, Scott, JM. Effect of increasing dietary folate on red-cell folate: Implications for prevention of neural tube defects. *Lancet* 1996; 347: 657–59.

42. Davidson, GP, Townley, RR. Structural and functional abnormalities of the small intestine due to nutritional folic acid deficiency in infancy. *J Pediatr* 1977; 90: 590–94.

43. Dawson, DW. Partial villous atrophy in nutritional megaloblastic anaemia corrected by folic acid therapy. *J Clin Pathol* 1971; 24: 131–35.

44. de Groot, LCPGM, Hautvast, JGAL, van Staveren, WA. Nutrition and health of elderly people in Europe: The EURONUT-SENECA study. *Nutr Rev* 1992; 50: 185–92.

45. De Laut, C, Wautrecht, JC, Brasseur, D, Dramaix, M, Boeynaems, JM, Decuyper, J, Kahn, A. Plasma homocysteine concentrations in a Belgian school-age population. *Am J Clin Nutr* 1999; 69: 968–72.

46. den Heijer, M, Brouwer, IA, Bos, GMJ, Blom, HJ, van der Put, NMJ, Spaans, AP, Rosendaal, FR, Thomas, CMG, Haak, HL, Wijermans, PW, Gerrits, WBJ. Vitamin supplementation reduces blood homocysteine levels. A controlled trial in patients with venous thrombosis and healthy volunteers. *Arterioscler Thromb Vasc Biol* 1998; 18: 356–61.

47. Ebly, EM, Schaefer, JP, Campbell, NRC, Hogan, DB. Folate status, vascular disease and cognition in elderly Canadians. *Age Ageing* 1999; 27: 485–91.

48. Eikelboom, JW, Lonn, E, Genest, J Jr, Hankey, G, Yusuf, S. Homocyst(e)ine and cardiovascular disease: A critical review of the epidemiologic evidence. *Ann Intern Med* 1999; 131: 363–75.

49. Elwood, PC, Shinton, NK, Wilson, CID, Sweetnam, P, Frazer, AC. Haemoglobin, vitamin B12 and folate levels in the elderly. *Br J Haematol* 1971; 21: 557–63.

50. Food and Drug Administration. Food standards: Amendment of standards of identity for enriched grain products to require addition of folic acid. *Fed Reg* 1996; 61: 8781–97.

51. Ford, ES, Bowman, BA. Serum and red blood cell folate concentrations, race, and education: Findings from the third National Health and Nutrition Examination Survey. *Am J Clin Nutr* 1999; 69: 476–81.

52. Franklin, JL, Rosenberg, IH. Impaired folic acid absorption in inflammatory bowel disease: Effects of salicylazosulfapyridine (azulfidine). *Gastroenterology* 1973; 64: 517–25.

53. Garry, PJ, Goodwin, JS, Hunt, WC. Folate and vitamin B12 status in a healthy elderly population. *J Am Geriatr Soc* 1984; 32: 719–26.

54. Gerhard, GT, Malinow, MR, DeLoughery, TG, Evans, AJ, Sexton, G, Connor, SL, Wander, RC, Connor, WE. Higher total homocysteine concentrations and lower folate concentrations in premenopausal black women than in premenopausal white women. *Am J Clin Nutr* 1999; 70: 252–60.

55. Giovannucci, E, Stampfer, MJ, Colditz, GA, Hunter, DJ, Fuchs, C, Rosner, BA, Speizer, FE, Willett, WC. Multivitamin use, folate, and colon cancer in women in the Nurses' Health Study. *Ann Intern Med* 1998; 129: 517–24.

56. Glynn, SA, Albanes, D. Folate and cancer: A review of the literature. *Nutr Cancer* 1994; 22: 101–19.

57. Glynn, SA, Albanes, D, Pietinen, P, Brown, CC, Rautalahti, M, Tangrea, JA, Gunter, EW, Barrett, MJ, Virtamo, J, Taylor, PR. Colorectal cancer and folate status: A nested case-control study among male smokers. *Cancer Epidemiol Biomarkers Prev* 1996; 5: 487–94.

58. Goulian, M, Bleile, B, Tseng, BY. Methotrexate-induced misincorporation of uracil into DNA. *Proc Natl Acad Sci USA* 1980; 77: 1956–60.

59. Green, R, Miller, JW. Folate deficiency beyond megaloblastic anemia: Hyperhomocysteinemia and other manifestations of dysfunctional folate status. *Semin Hematol* 1999; 36: 47–64.

60. Griffiths, HJL, Nicholson, WJ, O'Gorman, P. A haematological study of 500 elderly females. *Gerontology Clin* 1970; 12: 18–32.

61. Guttormsen, AB, Schneede, J, Ueland, PM, Refsum, H. Kinetics of total plasma homocysteine in subjects with hyperhomocysteinemia due to folate or cobalamin deficiency. *Am J Clin Nutr* 1996; 63: 194–202.

62. Guttormsen, AB, Ueland, PM, Nesthus, I, Nygård, O, Schneede, J, Vollset, SE, Refsum, H. Determinants and vitamin responsiveness of intermediate hyperhomocysteinemia (>40 µmol/L). The Hordaland Homocysteine Study. *J Clin Invest* 1996; 98: 2174–83.

63. Guynn, RW, Labaume, LB, Henkin, J. Equilibrium constants under physiological conditions for the condensation of acetaldehyde with tetrahydrofolic acid. *Arch Biochem Biophys* 1982; 217: 181–90.

64. Hall, CA, Chu, RC. Serum homocysteine in routine evaluation of potential vitamin B12 and folate deficiency. *Eur J Haematol* 1990; 45: 143–49.

65. Hallert, C, Tobiasson, P, Walan, A. Serum folate determinations in tracing adult coeliacs. *Scand J Gastroenterol* 1981; 16: 263–67.

66. Halsted, CH, Robles, EA, Mezey, E. Intestinal malabsorption in folate-deficient alcoholics. *Gastroenterology* 1973; 64: 526–32.

67. Hanger, HC, Sainsbury, R, Gilchrist, NL, Beard, MEJ, Duncan, JM. A community study of vitamin B12 and folate levels in the elderly. *J Am Geriatr Soc* 1991; 39: 1155–59.

68. Hayes, AN, Willans, DJ, Skelton, D. Vitamin B12 (cobalamin) and folate blood levels in geriatric reference groups as measured by two kits. *Clin Biochem* 1985; 18: 56–61.

69. Herbert, V. Experimental nutritional folate deficiency in man. *Trans Assoc Am Physicians* 1962; 75: 307–20.

70. Herrmann, W, Quast, S, Ullrich, M, Schultze, H, Bodis, M, Geisel, J. Hyperhomocysteinemia in high-aged subjects: Relation of B-vitamins, folic acid, renal function and the methylenetetrahydrofolate reductase mutation. *Atherosclerosis* 1999; 144: 91–101.

71. Hitchings, GH. Biochemical background of trimethoprim-sulphamethoxazole. *Med J Aust* 1973; 1(Suppl 2): 5–9.

72. Homocysteine Lowering Trialists' Collaboration. Lowering blood homocysteine with folic acid based supplements: meta-analysis of randomized trials. *Br Med J* 1998; 316: 894–98.

72a. Hustad, S, Ueland, PM, Vollset, SE, Zhang, Y, Bjørke-Monesen, AL, Schneede, J. Riboflavin as a determinant of plasma total homocysteine: effect modification by the methylenetetrahydrofolate reductase C677T polymorphism. *Clin Chem* 2000; 46: 1065–71.

73. Hultberg, B, Berglund, M, Andersson, A, Frank, A. Elevated plasma homocysteine in alcoholics. *Alcohol Clin Exp Res* 1993; 17: 687–89.

74. Hutto BR. Folate and cobalamin in psychiatric illness. *Compr Psychiatry* 1997; 38: 305–14.

75. Ingram, CF, Davidoff, AN, Marais, E, Sherman, GG, Mendelow, BV. Evaluation of DNA analysis for evidence of apoptosis in megaloblastic anaemia. *Br J Haematol* 1997; 96: 576–83.

76. Institute of Medicine, Panel on Folate, Other B Vitamins, and Choline. *Dietary Reference Intakes: Thiamin, Riboflavin, Niacin, Vitamin B6, Folate, Vitamin B12, Pantothenic Acid, Biotin and Choline*. National Academy Press, Washington DC, 1998; pp. 196–305.

77. Israelsson, B, Brattström, LE, Hultberg, BL. Homocysteine and myocardial infarction. *Atherosclerosis* 1988; 71: 227–33.

78. Iyengar, L, Rajalakshmi, K. Effect of folic acid supplement on birth weights of infants. *Am J Obstet Gynecol* 1975; 122: 332–36.

79. Jacob, RA, Wu, MM, Henning, SM, Swendseid, ME. Homocysteine increases as folate decreases in plasma of healthy men during short-term dietary folate and methyl group restriction. *J Nutr* 1994; 124: 1072–80.

80. Jacobsen, DW, Gatautis, VJ, Green, R, Robinson, K, Savon, SR, Secic, M, Ji, J, Otto, JM, Taylor, LM Jr. Rapid HPLC detection of total homocysteine and other thiols in serum and plasma: Sex differences and correlation with cobalamin and folate concentrations in healthy subjects. *Clin Chem* 1994; 40: 873–81.

81. Jacques, PF, Bostom, AG, Williams, RR, Ellison, RC, Eckfeldt, JH, Rosenberg, IH, Selhub, J, Rosen, R. Relation between folate status, a common mutation in methylenetetrahydrofolate reductase, and plasma homocysteine concentrations. *Circulation* 1996; 93: 7–9.

82. Jacques, PF, Selhub, J, Bostom, AG, Wilson, PWF, Rosenberg, IH. The effect of folic acid fortification on plasma folate and total homocysteine concentrations. *N Engl J Med* 1999; 340: 1449–54.

83. Jaffe, JP, Schilling, RF. Erythrocyte folate levels: A clinical study. *Am J Hematol* 1991; 36: 116–21.

84. Joosten, E, van den Berg, A, Riezler, R, Naurath, HJ, Lindenbaum, J, Stabler, SP, Allen, RH. Metabolic evidence that deficiencies of vitamin B12 (cobalamin), folate, and vitamin B6 occur commonly in elderly people. *Am J Clin Nutr* 1993; 58: 468–76.

85. Joosten, E, Lesaffre, E, Riezler, R, Ghekiere, V, Dereymaeker, L, Pelemans, W, Dejaeger, E. Is metabolic evidence for vitamin B-12 and folate deficiency more frequent in elderly patients with Alzheimer's disease? *J Gerontol* 1997; 52A: M76–9.

86. Kane, MA, Elwood, PC, Portillo, RM, Antony, AC, Kolhouse, JF. The interrelationship of the soluble and membrane-associated folate-binding proteins in human KB cells. *J Biol Chem* 1986; 261: 15625–31.

87. Kang, SS, Wong, PWK, Norusis, M. Homocysteinemia due to folate deficiency. *Metabolism* 1987; 36: 458–62.

88. Killmann, SA. Effect of deoxyuridine on incorporation of tritiated thymidine: Difference between normoblasts and megaloblasts. *Acta Med Scand* 1964; 175: 483–88.

89. Kim, Y-I. Folate and carcinogenesis: Evidence, mechanisms, and implications. *J Nutr Biochem* 1999; 10: 66–88.

90. Koehler, KN, Romero, LJ, Stauber, PN, Pareo-Tibbeh, SL, Liang, HC, Baumgartner, RN, Garry, PJ, Allen, RH, Stabler, SP. Vitamin supplementation and other variables affecting serum homocysteine and methylmalonic acid concentrations in elderly men and women. *J Am Coll Nutr* 1996; 15: 364–76.

91. Komaromy-Hiller, G, Nuttall, KL. Folic acid fortification. *Lancet* 1999; 354: 2167–68.

92. Koury, MJ, Horne, DW. Apoptosis mediates and thymidine prevents erythroblast destruction in folate deficiency anemia. *Proc Natl Acad Sci USA* 1994; 91: 4067–71.

93. Lawrence, JM, Petitti, DB, Watkins, M, Umekubo, MA. Trends in serum folate after food fortification. *Lancet* 1999; 354: 915–16.

94. Lehmann, M, Gottfries, CG, Regland, B. Identification of cognitive impairment in the elderly: Homocysteine is an early marker. *Dement Geriatr Cogn Disord* 1999; 10: 12–20.

95. Levitt, AJ, Karlinsky, H. Folate, vitamin B12 and cognitive impairment in patients with Alzheimer's disease. *Acta Psychiatr Scand* 1992; 86: 301–5.

96. Lewis, CJ, Crane, NT, Wilson, DB, Yetley, EA. Estimated folate intakes: Data updated to reflect food fortification, increased bioavailability, and dietary supplement use. *Am J Clin Nutr* 1999; 70: 198–207.

97. Lindenbaum, J, Nath, BJ. Megaloblastic anaemia and neutrophil hypersegmentation. *Br J Haematol* 1980; 44: 511–13.

98. Lindenbaum, J, Rosenberg, IH, Wilson, PWF, Stabler, SP, Allen, RH. Prevalence of cobalamin deficiency in the Framingham elderly population. *Am J Clin Nutr* 1994; 60: 2–11.

99. Lolin, YI, Sanderson, JE, Cheng, SK, Chan, CF, Pang, CP, Woo, KS, Masarei, JRL. Hyperhomocysteinaemia and premature coronary artery disease in the Chinese. *Heart* 1996; 76: 117–22.

100. Luhrs, CA, Slomiany, BL. A human membrane-associated folate binding protein is anchored by a glycosyl-phosphatidyl inositol tail. *J Biol Chem* 1989; 264: 21446–49.

101. Lumb, M, Sharer, N, Deacon, R, Jennings, P, Purkiss, P, Perry, J, Chanarin, I. Effect of nitrous oxide-induced inactivation of cobalamin on methionine and *S*-adenosylmethionine metabolism in the rat. *Biochim Biophys Acta* 1983; 756: 354–59.

102. Lussier-Cacan, S, Xhignesse, M, Piolot, A, Selhub, J, Davignon, J, Genest, J Jr. Plasma total homocysteine in healthy subjects: Sex-specific relation with biological traits. *Am J Clin Nutr* 1996; 64: 587–93.

103. Mackey, AD, Picciano, MF. Maternal folate status during extended lactation and the effect of supplemental folic acid. *Am J Clin Nutr* 1999; 69: 285–92.

104. Magnus, EM, Bache-Wiig, JE, Aanderson, TR, Melbostad, E. Folate and vitamin B12 (cobalamin) blood levels in elderly persons in geriatric homes. *Scand J Haematol* 1982; 28: 360–66.

105. Malinow, MR, Duell, PB, Hess, DL, Anderson, PH, Kruger, WD, Phillipson, BE, Gluckman, RA, Block, PC, Upson, BM. Reduction of plasma homocyst(e)ine levels by breakfast cereal fortified with folic acid in patients with coronary heart disease. *N Engl J Med* 1998; 338: 1009–15.

106. Maree, KA, van der Westhuyzen, J, Metz, J. Interrelationship between serum concentrations of methionine, vitamin B12 and folate. *Int J Vitam Nutr Res* 1989; 59: 136–41.

107. Matthews, JH, Clark, DM, Abrahamson, GM. Effect of therapy with vitamin B12 and folic acid on elderly patients with low concentrations of serum vitamin B12 or erythrocyte folate but normal blood counts. *Acta Haematol* 1988; 79: 84–7.

108. Meindok, H, Dvorsky, R. Serum folate and vitamin B12 levels in the elderly. *J Am Geriatr Soc* 1970; 18: 317–26.

109. Metz, J. The deoxyuridine suppression test. *CRC Crit Rev Clin Lab Sci* 1984; 20: 205–41.

110. Metz, J, Kelly, A, Swett, VC, Waxman, S, Herbert, V. Deranged DNA synthesis by bone marrow from vitamin B12-deficient humans. *Br J Haematol* 1968; 14: 575–92.

111. Meyer, RE, Oakley, GP Jr. Folic acid fortification. *Lancet* 1999; 354: 2167–68.

112. Michie, CA, Chambers, J, Abramsky, L, Kooner, JS. Folate deficiency, neural tube defects, and cardiac disease in UK Indians and Pakistanis. *Lancet* 1998; 351: 1105.

113. Munasinghe, DR, Pritchard, JG. The relationship between mean corpuscular volume, serum B12 and serum folate status in aged persons admitted to a geriatric unit. *Br J Clin Pract* 1978; 32: 16–8.

114. Nelen, WLDM, Blom, HJ, Thomas, CMD, Steegers, EAP, Boers, GHJ, Eskes, TKAB. Methylenetetrahydrofolate reductase polymorphism affects the change in homocysteine and folate concentrations resulting from low dose folic acid supplementation in women with unexplained recurrent miscarriages. *J Nutr* 1998; 128: 1336–41.

115. Nilsson, K, Gustafson, L, Fäldt, R, Andersson, A, Hultberg, B. Plasma homocysteine in relation to serum cobalamin and blood folate in a psychogeriatric population. *Eur J Clin Invest* 1994; 24: 600–6.

116. Nygård, O, Refsum, H, Ueland, PM, Vollset, SE. Major lifestyle determinants of plasma homocysteine distribution: The Hordaland Homocysteine Study. *Am J Clin Nutr* 1998; 67: 263–70.

117. Obeid, OA, Mannan, N, Perry, G, Iles, RA, Boucher, BJ. Homocysteine and folate in healthy east London Bangladeshis. *Lancet* 1998; 352: 1829–30.

118. Ortega, RM, Redondo, R, Andres, P, Eguileor, I. Nutritional assessment of folate and cyanocobalamin status in a Spanish elderly group. *Int J Vit Nutr Res* 1993; 63: 17–21.

119. Osganian, SK, Stampfer, MJ, Spiegelman, D, Rimm, E, Cutler, JA, Feldman, HA, Montgomery, DH, Webber, LS, Lytle, LA, Bausserman, L, Nader, PR. Distribution of and factors associated with serum homocysteine levels in children. Child and Adolescent Trial for Cardiovascular Health. *JAMA* 1999; 281: 1189–96.

120. Pancharuniti, N, Lewis, CA, Sauberlich, HE, Perkins, LA, Go, RCP, Alvarez, JO, Macaluso, M, Acton, RT, Copeland, RB, Cousins, AL, Gore, TB, Cornwell, PE, Roseman, JM. Plasma homocyst(e)ine, folate and vitamin B12 concentrations and risk for early-onset coronary artery disease. *Am J Clin Nutr* 1994; 59: 940–48.

121. Pelliniemi, TT, Beck, WS. Biochemical mechanisms in the Killmann experiment: Critique of the deoxyuridine suppression test. *J Clin Invest* 1980; 65: 449–60.

122. Pfeiffer, CM, Rogers, LM, Bailey, LB, Gregory, JF III. Absorption of folate from fortified cereal-grain products and of supplemental folate consumed with or without

food determined by using a dual-label stable-isotope protocol. *Am J Clin Nutr* 1997; 66: 1388–97.

123. Rabb, LM, Grandison, Y, Mason, K, Hayes, RJ, Serjeant, B, Serjeant, GR. A trial of folate supplementation in children with homozygous sickle cell disease. *Br J Haematol* 1983; 54: 589–94.

124. Rasmussen, K, Möller, J, Lyngbak, M, Holm Pedersen, AM, Dybkjaer, L. Age- and gender-specific reference intervals for total homocysteine and methylmalonic acid in plasma before and after vitamin supplementation. *Clin Chem* 1996; 42: 630–36.

125. Richens, A, Waters, AH. Acute effect of phenytoin on serum folate concentration. *Br J Pharmacol* 1971; 41: 414.

126. Riggs, KM, Spiro, A III, Tucker, K, Rush, D. Relations of vitamin B-12, vitamin B-6, folate, and homocysteine to cognitive performance in the Normative Aging Study. *Am J Clin Nutr* 1996; 63: 306–14.

127. Rodriguez-Cortes, HM, Griener, JC, Hyland, K, Bottiglieri, T, Bennett, MJ, Kamen, BA, Buchanan, GR. Plasma homocysteine levels and folate status in children with sickle cell anemia. *J Pediatr Hematol Oncol* 1999; 21: 219–23.

128. Rosenberg, IH, Bowman, BB, Cooper, BA, Halsted, CH, Lindenbaum, J. Folate nutrition in the elderly. *Am J Clin Nutr* 1982; 36: 1060–66.

129. Russell, RM, Dutta, SK, Oaks, EV, Rosenberg, IH, Giovetti, AC. Impairment of folic acid absorption by oral pancreatic extracts. *Digest Dis Sci* 1980; 25: 369–73.

130. Said, HM, Nguyen, TT, Dyer, DL, Cowan, KH, Rubin, SA. Intestinal folate transport: Identification of a cDNA involved in folate transport and the functional expression and distribution of its mRNA. *Biochim Biophys Acta* 1996; 1281: 164–72.

131. Sauberlich, HE. Detection of folic acid deficiency in populations. In *Folic Acid. Biochemistry and Physiology in Relation to the Human Nutritional Requirement.* National Academy of Sciences, Washington DC, 1977; pp. 213–31.

132. Sauberlich, HE, Kretch, MJ, Skala, JH, Johnson, HL, Taylor, PC. Folate requirement and metabolism in nonpregnant women. *Am J Clin Nutr* 1987; 46: 1016–28.

133. Savage, DG, Lindenbaum, J, Stabler, SP, Allen, RH. Sensitivity of serum methylmalonic acid and total homocysteine determinations for diagnosis of cobalamin and folate deficiencies. *Am J Med* 1994; 96: 239–46.

134. Scholl, TO, Johnson, WG. Folic acid: Influence on the outcome of pregnancy. *Am J Clin Nutr* 2000; 71(suppl): 1295S–1303S.

135. Selhub, J, Dhar, GJ, Rosenberg, IH. Inhibition of folate enzymes by sulfasalazine. *J Clin Invest* 1978; 61: 221–24.

136. Selhub, J, Nakamura, S, Carone, FA. Renal folate absorption and the kidney folate binding protein. II. Microinfusion studies. *Am J Physiol* 1987; 252: F757–60.

137. Selhub, J, Jacques, PF, Wilson, PWF, Rush, D, Rosenberg, IH. Vitamin status and input as primary determinants of homocysteinemia in an elderly population. *JAMA* 1993; 270: 2693–98.

138. Selhub, J, Jacques, PF, Rosenberg, IH, Rogers, G, Bowman, BA, Gunter, EW, Wright, JD, Johnson, CL. Serum total homocysteine concentrations in the Third National Health and Nutrition Survey (1991–1994): Population reference ranges and contribution of vitamin status to high serum concentrations. *Ann Intern Med* 1999; 131: 331–39.

139. Shane, B. Folylpolyglutamate synthesis and role in the regulation of one-carbon metabolism. *Vitam Horm* 1989; 45: 263–335.

140. Shapiro, WR, Allen, GC, Horten, BC. Chronic methotrexate toxicity to the central nervous system. *Clin Bull* 1980; 10: 49–52.

141. Shaw, S, Jayatilleke, E, Herbert, V, Colman, N. Cleavage of folates during ethanol metabolism. Role of acetaldehyde/xanthine oxidase-generated superoxide. *Biochem J* 1989; 257: 277–80.

142. Shojania, AM. Oral contraceptives: effect of folate and vitamin B12 metabolism. *Canad Med Assoc* 1982; 126: 244–47.

143. Shorvon, SD, Carney, MWP, Chanarin, I, Reynolds, EH. The neuropsychiatry of megaloblastic anaemia. *Br Med J* 1980; 281: 1036–38.

144. Sirotnak, FM, Tolner, B. Carrier-mediated membrane transport of folates in mammalian cells. *Annu Rev Nutr* 1999; 19: 91–122.

145. Smith, AM, Picciano, MF, Deering, RH. Folate intake and blood concentrations of term infants. *Am J Clin Nutr* 1985; 41: 590–98.

146. Smulders, YM, de Man, AME, Stehouwer, CDA, Slaats, EH. Trimethoprim and fasting plasma homocysteine. *Lancet* 1998; 352: 1827–28.

147. Snowdon, DA, Tully, CL, Smith, CD, Riley, KP, Markesberry, WR. Serum folate and the severity of atrophy of the neocortex in Alzheimer disease: Findings from the Nun Study. *Am J Clin Nutr* 2000; 71: 993–98.

148. Stabler, SP, Marcell, PD, Podell, ER, Allen, RH, Savage, DG, Lindenbaum, J. Elevation of total homocysteine in the serum of patients with cobalamin or folate deficiency detected by capillary gas chromatography/mass spectrometry. *J Clin Invest* 1988; 81: 466–74.

149. Stabler, SP, Lindenbaum, J, Savage, DG, Allen, RH. Elevation of serum cystathionine levels in patients with cobalamin and folate deficiency. *Blood* 1993; 81: 3404–13.

150. Stabler, SP, Allen, RH, Fried, LP, Pahor, M, Kittner, SJ, Penninx, BWJH, Guralnik, JM. Racial differences in prevalence of cobalamin and folate deficiencies in disabled elderly women. *Am J Clin Nutr* 1999; 70: 911–19.

151. Steinberg, SE, Campbell, CL, Hillman, RS. Kinetics of the normal folate enterohepatic cycle. *J Clin Invest* 1979; 64: 83–8.

152. Tonstad, S, Refsum, H, Sivertsen, M, Christophersen, B, Ose, L, Ueland, PM. Relation of total homocysteine and lipid levels in children to premature cardiovascular death in male relatives. *Pediatr Res* 1996; 40: 47–52.

153. Ubbink, JB, Vermaak, WJH, van der Merwe, A, Becker, PJ. Vitamin B12, vitamin B6, and folate nutritional status in men with hyperhomocysteinemia. *Am J Clin Nutr* 1993; 57: 47–53.

154. Ubbink, JB, Delport, R, Vermaak, WJH. Plasma homocysteine concentrations in a population with low coronary disease prevalence. *J Nutr* 1996; 126: 1254S–57S.

155. van der Dijs, FPL, Schnoog, JJB, Brouwer, DAJ, Velvis, HJR, van den Berg, GA, Bakker, AJ, Duits, AJ, Muskiet, FD, Muskiet, FAJ. Elevated homocysteine levels indicate suboptimal folate status in pediatric sickle cell patients. *Am J Hematol* 1998; 59: 192–98.

156. Verhoef, P, Stampfer, MJ, Buring, JE, Gaziano, JM, Allen, RH, Stabler, SP, Reynolds, RD, Kok, FJ, Hennekens, CH, Willett, WC. Homocysteine metabolism and risk of myocardial infarction: Relation with vitamin B6, B12, and folate. *Am J Epidemiol* 1996; 143: 845–59.

157. Ward, M, McNulty, H, McPartlin, J, Strain, JJ, Weir, DG, Scott, JM. Plasma homocysteine, a risk factor for cardiovascular disease, is lowered by physiological doses of folic acid. *Q J Med* 1997; 90: 519–24.

158. Weir, DG, McGing, PG, Scott, JM. Folate metabolism, the enterohepatic circulation and alcohol. *Biochem Pharmacol* 1985; 34: 1–7.

159. White, E, Shannon, JS, Patterson, RE. Relationship between vitamin and calcium supplement use and colon cancer. *Cancer Epidemiol Biomarkers Prev* 1997; 6: 769–74.

160. Wickramasinghe, SN. Morphology, biology and biochemistry of cobalamin- and folate-deficient bone marrow cells. *Baillieres Clin Haematol* 1995; 8: 441–59.

161. Wickramasinghe, SN. The wide spectrum and unresolved issues of megaloblastic anemia. *Semin Hematol* 1999; 36: 3–18.

162. Wickramasinghe, SN, Saunders, JE. Results of three years' experience with the deoxyuridine suppression test. *Acta Haematol* 1977; 58: 193–206.

163. Wilcken, DEL, Gupta, VJ, Betts, AK. Homocysteine in the plasma of renal transplant patients: The effect of cofactors for methionine metabolism. *Clin Sci* 1981; 61: 743–49.

164. Wilcken, DEL, Reddy, GSR, Gupta, VJ. Homocysteinemia, ischemic heart disease, and the carrier state for homocystinuria. *Metabolism* 1983; 32: 363–70.

165. Wilcken, DEL, Dudman, NPD, Tyrrell, PA, Robertson, MR. Folic acid lowers plasma homocysteine in chronic renal insufficiency: Possible implications for prevention of vascular disease. *Metabolism* 1988; 37: 697–701.

166. Winawer, SJ, Sullivan, LW, Herbert, V, Zamcheck, N. The jejunal mucosa in patients with nutritional folate deficiency and megaloblastic anemia. *N Engl J Med* 1965; 272: 892–95.

167. Wouters, MGAJ, Moorrees, MTEC, van der Mooren, MJ, Blom, HJ, Boers, GHJ, Schellekens, LA, Thomas, CMG, Eskes, TKAB. Plasma homocysteine and menopausal status. *Eur J Clin Invest* 1995; 25: 801–5.

168. Wu, A, Chanarin, I, Levi, AJ. Macrocytosis of chronic alcoholism. *Lancet* 1974; 1: 829–31.

169. Wu, A, Chanarin, I, Slavin, G, Levi, A. Folate deficiency in the alcoholic: Its relationship to clinical and haematological abnormalities, liver disease, and folate stores. *Br J Haematol* 1975; 29: 269–78.

170. Zhang, S, Hunter, DJ, Hankinson, SE, Giovannucci, EL, Rosner, BA, Colditz, GA, Speizer, FE, Willett, WC. A prospective study of folate intake and the risk of breast cancer. *JAMA* 1999; 281: 1632–37.

171. Zittoun, J, Marquet, J, Zittoun, R. Effect of folate and cobalamin compounds on the deoxyuridine suppression test in vitamin B$_{12}$ and folate deficiency. *Blood* 1978; 51: 119–28.

24

Cobalamin Deficiency

RALPH CARMEL

Cobalamin Metabolism and Physiology

Cobalamin is a corrinoid tetrapyrrole to whose central cobalt atom are linked the 5,6-dimethylbenzimidazole nucleotide in the α-axial position below the corrin plane and any one of several ligands in the β-axial position above the plane (Figure 24.1). The more common β-linked ligands found in humans are CH_3 (methylcobalamin), 5'-deoxyadenosyl (adenosylcobalamin), OH (hydroxocobalamin), H_2O (aquocobalamin), and CN (cyanocobalamin). Cyanocobalamin, the cobalamin to which the specific name of "vitamin B_{12}" is given, is largely a pharmaceutical creation. Bacteria are the only known synthesizers of cobalamin. Bacteria also synthesize noncobalamin corrinoids that are not functional in humans.

Cobalamin and Diet

Cobalamin in the human diet derives from animals that ingest and store bacterial cobalamin. Meat, poultry, and seafood are the major food sources, but eggs and dairy products are also important. A study of 2,156 adults found that those in the highest tertile of consumption of dairy products and fortified cereals had lower frequencies of low cobalamin levels than did those in the lowest tertile, whereas tertiles of meat

consumption did not show significant differences in cobalamin levels (135). This finding suggests variations in cobalamin availability among food sources. Plants, other than higher forms such as certain algae, do not contain cobalamin.

The Institute of Medicine recently proposed that the daily intake of cobalamin be increased to 2.4 µg from the Recommended Daily Allowance of 2 µg (68). A recent American survey found a mean daily intake of 6.2 µg in adults of all ages (135); another noted a mean intake of 8.4 µg in elderly persons with normal cobalamin status and 6.7 µg in those with abnormal status, a difference that was not significant (66). A Dutch survey of elderly people found a mean intake of 5.3 µg daily and suggested that Europeans ingest less cobalamin than Americans (138). The use of oral supplements has become increasingly common in recent years, especially in the United States (66, 88, 135).

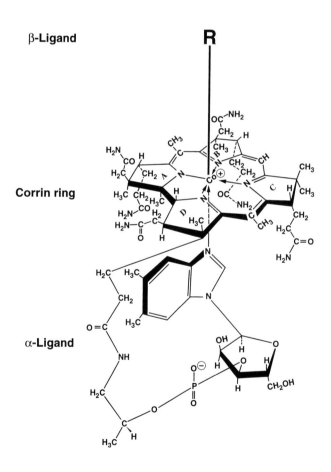

Fig. 24.1. The chemical structure of cobalamin. Different cobalamins are formed by substituting various ligands for the R in the β-axial plane above the tetrapyrrole plane (see text).

Ralph Carmel and Donald W. Jacobsen, eds. *Homocysteine in Health and Disease.* © Cambridge University Press 2001. All rights reserved. Printed in the United States of America.

289

Unlike folate, dietary cobalamin is relatively stable. Losses are small with most routine methods of food preparation (37). If the intrinsic factor-based mechanism of absorption is intact, 60% to 70% of dietary cobalamin is absorbed. Only 1% is thought to be absorbed by diffusion if the intrinsic factor mechanism is inoperative. The presumably milder reduction in absorption when dietary cobalamin release from food binding is impaired has not been quantitated.

Cobalamin Absorption and Excretion

The absorption of cobalamin is a tightly regulated process, involving several binding proteins and specifically targeted uptake (Figure 24.2). Once ingested, food-bound cobalamin is released in the stomach by pepsin in the presence of acid (45). It is thereupon bound by R binder (haptocorrin), a cobalamin-binding protein in saliva and other secretions. The later introduction of pancreatic enzymes, chiefly trypsin, into the duodenum degrades R binder, which allows the released cobalamin to be bound by intrinsic factor. In the ileum, the intrinsic factor-cobalamin complex attaches to cubilin, the receptor for intrinsic factor (81). The endocytosed complex releases its cobalamin, which is exported with transcobalamin II from the ileal cell into the portal circulation several hours later.

The circulating cobalamin-transcobalamin II complex is taken up by receptors for transcobalamin II in tissues throughout the body within 60 to 90 minutes (56). Next to the liver, the kidney, which is rich in transcobalamin II receptors as well as cubilin, accumulates the largest proportions of cobalamin (108). The kidney receptors help limit the urinary loss of cobalamin to <1 μg daily. The liver, in a poorly understood process, allows an estimated average of 1.4 μg/day to be excreted in the bile (49). About 1 μg of this cobalamin is reabsorbed in the ileum in a process presumably mediated by intrinsic factor.

Cobalamin Transport and Binding Proteins

Three binding proteins, which share several regions of structural homology (84), participate in the transport of cobalamin (Table 24.1). Intrinsic factor, via its receptor-mediated endocytosis by ileal epithelium, facilitates cobalamin absorption, while transcobalamin II is critical for uptake of absorbed cobalamin by all cells (Figure 24.2). Little unattached cobalamin can enter the cell by nonspecific mechanisms.

Transcobalamin I is the plasma representative of the R binders, which vary only in their glycosylation. With a few exceptions in some diseases (16), most circulating cobalamin in the plasma is carried at any given moment by transcobalamin I, which does not promote cellular uptake of its cobalamin, whereas the transcobalamin II-cobalamin complex is cleared rapidly (56). It has been suggested that R binder, which binds noncobalamin corrinoids as well as cobalamin, thereby prevents cellular uptake of nonfunctional cobalamin analogs.

Cellular Uptake and Metabolism

After endocytosis, cobalamin is released in the cell and transcobalamin II is degraded in lysosomes (Figure 24.2). Cobalamin becomes available for methylation in the cytoplasm as a cofactor for methionine synthase. It also becomes available to methylmalonyl CoA mutase in mitochondria as 5′-deoxyadenosylcobalamin. The mutase mediates the isomerization reaction in propionate metabolism whereby methylmalonyl CoA is converted to succinyl CoA. Cobalamin mediates no other known reactions in humans.

Cobalamin Deficiency

Cobalamin deficiency is more often an isolated, pure deficiency state than is folate deficiency, which is commonly part of a complex of deficiencies. Nevertheless, its diagnosis is sometimes difficult, in part because it suffers from the lack of a diagnostic "gold standard." Table 24.2 lists the common diagnostic criteria for cobalamin deficiency, as well as the common confounders for the abnormal "diagnostic" findings. Virtually every test, including serum cobalamin and metabolite levels, has confounders that produce falsely negative results as well. The reliability of each finding may vary with the patient and the nature of the problem, and this must be borne in mind when reading the literature, as well as in clinical encounters. Different levels of proof may be required, especially in persons who lack the typical symptoms and signs of deficiency. It is wise to insist on at least two separate diagnostic findings that do not share confounding factors.

Low Cobalamin Levels

The chief index of cobalamin deficiency has traditionally been the low serum cobalamin level. Clinically severe deficiency tends to be accompanied by particularly low levels. For example, hemoglobin levels tend to fall at cobalamin levels <70 pmol/L (141); moreover, in patients with the classical, cobalamin-malabsorptive disorder named pernicious anemia, 40% of those who had only slightly low cobalamin levels (148 to 184 pmol/L, or 200 to 250 ng/L; 0.738 pmol = 1 ng) had no anemia, in contrast with only 11% of those who had very low cobalamin levels (<74 pmol/L) (17). Moderately subnormal levels tend to accompany clinically less severe deficiency.

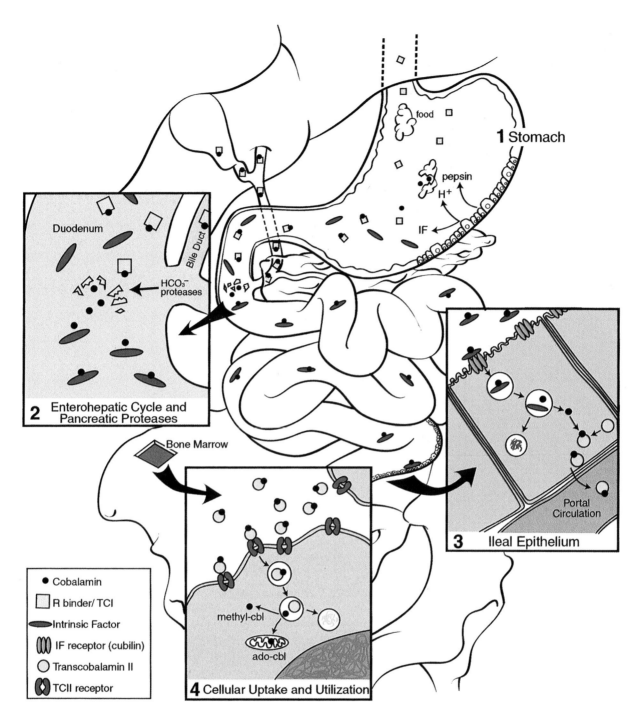

1 Stomach

food

pepsin

H^+

IF

2 Enterohepatic Cycle and Pancreatic Proteases

Duodenum

Bile Duct

HCO_3^- proteases

3 Ileal Epithelium

Portal Circulation

Bone Marrow

4 Cellular Uptake and Utilization

methyl-cbl

ado-cbl

- Cobalamin
- R binder/ TCI
- Intrinsic Factor
- IF receptor (cubilin)
- Transcobalamin II
- TCII receptor

Fig. 24.2. Absorption and cellular uptake cycle of cobalamin in humans. (Illustration by Jill K. Gregory.)

Table 24.1.   Binding Proteins of Cobalamin

	Intrinsic Factor	TC II	TC I; R Binder
Structure	Glycoprotein 48 kDa	Single-chain peptide 43 kDa	Glycoprotein 66 kDa
Gene location	11q12-q13	22q11.2-qter	11p11.11-q11
Distribution	GI tract ? Plasma[a]	Plasma CSF Semen	Plasma Exocrine secretions CSF Semen
Cell origin	Gastric parietal cell ? Pancreas[b]	Endothelial cell Fibroblast Ileal cell ? Hepatocyte	Neutrophil SG Exocrine gland epithelial cell
Cbl binding specificity	Very high	High	Also binds analogs
Receptor	Cubilin: ileum renal tubule yolk sac	TC II receptor: all cells	None identified
Function	Promotes ileal uptake of Cbl	Promotes cellular uptake of Cbl Facilitates Cbl exit from ileal cell	Unknown Carries most Cbl in plasma ? Enterohepatic cycle ? Antimicrobial role
Sequelae of deficiency	Malabsorption of Cbl	Severe cellular Cbl deficiency	Low serum Cbl level
Disorders	Addisonian PA Congenital PA	Congenital TC II deficiency Congenital TC II abnormality	Congenital TC I deficiency TC I/lactoferrin deficiency

TC, transcobalamin; Cbl, cobalamin; GI, gastrointestinal; CSF, cerebrospinal fluid; SG, specific granule; PA, pernicious anemia.
[a] Trace amounts have been detected immunologically.
[b] Occurs in some animals.

Many seemingly healthy people have low serum cobalamin levels. The low levels were regarded originally as spurious (67, 144) because most of these levels are only slightly low (80 to 150 pmol/L), clinical signs and symptoms of deficiency are infrequent, malabsorption is rarely found, and cobalamin therapy generally produces no discernible improvement. The phenomenon is especially common in the elderly, although by no means limited to them. It has also been noted that whites have lower cobalamin levels than blacks (22, 35, 115).

However, metabolic evidence, first provided with the deoxyuridine suppression test in bone marrow cells, showed that 50% to 72% of persons with seemingly innocuous, low cobalamin levels had cellular cobalamin insufficiency despite their asymptomatic state (18, 26, 28, 31, 32, 75). This metabolic evidence was soon buttressed by measurements of serum homocysteine and methylmalonic acid (18, 31, 32, 34, 107, 125). The deoxyuridine suppression and serum metabolite abnor-

malities in these patients were often mild, but they usually improved after cobalamin therapy; hematological improvement was inconsistent, in large part because anemia was absent to begin with (28, 31). This condition has been dubbed *mild or preclinical cobalamin deficiency* and has been reviewed recently (23).

Further expansion of the scope of cobalamin deficiency followed the metabolic evidence that deficiency can occur even in patients whose serum cobalamin levels are normal (i.e., > 150 or 200 pmol/L) (87, 95, 107). Some of these patients have clinically obvious deficiency with anemia and/or neurological dysfunction, but most do not. Lindenbaum et al. (87) estimated that 5.2% of cobalamin-deficient patients have normal serum cobalamin levels. They further suggested that the cutoff point between abnormal and normal cobalamin levels be moved up to 300 or 350 pmol/L. The recommendation has been questioned (23, 35), however, and is discussed later in this chapter.

Table 24.2. Findings Used to Diagnose Cobalamin Deficiency and Confounders Also Capable of Producing Abnormal Results.[a]

Diagnostic Finding	Major Confounders Producing Abnormal Results
Biochemical	
1. Low serum cobalamin level	Folate deficiency Transcobalamin I deficiency Pregnancy
2. Low-normal serum cobalamin level	Most low-normal levels do not represent deficiency
3. High homocysteine level	Folate deficiency Renal insufficiency Enzyme defects
4. High methylmalonic acid level	Renal insufficiency
5. Abnormal deoxy- uridine suppression	Folate deficiency (if effect of vitamin additives is not tested)
Hematological	
6. Anemia and/or macrocytosis[b]	Other causes are more common
7. Megaloblastic changes[b]	Folate deficiency
Clinical	
8. Neurological dysfunction[b]	Other causes are common
9. Presence of disorders known to cause cobalamin deficiency[b]	Deficiency is not invariable Long interval before deficiency ensues
10. Response of any of #1–9 to cobalamin therapy[c]	Some abnormalities always "improve", whether or not deficiency was present (#1,2) Coincidence; regression to the mean

[a] Many confounders producing falsely negative or normal findings also exist but are not listed here.
[b] Often not present in mild or preclinical deficiency.
[c] Response to a multivitamin supplement containing cobalamin cannot be interpreted.

A final point about cobalamin levels is important. Despite the growing interest in and emphasis on mild deficiency, not all low levels—and not all abnormal metabolic results—represent cobalamin deficiency (Table 24.2). Low cobalamin levels without evidence of deficiency have been described in patients with transcobalamin I deficiency (14, 33), AIDS (111), and multiple myeloma (59). Cobalamin levels also decline progressively during pregnancy and are often subnor-

mal by the third trimester, but have no associated homocysteine or methylmalonic acid abnormalities (although high methylmalonic acid levels unrelated to low cobalamin levels have been noted) (94). Most important from a clinical perspective, serum cobalamin levels decline as folate deficiency develops and may become subnormal (37); treating such folate-deficient patients with folic acid alone raises their cobalamin levels. Therefore, clinical assessment should usually include measuring both vitamins. It has been estimated that 5% to 10% of low cobalamin levels reflect folate deficiency rather than cobalamin deficiency.

Consequences of Deficiency

Hematological Consequences Impairment of homocysteine remethylation by cobalamin deficiency traps 5-methyltetrahydrofolate. Endproduct deficiency of S-adenosylmethionine stimulates 5,10-methylene- tetrahydrofolate reductase (MTHFR), further diverting 5,10-methylenetetrahydrofolate to form 5-methyltetrahydrofolate (Metabolic Diagram, Reaction 9). The diminished availability of 5,10-methylenetetrahydrofolate for thymidylate synthesis produces a megaloblastic anemia indistinguishable from that found in folate deficiency (see Chapter 23 and Figure 23.2). If folate therapy is given instead of cobalamin to a cobalamin-deficient patient, the megaloblastic anemia will improve as fresh 5,10-methylenetetrahydrofolate is generated.

Considered to be the classic feature of cobalamin deficiency, anemia is nevertheless not invariable (17, 86). Although many nonanemic patients have subtle megaloblastic changes in blood cells if carefully sought, sometimes no changes are present. It is noteworthy that cobalamin-deficient animals never develop megaloblastic anemia. Macrocytosis, which precedes anemia by months, resulting in many patients having mild macrocytosis without anemia, is also not invariable (17); 14% to 28% of patients with the classic malabsorptive disorder of cobalamin deficiency, pernicious anemia, have neither anemia nor macrocytosis when first diagnosed (17, 86, 114).

Neurological Consequences Most cobalamin-deficient patients develop some neurological dysfunction, but many do not. Accurate data on its frequency are not available. A detailed clinical and metabolic study (86) confirmed that neurological deficits often occur without anemia or macrocytosis (3, 70, 129). It is not clear why some patients develop predominantly neurological symptoms, whereas others develop primarily hematological ones (60, 86).

Cobalamin deficiency produces widespread, patchy demyelination throughout the central nervous system and can affect peripheral nerves. A roughly symmetrical demyelinating myelopathy involving the posterior and lateral columns of the spinal cord ("subacute combined degeneration") is classic. Symptoms usually begin in the feet and ascend as the lesions progress. The deficits are largely sensory, with little motor impairment other than that which results from hyperreflexia and spasticity. Cerebral abnormalities include cognitive, memory, and mood disorders and, rarely, optic atrophy.

The most common neurological symptoms described in a series from New York were paresthesias, numbness, and ataxia (60). The most common physical findings were decreased vibratory, proprioceptive, touch, and pain senses. In addition, electroencephalographic and evoked response abnormalities are common (50, 143); both are often demonstrable even in mild, preclinical deficiency when no neurological symptoms can be found (28, 31, 76). Mild cognitive defects and neuropathy have also been noted in mild, preclinical deficiency (7, 11, 28, 31, 52, 76, 88a, 113). Nevertheless, not all neurological symptoms in patients with low cobalamin levels and metabolic abnormalities are necessarily attributable to the deficiency (100).

Considerable attention has been paid to the high frequency of low cobalamin levels in patients with primary dementia compared with those having secondary dementias (42, 75), although some have not found the frequency to be increased (73, 83). The nature of the association, if any, remains unclear. In most cases, the cobalamin deficiency appears to be of the mild, subclinical variety, although electrophysiological changes and evidence of neuropathy were demonstrated in 11 of 15 patients in one study (31). Cobalamin therapy has produced no cognitive improvement in patients with presumed Alzheimer's disease who had mild cobalamin deficiency (31, 61), although metabolic and electrophysiological improvement occurred (31). A pilot trial suggested that earlier intervention might be effective, before cognitive deficit irreversibility has set in (92), but this finding awaits confirmation.

The mechanism whereby cobalamin deficiency produces neurological dysfunction remains unknown. Currently favored hypotheses center on the diminished generation of methionine and *S*-adenosylmethionine and decreased *S*-adenosylmethionine:*S*-adenosylhomocysteine ratios (see Chapter 17 for a detailed discussion of this subject).

Whereas the hematological abnormalities always reverse completely with therapy, neurological ones may not if they are extensive or have persisted for too long before treatment is begun (37). This makes neurological dysfunction a much more feared complication than the readily reversible megaloblastic anemia.

Other Organ Systems   All cells are affected by cobalamin deficiency, but the consequences are rarely clinically obvious outside of the blood and the nervous system. A few patients develop soreness of the tongue and mouth, which can be severe sometimes. Infertility has been attributed anecdotally to cobalamin deficiency. Osteoblast-related proteins decline with cobalamin deficiency (29), but no evidence linking cobalamin deficiency to osteoporosis has emerged.

Metabolic Changes   Metabolic changes characteristic of cobalamin deficiency precede clinical deficiency. The first demonstrations of metabolic changes in preclinical deficiency used the deoxyuridine suppression test, which is described in Chapter 23. In this test, cobalamin deficiency can be differentiated from folate deficiency by observing the effect of vitamins added to aliquots of the cells (145, 146). Methylmalonic acid can be measured reliably in serum or urine by gas chromatography–mass spectrometry. The levels are consistently elevated in cobalamin-deficient patients (1, 109, 114), but only infrequently in folate-deficient ones (114, 124). Methylmalonic acid elevation responds to cobalamin therapy and sometimes, for unknown reasons, to antibiotics (87). As with homocysteine, serum methylmalonic acid levels increase with renal insufficiency. The homocysteine issues pertinent to cobalamin deficiency are discussed in the last part of this chapter.

Causes of Deficiency

The vast majority of patients who come to medical attention because of clinical signs of cobalamin deficiency have malabsorption as the underlying cause (37, 113). In contrast, malabsorption is found in only 25% to 50% of the much larger number of people who have only preclinical cobalamin deficiency, and the malabsorption appears more often to be limited food-cobalamin malabsorption, rather than the classic malabsorption of free cobalamin caused by a failure of intrinsic factor-mediated absorption (28, 30, 138). The importance of food-cobalamin malabsorption as a cause of mild cobalamin deficiency was foreshadowed by the observation in 82 subjects that cobalamin levels declined in parallel with a decline in gastric acid secretion and not with any measurable decline in the intrinsic factor-mediated ability to absorb free cobalamin (48).

Whatever the underlying disorder, it must be present for years before the cobalamin depletion that it causes becomes great enough to produce symptomatic deficiency. Figure 24.3 illustrates several hypothetical time courses from the onset of the disorder responsible for cobalamin depletion to the appearance of clinical

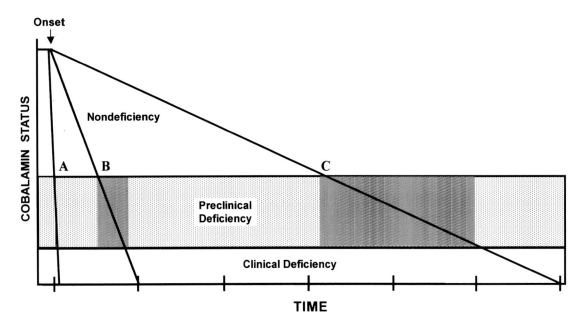

Fig. 24.3. Idealized progression of cobalamin depletion through preclinical and clinical deficiency stages. The rate of depletion determines how quickly each stage of deficiency is reached and how long the patient spends in each stage. (Slope A) Rapid onset of insufficiency, such as occurs in disorders of cellular metabolism. (Slope B) Several-year course typical for classic malabsorptive disorders such as pernicious anemia. (Slope C) Much longer course (duration unknown) when malabsorption is partial, such as occurs in food-cobalamin malabsorption, or when poor dietary intake is the cause (in which case, the slope may be even shallower). The comparative lengths of the shaded areas within the "preclinical deficiency stage" under each line illustrate why patients spend more time in, and are more likely to be encountered with, mild preclinical deficiency when they have disorders characterized by line C than line B (or line A). (Modified from Carmel [21].)

evidence of cobalamin deficiency; these slopes are probably dictated largely by the nature of the underlying process causing deficiency. The varying time curves may explain why partial malabsorption, such as in food-cobalamin malabsorption (line C), or even slower courses such as in dietary insufficiency, are more often associated with mild, preclinical cobalamin deficiency than is severe malabsorption (line B), such as pernicious anemia, or disorders of cellular metabolism (line A).

Table 24.3 lists the causes of cobalamin deficiency in the order of the sequence of events in cobalamin assimilation and utilization shown in Figure 24.2.

Dietary Disorders Because of the rather specific dietary sources of cobalamin and the small daily turnover of cobalamin in relation to its body stores, deficiency on a dietary basis is unusual. Neither general malnutrition nor dietary insufficiency lasting only a few

weeks or months will produce cobalamin deficiency. The diet must be nearly devoid of animal-derived foods for many years to produce clinically apparent deficiency. Even then, a coexisting malabsorptive disorder is often found to be responsible (13, 117).

Nevertheless, subclinical deficiency may exist in some vegetarians. Elevated methylmalonic acid levels have been described (98). Children display signs of deficiency, including hyperhomocysteinemia, more often than do adults (118, 140). A Norwegian study showed low cobalamin and high homocysteine levels in 83% of infants raised on a macrobiotic diet (118). Clinical problems are especially notable in infants born to and breast-fed by vegetarian mothers (43, 51, 53, 63, 69, 118). These infants often have severe neurological and developmental problems. The mothers, despite their usually low serum cobalamin levels, are asymptomatic.

Gastrointestinal Disorders Most clinically overt deficiencies arise from the failure of intrinsic factor–mediated absorption. This failure is usually detected with the Schilling test, a test of absorption of crystalline cobalamin in which urinary excretion of an oral dose of radioactive cobalamin is measured.

The loss of gastric intrinsic factor secretion, which has the misleadingly hematological name *pernicious anemia* even though many patients have little or no anemia, accounts for > 80% of clinically symptomatic cases of cobalamin deficiency (37, 85). Classic or addisonian pernicious anemia arises in the setting of atrophic gastritis, usually type A gastritis with antral sparing. It is most common in elderly people but can occur in younger individuals, especially among black women (24). Immune features are common, including

Table 24.3. Causes of Cobalamin Deficiency

Inadequate intake

   Strict vegetarianism/veganism[a]

   Babies born to and breastfed by cobalamin-deficient
     mothers[b]

Malabsorption[c]

  Failure of intrinsic factor-mediated absorption

   Pernicious anemia (loss of intrinsic factor secretion)
     Addisonian pernicious anemia
     Congenital pernicious anemia
   Parasitization of cobalamin
     Bacterial contamination of the small bowel
     Parasite infestation (*Diphyllobothrium latum*)
   Failure of intrinsic-factor/cobalamin uptake
     Acquired diseases of the ileum (e.g., sprue)
     Surgery of the ileum (resection, isolation)
     Congenital cobalamin malabsorption (receptor
       defect)
     Interference with ileal uptake
       Drugs (e.g., colchicine)
       Zollinger-Ellison syndrome

  Failure to release cobalamin from its binders in food

   Food-cobalamin malabsorption
     Atrophic gastritis
     Gastric surgery
     Inhibition of gastric acid secretion

Metabolic and transport disorders[b]

   Acquired
     Nitrous oxide exposure[d]
   Congenital[e]
     Transcobalamin II deficiency
     Cbl mutations

---

[a] Of all the disorders in this table, this carries the longest time to onset of cobalamin depletion (often more than a decade) because absorption (and reabsorption) of cobalamin is intact.
[b] Onset of cobalamin deficiency is relatively rapid (several days to several months).
[c] Must persist for many years to deplete cobalamin stores (duration varies depending on nature of the malabsorption, e.g., whether it also affects enterohepatic cycle reabsorption).
[d] Deficiency occurs only with chronic, repeated exposure or with coexistence of an unrecognized second cause of deficiency.
[e] See Chapter 21.

autoantibodies directed at intrinsic factor or the H+,K+-ATPase pump on the parietal cell membrane (134). In the rarer congenital pernicious anemia, intrinsic factor synthesis is defective, but the stomach is otherwise normal (15).

Gastric surgery of many types, especially partial gastrectomy, frequently leads to cobalamin deficiency (132). The mechanisms can be multiple.

Many bacteria take up cobalamin avidly. Inadequate absorption results when large numbers of bacteria are present in the small bowel, such as occurs when intestinal motility is impaired or in sites of stasis such as blind pouches after surgery or diverticuli.

Most diseases involving enough ileum, such as sprue, interfere with the normal uptake of the intrinsic factor–cobalamin complex. The cubilin receptor is absent or defective in congenital malabsorption of cobalamin (2).

A subtle but common disorder of cobalamin absorption, food-cobalamin malabsorption, occurs despite an intact intrinsic factor mechanism (19, 28, 30, 44, 47, 71, 97, 130). It arises when cobalamin cannot be released normally from its binders in food. This release process, dependent on gastric acid and pepsin, is impaired in gastritis, after gastric surgery, and when gastric acid secretion is suppressed by medication, such as omeprazole. However, it also occurs in some patients with little gastritis or achlorhydria (41). Most patients with food-cobalamin malabsorption have only mild, usually subclinical cobalamin deficiency, but some have severe deficiency (19, 71, 80, 131).

Metabolic and Transport Disorders Acquired and hereditary metabolic disorders are both uncommon. Nitrous oxide, a widely used inhalant in general anesthesia, oxidizes cobalamin and inactivates the methionine synthase to which oxidized cobalamin is bound (54, 80). Clinical manifestations, which are predominantly neurological, arise only when exposure is chronic (54, 82). Because exposure during surgery is transient, cobalamin deficiency does not result in that setting. However, some patients who had coexisting but unrecognized cobalamin deficiency before surgery have developed serious symptoms after intraoperative exposure to nitrous oxide (116).

The hereditary disorders of cobalamin metabolism, including transcobalamin II deficiency, are described in Chapter 21. Deficiency of transcobalamin I produces low serum cobalamin levels but does not cause cobalamin deficiency (14, 33).

Cobalamin and Aging

The reported prevalence of subnormal cobalamin levels among elderly persons has varied from 0 to 40.5%, depending on the subjects chosen, the assay methods, and the reference range used (21). However, most surveys report prevalences of 5% to 15%. Low levels appear to be more common in whites than in blacks (35, 128) and in men than in women (121). Some authors have adopted lower reference ranges for elderly persons, but this practice, based on the premise that it is normal for the aged to have low cobalamin levels, seems inappropriate.

The longitudinal study of community-dwelling Swedish elderly by Nilsson-Ehle et al. (105) is particularly valuable because nearly all other studies on aging have been cross-sectional. The prevalence of low cobalamin levels (< 130 pmol/L) increased from 4.6% to 7.2%, exclusive of persons already taking supplements, as the subjects aged from 70 to 81 years. Subnormal cobalamin levels predominated among those with somewhat lower initial levels, whereas those with initially higher levels tended to maintain normal levels.

Although metabolic evidence of cobalamin deficiency is common in elderly people, symptoms and clinical signs of deficiency are not. Nevertheless, electrophysiological neurological changes that reverse with cobalamin therapy are often seen (31, 52). Marginally poorer cognitive function, memory, and complex cerebral function have also been described in elderly people and other adults with low cobalamin levels (7, 11, 113).

About 40% of subjects with low cobalamin levels have food-cobalamin malabsorption (21), which seems to be more common in the elderly population (36). An additional 5% to 10% of those with low cobalamin levels have malabsorption of free cobalamin (21). Unrecognized pernicious anemia was found in 1.9% of 729 presumably healthy, elderly volunteers in California, and they were usually asymptomatic (20). Poor dietary intake rarely causes low cobalamin levels in elderly individuals (35, 57, 66, 138). Many reviews have summarized the extensive information on the subject of cobalamin and aging (4, 21, 104, 127).

Treatment of Cobalamin Deficiency

Megaloblastic anemia can be reversed easily with just 1 µg of cobalamin by injection, or even as little as 0.1 µg, but larger doses are commonly used. Treatment is usually given parenterally because most symptomatic deficiencies are malabsorptive in origin. However, about 1% of an oral dose may be absorbed passively even when the intrinsic factor mechanism is inoperative (6). Oral therapy, therefore, can be used even in malabsorptive disorders, but large doses (eg, 1 mg/day) must be given daily in place of the monthly injections. Because most underlying causes of cobalamin deficiency are malabsorptive and irreversible, treatment must usually be continued for life.

It is less clear how to treat the many asymptomatic people, especially elderly people, who are found often almost by accident to have preclinical deficiency—or indeed whether to treat them at all (21). Because most of them have no readily obvious cause or have only

food-bound cobalamin malabsorption, small oral doses of cobalamin, such as the 4 to 6 µg that is common to many multivitamin preparations, should suffice but may not always do so (35, 128).

Supplement Use

Self-directed use of oral cobalamin supplements has increased dramatically. Two American surveys found that 28% to 40.6% of elderly persons used cobalamin supplements (66, 88), and a Dutch study noted such use by 14.3% of elderly subjects (138). Supplement users have significantly higher cobalamin and lower homocysteine and methylmalonic acid levels than nonusers (35, 66, 79, 117, 138). Nevertheless, some supplement users continue to show metabolic abnormalities. One study reported abnormal metabolite levels in 18.6% of users, compared with 37.2% of nonusers (35). The dose may be important. None of the disabled elderly women taking supplements containing ≥9 µg cobalamin daily had low cobalamin levels, compared with 4.9% of those taking ≤6 µg (128).

Effect of Folic Acid Use in Cobalamin Deficiency

Problems arise if cobalamin-deficient patients are treated with folic acid instead of cobalamin. Hematological abnormalities often improve when > 0.2 mg of folic acid is given (58); however, neurological symptoms tend not to respond. The clinical concern is that the diagnosis of cobalamin deficiency may be delayed by the masking of anemia by folate therapy, thus allowing neurological dysfunction to develop or, if already present, to progress. Even greater concern has been generated by anecdotal suggestions that folate could sometimes accelerate progression of neurological dysfunction. These concerns have led to limitations on the extent of fortification of the food supply with folic acid that was mandated in the United States to decrease the incidence of neural tube defect births. It is worth noting, incidentally, that a study in 1986 found that 13% of patients with low cobalamin levels at an academic center were nevertheless treated with folic acid instead of cobalamin (27).

Nearly all of the data on the effects of folic acid in cobalamin deficiency were obtained about 50 years ago, when folic acid was tried in many patients with pernicious anemia as a substitute for liver extract therapy. Very high doses of folic acid were used, usually 10 to 50 mg daily. Dickinson (46) analyzed the published record and concluded that the induction of accelerated neurological deterioration by folic acid was unproven.

Whether or not one agrees fully with Dickinson's analysis and conclusions, it is clear that the record is much more complex than has been widely assumed. A careful argument outlining some of the complexities was presented by Reynolds (112). It is appropriate to note several facts. Although many cobalamin-deficient patients worsened neurologically when treated with folic acid, not all did. In fact, some patients improved, albeit temporarily (55). Moreover, hematological improvement with folic acid treatment was also often incomplete and transient (8, 55, 96, 119). For example, the largest study of folic acid therapy in cobalamin deficiency found that 23 of 98 patients treated with 5 mg folic acid for 3.5 years relapsed neurologically, but an equal number relapsed hematologically (119); 9 other patients relapsed both neurologically and hematologically; 12 of the 98 patients remained stable throughout the 3.5-year study.

In summary, there is no doubt that using folic acid without also giving cobalamin to cobalamin-deficient patients is poor practice. Nevertheless, reliable data do not exist on the sequelae of such practice, what dose of folic acid engenders the neurological worsening, how often and to whom it happens, and whether folate has any directly deleterious effect on the nervous system. Ethical considerations do not permit prospective study of the question. In terms of sheer numbers of subjects potentially affected, an important but still unaddressed question is whether widespread folic acid supplementation will have any adverse effects on the many people who have undiagnosed subclinical cobalamin deficiency.

Cobalamin and Homocysteine

Total Homocysteine Levels in Patients with Cobalamin Deficiency

In 1969, Hollowell et al. (65) described a child with malabsorption whose homocystinuria and methylmalonic aciduria cleared with cobalamin therapy and first suggested that cobalamin deficiency may cause high homocysteine levels. Similar metabolic findings in infants born to and breastfed by vegetarian mothers or mothers with malabsorption supported this concept (43, 51, 63, 64), long before the introduction of modern homocysteine and methylmalonic acid assay technology. Kass (77) attributed positive nickel chloride staining of bone marrow cells from cobalamin-deficient patients to excess intracellular homocysteine, although the reaction lacked specificity. The technical difficulty of detecting all but the most elevated levels of homocysteine in the blood limited the routine documentation of hyperhomocysteinemia in cobalamin deficiency for a long time. The first study showing an inverse relationship between homocysteine and cobalamin levels appeared in 1986 (133).

As a result of the advent of several sensitive methods of measuring homocysteine in the 1980s, it is now clear that its levels are elevated in most cobalamin-deficient patients (Table 24.4). In the largest study of clinically symptomatic cobalamin deficiency to date, hyperhomocysteinemia was found in 95.9% of 434 patients (114). The homocysteine elevation tends to be more pronounced in cobalamin deficiency than in folate deficiency (12, 114) or in heterozygosity for cystathionine β-synthase deficiency (12). However, the specificity and sensitivity of hyperhomocysteinemia for cobalamin deficiency are both lower than those of methylmalonic acidemia (87, 114), which is not affected by folate or vitamin B_6 deficiency.

It is not clear why hyperhomocysteinemia is absent in 5% of cobalamin-deficient patients. "Normal" homocysteine levels could represent relative hyperhomocysteinemia in certain individuals. Homocysteine transsulfuration or betaine-mediated remethylation might also compensate to a greater degree in some patients than others for the failure of the methionine synthase step.

At the same time, some clinically impaired patients have evidence of cobalamin deficiency despite normal cobalamin levels (87). This phenomenon had been suspected in scattered case reports before the advent of metabolic testing, and it was demonstrated with the deoxyuridine suppression test in one case (10). The Denver-New York group showed the problem to be

Table 24.4. Summary of Data from Large Surveys that Evaluated Homocysteine and Methylmalonic Acid (MMA) Abnormalities in Patients with Clinical Cobalamin Deficiency

Study (ref.)	Low cobalamin level cut-off (pmol/L)	Proportion of Subjects with Low Cobalamin Levels Who Have Abnormality of:		
		Homocysteine	MMA	Homocysteine and/or MMA
United States, 1988 (124)	<148	77/78 (98.7%)	74/78 (94.9%)	77/78 (98.7%)
United States, 1994 (114)	<148	416/434 (95.9%)	427/434 (98.4%)	433/434 (99.8%)

more common than suspected and, together with others, demonstrated that elevated homocysteine and methylmalonic acid levels often fell after cobalamin therapy whether or not clinical symptoms were present (87, 102, 107). They concluded that 5.2% of patients with clinical cobalamin deficiency have normal cobalamin levels and can be diagnosed only by their abnormal metabolite levels (87). They also noted that metabolite levels rose more than a year before the cobalamin levels fell when treated patients relapsed after stopping treatment (107).

Lindenbaum et al. (88) suggested that cobalamin deficiency be redefined to include all patients with low-normal cobalamin levels (i.e., up to 258 pmol/L) rather than adhering to the typical cutoff point for subnormal levels of 150 pmol/L. Although this concept has been adopted by some other investigators and is clearly relevant in patients with clinical signs of deficiency, its application to the entire asymptomatic population may be counterproductive, as discussed in the next section.

Total Homocysteine Levels and Cobalamin Status in the General Population

Studies of the general population have shown that mild cobalamin deficiency is more common than suspected, especially among the elderly subpopulation. When largely asymptomatic subjects who were found to have low cobalamin levels (<148 pmol/L) during untargeted surveys were tested further, 38.5% to

63.8% had hyperhomocysteinemia (Table 24.5). High methylmalonic acid levels were found in 48.0% to 55.1%, and one or both of the metabolite levels were high in 61.5% to 78.3%. These rates of abnormality closely match the slightly more sensitive deoxyuridine suppression test findings (34), which showed abnormal results in 18 of 25 asymptomatic persons with low cobalamin levels (72%) (28). All the data thus suggest that half or more of persons with unsuspected low cobalamin levels, most of whom have no clinical signs of deficiency, have metabolic evidence of deficiency. These rates of metabolic abnormality are much lower than the 95% or greater rates found in patients who have clear clinical evidence of deficiency (Table 24.4).

Pennypacker et al. (107) suggested in a small survey in elderly people that the frequency of abnormal metabolite levels was as high in persons whose cobalamin levels were within the low-normal range (148 to 258 pmol/L), as in those with subnormal cobalamin levels (< 148 pmol/L). However, a much larger study of elderly people in Los Angeles showed significantly fewer metabolite abnormalities in the subjects with low-normal cobalamin levels (35). Data from these and other surveys are summarized in Table 24.5. Homocysteine levels were elevated in only 14.0% to 28.8% of subjects with low-normal cobalamin levels (148 to 221 or 140 to 258 pmol/L). Methylmalonic acid levels were elevated in only 12.4% to 48.0% and one or both metabolites in only 32.4% to 56.0%, the highest of the rates of abnormality being reported each time from one survey of only 25 subjects (107).

Table 24.5.   Surveys Evaluating Homocysteine and Methylmalonic Acid (MMA) Abnormalities in Subjects, Usually Asymptomatic, Found to Have Low Cobalamin Levels During General Population Surveys[a]

| Study (ref.) | Cobalamin level cut-off (pmol/L) | Proportion of Subjects with Low or Low-Normal Cobalamin Levels Who Have Abnormality of | | |
		Homocysteine	MMA	Homocysteine and/or MMA
United States, 1990 (125)[b]	<148	153/300 (51.0%)	142/300 (47.3%)	186/300 (62.0%)
United States, 1992 (107)[b]	<148	5/13 (38.5%)	7/13 (53.8%)	8/13 (61.5%)
	148–221[c]	7/25 (28.0%)	12/25 (48.0%)	14/25 (56.0%)
South Africa, 1993 (136)	<200	25/102 (24.8%)	—	—
United States, 1994 (88)[b]	<258	31/222 (14.0%)	62/222 (27.9%)	72/222 (32.4%)
United States, 1996 (34)[d]	<140	25/50 (50.0%)	20/50 (40.0%)	30/50 (60.0%)
United States, 1999 (35)	<140	44/69 (63.8%)	38/69 (55.1%)	54/69 (78.3%)
	140–258[c]	65/226 (28.8%)	28/226 (12.4%)	80/226 (35.4%)

[a] Includes, one study of patients with known preclinical cobalamin deficiency. Studies vary in their handling of subjects with elevated creatinine levels and in their definitions of abnormal homocysteine and MMA levels.

[b] Studies came from the same group of investigators, but different populations were tested and different cutoff points were used.

[c] Low-normal, rather than subnormal, cobalamin levels.

[d] Study of patients with known preclinical, asymptomatic deficiency. Results may also be compared with the higher frequency of abnormality in deoxyuridine suppression test results (abnormal results in 38/50; 76.0%).

Because the total numbers of elderly in the low-normal cobalamin range greatly exceed those with low levels and may constitute one third of the entire population (35), the extended low-normal cobalamin range would cast the net of suspicion of deficiency on a huge number of people. Labeling so much of the population as abnormal may be clinically undesirable, given that the entity in question is subclinical in most cases and the tangible benefits of therapy still await proof. Moreover, > 70% of the persons so labeled turn out not to have metabolic evidence of deficiency when tested (Table 24.5).

Although high homocysteine and/or methylmalonic acid levels are considerably more common than low cobalamin levels in the population, they are often due to causes other than cobalamin deficiency (35, 72, 122) and do not constitute, in themselves, proof of vitamin deficiency (Table 24.2). Renal insufficiency and high creatinine levels are common confounders, especially among elderly individuals (35, 95).

To sum up, it appears that at least half of all seemingly healthy persons who are found to have subnormal cobalamin levels have matching metabolic evidence of cobalamin deficiency (although not every high homocysteine or methylmalonic acid level is due to cobalamin deficiency). The explanation for the low cobalamin levels in the remainder, who do not have metabolic evidence of deficiency, is unknown. The suggestion that the cobalamin range of suspicion be expanded to include low-normal levels has merit when testing symptomatic patients, but remains uncertain in the much larger number of people in the general population who are asymptomatic. The issue is made even more complicated by observations such as those by Nilsson et al. (103), who found that even normal homocysteine levels declined when elderly subjects with normal cobalamin levels were given cobalamin.

Effects of Hyperhomocysteinemia in Relation to Cobalamin

Despite the association of hyperhomocysteinemia with cobalamin deficiency, no evidence exists for an increased prevalence of vascular disease as part of clinical cobalamin deficiency. An autopsy study in 1964 found similar prevalences of atherosclerosis in patients with recent pernicious anemia and in control patients (99). A study in cobalamin-deficient sheep reported cardiac lesions (101), but they were not thrombotic.

An association between various types of cognitive impairment and high homocysteine levels along with low cobalamin and other vitamin levels has been suggested (113), but the Rotterdam Study showed no association between homocysteine and abnormal Mini-Mental State Examination scores (74). Associations

between homocysteine levels and both primary dementia and dementia of vascular origin have also appeared (39, 83, 93). A brief review by Selhub et al. (123) provided a useful, detailed table summarizing 17 published studies. Clarke et al. (39) found an odds ratio of 4.5 (95% confidence interval, 2.2 to 9.2) for confirmed Alzheimer's disease in the highest tertile of homocysteine levels in a case-control study of 164 patients. Radiological suggestion of progression was higher in these patients on follow-up evaluation as well. Similar odds ratios were found for low cobalamin and folate levels, suggesting that vitamin deficiencies underlay the homocysteine elevations, but the odds ratios were no longer significant once homocysteine was included in the analysis. Interestingly, the dementia or cognitive dysfunction was sometimes more strongly associated with abnormal folate and homocysteine levels than with abnormal cobalamin levels (39, 113). This important area of investigation has just begun, and future studies must resolve questions concerning the directness of the role of homocysteine and the relationship to underlying vitamin deficiencies.

Homocysteine has no demonstrable direct effect on cobalamin and folate-related deoxyuridine suppression in human bone marrow cells, aside from a toxic depression of DNA synthesis at very high concentrations (25, 38). Although methionine deficiency has not been shown to have direct effects on cobalamin metabolism, beneficial effects of methionine on neurological dysfunction have been found in cobalamin-deficient animals (120, 139).

Cobalamin Levels in Relation to Hyperhomocysteinemia

Hyperhomocysteinemic persons tend to have lower cobalamin levels than do those with normal homocysteine levels (121, 136). As shown by the analysis of elderly subjects from Framingham, a sharp increase of mean homocysteine levels to 15.4 µmol/L occurs in subjects in the lowest decile of cobalamin levels (121) (Figure 23.1 in Chapter 23). Surveys of homocysteine status have shown an inverse correlation between cobalamin and homocysteine levels (5, 12, 35, 40, 79, 88, 89, 142). This correlation was independent of the associations of homocysteine with age, serum creatinine, folate level, and male sex.

The significant association of hyperhomocysteinemia with poor dietary intake of folate is not replicated with cobalamin intake (5, 121). This difference might be explainable by the much greater role of malabsorption in cobalamin deficiency than in folate deficiency and the much smaller impact of daily intake in relation to body stores on cobalamin status than folate status.

Although B vitamin status was reported to account for 67% of hyperhomocysteinemia (121), the serum folate level is a stronger predictor of hyperhomocysteinemia than is the cobalamin level (12, 121, 122, 136). This is especially true in younger adults, in whom folate deficiency is more common than cobalamin deficiency (122). The balance shifts somewhat in the elderly in whom cobalamin deficiency becomes more common (35, 88, 122). Surveys in the elderly have reported prevalences of 1% to 7.8% for folate deficiency, compared with 6.3% to 20% for cobalamin deficiency (35, 57, 62, 72, 88).

Response of Total Homocysteine Levels to Cobalamin Therapy

When cobalamin-deficient patients are given cobalamin their homocysteine levels decrease to normal (1, 12, 102); it is noteworthy, however, that homocysteine levels also decrease in 20% of placebo-treated subjects (102). The homocysteine levels begin to decline by day 2 after cobalamin treatment and reach the normal range by day 4 (1). A study using cobalamin together with other vitamins noted that homocysteine levels were lower when retested on day 5, with a maximal lowering seen at day 12 (102). In contrast, the homocysteine levels do not fall if cobalamin deficiency is treated with folate, even if blood cell counts improve (1).

Application of homocysteine assay to monitor a patient's response to therapy may sometimes have clinical value, particularly when the nature of the deficiency is in doubt. Homocysteine levels are more useful to monitor in such cases than are cobalamin levels, which rise with cobalamin therapy regardless of the correct diagnosis. However, they are probably less useful to monitor than are methylmalonic acid levels.

In the general population, as discussed earlier, oral cobalamin supplementation tends to have a lesser effect on homocysteine levels than does folic acid supplementation (110, 137). Only 14.8% of hyperhomocysteinemic men responded to 0.4 mg cobalamin, compared with 49.8% who responded to 0.65 mg of folic acid (137). However, the addition of oral cobalamin to folic acid supplementation in healthy young women enhanced the lowering of homocysteine levels from 11% with folic acid alone to 15% to 18% in another study (9). Cobalamin supplementation may be more important in elderly persons, among whom cobalamin insufficiency is more common than in younger adults.

Homocysteine-Related Metabolites and Cobalamin

Initial reports suggested that methionine levels were low in cobalamin deficiency (106), but more recent data indicate that the levels are usually normal (12, 91, 117). In contrast cystathionine levels, were elevated in 87% of cobalamin-deficient patients (126). Data on cysteine levels conflict; both decreased (90, 124) and increased levels (12) were reported, although in the latter report, the levels increased further after therapy.

REFERENCES

1. Allen, RH, Stabler, SP, Savage, DG, Lindenbaum, J. Diagnosis of cobalamin deficiency. I. Usefulness of serum methylmalonic acid and total homocysteine concentrations. *Am J Hematol* 1990; 34: 90–8.
2. Aminoff, M, Carter, JE, Chadwick, RB, Johnson, C, Gräsbeck, R, Abdelaal, MA, Broch, H, Jenner, LB, Verroust, PJ, Moestrup, SK, de la Chapelle, A, Krahe, R. Mutations in *CUBN,* encoding the intrinsic factor-vitamin B12 receptor, cubilin, cause hereditary megaloblastic anaemia 1. *Nat Genet* 1999; 21: 309–13.
3. Arias, IM, Apt, L, Pollycove, M. Absorption of radioactive vitamin B12 in nonanemic patients with combined-system disease. *N Engl J Med* 1955; 253: 1005–10.
4. Baik, HW, Russell, RM. Vitamin B12 deficiency in the elderly. *Annu Rev Nutr* 1999; 19: 357–77.
5. Bates, CJ, Mansoor, MA, van der Pols, J, Prentice, A, Cole, TJ, Finch, S. Plasma total homocysteine in a representative sample of 972 British men and women aged 65 and over. *Eur J Clin Nutr* 1997; 51: 691–97.
6. Berlin, H, Berlin, R, Brante, G. Oral treatment of pernicious anemia with high doses of vitamin B12 without intrinsic factor. *Acta Med Scand* 1968; 184: 247–58.
7. Bernard, MA, Nakonezny, PA, Kashner, TM. The effect of vitamin B$_{12}$ deficiency on older veterans and its relationship to health. *J Am Geriatr Soc* 1998; 46: 1199–1206.
8. Bethell, FH, Sturgis, CC. The relation of therapy in pernicious anemia to changes in the nervous system. Early and late results in a series of cases observed for periods of not less than ten years, and early results of treatment with folic acid. *Blood* 1948; 3: 57–67.
9. Björnstrup, A, Hages, M, Prinz-Langenohl, R, Peitrzik, K. Effects of folic acid and combinations of folic acid and vitamin B-12 on plasma homocysteine concentrations in healthy, young women. *Am J Clin Nutr* 1998; 68: 1104–10.
10. Blundell, EL, Matthews, JH, Allen, SM, Middleton, AM, Morris, JE, Wickramasinghe, SN. Importance of low serum vitamin B12 and red cell folate concentrations in elderly hospital inpatients. *J Clin Pathol* 1985; 38: 1179–84.
11. Bohnen, N, Jolles, J, Degenaar, CP. Lower blood levels of vitamin B12 are related to decreased performance of healthy subjects in the Stroop color-word test. *Neurosci Res Comm* 1992; 11: 53–6.
12. Brattström, L, Israelsson, B, Lindegarde, F, Hultberg, B. Higher total plasma homocysteine in vitamin B12 deficiency than in heterozygosity for homocystinuria due to cystathionine β-synthase deficiency. *Metabolism* 1988; 37: 175–8.

13. Carmel, R. Nutritional vitamin B_{12} deficiency: Possible contributory role of subtle vitamin B_{12} malabsorption. *Ann Intern Med* 1978; 88: 647–49.

14. Carmel, R. R binder deficiency: A clinically benign cause of cobalamin pseudo-deficiency. *JAMA* 1983; 250: 1886–90.

15. Carmel, R. Gastric juice in congenital pernicious anemia contains no immunoreactive intrinsic factor molecule: Study of three kindreds with variable ages at presentation, including a patient first diagnosed in adulthood. *Am J Hum Genet* 1983; 35: 67–77.

16. Carmel, R. The distribution of endogenous cobalamin among cobalamin-binding proteins in the blood in normal and abnormal states. *Am J Clin Nutr* 1985; 41: 713–19.

17. Carmel, R. Pernicious anemia: The expected findings of very low serum cobalamin levels, anemia and macrocytosis are often lacking. *Arch Intern Med* 1988; 148: 1712–14.

18. Carmel, R. Reversal by cobalamin therapy of minimal defects in the deoxyuridine suppression test in patients without anemia: Further evidence for a subtle metabolic cobalamin deficiency. *J Lab Clin Med* 1992; 119: 240–44.

19. Carmel, R. Malabsorption of food cobalamin. *Baillieres Clin Haematol* 1995; 8: 639–55.

20. Carmel, R. Prevalence of undiagnosed pernicious anemia in the elderly. *Arch Intern Med* 1996; 156: 1097–1100.

21. Carmel, R: Cobalamin, the stomach and aging. *Am J Clin Nutr* 1997; 66: 350–59.

22. Carmel, R. Ethnic and racial factors in cobalamin metabolism and its disorders. *Semin Hematol* 1999; 36: 88–100.

23. Carmel, R. Current concepts in cobalamin deficiency. *Annu Rev Med* 2000; 51: 357–75.

24. Carmel, R, Johnson, CS. Racial patterns in pernicious anemia: Early age at onset and increased frequency of intrinsic-factor antibody in black women. *N Engl J Med* 1978; 298: 647–50.

25. Carmel, R, Bedros, AA, Mace, JW, Goodman, SI. Congenital methylmalonic aciduria-homocystinuria with megaloblastic anemia: Observations on response to hydroxocobalamin and on effect of homocysteine and methionine on the deoxyuridine suppression test. *Blood* 1980; 55: 570–79.

26. Carmel, R, Karnaze, DS. The deoxyuridine suppression test identifies subtle cobalamin deficiency in patients without typical megaloblastic anemia. *JAMA* 1985; 253: 1284–87.

27. Carmel, R, Karnaze, DS. Physician response to low serum cobalamin levels. *Arch Intern Med* 1986; 146: 1161–65.

28. Carmel, R, Sinow, RM, Karnaze, DS: Atypical cobalamin deficiency: Subtle biochemical evidence of deficiency is commonly demonstrable in patients without megaloblastic anemia and is often associated with protein-bound cobalamin malabsorption. *J Lab Clin Med* 1987; 109: 454–63.

29. Carmel, R, Lau, KHW, Baylink, DJ, Saxena, S, Singer, FR. Cobalamin and osteoblast-specific proteins. *N Engl J Med* 1988; 319: 70–5.

30. Carmel, R, Sinow, RM, Siegel, ME, Samloff, IM. Food cobalamin malabsorption occurs frequently in patients with unexplained low serum cobalamin levels. *Arch Intern Med* 1988; 148: 1715–19.

31. Carmel, R, Gott, PS, Waters, CH, Cairo, K, Green, R, Bondareff, W, DeGiorgio, CM, Cummings, JL, Jacobsen, DW, Buckwalter, G, Henderson, VW. The frequently low cobalamin levels in dementia usually signify treatable metabolic, neurologic and electrophysiologic abnormalities. *Eur J Haematol* 1995; 54: 245–53.

32. Carmel, R, Cairo, K, Bondareff, W, Gott, PS, Cummings, JL, Henderson, VW. Spouses of demented patients with low cobalamin levels: A new risk group for cobalamin deficiency. *Eur J Haematol* 1996; 57: 62–7.

33. Carmel, R, Montes-Garces, R, Wardinsky, T, Liebman, H. Mild transcobalamin I deficiency is common and may be responsible for many low serum cobalamin levels: Observations in a family and survey of 106 patients with low serum cobalamin levels not explained by malabsorption. *Blood* 1996; 88 (suppl 1): 646a.

34. Carmel, R, Rasmussen, K, Jacobsen, DW, Green, R. Comparison of deoxyuridine suppression test with serum levels of methylmalonic acid and homocysteine in mild cobalamin deficiency. *Br J Haematol* 1996; 93: 311–18.

35. Carmel, R, Green, R, Jacobsen, DW, Rasmussen, K, Florea, M, Azen, C. Serum cobalamin, homocysteine, and methylmalonic acid concentrations in a multiethnic elderly population: Ethnic and sex differences in cobalamin and metabolite abnormalities. *Am J Clin Nutr* 1999; 70: 904–10.

36. Carmel, R, Aurangzeb, I, Qian, D. Associations of food-cobalamin malabsorption with ethnic origin, age, *Helicobacter pylori* infection and serum markers of gastritis. *Am J Gastroenterol* 2001; 96: 63–70.

37. Chanarin, I. *The Megaloblastic Anaemias*, 2nd ed. Blackwell Scientific, Oxford, 1979.

38. Cheng, FW, Shane, B, Stokstad, ELR. The antifolate effect of methionine on bone marrow of normal and vitamin B12-deficient rats. *Br J Haematol* 1975; 31: 323–36.

39. Clarke, R, Smith, AD, Jobst, KA, Refsum, H, Sutton, L, Ueland, PM. Folate, vitamin B_{12}, and serum total homocysteine levels in confirmed Alzheimer disease. *Arch Neurol* 1988; 55: 1449–55.

40. Clarke, R, Woodhouse, P, Ulvik, A, Frost, C, Sherliker, P, Refsum, H, Ueland, PM, Khaw, K-T. Variability and determinants of total homocysteine concentrations in plasma in an elderly population. *Clin Chem* 1998; 44: 102–7.

41. Cohen, H, Weinstein, WM, Carmel, R. The heterogeneity of gastric histology and function in food-cobalamin malabsorption: Absence of atrophic gastritis and achlorhydria in some patients with severe malabsorption. *Gut*, 2000; 47: 638–45.

42. Cole, MG, Prchal, JF. Low serum vitamin B12 in Alzheimer-type dementia. *Age Ageing* 1984; 13: 101–5.

43. Davis, JR Jr, Goldenring, J, Lubin, BH. Nutritional vitamin B12 deficiency in infants. *Am J Dis Child* 1981; 135: 566–67.

44. Dawson, DW, Sawers, AH, Sharma, RK. Malabsorption of protein-bound vitamin B_{12}. *Br Med J* 1984; 288: 675–78.

45. del Corral, A, Carmel, R. Transfer of cobalamin from the cobalamin-binding protein of egg yolk to R binder of human saliva and gastric juice. *Gastroenterology* 1990; 98: 1460–66.

46. Dickinson, CJ. Does folic acid harm people with vitamin B12 deficiency? *Q J Med* 1995; 88: 357–64.

47. Doscherholmen, A, Swaim, WR. Impaired assimilation of egg Co^{57} vitamin B_{12} in patients with hypochlorhydria and achlorhydria and after gastric resection. *Gastroenterology* 1973; 64: 913–19.

48. Doscherholmen, A, Ripley, D, Chang, S, Silvis, SE. Influence of age and stomach function on serum vitamin B12 concentration. *Scand J Gastroenterol* 1977; 12: 313–19.

49. el Kholty, S, Guéant, JL, Bressler, L, Djalali, M, Boissel, P, Gerard, P, Nicolas, JP. Portal and biliary phases of enterohepatic circulation of corrinoids in humans. *Gastroenterology* 1991; 101: 1399–1408.

50. Fine, EJ, Soria, E, Paroski, MW, Petryk, D, Thomasula, L. The neurophysiological profile of vitamin B12 deficiency. *Muscle Nerve* 1990; 13: 158–64.

51. Frader, JO, Reibman, B, Turkewitz, D. Vitamin B12 deficiency in strict vegetarians. *N Engl J Med* 1978; 299: 1319.

52. Gott, PS, Degiorgio, CM, Schreiber, SS, McCleary, CA, Qian, D, Carmel, R. P300 event-related potentials in elderly patients with subtle preclinical cobalamin (B12) deficiency. *J Clin Neurophysiol* 1997; 14: 447.

53. Graham, SM, Arvela, OM, Wise, GA. Long-term neurologic consequences of nutritional vitamin B12 deficiency in infants. *J Pediatr* 1992; 121: 710–14.

54. Guttormsen, AB, Refsum, H, Ueland, PM. The interaction between nitrous oxide and cobalamin. Biochemical events and clinical consequences. *Acta Anaesthesiol Scand* 1994; 38: 753–56.

55. Hall, BE, Watkins, CH. Experience with pteroylglutamic (synthetic folic) acid in the treatment of pernicious anemia. *J Lab Clin Med* 1947; 32: 622–34.

56. Hall, CA. The plasma transport of vitamin B12. *Br J Haematol* 1976; 33: 161–71.

57. Hanger, HC, Sainsbury, R, Gilchrist, NL, Beard, MEJ, Duncan, JM. A community study of vitamin B_{12} and folate levels in the elderly. *J Am Geriatr Soc* 1991; 39: 1155–59.

58. Hansen, HA, Weinfeld, A. Metabolic effects and diagnostic value of small doses of folic acid and B12 in megaloblastic anemias. *Acta Med Scand* 1962; 172: 427–43.

59. Hansen, OP, Drivsholm, A, Hippe, E. Vitamin B12 metabolism in myelomatosis. *Scand J Haematol* 1977; 18: 395–402.

60. Healton, EB, Savage, DG, Brust, JCM, Garrett, TJ, Lindenbaum, J. Neurologic aspects of cobalamin deficiency. *Medicine* 1991; 70: 229–245.

61. Hector, M, Burton, JR. What are the psychogeriatric manifestations of vitamin B_{12} deficiency? *J Am Geriatr Soc* 1988; 36: 1105–12.

62. Herrmann, W, Quast, S, Ullrich, M, Schultze, H, Bodis, M, Geisel, J. Hyperhomocysteinemia in high-aged subjects: Relation of B-vitamins, folic acid, renal function and the methylenetetrahydrofolate reductase mutation. *Atherosclerosis* 1999; 144: 91–101.

63. Higginbottom, MC, Sweetman, L, Nyhan, WL. A syndrome of methylmalonic aciduria, homocystinuria, megaloblastic anemia and neurologic abnormalities in a vitamin B12-deficient, breast-fed infant of a strict vegetarian. *N Engl J Med* 1978; 299: 317–23.

64. Hoey, H, Linnell, JC, Oberholzer, VG, Laurance, BM. Vitamin B12 deficiency in a breast fed infant of a mother with pernicious anaemia. *J R Soc Med* 1982; 75: 656–58.

65. Hollowell, JG Jr, Hall, WK, Coryell, ME, McPherson, J Jr, Hahn, DA. Homocystinuria and organic aciduria in a patient with vitamin-B12 deficiency. *Lancet* 1969; 2: 1428.

66. Howard, JM, Azen, C, Jacobsen, DW, Green, R, Carmel, R. Dietary intake of cobalamin in elderly people who have abnormal serum cobalamin, methylmalonic acid and homocysteine levels. *Eur J Clin Nutr* 1998; 52: 582–87.

67. Hughes, D, Elwood, PC, Shinton, NK, Wrighton, RJ. Clinical trial of the effect of vitamin B_{12} in elderly subjects with low serum B_{12} levels. *Br Med J* 1970; 2: 458–60.

68. Institute of Medicine, Panel on Folate, Other B Vitamins, and Choline. *Dietary Reference Intakes: Thiamin, Riboflavin, Niacin, Vitamin B6, Folate, Vitamin B12, Pantothenic Acid, Biotin and Choline.* National Academy Press, Washington DC, 1998; pp. 306–56.

69. Jadhav, M, Webb, JKG, Vaishnava, S, Baker, S. Vitamin B_{12} deficiency in Indian infants: A clinical syndrome. *Lancet* 1962; 2: 903–7.

70. Jewesbury, ECO. Subacute combined degeneration of the cord and achlorhydric peripheral neuropathies without anaemia. *Lancet* 1954; 3: 307–12.

71. Jones, BP, Broomhead, AF, Kwan, YL, Grace, CS. Incidence and clinical significance of protein-bound vitamin B12 malabsorption. *Eur J Haematol* 1987; 38: 131–36.

72. Joosten, E, van den Berg, A, Riezler, R, Naurath, HJ, Lindenbaum, J, Stabler, SP, Allen, RH. Metabolic evidence that deficiencies of vitamin B12 (cobalamin), folate, and vitamin B6 occur commonly in elderly people. *Am J Clin Nutr* 1993; 58: 468–76.

73. Joosten, E, Lesaffre, E, Riezler, R, Ghekiere, V, Dereymaeker, L, Pelemans, W, Dejaeger, E. Is metabolic evidence for vitamin B-12 and folate deficiency more frequent in elderly patients with Alzheimer's disease? *J Gerontol* 1997; 52A: M76–9.

74. Kalmijn, S, Launer, LJ, Lindemans, J, Bots, ML, Hofman, A, Breteler, MMB. Total homocysteine and cognitive decline in a community-based sample of elderly subjects. The Rotterdam Study. *Am J Epidemiol* 1999; 150: 283–89.

75. Karnaze, DS, Carmel, R. Low serum cobalamin levels in primary degenerative dementia: Do some patients harbor atypical cobalamin deficiency states? *Arch Intern Med* 1987; 147: 429–31.

76. Karnaze, DS, Carmel, R. Neurologic and evoked potential abnormalities in subtle cobalamin deficiency states, including deficiency without anemia and with normal absorption of free cobalamin. *Arch Neurol* 1990; 47: 1008–12.

77. Kass, L. Cytochemical detection of homocysteine in pernicious anemia and erythremic myelosis. *Am J Clin Pathol* 1977; 67: 53–6.

78. King, CE, Leibach, J, Toskes, PP. Clinically significant vitamin B$_{12}$ deficiency secondary to malabsorption of protein-bound vitamin B$_{12}$. *Digest Dis Sci* 1979; 24: 397–402.

79. Koehler, KN, Romero, LJ, Stauber, PN, Pareo-Tibbeh, SL, Liang, HC, Baumgartner, RN, Garry, PJ, Allen, RH, Stabler, SP. Vitamin supplementation and other variables affecting serum homocysteine and methylmalonic acid concentrations in elderly men and women. *J Am Coll Nutr* 1996; 15: 364–76.

80. Kondo, H, Osborne, ML, Kolhouse, JF, Binder, MJ, Podell, ER, Utley, CS, Abrams, RS, Allen, RH. Nitrous oxide has multiple deleterious effects on cobalamin metabolism and causes decreases in activities of both mammalian cobalamin-dependent enzymes in rats. *J Clin Invest* 1981; 67: 1270–83.

81. Kozyraki, R, Kristiansen, M, Silahtaroglu, A, Hansen, C, Jacobsen, C, Tommerup, N, Verroust, PJ, Moestrup, SK. The human intrinsic factor-vitamin B12 receptor, *cubilin:* Molecular characterization and chromosomal mapping of the gene to 10p within the autosomal recessive megaloblastic anemia *(MGA1)* region. *Blood* 1998; 91: 3593–3600.

82. Layzer, RB. Myeloneuropathy after prolonged exposure to nitrous oxide. *Lancet* 1978; 2: 1227–1230.

83. Lehmann, M, Gottfries, CG, Regland, B. Identification of cognitive impairment in the elderly: homocysteine is an early marker. *Dement Geriatr Cogn Disord* 1999; 10: 12–20.

84. Li, N, Seetharam, S, Seetharam, B. Genomic structure of human transcobalamin II: Comparison to human intrinsic factor and transcobalamin I. *Biochem Biophys Res Comm* 1995; 208: 756–64.

85. Lindenbaum, J. Aspects of vitamin B12 and folate metabolism in malabsorption syndromes. *Am J Med* 1979; 67: 1037–48.

86. Lindenbaum, J, Healton, EB, Savage, DG, Brust, JCM, Garrett, TJ, Podell, ER, Marcell, PD, Stabler, SP, Allen, RH. Neuropsychiatric disorders caused by cobalamin deficiency in the absence of anemia or macrocytosis. *N Engl J Med* 1988; 318: 1720–28.

87. Lindenbaum, J, Savage, DG, Stabler, SP, Allen, RH. Diagnosis of cobalamin deficiency. II. Relative sensitivities of serum cobalamin, methylmalonic acid, and total homocysteine concentrations. *Am J Hematol* 1990; 34: 99–107.

88. Lindenbaum, J, Rosenberg, IH, Wilson, PWF, Stabler, SP, Allen, RH. Prevalence of cobalamin deficiency in the Framingham elderly population. *Am J Clin Nutr* 1994; 60: 2–11.

88a. Louwman, MWJ, van Dusseldorp, M, van de Vijver, FJR, Thomas, CMG, Schneede, J, Ueland PM, Refsum, H, van Staveren, WA. Signs of impaired cognitive function in adolescents with marginal cobalamin status. *Am J Clin Nutr* 2000; 72: 762–9.

89. Lussier-Cacan, S, Xhignesse, M, Piolot, A, Selhub, J, Davignon, J, Genest, J Jr. Plasma total homocysteine in healthy subjects: Sex-specific relation with biological traits. *Am J Clin Nutr* 1996; 64: 587–93.

90. Mansoor, MA, Ueland, PM, Svardal, AM. Redox status and protein binding of plasma homocysteine and other aminothiols in patients with hyperhomocysteinemia due to cobalamin deficiency. *Am J Clin Nutr* 1994; 59: 631–35.

91. Maree, KA, van der Westhuyzen, J, Metz, J. Interrelationship between serum concentrations of methionine, vitamin B12 and folate. *Int J Vitamin Nutr Res* 1989; 59: 136–41.

92. Martin, DC, Francis, J, Protetch, J, Huff, FJ. Time dependency of cognitive recovery with cobalamin replacement: Report of a pilot study. *J Am Geriatr Soc* 1992; 40: 168–72.

93. McCaddon, A, Davies, G, Hudson, P, Tandy, S, Cattell, H. Total serum homocysteine in senile dementia of the Alzheimer type. *Int J Geriatr Psychiatry* 1998; 13: 235–39.

94. Metz, J, McGrath, K, Bennett, M, Hyland, K, Bottiglieri, T. Biochemical indices of vitamin B$_{12}$ nutrition in pregnant patients with subnormal serum vitamin B$_{12}$ levels. *Am J Hematol* 1995; 48: 251–55.

95. Metz, J, Bell, AH, Flicker, L, Bottiglieri, T, Ibrahim, J, Seal, E, Schultz, D, Savoia, H, McGrath, KM. The significance of subnormal serum vitamin B$_{12}$ concentration in older people: A case control study. *J Am Geriatr Soc* 1996; 44: 1355–61.

96. Meyer, LM. Folic acid in the treatment of pernicious anemia. *Blood* 1947; 2: 50–62.

97. Miller, A, Furlong, D, Burrows, BA, Slingerland, DW. Bound vitamin B$_{12}$ absorption in patients with low serum B$_{12}$ levels. *Am J Hematol* 1992; 40: 163–66.

98. Miller, DR, Specker, BL, Ho, ML, Norman, EJ. Vitamin B-12 status in a macrobiotic community. *Am J Clin Nutr* 1991; 53: 524–29.

99. Mitchell, IA, Mitchell, SG. "The protective effect" of pernicious anemia on the development of atherosclerosis: A comparative study. *Am J Med Sci* 1964; 246: 36–41.

100. Moelby, L, Nielsen, G, Rasmussen, K, Jensen, MK, Pedersen, KO. Metabolic cobalamin deficiency in patients with low to low-normal plasma cobalamins. *Scand J Clin Lab Invest* 1997; 57: 209–16.

101. Mohammed, R, Lamand, M. Cardiovascular lesions in cobalt-vitamin B12 deficient sheep. *Ann Rech Vet* 1986; 17: 447–50.

102. Naurath, HJ, Joosten, E, Riezler, R, Stabler, SP, Allen, RH, Lindenbaum, J. Effects of vitamin B12, folate, and vitamin B6 supplements in elderly people with normal serum concentrations. *Lancet* 1995; 346: 85–9.

103. Nilsson, K, Gustafson, L, Fäldt, R, Andersson, A, Hultberg, B. Plasma homocysteine in relation to serum cobalamin and blood folate in a psychogeriatric population. *Eur J Clin Invest* 1994; 24: 600–6.

104. Nilsson-Ehle, H. Age-related changes in cobalamin (vitamin B12) handling. Implications for therapy. *Drugs Aging* 1998; 12: 277–92.

105. Nilsson-Ehle, H, Jagenburg, R, Landahl, S, Lindstaedt, S, Svanborg, A, Westin, J. Serum cobalamins in the elderly:

A longitudinal study of a representative population sample from age 70 to 81. *Eur J Haematol* 1991; 47: 10–6.

106. Parry, TE. Serum valine and methionine levels in pernicious anaemia under treatment. *Br J Haematol* 1969; 16: 1–9.

107. Pennypacker, LC, Allen, RH, Kelly, JP, Matthews, LM, Grigsby, J, Kaye, K, Lindenbaum, J, Stabler, SP. High prevalence of cobalamin deficiency in elderly outpatients. *J Am Geriatr Soc* 1992; 40: 1197–1204.

108. Rappazzo, ME, Salmi, HA, Hall, CA. The content of vitamin B12 in adult and foetal tissue: A comparative study. *Br J Haematol* 1970; 18: 425–33.

109. Rasmussen, K, Moelby, L, Jensen, MK. Studies on methylmalonic acid in humans. II. Relationships between concentrations in serum and urinary excretion and the correlation between cobalamin and accumulation of MMA. *Clin Chem* 1989; 35: 77–80.

110. Rasmussen, K, Möller, J, Lyngbak, M, Holm Pedersen, AM, Dybkjaer, L. Age- and gender-specific reference intervals for total homocysteine and methylmalonic acid in plasma before and after vitamin supplementation. *Clin Chem* 1996; 42: 630–36.

111. Remacha, AF, Cadafalch, J. Cobalamin deficiency in patients infected with the human immunodeficiency virus. *Semin Hematol* 1999; 36: 75–87.

112. Reynolds, EH. Interrelationships between the neurology of folate and vitamin B12 deficiency. In *Folic Acid in Neurology, Psychiatry and Internal Medicine.* (Botez, MI, Reynolds, EH, eds.). Raven Press, New York, 1979; pp. 501–15.

113. Riggs, KM, Spiro, A III, Tucker, K, Rush, D. Relations of vitamin B_{12}, vitamin B_6, folate, and homocysteine to cognitive performance in the Normative Aging Study. *Am J Clin Nutr* 1996; 63: 306–14.

114. Savage, DG, Lindenbaum, J, Stabler, SP, Allen, RH. Sensitivity of serum methylmalonic acid and total homocysteine determinations for diagnosis of cobalamin and folate deficiencies. *Am J Med* 1994; 96: 239–46.

115. Saxena, S, Carmel, R. Racial differences in vitamin B12 levels in the United States. *Am J Clin Pathol* 1987; 88: 95–7.

116. Schilling, RF. Is nitrous oxide a dangerous anesthetic for vitamin B12-deficient subjects? *JAMA* 1986; 255: 1605–6.

117. Schloesser, LL, Schilling, RF. Vitamin B12 absorption studies in a vegetarian with megaloblastic anemia. *Am J Clin Nutr* 1963; 12: 70–4.

118. Schneede, J, Dagnelie, PC, van Staveren, WA, Vollset, SE, Refsum, H, Ueland, PM. Methylmalonic acid and homocysteine in plasma as indicators of functional cobalamin deficiency in infants on macrobiotic diets. *Pediatr Res* 1994; 36: 194–201.

119. Schwartz, SO, Kaplan, SR, Armstrong, BE. The long-term evaluation of folic acid in the treatment of pernicious anemia. *J Lab Clin Med* 1950; 35: 894–98.

120. Scott, JM, Dinn, JJ, Wilson, P, Weir, DG. Pathogenesis of subacute combined degeneration: A result of methyl group deficiency. *Lancet* 1981; 2: 334–37.

121. Selhub, J, Jacques, PF, Wilson, PWF, Rush, D, Rosenberg, IH. Vitamin status and input as primary determinants of homocysteinemia in an elderly population. *JAMA* 1993; 270: 2693–98.

122. Selhub, J, Jacques, PF, Rosenberg, IH, Rogers, G, Bowman, BA, Gunter, EW, Wright, JD, Johnson, CL. Serum total homocysteine concentrations in the Third National Health and Nutrition Survey (1991–1994): Population reference ranges and contribution of vitamin status to high serum concentrations. *Ann Intern Med* 1999; 131: 331–39.

123. Selhub, J, Bagley, LC, Miller, J, Rosenberg, IH. B vitamins, homocysteine, and neurocognitive function in the elderly. *Am J Clin Nutr* 2000; 71 (suppl): 614S–20S.

124. Stabler, SP, Marcell, PD, Podell, ER, Allen, RH, Savage, DG, Lindenbaum, J. Elevation of total homocysteine in the serum of patients with cobalamin or folate deficiency detected by capillary gas chromatography/mass spectrometry. *J Clin Invest* 1988; 81: 466–74.

125. Stabler, SP, Allen, RH, Savage, DG, Lindenbaum, J. Clinical spectrum and diagnosis of cobalamin deficiency. *Blood* 1990; 76: 871–81.

126. Stabler, SP, Lindenbaum, J, Savage, DG, Allen, RH. Elevation of serum cystathionine levels in patients with cobalamin and folate deficiency. *Blood* 1993; 81: 3404–13.

127. Stabler, SP, Lindenbaum, J, Allen, RH. Vitamin B-12 deficiency in the elderly: Current dilemmas. *Am J Clin Nutr* 1997; 66: 741–49.

128. Stabler, SP, Allen, RH, Fried, LP, Pahor, M, Kittner, SJ, Penninx, BWJH, Guralnik, JM. Racial differences in prevalence of cobalamin and folate deficiencies in disabled elderly women. *Am J Clin Nutr* 1999; 70: 911–19.

129. Strachan, RW, Henderson, JG. Psychiatric syndromes due to avitaminosis B12 with normal blood and marrow. *Q J Med* 1965; 34: 303–17.

130. Streeter, AM, Duraiappah, B, Boyle, R, O'Neill, BJ, Pheils, MT. Malabsorption of vitamin B_{12} after vagotomy. *Am J Surg* 1974; 128: 340–43.

131. Streeter, AM, Shum, HY, Duncombe, VM, Hewson, JW, Thorpe, MEC. Vitamin B12 malabsorption associated with a normal Schilling test result. *Med J Aust* 1976; 1: 54–5.

132. Sumner, AE, Chin, MM, Abrahm, JL, Berry, GT, Gracely, EJ, Allen, RH, Stabler, SP. Elevated methylmalonic acid and total homocysteine levels show high prevalence of vitamin B12 deficiency after gastric surgery. *Ann Intern Med* 1996; 124: 469–76.

133. Swift, ME, Schultz, TD. Relationship of vitamins B6 and B12 to homocysteine level: Risk for coronary heart disease. *Nutr Rep Int* 1986; 34: 1–14.

134. Toh, B-H, van Driel, IR, Gleeson, PA. Pernicious anemia. *N Engl J Med* 1997; 337: 1441–48.

135. Tucker, KL, Rich, S, Rosenberg, I, Jacques, P, Dallal, G, Wilson, PWF, Selhub, J. Plasma vitamin B-12 concentrations relate to intake source in the Framingham Offspring Study. *Am J Clin Nutr* 2000; 71: 514–22.

136. Ubbink, JB, Vermaak, WJH, van der Merwe, A, Becker, PJ. Vitamin B12, vitamin B6, and folate nutritional status in men with hyperhomocysteinemia. *Am J Clin Nutr* 1993; 57: 47–53.

137. Ubbink, JB, Vermaak, WJH, van der Merwe, A, Becker, PJ, Delport, R, Potgieter, HC. Vitamin requirements for the treatment of hyperhomocysteinemia in humans. *J Nutr* 1994; 124: 1927–33.

138. van Asselt, DZB, de Groot, LCPGM, van Staveren, WA, Blom, HJ, Wevers, RA, Biemond, I, Hoefnagels, WHL. Role of cobalamin intake and atrophic gastritis in mild cobalamin deficiency in older Dutch subjects. *Am J Clin Nutr* 1998; 68: 328–34.

139. van der Westhuyzen, J, Fernandes-Costa, F, Metz, J. Cobalamin inactivation by nitrous oxide produces severe neurological impairment in fruit bats: Protection by methionine and aggravation by folates. *Life Sci* 1982; 31: 2001–10.

140. van Dusseldorp, M, Schneede, J, Refsum, H, Ueland, PM, Thomas, CMG, de Boer, E, van Staveren, WA. Risk of persistent cobalamin deficiency in adolescents fed a macrobiotic diet in early life. *Am J Clin Nutr* 1999; 69: 664–71.

141. vant Sant, P, Küsters, PFMM, Harthoorn-Lasthuzen, EJ. Dependency of MCV and haemoglobin concentration on plasma vitamin B12 levels in relation to sex and age. *Clin Lab Haematol* 1997; 19: 27–31.

142. Verhoef, P, Stampfer, MJ, Buring, JE, Gaziano, JM, Allen, RH, Stabler, SP, Reynolds, RD, Kok, FJ, Hennekens, CH, Willett, WC. Homocysteine metabolism and risk of myocardial infarction: Relation with vitamin B6, B12, and folate. *Am J Epidemiol* 1996; 143: 845–59.

143. Wallace, PW, Westmoreland, BF. The electroencephalogram in pernicious anemia. *Mayo Clin Proc* 1976; 51: 281–85.

144. Waters, WE, Withey, JL, Kilpatrick, GS, Wood, PHN. Serum vitamin B12 concentrations in the general population: A ten-year follow-up. *Br J Haematol* 1971; 20: 521–6.

145. Wickramasinghe, SN, Matthews, JH. Deoxyuridine suppression: Biochemical basis and diagnostic applications. *Blood Rev* 1988; 2: 168–77.

146. Zittoun, J, Marquet, J, Zittoun, R. Effect of folate and cobalamin compounds on the deoxyuridine suppression test in vitamin B_{12} and folate deficiency. *Blood* 1978; 51: 119–28.

25

Vitamin B$_6$ Deficiency

JESSE F. GREGORY III

History and Overview of Vitamin B$_6$ in Nutrition and Metabolism

Although the existence of vitamin B$_6$ has been known for more than 60 years, the role of vitamin B$_6$ in human nutrition is still not completely understood, nor is there consensus regarding optimal intake. This chapter summarizes current knowledge regarding the nature of vitamin B$_6$, its metabolic function, assessment of vitamin B$_6$ nutritional status, and evidence of vitamin B$_6$ requirements. Attention is then focused on the evidence of dietary adequacy with respect to vitamin B$_6$, as well as the metabolic consequences of inadequate nutritional status and association with adverse effects on health.

Vitamin B$_6$ was first described by Gyorgy (39) and was identified as the component of rice bran that prevented the nutritional deficiency syndrome known as acrodynia in rats (7). Shortly thereafter, five laboratories independently isolated and crystallized the nutritionally active material, which was termed *pyridoxine* (Figure 25.1) (40, 47, 52, 56, 60). Two research groups reported the synthesis and proof of structure of pyridoxine as 2-methyl-3-hydroxy-4,5-bis(hydroxymethyl)pyridine in 1939. In the early 1940s, pyridoxal and pyridoxamine were identified in studies with bacterial assay systems (95). Coenzymatic activity of a

phosphorylated form of pyridoxal, later identified as pyridoxal 5′-phosphate, was identified in 1944 (37). Studies of the function of pyridoxal 5′-phosphate in enzymatic transamination reactions led to the observation that pyridoxamine 5′-phosphate and pyridoxal 5′-phosphate play a coenzymatic role in most aminotransferases (71). Most of the coenzymatic function of pyridoxal 5′-phosphate involves condensation of the pyridoxal 5′-phosphate carbonyl group with the α-amino group of an amino acid substrate to form a Schiff base that promotes enzymatic reactions by facile double-bond migration to facilitate further reaction (e.g., hydrolysis). Reviews by Snell (93–95) provide a more detailed summary of the discovery and early history of vitamin B$_6$.

An adequate intake of vitamin B$_6$ is needed to allow sufficient synthesis of its coenzyme forms, pyridoxal 5′-phosphate and pyridoxamine phosphate. Vitamin B$_6$-dependent enzymes catalyze many reactions in the interconversion and catabolism of amines and amino acids, including transamination, decarboxylation, desulfhydration, dehydration, and various reactions involving substitution, transfer, or other modifications of amino acid side chains. Pyridoxal 5′-phosphate exhibits a different form of coenzymatic function in glycogen phosphorylase, apparently with its 5′-phosphate involved in general acid catalysis (43). Pyridoxal 5′-phosphate may also participate in governing the expression of certain genes (102), although the physiological significance of this proposed genetic regulatory function is unclear.

Chemistry and Nomenclature

Vitamin B$_6$ is the preferred generic term for the class of 2-methyl-3-hydroxy-4,5-bis(hydroxymethyl)pyridines (Figure 25.1) that has the qualitative vitamin activity of pyridoxine (1). Confusion exists because the term pyridoxine is used generically in some clinically oriented contexts. In this book, vitamin B$_6$, not pyridoxine, is used as the generic descriptor.

The vitamin B$_6$ group includes three subclasses that differ in the substituent at the fourth position of the pyridine ring. Pyridoxine (once also called pyridoxol) is an alcohol, pyridoxal is an aldehyde, and pyridoxamine is a primary amine with respect to the 4′-carbon. Each form also exists with a phosphate ester on the 5′-hydroxymethyl group. The primary vitamin B$_6$ catabolic product in humans is 4-pyridoxic acid, in which the 4′-carbon is a carboxyl group. Many plant tissues contain pyridoxine with one or more glucose units linked to the 5′-hydroxymethyl group through a

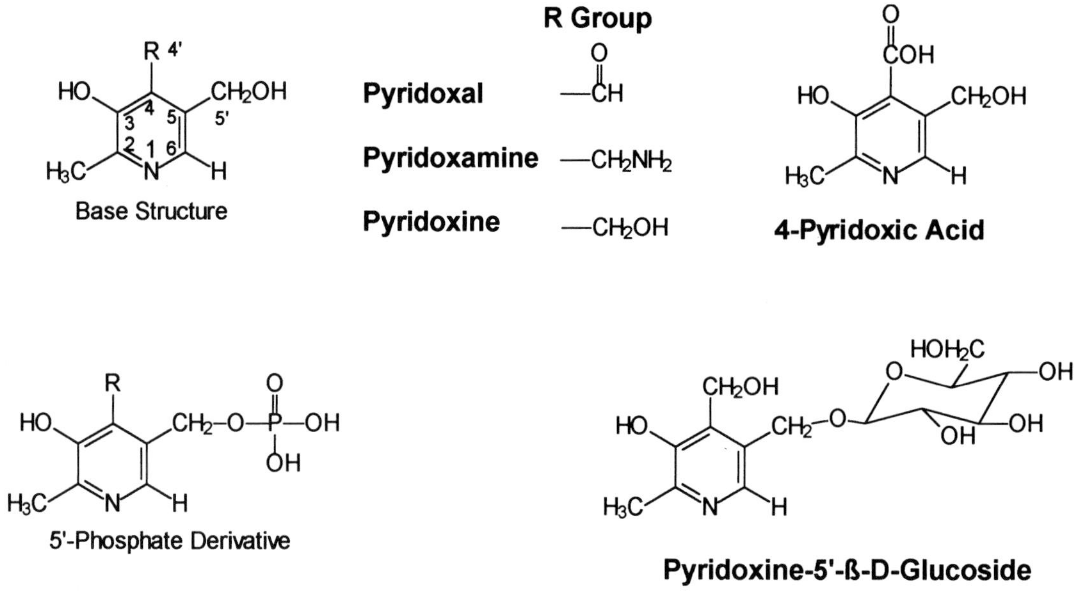

Fig. 25.1. Chemical structures of vitamin B_6 compounds.

β-glycosidic bond (34). Pyridoxine-5′-β-D-glucoside (35, 114) is generally the major glycosylated form of vitamin B_6 (Figure 25.1).

Overview of Vitamin B_6 Metabolism

Intestinal absorption takes place mainly in the jejunum by nonsaturable, passive diffusion of the nonphosphorylated forms of the vitamin (45). Dietary pyridoxal 5′-phosphate and pyridoxamine phosphate undergo enzymatic dephosphorylation before absorption. As summarized in Figure 25.2, postabsorptive phosphorylation of pyridoxal, pyridoxine, and pyridoxamine is catalyzed by pyridoxal kinase. Phosphorylation of these forms of vitamin B_6 constitutes a form of cellular metabolic trapping in intestinal mucosal cells and in other tissues (e.g., liver, muscle, brain) because the charge on the phosphate hinders efflux through the cell membrane. The uptake of nonphosphorylated forms of vitamin B_6 is mediated by a specific saturable transporter in the plasma membrane of hepatocytes and potentially other cells (54). Conversion of pyridoxine phosphate and pyridoxamine phosphate is catalyzed by flavin mononucleotide-dependent pyridoxine (pyridoxamine) 5′-phosphate oxidase to yield pyridoxal 5′-phosphate. Aside from the phosphorylation of pyridoxamine to form pyridoxamine phosphate, pyridoxamine phosphate also is formed as an intermediate of enzymatic transamination reactions in which aminotransferases catalyze pyridoxal 5′-phosphate-mediated movement of an NH_2 group from an amino acid to a keto acid. Pyridoxine (pyridoxamine) 5′-phosphate oxidase exhibits strong inhibition by its product, pyri-

doxal 5′-phosphate (74). This inhibition tends to protect cells from accumulating potentially toxic concentrations of pyridoxal 5′-phosphate even when vitamin B_6 intake is relatively high. The coenzymatic function of pyridoxal 5′-phosphate and its interconversion with pyridoxamine phosphate in aminotransferases are based on formation of a Schiff base between the amino group of the substrate and pyridoxal 5′-phosphate, generally followed by shifting of double bonds to facilitate the catalyzed reaction (e.g., transfer of the amino group to form pyridoxamine phosphate). This general type of mechanism is typical of most pyridoxal 5′-phosphate-mediated enzymatic processes.

The ratios of phosphorylated and nonphosphorylated forms of vitamin B_6 vary depending on the particular tissue, although pyridoxal 5′-phosphate and pyridoxamine phosphate predominate in most tissues. Dephosphorylation of pyridoxal 5′-phosphate and pyridoxamine phosphate occurs in mammalian cells by nonspecific phosphatase activity, as well as by a B_6-specific form of alkaline phosphatase (27). There are no true storage forms of vitamin B_6 in mammalian tissues. All forms of vitamin B_6 either serve as functional coenzymes (i.e., pyridoxal 5′-phosphate and pyridoxamine phosphate) or are metabolic intermediates in the dynamically interconnected reactions constituting vitamin B_6 metabolism. The most common form of vitamin B_6 catabolism is the oxidation of pyridoxal to 4-pyridoxic acid catalyzed by aldehyde oxidase and aldehyde dehydrogenase enzymes (98).

The liver is the major site of vitamin B_6 metabolism in the body. A model of vitamin B_6 metabolism in liver has been devised based on in vivo assays of enzymatic reactions measured under physiologically relevant conditions (65) that indicates the following:

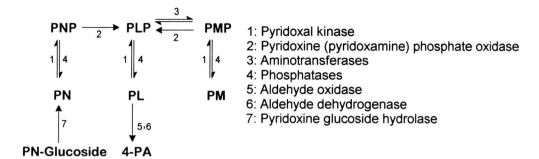

Fig. 25.2. Overview of vitamin B$_6$ metabolism. (PN, pyridoxine; PNP, pyridoxine phosphate; PL, pyridoxal; PLP, pyridoxal 5'-phosphate; PA, pyridoxic acid; PM, pyridoxamine; PMP, pyridoxamine phosphate.)

1. The hepatic rate of vitamin B$_6$ phosphorylation exceeds that of dephosphorylation.
2. The rate of oxidation of pyridoxal to 4-pyridoxic acid is comparable to the rate of pyridoxal phosphorylation, which suggests rapid conversion of pyridoxal to 4-pyridoxic acid as well as to pyridoxal 5'-phosphate.
3. Essentially all tissues can phosphorylate pyridoxal, pyridoxine, and pyridoxamine, whereas liver is the main tissue that can convert pyridoxine phosphate and pyridoxamine phosphate to pyridoxal 5'-phosphate. This supports the belief that the liver is the main site of conversion of pyridoxine and pyridoxamine to pyridoxal 5'-phosphate.

Interorgan transport of vitamin B$_6$ appears to occur via plasma pyridoxal. Although the primary form of vitamin B$_6$ in plasma is pyridoxal 5'-phosphate bound to albumin, its uptake into cells would be less favorable than that of the nonphosphorylated forms.

Forms of Vitamin B$_6$ in Foods and Supplements

Vitamin B$_6$ is found in many types of foods. Meats (including fish) are excellent sources, as are legumes and bananas; potatoes, whole grain cereal products, and many vegetables are good sources. Fortified breakfast cereals and vitamin supplements are also significant sources (28, 51). The major forms of vitamin B$_6$ in foods of animal origin (meats, dairy products, and eggs) include pyridoxal 5'-phosphate, pyridoxamine phosphate, pyridoxal, and pyridoxamine. Pyridoxal 5'-phosphate and pyridoxamine phosphate typically are the most abundant in vivo forms of vitamin B$_6$ in most animal tissues. Pyridoxine accounts for a small fraction of the total vitamin B$_6$ in animal tissues and products (meats, dairy products, and eggs). Glycosylated forms of vitamin B$_6$ do not exist in significant quanti-

ties in animal tissues and products; however, foods of plant origin (e.g., fruits, vegetables, grains, legumes) contain from 5% to 75% of their vitamin B$_6$ in glycosylated form. The total concentration and relative proportions of aldehyde (pyridoxal 5'-phosphate and pyridoxal) and amine (pyridoxamine phosphate and pyridoxamine) forms of vitamin B$_6$ differ among tissues. Nonenzymatic transamination reactions that occur during the cooking, storage, or thermal processing of foods can dramatically alter the ratios of aldehyde and amine forms of the vitamin (33). Pyridoxine β-D-glucoside accounts for a high proportion of total vitamin B$_6$ in many common plant-derived foods, with a mean of perhaps one third of total vitamin B$_6$ (34, 35, 58). Glycosylated vitamin B$_6$ constitutes approximately 15% of the vitamin B$_6$ in many common diets, with a wide range depending on food selection patterns. A typical mixed diet may include all of the various forms of vitamin B$_6$ except pyridoxine phosphate, which is a quantitatively minor intermediate in vitamin B$_6$ metabolism. Differences in in vivo kinetics among pyridoxine, pyridoxal, and pyridoxamine have been reported (113), but all are effectively absorbed and metabolically utilized.

Vitamin B$_6$ in food exhibits generally good stability during many forms of storage and handling, although large losses can occur during prolonged cooking or thermal processing (33). Pyridoxine exhibits greater stability than other forms of vitamin. Perhaps the most notable case of nutritionally important loss of vitamin B$_6$ in thermal processing is the frequently cited incident in which a nonfortified canned infant formula was associated with the onset of convulsive seizures in infants (24). The addition of pyridoxine to infant formulas alleviated the problem because of its greater thermal stability compared with the naturally occurring forms of vitamin B$_6$ in the milk-based formula (42).

Pyridoxine, as the hydrochloride salt, is used in dietary supplements and in food fortification because of its stability, relative lack of chemical reactivity, comparative ease of manufacture, and low cost. Addition of pyridoxine to foods is mainly limited to breakfast cereals and meal replacement products. Despite a recommendation that pyridoxine be included in enriched flour (29), this practice has never been adopted in the United States. Only thiamin, niacin, riboflavin, and, more recently, folic acid are added under current flour enrichment policy.

Occasionally, pyridoxal or pyridoxal 5′-phosphate are marketed or used experimentally as nutritional supplements. The metabolic benefit of pyridoxal or pyridoxal 5′-phosphate supplements relative to pyridoxine, if any, is unclear. Another minor form of supplemental vitamin B_6 is a pyridoxine α-ketoglutarate complex. In a study cited in support of pyridoxine α-ketoglutarate supplements, administration of pyridoxine α-ketoglutarate at 30 mg pyridoxine α-ketoglutarate/kg body weight (corresponding to 1,125 mg pyridoxine and 973 mg α-ketoglutarate in a 70 kg man) reduced peak blood lactate in trained nonathletic subjects and slightly increased maximal oxygen consumption (67). However, a later study of trained cyclists given pyridoxine α-ketoglutarate at 50 mg/kg showed no significant effect of the supplement on blood lactate concentration or power output during exercise (61). Thus, evidence of metabolic benefit of pyridoxine α-ketoglutarate in exercise is at best equivocal, and doses used in these studies would now be considered as causing risk of pyridoxine toxicity, as discussed later in this chapter.

Bioavailability of Vitamin B_6

The bioavailability of nutrients in foods and supplements is an important issue in evaluating the adequacy of diets and the efficacy of supplements in meeting nutritional requirements and resolving inadequate status. The bioavailability of vitamin B_6 has been reviewed (34). Initial interest in this topic arose largely in response to the infant formula incident discussed previously. Tomarelli et al. (100) examined milk-based, unfortified formulas that had been heat-sterilized during the canning process. They found different responses when assaying for vitamin B_6 by microbial and rat bioassays, which were interpreted as evidence that the heat sterilization had reduced the bioavailability of the vitamin B_6. Reexamination of this issue suggested that thermal destruction or other reactions of the naturally occurring forms of vitamin B_6, not the hypothesized reduced bioavailability of the remaining vitamin B_6, caused nutritional inferiority of the unfortified formula (34).

The overall bioavailability of vitamin B_6 in a mixed diet is approximately 75% (99). Incomplete bioavailability is probably due to several factors including entrapment in cellular structure and nondigestible residue and partial utilization of glycosylated forms of vitamin B_6 (34), primarily pyridoxine-5′-β-D-glucoside (35, 114). Isotopic studies in rats and humans have indicated effective absorption of pyridoxine-glucoside but incomplete enzymatic hydrolysis to release

the pyridoxine moiety for metabolic utilization (36, 48, 79). This hydrolysis is catalyzed primarily by a novel intestinal mucosal cytosolic enzyme designated pyridoxine-β-D-glucoside hydrolase (70). Purified pyridoxine-glucoside exhibits approximately 50% bioavailability relative to pyridoxine in humans (36, 79), which exceeds bioavailability in rats (34, 36, 48). Incomplete bioavailability of naturally occurring glycosylated vitamin B_6 in foods also has been demonstrated in humans (41, 50, 58). In summary, vitamin B_6 bioavailability is incomplete in typical human diets and is expected to vary depending on food selection.

In Vivo Kinetics of Vitamin B_6

Many studies of in vivo kinetics have been conducted with the objective of determining the size of the various body vitamin B_6 pools and their rate of turnover (19). Interpretation of studies of short-term kinetics is complicated by the fact that a high percentage of the vitamin B_6 exists as pyridoxal 5′-phosphate associated with glycogen phosphorylase in muscle, a pool that turns over very slowly relative to the vitamin B_6 compounds in other tissues. A novel estimate was based on estimates of total muscle mass and direct analysis of muscle sampled from volunteers (20). This analysis indicated total muscle vitamin B_6 pools of 917 ± 319 μmol for women and 850 ± 216 μmol for men. Assuming that muscle accounts for approximately 80% of the vitamin B_6 in the body, the estimated total body B_6 pool is approximately 1,000 μmol (~170 mg total vitamin B_6, expressed as pyridoxine equivalents). One can estimate that at an intake of 1.8 mg total dietary B_6 per day and 75% bioavailability, approximately 0.8% of the whole body vitamin B_6 pool is lost daily by excretion or catabolism and is replaced by newly absorbed vitamin B_6. During periods of rapid growth and development, much of the vitamin B_6 requirement provides coenzymes needed in new tissues (18). Another interesting finding regarding the behavior of in vivo vitamin B_6 is that there is little or no loss of muscle vitamin B_6 during periods of moderate dietary deficiency (21). Extensions in the use of stable-isotope labeled tracers will allow an expanded understanding of whole-body vitamin B_6 metabolism in various conditions of nutritional adequacy, physiological states (e.g., pregnancy and lactation), and disease states (19).

Vitamin B_6 Nutrition and Health

Assessment of Vitamin B_6 Nutritional Status and Recommended Allowances

Many biochemical criteria have been devised for the assessment of vitamin B_6 status (57, 58, 86). The more commonly used approaches include pyridoxal 5′-phosphate concentration in plasma or erythrocytes, total vitamin B$_6$ concentration in plasma, urinary 4-pyridoxic acid or total vitamin B$_6$ excretion, the activity of aminotransferases (aspartate or alanine) in erythrocytes, and the degree of stimulation of these enzymes by the in vitro addition of pyridoxal 5′-phosphate (Table 25.1). The latter methods are based on the principle that cellular vitamin B$_6$ status (at least in erythrocytes) is reflected closely by the degree of stimulation of enzyme activity when assayed with and without added pyridoxal 5′-phosphate. Such methods provide functional information by indirectly reflecting pyridoxal 5′-phosphate concentration within the erythrocytes relative to the pyridoxal 5′-phosphate affinity of the apoenzyme, but their use is declining because of cumbersome methods and lack of standardization.

By far the most commonly used criterion for status assessment is plasma pyridoxal 5′-phosphate. Its use is based on observations that plasma pyridoxal 5′-phosphate concentration is closely related to the concentration of pyridoxal 5′-phosphate in tissues (30, 66) and, thus, provides a measure of long-term nutritional status. Pyridoxal 5′-phosphate can be readily measured with appropriately validated chromatographic or enzymatic methods, although methods based on direct analysis of plasma without deproteination would underestimate pyridoxal 5′-phosphate concentration. Although plasma pyridoxal 5′-phosphate is appropriate for status assessment in most cases, plasma pyridoxal 5′-phosphate concentration is not an accurate indicator of vitamin B$_6$ status in individuals with altered activity of plasma phosphatase (111). In this regard, tests of urinary 4-pyridoxic acid excretion or activities of erythrocyte aminotransferases are potential alternatives (Table 25.1) (58, 59, 86). It should be recognized that 4-pyridoxic acid excretion is more sensitive to recent vitamin B$_6$ intake than is plasma pyridoxal 5′-phosphate. Although urinary 4-pyridoxic acid excretion is generally based on a 24-hour urine collection, measurement of the 4-pyridoxic acid/creatinine ratio in random urine collections appears to be equally informative (88).

The need also exists for functional indicators for conclusive nutritional assessment. Conclusions based on the use of functional indicators do not always agree with static indices such as plasma pyridoxal 5′-phosphate concentration. For example, a study of patients with cirrhosis indicated effective utilization of pyridoxine supplements based on the response of plasma forms of vitamin B$_6$ despite the fact that abnormalities of amino acid metabolism were not normalized (44).

Because of the many metabolic functions of vitamin B$_6$, many metabolites can be functional indicators of vitamin B$_6$ status. Changes in plasma concentration or urinary excretion of tryptophan metabolites derived

Table 25.1. Indices for Assessment of Vitamin B$_6$ Status and Suggested Minimal Values for Adequate Status.[a]

Index	Adequate Status
Direct	
Plasma pyridoxal 5′-phosphate	> 30 nmol/L[b]
Plasma total vitamin B$_6$	> 40 nmol/L
Urinary 4-pyridoxic acid	> 3 μmol/day
Urinary total vitamin B$_6$	> 0.5 μmol/day
Indirect	
Erythrocyte alanine aminotransferase coenzyme stimulation index[c]	< 1.25
Erythrocyte aspartate aminotransferase coenzyme stimulation index[c]	< 1.80
2 g L-tryptophan load, urinary xanthurenic acid	< 65 μmol/day
3 g L-methionine load, urinary cystathionine	< 350 μmol/day
Dietary Intake	
Vitamin B$_6$ intake, weekly average	> 1.25–1.5 mg/day
Vitamin B$_6$:protein ratio	≥ 0.016 mg/g

[a] Adapted from Leklem (57), with permission.
[b] Plasma pyridoxal 5′-phosphate < 20 nmol/L is considered indicative of deficiency.
[c] Coenzyme stimulation index is the ratio of enzyme activity values measured with and without preincubation of the erythrocyte hemolysate with added pyridoxal 5′-phosphate. This index is proportional to the fraction of enzyme in apoenzyme form.

from pyridoxal 5′-phosphate-dependent reactions were the first functional indicators used (58). As discussed in other chapters, plasma homocysteine levels are governed by several factors including the rate and extent of methyl group generation (as 5-methyltetrahydrofolate), rate of synthesis of homocysteine, rates of homocysteine catabolism and remethylation processes, and efficiency of renal handling of homocysteine.

Fasting homocysteine concentration is only a weak function of vitamin B$_6$ status (17, 77, 96, 97). Under fasting conditions, remethylation reactions apparently have sufficient capacity so that the steady-state plasma concentration of homocysteine is relatively unchanged by the reduced efficiency of the pyridoxal 5′-phosphate-dependent transsulfuration reactions. Because fasting homocysteine levels are much less sensitive to vitamin B$_6$ deficiency than to folate deficiency (and, presumably, cobalamin deficiency), fasting homocysteine is not a good indicator of vitamin B$_6$ status. In contrast, elevation of homocysteine following a methionine load is diagnostic primarily for effects of inadequate vitamin B_6 status (76, 104). The methionine load test is discussed in Chapter 19. Other metabolites in plasma that may provide functional markers of vitamin B_6 deficiency include elevated cystathionine and intermediates of other pyridoxal 5′-phosphate-dependent pathways (104). Cystathionine elevation in vitamin B_6 deficiency may also be influenced with faster turnover of γ-cystathionase (104). The use of cystathionine or other such metabolites in the assessment of vitamin B_6 status requires further study and standardization.

What Is an Adequate Intake of Vitamin B_6?

The Institute of Medicine/National Academy of Sciences has thoroughly reviewed and reassessed requirements for B vitamins, including vitamin B_6 (28). They proposed an Estimated Average Requirement for total vitamin B_6 in men and women (19 to 50 years) of 1.1 mg/day and a Recommended Dietary Allowance of 1.3 mg/day, which is the Estimated Average Requirement adjusted upward by an assumed coefficient of variation. Many studies have shown an apparent increase of vitamin B_6 requirement with increasing protein intake, although some have argued that the precision of the requirement is not improved by including an adjustment for protein intake (28). This assessment of the Estimated Average Requirement was supported, in part, by an observation that 0.5 mg/day was sufficient to prevent the observed electroencephalographic changes associated with pronounced dietary depletion (55).

Some comment is needed regarding the apparent requirements determined in several other studies that differ somewhat from the new Recommended Dietary Allowance. A well-conducted depletion-repletion study indicated that a mean of 1.94 mg/day was needed to return several B_6 status indicators to predepletion levels (46), although this amount exceeds an optimal intake under steady-state conditions. A depletion-repletion study evaluating immune function in elderly subjects indicated that intakes of 1.90 ± 0.18 mg/day for women and 2.88 ± 0.17 mg/day for men were necessary to return interleukin-2 production and lymphocyte proliferation to predepletion levels (75), which suggests that steady-state had not been reached in vitamin B_6 status. Examination of plasma pyridoxal 5′-phosphate values and estimated dietary intakes in subjects from the Framingham study indicated that plasma homocysteine was significantly elevated in the lowest decile of vitamin B_6 intake (mean, 1.33 mg/day) but was not significantly elevated in the second lowest decile (mean, 1.57 mg/day) (90). Interpretation of this study is complicated somewhat by the uncertain absolute accuracy of estimations of vitamin B_6 intake.

What is the Vitamin B_6 Status of American and Other Populations?

Vitamin B_6 Intake Dietary intake data from national surveys have been summarized recently (28). An aggregate evaluation of surveys indicated a median vitamin B_6 intake of approximately 2.0 mg/day for men and 1.5 mg/day for women (28). Although the median values appear reasonably adequate, the data also indicated a high proportion of individuals at risk from very low intakes. The following percentages of population groups were estimated to consume less vitamin B_6 than the Estimated Average Requirement: males > 50 years, 10% to 25%; women > 50 years, 25% to 50%; women 19 to 50 years, 15%; pregnant women, 25% to 50%; lactating women, 10% to 15%. Earlier data from the Second National Health and Nutrition Examination Survey indicated that mean intake of vitamin B_6 was 1.48 mg/day for the total population, 1.85 for males, and 1.14 for females (51). Estimates of dietary vitamin B_6 intake of ~80,000 women in the Nurse's Health Study indicated a median intake of 1.1 mg/day in the lowest quintile (82).

A consistent finding among studies such as these is that a substantial proportion of subjects sampled, especially women, consumed low amounts of vitamin B_6 relative to recommended intakes. A study involving direct analysis of diet composites from pregnant and postpartum women (81) showed vitamin B_6 intakes of approximately 50% of respective Recommended Dietary Allowance values. These low intakes were confirmed in a further analysis of diet composites collected from lactating women (2). In total, these studies clearly indicate that dietary intake of vitamin B_6 is inadequate in significant portions of the US population. Data from European studies yield a similar conclusion (13, 64, 107).

Assessment of Vitamin B_6 Nutritional Status The most commonly accepted criteria for interpretation of vitamin B_6 status are presented in Table 25.1. Most recent assessments of nutritional status of populations have been conducted using plasma pyridoxal 5′-phosphate < 20 nmol/L as the primary indicator of inadequacy (58). A study of elderly subjects from Framingham indicated a mean plasma pyridoxal 5′-phosphate of 18.1 nmol/L in the lowest decile (see Figure 23.1 in Chapter 23), which indicates inadequate status in approximately 10% of subjects (90). These data are similar to those reported in other studies. Analysis of metabolites providing functional indices of vitamin B_6, cobalamin, and folate status in elderly individuals indicated that poor status is prevalent for all three vitamins (49).

Clinical Causes of Vitamin B_6 Deficiency

Aside from dietary inadequacy, vitamin B_6 deficiency can be caused by several clinical defects in absorption of dietary forms of vitamin B$_6$, impaired metabolic activation to pyridoxal 5'-phosphate, or excessive clearance (72). Celiac disease is an example of a generalized malabsorption syndrome associated with poor vitamin B$_6$ status. Vitamin B$_6$ nutriture, as indicated by plasma pyridoxal 5'-phosphate concentration and functional indices, improves when the disease is in remission (80).

Evidence of low vitamin B$_6$ status has been reported in patients with cirrhosis, cancer, diabetes, renal disease, Hodgkin's disease, and sickle cell disease (59). In most cases, it is unclear whether these observations reflect impaired formation of pyridoxal 5'-phosphate, increased metabolic needs, altered catabolism, or inadequate intake. Perhaps the only situation in which this question has been examined is in alcoholic cirrhosis, in which conversion of pyridoxine to pyridoxal 5'-phosphate is impaired (44).

During pregnancy, many indicators of vitamin B$_6$ nutritional status frequently decline even with adequate intake. For example, an intake between 5.5 and 7.6 mg pyridoxine/day is needed to maintain plasma pyridoxal 5'-phosphate at prepregnancy levels (89), although an intake of 1.9 mg/day appears to be adequate to meet maternal and fetal needs (28).

Interpretation of vitamin B$_6$ nutritional status is also complicated in aging, which is associated with a general decline in plasma pyridoxal 5'-phosphate concentrations and other indicators. Bates et al. (5) reported that both plasma pyridoxal 5'-phosphate and urinary pyridoxic acid declined with increasing age and frailty in Great Britain. This decline was partly attributable to reduced intake of vitamin B$_6$, but inflammation, acute phase response, and renal function were also confounding variables.

As discussed previously, individuals with hypophosphatasia exhibit markedly elevated plasma pyridoxal 5'-phosphate concentration because of a lack of the tissue nonspecific alkaline phosphatase (111). Analysis of tissues from patients with hypophosphatasia indicated unremarkable concentrations of total vitamin B$_6$ and distributions of vitamer forms, which suggests that the elevation in plasma pyridoxal 5'-phosphate is not an indicator of high vitamin B$_6$ nutritional status (110). The authors concluded that tissue nonspecific alkaline phosphatase missing in hypophosphatasia regulates only extracellular pyridoxal 5'-phosphate concentrations. Although severe hypophosphatasia is a rare inborn error, milder forms may be more prevalent, which may complicate the use of plasma pyridoxal 5'-phosphate as an indicator of vitamin B$_6$ status in the general population. Because of the growing awareness of nonnutritional factors that can influence the concentration of plasma pyridoxal 5'-phosphate, many nutritionists feel that assessment of vitamin B$_6$ status

should not be based solely on the measurement of plasma pyridoxal 5'-phosphate.

Clinical Consequences of Inadequate Vitamin B$_6$ Status

Overt deficiency of vitamin B$_6$ is rare or nonexistent in most developed countries. The consequences of chronic inadequacy of vitamin B$_6$ have been reviewed previously (58). Chronically marginal vitamin B$_6$ status can cause a microcytic anemia owing to the pyridoxal 5'-phosphate-dependence of δ-aminolevulinic acid synthase in heme synthesis. In most cases of vitamin B$_6$ inadequacy, low plasma pyridoxal 5'-phosphate and other biochemical parameters, including abnormal methionine load test results, are the only detectable indices of deficiency. Severe deficiency can cause abnormalities in neurological function, as illustrated by convulsions observed in a small percentage of infants consuming a vitamin B$_6$-deficient formula (24). Abnormal electroencephalographic patterns have been seen in experimentally depleted women and men (15, 55) but not in a similar study with men at similar levels of intake (32). It is unlikely that neurological dysfunction would be a concern in most levels of dietary vitamin B$_6$ deficiency. Most attention currently is on vitamin B$_6$ as a component of the group of vitamins affecting one-carbon metabolism and homocysteine metabolism.

Adequate vitamin B$_6$ is essential for maternal and fetal well-being during pregnancy (28). A possible direct connection with neonatal status is the finding that infants exhibited poorer condition at birth (i.e., lower Apgar scores) when mothers had low vitamin B$_6$ status (89).

Vitamin B$_6$ Antagonists: Natural Antagonists and Drug-B$_6$ Interactions

Several types of naturally occurring antagonists of vitamin B$_6$ have been identified (53). These compounds apparently have little impact on the vitamin B$_6$ nutritional status of individuals consuming typical diets.

Several pharmaceuticals exhibit antivitamin B$_6$ properties (4, 105). The mechanism of drug effects on vitamin B$_6$ most frequently involves formation of a stable complex typically involving condensation of a reactive amino group of the drug or a metabolite with the carbonyl group of pyridoxal 5'-phosphate. Such interactions cause depletion of pyridoxal 5'-phosphate available for coenzymatic function, and the drug-pyridoxal 5'-phosphate complex is itself an inhibitor of certain enzymes. Isoniazid, which is used to treat tuberculosis, is a well-known vitamin B$_6$ antagonist by virtue of its ability to complex with pyridoxal 5'-phosphate in vivo (91). There is no direct interaction between pyridoxine and isoniazid or related drugs having reactive amino groups; their antagonistic effect is solely mediated through complexing with pyridoxal 5'-phosphate. Persons who acetylate isoniazid slowly are at increased risk for the neurological toxicity of vitamin B_6 deficiency. Similar B_6 antagonism has been reported with cycloserine, hydralazine, dopamine, phenelzine, and gentamycin. Supplementation with pyridoxine usually can prevent or alleviate deficiency symptoms without lessening the therapeutic benefit of the drug (6). Theophylline, used in asthma therapy, acts through an apparently different mechanism. Rather than directly complexing with pyridoxal 5'-phosphate, theophylline exerts its antivitamin effect by inhibiting pyridoxal kinase, an enzyme critical in the conversion of pyridoxine to pyridoxal 5'-phosphate (103).

Probably the most commonly used vitamin B_6 antagonist is ethanol. Chronic alcohol abuse is frequently associated with poor vitamin B_6 status owing to poor diet and is probably aggravated by antagonism from the ethanol metabolite, acetaldehyde. Acetaldehyde competes with and displaces pyridoxal 5'-phosphate from binding sites, which increases its susceptibility to dephosphorylation and catabolism (65). Consequently, pyridoxine at moderate levels is a logical component in the nutritional management of alcoholism. Alcoholics, especially those with poor vitamin B_6 nutritional status, are at risk for the development of sideroblastic anemia (62).

Sideroblastic anemia and sideroblastic bone marrow are characterized by the accumulation of non-heme iron in mitochondria and impairment of normal mitochondrial heme synthesis. In their thorough review, Lindenbaum and Roman (62) concluded that there is no clear evidence linking vitamin B_6 depletion causally in the etiology of sideroblastic anemia. Sideroblastic anemias can be hereditary, induced by acquired clonal mutations of blood cells, or drug- or toxin-induced in origin but are nevertheless often at least partially pyridoxine-responsive. The "pyridoxine-responsive" nature of sideroblastic anemia apparently is bifunctional: 1) cellular pyridoxal 5'-phosphate levels can be partially increased by a mass-action effect overcoming the antagonistic effect of ethanol on pyridoxal 5'-phosphate synthesis, and 2) this increase in coenzyme concentration can partially increase the activity of pyridoxal 5'-phosphate-dependent erythroid δ-aminolevulinate synthase. Polymorphism of the gene encoding this enzyme has been identified, with several of the gene products having reduced enzymatic activity and apparently altered pyridoxal 5'-phosphate-binding affinity (23, 69). Sideroblastic anemia does not always respond to pharmacological therapy with pyridoxine. Reduction or prevention of excessive iron accumulation often helps to improve the response to pyridoxine treatment (23).

Shortly after the introduction of oral contraceptives in the mid-1960s, reports of impairment of vitamin B_6 nutritional status or functional indicators of pyridoxal 5'-phosphate-dependent metabolic processes were published (58, 59). However, a more recent report that compared seven low-dose oral contraceptives showed no significant effect on vitamin B_6 status and no significant difference among the seven oral contraceptive formulations tested (108). These results suggest that low-dose combined formulations (i.e., ethinylestradiol plus a progestogen) may be less antagonistic toward vitamin B_6 than earlier preparations. Further studies are needed to assess effects of newer steroidal contraceptives on vitamin B_6 metabolism and function.

Vitamin B_6 Toxicity

It is essential to recognize the potential toxicity of excessive intake of vitamin B_6 when supplements are taken (e.g., recommended sometimes for pyridoxine-responsive anemia as discussed previously, premenstrual syndrome, and carpal tunnel syndrome). The effect of pyridoxine supplements in such disorders appears to be pharmacological and not indicative of a nutritional deficiency, and therapeutic benefit has been difficult to demonstrate clearly (58, 59). Excessive pyridoxine intake can cause neurotoxicity manifested as sensory neuropathy (87), which apparently occurs as direct toxicity of unmetabolized pyridoxine. Reviews of dose-response relationships indicate that greatest risk occurs in the range of > 1000 mg/day (22, 28). The Institute of Medicine (28) defined the no-observed-adverse-effect level of 200 mg/day based on dose-response data and the widespread use of pyridoxine in the range of ~100 to 200 mg/day with little or no incidence of peripheral neuropathy. It should also be recognized that tissue concentrations of vitamin B_6 coenzymes would be maximized at far lower intakes owing to the saturability of kinase and oxidase enzymes involved in their synthesis. Thus, the clinical benefit of pyridoxine supplementation in the range of ≥ 100 mg/day is questionable.

Vitamin B_6 in Homocysteine Metabolism and Its Role in Human Health

Influence of Vitamin B_6 Nutritional Status on Homocysteine and One-Carbon Metabolism

As discussed previously, the concentration of homocysteine in fasting plasma is weakly related to vitamin B_6 status. Apparently impairment in the transsulfuration pathway in vitamin B_6 deficiency has little effect during fasting conditions because remethylation reactions are sufficient to maintain near-normal homocysteine levels. The principle of the methionine load test is that the bolus of exogenous methionine causes an elevation in plasma homocysteine because remethylation reactions cannot accommodate the entire load of substrate. Thus, the rise in plasma homocysteine is inversely related to the flux through the transsulfuration pathway. This effect is accentuated in pronounced vitamin B$_6$ deficiency by the fact that S-adenosylmethionine tends to be reduced, which may secondarily alter homocysteine remethylation (76). The importance of the methionine load test as a diagnostic procedure is best illustrated by the findings of Bostom et al. (9), in which more than 40% of individuals with postmethionine hyperhomocysteinemia did not exhibit elevated fasting plasma homocysteine.

The influence of vitamin B$_6$ status on cytosolic and mitochondrial serine hydroxymethyltransferase isozymes is unclear. A preliminary study in the author's laboratory with rats indicated that vitamin B$_6$ deficiency caused reduced flux of carbon from serine to remethylate homocysteine (i.e., via serine hydroxymethyltransferase), whereas total hepatic serine hydroxymethyltransferase activity was correspondingly reduced and homocysteine concentration in liver and plasma was elevated (68). Thus, inadequate vitamin B$_6$ status may suppress the acquisition and processing of one-carbon units, as well as interfere with transsulfuration. It appears prudent that any vitamin supplementation regimen intended to control homocysteine levels include pyridoxine, as well as folic acid and cobalamin.

Asthmatic patients treated with theophylline exhibit abnormal postmethionine load homocysteine response owing to the drug-induced reduction in vitamin B$_6$ status (104). Supplementation with 20 mg/day pyridoxine yielded a reduction in postmethionine load homocysteine in individuals taking theophylline, but not in apparently adequately nourished control subjects (104). A previous study also indicated that vitamin B$_6$ supplementation lessens the neurological side effects of theophylline (4).

Hyperhomocysteinemia commonly occurs in end-stage renal disease and may contribute to an increased risk of vascular disease (8, 84, 92). Patients with end-stage renal disease frequently exhibit vitamin B$_6$ and folate deficiency (10–12, 84). Bostom et al. (10) examined fasting and postmethionine load homocysteine levels in renal transplant recipients and found that renal function was related to both forms of hyperhomocysteinemia, which suggests inadequate status with respect to both folate and vitamin B$_6$. A study of vitamin supplementation in renal transplant recipients indicated that a mixed dose of 50 mg/day pyridoxine,

5 mg/day folic acid, and 0.4 mg/day cobalamin yielded a 26.2% reduction in fasting plasma homocysteine and a 22.1% reduction in postmethionine load plasma homocysteine concentration (9). These effects are similar to those reported in a study of supplementation (folic acid plus pyridoxine) of patients with cardiovascular disease and mild hyperhomocysteinemia (107). A high incidence of mild hyperhomocysteinemia concurrent with low folate and vitamin B$_6$ status also has been observed in heart transplant patients and is associated with vascular disease complications (38).

Vitamin B$_6$ Status and Risk of Vascular Disease Associated with Aberrant One-Carbon Metabolism

Although hyperhomocysteinemia under fasting and postmethionine load conditions is a risk factor for various forms of vascular disease and folate and vitamin B$_6$ status affects each dramatically (25), such data do not definitively establish a causal relationship. The data also do not establish whether reduction of plasma homocysteine concentration by vitamin supplementation would reduce the risk of disease. However, several epidemiological studies provide strong evidence of links between vitamin B$_6$ nutritional status and health.

Rimm et al. (82) examined data regarding coronary heart disease and vitamin intake from more than 80,000 women in the Nurse's Health Study. Women in the highest quintile of intake of vitamin B$_6$, folate, or vitamin B$_6$ plus folate exhibited a significantly lower incidence of coronary heart disease compared with women in the lowest quintile of intake. This relationship was equally robust for total intake of each vitamin (i.e., diet plus supplements) and intake from dietary sources alone. Interpretation of the individual effects of each vitamin was complicated somewhat because of the close correlation between intake of folate and vitamin B$_6$ owing to their presence in supplements and fortified cereals. These data extend the findings of Verhoef et al. (109), who reported that dietary intake and plasma concentrations of vitamin B$_6$ (plasma pyridoxal 5'-phosphate) and folate were lower in patients with myocardial infarction than in control subjects and that both vitamins were inversely associated with the risk.

The results of a multicenter trial examining fasting and postmethionine load plasma homocysteine, plasma pyridoxal 5'-phosphate concentration, and incidence of vascular disease were reported by Robinson et al. (83). Consistent with the conclusions of Rimm et al. (82), in healthy control subjects low folate or vitamin B$_6$ status increased risk of vascular disease. This study yielded the unexpected finding that the risk of vascular disease in subjects with low vitamin B$_6$ status was independent of *both* fasting and postmethionine load homocysteine concentration. These findings suggest that vitamin B_6 deficiency also contributes to the risk of vascular disease by a mechanism independent of the concurrent impairment of the transsulfuration pathway.

Can Nutritional Intervention Reduce Plasma Homocysteine Concentration and Risk of Disease?

Most intervention studies that have included vitamin B_6 have involved multivitamin supplementation regimens. In view of the possible association of vitamin B_6 status with cardiovascular risk, it is prudent to maintain adequate nutritional status through an adequate diet and possibly with supplements providing an intake in the range of the Recommended Dietary Allowance value. Intakes of this magnitude will optimize static and functional indicators of vitamin B_6 status. At present there is no dose-response information regarding vitamin B_6 intakes and response of postmethionine load homocysteine. In addition, it is not known whether reduction of fasting plasma homocysteine or normalization of postmethionine load homocysteine response by vitamin supplementation will lessen the risk of vascular disease. A wide range of supplementation regimens has been used experimentally. These should not be viewed as optimal daily doses to normalize homocysteine metabolism in clinical studies and may be excessive: 0.4 to 5 mg folic acid with 0.5 mg cobalamin and 12.5 mg pyridoxine (63); 5 mg folic acid, 0.4 mg cobalamin, and 50 mg pyridoxine (26); 50 mg pyridoxine with or without 5 mg folic acid and/or 0.4 mg cobalamin (8); 250 mg pyridoxine and 5 mg folic acid (106); 240 mg pyridoxine and 10 mg folic acid (14).

Genetic Aspects of Vitamin B_6 in One-Carbon Metabolism

Genetic polymorphisms affect several enzymes of one-carbon metabolism, ranging from common polymorphisms (3) to much more deleterious mutations of 5,10-methylenetetrahydrofolate reductase (31) and cystathionine β-synthase (78). When Irish subjects were classified according to genotype for the 677C→T methylenetetrahydrofolate reductase polymorphism, values for plasma pyridoxal 5′-phosphate were within adequate ranges, and there was no significant relationship between genotype and pyridoxal 5′-phosphate values (112). Although evidence of genetic polymorphisms of pyridoxal 5′-phosphate-dependent serine hydroxymethyltransferase has been reported (3), the metabolic impact and the interrelationships with vitamin B_6 nutrition are unknown. The genetic basis, etiology, and pyridoxine-responsiveness of cystathionine

β-synthase deficiency disorders have been reviewed recently (78) and are discussed in Chapter 20.

REFERENCES

1. American Institute of Nutrition. Nomenclature policy: Generic descriptors and trivial names for vitamins and related compounds. *J Nutr* 1990; 120: 12–9.
2. Andon, MB, Reynolds, RD, Moser-Veillon, PB, Howard, MP. Dietary intake of total and glycosylated vitamin B_6 and the vitamin B_6 nutritional status of unsupplemented lactating women and their infants. *Am J Clin Nutr* 1989; 50: 1050–58.
3. Bailey, LB, Gregory, JF. Polymorphisms of methylenetetrahydrofolate reductase and other enzymes: Metabolic significance, risks and impact on folate requirement. *J Nutr* 1999; 129: 919–22.
4. Bartel, PR, Ubbink, JB, Delport, R, Lotz, BP, Becker, PJ. Vitamin B_6 supplementation and theophylline-related effects in humans. *Am J Clin Nutr* 1994; 60: 93–9.
5. Bates, CJ, Pentieva, KD, Prentice, A, Mansoor, MA, Finch, S. Plasma pyridoxal phosphate and pyridoxic acid and their relationship to plasma homocysteine in a representative sample of British men and women aged 65 years and over. *Br J Nutr* 1999; 81: 191–201.
6. Bhagavan, HN, Brin, M. Drug-vitamin B_6 interaction. *Curr Concepts Nutr* 1983; 12: 1–12.
7. Birch, TW, Gyorgy, P. Vitamin B_6 and methods for preparation in a concentrated state. *Biochem J* 1936; 30: 304–7.
8. Bostom, AG, Gohh, R, Beaulieu, AJ, Nadeau, MR, Hume, AL, Jacques, PF, Selhub, J, Rosenberg, IH. Treatment of hyperhomocysteinemia in renal transplant recipients. *Ann Intern Med* 1997; 127: 1089–92.
9. Bostom, AG, Gohh, RY, Tsai, MY, Hopkins-Garcia, BJ, Nadeau, MR, Bianchi, LA, Jacques, PF, Rosenberg, IH, Selhub, J. Excess prevalence of fasting and postmethionine-loading hyperhomocysteinemia in stable renal transplant recipients. *Arterioscler Thromb Vasc Biol* 1997; 17: 1894–1900.
10. Bostom, AG, Jacques, PF, Nadeau, MR, Williams, RR, Ellison, RC, Selhub, J. Post-methionine load hyperhomocysteinemia in persons with normal fasting total plasma homocysteine: Initial results from the NHLBI Family Heart Study. *Atherosclerosis* 1995; 116: 147–51.
11. Bostom, AG, Shemin, D, Gohh, RY, Verhoef, P, Nadeau, MR, Bianchi, LA, Hopkins-Garcia, BJ, Jacques, PF, Selhub, J, Dworkin, L, Rosenberg, IH. Lower fasting total plasma homocysteine levels in stable renal transplant recipients versus maintenance dialysis patients. *Transplant Proc* 1998; 30: 160–62.
12. Bostom, AG, Shemin, D, Verhoef, P, Nadeau, MR, Jacques, PF, Selhub, J, Dworkin, L, Rosenberg, IH. Elevated fasting total plasma homocysteine levels and cardiovascular disease outcomes in maintenance dialysis patients. A prospective study. *Arterioscler Thromb Vasc Biol* 1997; 17: 2554–58.
13. Brants, HA, Brussaard, JH, Bouman, M, Lowik, MR. Dietary intake among adults with special reference to vitamin B_6. *Eur J Clin Nutr* 1997; 51(Suppl 3): S25–31.

14. Brattstrom, L, Israelsson, B, Norrving, B, Bergqvist, D, Thorne, J, Hultberg, B, Hamfelt, A. Impaired homocysteine metabolism in early-onset cerebral and peripheral occlusive arterial disease. Effects of pyridoxine and folic acid treatment. *Atherosclerosis* 1990; 81: 51–60.

15. Canham, JE, Baker, EM, Harding, RS, Sauberlich, HE, Plough, IC. Dietary protein—its relationship to vitamin B$_6$ requirements and function. *Ann N Y Acad Sci* 1969; 166: 16–29.

16. Chanarin, I. Nutritional aspects of hematologic disorders. In *Modern Nutrition in Health and Disease,* 9th ed. (Shils, ME, Olson, JA, Shihe, M, Ross, AC, eds.). Williams & Wilkins, Baltimore, 1998; pp. 1719–37.

17. Clarke, R. Lowering blood homocysteine with folic acid supplements: Meta-analysis of randomised trials. *Br Med J* 1998; 316: 894–98.

18. Coburn, SP. A critical review of minimal vitamin B$_6$ requirements for growth in various species with a proposed method of calculation. *Vitam Horm* 1994; 48: 259–300.

19. Coburn, SP. Modeling vitamin B$_6$ metabolism. *Adv Food Nutr Res* 1996; 40: 107–32.

20. Coburn, SP, Lewis, DL, Fink, WJ, Mahuren, JD, Schaltenbrand, WE, Costill, DL. Human vitamin B$_6$ pools estimated through muscle biopsies. *Am J Clin Nutr* 1988; 48: 291–94.

21. Coburn, SP, Ziegler, PJ, Costill, DL, Mahuren, JD, Fink, WJ, Schaltenbrand, WE, Pauly, TA, Pearson, DR, Conn, PS, Guilarte, TR. Response of vitamin B$_6$ content of muscle to changes in vitamin B$_6$ intake in men. *Am J Clin Nutr* 1991; 53: 1436–42.

22. Cohen, M, Bendich, A. Safety of pyridoxine: A review of human and animal studies. *Toxicol Lett* 1986; 34: 129–39.

23. Cotter, PD, May, A, Li, L, Al-Sabah, AI, Fitzsimons, EJ, Cazzola, M, Bishop, DF. Four new mutations in the erythroid-specific 5-aminolevulinate synthase (ALAS2) gene causing X-linked sideroblastic anemia: Increased pyridoxine responsiveness after removal of iron overload by phlebotomy and coinheritance of hereditary hemochromatosis. *Blood* 1999; 93(5): 1757–69.

24. Coursin, DB. Convulsive seizures in infants with pyridoxine-deficient diet. *J Am Med Assoc* 1954; 154: 406–8.

25. Dalery, K, Lussier-Cacan, S, Selhub, J, Davignon, J, Latour, Y, Genest, J. Homocysteine and coronary artery disease in French Canadian subjects: Relation with vitamins B$_{12}$, B$_6$, pyridoxal phosphate, and folate. *Am J Cardiol* 1995; 75: 1107–11.

26. den Heijer, M, Brouwer, IA, Bos, GMJ, Blom, HJ, van der Put, NMJ, Spaans, AP, Rosendaal, FR, Thomas, CMG, Haak, HL, Wijermans, PW, Gerrits, WBJ. Vitamin supplementation reduces blood homocysteine levels. A controlled trial in patients with venous thrombosis and healthy volunteers. *Arterioscler Thromb Vasc Biol* 1998; 18: 356–61.

27. Fonda, ML. Purification and characterization of vitamin B$_6$-phosphate phosphatase from human erythrocytes. *J Biol Chem* 1992; 267: 15978–83.

28. Food and Nutrition Board, Institute of Medicine. Vitamin B$_6$. In *Dietary Reference Intakes for Thiamin, Riboflavin, Niacin, Vitamin B$_6$, Folate, Vitamin B$_{12}$, Pantothenic Acid, Biotin, and Choline. A Report of the Standing Committee on the Scientific Evaluation of Dietary Reference Intakes and Its Panel on Folate, Other B Vitamins, and Choline and Subcommittee on Upper Reference Levels of Nutrients.* National Academy Press, Washington DC, 1998; pp. 150–95.

29. Food and Nutrition Board, National Research Council. *Proposed Fortification Policy for Cereal-Grain Products* National Academy of Sciences, Washington DC, 1974.

30. Furth-Walker, D, Leibman, D, Smolen, A. Relationship between blood, liver and brain pyridoxal phosphate and pyridoxamine phosphate concentrations in mice. *J Nutr* 1990; 120: 1338–43.

31. Goyette, P, Frosst, P, Rosenblatt, DS, Rozen, R. Seven novel mutations in the methylenetetrahydrofolate reductase gene and genotype/phenotype correlations in severe methylenetetrahydrofolate reductase deficiency. *Am J Hum Genet* 1995; 56: 1052–59.

32. Grabow, JD, Linkswiler, H. Electroencephalographic and nerve-conduction studies in experimental vitamin B$_6$ deficiency in adults. *Am J Clin Nutr* 1969; 22: 1429–34.

33. Gregory, JF. Vitamins. In *Food Chemistry,* 3rd ed. (Fennema OR, ed.). M. Dekker, Inc, New York, 1996; pp. 531–616.

34. Gregory, JF. Bioavailability of vitamin B$_6$. *Eur J Clin Nutr* 1997; 51(suppl): S43–8.

35. Gregory, JF, Ink, SL. Identification and characterization of pyridoxine-β-glucoside as a major form of vitamin B$_6$ in plant-derived foods. *J Agric Food Chem* 1987; 35: 76–82.

36. Gregory, JF, Trumbo, PR, Bailey, LB, Toth, JP, Baumgartner, TG, Cerda, JJ. Bioavailability of pyridoxine-5'-β-D-glucoside determined in humans by stable-isotopic methods. *J Nutr* 1991; 121: 177–86.

37. Gunsalus, IC, Bellamy, WD, Umbreit, WW. A phosphorylated derivative of pyridoxal as coenzyme of tyrosine decarboxylase. *J Biol Chem* 1944; 155: 685–86.

38. Gupta, A, Moustapha, A, Jacobsen, DW, Goormastic, M, Tuzcu, EM, Hobbs, R, Young, J, James, K, McCarthy, P, Van Lente, F, Green, R, Robinson, K. High homocysteine, low folate, and low vitamin B$_6$ concentrations. Prevalent risk factors for vascular disease in heart transplant recipients. *Transplantation* 1998; 65: 544–50.

39. Gyorgy, P. Vitamin B$_2$ and the pellagra-like dermatitis of rats. *Nature* 1934; 133: 448–49.

40. Gyorgy, P. Crystalline vitamin B$_6$. *J Am Chem Soc* 1938; 60: 983–84.

41. Hansen, CM, Leklem, JE, Miller, LT. Vitamin B$_6$ status indicators decrease in women consuming a diet high in pyridoxine glucoside. *J Nutr* 1996; 126: 2512–18.

42. Hassinen, JB, Durbin, GT, Bernhart, FW. The vitamin B$_6$ content of milk products. *J Nutr* 1954; 53: 249–57.

43. Helmreich, EJ. How pyridoxal 5'-phosphate could function in glycogen phosphorylase catalysis. *Biofactors* 1992; 3: 159–72.

44. Henderson, JM, Scott, SS, Merrill, AH, Hollins, B, Kutner, MH. Vitamin B$_6$ repletion in cirrhosis with oral pyridoxine: Failure to improve amino acid metabolism. *Hepatology* 1989; 9: 582–88.

45. Henderson, LM. Intestinal absorption of B$_6$ vitamers. In *Vitamin B$_6$: Its Role in Health and Disease.* (Reynolds,

RD, Leklem, JE, eds.). Alan R. Liss, Inc, New York, 1985; pp. 25–33.

46. Huang, Y-C, Chen, W, Evans, MA, Mitchell, ME, Shultz, TD. Vitamin B_6 requirement and status assessment of young women fed a high-protein diet with various levels of vitamin B_6. *Am J Clin Nutr* 1998; 67: 208–20.

47. Ichiba, A, Michi, K. Isolation of vitamin B_6. *Scientific Papers of the Institute of Physical and Chemical Research. (Tokyo) Japan* 1938; 34: 623–26.

48. Ink, SL, Gregory, JF, Sartain, DB. The determination of pyridoxine-β-glucoside bioavailability in the rat. *J Agric Food Chem* 1986; 34: 857–62.

49. Joosten, E, van den Berg, A, Riezler, R, Naurath, HJ, Lindenbaum, J, Stabler, SP, Allen, RH. Metabolic evidence that deficiencies of vitamin B_{12} (cobalamin), folate, and vitamin B_6 occur commonly in elderly people. *Am J Clin Nutr* 1993; 58: 468–76.

50. Kabir, H, Leklem, JE, Miller, LT. Relationship of the glycosylated vitamin B_6 content of foods to vitamin B_6 bioavailability in humans. *Nutr Rept Int* 1983; 28: 709–16.

51. Kant, AK, Block, G. Dietary vitamin B_6 intake and food sources in the US population: NHANES II, 1976–1980. *Am J Clin Nutr* 1990; 52: 707–16.

52. Keresztesy, JC, Stevens, JR. Vitamin B_6. *Proc Soc Exp Biol Med* 1938; 38: 64–5.

53. Klosterman, HJ. Vitamin B_6 antagonists of natural origin. *J Agric Food Chem* 1974; 22: 13–6.

54. Kozik, A, McCormick, DB. Mechanism of pyridoxine uptake by isolated rat liver cells. *Arch Biochem Biophys* 1984; 229: 187–93.

55. Kretsch, MJ, Sauberlich, HE, Newbrun, E. Electroencephalographic changes and periodontal status during short-term vitamin B_6 depletion of young nonpregnant women. *Am J Clin Nutr* 1991; 53: 1266–74.

56. Kuhn, R, Wendt, G. Uber das antidermatitisch vitamin der hefe. *Berichte der Deutschen Chemischen Gesselschaft.* 1938; 71B: 780–82.

57. Leklem, JE. Vitamin B_6: A status report. *J Nutr* 1990; 120(Suppl 11): 1503–7.

58. Leklem, JE. Vitamin B_6. In *Handbook of Vitamins*, 2nd ed. (Machlin, LJ, ed.). Marcel Dekker, Inc, New York, 1991; pp. 341–92.

59. Leklem, JE. Vitamin B_6. In *Modern Nutrition in Health and Disease,* 9th ed. (Shils, ME, Olson, JA, Shihe, M, Ross, AC, eds.). Williams & Wilkins, Baltimore, 1998; pp. 1413–21.

60. Lepkovsky, S. Crystalline factor I. *Science* 1938; 87: 169–70.

61. Linderman, J, Kirk, L, Musselman, J, Dolinar, B, Fahey, TD. The effects of sodium bicarbonate and pyridoxine-alpha-ketoglutarate on short-term maximal exercise capacity. *J Sports Sci* 1992; 10: 243–53.

62. Lindenbaum, J, Roman, MJ. Nutritional anemia in alcoholism. *Am J Clin Nutr* 1980; 33: 2727–35.

63. Lobo, A, Naso, A, Arheart, K, Kruger, WD, Abou-Ghazala, T, Alsous, F, Nahlawi, M, Gupta, A, Moustapha, A, van Lente, F, Jacobsen, DW, Robinson, K. Reduction of homocysteine levels in coronary artery disease by low-dose folic acid combined with vitamins B_6 and B_{12}. *Am J Cardiol* 1999; 83: 821–25.

64. Lowik, MR, Schrijver, J, van den Berg, H, Hulshof, KF, Wedel, M, Ockhuizen, T. Effect of dietary fiber on the vitamin B_6 status among vegetarian and nonvegetarian elderly (Dutch nutrition surveillance system). *J Am Coll Nutr* 1990; 9: 241–49.

65. Lumeng, L. The role of acetaldehyde in mediating the deleterious effect of ethanol on pyridoxal 5′-phosphate metabolism. *J Clin Invest* 1978; 62: 286–93.

66. Lumeng, L, Ryan, MP, Li, TK. Validation of the diagnostic value of plasma pyridoxal 5′-phosphate measurements in vitamin B_6 nutrition of the rat. *J Nutr* 1978; 108: 545–53.

67. Marconi, C, Sassi, G, Cerretelli, P. The effect of an alpha-ketoglutarate-pyridoxine complex on human maximal aerobic and anaerobic performance. *Eur J Appl Physiol* 1982; 49: 307–17.

68. Martinez, M, Toth, JP, Williamson, J, Gregory, JF. Effects of vitamin B_6 deficiency on one-carbon metabolism using stable isotope infusion of serine. *FASEB J* 1999; 13: A227 (Abstract 208.1).

69. May, A, Bishop, DF. The molecular biology and pyridoxine responsiveness of X-linked sideroblastic anaemia. *Haematologica* 1998; 83(1): 56–70.

70. McMahon, LG, Nakano, H, Levy, MD, Gregory, JF. Cytosolic pyridoxine-β-D-glucoside hydrolase from porcine jejunal mucosa. Purification, properties, and comparison with broad specificity β-glucosidase. *J Biol Chem* 1997; 272: 32025–33.

71. Meister, A, Sober, HA, Peterson, EA. Activation of purified glutamic-aspartic apotransaminase by crystalline pyridoxamine phosphate. *J Am Chem Soc* 1954; 74: 2385–89.

72. Merrill, AH, Henderson, JM. Diseases associated with defects in vitamin B_6 metabolism or utilization. *Annu Rev Nutr* 1987; 7: 137–56.

73. Merrill, AH, Henderson, JM. Vitamin B_6 metabolism by human liver. *Ann N Y Acad Sci* 1990; 585: 110–17.

74. Merrill, AH, Horiike, K, McCormick, DB. Evidence for the regulation of pyridoxal 5-phosphate formation in liver by pyridoxamine (pyridoxine) 5′-phosphate oxidase. *Biochem Biophys Res Commun* 1978; 83: 984–90.

75. Meydani, SN, Ribaya-Mercado, JD, Russell, RM, Sahyoun, N, Morrow, FD, Gershoff, SN. Vitamin B_6 deficiency impairs interleukin 2 production and lymphocyte proliferation in elderly adults. *Am J Clin Nutr* 1991; 53: 1275–80.

76. Miller, JW, Nadeau, MR, Smith, D, Selhub, J. Vitamin B_6 deficiency vs folate deficiency: Comparison of responses to methionine loading in rats. *Am J Clin Nutr* 1994; 9: 1033–39.

77. Miller, JW, Ribaya-Mercado, JD, Russell, RM, Shepard, DC, Morrow, FD, Cochary, EF, Sadowski, JA, Gershoff, SN, Selhub, J. Effect of vitamin B_6 deficiency on fasting plasma homocysteine concentrations. *Am J Clin Nutr* 1992; 55: 1154–60.

78. Mudd, SH, Levy, HL, Skovby, F. Disorders of transsulfuration. In *The Metabolic and Molecular Basis of Inherited Disease.* (Scriver, CR, Beaudet, AL, Sly, WS, Vall, D, eds.). McGraw Hill, Inc, New York, 1995; pp. 1279–1327.

79. Nakano, H, McMahon, LG, Gregory, JF. Pyridoxine-5′-beta-glucoside exhibits incomplete bioavailability as a source of vitamin B$_6$ and partially inhibits the utilization of co-ingested pyridoxine in humans. *J Nutr* 1997; 127: 1508–13.

80. Reinken, L, Zieglauer, H, Berger, H. Vitamin B$_6$ nurture of children with acute celiac disease, celiac disease in remission, and of children with normal duodenal mucosa. *Am J Clin Nutr* 1976; 29: 750–53.

81. Reynolds, RD, Polansky, M, Moser, PB. Analyzed vitamin B$_6$ intakes of pregnant and postpartum lactating and nonlactating women. *J Am Diet Assoc* 1984; 84: 1339–44.

82. Rimm, EB, Willett, WC, Hu, FB, Sampson, L, Colditz, GA, Manson, JE, Hennekens, C, Stampfer, MJ. Folate and vitamin B$_6$ from diet and supplements in relation to risk of coronary heart disease among women. *J Am Med Assoc* 1998; 279: 359–64.

83. Robinson, K, Arheart, K, Refsum, H, Brattstrom, L, Goers, G, Ueland, P, Rubba, P, Palma-Reis, R, Meleady, R, Daly, L, Witteman, J, Graham, I. Low circulating folate and vitamin B$_6$ concentrations. Risk factors for stroke, peripheral vascular disease, and coronary artery disease. European COMAC Group. *Circulation* 1998; 97: 437–43.

84. Robinson, K, Gupta, A, Dennis, V, Arheart, K, Chaudhary, D, Green, R, Vigo, P, Mayer, EL, Selhub, J, Kutner, M, Jacobsen, DW. Hyperhomocysteinemia confers an independent increased risk of atherosclerosis in end-stage renal disease and is closely linked to plasma folate and pyridoxine concentrations. *Circulation* 1996; 94: 2743–48.

85. Sato, A, Nishioka, M, Awata, S, Nakayama, K, Okada, M, Horiuchi, S, Okabe, N, Sass, T, Oka, T, Natori, Y. Vitamin B$_6$ deficiency accelerates metabolic turnover of cystathionase in rat liver. *Arch Biochem Biophys* 1996; 330: 409–13.

86. Sauberlich, HE, Dowdy, RP, Skala, JH. *Laboratory Tests for the Assessment of Nutritional Status*. CRC Press, Inc, Cleveland, 1974: pp. 37–49.

87. Schaumberg, H, Kaplan, J, Windebank, A, Vick, N, Rasmus, S, Pleasure, D, Brown, MJ. Sensory neuropathy from pyridoxine abuse. A new megavitamin syndrome. *N Engl J Med* 1983; 309: 445–48.

88. Schuster, K, Bailey, LB, Cerda, JJ, Gregory, JF. Urinary 4-pyridoxic acid excretion in 24-hour versus random urine samples as a measurement of vitamin B$_6$ status in humans. *Am J Clin Nutr* 1984; 39: 466–70.

89. Schuster, K, Bailey, LB, Mahan, CS. Effect of maternal pyridoxine HCl supplementation on the vitamin B$_6$ status of mother and infant and on pregnancy outcome. *J Nutr* 1984; 114: 977–88.

90. Selhub, J, Jacques, PF, Wilson, PWF, Rush, D, Rosenberg, IH. Vitamin status and intake as primary determinants of homocysteinemia in an elderly population. *J Am Med Assoc* 1993; 70: 2693–98.

91. Sevigny, SJ de J, White, SL, Halsey, ML, Johnston, FA. Effect of isoniazid on the loss of pyridoxal phosphate from, and its distribution in, the body of the rat. *J Nutr* 1966; 88: 45–50.

92. Shemin, D, Lapane, KL, Bausserman, L, Kanaan, E, Kahn, S, Dworkin, L, Bostom, AG. Plasma total homocysteine and hemodialysis access thrombosis: A prospective study. *J Am Soc Nephrol* 1999; 10: 1095–99.

93. Snell, EE. Vitamin B$_6$ analysis: Some historical aspects. In *Methods in Vitamin B$_6$ Nutrition. Analysis and Status Assessment.* (Leklem, JE, Reynolds, RD, eds.). Plenum Press, New York, 1981; pp. 1–18.

94. Snell, EE. Pyridoxal phosphate: History and nomenclature. In *Vitamin B$_6$ Pyridoxal Phosphate. A. Chemical, Biochemical, and Medical Aspects.* (Dolphin, D, Poulson, R, Avramovic, O, eds.). John Wiley, New York, 1986; pp. 1–11.

95. Snell, EE. Nutrition research with lactic acid bacteria. *Annu Rev Nutr* 1989; 9: 1–19.

96. Smolin, LA, Benevenga, NJ. Accumulation of homocyst(e)ine in vitamin B$_6$ deficiency: A model for the study of cystathionine beta-synthase deficiency. *J Nutr* 1982; 112: 1264–72.

97. Smolin, LA, Benevenga, NJ. Factors affecting the accumulation of homocyst(e)ine in rats deficient in vitamin B$_6$. *J Nutr* 1984; 114: 103–11.

98. Stanulovic, M, Jeremic, V, Leskovac, V, Chaykin, S. New pathway of conversion of pyridoxal to 4-pyridoxic acid. *Enzyme* 1976; 21: 357–69.

99. Tarr, JB, Tamura, T, Stokstad, ELR. Availability of vitamin B$_6$ and pantothenate in an average American diet in man. *Am J Clin Nutr* 1981; 34: 1328–37.

100. Tomarelli, RM, Spence, ER, Bernhart, FW. Biological availability of vitamin B$_6$ in heated milk. *J Agric Food Chem* 1955; 3: 338–41.

101. Trumbo, PR, Gregory, JF, Sartain, DB. Incomplete utilization of pyridoxine-beta-glucoside as vitamin B$_6$ in the rat. *J Nutr* 1988; 118: 170–75.

102. Tully, DB, Allgood, VE, Cidlowski, JA. Modulation of steroid receptor-mediated gene expression by vitamin B$_6$. *FASEB J* 1994; 8: 343–49.

103. Ubbink, JB, Delport, R, Becker, PJ, Bissbort, S. Evidence of a theophylline-induced vitamin B$_6$ deficiency caused by noncompetitive inhibition of pyridoxal kinase. *J Lab Clin Med* 1989; 113: 15–22.

104. Ubbink, JB, van der Meere, A, Delport, R, Allen, RH, Stabler, SP, Riezler, R, Vermaak, WJH. The effect of a subnormal vitamin B$_6$ status on homocysteine metabolism. *J Clin Invest* 1996; 98: 177–84.

105. Utermohlen, V. Diet, nutrition, and drug interactions. In *Modern Nutrition in Health and Disease*, 9th ed. (Shils, ME, Olson, JA, Shihe, M, Ross, AC, eds.). Williams & Wilkins, Baltimore, 1999; pp. 1619–41.

106. van den Berg, M, Franken, DG, Boers, GH, Blom, HJ, Jakobs, C, Stehouwer, CD, Rauwerda, JA. Combined vitamin B$_6$ plus folic acid therapy in young patients with arteriosclerosis and hyperhomocysteinemia. *J Vasc Surg* 1994; 20: 933–40.

107. van der Vange, N, van den Berg, H, Klosterboer, HJ, Haspels, AA. Effects of seven low-dose combined contraceptives on vitamin B$_6$ status. *Contraception* 1989; 40: 377–84.

108. van der Wielen, RP, Lowik, MR, Haller, J, van den Berg, H, Ferry, M, van Staveren, WA. Vitamin B$_6$ malnutrition

among elderly Europeans: The SENECA study. *J Gerontol, A. Biol Sci Med Sci* 1996; 51: B417–24.

109. Verhoef, P, Stampfer, MJ, Buring, JE, Gaziano, JM, Allen, RH, Stabler, SP, Reynolds, RD, Kok, FJ, Hennekens, CH, Willett, WC. Homocysteine metabolism and risk of myocardial infarction: Relation with vitamins B$_6$, B$_{12}$, and folate. *Am J Epidemiol* 1996; 143: 845–59.

110. Whyte, MP, Mahuren, JD, Fedde, KN, Cole, FS, McCabe, ER, Coburn, SP. Perinatal hypophosphatasia: Tissue levels of vitamin B$_6$ are unremarkable despite markedly increased circulating concentrations of pyridoxal-5'-phosphate. Evidence for an ectoenzyme role for tissue-nonspecific alkaline phosphatase. *J Clin Invest* 1988; 81: 1234–39.

111. Whyte, MP, Mahuren, JD, Vrabel, LA, Coburn, SP. Markedly increased circulating pyridoxal-5'-phosphate levels in hypophosphatasia. Alkaline phosphatase acts in vitamin B$_6$ metabolism. *J Clin Invest* 1985; 76: 752–56.

112. Woodside, JV, Yarnell, JWG, McMaster, D, Young, IS, McCrum, EE, Evans, AE, Gey, KF, Harmon, DL, Whitehead, AS. Vitamin B$_6$ status, MTHFR and hyperhomocysteinemia, *Q J Med* 1997; 90: 551–52.

113. Wozenski, JR, Leklem, JE, Miller, LT. The metabolism of small doses of vitamin B$_6$ in men. *J Nutr* 1980; 110: 275–85.

114. Yasumoto, K, Tsuji, H, Iwami, K, Mitsuda, H. Isolation from rice bran of a bound form of vitamin B$_6$ and its identification as 5'-O-(β-D-glucopyranosyl)pyridoxine. *Agric Biol Chem* 1997; 41: 1061–67.

26

Homocysteine in Renal Disease

MARGRET ARNADOTTIR
BJÖRN HULTBERG

In the early 1970s, Condon and Asatoor (27) as well as Robins et al. (68) reported a peak in the isoleucine region of the amino acid chromatogram of uremic plasma not seen in that of normal plasma. This peak probably represented cysteine-homocysteine mixed disulfide, reported by Wilcken and Gupta (85) to be increased in patients with renal failure. Since then, increases in the plasma concentrations of mixed disulfides, protein-bound homocysteine and, in particular, total homocysteine have been confirmed many times (18, 29). By now, it is generally recognized that moderate hyperhomocysteinemia accompanies renal failure. This finding is of special interest owing to the greatly increased mortality from cardiovascular disease among uremic patients (66) that represents one of the major challenges of modern nephrology. The hope of bringing the atherothrombotic processes under control has stimulated research in homocysteine metabolism in renal disease. Most of the studies have recruited patients on chronic dialysis because these patients manifest the full-blown metabolic abnormality.

Homocysteine Concentrations in Relation to Renal Function

In clinical practice and research, the creatinine concentration in serum is the most frequently applied marker

for renal function. Accordingly, when studying the relationship between plasma homocysteine concentrations and renal function, most investigators have used the serum creatinine concentration. They generally found a significant direct correlation between the two concentrations, not only in patients with different degrees of renal failure (4) but also in the healthy population (77). However, such a relationship may not accurately reflect the influence of renal function on homocysteine metabolism. First, the serum creatinine concentration is an imprecise predictor of the glomerular filtration rate because it depends not only on the rate of creatinine excretion but also on the rate of creatinine production. Creatinine originates from metabolism in skeletal muscle, and the amount of creatinine released is therefore determined by muscle mass. Second, there is a direct metabolic relationship between creatinine and homocysteine. The formation of creatine, the precursor of creatinine, depends on methyl donation by *S*-adenosylmethionine (60), leading to the formation of homocysteine. Thus ultimately, the homocysteine concentration would be expected to reflect muscle mass much as the creatinine concentration does. This is probably the reason why men generally have higher concentrations of both creatinine and homocysteine than women (77). Indeed, within a narrow "normal" creatinine interval, there was no difference between the homocysteine concentrations of the sexes (62).

Studies using plasma clearance methods for estimation of renal function showed a significant and inverse correlation between the plasma homocysteine concentrations and the glomerular filtration rates through almost the entire renal functional range in health and disease (4, 87). In 64 nondiabetic patients who had glomerular filtration rates in the range of 6 to 106 mL/min/1.73 m^2 but who manifested a minimum of other confounding factors for homocysteine metabolism, the correlation coefficient was −0.70 (Figure 26.1) (4). In 80 patients with insulin-dependent-diabetes, with glomerular filtration rates ranging between 47 and 165 mL/min/1.73 m^2 but without overt proteinuria, the correlation coefficient was −0.44 (87). Multivariate analysis of both patient samples showed that only the glomerular filtration rate and not the serum creatinine concentration independently predicted the homocysteine concentration (4, 87).

Considering the high plasma homocysteine concentrations in patients undergoing dialysis reported by numerous authors, a steep rise seems to occur at this end of the renal functional range. Notably, no homocysteine study has measured the residual renal function

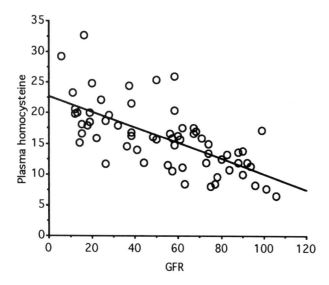

Fig. 26.1. Plasma homocysteine concentrations (μmol/L) plotted against glomerular filtration rates (GFR) (mL/min). The univariate correlation coefficient was −0.70 (7). (Reproduced from Arnadottir et al. [4], with permission.)

of dialysis patients by a plasma clearance method, but in two studies the creatinine clearances did not correlate with the homocysteine concentrations (8, 15).

Potential Mechanisms Underlying the Uremic Hyperhomocysteinemia

Unique Pathogenetic Mechanisms

The serum concentrations of the B vitamins that act as substrates or cofactors in homocysteine metabolism and the genetic mutations of relevant enzymes help predict the homocysteine concentration in the general population (22, 77). In patients with renal failure, the same factors operate. Significant inverse correlations between homocysteine concentrations and plasma folate, red cell folate and serum cobalamin, as well as vitamin B_6 concentrations have been reported in patients with different degrees of renal failure (4, 15, 69, 73). Polymorphism of the 5,10-methylenetetrahydrofolate reductase gene involving the 677C→T mutation affects the homocysteine concentration of uremic patients in a manner similar to that of healthy individuals, leading to an increase in those who are homozygous for the mutation, at least in those whose folate concentrations are below the median (35).

The influence of the previously mentioned factors on homocysteine metabolism is comparable in patients with renal failure and healthy individuals. Because these factors are similarly represented in both groups, they cannot explain the uremic hyperhomocysteine-

mia. Folate or cobalamin deficiency is not especially common in uremic patients (69), and the frequency of the 677C→T mutation seems to be of the same magnitude as in the general population (35). Only vitamin B_6 deficiency is frequently reported in uremic patients (4, 69), but this is probably not of major importance for the fasting homocysteine concentration because vitamin B_6 supplementation does not affect the fasting concentration (3).

The inverse relationship between homocysteine concentrations and glomerular filtration rates, the absence of deviations in the major determinants of homocysteine metabolism, and the relative resistance to treatment as discussed later strongly indicate that uremic hyperhomocysteinemia is caused by unique pathogenetic mechanisms that are still largely unknown.

Increased Cellular Production or Delayed Plasma Clearance

On a daily basis, approximately 1,200 μmol of homocysteine are transported through cell membranes into plasma (43), the hepatocyte probably being the main source of the amino acid (52). To maintain a steady state (42), the same amount of homocysteine must be cleared from plasma. Theoretically, hyperhomocysteinemia can be induced either by increased cellular release or by decreased plasma clearance. A study based on the homocysteine loading test revealed that, compared with healthy control subjects, uremic patients had about four times as high homocysteine half-life and area under the time-concentration curve, while the plasma clearance was reduced to about 30% (44). These results indicate that delayed plasma clearance is a dominating influence on homocysteine metabolism in patients with advanced renal failure (44). This and related issues are discussed in greater detail in Chapter 16.

Site of Clearance

The homocysteine loading test (44) could not distinguish between renal and extrarenal clearance. For obvious reasons, research has focused on renal clearance. In healthy individuals, the urinary excretion of homocysteine is less than 10 μmol/day (67). Because this amounts to less than 1% of the daily homocysteine turnover in plasma, the loss of the urinary excretion of homocysteine is not important for the regulation of the plasma concentration. In contrast, the prerequisites for homocysteine removal by metabolism are present in the renal parenchyma; homocysteine can be taken up from the glomerular filtrate by the proximal renal tubular cells (37), and the enzymes of transsulfuration as well as remethylation are present in these cells (37, 58). However, current evidence seems to favor impaired extrarenal clearance of homocysteine as the main pathogenetic mechanism behind uremic hyperhomocysteinemia in humans (see Chapter 16).

Delayed Cellular Reuptake

For removal by metabolism, circulating homocysteine must be taken up again by cells because the relevant enzymes are located intracellularly (58). Conceivably, cellular reuptake could be impaired. Although plasma concentrations of total and free (not protein-bound) homocysteine are increased in renal failure, that of reduced homocysteine is not (2, 50). Thus, reduced homocysteine must be specifically controlled by other mechanisms, most likely the redox status of the plasma (38). Indeed, there is evidence of increased oxidative stress in uremic plasma (23, 24), which may explain the tendency of homocysteine to undergo oxidation, leaving less homocysteine in the reduced form. Because homocysteine is most bioavailable in its reduced form (49), the high oxidative capacity of uremic plasma may slow the cellular reuptake of circulating homocysteine.

What Happens in the Metabolizing Cell?

Studies that applied the methionine loading test observed an excessive increase in the postload homocysteine concentration, suggesting a disturbed transsulfuration pathway in uremic patients (50, 81). However, normal hepatic activities of cystathionine β-synthase and γ-cystathionase, the rate-limiting enzymes of the transsulfuration pathway, were found in uremic rats (12). Moreover, a double-isotope study in hemodialysis patients indicated a decrease in the remethylation but not in the transsulfuration process (82), a disturbance that would explain the increased plasma cysteine concentration generally reported in uremic patients (4, 72).

The existence of enzyme inhibitors in uremic plasma is well documented (39, 61). Thus, it is conceivable that the removal of homocysteine, whether by renal or extrarenal cells, is hampered by substances that accumulate in renal failure. Indeed, uremic plasma and normal urine from humans contain a heat-stable inhibitory activity (possibly sulfate) against folate conjugase (54), the enzyme that cleaves glutamyl residues of polyglutamyl folates. At present, this constitutes the only experimental evidence of inhibitory activities against an enzyme that is relevant to homocysteine metabolism. However, the finding in a small group of patients that the homocysteine concentration was stable for 8 hours after a hemodialysis procedure (8) can be explained by dialyzable inhibitory activities in uremic plasma. The amount of homocysteine in dialysate was negligible (less than 5% of expected daily turnover).

Plasma Homocysteine Concentrations in Dialysis Patients

Reported Levels and Prevalence of Hyperhomocysteinemia

A study of hemodialysis patients and some peritoneal dialysis patients observed that 85% of the participants were hyperhomocysteinemic and that the mean homocysteine concentration was almost three times higher than that of the general population (69). Folate concentrations varied widely and, in agreement with others, the authors concluded that the folate concentration was the most important independent determinant of the homocysteine concentration in this population (15, 69). Indeed, most studies report an inverse correlation between homocysteine and folate concentrations in dialysis patients (3, 15, 69, 73). In many studies, the same patterns apply to cobalamin and vitamin B_6 (less often analyzed) concentrations.

B vitamins are commonly given to dialysis patients even though the need for this practice and the appropriate doses are debated (63). Practice ranges from giving no supplementation at all, to physiological replacement of losses, to pharmacological treatment. Obviously, information about the level of B-vitamin supplementation is of considerable importance for the evaluation of the homocysteine concentrations in these patients.

Dialysis-Specific Influence

A decrease of 25% to 50% in the plasma homocysteine concentration during a hemodialysis session has been demonstrated repeatedly (8, 48, 72, 73). This finding has stimulated interest in the possible role of dialysis itself in regulating the homocysteine concentration. One study did not find a relationship between homocysteine concentrations and urea reduction ratios in hemodialysis patients (15). In another study of folate-loaded patients, homocysteine concentrations and indices of dialysis adequacy correlated significantly (8). However, in a multivariate analysis of those data, only the albumin concentration was an independent predictor of the homocysteine concentration. These results are in accord with previous studies of dialysis patients showing a direct correlation between the concentrations of homocysteine and albumin (35, 48), and they suggest that increased dialysis results in better nutritional status and a higher albumin concentration, which, in turn, leads to a higher homocysteine concentration.

Only the 25% to 30% of circulating homocysteine that is not bound to albumin (50, 72) can be expected to pass the dialyzer membranes. Indeed, it has been shown that the free homocysteine fraction declines more than the protein-bound fraction during dialysis (72). The total amount of homocysteine that is recovered in the dialysate (<100 μmol) is small compared with daily cellular export, which indicates that there is no major flux of homocysteine among fractions or compartments and that this loss of homocysteine plays a minor regulatory role (8). The ability of dialysis to remove metabolic waste products may be more important in this regard. Such waste products may inhibit enzyme activities, and removal of waste products would be expected to facilitate the function of the relevant pathway of homocysteine metabolism.

A cross-sectional study of peritoneal dialysis patients showed no relationship between total homocysteine concentrations and parameters of dialysis adequacy (83), and another study found no effect of the mode of dialysis on the homocysteine concentration (15). However, a recent prospective study showed that during the first month after starting peritoneal dialysis, the homocysteine concentration declined significantly (34). The decreases in homocysteine concentration correlated significantly with the peritoneal dialysis creatinine clearances but not with the changes in albumin concentration (34). It is still not clear whether peritoneal dialysis is associated with lower homocysteine concentrations than is hemodialysis. In any case, the comparison is difficult because peritoneal dialysis is given continuously and hemodialysis intermittently.

Potential Adverse Effects of Hyperhomocysteinemia

Meta-analysis showed that the odds ratio for coronary artery disease for every 5 μmol/L increment of the total homocysteine concentration was 1.6 for men and 1.8 for women (21). If extrapolated directly to dialysis patients, the odds ratio increase associated with their hyperhomocysteinemia would explain much of the excess cardiovascular disease in these patients. However, such an extrapolation is not justified because dialysis patients differ in many respects from the general population. They have a multitude of other cardiovascular risk factors such as hypertension, dyslipoproteinemia, ventricular hypertrophy, and hyperparathyroidism, the interplay and relative importance of which have not yet been adequately described.

Therefore, the cardiovascular risk associated with hyperhomocysteinemia must be evaluated separately in this special patient category. Several studies have addressed the question (10, 15, 19, 59, 69) but, like most studies of dialysis patients, were rather small. A cross-sectional study of 176 patients found an odds ratio of 2.9 for the association between vascular events and homocysteine concentrations when the upper two quintiles of homocysteine concentrations were compared with the lower three quintiles (69). A prospective study that followed 167 dialysis patients for 17.4 ± 6.4 months concluded that hyperhomocysteinemia is an independent cardiovascular risk factor, with an increased relative risk of 1% per μmol/L increase in the homocysteine concentration (59). Another prospective study of 73 dialysis patients, monitored for a median of 17 months, reported comparable results (19). Taken together, hyperhomocysteinemia seems to indicate a cardiovascular risk in dialysis patients similar to that in the general population, the causal association remaining unproven. However, during a short-term follow-up study of 88 patients, a higher mortality rate was noted among those who had the lowest homocysteine concentrations (70). Malnutrition, common among dialysis patients (40), may complicate the evaluation of the homocysteine-associated risk.

The maintenance of a patent arteriovenous fistula or graft is a unique feature of the care of hemodialysis patients. These nonphysiological arteriovenous connections are prone to clotting, especially on the venous side. Because hyperhomocysteinemia has been associated with venous thrombosis also (28), theoretical grounds exist for assuming that hyperhomocysteinemia may be a risk factor for thrombosis of the vascular access of hemodialysis patients. However, only one small cross-sectional study has found evidence for such an association (32), whereas three larger studies did not (56, 70, 74).

The *S*-adenosylmethionine:*S*-adenosylhomocysteine ratio is important for the regulation of transmethylation reactions. *S*-adenosylhomocysteine is hydrolyzed to adenosine and homocysteine, but if homocysteine is not rapidly removed, the reaction favors the accumulation of *S*-adenosylhomocysteine. The delayed plasma homocysteine clearance in uremia results in a reduced *S*-adenosylmethione:*S*-adenosylhomocysteine ratio, which is demonstrated both in plasma (55) and red blood cells (64). Therefore, impaired transmethylation capacity is probably one of the ultimate consequences of the disturbed homocysteine metabolism in renal failure influencing the biosynthesis of a wide range of compounds.

Homocysteine-Lowering Treatment

In individuals with normal renal function, B-vitamin treatment almost invariably leads to normalization of the homocysteine concentration (76). A meta-analysis of homocysteine-lowering trials quantified this response. After pretreatment standardization of homocysteine and folate concentrations, administration of folic acid resulted in a decline in the homocysteine concentration by 25%, with similar effects in the dose range of 0.5 to 5.0 mg daily (45). Treatment with cobalamin (mean dose of 0.5 mg daily) gave an additional decrease of 7%, whereas vitamin B_6 seemed to produce no effect (45). In many respects, dialysis (and predialytic) patients respond similarly to B-vitamins. Several treatment trials with folic acid showed a homocysteine-lowering effect of 30% to 40% (3, 16, 25, 30, 51, 65) (Table 26.1), but two studies did not find vitamin B_6 to be effective (3, 25). Cobalamin treatment has not been investigated separately in cobalamin-replete patients undergoing dialysis. However, as discussed later, the response of dialysis patients to B-vitamin treatment deviates in many ways from that observed in healthy individuals.

Even the administration of supraphysiological B-vitamin doses does not normalize the homocysteine concentration in most dialysis patients. Of 15 patients given 16 mg of folic acid, 1,012 μg of cobalamin, and 110 mg of vitamin B_6 daily, only five achieved homocysteine concentrations below 15 μmol/L (16). This relative inefficiency has prompted a search for alternative therapies. Substances such as betaine (14) and serine (13, 53), of theoretical interest because they are known to be deficient in renal failure, have been tried without benefit. Lower homocysteine concentrations could possibly result from a wider use of convective treatment methods or daily hemodialysis, which more effectively remove putative enzyme inhibitors (8, 75). However, there is little evidence for this at present.

Until quite recently, it has been assumed that a large dose of folic acid is needed for maximal homocysteine-lowering response in dialysis patients. More than 1 mg daily seemed to be required for maximal effect; an additional homocysteine-lowering effect of 26% to 30% was observed when the daily dose of folic acid was increased from 1 mg to 16 mg (16). Although the doses of cobalamin and vitamin B_6 were also markedly increased in that study, most of the homocysteine-lowering response probably was caused by the increase of folic acid. A recent study observed no difference between the homocysteine-lowering effects of folic acid, 7.5 mg/week (2.5 mg after each dialysis session), and folic acid, 15 mg/week (30). Thus, the optimal dose of folic acid in dialysis patients is probably in the range of 1 to 2 mg/day. It is still not known whether the addition of cobalamin to the regimen makes any difference, but, as in the general population, such supplementation could also prevent any masked cobalamin deficiency.

When given in supraphysiological doses to dialysis patients, folate accumulates in the body as evidenced by high concentrations of red blood cell folate (3). After discontinuation of treatment with 5 mg of folic acid daily, it takes at least 8 to 9 months for the red cell folate concentration to reach nontreatment levels, whether or not erythropoietin (3) is given (84).

It is not known whether homocysteine-lowering treatment reduces cardiovascular morbidity and mortality. In dialysis patients, it has been shown that treatment with high doses of folic acid does not improve the endothelial dysfunction, determined by endothelium-dependent vasodilatation (79, 80), which is common in this patient population (78).

Table 26.1.   Plasma Homocysteine Concentrations in Dialysis Patients Before and After Different Treatment Regimens

Baseline Treatment	Study Treatment	Homocysteine (μmol/L)		Relative Response	Reference
		Pretreatment	Post-treatment		
Folic acid 1 mg/day Cobalamin 12 μg/day Vitamin B_6 10 mg/day	Folic acid 15 mg/day Cobalamin 1 mg/day Vitamin B_6 100 mg/day	29.5 ± 10.0	21.9 ± 7.7	26%	16[a]
None	Methyltetrahydrofolate 15 mg/day	68.0 ± 14.9	18.9 ± 2.4	NG	65
None	Folic acid 7.5 mg/week	34.4 (19.8 – 85.4)	25.1 (12.5 – 37.4)	≈35%	30[b]
None	Folic acid 15 mg/week	32.4 (20.1 – 56.9)	21.1 (12.9 – 33.6)	≈35%	
?	Folic acid 5 mg/day	55.7 ± 10.1	24.0 ± 1.8	NG	51

NG, not given.
[a] Randomized and placebo-controlled.
[b] Randomized.

Plasma Homocysteine Concentrations in Renal Transplant Recipients

Prevalence and Magnitude of Hyperhomocysteinemia

The homocysteine concentrations in renal transplant recipients were compared with those of healthy control subjects for the first time in 1981 (86). These patients, immunosuppressed with azathioprine and prednisolone, had significantly increased concentrations of free homocysteine (86). Since then, elevated total homocysteine concentrations have been reported in as many as 85% of renal transplant recipients treated with different immunosuppressive regimens (5, 7, 19, 33, 57). The transplant recipients generally manifested mean homocysteine concentrations approximately twice those of healthy control subjects (5, 19).

Transplantation-Specific Influence

Metabolic disturbances in renal transplant recipients are most often the result of inadequate renal function alone or in combination with toxic effects of the obligatory immunosuppressive drugs. Normal homocysteine concentrations would not be expected in renal transplant recipients because these patients generally manifest moderate renal insufficiency. Indeed, most authors report significant correlations between measures of renal function and homocysteine concentrations in these patients (5, 7, 19, 33). However, the residual renal insufficiency does not seem to be the sole or even the most important cause of disturbances in homocysteine metabolism; homocysteine concentrations were higher in renal transplant recipients than in patients with matched renal function who had not received a renal transplant (5, 7) and declined by only 14% 6 months after transplantation (7). In this study, the changes in the homocysteine concentration after transplantation varied widely, from a reduction of 85% to an increase of 142% (7). The only independent, positive predictors of the post-transplant homocysteine changes were the post-transplant changes in the albumin concentration and the trough concentration of cyclosporine. Multiple regression analysis also showed that the higher pretransplant homocysteine concentrations were associated with greater post-transplant changes, but neither the changes in the folate concentration nor the post-transplant creatinine clearances correlated independently with the post-transplant changes in the homocysteine concentration (7).

Because this investigation measured neither cobalamin nor vitamin B_6 concentrations, vitamin status needs to be studied further. It seems likely that other influences are operating in these patients. This notion is supported by reports on homocysteine metabolism in heart transplant recipients, whose situation closely reflects that of renal transplant recipients in most relevant aspects (i.e., organ transplant reception, treatment with immunosuppressive drugs, reduced renal function, and a tendency to B-vitamin deficiency) (1, 41). A prospective study of heart transplant recipients found a mean post-transplant increase in the homocysteine concentration of 70%, but the changes did not correlate significantly with changes in B-vitamin concentrations or renal function (11). In another study of heart transplant recipients, more than 50% of the variation in the homocysteine concentration could be explained by the positive predictors, serum creatinine concentration and trough blood cyclosporine concentration, as well as the negative predictors, serum folate concentration and time since transplantation (26).

Thus, there is evidence from two studies that cyclosporine itself interferes with the metabolism of homocysteine, causing a mild increase in the homocysteine concentration (1.75 µmol/L per 100 µg/L increase in the cyclosporine concentration in reference 26) (7, 26). In addition, cyclosporine probably influences homocysteine by its adverse effect on renal function (33). There is less evidence for the other immunosuppressants, but a correlation has been shown between homocysteine concentrations and cumulative steroid doses (57). Moreover, the possible influence of immunologically activated processes cannot be excluded. However, because of the similarities between the heart and renal transplant situations, the presence of a specific renal factor seems unlikely.

Potential Adverse Effects of Hyperhomocysteinemia

Only a few studies with small numbers of patients have addressed the question of cardiovascular risk associated with hyperhomocysteinemia in renal transplant recipients. Men, but not women, who had suffered from cardiovascular accidents had a tendency toward higher homocysteine concentrations in samples collected before the incident (57). The homocysteine concentration was also significantly higher in renal transplant recipients with a history of atherosclerotic complications than in those without such a history (5, 33) in studies that suffered from survivorship effects among other flaws. These tenuous data tend to support the role of homocysteine as a cardiovascular risk factor in renal transplant recipients.

Vascular graft rejection is associated with endothelial dysfunction, and in chronic cases the histopathological picture resembles that of atherosclerosis (36). Accordingly, there are theoretical grounds for the hypothesis that hyperhomocysteinemia adversely influences renal graft outcome. However, in a study including 81 patients monitored for 5 years, no relationship was observed between the homocysteine concentrations and the parameters of graft function, graft survival, or graft histopathology (31).

Homocysteine-Lowering Treatment

Daily treatment with 5 mg of folic acid was associated with a reduction of about 25% in the homocysteine concentration in three studies (6, 17, 86), two of which included cyclosporine-treated patients (6, 17). Moreover, the postmethionine load elevation of the homocysteine concentration, which is greater in renal transplant recipients than in healthy control subjects (20), decreased by 22% after daily treatment with 50 mg of vitamin B_6 (17); in another study, vitamin B_6 did not influence the fasting homocysteine concentration (86).

Plasma Homocysteine Concentrations in Patients with Proteinuria

The data in proteinuric renal disease are scant. Only one study was primarily designed to investigate the association between homocysteine concentrations and proteinuria (46). This large, population-based study focused on microalbuminuria, for which the odds ratio per increment in homocysteine concentration of 5 μmol/L was found to be 1.33 (95% confidence interval: 1.08 to 1.63), after adjustment for renal function and known risk factors for microalbuminuria (46). Hence, hyperhomocysteinemia may be causally related to microalbuminuria. If so, the effect is probably mediated through glomerular endothelial dysfunction leading to urinary protein leakage.

A significant direct correlation between homocysteine concentrations and low-moderate urinary albumin excretion has been reported (4). This correlation appeared in a simple linear regression analysis but disappeared after adjustment for glomerular filtration rates. Higher homocysteine concentrations were observed in diabetic patients with overt nephropathy than in those with incipient nephropathy, again probably explained by differences in glomerular filtration rates (47). Little is known about the influence of severe proteinuria itself on homocysteine metabolism. The hypoalbuminemia that is integral to the nephrotic syndrome is probably associated with decreased homocysteine concentrations owing to reduced homocysteine-binding capacity. Accordingly, the ratio between non-protein-bound and total concentrations of homocysteine was increased in a small group of nephrotic patients (50). The nephrotic syndrome is characterized not only by increased urinary protein loss but also by overcompensated hepatic synthesis of many proteins. Thus, there may be changes in the kinetics of proteins, such as enzymes or vitamin-binding proteins, that are important for homocysteine metabolism.

Areas for Future Research

As discussed here and in Chapter 16, the pathogenetic mechanisms behind uremic hyperhomocysteinemia have not been elucidated. However, it seems likely that accumulated waste products of protein breakdown interfere with homocysteine metabolism, for example, by inhibiting enzyme activities. It is of theoretical and practical interest to clarify these processes. Unfortunately, pinpointing specific substances in uremic plasma and their adverse effects has proven singularly difficult, and this will probably also be the case for the influence of uremia on homocysteine metabolism.

Several issues regarding optimal homocysteine-lowering treatment in uremic patients remain unanswered. It is not clear whether the administration of cobalamin has a homocysteine-lowering effect in the cobalamin-replete subject or whether supraphysiological doses of vitamin B_6 lower the excessive increase in the homocysteine concentration after methionine load. The administration of antioxidants possibly leads to an increase in the reduced species of homocysteine and thereby facilitates the cellular reuptake and metabolism of homocysteine. Treatment studies will provide answers to these questions.

The question of whether homocysteine-lowering treatment results in reduced cardiovascular morbidity and mortality is of great general importance. It is a matter of debate whether the nephrological community should rely on results from intervention studies on the general population that will emerge in the coming years, or whether separate studies should be carried out on the uremic population. Arguments favoring the latter alternative include the high prevalence of both cardiovascular disease and hyperhomocysteinemia in combination with the unique internal environment of uremia.

The influence of renal function on plasma homocysteine may have consequences beyond the nephrological clientele. The generally reported differences in the mean homocysteine concentrations between cardiovascular patients and control subjects in large epidemiological studies may have been at least partially due to worse renal function in cardiovascular patients, who probably were at higher risk for nephrosclerosis (22). These differences in the homocysteine concentrations between the groups were rather small, amounting to about 1 μmol/L (9, 71), which corresponded to eventual differences in the glomerular filtration rates of less than 10 mL/min (4, 87). A more precise indicator of renal function than the serum creatinine concentration should obviously be applied in future epidemiological studies on homocysteine.

REFERENCES

1. Ambrosi, P, Barlatier, A, Habib, G, Garcon, D, Kreitman, B, Roland, PH, Saingra, S, Metras, D, Luccioni R. Hyperhomocysteinaemia in heart transplant recipients. *Eur Heart J* 1994; 15: 1191–95.

2. Andersson, A, Lindgren, A, Arnadottir, M, Prytz, H, Hultberg, B. Thiols as a measure of plasma redox status in healthy subjects and in patients with renal or liver failure. *Clin Chem* 1999; 45: 1084–86.

3. Arnadottir, M, Brattström, L, Simonsen, O, Thysell, H, Hultberg, B, Andersson, A, Nilsson-Ehle, P. The effect of high-dose pyridoxine and folic acid supplementation on serum lipid and plasma homocysteine concentrations in dialysis patients. *Clin Nephrol* 1993; 40: 236–40.

4. Arnadottir, M, Hultberg, B, Nilsson-Ehle, P, Thysell, H. The effect of reduced glomerular filtration rate on plasma total homocysteine concentration. *Scand J Clin Lab Invest* 1996; 56: 41–6.

5. Arnadottir, M, Hultberg, B, Vladov, V, Nilsson-Ehle, P, Thysell, H. Hyperhomocysteinemia in cyclosporine-treated renal transplant recipients. *Transplantation* 1996; 61: 509–12.

6. Arnadottir, M, Hultberg, B. Treatment with high-dose folic acid effectively lowers plasma homocysteine concentration in cyclosporine-treated renal transplant recipients. *Transplantation* 1997; 64: 1087–88.

7. Arnadottir, M, Hultberg, B, Wahlberg, J, Fellström, B, Dimény, E. Serum total homocysteine concentration before and after renal transplantation. *Kidney Int* 1998; 54: 1380–84.

8. Arnadottir, M, Berg, AL, Hegbrant, J, Hultberg, B. Influence of haemodialysis on plasma total homocysteine concentration. *Nephrol Dial Transplant* 1999; 14: 142–46.

9. Arnesen, E, Refsum, H, Bönå, KH, Ueland, PM, Förde, OH, Nordrehaug, JE. Serum total homocysteine and coronary heart disease. *Int J Epidemiol* 1995; 24: 704–9.

10. Bachmann, J, Tepel, M, Raidt, H, Riezler, R, Graefe, U, Langer, K, Zidek, W. Hyperhomocysteinemia and the risk for vascular disease in hemodialysis patients. *J Am Soc Nephrol* 1995; 6: 121–25.

11. Berger, PB, Jones, JD, Olson, LJ, Edwards, BS, Frantz, RP, Rodeheffer, RJ, Kottke, BA, Daly, RC, McGregor, CG. Increase in total plasma homocysteine concentration after cardiac transplantation. *Mayo Clin Proc* 1995; 70: 125–31.

12. Bocock, MA, Zlotkin, SH. Hepatic sulfur amino acid metabolism in rats with chronic renal failure. *J Nutr* 1990; 120: 691–99.

13. Bostom, AG, Shemin, D, Lapane, KL, Miller, JW, Sutherland, P, Nadeau, M, Seyoum, E, Hartman, W, Prior, R, Wilson, PW. Hyperhomocysteinemia and traditional cardiovascular disease risk factors in end-stage renal disease patients on dialysis: A case control study. *Atherosclerosis* 1995; 114: 93–103.

14. Bostom, AG, Shemin, D, Nadeau, MR, Shih, V, Stabler, S, Allen, RH, Selhub, J. Short-term betaine therapy fails to lower elevated fasting total plasma homocysteine concentrations in hemodialysis patients maintained on chronic folic acid supplementation. *Atherosclerosis* 1995; 113: 129–32.

15. Bostom, AG, Shemin, D, Lapane, KL, Nadeau, M, Sutherland, P, Chan, J, Rozen, R, Yoburn, D, Jacques, PF, Selhub, J, Rosenberg, IH. Folate status is the major deter-

minant of fasting total plasma homocysteine levels in maintenance dialysis patients. *Atherosclerosis* 1996; 123: 193–202.

16. Bostom, AG, Shemin, D, Lapane, KL, Hume, AL, Yoburn, D, Nadeau, M, Bendich, A, Selhub, J, Rosenberg, IH. High dose B-vitamin treatment of hyperhomocysteinemia in dialysis patients. *Kidney Int* 1996; 49: 147–52.

17. Bostom, AG, Gohh, RY, Beaulieu, A, Nadeau, MR, Hume, AL, Jacques, PF, Selhub, J, Rosenberg, IH. Treatment of hyperhomocysteinemia in renal transplant recipients: A randomized, placebo-controlled trial. *Ann Int Med* 1997; 127: 1089–92.

18. Bostom, AG, Lathrop, L. Hyperhomocysteinemia in end-stage renal disease: Prevalence, etiology, and potential relationship to arteriosclerotic outcomes. *Kidney Int* 1997; 52: 10–20.

19. Bostom, AG, Shemin, D, Verhoef, P, Nadeau, M, Jacques, PF, Selhub, J, Dworkin, L, Rosenberg, IH. Elevated fasting total plasma homocysteine levels and cardiovascular disease outcomes in maintenance dialysis patients: A prospective study. *Arterioscler Thromb Vasc Biol* 1997; 17: 2554–58.

20. Bostom, AG, Gohh, RY, Tsai, MY, Hopkins-Garcia, BJ, Nadeau, MR, Bianchi, LA, Jacques, PF, Rosenberg, IH, Selhub, J. Excess prevalence of fasting and postmethionine-loading hyperhomocysteinemia in stable renal transplant recipients. *Arterioscler Thromb Vasc Biol* 1997; 17: 1894–1900.

21. Boushey, CJ, Beresford, SAA, Omenn, GS, Motulsky, AG. A quantitative assessment of plasma homocysteine as a risk factor for vascular disease: Probable benefits of increasing folic acid intakes. *JAMA* 1995; 274: 1049–57.

22. Brattström, L, Wilcken, DEL, Öhrvik, J, Brudin, L. Common methylenetetrahydrofolate reductase gene mutation leads to hyperhomocysteinemia but not to vascular disease: The result of a meta-analysis. *Circulation* 1998; 98: 2520–26.

23. Canestrari, F, Buoncristiani, U, Galli, F, Giorgini, A, Albertini, MC, Carobi, C, Pascucci, M, Bossu, M. Redox state, antioxidative activity and lipid peroxidation in erythrocytes and plasma of chronic ambulatory peritoneal dialysis patients. *Clin Chim Acta* 1995; 234: 127–36.

24. Ceballos-Picot, I, Witko-Sarsat, V, Merad-Boudia, M, Nguyen, AT, Thevenin, M, Jaubon, MC, Zingraff, J, Verger, C, Jungers, P, Deschamps-Latscha, B. Glutathionine antioxidant system as a marker of oxidative stress in chronic renal failure. *Free Radic Biol Med* 1996; 21: 845–53.

25. Chauveau, P, Chadefaux, B, Coudé, M, Aupetit, J, Kamoun, P, Jungers, P. Long-term folic acid (but not pyridoxine) supplementation lowers elevated plasma homocysteine level in chronic renal failure. *Miner Electrolyte Metab* 1996; 22: 106–9.

26. Cole, DEC, Ross, HJ, Evrovski, J, Langman, CJ, Miner, SE, Daly, PA, Wong, PY. Correlation between total homocysteine and cyclosporine concentrations in cardiac transplant recipients. *Clin Chem* 1998; 44: 2307–12.

27. Condon, JR, Asatoor, AM. Amino acid metabolism in uraemic patients. *Clin Chim Acta* 1971; 32: 333–37.

28. den Heijer, M, Koster, T, Blom, HJ, Bos, GMJ, Briet, E, Reitsma, PH, Vandenbroucke, JP, Rosendaal, FR. Hyperhomocysteinemia as a risk factor for deep-vein thrombosis. *N Engl J Med* 1996; 334: 759–62.

29. Dennis, VW, Robinson, K. Homocysteinemia and vascular disease in end-stage renal disease. *Kidney Int* 1996; 50: S-11–17.

30. Dierkes, J, Domröse, U, Ambrosch, A, Bosselmann, HP, Neumann, KH, Luley, C. Response of hyperhomocysteinemia to folic acid supplementation in patients with end-stage renal disease. *Clin Nephrol* 1999; 51: 108–15.

31. Diménÿ, E, Hultberg, B, Wahlberg, J, Fellström, B, Arnadottir, M. Serum total homocysteine concentration does not predict outcome in renal transplant recipients. *Clin Transplant* 1998; 12: 563–68.

32. Ducloux, D, Pascal, B, Jamali, M, Gibey, R, Chalopin, JM. Is hyperhomocysteinemia a risk factor for recurrent vascular access thrombosis in haemodialysis patients? *Nephrol Dial Transplant* 1997; 12: 2037–38.

33. Ducloux, D, Ruedin, C, Gibey, R, Vautrin, P, Bresson-Vautrin, C, Rebibou, JM, Chalopin, JM. Prevalence, determinants, and clinical significance of hyperhomocyst(e)inaemia in renal-transplant recipients. *Nephrol Dial Transplant* 1998; 13: 2890–93.

34. Ducloux, D, Heuzé-Lecornu, L, Gibey, R, Bresson-Vautrin, C, Vautrin, P, Chalopin, JM. Dialysis adequacy and homocyst(e)ine concentrations in peritoneal dialysis patients. *Nephrol Dial Transplant* 1999; 14: 728–31.

35. Födinger, M, Mannhalter, C, Gabriele, W, Pabinger, I, Muller, E, Schmid, R, Hörl, W, Sunder-Plassmann, G. Mutation (677 C to T) in the methylenetetrahydrofolate reductase gene aggravates hyperhomocysteinemia in hemodialysis patients. *Kidney Int* 1997; 52: 517–23.

36. Foegh, ML. Chronic rejection—graft arteriosclerosis. *Transplant Proc* 1990; 22: 119–22.

37. Foreman, JW, Wald, H, Blumberg, G, Pepe, LM, Segal, S. Homocysteine uptake in isolated rat renal cortical tubules. *Metabolism* 1982; 31: 613–19.

38. Frei, B, Stocker, R, Ames, BN. Antioxidant defenses and lipid peroxidation in human blood plasma. *Proc Natl Acad Sci USA* 1988; 85: 9748–53.

39. Gallice, PM, Kovacic, HN, Brunet, PJ, Berland, YF, Crevat, AB. A non-ouabain-like inhibitor of the sodium pump in uremic plasma ultrafiltrate and urine from healthy subjects. *Clin Chim Acta* 1993; 273: 149–60.

40. Guarnieri, G, Toigo, G, Fiotti, N, Ciocchi, B, Situlin, R, Giansante, G, Vasile, A, Carraro, M, Faccini, L, Biolo, G. Mechanisms of malnutrition in uremia. *Kidney Int* 1997; 62: S-41–4.

41. Gupta, A, Moustapha, A, Jacobsen, DW, Goormastic, M, Tuzcu, EM, Hobbs, R, Young, J, James, K, McCarthy, P, van Lente, F, Green, R, Robinson, K. High homocysteine, low folate, and low vitamin B_6 concentrations: Prevalent risk factors for vascular disease in heart transplant recipients. *Transplantation* 1998; 65: 544–50.

42. Guttormsen, AB, Schneede, J, Fiskerstrand, T, Ueland, PM, Refsum, H. Plasma concentrations of homocysteine and other aminothiol compounds are related to food intake in healthy subjects. *J Nutr* 1994; 124: 1934–41.

43. Guttormsen, AB, Schneede, J, Ueland, P, Refsum, H. Kinetics of total plasma homocysteine in subjects with hyperhomocysteinemia due to folate or cobalamine deficiency. *Am J Clin Nutr* 1996; 63: 194–202.

44. Guttormsen, AB, Ueland, PM, Svarstad, E, Refsum, H. Kinetic basis of hyperhomocysteinemia in patients with chronic renal failure. *Kidney Int* 1997; 52: 495–502.

45. Homocysteine Lowering Trialists collaboration. Lowering blood homocysteine with folic acid based supplements. *BMJ* 1998; 316: 894–98.

46. Hoogeveen, EK, Kostense, PJ, Jager, A, Heine, RJ, Cornelis, J, Bouter, LM, Donker, AJM, Stehouwer, CDA. Serum homocysteine level and protein intake are related to risk of microalbuminuria: The Hoorn study. *Kidney Int* 1998; 54: 203–9.

47. Hultberg, B, Agardh, E, Andersson, A, Brattström, L, Isakson, A, Israelsson, B, Agardh, CD. Increased levels of plasma homocysteine are associated with nephropathy, but not severe retinopathy in type 1 diabetes mellitus. *Scand J Clin Lab Invest* 1991; 51: 277–82.

48. Hultberg, B, Andersson, A, Sterner, G. Plasma homocysteine in renal failure. *Clin Nephrol* 1993; 40: 230–34.

49. Hultberg, B, Andersson, A, Masson, P, Larsson, M, Tunek, A. Plasma homocysteine and thiol compound fractions after oral administration of N-acetylcysteine. *Scand J Clin Lab Invest* 1994; 54: 417–22.

50. Hultberg, B, Andersson, A, Arnadottir, M. Reduced, free and total fractions of homocysteine and other thiol compounds in plasma from patients with renal failure. *Nephron* 1995; 70: 62–7.

51. Janssen, MJFM, van Guldener, C, de Jong, GM, van den Berg, M, Stehouwer, CDA, Donker, AJM. Folic acid treatment of hyperhomocysteinemia in dialysis patients. *Miner Electrolyte Metab* 1996; 22: 110–14.

52. Kotb, M, Geller, AM. Methionine adenosyltransferase: Structure and function. *Pharm Ther* 1993; 59: 125–43.

53. Laidlaw, SA, Berg, RL, Kopple, JD, Naito, H, Walker, WG, Walser, M. Patterns of fasting plasma amino acid levels in chronic renal insufficiency: Results from the feasibility phase of the Modification of Diet in Renal Disease Study. *Am J Kidney Dis* 1994; 23: 504–13.

54. Livant, EJ, Tamura, T, Johnston, KE, Vaughn, H, Bergman, SM, Forehand, J, Walthaw, J. Plasma folate conjugase activities and folate concentrations in patients receiving hemodialysis. *J Nutr Biochem* 1994; 5: 504–8.

55. Loehrer, FMT, Angst, CP, Brunner, FP, Haefeli, WE, Fowler, B. Evidence for disturbed S-adenosylmethionine: S-adenosylhomocysteine ratio in patients with end-stage renal failure: A cause for disturbed methylation reactions? *Nephrol Dial Transplant* 1998; 13: 656–61.

56. Manns, BJ, Burgess, ED, Parsons, HG, Schaefer, JP, Hyndman, ME, Scott-Douglas, NW. Hyperhomocysteinemia, anticardiolipin antibody status, and risk for vascular access thrombosis in hemodialysis patients. *Kidney Int* 1999; 55: 315–20.

57. Massy, ZA, Chadefaux-Vekemans, B, Chevalier, A, Bader, CA, Drueke, TB, Legendre, C, Lacour, B, Kamoun, P, Kreis, M. Hyperhomocysteinaemia: A significant risk factor for cardiovascular disease in renal transplant recipients. *Nephrol Dial Transplant* 1994; 9: 1103–8.

58. McKeever, MP, Weir, DG, Molloy, A, Scott, JM. Betaine-homocysteine methyltransferase: Organ distribution in man, pig and rat and subcellular distribution in the rat. *Clin Sci* 1991; 81: 551–56.

59. Moustapha, A, Naso, A, Nahlawi, M, Gupta, A, Arheart, KL, Jacobsen, DW, Robinson, K, Dennis, VW. Prospective study of hyperhomocysteinemia as an adverse cardiovascu-

lar risk factor in end-stage renal disease. *Circulation* 1998; 97: 138–41.

60. Mudd, SH, Poole, JR. Labile methyl balances for normal humans on various dietary regimens. *Metabolism* 1975; 24: 721–35.

61. Murase, T, Cattran, DC, Rubenstein, B, Steiner, G. Inhibition of lipoprotein lipase by uremic plasma, a possible cause of hypertriglyceridemia. *Metabolism* 1975; 24: 1279–86.

62. Norlund, L, Grubb, A, Fex, G, Leksell, H, Nilsson, JE, Schenck, H, Hultberg, B. The increase of plasma homocysteine concentrations with age is partly due to the deterioriation of renal function as determined by plasma cystatin C. *Clin Chem Lab Med* 1998; 36: 175–78.

63. Ono, K, Hisasue, Y. Is folate supplementation necessary in hemodialysis patients on erythropoietin therapy? *Clin Nephrol* 1992; 38: 290–92.

64. Perna, AF, Ingrosso, D, Galletti, P, Zappia, V, De Santo, NG. Membrane protein damage and methylation reactions in chronic renal failure. *Kidney Int* 1996; 50: 358–66.

65. Perna, AF, Ingrosso, D, De Santo, NG, Galletti, P, Brunone, M, Zappia, V. Metabolic consequences of folate-induced reduction of hyperhomocysteinemia in uremia. *J Am Soc Nephrol* 1997; 8: 1899–1905.

66. Raine, AEG, Margreiter, R, Brunner, FP, Ehrich, JHH, Geerlings, W, Landais, P, Loirat, C, Mallick, NP, Selwood, NH, Tufveson, G, Valderrabano, F. Report on management of renal failure in Europe, XXII, 1991. *Nephrol Dial Transplant* 1992; 7(suppl 2): 7–35.

67. Refsum, H, Helland, S, Ueland, PM. Radioenzymatic determination of homocysteine in plasma and urine. *Clin Chem* 1985; 31: 624–28.

68. Robins, AJ, Milewczyk, BK, Booth, EM, Mallick, NP. Plasma amino acid abnormalities in chronic renal failure. *Clin Chim Acta* 1972; 42: 215–17.

69. Robinson, K, Gupta, A, Dennis, V, Arheart, K, Chaudhary, D, Green, R, Vigo, P, Mayer, EM, Selhub, J, Kutner, M, Jacobsen, DW. Hyperhomocysteinemia confers an independent increased risk of atherosclerosis in end-stage renal disease and is closely linked to plasma folate and pyridoxine concentrations. *Circulation* 1996; 94: 2743–48.

70. Sirrs, S, Duncan, L, Djurdjev, O, Nussbaumer, G, Ganz, G, Frohlich, J, Levin, A. Homocyst(e)ine and vascular access complications in hemodialysis patients: Insights into a complex metabolic relationship. *Nephrol Dial Transplant* 1999; 14: 738–43.

71. Stampfer, MJ, Malinow, MR, Willett, WC, Newcomer, LM, Upson, B, Ullmann, D, Tishler, PV, Hennekens, CH. A prospective study of plasma homocyst(e)ine and risk of myocardial infarction in US physicians. *JAMA* 1992; 268: 877–81.

72. Suliman, ME, Anderstam, B, Lindholm, B, Bergström, J. Total, free, and protein-bound sulphur amino acids in uraemic patients. *Nephrol Dial Transplant* 1997; 12: 2332–38.

73. Tamura, T, Johnston, KE, Bergman, SM. Homocysteine and folate concentrations in blood from patients treated with hemodialysis. *J Am Soc Nephrol* 1996; 7: 2414–18.

74. Tamura, T, Bergman, S, Morgan, SL. Homocysteine, B vitamins, and vascular-access thrombosis in patients treated with hemodialysis. *Am J Kidney Dis* 1998; 32: 475–81.

75. Tamura, T, Bergman, SM, Morgan, SL. Hyperhomocysteinemia as a cause of vascular occlusion in end-stage-renal disease. *Int J Artif Organs* 1998; 21: 72–4.

76. Ubbink, JB, Hayward, WJ, van der, Merwe, A, Becker, PJ, Delport, R, Potgieter, HC. Vitamin requirements for the treatment of hyperhomocysteinemia in humans. *J Nutr* 1994; 124: 1927–33.

77. Ueland, PM, Refsum, H. Brattström, L. Plasma homocysteine and cardiovascular disease. In *Atherosclerotic Cardiovascular Disease, Hemostasis, and Endothelial Function.* (Francis, RB Jr, ed.). Marcel Dekker, New York, 1992, pp. 183–235.

78. van Guldener, C, Lambert, J, Janssen, MJFM, Donker, AJM, Stehouwer, CDA. Endothelium-dependent vasodilatation and distensibility of large arteries in chronic haemodialysis patients. *Nephrol Dial Transplant* 1997; 12(Suppl 2): 14–8.

79. van Guldener, C, Janssen, MJFM, Lambert, J, ter Wee, PM, Jakobs, C, Donker, AJM, Stehouwer, CDA. No change in impaired endothelial function after long-term folic acid therapy of hyperhomocysteinaemia in haemodialysis patients. *Nephrol Dial Transplant* 1998; 13: 106–12.

80. van Guldener, C, Janssen, MJFM, Lambert, J, ter Wee, PM, Donker, AJM, Stehouwer, CDA. Folic acid treatment of hyperhomocysteinaemia in peritoneal dialysis patients: No change in endothelial function after long-term therapy. *Perit Dial Int* 1998; 18: 282–89.

81. van Guldener, C, Janssen, MJFM, de Meer, K, Donker, AJM, Stehouwer, CDA. Effect of folic acid and betaine on fasting and post-methionine-loading plasma homocysteine and methionine levels in chronic haemodialysis patients. *J Intern Med* 1999; 245: 173–83.

82. van Guldener, C, Kulik, W, Berger, R, Dijkstra, DA, Jakobs, C, Reijngoud, DJ, Donker, AJM, Stehouwer, CDA, de Meer, K. Homocysteine remethylation and methionine transmethylation are proportionally decreased in end-stage renal disease: A stable isotope study with L-[^{2}H$_3$-methyl-1-^{13}C]methionine. Vrije Universiteit (dissertation), Amsterdam, The Netherlands, 1999; pp. 93–100.

83. Vychytil, A, Födinger, M, Wölfl, G, Enzenberger, B, Auinger, M, Prischl, F, Buxbaum, M, Wiesholzer, M, Mannhalter, C, Hörl, WH, Sunder-Plassmann, G. Major determinants of hyperhomocysteinemia in peritoneal dialysis patients. *Kidney Int* 1998; 53: 1775–82.

84. Westhuyzen, J, Matherson, K, Tracey, R, Fleming, SJ. Effect of withdrawal of folic acid supplementation in maintenance hemodialysis patients. *Clin Nephrol* 1993; 40: 96–9.

85. Wilcken, DEL, Gupta, V. Sulphur containing amino acids in chronic renal failure with particular reference to homocystine and cysteine-homocysteine mixed disulphide. *Eur J Clin Invest* 1979; 9: 301–7.

86. Wilcken, DEL, Gupta, VJ, Betts, AK. Homocysteine in the plasma of renal transplant recipients: Effects of cofactors for methionine metabolism. *Clin Sci* 1981; 61: 743–49.

87. Wollesen, F, Brattström, L, Refsum, H, Ueland, PM, Berglund, L, Berne, C. Plasma total homocysteine and cysteine in relation to glomerular filtration rate in diabetes mellitus. *Kidney Int* 1999; 55: 1028–35.

27

Diseases and Drugs Associated with Hyperhomocysteinemia

HENK J. BLOM

The diseases and drugs associated with hyperhomocysteinemia can be separated into those presumed to be the consequence of hyperhomocysteinemia (see Section 7) and those causing hyperhomocysteinemia (see Section 6). Many retrospective and prospective studies have associated hyperhomocysteinemia with a twofold to fourfold increased risk for arterial occlusive disease. Increasing numbers of studies also relate hyperhomocysteinemia to an increased risk for thrombosis, neural tube defects (and possibly other midline congenital disorders), cognitive dysfunction, and complications of pregnancy, such as recurrent spontaneous abortion, preeclampsia, and placental pathology. Folate effectively lowers homocysteine, but randomized controlled trials of folate have been performed only for the prevention of neural tube defects. Whether folate, alone or in combination with vitamin B_6 and cobalamin, will prevent the other diseases mentioned remains to be clarified before a causal relation can be accepted. The retrospective and prospective case/control studies do not prove causality; they merely demonstrate an association. Theoretically, it may still be that arteriosclerosis, thrombosis, complications of pregnancy, and cognitive dysfunction are causes of hyperhomocysteinemia instead of consequences.

Diseases Associated with Hyperhomocysteinemia

Kidney Dysfunction

The plasma total homocysteine concentration strongly correlates with kidney function (see Chapters 16 and 26). Patients with severe renal failure have obviously elevated plasma homocysteine levels, but even incipient renal insufficiency is associated with an increase in plasma homocysteine. Excretion of homocysteine is very low. Therefore, either kidney function influences or even regulates homocysteine metabolism in the body, or the kidney itself converts a major amount of homocysteine present in blood. Homocysteine in plasma is 99% bound as disulfides to proteins and other thiol-group-containing components. These disulfides need to be reduced to liberate homocysteine and so become available for conversion to methionine or cysteine. In the kidney, the nonprotein-bound fraction of homocysteine in plasma (about 30% of the total plasma homocysteine concentration) is taken up by renal tubular cells. Due to the low redox state in the cells, the disulfides are reduced, which will make homocysteine available for transsulfuration or remethylation. The efficient uptake and metabolism of homocysteine by tubular cells can explain the strong correlation between kidney function and plasma homocysteine concentration.

Proliferating Diseases

Patients with proliferating disease such as cancer or psoriasis have elevated total homocysteine concentrations in their body fluids (22, 71, 73). Presumably, the rapidly dividing cells take up the methionine required for protein synthesis and in particular for S-adenosylmethionine synthesis. After S-adenosylmethionine methylates vital cell components, the product S-adenosylhomocysteine is hydrolyzed to homocysteine and adenosine. Because the equilibrium of this reaction favors synthesis of S-adenosylhomocysteine, which inhibits most methylation reactions, export of homocysteine out of the cell will keep the intracellular S-adenosylhomocysteine concentrations low. In vitro many different types of cancer cells lack functional homocysteine remethylation (39), leaving homocysteine export as the only way to eliminate homocysteine from the cell. Rapidly dividing cells seem to divert all one-carbon units of tetrahydrofolates for the synthesis of purines and thymidine, the building blocks of DNA and RNA, at the expense of homocysteine remethylation. On the basis of this mechanism, proliferating diseases may cause hyperhomocysteinemia. However, folate deficiency or even hyperhomocysteinemia itself may theoretically predispose to proliferating disease (32).

The presence of hyperhomocysteinemia in patients with cancer has led to the speculation that the increased thromboembolic risk in this population may in part be attributable to their elevated homocysteine.

Rheumatoid Arthritis

Recent studies demonstrated increased total homocysteine in the blood of patients with rheumatoid arthritis in the fasting state, as well as after methionine loading (37, 68, 75), independent of the use of methotrexate. No clear explanation for this hyperhomocysteinemia in rheumatoid arthritis is available. It is possible that gastrointestinal dysfunction in some patients with rheumatoid arthritis leads to cobalamin deficiency, which is indicated by elevated methylmalonic acid (65). It has also been suggested that the presence of hyperhomocysteinemia in patients with rheumatoid arthritis may play a role in the increased prevalence of cardiovascular disease in them.

Hypothyroidism

Several studies have described increased plasma homocysteine concentrations in hypothyroid patients (25, 42, 43, 57, 67), which may be attributed in part to reduced renal function in hypothyroidism (57, 93). In hyperthyroid patients normal homocysteine concentrations have been observed (67). However, Diekman et al. (25) found an increase of homocysteine during the transition from the hyperthyroid to the euthyroid state. The latter study demonstrated a strong inverse correlation between changes in plasma free thyroid hormone and homocysteine concentrations, independent of changes in plasma creatinine and folate, and independent of 5,10-methylenetetrahydrofolate reductase (MTHFR) 677C→T genotypes. Homocysteine concentrations fell after treatment of hypothyroidism (42).

Hypothyroid rats had reduced MTHFR but increased methionine synthase activities, which may influence the homocysteine concentration (66). It may be that the hyperhomocysteinemia of hypothyroid patients contributes to their increased risk for arteriosclerosis.

Drugs

Hormones

Sex Hormones Sex hormones seem to affect plasma homocysteine concentrations. The influences can be categorized by endogenous and exogenous sex hormones.

ENDOGENOUS SEX HORMONES Several studies have reported gender differences in homocysteine concentrations. Homocysteine concentrations are higher in men than in premenopausal women (12, 13). As discussed in Chapter 37, blood homocysteine concentrations are decreased during pregnancy, a condition characterized by elevated estrogen levels (5, 48). After menopause, when endogenous estrogen production ceases, homocysteine concentrations are higher than before menopause (13, 15, 47). However, others have reported nonsignificant differences (4) or no difference at all (26) between premenopausal and postmenopausal women. Our group has observed clear differences in plasma homocysteine concentrations between these two groups of women, both fasting and after methionine loading (12, 13, 95), and homocysteine concentrations were negatively correlated with estrogen levels in premenopausal women. Still, these effects on homocysteine concentrations are blurred by the influence of age. It remains to be established whether menopause influences homocysteine concentration. Theoretically, the more efficient methionine metabolism in premenopausal women (13) may explain in part the lower incidence of cardiovascular morbidity and mortality observed in this population group.

EXOGENOUS SEX HORMONES Changes in homocysteine concentrations have been described during administration of oral contraceptives, postmenopausal hormone replacement, and antiestrogen therapy, which is more extensively discussed in Chapter 37. In short, oral contraceptives, containing the synthetic hormone ethinyl-estradiol in combination with a progesterone, may increase homocysteine (82); however, this is not a consistent observation (16). The reported increase was detected in the pill-free interval of the oral contraceptive cycle, whereas no significant fluctuations were found during the normal menstrual cycle. Increased thromboembolic disorders during oral contraceptive use may thus be explained in part by the increased homocysteine concentrations.

In contrast to these observations, homocysteine concentrations decrease during postmenopausal hormone replacement therapy. Several oral and transdermal hormone replacement regimens containing estrogen alone or combined estrogen/progestogen reduced fasting homocysteine concentrations (7, 34, 59–61, 89, 90). The decrease in cardiovascular risk in postmenopausal women using hormone replacement therapy may be attributable in part to a decrease of homocysteine.

Giltay et al. (33) observed a homocysteine decrease in male-to-female transsexuals after estrogen and antiandrogen administration. Supraphysiological doses of testosterone do not seem to affect homocysteine in normal men (97). Estradiol-treated rats had lower plasma homocysteine than control animals (51). Taken together, estradiol-like substances are believed to reduce homocysteine. Tamoxifen, an antiestrogen drug used as adjuvant therapy in women with breast cancer, also reduces plasma homocysteine, underlining that manipulation of estrogen metabolism influences homocysteine metabolism (6, 20).

Insulin The relationship between homocysteine and insulin is unclear. One study reported an inverse relation between plasma homocysteine and insulin concentrations in a normoinsulinemic, nondiabetic Jewish population (8a). Another study found no relation between homocysteine and insulin or proinsulin concentrations in men (68a), whereas in a third study insulin was a major determinant of homocysteine in children and adolescents (32a). Fonseca et al. (31) reported that insulin reduced homocysteine in normal subjects but had no effect on homocysteine concentrations in patients with insulin-resistant diabetes mellitus. Rats that were made diabetic by administration of streptozotocin had 30% lower plasma homocysteine concentrations (44). Insulin administration returned these concentrations to normal. These studies indicate that insulin status may influence homocysteine metabolism via an unknown mechanism.

Antiepileptic Drugs

Antiepileptic drugs such as phenobarbital, carbamazepine, primidone and, in particular, valproate and phenytoin appear to be inhibitors of enzymes of folate metabolism and may cause folate deficiency (38, 56, 72). The association between the use of antiepileptics and the increased risk of having a child with a neural tube defect may be based on this inhibition of folate metabolism.

Data on the possible relation between the use of antiepileptic drugs and plasma homocysteine in humans are scarce. Schwaninger et al. (79) observed an increase of homocysteine and a reduction of folate and vitamin B_6 concentrations in the serum of patients using anticonvulsants. In particular, carbamazepine (79) and phenytoin (45) were associated with an increase in plasma homocysteine. Treatment of pregnant mice with valproate increased plasma homocysteine, which was normalized by coadministration of folate (38). In rats, valproate did not influence the homocysteine concentration but reduced plasma methionine (3). Taken together, data are accumulating that antiepileptic drugs reduce homocysteine remethylation and possibly also transsulfuration and therefore can cause hyperhomocysteinemia.

Methotrexate

The inhibition of dihydrofolate reductase (Metabolic Diagram, Reaction 11) by methotrexate decreases purine and in particular thymidine synthesis, owing to the accumulation of unreduced folates and the diminished availability of tetrahydrofolates required for the synthesis of these DNA building blocks. This inhibition of dihydrofolate reductase therefore should also decrease homocysteine remethylation by methionine synthase. Indeed, many studies have established that high-dose methotrexate therapy for cancer increases homocysteine in urine, blood (17, 35, 50, 70, 73), and cerebrospinal fluid (69). Even the use of low-dose methotrexate for the treatment of psoriasis (71) or rheumatoid arthritis (36, 64, 65, 92) elevates plasma homocysteine.

The toxic side effects of high-dose methotrexate in the treatment for cancer are counteracted by administration of high amounts of folate, mainly in the form of 5-formyltetrahydrofolate as a rescue agent. The toxic side effects of long term administration of low-dose methotrexate used for treatment of rheumatoid arthritis also seem to be preventable by the use of low amounts of folate, without affecting methotrexate's clinical efficacy (92). The toxicity of low-dose methotrexate may be related to the increase of homocysteine (36, 92). If that is the case, then betaine may be considered as a possible prophylactic agent, in addition to folate, because betaine remethylates homocysteine via a folate-independent pathway.

Other antifolates such as raltitrexed, trimetrexate, or trimethoprim may also increase plasma homocysteine. Indeed, Smulders et al. (81) observed a large increase of plasma homocysteine in healthy volunteers taking trimethoprim.

Nitrous Oxide (N_2O)

Nitrous oxide or "laughing gas" is used in many general anesthetics. Several studies showed an increase of homocysteine in plasma or urine by nitrous oxide use (21, 27). A randomized, controlled study demonstrated that homocysteine concentrations increased by about 10 μmol/L after nitrous oxide use (8). The homocysteine concentration did not increase if more isoflurane was supplied to replace nitrous oxide. Even 7 days after nitrous oxide exposure, the homocysteine concentrations were still increased by about 30% (21).

The cause of this homocysteine increase is the well-known inactivation of methionine synthase by nitrous oxide. In a set of elegant in vitro and in vivo studies, Refsum et al. (21, 28, 30) demonstrated that nitrous oxide can inactivate methionine synthase only if this enzyme is catalytically active. During catalytic turnover, the methyl group bound to the cobalamin attached to methionine synthase is transferred to homocysteine, which leaves the cobalamin free to react with nitrous oxide, resulting in inactivation of methionine synthase. Thus, if there is no catalytic turnover of methionine synthase, it will not be inactivated by nitrous oxide. Methionine loading reduces the catalytic turnover of methionine synthase and thus its inactivation by nitrous oxide (21), but the methionine loading itself will increase plasma homocysteine. Preoperative use of folate will reduce plasma homocysteine, but it also activates methionine synthase, thus making it susceptible to inactivation. Preoperative administration of betaine may be the best choice, because it remethylates homocysteine independently methionine synthase. In fruit bats, administration of betaine delayed neurological impairment by nitrous oxide (91).

The increased postoperative risk for myocardial infarction and thrombosis may in part be related to the 30% to 100% increase of plasma homocysteine concentrations after nitrous oxide use. In addition, patients with unrecognized cobalamin deficiency may be particularly susceptible to nitrous oxide exposure, resulting in neurological deterioration (52). In this respect it is of importance to note that about 10% to 30% of elderly persons in North America and Western Europe are considered cobalamin deficient (19, 88) (see also Chapter 24).

Lipid-Lowering Drugs

Beyond their effects on blood lipids, lipid-lowering drugs may influence other risk factors for cardiovascular disease, such as homocysteine. However, data on the effect of statins, niacin, cholestyramine, and fibric acid on plasma homocysteine are scarce (85). The combination of niacin and colestipol increased homocysteine in plasma (11). In rats, niacin administration caused hyperhomocysteinemia, hypermethioninemia, hypocysteinemia, and reduced plasma concentrations of vitamin B_6 (9). Addition of vitamin B_6 normalized these abnormalities without affecting the hypolipidemic action of niacin. In children with familial hypercholesterolemia, the use of cholestyramine did not clearly affect homocysteine in plasma, although it may cause folate deficiency (86). Recently, de Lorgeril et al. (24) found that simvastatin did not influence plasma homocysteine in dyslipidemic patients with coronary heart disease. However, the fibric acid derivative fenofibrate increased plasma homocysteine concentrations about 5 μmol/L, which may reduce the clinical benefits of fibric acid.

Metformin

Metformin is known to influence several risk factors for cardiovascular disease, such as blood lipids, body weight, and insulin in diabetic as well as nondiabetic individuals. Because insulin might influence methionine metabolism (see Insulin section), metformin may also affect plasma homocysteine concentrations. In patients with noninsulin-dependent diabetes mellitus, metformin treatment increased plasma homocysteine (1, 40), which was counteracted by folate administration. Metformin is also related to an increase of plasma homocysteine in nondiabetic individuals (18, 80). Metformin decreased serum cobalamin, without affecting the methylmalonic acid concentration, and, to a lesser extent, serum folate (18), which may also explain its homocysteine-increasing property. The clinical benefit of metformin may be offset by this homocysteine increase. Coadministration of cobalamin and folate could be considered in order to eliminate this side effect.

Disulfide exchangers

Compounds with a free thiol function (R-SH) such as N-acetylcysteine, D-penicillamine, or cysteamine can react with disulfide forms of homocysteine, which account for 99% of the total amount of homocysteine in plasma, via a disulfide exchange reaction:

$$R_1\text{-SH} + R_2\text{-S-S-homocysteine} \longleftrightarrow R_1\text{-S-S-homocysteine} + R_2\text{-SH}$$

$$\text{or } R_1\text{-SS-}R_2 + \text{Homocysteine-SH}$$

Such a reaction can liberate homocysteine from plasma proteins, making homocysteine available for cellular uptake and metabolic conversion and possibly excretion. Indeed, Kang et al. (48) observed an approximately 60% reduction of protein-bound homocysteine by the use of D-penicillamine. Administration of N-acetylcysteine reduced total homocysteine in plasma by 20% to 50% (41, 94). Homocysteine was not reduced by N-acetylcysteine in patients with chronic hepatitis C (10), however, possibly because of a lack of metabolic capacity for homocysteine conversion by the liver. Plasma homocysteine in patients undergoing hemodialysis was reduced by 16% by N-acetylcysteine administration, but no increased dialytic removal of homocysteine was found (14). These studies indicate that N-acetylcysteine does not increase homocysteine excretion but rather improves the metabolic availability of homocysteine. High-dose N-acetylcysteine is well tolerated, and homocysteine can be reduced substantially via disulfide exchange reactions in a dose-dependent manner. Therefore, N-acetylcysteine and possibly cysteamine may be clinically relevant in patients with different forms of hyperhomocysteinemia, particularly those resistant to folate, cobalamin, vitamin B_6, and betaine administration as seen in kidney disease with severe hyperhomocysteinemia.

Gastric Proton Pump Inhibition

As discussed in Chapter 24, cobalamin is bound to proteins in food, from which it needs to be released before it can be taken up by a cobalamin-specific process. Gastric acidity plays an important role in this process. Indeed, proton pump inhibitors such as omeprazole reduced cobalamin uptake, as measured by the protein-bound cobalamin absorption test (53, 54, 58, 76, 77). These proton pump inhibitors probably need to be used over a very long period (> 4 years) before an effect on plasma cobalamin is observed (55, 77, 84), perhaps owing to the relatively large stores of cobalamin under normal conditions and because cobalamin absorption is only partly reduced.

No data are available on the effect of proton pump inhibitors on plasma homocysteine concentrations of individuals prone to develop cobalamin deficiency, such as elderly people. Studies are needed to examine whether, in such populations, the use of proton pump inhibitors may be an additional risk factor for developing cobalamin deficiency and thus hyperhomocysteinemia.

Vitamin B_6 Antagonists

As discussed in Chapter 25, vitamin B_6 in the form of pyridoxal 5′-phosphate is an essential cofactor for cystathionine β-synthase activity. Antagonists of vitamin B_6 can cause hyperhomocysteinemia, in particular after methionine loading. The vitamin B_6 antagonist, 6-azauridine, which was withdrawn by the Food and Drug Administration in 1976, decreased serum pyridoxal 5′-phosphate and increased plasma homocysteine, an effect that was counteracted by vitamin B_6 administration (46).

The bronchodilator, theophylline inhibits pyridoxal kinases, resulting in low levels of pyridoxal 5′-phosphate. Ubbink et al. (87) demonstrated that theophylline treatment of patients with asthma reduced their plasma pyridoxal 5′-phosphate, but fasting homocysteine concentrations remained normal. However, after methionine loading, theophylline users had about 30% higher homocysteine concentrations than control subjects. Vitamin B_6 administration (20 mg/day) reduced, but did not normalize, these elevated postmethionine load homocysteine concentrations.

Several other drugs, such as isoniazid, cycloserine, hydralazine, phenelzine, and procarbazine, may also interfere with vitamin B_6 metabolism and thus elevate homocysteine levels (72).

Methyl Group Acceptors

S-Adenosylmethionine donates its methyl group in more than 100 different reactions (see Chapter 7), resulting in the formation of S-adenosylhomocysteine, which is quickly hydrolyzed to homocysteine and adenosine under normal conditions. Administration of high doses of drugs that require methylation for activation or detoxification produces substantial amounts of S-adenosylhomocysteine and thus may cause hyperhomocysteinemia.

L-dopa, which is O-methylated by S-adenosyl methionine to 3-O-methyldopa, is given in high doses for the treatment of Parkinson's disease. Homocysteine concentrations in plasma were higher in such patients than in control subjects (2), especially in those patients with the 5,10-methylenetetrahydrofolate reductase 677TT genotype (96). Rats treated with L-dopa had decreased S-adenosylmethionine and increased S-adenosylhomocysteine concentrations in all brain regions and peripheral tissues, and their plasma homocysteine was elevated (23, 62). The homocysteine concentration was higher after 1 day of L-dopa treatment than after 17 days, suggesting some attenuation of the effect of chronic L-dopa administration on homocysteine (23).

The anticancer drug, 6-mercaptopurine, is metabolized to a large extent by methylation in vitro and in vivo (50, 83). Children with acute lymphoblastic leukemia treated with 6-mercaptopurine have markedly decreased S-adenosylmethionine but normal S-adenosylhomocysteine concentrations in their red blood cells and normal homocysteine concentrations in plasma. High-dose 6-mercaptopurine not only consumes the methyl group of S-adenosylmethionine, but also depletes adenosine triphosphate, which is required for S-adenosylmethionine synthesis from methionine. This reduced S-adenosylmethionine synthesis may explain the lack of influence of 6-mercaptopurine on the plasma homocysteine concentration, despite the extensive methylation of 6-mercaptopurine.

Other Drugs

Sulfasalazine may also increase plasma homocysteine (36, 78), owing to its effect on folate metabolism (see Chapter 23) or because of an unknown mechanism. Megadoses of vitamin C (500 to 1,000 mg) may compromise cobalamin and folate metabolism, leading to hyperhomocysteinemia (63).

Little attention has been given to drugs that may decrease homocysteine or even cause hypohomocysteinemia, including some antiviral drugs and adenosine analogs, which inhibit S-adenosylhomocysteine hydrolysis (72). Exploration of their homocysteine-

Table 27.1.   Diseases and Drugs Associated with Hyperhomocysteinemia and Hypohomocysteinemia[a]

	Effect[b]
Inherited	
Cystathionine β-synthase deficiency	↑↑↑↑
MTHFR:	
deficiency	↑↑↑↑
677C→T (thermolabile)	↑↑
1298A→G	↑
Inborn errors of folate and cobalamin metabolism	↑↑↑↑
Acquired	
Deficiencies	
Cobalamin	↑↑↑↑
Folate	↑↑↑
Vitamin B$_6$	↑↑[c]
Diseases	
Renal failure	↑↑↑
Proliferating diseases	↑↑
Rheumatoid arthritis	↑↑
Hypothyroidism	↑↑
Hyperthyroidism	↓
Drugs	
Estrogen, insulin	↓
Antiepileptics	↑↑
Methotrexate	↑↑
Nitrous oxide	↑↑↑
Lipid lowering drugs	↑↑
Metformin	↑↑
Disulfide exchangers	↓
Gastric proton pump inhibitors	?
Vitamin B$_6$ antagonists	↑↑[c]
Methyl group acceptors (L-dopa and 6-mercaptopurine)	↑↑
Miscellaneous	
Increasing age	↑
Male sex	↑
Increased muscle mass	↑
Exercise	↓
Gastroplasty	↑
Carbon monoxide, cyanide	↑
Coffee intake	↑
Smoking	↑
Alcohol consumption	↑ and ↓
Down syndrome	↓

[a] These entities are discussed in this chapter and in other chapters in the book. Modified from Refsum et al. [74].
[b] ↓ is a decrease of plasma homocysteine concentration, ↑ is increase within normal range (5 to 15 μmol/L), ↑↑ is mild or moderate hyperhomocysteinemia (15 to 30 μmol/L), ↑↑↑ is intermediate hyperhomocysteinemia (30 to 100 μmol/L), and ↑↑↑↑ is severe hyperhomocysteinemia (>100 μmol/L).
[c] Especially after methionine loading

lowering potential may lead to novel approaches of homocysteine-lowering therapy.

Miscellaneous

Additional factors that influence plasma homocysteine concentrations, including age, sex, chromosomal abnormalities, exercise, coffee intake, smoking, and alcohol consumption, are given in Table 27.1, but are beyond the scope of this chapter. They are extensively described in other chapters.

Possible interactions between homocysteine and other diseases and drugs have not been studied extensively. Plasma homocysteine is 1) a sensitive marker of folate and cobalamin status, 2) related to the redox state of the cell, 3) dependent on methylation by S-adenosylmethionine, and 4) strongly influenced by liver and kidney function. Because many diseases and drugs interrelate with one or more of these four characteristics, many more factors that affect homocysteine metabolism have yet to be discovered.

REFERENCES

1. Aarsand, AK, Carlsen, SM. Folate administration reduces circulating homocysteine levels in NIDDM patients on long-term metformin treatment. *J Intern Med* 1998; 244: 169–74.
2. Allain, P, Le Bouil, A, Cordillet, E, Le Quay, L, Bagheri, H, Montastruc, JL. Sulfate and cysteine levels in the plasma of patients with Parkinson's disease. *Neurotoxicology* 1995; 16: 527–29.
3. Alonso Aperte, E, Ubeda, N, Achon, M, Perez de Miguelsanz, J, Varela Moreiras, G. Impaired methionine synthesis and hypomethylation in rats exposed to valproate during gestation. *Neurology* 1999; 52: 750–56.
4. Andersson, A, Brattström, L, Israelsson, B, Isaksson, A, Hamfelt, A, Hultberg, B. Plasma homocysteine before and after methionine loading with regard to age, gender, and menopausal status. *Eur J Clin Invest* 1992; 22: 79–87.
5. Andersson, A, Hultberg, B, Brattström, L, Isaksson, A. Decreased serum homocysteine in pregnancy. *Eur J Clin Chem Clin Biochem* 1992; 30: 377–79.
6. Anker, G, Lonning, PE, Ueland, PM, Refsum, H, Lien, EA. Plasma levels of the atherogenic amino acid homocysteine in post-menopausal women with breast cancer treated with tamoxifen. *Int J Cancer* 1995; 60: 365–68.
7. Anker, GB, Refsum, H, Ueland, PM, Johannessen, DC, Lien, EA, Lonning, PE. Influence of aromatase inhibitors on plasma total homocysteine in postmenopausal breast cancer patients. *Clin Chem* 1999; 45: 252–56.
8. Badner, NH. The use of intraoperative nitrous oxide leads to postoperative increases in plasma homocysteine. *Anesth Analg* 1998; 87: 711–13.
8a. Bar-On, H, Kidron, M, Friedlander, Y, Ben-Yehuda, A, Selhub, J, Rosenberg, IH, Friedman, G. Plasma total homocysteine levels in subjects with hyperinsulinemia. *J Intern Med* 2000; 247: 287–94.

9. Basu, TK, Mann, S. Vitamin B-6 normalizes the altered sulfur amino acid status of rats fed diets containing pharmacological levels of niacin without reducing niacin's hypolipidemic effects. *J Nutr* 1997; 127: 117–21.

10. Bernhard, MC, Junker, E, Hettinger, A, Lauterburg, BH. Time course of total cysteine, glutathione and homocysteine in plasma of patients with chronic hepatitis C treated with interferon-alpha with and without supplementation with N-acetylcysteine. *J Hepatol* 1998; 28: 751–55.

11. Blankenhorn, DH, Malinow, MR, Mack, WJ. Colestipol plus niacin therapy elevates plasma homocyst(e)ine levels. *Coron Art Dis* 1991; 2: 357–60.

12. Blom, HJ, Boers, GH, van den Elzen, JP, van Roessel, JJ, Trijbels, JM, Tangerman, A. Differences between premenopausal women and young men in the transamination pathway of methionine catabolism, and the protection against vascular disease. *Eur J Clin Invest* 1988; 18: 633–38.

13. Boers, GH, Smals, AG, Trijbels, FJ, Leermakers, AI, Kloppenborg, PW. Unique efficiency of methionine metabolism in premenopausal women may protect against vascular disease in the reproductive years. *J Clin Invest* 1983; 72: 1971–76.

14. Bostom, AG, Shemin, D, Yoburn, D, Fisher, DH, Nadeau, MR, Selhub, J. Lack of effect of oral N-acetylcysteine on the acute dialysis-related lowering of total plasma homocysteine in hemodialysis patients. *Atherosclerosis* 1996; 120: 241–44.

15. Brattström, LE, Hultberg, BL, Hardebo, JE. Folic acid responsive postmenopausal homocysteinemia. *Metabolism* 1985; 34: 1073–77.

16. Brattström, L, Israelsson, B, Olsson, A, Andersson, A, Hultberg, B. Plasma homocysteine in women on oral oestrogen-containing contraceptives and in men with oestrogen-treated prostatic carcinoma. *Scand J Clin Lab Invest* 1992; 52: 283–87.

17. Broxson, EH, Jr, Stork, LC, Allen, RH, Stabler, SP, Kolhouse, JF. Changes in plasma methionine and total homocysteine levels in patients receiving methotrexate infusions. *Cancer Res* 1989; 49: 5879–83.

18. Carlsen, SM, Folling, I, Grill, V, Bjerve, KS, Schneede, J, Refsum, H. Metformin increases total serum homocysteine levels in non-diabetic male patients with coronary heart disease. *Scand J Clin Lab Invest* 1997; 57: 521–27.

19. Carmel, R, Green, R, Jacobsen, DW, Rasmussen, K, Florea, M, Azen, C. Serum cobalamin, homocysteine, and methylmalonic acid concentrations in a multiethnic elderly population: Ethnic and sex differences in cobalamin and metabolite abnormalities. *Am J Clin Nutr* 1999; 70: 904–10.

20. Cattaneo, M, Baglietto, L, Zighetti, ML, Bettega, D, Robertson, C, Costa, A, Mannucci, PM, Decensi, A. Tamoxifen reduces plasma homocysteine levels in healthy women. *Br J Cancer* 1998; 77: 2264–66.

21. Christensen, B, Guttormsen, AB, Schneede, J, Riedel, B, Refsum, H, Svardal, A, Ueland, PM. Preoperative methionine loading enhances restoration of the cobalamin-dependent enzyme methionine synthase after nitrous oxide anesthesia. *Anesthesiology* 1994; 80: 1046–56.

22. Corona, G, Toffoli, G, Fabris, M, Viel, A, Zarrelli, A, Donada, C, Boiocchi, M. Homocysteine accumulation in human ovarian carcinoma ascitic/cystic fluids possibly caused by metabolic alteration of the methionine cycle in ovarian carcinoma cells. *Eur J Cancer* 1997; 33: 1284–90.

23. Daly, D, Miller, JW, Nadeau, MR, Selhub, J. The effect of L-dopa administration and folate deficiency on plasma homocysteine concentrations in rats. *J Nutr Biochem* 1997; 8: 634–40.

24. de Lorgeril, M, Salen, P, Paillard, F, Lacan, P, Richard, G. Lipid-lowering drugs and homocysteine [letter]. *Lancet* 1999; 353: 209–10.

25. Diekman, MJM, van der Put, NM, Blom, HJ, Tijssen, JGP, Wiersinga, WM. Plasma homocysteine concentrations in relation to thyroid function disorders. *Clin Endocrinol*, in press.

26. Dudman, NP, Wilcken, DE, Wang, J, Lynch, JF, Macey, D, Lundberg, P. Disordered methionine/homocysteine metabolism in premature vascular disease. Its occurrence, cofactor therapy, and enzymology. *Arterioscler Thromb* 1993; 13: 1253–60.

27. Ermens, AA, Refsum, H, Rupreht, J, Spijkers, LJ, Guttormsen, AB, Lindemans, J, Ueland, PM, Abels, J. Monitoring cobalamin inactivation during nitrous oxide anesthesia by determination of homocysteine and folate in plasma and urine. *Clin Pharmacol Ther* 1991; 49: 385–93.

28. Fiskerstrand, T, Christensen, B, Tysnes, OB, Ueland, PM, Refsum, H. Development and reversion of methionine dependence in a human glioma cell line: Relation to homocysteine remethylation and cobalamin status. *Cancer Res* 1994; 54: 4899–906.

29. Fiskerstrand, T, Ueland, PM, Refsum, H. Response of the methionine synthase system to short-term culture with homocysteine and nitrous oxide and its relation to methionine dependence. *Int J Cancer* 1997; 72: 301–6.

30. Fiskerstrand, T, Ueland, PM, Refsum, H. Folate depletion induced by methotrexate affects methionine synthase activity and its susceptibility to inactivation by nitrous oxide. *J Pharmacol Exp Ther* 1997; 282: 1305–11.

31. Fonseca, VA, Mudaliar, S, Schmidt, B, Fink, LM, Kern, PA, Henry, RR. Plasma homocysteine concentrations are regulated by acute hyperinsulinemia in nondiabetic but not type 2 diabetic subjects. *Metabolism* 1998; 47: 686–89.

32. Fritzer-Szekeres, M, Blom, HJ, Boers, GH, Szekeres, T, Lubec, B. Growth promotion by homocysteine but not by homocysteic acid: A role for excessive growth in homocystinuria or proliferation in hyperhomocysteinemia? *Biochim Biophys Acta* 1998; 1407: 1–6.

32a. Gallistl, S, Sudi, K, Mangge, H, Erwa, W, Borkenstein, M. Insulin is an independent correlate of plasma homocysteine levels in obese children and adolescents. *Diabetes Care* 2000; 23: 1348–52.

33. Giltay, EJ, Hoogeveen, EK, Elbers, JM, Gooren, LJ, Asscheman, H, Stehouwer, CD. Effects of sex steroids on plasma total homocysteine levels: A study in transsexual males and females. *J Clin Endocrinol Metab* 1998; 83: 550–53.

34. Giri, S, Thompson, PD, Taxel, P, Contois, JH, Otvos, J, Allen, R, Ens, G, Wu, AH, Waters, DD. Oral estrogen

improves serum lipids, homocysteine and fibrinolysis in elderly men. *Atherosclerosis* 1998; 137: 359–66.

35. Guttormsen, AB, Ueland, PM, Lonning, PE, Mella, O, Refsum, H. Kinetics of plasma total homocysteine in patients receiving high-dose methotrexate therapy. *Clin Chem* 1998; 44: 1987–9.

36. Haagsma, CJ, Blom, HJ, Van Riel, PLCM, Van't Hof, MA, Giesendorf, BA, van Oppenraaij, D, Van de Putte, LBA. Influence of sulphasalazine, methotrexate, and the combination of both on plasma homocysteine concentrations in patients with rheumatoid arthritis. *Ann Rheum Dis* 1999; 58: 79–84.

37. Hernanz, A, Plaza, A, Martin-Mola, E, De Miguel, E. Increased plasma levels of homocysteine and other thiol compounds in rheumatoid arthritis women. *Clin Biochem* 1999; 32: 65–70.

38. Hishida, R, Nau, H. VPA-induced neural tube defects in mice. I. Altered metabolism of sulfur amino acids and glutathione. *Teratog Carcinog Mutagen* 1998; 18: 49–61.

39. Hoffman, RM. Altered methionine metabolism and transmethylation in cancer. *Anticancer Res* 1985; 5: 1–30.

40. Hoogeveen, EK, Kostense, PJ, Jakobs, C, Bouter, LM, Heine, RJ, Stehouwer, CDA. Does metformin increase the serum total homocysteine level in non-insulin-dependent diabetes mellitus? *J Intern Med* 1997; 242: 389–94.

41. Hultberg, B, Andersson, A, Masson, P, Larson, M, Tunek, A. Plasma homocysteine and thiol compound fractions after oral administration of N-acetylcysteine. *Scand J Clin Lab Invest* 1994; 54: 417–22.

42. Hussein, WI, Green, R, Jacobsen, DW, Faiman, C. Normalization of hyperhomocysteinemia with levothyroxine in hypothyroidism. *Ann Intern Med* 1999; 131: 348–51.

43. Ingenbleek, Y, Barclay, D, Dirren, H. Nutritional significance of alterations in serum amino acid patterns in goitrous patients. *Am J Clin Nutr* 1986; 43: 310–19.

44. Jacobs, RL, House, JD, Brosnan, ME, Brosnan, JT. Effects of streptozotocin-induced diabetes and of insulin treatment on homocysteine metabolism in the rat. *Diabetes* 1998; 47: 1967–70.

45. James, GK, Jones, MW, Pudek, MR. Homocyst(e)ine levels in patients on phenytoin therapy. *Clin Biochem* 1997; 30: 647–49.

46. Juszko, J, Kubalska, J, Kanigowska, K. [Ocular problems in children with homocystinuria] Problemy okulistyczne u dzieci z homocystynuria. *Klin Oczna* 1994; 96: 212–15.

47. Kang, SS, Wong, PW, Cook, HY, Norusis, M, Messer, JV. Protein-bound homocyst(e)ine. A possible risk factor for coronary artery disease. *J Clin Invest* 1986; 77: 1482–86.

48. Kang, SS, Wong, PW, Glickman, PB, MacLeod, CM, Jaffe, IA. Protein-bound homocyst(e)ine in patients with rheumatoid arthritis undergoing D-penicillamine treatment. *J Clin Pharmacol* 1986; 26: 712–15.

49. Kang, SS, Wong, PW, Zhou, JM, Cook, HY. Total homocyst(e)ine in plasma and amniotic fluid of pregnant women. *Metabolism* 1986; 35: 889–91.

50. Keuzenkamp Jansen, CW, De Abreu, RA, Blom, HJ, Bokkerink, JP, Trijbels, JM. Effects on transmethylation by high-dose 6-mercaptopurine and methotrexate infusions during consolidation treatment of acute lym-

phoblastic leukemia. *Biochem Pharmacol* 1996; 51: 1165–71.

51. Kim, MH, Kim, E, Passen, EL, Meyer, J, Kang, SS. Cortisol and estradiol: Nongenetic factors for hyperhomocyst(e)inemia. *Metabolism* 1997; 46: 247–49.

52. Kinsella, LJ, Green, R. Anesthesia paresthetica: Nitrous oxide-induced cobalamin deficiency. *Neurology* 1995; 45: 1608–10.

53. Kittang, E, Aadland, E, Schjonsby, H, Rohss, K. The effect of omeprazole on gastric acidity and the absorption of liver cobalamins. *Scand J Gastroenterol* 1987; 22: 156–60.

54. Kittang, E, Schjonsby, H. Effect of gastric anacidity on the release of cobalamins from food and their subsequent binding to R-protein. *Scand J Gastroenterol* 1987; 22: 1031–37.

55. Koop, H, Bachem, MG. Serum iron, ferritin, and vitamin B_{12} during prolonged omeprazole therapy. *J Clin Gastroenterol* 1992; 14: 288–92.

56. Lambie, DG, Johnson, RH. Drugs and folate metabolism. *Drugs* 1985; 30: 145–55.

57. Lien, EA, Nedrebø, BG, Varhaug, JE, Nygård, O, Aakvaag, A, Ueland, PM. Plasma total homocysteine levels during short-term iatrogenic hypothyroidism. *J Clin Endocrinol Metab* 2000; 85: 1049–53.

58. Marcuard, SP, Albernaz, L, Khazanie, PG. Omeprazole therapy causes malabsorption of cyanocobalamin. *Ann Intern Med* 1994; 120: 211–15.

59. Mijatovic, V, Kenemans, P, Jakobs, C, van Baal, WM, Peters-Muller, ER, van der Mooren, MJ. A randomized controlled study of the effects of 17-β-estradiol-dydrogesterone on plasma homocysteine in postmenopausal women. *Obstet Gynecol* 1998; 91: 432–36.

60. Mijatovic, V, Kenemans, P, Netelenbos, C, Jakobs, C, Popp-Snijders, C, Peters-Muller, ER, van der Mooren, MJ. Postmenopausal oral 17-β-estradiol continuously combined with dydrogesterone reduces fasting serum homocysteine levels. *Fertil Steril* 1998; 69: 876–82.

61. Mijatovic, V, Netelenbos, C, van der Mooren, MJ, de Valk de Roo, GW, Jakobs, C, Kenemans, P. Randomized, double-blind, placebo-controlled study of the effects of raloxifene and conjugated equine estrogen on plasma homocysteine levels in healthy postmenopausal women. *Fertil Steril* 1998; 70: 1085–89.

62. Miller, JW, Shukitthale, B, Villalobosmolina, R, Nadeau, MR, Selhub, J, Joseph, JA. Effect of L-dopa and the catechol-O-methyltransferase inhibitor Ro 41-0960 on sulfur amino acid metabolites in rats. *Clin Neuropharmacol* 1997; 20: 55–66.

63. Mix, JA. Do megadoses of vitamin C compromise folic acid's role in the metabolism of plasma homocysteine? *Nutr Res* 1999; 19: 161–65.

64. Morgan, SL, Baggott, JE, Refsum, H, Ueland, PM. Homocysteine levels in patients with rheumatoid arthritis treated with low-dose methotrexate. *Clin Pharmacol Ther* 1991; 50: 547–56.

65. Morgan, SL, Baggott, JE, Lee, JY, Alarcon, GS. Folic acid supplementation prevents deficient blood folate levels and hyperhomocysteinemia during long-term, low dose methotrexate therapy for rheumatoid arthritis: Implications for cardiovascular disease prevention. *J Rheumatol* 1998; 25: 441–46.

66. Nair, CPP, Viswanathan, G, Noronha, JM. Folate-mediated incorporation of ring-2-carbon of histidine into nucleic acids: Influence of thyroid hormone. *Metabolism* 1994; 43: 1575–78.

67. Nedrebøo, BG, Ericsson, UB, Nygard, O, Refsum, H, Ueland, PM, Aakvaag, A, Aanderud, A, Lien, EA. Plasma total homocysteine levels in hyperthyroid and hypothyroid patients. *Metabolism* 1998; 47: 89–93.

68. Pettersson, T, Friman, C, Abrahamsson, L, Nilsson, B, Norberg, B. Serum homocysteine and methylmalonic acid in patients with rheumatoid arthritis and cobalaminopenia. *J Rheumatol* 1998; 25: 859–63.

68a. Pixa, A, Pietzsch, J, Julius, U, Menschikowski, M, Hanefeld, M. Impaired glucose tolerance (IGT) is not associated with disturbed homocysteine metabolism. *Amino Acids* 2000; 18: 289–98.

69. Quinn, CT, Griener, JC, Bottiglieri, T, Hyland, K, Farrow, A, Kamen, BA. Elevation of homocysteine and excitatory amino acid neurotransmitters in the CSF of children who receive methotrexate for the treatment of cancer. *J Clin Oncol* 1997; 15: 2800–6.

70. Refsum, H, Ueland, PM, Kvinnsland, S. Acute and long-term effects of high-dose methotrexate treatment on homocysteine in plasma and urine. *Cancer Res* 1986; 46: 5385–91.

71. Refsum, H, Helland, S, Ueland, PM. Fasting plasma homocysteine as a sensitive parameter of antifolate effect: A study of psoriasis patients receiving low-dose methotrexate treatment. *Clin Pharmacol Ther* 1989; 46: 510–20.

72. Refsum, H, Ueland, PM. Clinical significance of pharmacological modulation of homocysteine metabolism. *Trends Pharmacol Sci* 1990; 11: 411–16.

73. Refsum, H, Wesenberg, F, Ueland, PM. Plasma homocysteine in children with acute lymphoblastic leukemia: Changes during a chemotherapeutic regimen including methotrexate. *Cancer Res* 1991; 51: 828–35.

74. Refsum, H, Ueland, PM, Nygard, O, Vollset, SE. Homocysteine and cardiovascular disease. *Annu Rev Med* 1998; 49: 31–62.

75. Roubenoff, R, Dellaripa, P, Nadeau, MR, Abad, LW, Muldoon, BA, Selhub, J, Rosenberg, IH. Abnormal homocysteine metabolism in rheumatoid arthritis. *Arthritis Rheum* 1997; 40: 718–22.

76. Saltzman, JR, Kemp, JA, Golner, BB, Pedrosa, MC, Dallal, GE, Russell, RM. Effect of hypochlorhydria due to omeprazole treatment or atrophic gastritis on protein-bound vitamin B12 absorption. *J Am Coll Nutr* 1994; 13: 584–91.

77. Schenk, BE, Festen, HP, Kuipers, EJ, Klinkenberg-Knol, EC, Meuwissen, SG. Effect of short- and long-term treatment with omeprazole on the absorption and serum levels of cobalamin. *Aliment Pharmacol Ther* 1996; 10: 541–45.

78. Schieken, RM. Hypertension and atherosclerosis in children. *Curr Opin Cardiol* 1994; 9: 130–6.

79. Schwaninger, M, Ringleb, P, Winter, R, Kohl, B, Fiehn, W, Rieser, PA, Walter-Sack, I. Elevated plasma concentrations of homocysteine in antiepileptic drug treatment. *Epilepsia* 1999; 40: 345–50.

80. Shaw, JT, McWhinney, B, Tate, JR, Kesting, JB, Marczak, M, Purdie, D, Gibbs, H, Cameron, DP, Hickman, PE. Plasma homocysteine levels in indigenous Australians. *Med J Aust* 1999; 170: 19–22.

81. Smulders, YM, de Man, AM, Stehouwer, CD, Slaats, EH. Trimethoprim and fasting plasma homocysteine [letter]. *Lancet* 1998; 352: 1827–28.

82. Steegers Theunissen, RP, Boers, GH, Steegers, EA, Trijbels, FJ, Thomas, CM, Eskes, TK. Effects of sub-50 oral contraceptives on homocysteine metabolism: A preliminary study. *Contraception* 1992; 45: 129–39.

83. Stet, EH, De Abreu, RA, Bokkerink, JP, Blom, HJ, Lambooy, LH, Vogels Mentink, TM, de Graaf Hess, AC, van Raay Selten, B, Trijbels, FJ. Decrease in S-adenosylmethionine synthesis by 6-mercaptopurine and methylmercaptopurine ribonucleoside in Molt F4 human malignant lymphoblasts. *Biochem J* 1994; 304: 163–68.

84. Termanini, B, Gibril, F, Sutliff, VE, Yu, F, Venzon, DJ, Jensen, RT. Effect of long-term gastric acid suppressive therapy on serum vitamin B12 levels in patients with Zollinger-Ellison syndrome. *Am J Med* 1998; 104: 422–30.

85. Tonstad, S. Correlates of plasma total homocysteine in patients with hyperlipidaemia. *Eur J Clin Invest* 1997; 27: 1025–29.

86. Tonstad, S, Knudtzon, J, Sivertsen, M, Refsum, H, Ose, L. Efficacy and safety of cholestyramine therapy in peripubertal and prepubertal children with familial hypercholesterolemia. *J Pediatr* 1996; 129: 42–9.

87. Ubbink, JB, van der Merwe, A, Delport, R, Allen, RH, Stabler, SP, Riezler, R, Vermaak, WJ. The effect of a subnormal vitamin B-6 status on homocysteine metabolism. *J Clin Invest* 1996; 98: 177–84.

88. van Asselt, DZ, de Groot, LC, van Staveren, WA, Blom, HJ, Wevers, RA, Biemond, I, Hoefnagels, WH. Role of cobalamin intake and atrophic gastritis in mild cobalamin deficiency in older Dutch subjects. *Am J Clin Nutr* 1998; 68: 328–34.

89. van der Mooren, MJ, Wouters, MG, Blom, HJ, Schellekens, LA, Eskes, TK, Rolland, R. Hormone replacement therapy may reduce high serum homocysteine in postmenopausal women. *Eur J Clin Invest* 1994; 24: 733–36.

90. van der Mooren, MJ, Demacker, PNM, Blom, HJ, De Rijke, YB, Rolland, R. The effect of sequential three-monthly hormone replacement therapy on several cardiovascular risk estimators in postmenopausal women. *Fertil Steril* 1997; 67: 67–73.

91. van der Westhuyzen, J, Metz, J. Betaine delays the onset of neurological impairment in nitrous oxide-induced vitamin B-12 deficiency in fruit bats. *J Nutr* 1984; 114: 1106–11.

92. Van Ede, AE, Laan, RFJM, Blom, HJ, De Abreu, RA, Van de Putte, LBA. Methotrexate in rheumatoid arthritis: An update with focus on mechanisms involved in toxicity. *Semin Arthritis Rheum* 1998; 27: 277–92.

93. Weis, D. Hyperhomocysteinemia in hypothyroidism (Letter; response by Faiman, C, Jacobsen, DW, Green R). *Ann Intern Med* 2000; 132: 677.

94. Wiklund, O, Fager, G, Andersson, A, Lundstam, U, Masson, P, Hultberg, B. N-acetylcysteine treatment lowers plasma homocysteine but not serum lipoprotein(a) levels. *Atherosclerosis* 1996; 119: 99–106.

95. Wouters, MG, Moorrees, MT, van der Mooren, MJ, Blom, HJ, Boers, GH, Schellekens, LA, Thomas, CM,

Eskes, TK. Plasma homocysteine and menopausal status. *Eur J Clin Invest* 1995; 25: 801–5.

96. Yasui, K, Kowa, H, Nakaso, K, Takeshima, T, Nakashima, K. Plasma homocysteine and MTHFR C677T genotype in levodopa-treated patients with PD. *Neurology* 2000; 55: 437–40.

97. Zmuda, JM, Bausserman, LL, Maceroni, D, Thompson, PD. The effect of supraphysiologic doses of testosterone on fasting total homocysteine levels in normal men. *Atherosclerosis* 1997; 130: 199–202.

28

Lifestyle Factors Associated with Hyperhomocysteinemia

STEIN EMIL VOLLSET
HELGA REFSUM
OTTAR NYGÅRD
PER MAGNE UELAND

Hyperhomocysteinemia has somewhat arbitrarily been divided into *mild* (15 to 30 μmol/L), *intermediate* (30 to 100 μmol/L), or *severe* (≥ 100 μmol/L) forms. Causes of severe hyperhomocysteinemia include inborn errors of metabolism (homocystinuria) and severe cobalamin deficiency. Intermediate hyperhomocysteinemia is often caused by severe renal failure, moderate cobalamin deficiency, cobalamin antagonists (e.g., nitrous oxide), severe folate deficiency, or thermolabile 5,10-methylenetetrahydrofolate reductase (MTHFR) combined with low folate status. Finally, mild hyperhomocysteinemia is associated with drug use (antiepileptic drugs, methotrexate), renal failure, hypothyroidism, hyperproliferative disorders, thermolabile MTHFR, and subtle to moderate folate or cobalamin deficiencies (76).

A series of lifestyle factors, such as dietary habits, smoking, coffee drinking, alcohol consumption, and physical activity, are also associated with total homocysteine level differences and may predispose to hyperhomocysteinemia. This chapter reviews the epidemiological evidence regarding the relationship between these lifestyle factors and total homocysteine levels.

The Distribution of Total Homocysteine

The typical distribution of total homocysteine in the general adult population is skewed with a long thin tail toward high values. The largest data set on total homocysteine is the Hordaland Homocysteine Study, which collected data in Hordaland County, Norway, in 1992–1993 (66). Summary measures of the distribution of homocysteine in this population-based sample of 18,044 men and women aged 40 to 67 years are

Table 28.1   Characteristics of the Plasma Total Homocysteine Distribution in the Hordaland Homocysteine Study, 1992–1993

| | Number of Subjects | Proportion with Hyperhomocysteinemia (%) | | | Percentiles of the Plasma Total Homocysteine (μmol/L) Distributions | | | | | |
		Mild (15–29.99 μmol/L)	Intermediate (30–99.99 μmol/L)	Severe (≥100 μmol/L)	2.5th	5th	50th (median)	95th	97.5th	99th
All	18,044	8.5	0.80	0.017	6.2	6.7	10.2	17.1	20.3	28.3
Women										
40–42 y	6,485	4.3	0.52	0	5.6	6.0	8.9	14.8	17.7	24.5
43–64 y	347	5.2	1.15	0	5.8	6.5	9.5	16.5	19.4	a
65–67 y	2,639	11.6	0.80	0	6.8	7.3	10.8	17.7	20.8	26.7
Men										
40–42 y	6,110	8.1	0.98	0.016	7.0	7.5	10.5	17.0	20.9	29.9
43–64 y	336	8.0	1.19	0	7.3	7.7	11.0	17.9	21.4	a
65–67 y	2,127	18.9	1.03	0.094	8.0	8.4	12.1	19.7	23.3	33.1

[a] Number of observations too low to allow precise estimate of 99th percentile.

given in Table 28.1 and show that concentrations increase with age and are higher in men than in women. Mild hyperhomocysteinemia was present in 8.5% of the subjects, intermediate hyperhomocysteinemia in 0.8%, and severe in 0.02%. Whereas the prevalence of mild hyperhomocysteinemia was higher in men than in women, and more than twice as high in those 65 to 67 years old compared with those 40 to 42 years old, the prevalence of intermediate hyperhomocysteinemia showed a weaker relation to gender and almost no relation to age. Detailed data on the distribution of total homocysteine have also been reported from the Third US National Health and Nutrition Examination Survey (43) and in a large study of American schoolchildren (69).

Lifestyle Factors and Total Homocysteine Levels

This section concerns the epidemiological evidence regarding the associations between lifestyle factors and serum/plasma total homocysteine levels. Results are pre-

sented separately for each factor. The review of homocysteine and diet is confined to studies that estimated intake of nutrients, foods, or food groups and does not include vitamin trials or correlation studies based on blood levels of vitamins or nutrients only, which are presented in other chapters. Table 28.2 lists the design features of large cross-sectional and other studies that have reported on lifestyle factors and homocysteine.

Smoking

A rationale for assessing the relationship between smoking and total homocysteine levels is provided by the association between B-vitamin status and smoking (68, 72, 94). Some (6, 10, 19, 28, 54, 57, 66, 69, 80, 82, 85, 87, 91), but not all (1, 3, 4, 13, 26, 29, 32, 52, 71), studies have shown an association between smoking and homocysteine. Only a few of these studies have accounted for potential confounding by folate intake, age, gender, and other factors that are associated with both homocysteine and smoking.

Table 28.2. Studies of Total Homocysteine and Lifestyle Factors

Study Description	n[a]	Key Characteristics	Key Variables	References
The Atherosclerosis Risk in Communities Study. The cohort was established in 1987–1989 to investigate atherosclerotic disease in middle-aged individuals. The study recruited 15,792 men and women from four US communities. Diet was assessed by a 66-food item, semiquantitative food frequency questionnaire (98). Total homocysteine was measured in subsamples in connection with a case-control and a case-cohort study.	318[b] 537[c]	M+F 45–64 y	Diet Smoking Nutrient intakes Coffee	82 26 62
The Boston Area Health Study. A case-control study included 340 cases of first myocardial infarction in 1982–1983 and 339 matched controls. Homocysteine and related metabolites were determined in 130 cases and 118 matched controls in 1993. Diet was assessed by a 116-item food frequency questionnaire (98).	118[a]	M+F <76 y	Diet Nutrient intakes	93
The Caerphilly cohort. The cohort of 2,512 participants was established in 1979–1983 by inviting all men of Caerphilly and surrounding villages in South Wales. Willing subjects were seen again in 5 years, and the cohort was augmented with men who had moved to the area, totaling 2,398 men in 1988. A detailed food frequency questionnaire (100) was used.	2,290	M adults	Diet Smoking Alcohol Nutrient intakes	91
The Child and Adolescent Trial for Cardiovascular Health. The cohort of 5,016 children was established in 1991–1992 from 96 public elementary schools in four US states. Total homocysteine was measured in a subsample of children.	3,524	M+F 13–14 y	Smoking Vitamins	69
European Atherosclerosis Research Study II. The study recruited male university students in 1993 whose fathers had suffered myocardial infarction before the age of 55, along with age-matched control subjects.	788	M 22–25 y	Smoking Alcohol Physical activity	32

Study Description	n[a]	Key Characteristics	Key Variables	References
Children with familial hypercholesterolemia study. Children with familial hypercholesterolemia were studied and diet assessed with a 190-food item quantitative food frequency questionnaire (27).	154	M+F 7–17 y FH	Diet Nutrient intakes	89
The Framingham Heart Study. The cohort consisted initially (1948–1950) of 5,209 men and women aged 30–62 years in Massachusetts. The participants were examined biennially. In 1988–1989, new blood samples were drawn and diet was assessed in 887 individuals by a 126-item food frequency questionnaire (77).	1,160	M+F 67–96 y	Diet Nutrient intakes	78 90
As part of a case-control study of premature coronary artery disease, control subjects were recruited by random selection from telephone numbers in Georgia. Diet was assessed by a food-frequency questionnaire (7).	108	M 30–50	Smoking Alcohol Physical activity Diet	71
The Hordaland Homocysteine Study. The cohort was established in 1992–1993 as part of a population-based cardiovascular screening in the county of Hordaland, Norway. Diet was assessed by questions on frequency of use of 41 food items/food groups.	18,044	M+F 40–67 y	Age/gender Smoking Coffee Alcohol Physical activity Diet	66 34 75 64 95 65
A sample of 380 men and 204 women was selected among white-collar employees of Hydro-Quebec in Montréal.	584	M+F 23–59 y	Smoking Alcohol Physical activity Diet	52
The Malmø study recruited a population-based sample of adults in the southern Swedish cities of Malmø and Lund.	244	M+F 35–95 y	Vitamins Smoking	13
The UK National Diet and Nutrition Survey. Participants, aged 65 years and over, were recruited in 1994–1995 from randomly selected postal code sectors with substratification by age and gender. Homocysteine was measured in a subgroup who gave diet information (4-day weighted dietary record with data on supplemental vitamin intake).	972	M+F 65 y and older	Diet Smoking Nutrient intakes	3
The National Health and Nutrition Examination Survey III. During 1988–1994, nationally representative information was obtained on health and nutritional status from about 40,000 individuals in the United States. Homocysteine was measured in surplus sera obtained from a subset in a later phase.	8,585	M+F 12 y and older	Age/gender Race/ethnicity Educational level Smoking	28 43
The New Mexico Aging Process Study. Participants were selected from the study cohort. Food frequency information was assessed by a slight modification of the Health Habits and History Questionnaire (8).	88	M+F 68–96 y	Diet Nutrient intakes	48
The North Sea Study. A cross-sectional study of oil production platform workers in the Norwegian sector of the North Sea assessed diet by the 24-hour recall method and a questionnaire on frequency of intake both during the periods the the men lived at home and on the platform.	310	M 21–59 y	Diet Nutrient intakes Smoking	70
The Ontario Study. Adolescent females were recruited from various sources to study relations between B-vitamin/ homocysteine status and use of oral contraceptives, alcohol, and smoking. Diet was assessed using a 3-day weighed food record.	229	F 14–20 y	Diet Nutrient intakes Smoking Alcohol	29
The Oslo Hyperlipidemic Smokers Trial. Male hyperlipidemic smokers were recruited to a randomized double-blind	42 × 2	M 40–60 y	Diet Nutrient intakes	15

(Continues)

Table 28.2.   *(Continued)*

Study Description	n^a	Key Characteristics	Key Variables	References
factorial intervention trial with ω-3 fatty acids and antioxidants (vitamin E,C, β-carotene and coenzyme Q10). Diet was assessed with a self-administered, quantitative, food frequency questionnaire (27). Total homocysteine was measured before and after 6 weeks of intervention.		Smokers Hyperlipidemia		
The Physicians' Health Study. During 1982–84, 22,071 US male physicians were recruited for a randomized 2 × 2 factorial trial with aspirin and β-carotene. Lifestyle assessment included information on vitamin supplements and breakfast cereals. Use of other dietary items was assessed by a limited food-frequency questionnaire focusing on vitamin A and carotene. Plasma samples were obtained from 14,916 of the participants and homocysteine levels were determined in subsamples in connection with case-control studies.	290^b 427^b	M 40–84 y	Diet Smoking Nutrient intakes Alcohol	83 92 54
The Vitamin, Teachers, and Longevity Study. The pilot study enrolled 297 men and women from 4,774 retired teachers who were approached for a trial of antioxidant vitamin supplements. Diet history was obtained with the 1992 version of the Health Habits and History Questionnaire, a semiquantitative food frequency questionnaire (8).	260	M+F Retired teachers	Diet Nutrient intakes Coffee	86

^{a} Number of homocysteine measurements.
^{b} Number of controls in case-control study.
^{c} Size of cohort sample from a case-cohort study.
M, male; F, female; y, years; FH, familial hypercholesterolemia.

The first large study to address these issues was the Hordaland Homocysteine Study, where the relation between cigarette smoking and total homocysteine was studied in 16,176 men and women aged 40 to 67 years (66). There was a strong and graded association between the daily number of cigarettes smoked and homocysteine levels. The association was stronger in women than in men and stronger among elderly subjects. Former smokers had homocysteine levels similar to those of persons who never smoked. The age- and gender-adjusted estimated difference in mean total homocysteine between heavy smokers (≥20 cigarettes/day) and those who never smoked was 1.9 μmol/L. Further adjustment for intake of fruit and vegetables, use of vitamin supplements, and other possible confounders attenuated the estimated difference to 1.7 μmol/L (p-trend <0.001) (66).

A multiple regression analysis based on 293 cases of myocardial infarction and 290 control cases within the Physicians' Health Study showed a similar association between smoking and homocysteine (54). The contrast between current smokers and nonsmokers was 2.3 μmol/L before and 1.9 μmol/L after adjustment for multivitamin use and plasma folate status.

A third study was a population-based survey carried out in indigenous Australians (80). In this study of 365 men and women, the crude mean difference in total homocysteine levels between current smokers and those who never smoked was 1.5 μmol/L. The mean total homocysteine level of ex-smokers was intermediate. The smoking-homocysteine relation was strengthened by adjustment for age, sex, levels of folate and cobalamin, and other determinants of homocysteine.

In summary, although a relationship between smoking and homocysteine levels is not a consistent finding across studies, it is well supported by a series of investigations. Several detailed analyses have shown that smoking may be associated with a 1.5 to 2.0 μmol/L elevation of homocysteine levels. This is compatible with reports of low folate, vitamin B_6, and cobalamin status in smokers compared with nonsmokers (68, 72, 94). Because smokers usually eat less fruit and vegetables and use fewer vitamin supplements than do nonsmokers (5, 51, 61, 101), confounding with folate intake is likely to contribute to at least part of the smoking-homocysteine association. However, since the association remained in the studies after adjusting for these factors, a diet-independent smoking effect on total homocysteine may exist.

Coffee Consumption

An unexpected finding in the Hordaland Homocysteine Study (64) was a strong, graded relation between the number of cups of coffee consumed per day and plasma total homocysteine. The participants were characterized by a high intake of predominantly filtered coffee. An age-gender adjusted difference of 2.5 μmol/L was observed between consumers of nine or more cups of coffee per day (974 individuals, or 6%) and subjects not drinking coffee. The association was observed among nonsmokers as well as smokers and remained strong after additional adjustments for smoking and intake of fruit, vegetables, and vitamin supplements (adjusted difference 1.7 μmol/L, p-trend < 0.005).

The coffee-homocysteine relationship was investigated in two other populations. In 537 participants of the Atherosclerosis Risk in Communities Study cohort, no association between coffee consumption and total homocysteine was found (62). In contrast, a significant trend (p = 0.01) of increasing homocysteine levels with coffee consumption was reported in a study of 260 retired schoolteachers in Baltimore (86). In a regression model accounting for folate intake, dietary protein, and serum creatinine, the contrast between the users of 3 to 9 cups/day and nonusers of coffee was 1.3 μmol/L. Like the participants of the Atherosclerosis Risk in Communities Study, these individuals were characterized by a lower consumption of coffee than the Hordaland cohort members.

In conclusion, two studies have found that high consumption of coffee is associated with a 1.3 to 1.7 μmol/L elevation in homocysteine after adjustment for folate and other lifestyle factors (64, 86). Although coffee use and smoking are highly correlated (42, 64), the latter is not an important confounder, because in the Hordaland Study, the association was also observed in nonsmokers, and very few of the Baltimore study (86) subjects smoked. However, as coffee drinking is negatively associated with intake of fruit and vegetables and vitamin supplements (5, 42, 64), residual confounding by folate intake cannot be ruled out.

Alcohol Consumption

The relationship between alcohol consumption and homocysteine levels was first studied in alcohol abusers. Total homocysteine levels were 10.5 to 11 μmol/L higher in 42 alcoholics hospitalized for alcohol detoxification than in 16 abstinent alcohol-dependent individuals or 23 control subjects (41). The findings were similar in a study of 32 chronic alcoholics and 31 healthy volunteers where mean levels were about 10 μmol/L higher in the former group (p for difference in means < 0.001) (20). The latter study found lower homocysteine levels in beer drinkers than in wine/spirits consumers (mean of 13.8 μmol/L vs 21.2 μmol/L, p = 0.05). B-vitamin status was assessed, and, whereas red blood cell folate and serum vitamin B_6 levels were lower in alcoholics than in control subjects, serum folate and cobalamin levels were higher (20).

The large population-based Caerphilly cohort showed a highly significant but decreasing trend in total homocysteine levels as alcohol consumption increased (91). After adjustment for age, social class, body mass index, smoking, total energy intake, and prevalent heart disease, mean homocysteine level was 1.8 μmol/L higher in alcohol abstainers than in men in the highest quartile of alcohol intake (p-trend < 0.0005). Standardization for folate intake, which was 0.13 mg/day lower among abstainers than among those in the upper intake quartile, greatly diminished the alcohol-homocysteine relationship. The authors attributed the association to the folate content of beer (0.09 mg/L), which was the predominant alcoholic beverage consumed by the cohort members.

The Hordaland Study found weak and quite complex associations between alcohol consumption and homocysteine levels (95). Overall, a shallow U-shaped relation was seen with a maximum homocysteine difference of 0.5 μmol/L between nondrinkers and consumers of 7 to 13 drinks of alcohol per week. After additional adjustment for smoking and intake of fruit and vegetables, the U-shape disappeared and homocysteine was 0.7 μmol/L lower in the maximum alcohol intake group (≥ 14 drinks per week) than among nondrinkers (p-trend < 0.0001). The inverse relationship between alcohol use and homocysteine was significantly stronger among smokers than nonsmokers.

A Canadian study of young women found 13% higher total homocysteine concentrations among alcohol users (29). Other studies have reported either a weak positive (26, 92) or no association (32, 52, 82) between alcohol intake and homocysteine levels.

To summarize, the conflicting results among studies (inverse, no, U-shaped, or positive associations) indicate that the relationship between alcohol consumption and total homocysteine is complex. Two small studies have shown that homocysteine levels are higher in chronic alcohol abusers than in control subjects (20, 41). Beer contains folate and two studies have shown that beer consumption is associated with lower homocysteine levels (20, 91). The latter observation is supported by a Dutch study showing a positive association between alcohol intake and serum folate levels (16). Future studies need to carefully assess the potential confounding by folate intake and nutritional deficiencies that may accompany alcohol abuse.

B-Vitamin Intake (see also Chapters 23–25)

The vitamins folate, B_6 and cobalamin play a key role in homocysteine regulation and metabolism. Most studies with diet information have quantified the associations between total homocysteine levels and the estimated intakes of these vitamins.

Among 1,160 participants, aged 67 to 96 years, in the Framingham study, plasma levels of folate, vitamin B_6, and cobalamin showed significant inverse relationships with total homocysteine (78). On the other hand, the estimated intakes of folate and vitamin B_6, but not cobalamin, were inversely associated with homocysteine. The analyses of the relation between the intake of each vitamin and homocysteine were adjusted for the intakes of the other two of the key B vitamins. After additional adjustment for age and sex, differences in mean homocysteine levels between the lower and upper intake deciles were 3.3 µmol/L for both folate and vitamin B_6.

Another thorough analysis was done within the Caerphilly cohort (91). After adjustment for age, social class, body mass index, smoking, total energy intake, and heart disease, differences in total homocysteine between lower and upper quintiles of folate, cobalamin, and vitamin B_6 intakes were 3.1, 1.8, and 2.5 µmol/L, respectively, all with highly significant trends ($p < 0.0005$).

Associations between total homocysteine levels and B-vitamin intakes have also been studied in a control group from the Atherosclerosis Risk in Communities Study cohort (82). Among nonusers of vitamin supplements, the difference in homocysteine (after adjustment for age, gender, and smoking) between the lower and upper intake tertiles was 0.9 µmol/L for folate ($p = 0.04$), 1.0 µmol/L for vitamin B_6 ($p = 0.02$), 1.4 µmol/L for cobalamin ($p < 0.01$), 1.1 µmol/L for vitamin B_1 ($p = 0.01$), and 2.1 µmol/L for vitamin B_2 ($p < 0.01$).

The UK National Diet and Nutrition Survey reported on a nationally representative sample of 972 elderly men and women (3). In a multiple regression model with nutrient intakes, age, gender, and domicile category (whether or not institutionalized), significant inverse relationships were found between total homocysteine and both folate and vitamin B_6 intake. The magnitude of the relationship was reported only for folate. The adjusted difference between lower and upper intake deciles was about 4.4 µmol/L after adjustment for confounders including creatinine and cobalamin levels (3).

In the Hordaland study, folate and cobalamin scores were constructed from data on the frequency of use of foods and vitamin supplements. Both combined food and supplement intake scores were significantly and inversely correlated with plasma homocysteine (r = −0.20 for the folate score, and r = −0.12 for the cobalamin score). Homocysteine differences between the lowest and highest decile of the folate score were 1.7 and 1.8 µmol/L in 40- to 42-year-old men and women, respectively, and 2.4 and 2.7 µmol/L, respectively, in men and women aged 65 to 67 years (65). The difference in total homocysteine between the extreme deciles of the cobalamin score was 0.8 to 2.3 µmol/L in the four main age-gender groups (65).

A laboratory-based study of 95 elderly individuals with abnormal or marginal cobalamin status and 78 control subjects included estimation of cobalamin intake using food frequency questionnaires (40). Although the study failed to show a significant association between cobalamin intake and serum homocysteine levels, the difference in total homocysteine was 2.5 µmol/L between the lower and upper quintiles of cobalamin intake.

Unadjusted analyses in 271 controls in the Physicians' Health Study (83) showed significant negative correlations ranging from −0.27 to −0.36 between homocysteine and the estimated intakes of vitamins B_1, B_2, B_6, cobalamin, folate, and niacin (all $p < 0.001$). Among 118 control subjects in a Boston area case-control study, homocysteine showed a weaker relationship with folate intake and no association with vitamin B_6 and cobalamin intakes (93). A study of 154 children with familial hypercholesterolemia found homocysteine to be inversely associated with folate intake (r = −0.23, $p = 0.007$) (89).

In summary, the observed differences in total homocysteine between contrasting intakes of the key B vitamins, folate, B_6, and cobalamin, range from 1 to 4 µmol/L and are strongest for folate and weakest for cobalamin. The homocysteine-lowering effects of folate and cobalamin, but not vitamin B_6, have been established in intervention trials (39). Intakes of the vitamins B_1, B_2, and niacin have also been shown to correlate with homocysteine levels (82, 83). Strong correlations between intakes of the various B vitamins (47, 93) should be taken into account when considering homocysteine associations with B vitamins other than folate and cobalamin.

Intake of Non-B Vitamins and Other Nutrients

Several studies have reported inverse association between homocysteine levels and intakes of vitamin A (15, 82, 83), vitamin C (15, 83, 89), and vitamin E (83). No associations between the intakes of any of these vitamins and homocysteine were seen in another study (71). Two studies have reported an inverse association between phosphorus intake and homocysteine levels (3, 82). We are aware of only single reports of associations between homocysteine levels and intakes of calcium (82), magnesium (3), and sodium (3). The reported association with calcium was inverse, and the positive associations between homocysteine and magnesium and sodium were adjusted for folate intake.

Intake of non-B vitamins and other nutrients may correlate with the intakes of folate and cobalamin, which have an established homocysteine lowering effect. Most studies did not account for this possible confounding, and the results have not been supported by intervention studies. Neither a trial with antioxidants (vitamin E, vitamin C, β-carotene, and coenzyme Q10) (15) nor a trial with high-dose vitamin C (9) showed any effect on homocysteine levels.

Protein Intake

Homocysteine in humans is formed from the essential amino acid methionine (23), and methionine or a protein-rich meal causes an acute increase in total homocysteine (33). Therefore, it was suspected that a diet rich in protein or methionine would be associated with elevated homocysteine levels.

The most careful study on long-term dietary protein intake and total homocysteine reported a strong inverse relation between energy-adjusted protein intake and homocysteine levels (86). The difference in total homocysteine levels between the lower and upper quintiles of protein intake was about 3.1 μmol/L (p = 0.008) after adjustment for energy-adjusted dietary folate intake, use of vitamin supplements, serum creatinine, dietary energy, and coffee use.

Other studies have also showed an inverse association between the usual dietary intake of protein or methionine and homocysteine levels. Among 49 individuals not taking B-vitamin supplements, an inverse association between protein intake and homocysteine existed that was nonsignificant overall (r = –0.23, p = 0.13) but highly significant among women (r = –0.45, p < 0.01) (48). A negative association between dietary methionine intake and homocysteine was also seen among 118 control subjects in a Boston area case-control study of myocardial infarction (93). The correlation between homocysteine levels and methionine intake was –0.27 (p = 0.003) before and –0.22 (p = 0.01) after adjustment for intake of vitamin B$_6$, cobalamin, and folate. Homocysteine levels also decreased across groups with increasing methionine and protein intake in nonusers of vitamin supplements among control subjects in the Atherosclerosis Risk in Communities Study (82). For both estimated methionine and total protein intake, homocysteine was 0.8 μmol/L lower in the upper compared with the lower

tertile (p = 0.07 for both comparisons after adjustment for age, race, gender, and cigarette smoking). Finally, intake of protein was inversely associated with homocysteine levels among 108 population-based control subjects in a case-control study of premature coronary artery disease (r = –0.20, p = 0.03) (71).

In summary, several studies have reported an inverse relation between dietary intake of protein and homocysteine levels. Whether dietary protein induces a more efficient homocysteine metabolism or the association is due to confounding with other homocysteine-lowering factors is not clear (86).

Consumption of Individual Food Items

Relatively few studies have addressed the relationships between the consumption of individual food items and total homocysteine levels. Such studies are important because the bioavailability of folate (2, 30) and, therefore, the homocysteine response, may vary substantially depending on the food source of folate.

Relations between food items and homocysteine were studied among 885 elderly subjects in the Framingham Heart Study (90). In this study, the three major sources of folate were cold cereals, multivitamins, and orange juice, each contributing 13.3%, 12.8% and 12.4%, respectively, of the total folate intake. The strongest associations with homocysteine were found for breakfast cereals and fruit and vegetables. Differences in mean homocysteine levels between the lower and upper intake quintiles (adjusted for age, sex, energy intake, and vitamin supplement use) were 1.4 μmol/L for breakfast cereals and 1.1 μmol/L for fruit and vegetables. Despite being a major source of dietary folate and significantly associated with plasma folate, consumption of orange juice was not associated with differences in homocysteine levels (78).

In a control set of the Atherosclerosis Risk in Communities study, the strongest associations with homocysteine were found for cereals and milk (82). Among nonusers of vitamin supplements, the difference between the lower and upper intake tertiles was 1.3 μmol/L (p < 0.01) for cold cereals and 1.4 μmol/L (p < 0.01) for milk. These analyses were adjusted for age, race, gender, and cigarette smoking.

The relationship between diet and homocysteine was studied in 310 oil workers in the North Sea (70). A multiple regression analysis showed that intake of bread (p = 0.01) and vegetables (p = 0.04) was negatively associated with total homocysteine, but intake of fat (p = 0.05) was positively correlated. After adjustment for age and smoking, differences in mean homocysteine levels between the no-intake group and the group with intake above the median were 1.0 μmol/L (p = 0.10) for bread, 0.7 μmol/L (p = 0.04) for skimmed milk, and 2.5

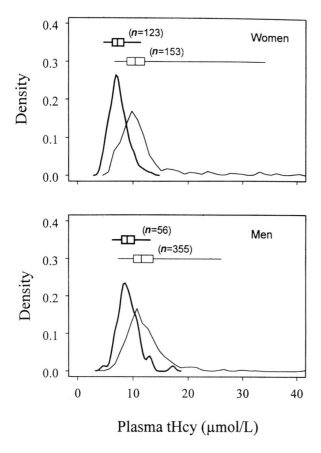

Fig. 28.1. The density distribution of plasma total homocysteine (tHcy) according to contrasting lifestyle groups in 40- to 42-year-old women (top) and men (bottom). The distributions of homocysteine (continuous curves) are shown in the main part of each figure and the same data are presented as box plots at the top of the figure. The curve in boldface represents nonsmokers with high folate intakes and consumption of <1 cup of coffee/day, whereas the thin line represents smokers drinking ≥5 cups of coffee/day and with low folate intakes. Each box plot shows the 25th to the 75th percentile interval, the vertical line inside the box is the median value, and the horizontal line indicates the 2.5th and 97.5th percentile interval. (Reproduced from Nygård et al. [65], with permission.)

μmol/L for vegetables (p = 0.008). The UK National Diet and Nutrition Survey observed significant, inverse associations between total homocysteine and consumption of breakfast cereals and liver but did not report the magnitude of the relationships (3).

The impact on homocysteine levels of the compulsory folate fortification of enriched grain products that started in the United States in 1997 was assessed in the Framingham Offspring Study (44). Among nonusers of B-vitamin supplements, mean homocysteine levels were 0.7 μmol/L (p < 0.001) lower after folate fortification, whereas among supplement users an increase of 0.6 μmol/L (p = 0.006) was observed.

To summarize, individual food items associated with homocysteine levels include breakfast cereals, fruit and vegetables, milk, liver, and bread. These foods are all important sources of folate (16, 90), and differences in homocysteine levels between low and high intakes ranged from 0.7 to 2.5 μmol/L. Orange juice is an example of a folate-rich food item that seems not to be associated with lower homocysteine levels. This may be related to poor bioavailability of folate in orange juice resulting from inhibition of folate deconjugation by organic acids (31). The strongest and most consistent association with homocysteine was found for breakfast cereals, which are commonly fortified with folate and other B-vitamins in the countries where the studies were conducted. Furthermore, a randomized, blinded trial of fortified cereals has shown that daily portions of cereals containing 0.13, 0.50, or 0.67 mg of folic acid taken for 5 weeks reduced homocysteine levels by 0.5 (p = 0.24), 1.7 (p < 0.001), and 2.8 μmol/L (p = 0.001), respectively (56).

Use of Multivitamins

Multivitamins often contain all three key B vitamins involved in homocysteine metabolism (vitamin B_6, cobalamin, and folic acid), along with several other B vitamins and vitamins A, C, D, and E. The composition and doses show considerable variation among products and countries, often as a consequence of legislation regulating the maximum doses of individual vitamins. For example, in the United States, the folate content of multivitamins is usually 0.4 to 0.8 mg, whereas in Norway, multivitamins contain no or, at most, 0.1 to 0.2 mg of folic acid.

In the Framingham Study, the strongest association between homocysteine and any single dietary component was reported for vitamin supplements containing folic acid. After adjustment for age, gender, and total energy intake, the difference in mean homocysteine levels between nonusers and users was 2.7 μmol/L (p < 0.0001) (90). In a Swedish population-based sample of 244 men and women, homocysteine levels were 3.0 μmol/L lower among 31 regular users of multivitamins (with folic acid) than among nonusers (13). In the New Mexico Aging Process Study, the difference in homocysteine levels between nonusers and users of vitamin supplements containing vitamin B_6, cobalamin, and folate was 1.7 μmol/L (48). The Atherosclerosis Risk in Communities study observed homocysteine levels about 1.5 μmol/L lower in users of vitamin supplements than in nonusers (82). In the main age and gender groups of the Hordaland Study, mean homocysteine levels were 1.5 to 2.2 μmol/L lower in nonusers compared with daily users of multivitamin supplements (65). The difference was larger in 65 to 67 year olds (2.0 in men and 2.2 μmol/L in women) than in the 40 to 42 year olds (1.5 μmol/L in both men and women) (65).

To summarize the data from observational studies, multivitamin supplement users have a mean total homocysteine level that is 1.5 to 3.0 μmol/L lower than among nonusers. This difference is slightly smaller than the typical reduction from 12 μmol/L to 8 to 9 μmol/L estimated from the combined evidence of placebo-controlled trials of folic acid alone or combined with other B vitamins (39).

Fish Oil Intake

A small, cross-over trial first suggested that fish oil may lower homocysteine levels in hyperhomocysteinemic men (67). Another small, cross-over trial reported a significant 10% decrease in homocysteine levels after administration of a mixture of fish oil and evening primrose oil (36). However, the participants also received folic acid and vitamin B_6. There was no difference in homocysteine levels between Greenland Inuits, who have higher intakes of fish oil, and Danes on a standard Western diet (60). A Norwegian trial in hyperlipidemic smokers found no effect of intervention with omega-3 fatty acids on homocysteine levels (15) despite an inverse, pretreatment association between omega-3 fatty acids in serum phospholipids and homocysteine levels (r = −0.37, $p < 0.05$). Thus, the current evidence for an effect of fish oil on homocysteine levels is limited and has not been supported by later research.

Weight Reduction

A mean increase of 0.8 μmol/L ($p < 0.0001$) in homocysteine levels was observed during a 3-week period with moderate weight reduction in 11 subjects. The same authors later showed that supplementation with B-vitamins prevented such an increase (37, 38). This evidence for a relationship between weight loss and homocysteine must be regarded as preliminary.

Physical Activity

The relationship between leisure-time physical activity, assessed by a four-category question, and homocysteine was studied in the Hordaland Homocysteine Study (66). A 1.2 μmol/L contrast between the no-activity and heavy-training groups was observed (p-trend < 0.001; adjusted for age and gender). This difference was reduced to 0.4 μmol/L (p-trend < 0.001) after additional adjustment for smoking, intake of fruit and vegetables, and vitamin supplements.

However, two other studies found no relation between physical activity and homocysteine (32, 52). Likewise, no significant relation was found between the maximum oxygen uptake capacity, a more objective measure of fitness, and homocysteine levels in a controlled study of 20 healthy men (99).

Lifestyle Patterns and the Homocysteine Distribution

The Hordaland Study compared homocysteine levels in individuals with contrasting lifestyle patterns. The homocysteine differences between individuals characterized by low folate intake, smoking, and high coffee consumption, on the one hand, and nonsmoking individuals with a high folate intake and low coffee consumption, on the other, ranged from 3.2 to 4.8 μmol/L in the four main gender and age groups (65). Similarly, among the elderly Framingham subjects, combining intake of the three main B vitamins—folate, cobalamin, and B_6—produced a contrast of 5.3 μmol/L between the low and high B-vitamin intake groups (78).

The large sample size of the Hordaland study has permitted study of lifestyle-associated differences in the shape of the homocysteine distribution. Figure 28.1 shows the distribution of homocysteine levels among 40- to 42-year-old subjects who smoked and who had high consumption of coffee and low folate intake. For such individuals, the distribution was skewed with a long tail toward high values (Figure 28.1; thin line). In contrast, in nonsmoking subjects with high folate intake and low or no coffee consumption, the homocysteine distribution not only was shifted toward lower values but was almost symmetrical with a much smaller upper tail (thick line).

Age, gender, and the major lifestyle determinants of homocysteine also show different associations with very low or very high homocysteine values (64, 75). Based on data from the Hordaland study, Figure 28.2 shows the associations between extreme values of homocysteine and age, gender, smoking, coffee consumption, and use of vitamin supplements. Only cigarette smoking and nonuse of vitamin supplements showed a relationship with *intermediate* hyperhomocysteinemia, whereas these two factors plus old age and male gender were associated with *mild* hyperhomocysteinemia. The figure also shows the relationships between these five factors and low (5.5 to 6.9 μmol/L) and very low homocysteine levels (< 5.5 μmol/L). These two low ranges of homocysteine values were chosen to contain similar proportions of the population values as mild and intermediate hyperhomocysteinemia, respectively. All five factors were inversely associated with the likelihood of having a low or very low homocysteine value. It is also noteworthy that

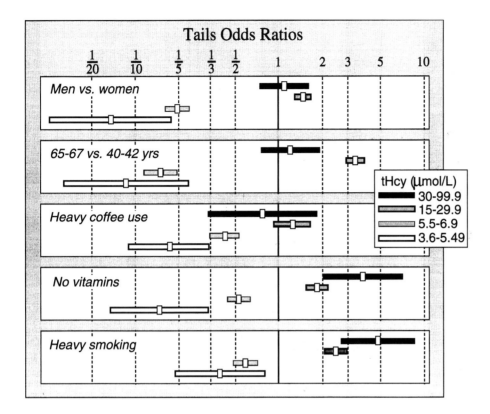

Fig. 28.2. Odds ratios (with 95% confidence limits) of having a high or low value of total homocysteine (tHcy), comparing contrasting categories of cigarette smoking (≥10/day vs. never smoked), use of vitamin supplements (no use vs. frequent use), coffee consumption (≥5 cups/day vs. no use), age (65 to 67 years vs. 40 to 42 years), and gender (men vs. women). Four definitions of high and low total homocysteine levels are used: intermediate (30 to 99.99 μmol/L) and mild hyperhomocysteinemia (15 to 29.99 μmol/L), and low (5.50 to 6.99 μmol/L) and very low (3.6 to 5.49 μmol/L) homocysteine levels, with 0.8%, 8%, 7%, and 0.7% of the population belonging to each of these four homocysteine groups, respectively. The estimated odds ratios are from logistic regression models with all factors present. These odds ratios are also denoted as tails odds ratios as they estimate the risk of having a very low (being in the lower tail of the distribution) or very high homocysteine value (being in the upper tail of the homocysteine distribution).

both old age and male gender decreased the likelihood of having a low homocysteine value more strongly than they increased the risk of hyperhomocysteinemia.

As to the lifestyle factors, the extremes of coffee use and cigarette smoking were associated with about the same contrast in mean homocysteine levels (64, 66). However, coffee use was associated only with a decreased probability of having a low value and not with high homocysteine values. On the other hand, heavy smoking was associated with both a decreased likelihood of having a low homocysteine value and an increased risk of hyperhomocysteinemia. Nonuse of

vitamin supplements showed a pattern similar to cigarette smoking. Smoking and nonuse of vitamins were more strongly associated with intermediate than with mild hyperhomocysteinemia, and more strongly with very low (< 5.5 μmol/L) than with low (5.5 to 6.99 μmol/L) homocysteine values. The implications of these differential associations with low and high homocysteine values are unclear, but they suggest different underlying biological mechanisms for the various factors. Furthermore, if hyperhomocysteinemia causes disease, and the lifestyle associations are causal, these results suggest that the effect of coffee on homocysteine levels may be more benign than that of smoking or low vitamin status.

The 677C→T MTHFR Polymorphism and Lifestyle

The 677C→T polymorphism in the MTHFR gene (see Chapter 22) has been studied extensively in relation to homocysteine and folate levels, and to diseases associated with them (14, 49, 53, 79, 81). The homozygous TT genotype is generally associated with reduced MTHFR enzyme activity and with about 25% higher total homocysteine levels than the more common CC genotype (14). Subjects with the TT genotype are susceptible to hyperhomocysteinemia under conditions of impaired folate status (14, 34, 56). They also attain particularly high homocysteine levels during renal failure (24, 25) and after intake of some drugs (35, 88). Notably, elevated homocysteine levels in subjects with the TT genotype are folate-responsive and are efficiently reduced by folate supplementation (34, 56).

In the Hordaland study, 73% of the 67 individuals found to have hyperhomocysteinemia ≥ 40 μmol/L were of the TT genotype, compared with only 10% of control subjects (33). However, the individuals with high homocysteine levels also had a different lifestyle, characterized by a higher proportion of current smokers (59% vs. 29% in control subjects) and less use of vitamin supplements (2% daily use vs. 13% in control subjects). These observations suggest that smoking may contribute to intermediate hyperhomocysteinemia in individuals with TT genotype. No studies have yet addressed the issue of differential effects by the MTHFR genotype on homocysteine response to smoking or other nondietary lifestyle factors.

Causality, Confounding, and Consequences

Diet, Other Lifestyle Factors, and Homocysteine

As discussed in Chapters 23 and 24, folate and cobalamin treatment lowers homocysteine levels. A meta-analysis of 12 randomized trials of B-vitamin therapy showed that, on average, folic acid lowers homocysteine levels by 25% and that cobalamin has an additional homocysteine lowering effect of about 7% (39). The observed associations between homocysteine and intake of individual food items that are important sources of folate (fruit, vegetables, liver, milk, bread) are likely to be causal. However, this has been proven and quantified only for fortified breakfast cereals (55).

Because of strong interrelations among age, gender, dietary patterns, smoking, coffee use, alcohol consumption, and physical activity (5, 42, 51, 61, 64, 101), efficient analytical adjustment for age, gender, and folate intake is of paramount importance to avoid confounding in the assessment of lifestyle determinants of homocysteine. Such adjustment is dependent on precise measurement of the confounders, which poses no problem with age and gender. The accurate quantification of folate intake, however, is problematic. Sources of error include both imperfect dietary assessment using food frequency questionnaires or other methods (97) and lack of standardized and precise food composition tables for folate (22).

Identification of nutritional factors that affect homocysteine levels is further complicated by the presence of strong correlations between the dietary intake of many nutrients (17, 47, 82, 86). For example, food items that provide folate frequently contain vitamin B_6 and cobalamin (47). Folate-rich vegetables are also rich in the vitamins A and C and in dietary fiber. Use of multivitamin preparations will further complicate the identification of the vitamins that are responsible

for the homocysteine reduction. The difficulty in discriminating between different nutrients was well illustrated in an Australian case-control study of neural tube defects and nutrient intake in early pregnancy. Before folate was included as an adjustment variable in the analyses, equally strong, inverse, and statistically significant relationships with neural tube defects were found for intakes of fiber, calcium, vitamin C, and carotene (12). Thus, correlations with folate may explain the relatively strong associations between intakes of vitamin B_6 and vitamin C and homocysteine levels that until now have been unsupported by intervention trials (9, 15, 39).

Reliable answers to these questions may be obtained only by manipulation of each potential homocysteine-lowering factor in controlled trials. Such studies are complex and expensive but could be carried out for coffee, selected food items, and vitamins. Valuable insight into the role of smoking on homocysteine levels could be obtained by monitoring subjects in smoking cessation programs.

Clinical Implications

Contrasting levels of the various lifestyle factors are associated with 0.5 to 3 μmol/L differences in homocysteine levels; the differences are smallest for physical activity, higher for coffee and smoking, and highest for use of vitamin supplements or foods fortified with folic acid (e.g., breakfast cereals). The combination of extreme settings of several of these factors may be associated with 4 to 5 μmol/L group differences in homocysteine levels, which may be of considerable clinical relevance. Among patients with coronary heart disease, subjects with a homocysteine level of 15 μmol/L have an estimated 60% higher overall mortality compared with those with a level of 10 μmol/L (63). Similar differences in risk have been reported from meta-analyses on homocysteine and ischemic heart disease, where the combined evidence suggests a highly significant 60% to 90% risk enhancement per 5 μmol/L homocysteine increase (11, 21, 96). When only prospective nested case-control studies were considered, the corresponding risk increase was 30% (95% confidence interval: 10% to 50%) (21). Results from ongoing clinical trials with homocysteine-lowering vitamin therapy in secondary prevention of heart disease (18) will provide valuable new information on the clinical importance of B vitamins and homocysteine. This knowledge is crucial to understanding the relevance of the lifestyle-homocysteine relationships.

Homocysteine levels have also been reported to be associated with an increased risk of Alzheimer's disease (19, 58), pregnancy complications (50, 73, 74), congenital malformations (59, 84), and colon cancer

(45); there are ongoing intervention trials with folate in subjects with colorectal adenomas (46). Depending on the still unclarified role of homocysteine in these diseases, the observed lifestyle-homocysteine relationships may contribute to the understanding of the etiology and to possible prevention of some of these clinical conditions.

REFERENCES

1. Alfthan, G, Pekkanen, J, Jauhiainen, M, Pitkäniemi, J, Karvonen, M, Tuomilehto, J, Salonen, JT, Ehnholm, C. Relation of serum homocysteine and lipoprotein(a) concentrations to atherosclerotic disease in a prospective Finnish population based study. *Atherosclerosis* 1994; 106: 9–19.

2. Bailey, LB. Dietary reference intakes for folate: The debut of dietary folate equivalents. *Nutr Rev* 1998; 56: 294–99.

3. Bates, CJ, Mansoor, MA, van der Pols, J, Prentice, A, Cole, TJ, Finch, S. Plasma total homocysteine in a representative sample of 972 British men and women aged 65 and over. *Eur J Clin Nutr* 1997; 51: 691–97.

4. Berg, K, Malinow, MR, Kierulf, P, Upson, B. Population variation and genetics of plasma homocyst(e)ine level. *Clin Genet* 1992; 41: 315–21.

5. Berger, J, Wynder, EL. The correlation of epidemiological variables. *J Clin Epidemiol* 1994; 47: 941–52.

6. Bergmark, C, Mansoor, MA, Swedenborg, J, de Faire, U, Svardal, AM, Ueland, PM. Hyperhomocysteinemia in patients operated for lower extremity ischaemia below the age of 50. Effect of smoking and extent of disease. *Eur J Vasc Surg* 1993; 7: 391–96.

7. Block, G. *A Data-Based Brief Diet Questionnaire for Epidemiologic Studies.* National Cancer Institute, Bethesda, MD, 1984.

8. Block, G, Hartman, AM, Dresser, CM, Carroll, MD, Gannon, J, Gardner, L. A data-based approach to diet questionnaire design and testing. *Am J Epidemiol* 1986; 124: 453–69.

9. Bostom, AG, Yanek, L, Hume, AL, Eaton, CB, McQuade, W, Nadeau, M, Perrone, G, Jacques, PF, Selhub, J. High dose ascorbate supplementation fails to affect plasma homocyst(e)ine levels in patients with coronary heart disease. *Atherosclerosis* 1994; 111: 267–70.

10. Bots, ML, Launer, LJ, Lindemans, J, Hoes, AW, Hofman, A, Witteman, JCM, Koudstaal, PJ, Grobbee, DE. Homocysteine and short-term risk of myocardial infarction and stroke in the elderly. *Arch Intern Med* 1999; 159: 38–44.

11. Boushey, CJ, Beresford, SAA, Omenn, GS, Motulsky, AG. A quantitative assessment of plasma homocysteine as a risk factor for vascular disease. Probable benefits of increasing folic acid intakes. *JAMA* 1995; 274: 1049–57.

12. Bower, C, Stanley, FJ. Dietary folate as a risk factor for neural-tube defects: Evidence from a case-control study in Western Australia. *Med J Aust* 1989; 150: 613–19.

13. Brattström, L, Lindgren, A, Israelsson, B, Andersson, A, Hultberg, B. Homocysteine and cysteine: Determinants of plasma levels in middle-aged and elderly subjects. *J Intern Med* 1994; 236: 633–41.

14. Brattström, L, Wilcken, DEL, Öhrvik, J, Brudin, L. Common methylenetetrahydrofolate reductase gene mutation leads to hyperhomocysteinemia but not to vascular disease. The result of a meta-analysis. *Circulation* 1998; 98: 2520–26.

15. Brude, IR, Finstad, HS, Seljeflot, I, Drevon, CA, Solvoll, K, Sandstad, B, Hjermann, I, Arnesen, H, Nenseter, MS. Plasma homocysteine concentration related to diet, endothelial function and mononuclear gene expression among male hyperlipidaemic smokers. *Eur J Clin Invest* 1999; 29: 100–8.

16. Brussaard, JH, Lowik, MRH, van den Berg, H, Brants, HAM, Goldbohm, RA. Folate intake and status among adults in the Netherlands. *Eur J Clin Nutr* 1997; 51: S46–S50.

17. Chasan-Taber, L, Selhub, J, Rosenberg, IH, Malinow, MR, Terry, P, Tishler, PV, Willett, W, Hennekens, CH, Stampfer, MJ. A prospective study of folate and vitamin B6 and risk of myocardial infarction in US physicians. *J Am Coll Nutr* 1996;5:36–43.

18. Clarke, R, Collins, R. Can dietary supplements with folic acid or vitamin B6 reduce cardiovascular risk? Design of clinical trials to test the homocysteine hypothesis of vascular disease. *J Cardiovasc Risk* 1998; 5: 249–55.

19. Clarke, R, Smith, AD, Jobst, KA, Refsum, H, Sutton, L, Ueland, PM. Folate, vitamin B12, and serum total homocysteine levels in confirmed Alzheimer disease. *Arch Neurol* 1998; 55: 1449–55.

20. Cravo, ML, Glória, LM, Selhub, J, Nadeau, MR, Camilo, ME, Resende, MP, Cardoso, JN, Leitão, CN, Mira, FC. Hyperhomocysteinemia in chronic alcoholism: Correlation with folate, vitamin B-12, and vitamin B-6 status. *Am J Clin Nutr* 1996; 63: 220–24.

21. Danesh, J, Lewington, S. Plasma homocysteine and coronary heart disease: Systematic review of published epidemiological studies. *J Cardiovasc Risk* 1998; 5: 229–32.

22. Deharveng, G, Charrondière, UR, Slimani, N, Southgate, DAT, Riboli, E. Comparison of nutrients in the food composition tables available in the nine European countries participating in EPIC. *Eur J Clin Nutr* 1999; 53: 60–79.

23. Finkelstein, JD. Methionine metabolism in mammals. *J Nutr Biochem* 1990; 1: 228–37.

24. Fodinger, M, Mannhalter, C, Wolfl, G, Pabinger, I, Muller, E, Schmid, R, Horl, WH, Sunder-Plassmann, G. Mutation (677 C to T) in the methylenetetrahydrofolate reductase gene aggravates hyperhomocysteinemia in hemodialysis patients. *Kidney Int* 1997; 52: 517–23.

25. Fodinger, M, Wolfl, G, Fischer, G, Rasoul-Rockenschaub, S, Schmid, R, Horl, WH, Sunder-Plassmann, G. Effect of MTHFR 677C>T on plasma total homocysteine levels in renal graft recipients. *Kidney Int* 1999; 55: 1072–80.

26. Folsom, AR, Nieto, FJ, McGovern, PG, Tsai, MY, Malinow, MR, Eckfeldt, JH, Hess, DL, Davis, CE. Prospective study of coronary heart disease incidence in relation to fasting total homocysteine, related genetic polymorphisms and B vitamins: The Atherosclerosis

Risk in Communities (ARIC) study. *Circulation* 1998; 98: 204–10.

27. Frost Andersen, L, Nes, M, Lillegaard, IT, Sandstad, B, Bjørneboe, GE, Drevon, CA. Evaluation of a quantitative food frequency questionnaire used in a group of Norwegian adolescents. *Eur J Clin Nutr* 1995; 49: 543–54.

28. Giles, WH, Croft, JB, Greenlund, KJ, Ford, ES, Kittner, SJ. Total homocyst(e)ine concentration and the likelihood of nonfatal stroke: Results from the third National Health and Nutrition Examination Survey, 1988–1994. *Stroke* 1998; 29: 2473–77.

29. Green, TJ, Houghton, LA, Donovan, U, Gibson, RS, O'Connor, DL. Oral contraceptives did not affect biochemical folate indexes and homocysteine concentrations in adolescent females. *J Am Diet Assoc* 1998; 98: 49–55.

30. Gregory, JF. The bioavailability of folate. In *Folate in Health and Disease.* (Bailey, LB, ed.). Marcel Dekker, Inc, New York, 1995; pp. 195–235.

31. Gregory, JF, Wei, MM. Organic acids in selected foods inhibit intestinal brush border pteroylpolyglutamate hydrolase in vitro: Potential mechanism affecting the bioavailability of dietary polyglutamyl folate. *J Agric Food Chem* 1998; 46: 211–19.

32. Gudnason, V, Stansbie, D, Scott, J, Bowron, A, Nicaud, V, Humphries, S, on behalf of the EARS group S. C677T (thermolabile alanine/valine) polymorphism in methylenetetrahydrofolate reductase (MTHFR): Its frequency and impact on plasma homocysteine concentration in different European populations. *Atherosclerosis* 1998; 136: 347–54.

33. Guttormsen, AB, Schneede, J, Fiskerstrand, T, Ueland, PM, Refsum, HM. Plasma concentrations of homocysteine and other aminothiol compounds are related to food intake in healthy human subjects. *J Nutr* 1994; 124: 1934–41.

34. Guttormsen, AB, Ueland, PM, Nesthus, I, Nygård, O, Schneede, J, Vollset, SE, Refsum, H. Determinants and vitamin responsiveness of intermediate hyperhomocysteinemia (≥40 µmol/liter). The Hordaland Homocysteine Study. *J Clin Invest* 1996; 98: 2174–83.

35. Haagsma, CJ, Blom, HJ, van Riel, PL, van't Hof, MA, Giesendorf, BA, van Oppenraaij-Emmerzaal, D, van de Putte, LB. Influence of sulphasalazine, methotrexate, and the combination of both on plasma homocysteine concentrations in patients with rheumatoid arthritis. *Ann Rheum Dis* 1999; 58: 79–84.

36. Haglund, O, Wallin, R, Wretling, S, Hultberg, B, Saldeen, T. Effects of fish oil alone and combined with long chain (n-6) fatty acids on some coronary risk factors in male subjects. *J Nutr Biochem* 1998; 9: 629–35.

37. Henning, BF, Tepel, M, Riezler, R, Doberauer, C. Unfavourable changes in homocysteine metabolism during weight reduction. *Med Sci Res* 1997; 25: 555–56.

38. Henning, BF, Tepel, M, Riezler, R, Gillessen, A, Doberauer, C. Vitamin supplementation during weight reduction—favourable effect on homocysteine metabolism. *Res Exp Med* 1998; 198: 37–42.

39. Homocysteine Lowering Trialists' Collaboration. Lowering blood homocysteine with folic acid based supplements: Meta-analysis of randomised trials. *BMJ* 1998; 316: 894–98.

40. Howard, JM, Azen, C, Jacobsen, DW, Green, R, Carmel, R. Dietary intake of cobalamin in elderly people who have abnormal serum cobalamin, methylmalonic acid and homocysteine levels. *Eur J Clin Nutr* 1998; 52: 582–87.

41. Hultberg, B, Berglund, M, Andersson, A, Frank, A. Elevated plasma homocysteine in alcoholics. *Alcohol Clin Exp Res* 1993; 17: 687–89.

42. Jacobsen, BK, Thelle, DS. The Tromsø Heart Study: Is coffee drinking an indicator of a life style with high risk for ischemic heart disease? *Acta Med Scand* 1987; 222: 215–21.

43. Jacques, PF, Rosenberg, IH, Rogers, G, Selhub, J, Bowman, BA, Gunter, EW, Wright, JD, Johnson, CL. Serum total homocysteine concentrations in adolescent and adult Americans: Results from the third National Health and Nutrition Examination Survey. *Am J Clin Nutr* 1999; 69: 482–89.

44. Jacques, PF, Selhub, J, Bostom, AG, Wilson, PWF, Rosenberg, IH. The effect of folic acid fortification on plasma folate and total homocysteine concentrations. *N Engl J Med* 1999; 340: 1449–54.

45. Kato, I, Dnistrian, AM, Schwartz, M, Toniolo, P, Koenig, K, Shore, RE, Akhmedkhanov, A, Zeleniuch-Jacquotte, A, Riboli, E. Serum folate, homocysteine and colorectal cancer risk in women: A nested case-control study. *Br J Cancer* 1999; 79: 1917–22.

46. Kim, YI. Folate and carcinogenesis: Evidence, mechanisms, and implications. *J Nutr Biochem* 1999;10: 66–88.

47. Koehler, KM, Pareo-Tubbeh, SL, Liang, HC, Romero, LJ, Baumgartner, RN, Garry, PJ. Some vitamin sources relating to plasma homocysteine provide not only folate but also vitamins B-12 and B-6. *J Nutr* 1997;27: 1534–35.

48. Koehler, KM, Romero, LJ, Stauber, PM, Pareo-Tubbeh, SL, Liang, HC, Baumgartner, RN, Garry, PJ, Allen, RH, Stabler, SP. Vitamin supplementation and other variables affecting serum homocysteine and methylmalonic acid concentrations in elderly men and women. *J Am Coll Nutr* 1996; 15: 364–76.

49. Kupferminc, MJ, Eldor, A, Steinman, N, Many, A, Bar-Am, A, Jaffa, A, Fait, G, Lessing, JB. Increased frequency of genetic thrombophilia in women with complications of pregnancy. *N Engl J Med* 1999; 340: 9–13.

50. Laivuori, H, Kaaja, R, Turpeinen, U, Viinikka, L, Ylikorkala, O. Plasma homocysteine levels elevated and inversely related to insulin sensitivity in preeclampsia. *Obstet Gynecol* 1999; 93: 489–93.

51. La Vecchia, C, Negir, E, Franceschi, S, Parazzini, F, Decarli, A. Differences in dietary intake with smoking, alcohol, and education. *Nutr Cancer* 1992; 17: 297–304.

52. Lussier-Cacan, S, Xhignesse, M, Piolot, A, Selhub, J, Davignon, J, Genest, J. Plasma total homocysteine in healthy subjects: Sex-specific relation with biological traits. *Am J Clin Nutr* 1996; 64: 587–93.

53. Ma, J, Stampfer, MJ, Giovannucci, E, Artigas, C, Hunter, DJ, Fuchs, C, Willett, WC, Selhub, J, Hennekens, CH, Rozen, R. Methylenetetrahydrofolate reductase poly-

morphism, dietary interactions, and risk of colorectal cancer. *Cancer Res* 1997; 57: 1098–102.

54. Ma, J, Stampfer, MJ, Hennekens, CH, Frosst, P, Selhub, J, Horsford, J, Malinow, MR, Willett, WC, Rozen, R. Methylenetetrahydrofolate reductase polymorphism, plasma folate, homocysteine, and risk of myocardial infarction in US physicians. *Circulation* 1996; 94: 2410–16.

55. Malinow, MR, Duell, PB, Hess, DL, Anderson, PH, Kruger, WD, Phillipson, BE, Gluckman, RA, Block, PC, Upson, BM. Reduction of plasma homocyst(e)ine levels by breakfast cereal fortified with folic acid in patients with coronary heart disease. *N Engl J Med* 1998; 338: 1009–15.

56. Malinow, MR, Nieto, FJ, Kruger, WD, Duell, PB, Hess, DL, Gluckman, RA, Block, PC, Holzgang, CR, Anderson, PH, Seltzer, D, Upson, B, Lin, QR. The effects of folic acid supplementation on plasma total homocysteine are modulated by multivitamin use and methylenetetrahydrofolate reductase genotypes. *Arterioscler Thromb Vasc Biol* 1997; 17: 1157–62.

57. Mansoor, MA, Bergmark, C, Svardal, AM, Lønning, PE, Ueland, PM. Redox status and protein binding of plasma homocysteine and other aminothiols in patients with early-onset peripheral vascular disease. *Arterioscler Thromb Vasc Biol* 1995; 15: 232–40.

58. McCaddon, A, Davies, G, Hudson, P, Tandy, S, Cattell, H. Total serum homocysteine in senile dementia of Alzheimer type. *Int J Geriatr Psychiatry* 1998; 13: 235–39.

59. Mills, JL, McPartlin, JM, Kirke, PN, Lee, YJ, Conley, MR, Weir, DG, Scott, JM. Homocysteine metabolism in pregnancies complicated by neural-tube defects. *Lancet* 1995; 345: 149–51.

60. Møller, JM, Nielsen, GL, Ekelund, S, Schmidt, EB, Dyerberg, J. Homocysteine in Greenland Inuits. *Thromb Res* 1997; 86: 333–35.

61. Morabia, A, Wynder, EL. Dietary habits of smokers, people who never smoked, and ex-smokers. *Am J Clin Nutr* 1990; 52: 933–37.

62. Nieto, FJ, Comstock, GW, Chambless, LE, Malinow, MR. Coffee consumption and plasma homocyst(e)ine: Results from the Atherosclerosis Risk in Communities Study. *Am J Clin Nutr* 1997; 66: 1475–76.

63. Nygård, O, Nordrehaug, JE, Refsum, H, Ueland, PM, Farstad, M, Vollset, SE. Plasma homocysteine levels and mortality in patients with coronary artery disease. *N Engl J Med* 1997; 337: 230–36.

64. Nygård, O, Refsum, H, Ueland, PM, Stensvold, I, Nordrehaug, JE, Kvåle, G, Vollset, SE. Coffee consumption and plasma total homocysteine: The Hordaland Homocysteine Study. *Am J Clin Nutr* 1997; 65: 136–43.

65. Nygård, O, Refsum, H, Ueland, PM, Vollset, SE. Major lifestyle determinants of plasma total homocysteine distribution: The Hordaland Homocysteine Study. *Am J Clin Nutr* 1998; 67: 263–70.

66. Nygård, O, Vollset, SE, Refsum, H, Stensvold, I, Tverdal, A, Nordrehaug, JE, Ueland, PM, Kvåle, G. Total plasma homocysteine and cardiovascular risk profile. The Hordaland Homocysteine Study. *JAMA* 1995; 274: 1526–33.

67. Olszewski, AJ, McCully, KS. Fish oil decreases serum homocysteine in hyperlipemic men. *Coron Artery Dis* 1993; 4: 53–60.

68. Ortega, RM, Lopez-Sobaler, AM, Gonzalez-Gross, MM, Redondo, RM, Marzana, I, Zamora, MJ, Andres, P. Influence of smoking on folate intake and blood folate concentrations in a group of elderly Spanish men. *J Am Coll Nutr* 1994; 13: 68–72.

69. Osganian, SK, Stampfer, MJ, Spiegelman, D, Rimm, E, Cutler, JA, Feldman, HA, Montgomery, DH, Webber, LS, Lytle, LA, Bausserman, L, Nader, PR. Distribution of and factors associated with serum homocysteine levels in children. Child and adolescent trial for cardiovascular health. *JAMA* 1999; 281: 1189–96.

70. Oshaug, A, Bugge, KH, Refsum, H. Diet, an independent determinant for plasma total homocysteine. A cross sectional study of Norwegian workers on platforms in the North Sea. *Eur J Clin Nutr* 1998; 52: 7–11.

71. Pancharuniti, N, Lewis, CA, Sauberlich, HE, Perkins, LL, Go, RCP, Alvarez, JO, Macaluso, M, Acton, RT, Copeland, RB, Cousins, AL, Gore, TB, Cornwell, PE, Roseman, JM. Plasma homocyst(e)ine, folate, and vitamin B-12 concentrations and risk for early-onset coronary artery disease. *Am J Clin Nutr* 1994; 59: 940–48.

72. Piyathilake, CJ, Macaluso, M, Hine, RJ, Richards, EW, Krumdieck, CL. Local and systemic effects of cigarette smoking on folate and vitamin B-12. *Am J Clin Nutr* 1994; 60: 559–66.

73. Powers, RW, Evans, RW, Majors, AK, Ojimba, JI, Ness, RB, Crombleholme, WR, Roberts, JM. Plasma homocysteine concentration is increased in preeclampsia and is associated with evidence of endothelial activation. *Am J Obstet Gynecol* 1998; 179: 1605–11.

74. Rajkovic, A, Catalano, PM, Malinow, MR. Elevated homocyst(e)ine levels with preeclampsia. *Obstet Gynecol* 1997; 90: 168–71.

75. Refsum, H, Nygård, O, Kvåle, G, Ueland, PM, Vollset, SE. The Hordaland Homocysteine Study: The opposite tails odds ratios reveal differential effects of gender and intake of vitamin supplements at high and low plasma total homocysteine concentrations. *J Nutr* 1996; 126: 1244S–48S.

76. Refsum, H, Ueland, PM, Nygård, O, Vollset, SE. Homocysteine and cardiovascular disease. *Annu Rev Med* 1998; 49: 31–62.

77. Rimm, ED, Giovannucci, EL, Stampfer, MJ, Colditz, GC, Litin, LB, Willett, WC. Reproducibility and validity of an expanded self-administered semiquantitative food frequency questionnaire among male health professionals. *Am J Epidemiol* 1992; 135: 1114–26.

78. Selhub, J, Jacques, PF, Wilson, PWF, Rush, D, Rosenberg, IH. Vitamin status and intake as primary determinants of homocysteinemia in an elderly population. *JAMA* 1993; 270: 2693–98.

79. Shaw, GM, Rozen, R, Finnell, RH, Wasserman, CR, Lammer, EJ. Maternal vitamin use, genetic variation of infant methylenetetrahydrofolate reductase, and risk for spina bifida. *Am J Epidemiol* 1998; 148: 30–7.

80. Shaw, JTE, McWhinney, B, Tate, JR, Kesting, JB, Marczak, M, Purdie, D, Gibbs, H, Cameron, DP,

Hickman, PE. Plasma homocysteine levels in indigenous Australians. *Med J Aust* 1999; 170: 19–22.

81. Shields, DC, Kirke, PN, Mills, JL, Ramsbottom, D, Molloy, AM, Burke, H, Weir, DG, Scott, JM, Whitehead, AS. The "thermolabile" variant of methylenetetrahydrofolate reductase and neural tube defects: An evaluation of genetic risk and the relative importance of the genotypes of the embryo and the mother. *Am J Hum Genet* 1999; 64: 1045–55.

82. Shimakawa, T, Nieto, FJ, Malinow, MR, Chambless, LE, Schreiner, PJ, Szklo, M. Vitamin intake: A possible determinant of plasma homocyst(e)ine among middle-aged adults. *Ann Epidemiol* 1997; 7: 285–93.

83. Stampfer, MJ, Malinow, MR, Willett, WC, Newcomer, LM, Upson, B, Ullmann, D, Tishler, PV, Hennekens, CH. A prospective study of plasma homocyst(e)ine and risk of myocardial infarction in US physicians. *JAMA* 1992; 268: 877–81.

84. Steegers-Theunissen, RP, Boers, GH, Trijbels, FJ, Finkelstein, JD, Blom, HJ, Thomas, CM, Borm, GF, Wouters, MG, Eskes, TK. Maternal hyperhomocysteinemia: A risk factor for neural-tube defects? *Metabolism* 1994; 43: 1475–80.

85. Stehouwer, CDA, Weijenberg, MP, van den Berg, M, Jakobs, C, Feskens, EJM, Kromhout, D. Serum homocysteine and risk of coronary heart disease and cerebrovascular disease in elderly men: A 10-year follow-up. *Arterioscler Thromb Vasc Biol* 1998; 18: 1895–901.

86. Stolzenberg-Solomon, RZ, Miller, ER, Maguire, MG, Selhub, J, Appel, LJ. Association of dietary protein intake and coffee consumption with serum homocysteine concentrations in an older population. *Am J Clin Nutr* 1999; 69: 467–75.

87. Taylor, LM, Moneta, GL, Sexton, GJ, Schuff, RA, Porter, JM. The Homocysteine and Progression of Atherosclerosis Study Investigators. Prospective blinded study of the relationship between plasma homocysteine and progression of symptomatic peripheral arterial disease. *J Vasc Surg* 1999; 29: 8–19.

88. Tonstad, S, Refsum, H, Ose, L, Ueland, PM. The C677T mutation in the methylenetetrahydrofolate reductase gene predisposes to hyperhomocysteinemia in children with familial hypercholesterolemia treated with cholestyramine. *J Pediatr* 1998; 132: 365–68.

89. Tonstad, S, Refsum, H, Ueland, PM. Association between plasma total homocysteine and parental history of cardiovascular disease in children with familial hypercholesterolemia. *Circulation* 1997; 96: 1803–8.

90. Tucker, KL, Selhub, J, Wilson, PWF, Rosenberg, IH. Dietary intake pattern relates to plasma folate and homocysteine concentrations in the Framingham Heart Study. *J Nutr* 1996; 126: 3025–31.

91. Ubbink, JB, Fehily, AM, Pickering, J, Elwood, PC, Vermaak, WJH. Homocysteine and ischaemic heart disease in the Caerphilly cohort. *Atherosclerosis* 1998; 140: 349–56.

92. Verhoef, P, Hennekens, CH, Malinow, MR, Kok, FJ, Willett, WC, Stampfer, MJ. A prospective study of plasma homocyst(e)ine and risk of ischemic stroke. *Stroke* 1994; 25: 1924–30.

93. Verhoef, P, Stampfer, MJ, Buring, JE, Gaziano, JM, Allen, RH, Stabler, SP, Reynolds, RD, Kok, FJ, Hennekens, CH, Willett, WC. Homocysteine metabolism and risk of myocardial infarction: Relation with vitamins B6, B12, and folate. *Am J Epidemiol* 1996; 143: 845–59.

94. Vermaak, WJH, Ubbink, JB, Barnard, HC, Potgieter, GM, van Jaarsveld, H, Groenewald, AJ. Vitamin B-6 nutrition status and cigarette smoking. *Am J Clin Nutr* 1990; 51: 1058–61.

95. Vollset, SE, Nygård, O, Kvåle, G, Ueland, PM, Refsum, H. The Hordaland Homocysteine Study: Lifestyle and total plasma homocysteine in western Norway. In *Homocysteine Metabolism: From Basic Science to Clinical Medicine*. (Graham, I, Refsum, H, Rosenberg IH, Ueland PM, eds.). Kluwer Academic Publishers, Boston, 1997. pp 177–82.

96. Wald, NJ, Watt, HC, Law, MR, Weir, DG, McPartlin, J, Scott, JM. Homocystine and ischemic heart disease. Results of a prospective study with implications regarding prevention. *Arch Intern Med* 1998; 158: 862–67.

97. Willett, WC. *Nutritional Epidemiology. Monographs in Epidemiology and Biostatistics,* 2nd ed. Oxford University Press, New York, 1998.

98. Willett, WC, Sampson, L, Stampfer, MJ, Rosner, B, Bain, C, Witschi, J, Hennekens, CH, Speizer, FE. Reproducibility and validity of a semi-quantitative food frequency questionnaire. *Am J Epidemiol* 1985; 122: 51–65.

99. Wright, M, Francis, K, Cornwell, P. Effect of acute exercise on plasma homocysteine. *J Sports Med Phys Fitness* 1998; 38: 262–65.

100. Yarnell, JWG, Fehily, AM, Milbank, JE, Sweetnam, PM, Walker, CL. A short dietary questionnaire for use in an epidemiological survey: Comparison with weighed dietary records. *Hum Nutr Appl Nutr* 1983; 37A: 103–12.

101. Zondervan, KT, Ocké, MC, Smit, HA, Seidell, JC. Do dietary and supplementary intakes of antioxidants differ with smoking status? *Int J Epidemiol* 1996; 25: 70–9.

29

Epidemiology of Vascular and Thrombotic Associations

PETRA VERHOEF
MEIR STAMPFER

Persons with the inborn, enzymatic disorder homocystinuria have extremely high levels of homocysteine (37). Affected subjects usually suffer from vascular occlusion and thrombosis in arteries and large veins. Coronary, cerebral, and peripheral vessels all may be affected (52). In the last 10 to 15 years, many cross-sectional and case-control studies have found that moderately elevated plasma levels of homocysteine were more common in patients with vascular disease than in control subjects (13, 47). Several prospective studies confirmed these findings (13, 47); however, some recent large prospective studies did not (22, 23). As prospective studies bear a greater potential of unraveling a cause-effect relationship than case-control studies, doubt on a causal role of homocysteine has grown. Further doubt arose when a recent meta-analysis suggested that homozygous carriers of a common 677C→T mutation in the gene encoding a key enzyme in homocysteine metabolism appeared to have no increased risk of vascular disease despite having elevated homocysteine levels (14).

The first section of this chapter addresses methodological issues that generally apply to observational studies of homocysteine and vascular disease, such as measurement error and confounding. It also describes specific advantages and disadvantages of retrospective case-control and prospective studies. The second sec-tion summarizes the data from observational studies on the relation between homocysteine and the risk of vascular disease in light of several current hypotheses.

Methodological Issues in Epidemiological Studies: Study Design and General Sources of Bias

The early investigations of homocysteine and vascular disease were case-control studies that measured homocysteine levels after the disease onset. A major limitation of this design is that one cannot rule out the possibility that homocysteine levels were increased by the disease or its treatment. One is always also concerned about the appropriateness of the control group in case-control studies. These issues pose much less of a problem in prospective studies. However, although prospective studies have some distinct advantages, they also have limitations (i.e., homocysteine in frozen plasma samples could deteriorate, or prolonged follow-up of subjects could lead to attenuation of the association). These advantages and disadvantages of both study designs are discussed, and the impact of error in the measurement of homocysteine and vitamins and aspects of confounding are reviewed.

Case-control Studies

Effect of an Acute Event on Plasma Homocysteine and Vitamins Several findings suggest that plasma total homocysteine levels are lower in the acute phase of a myocardial infarction or stroke than after 6 weeks or more (20, 31, 32, 68). For blood levels of folate (68), cobalamin, and serum creatinine (28), no such differences were observed.

It is difficult to interpret these findings given that plasma homocysteine was not measured *before* the clinical event in any of the studies. A plausible explanation for low homocysteine levels just after an event is an acute-phase reduction in homocysteine, perhaps owing to a decrease in plasma albumin (the main binding protein of homocysteine). Most likely the concentrations returned to preevent levels later on. However, we cannot exclude the possibility that homocysteine levels rise in the months after the event to a higher level than before the event. This could strengthten the apparent relationship between homocysteine and vascular disease. In the Multiple Risk Factor Intervention Trial (22), concentrations of C-reactive protein, an acute-phase protein that rises with inflammation and after a vascular event, were weakly but significantly directly associated with homocysteine levels.

Dietary Changes and Medication Besides the likelihood of alteration of homocysteine levels after an acute event, there are two other limitations of the case-control design: 1) medication prescribed for patients with cardiovascular disease may modify homocysteine levels, and 2) patients may have altered their diet or use of vitamin supplements as a reaction to their illness.

Diuretics have been associated with increased plasma homocysteine levels (58), which may lead to a spuriously higher level of homocysteine among patients than control subjects. In another study, however, homocysteine changes during follow-up evaluation after an acute event were not related to medications commonly used by patients with vascular disease (nitroglycerine, streptokinase, beta blockers, or acetylsalicylic acid) (31). With respect to dietary changes, some literature indicates that patients with myocardial infarction tend to make healthy diet changes (30, 38), such as frying food less, trimming fat from meat, and using more polyunsaturated fat. Similarly, it is not unlikely that patients increase their intake of fruits and vegetables or use of vitamin supplementation. These dietary changes would be more likely to induce lower rather than higher homocysteine levels and would lead to an attenuation of the association.

Control Group In a cohort study, one does not have the problem of selecting an appropriate control group, because an internal comparison group is used. However, in the case-control studies, the selection of a proper control group is of major importance. Improper selection can lead to serious bias. Because homocysteine levels are sensitive to diet and other lifestyle factors, selection of control subjects who do not well represent the population from which the cases arose could easily bias results in either direction.

Prospective Studies

Inclusion of Subjects with Preexisting Disease If homocysteine rises in the months after an acute event, inclusion of subjects with preexisting disease in prospective studies may strengthen the apparent relationship between plasma homocysteine and risk of vascular disease. This possibility is illustrated by data from the British Regional Heart Study (43), a prospective study of homocysteine and risk of ischemic stroke. In that study, men with earlier coronary disease were included (37.4% of patients vs. 5.1% of control subjects). As patients with preexisting disease had higher homocysteine levels than patients without, the association between homocysteine and risk of stroke was stronger before subjects with prior disease were excluded from analyses.

Prolonged Storage In nested case-control studies with prospectively collected samples, the blood has often been stored at $-20°C$ or $-80°C$ for an extended period. It is possible that samples may deteriorate during prolonged storage. Mereau-Richard et al. (35) reported that the plasma concentration of homocysteine decreased after prolonged storage, although they did not describe the storage conditions. However, plasma homocysteine is known to be stable for at least 1 year at $-20°C$, and the distribution of values from stored samples is generally similar to those from assays on freshly obtained plasma (62). Therefore, this seems an unlikely source of bias in prospective studies, especially in those that store plasma samples at even lower temperatures. Although homocysteine determination is usually performed relatively soon after blood samples have been drawn in case-control studies, there are case-control studies in which blood samples have been stored for several years before homocysteine determination, potentially leading to bias in case-control studies as well.

Prolonged Follow-up When the follow-up interval after baseline sampling becomes long, the relation between homocysteine levels and vascular events occurring many years afterward may become attenuated, owing to changes in homocysteine during the follow-up period that were not accounted for. Evidence for the attenuation of the predictive capability for a single homocysteine determination was present in the Physicians' Health Study (16) in which the relative risk of myocardial infarction for men with elevated homocysteine was reduced to 1.7 (95% confidence interval, 0.9 to 3.3) when an additional group of men who developed myocardial infarction 6 to 9 years after baseline was included (the initial analyses were based on a 5-year follow-up period) (55). Conversely, some data seem to indicate that the plasma homocysteine level is fairly stable in individuals over time. In the Physicians' Health Study, a second blood sample was drawn, 10 years after the first, from 49 participants who had remained free from diagnosed vascular disease. The Spearman correlation coefficient between homocysteine measured in the samples drawn 10 years apart was 0.68 ($p = 0.0001$), showing that the within-person variation, even over a long period, is moderate. Israelsson et al. (29) measured homocysteine in fresh plasma from 76 men and plasma that had been stored at $-20°C$ for a mean of 10.9 ± 2.5 (standard deviation) years. The mean plasma homocysteine level was higher in the fresh samples than in the stored samples, which may be related to increasing age in the subjects. However, values in fresh and stored samples correlated significantly ($r = 0.58$, $p <0.001$). This correlation was apparent in subjects who suffered a vascular event and in subjects who remained healthy. However, in other populations, changes in diet and vitamin supplement usage during the follow-up period might vary, altering homocysteine levels and possibly leading to an attenuation of the risk estimates.

Exposure Measurement Error

In general, when there is little exposure measurement error, the measured exposure comes close to the "true" exposure of interest. Measurement error may be caused by high intraindividual variation and imprecision of the determinations. The first aspect relates to the fact that homocysteine levels are usually measured only once in epidemiological studies. The second aspect refers to accurate blood sampling and handling. In general, different methods of homocysteine determinations are used within the studies, performed by several laboratories. The different methods tend to correlate well (62). The coefficients of variation for the homocysteine determinations vary between 3% and 7%, which is not considered a major source of measurement error.

Single Measurement Most epidemiological studies of homocysteine and vascular disease are based on a single homocysteine determination per individual. A large within-person variability will underestimate the true strength of risk associations. Clarke et al. (19) have reported that epidemiological studies based on a single homocysteine measurement may underestimate the magnitude of the risk association with disease by 10% to 15%. This magnitude of regression dilution for a single homocysteine measurement (1.14) was less than for serum cholesterol (1.18) and blood pressure (1.35). No epidemiological study has measured homocysteine levels two or more times, at various moments in time, to obtain a value closer to the "true" homocysteine level.

Blood Sampling and Handling Incorrect handling of blood samples may also lead to imprecise assessment of homocysteine exposure status of an individual. When whole blood is stored at room temperature for longer than 4 hours, homocysteine in plasma may increase by 35%. This increase can be avoided when blood is put on ice immediately after collection, or when plasma or serum is prepared within 1 hour after collection (62). In epidemiological studies that were not originally designed to study the relationship between homocysteine and risk of cardiovascular disease, this may be an important source of measurement error.

Most of the remarks made for homocysteine also apply to measurements of the vitamins in plasma,

serum, or whole blood. For example, after blood sampling, precautions must be taken to protect folate against oxidative destruction before assay (by adding a reducing agent such as ascorbate) (27). Plasma pyridoxal 5'-phosphate is probably stable at long storage, but for folate this is uncertain (75).

Finally, when biomarkers of dietary intake of folate and vitamin B_6 are measured in studies, the long-term exposure measurements (e.g., erythrocyte folate, which reflects body stores of folate) may be preferable to short-term exposure measurements (e.g., plasma folate, which measures recent intake), because they may refer to a more relevant time period (especially in case-control studies).

In general, it is hard to draw conclusions on the effect of these causes of measurement error. Effect attenuation will probably occur in most occasions, but a strengthening of the association is not unlikely (4).

Confounding

A confounder is a factor that is independently related to the exposure of interest (e.g., plasma total homocysteine) and to the outcome of interest (e.g., vascular disease). By definition, a confounder is not part of the causal pathway (i.e., it may not directly lead to the exposure factor or be the factor by which the exposure factor exerts its effect on the disease outcome).

For homocysteine and vascular disease, gender and age are important potential confounders, as men usually have higher homocysteine levels than women, both fasting and after methionine loading, and homocysteine tends to increase with advancing age (2, 40). Notably, male gender and increasing age are related to higher risk of vascular disease.

Other possible confounders are known risk factors for vascular disease: smoking, alcohol intake, blood pressure, serum cholesterol, and renal function. As discussed in Chapter 28, the use of tobacco is associated with lower blood levels of folate, cobalamin, and vitamin B_6 (47), which is a plausible explanation for observed higher total homocysteine levels among smokers than nonsmokers (40, 60). Also, in several studies, positive associations between plasma homocysteine and total and low-density lipoprotein cholesterol have been observed (40, 42). Similarly, blood pressure is positively associated with homocysteine levels (3, 40, 60). High-density lipoprotein cholesterol has been found to correlate inversely with homocysteine levels (60). Several studies have observed inverse associations between homocysteine levels and alcohol intake. In the Caerphilly Cohort Study (60), this association was explained by folate intake. The most widely consumed alcoholic beverage was beer, which contains about 9 µg of folate per 100 mL. Thus, alcohol may be a potential confounder, being related inversely to both coronary heart disease and homocysteine levels.

Confounding can be (partially) controlled for by stratified analyses according to categories of confounders, such as gender or age, or by multivariate adjustment. As many of the confounders may be measured with substantial error, control for confounding may be incomplete. Most epidemiological studies provided risk estimates that were controlled for most of the previously mentioned factors in multivariate analyses. Compared with crude estimates, effects generally remained present or became slightly weaker. However, there are examples of strong effect attenuation after adjustment for confounding (26, 34, 60).

Impaired kidney function, reflected by elevation of serum creatinine levels, may be an additional confounder, because it is associated with increased homocysteine levels (8) and may be related to cardiovascular disease as well. If there are more persons with diminished renal function among study subjects than control subjects, a spurious positive association between homocysteine and risk of vascular disease may be observed. Several epidemiological studies have controlled for creatinine levels in multivariate analyses, and associations between elevated homocysteine and risk of vascular disease remained.

Several of the mentioned confounders, such as age and hypertension, may also act as effect modifiers, factors that modify the association between plasma homocysteine and risk of vascular disease. These are discussed in a later section.

Conclusion

We have summarized methodological issues that apply to observational studies of homocysteine and vascular disease. Obviously, there is more risk of bias in retrospective studies (e.g., through effects of the disease on homocysteine levels or inappropriate choice of control subjects). However, findings from prospective studies could still be biased because of improper or incomplete control for confounding or inclusion of patients with preexisting disease.

Four Popular Hypotheses

This section summarizes the currently available data on the association between homocysteine and risk of vascular disease in light of four popular hypotheses among researchers in this field. Table 29.1 lists the four hypotheses. These hypotheses have been formulated mainly to explain why several studies, especially the prospective studies, find a weak or no association between plasma homocysteine and risk of vascular dis-

ease. For each hypothesis, Table 29.1 summarizes arguments in favor, the type of evidence that is missing, and our assessment of these hypotheses.

1. Elevated Homocysteine is Not a Cause of Vascular Disease

This hypothesis is based on the observation that prospective studies find weaker associations than retrospective studies and on the observed absence of an association between homozygosity for the 5,10-methylenetetrahydrofolate reductase (MTHFR) 677C→T mutation and risk of vascular disease. This latter observation has provoked intense discussion among researchers in the field, so we will start there.

Methylenetetrahydrofolate Reductase 677C→T Mutation and Risk of Vascular Disease The MTHFR enzyme is responsible for the reduction of 5,10-methylenetetrahydrofolate to 5-methyltetrahydrofolate, a required substrate for homocysteine remethylation (see Chapter 22). In 1995, a 677C→T mutation in the MTHFR gene was discovered (24). The mutation renders the enzyme thermolabile, thereby leading to elevation of homocysteine levels in homozygous subjects, especially in those with low folate status (66). This genotype can be regarded as a lifelong predisposition to moderately elevated homocysteine levels and, inherently, one would expect increased risk of vascular disease among these subjects. Several epidemiological studies have investigated this association.

Brattström et al. (14) reported a meta-analysis of 23 of these studies, in which they observed no significant increased risk of vascular disease among subjects with the TT genotype for the 677C→T polymorphism compared with those with the CC genotype. They concluded that mild hyperhomocysteinemia is not causally related to the pathogenesis of vascular disease. These investigators calculated that subjects with the TT genotype have a mean plasma homocysteine concentration that is 2.6 μmol/L higher than that of subjects with the CC genotype. Presuming that an increase in plasma homocysteine of 1 μmol/L is associated with approximately a 10% increase in risk of vascular disease (13, 47), the expected odds ratio for the TT genotype compared with the CC genotype is 1.26, well within the 95% confidence interval calculated by Brattström et al. (14) (OR: 1.12; 95% confidence interval, 0.92 to 1.37). Therefore, the meta-analysis does not rule out the possibility that TT genotype is associated with increased risk of vascular disease.

It is also possible that the TT genotype is beneficial in other ways. MTHFR regulates the availability of one-

Table 29.1. Four Popular Hypotheses Regarding the Association of Homocysteine with Vascular Disease

Hypotheses: Elevated Homocysteine is...	Arguments in Favor	Type of Evidence That is Missing	Overall Evidence for Support of Hypothesis
(1)... not a cause of vascular disease.	• Some prospective studies showed no association.	• Clinical trials, although they cannot distinguish between effect of vitamins and homocysteine	• Insufficient
	• MTHFR 677C→T mutation is not associated with increased risk in many studies.	• Studies that measure homocysteine before and after an acute event • Large studies on MTHFR 677C→T mutation that take into account effect modification by folate status	
(2)... a risk factor only in high risk groups.	• Several prospective studies are in line with this hypothesis.	• More studies that support this hypothesis	• Several indications
(3)... is related to thrombosis, not to atherosclerosis.	• None, although evidence for thrombosis is more coherent	• Clinical trials of homocysteine lowering that use pure atherosclerotic and thrombotic endpoints	• Insufficient
(4)... is a marker for low B-vitamin status, which confers the true risk.	• Some studies find association of B_6 with vascular disease, but not with homocysteine and vascular disease. • MTHFR 677C→T mutation is not associated with increased risk in many studies.	• Clinical trials intervening with nonvitamin, homocysteine-lowering agents	• Insufficient

carbon units of folate not only for remethylation of homocysteine, but also for synthesis of thymidine and purines. Reduced MTHFR activity hampers homocysteine remethylation but leads to higher availability of folate for DNA synthesis (6, 63). This effect may explain the marked reduction in risk of colon cancer among those with the TT genotype (17, 33). Increased DNA synthesis may also be beneficial during repair of endothelial damage. Hence, a higher risk due to elevated homocysteine might be counterbalanced, in part, by better endothelial function.

Furthermore, it is not unlikely that the TT genotype emerges as a risk factor for vascular disease mainly in populations with low-normal folate intake, considering that it results in moderate hyperhomocysteinemia mainly in subjects with suboptimal folate status (66). In fact, from the meta-analysis (14), it appears that this polymorphism is directly associated with vascular disease more often in European than in North American studies. This may be explained in part by the fact that use of multivitamin supplements and replete folate status are much more common in North America than in Europe.

Findings From Prospective Studies Generally, results from cross-sectional and case-control studies support the hypothesis that elevation of homocysteine is a risk factor for vascular disease (13, 47). However, the findings from several prospective studies have been less convincing (1, 22, 23, 64). As noted earlier, prospective studies have the advantage of measuring homocysteine levels before disease onset (although often in blood samples that were stored long term) and thus can directly address the direction of any potential causal relation between homocysteine and risk of vascular disease. A further advantage is that patients and control subjects are derived from the same study population.

Table 29.2 provides a comprehensive overview of 20 prospective studies on homocysteine and vascular disease and/or total mortality. Two of the studies with total mortality as an outcome were among patients with vascular disease (39, 59). Prospective studies with venous thrombosis as the disease endpoint are discussed later. We have not included prospective studies among patients with renal disease, as they are discussed in Chapter 26.

Table 29.2. Prospective Studies of Plasma Levels of Total Homocysteine and the Risk of Vascular Disease

Year (ref)	Study, Country	Study design; Follow-up	Outcome	#Cases/Controls or Events	Age (yr) and Gender	Outcome Direction and Magnitude[a]
1992 (55)	PHS, US	Nested case-control; 5 years	Acute MI or CHD death	271 case-control pairs matched for age and smoking	59 ± 9 M	(+) OR upper 5% vs. bottom 90%: 3.4 (1.3–8.8)
1994 (1)	North Karelia Project, Finland	Nested case-control; 9 years	MI or stroke	265 case-control pairs matched for age	40–64 M & F	(−) All ORs close to unity
1994 (65)	PHS, US	Nested case-control; 5 years	Ischemic stroke	109 cases 427 controls	60 ± 9 M	(+)[b] OR upper 20% vs. bottom 80%: 1.2 (0.7–2.0)
1995 (5)	Tromsø Health Study, Norway	Nested case-control; 4 years	CHD	122 cases 478 controls matched for age	51 ± 7 M & F	(+) Graded, OR per 4 µmol/L: 1.3 (1.1–1.7)
1995 (43)	BRHS Cohort, UK	Nested case-control; 12 years	Ischemic stroke	107 cases 118 controls matched for age	54 ± 5 M	(+) Graded, OR upper 25% vs. bottom 25%: 2.5 (1.1–6.1)
1996 (16)	PHS, US	Nested case-control; 7.5 years	MI	333 case-control pairs matched for age and smoking	40–84 M	(+)[b] OR upper 5% vs. bottom 90%: 1.7 (0.9–3.3)
1996 (45)	US	Prospective cohort study among 337 patients with SLE; mean 4.8 years	Stroke and thrombotic events	29 events of stroke 31 events of ATD 33 events of VTD	35 ± 12 mainly F	(+) RRs for > 14.1 µmol/L; Stroke: 2.4 (1.0–5.8); ATD: 3.5 (1.0–12.5); No association for VTD
1997 (22)	MRFIT, US	Nested case-control; 20 years	Nonfatal MI, fatal CHD	240 cases 472 controls matched for age, smoking, race	mean: 46 M	(−) OR upper 25% vs. bottom 25%: 0.8 (0.6–1.5)
1997 (39)	Norway	Prospective cohort study among 587 patients with CAD; median 4.6 years	Total mortality	64 deaths (50 from CVD)	median: 62 M & F	(+) Graded, mortality ratio upper 25% vs. bottom 25%: 4.5 (1.2–16.6)
1997 (64)	PHS, US	Nested case-control; 9 years	Angina pectoris with subsequent coronary bypass surgery	149 case-control pairs matched for age and smoking	58 ± 8 M	(−) All ORs close to unity
1998 (23)	ARIC, US	Case-cohort (n = 15,792); median 3.3 years	CHD	232 events 537 controls	45–64 M & F	(+/−)[b] RR upper 20% vs. bottom 20%: 1.3 (0.5–3.2); positive, graded association in women, and no association in men

Year (ref)	Study, Country	Study design; Follow-up	Outcome	#Cases/Controls or Events	Age (yr) and Gender	Outcome Direction and Magnitude[a]
1998 (57)	Zutphen Elderly Study, Netherlands	Prospective cohort study (n = 878); 10 years	CHD and stroke; death and first event	52 CHD deaths 28 stroke deaths 56 1st MI 49 1st stroke	mean: 71.5 M	(+/−) RR stroke mortality, highest vs. lowest tertile (normotensives only): 6.2 (2.3–17.0); weaker associations with other endpoints
1998 (60)	Caerphilly, UK	Prospective cohort study (n = 2,290); 5 years	Fatal and nonfatal ischemic heart disease (mostly MI)	56 deaths 98 MI	50–64 M	(+)[b] RR upper 20% vs. bottom 20%: 1.4 (0.8–2.3)
1998 (72)	BUPA, UK	Nested case-control; mean 8.7 years	Death from ischemic heart disease	229 cases 1,126 controls matched for age and duration of sample storage	35–64 M	(+) Graded, OR per 5 μmol/L: 1.3 (1.2–1.6)
1998 (74)	BRHS Cohort, UK	Nested case-control; 12 years	MI	386 cases 454 controls matched for age	40–59 M	(+) OR upper 30% vs. bottom 70%: 1.8 (1.3–2.4)
1999 (9)	Framingham Elderly Study, US	Prospective cohort study (n = 1,933); median 10 years	All-cause and CVD mortality	653 all cause 244 CVD	70 ± 7 M & F	(+) RR upper 25% vs. bottom 75% All: 1.5 (1.3–1.8) CVD: 1.5 (1.2–2.0)
1999 (11)	Rotterdam Study, Netherlands	Nested case-control; 1–4 years	MI and stroke	104 MI cases 120 stroke sases 533 controls	≥55 M & F	(+) OR upper 20% vs. bottom 20% MI: 2.4 (1.1–5.4) stroke: 2.5 (1.2–5.4)
1999 (49)	Women's Health Study, US	Nested case-control; 3 years	MI, stroke, coronary revascularization	122 cases 244 controls matched for age and smoking	mean: 59 F	(+) Graded, OR upper 25% vs. bottom 25%: 2.3 (1.2–4.3)
1999 (56)	Hoorn Study, Netherlands	Prospective study among NIDDM patients (n = 211); median 6.4 years	Total and CHD mortality	49 deaths (30 from CVD)	< 70 M & F	(+) Graded, only significant for all-cause mortality RR per 1 μmol/L: 1.11 (1.08–1.15)
1999 (59)	Homocysteine and Progression of Atherosclerosis Study, US[c]	Prospective cohort study (n = 351); mean 37 months	Total mortality	47 deaths (33 from CVD)	66 ± 9 M & F	(+) RR upper 20% vs. bottom 20%: 3.1 (1.7–6.6)

ARIC = Atherosclerosis Risk in Communities; ATD = arterial thrombotic disease; BRHS = British Regional Heart Study; BUPA = British United Provident Association; CHD = coronary heart disease; CVD = cardiovascular disease; DVT = deep-vein thrombosis; F = females; M = males; MI = myocardial infarction; NIDDM = non-insulin-dependent diabetes mellitus; OR = odds ratio; PHS = Physicians' Health Study; RR = relative risk; SLE = systemic lupus erythematosus; VTD = venous thrombotic disease; VTE = venous thromboembolism
[a] Multivariately adjusted ORs or RRs are shown with 95% confidence intervals in brackets.
[b] Not significant.
[c] We discuss total mortality and CVD mortality only. The study looked at clinical progression as well.

Table 29.2 provides the direction and magnitude of the association. If it was calculated, a risk estimate for the upper quartile or quintile versus the lowest quartile(s) is shown. When there was indication for a clear graded effect, this is stated in the table, and risk estimates are shown accordingly.

Three studies showed no association (1, 22, 64). Four studies showed weak, nonsignificant, direct associations (16, 23, 60, 65). The odds ratio for ischemic stroke in the Physicians' Health Study (65) was only 1.2 and not statistically significant. Similarly, a second article on homocysteine and risk of myocardial infarction in the Physicians' Health Study observed a nonsignificant association (16). The Atherosclerosis Risk in Communities study observed a direct, although not statistically significant, association in women, but not in men (23). Finally, in the Caerphilly Cohort Study, the relative risk was small and not statistically significant (60).

Thirteen other studies showed direct associations (5, 9, 11, 39, 43, 45, 49, 55–57, 59, 72, 74). Two of these studies consisted entirely of patients with vascular disease (39, 59). Two other studies included both healthy individuals and patients with vascular disease (43, 74). As there were more subjects with baseline vascular disease among the subjects who had a vascular event during follow-up evaluation than among those who remained free from disease, and subjects with baseline vascular disease tended to have higher homocysteine levels than those without, this led to overestimation of the effect.

The relationship between elevated homocysteine and risk of myocardial infarction in the Physicians' Health Study (55) became weaker after prolonged follow-up evaluation (16). The study with the longest follow-up time (20 years) observed no association (22). However, there is no clear trend that studies with the longest follow-up time tend to find the weakest associations.

Conclusion Based on the currently available evidence on the association between the MTHFR 677C→T polymorphism and vascular disease, there is no strong reason to assume that elevated homocysteine is not a causal risk factor for vascular disease. Furthermore, the findings of the majority of prospective studies favor a causal relationship between elevated homocysteine and risk of vascular disease.

2. Elevated Homocysteine is Associated with Increased Risk only Among High-risk Groups

Stated in other words, elevated homocysteine alone may not be harmful, but it may lead to an event only under conditions predisposing to vascular disease,

such as atherosclerosis, high blood pressure, or diabetes. The current evidence for this hypothesis is described next.

Special High-risk Populations PATIENTS WITH VASCULAR DISEASE In two prospective studies listed in Table 29.2, the association between elevated homocysteine and recurrence of vascular disease was investigated. One study examined all-cause mortality among 587 patients with coronary artery disease during a median follow-up period of 4.6 years, in which 64 patients died, 50 of them from vascular disease (39). Baseline homocysteine levels bore a strong, graded relationship to overall mortality; compared with subjects with homocysteine levels below 9 μmol/L (the reference group), those with levels above 20 μmol/L had a 4.5 times higher chance of dying during the follow-up period. The second report was a blinded prospective study of the influence of homocysteine and of other atherosclerotic risk factors on the progression of disease in patients with symptomatic cardiovascular disease, lower extremity disease, or both (59). After multivariate adjustment, each 1.0 μmol/L increase in the plasma homocysteine levels resulted in a 3.6% increase (95% confidence interval, 0.0% to 6.6%; $p = 0.06$) in the risk of death (all causes) at 3 years and a 5.6% increase (95% confidence interval, 2.2% to 8.5%; $p = 0.003$) in the risk of death from vascular disease.

OTHER SPECIAL GROUPS Several studies summarized in Table 29.2 examined specific populations; these included the elderly (9, 11, 57), women with systemic lupus erythematosus (45), and patients with non-insulin-dependent diabetes mellitus (56). These populations could be considered as having an elevated susceptibility for vascular disease. All of these studies showed positive associations between homocysteine levels and vascular disease. However, there was no indication that risk was particularly stronger than in several studies among healthy populations that showed positive associations, such as the British United Provident Association study (72).

Effect Modification GENDER Gender may modify the association between homocysteine and risk of vascular disease. One study in Table 29.2 was restricted to postmenopausal women—the Women's Health Study (49), the female counterpart of the Physicians' Health Study. Associations were stronger than in the Physician's Health Study, although the findings cannot be fully compared owing to the shorter follow-up period among the women than the men (3 years vs. 5 to 7 years). The effect modification by gender in 12 epidemiological studies has been reviewed (69). Seven of the 12 epidemiological studies that included both men and women, found that elevated homocysteine levels were a stronger risk factor in women than in men. Several of these studies estimated that the risk was about twice as high in women as in men. However, the interaction effect was statistically significant for only one study. Three studies observed no risk difference between men and women, and two observed a weaker association in women.

The stronger effect among women in some studies may be explained by aspects of the study design, such as young age at inclusion, or aspects of the data analysis, such as use of an overall instead of a gender-specific cutoff point. Also, one cannot exclude the possibility that women are somehow more susceptible to detrimental effects of homocysteine than men, although there is evidence from other studies that estrogens have a "protective" effect on the vascular wall and a favorable effect on hemostasis (69).

CONVENTIONAL RISK FACTORS Hypertension is a strong risk factor for ischemic stroke. The presence or absence of hypertension appears to modify the association between elevated homocysteine and ischemic stroke. In the Physicians' Health Study (65) and the Zutphen Elderly Study (57), the association between elevated homocysteine levels and stroke was stronger among normotensive subjects. It may be that homocysteine emerges as a risk factor for stroke only among those with an otherwise low risk. However, in the European multicenter study, there was a much stronger association between homocysteine and risk of vascular disease among hypertensive subjects than among normotensive ones, especially among women (26). These findings were confirmed in other studies (11, 34, 43). Furthermore, in the European multicenter study, there was a stronger association among smokers, but no interaction effect for serum cholesterol. In the Atherosclerosis Risk in Communities study, the relationship between elevated homocysteine and carotid artery wall thickness was weaker among smokers than among nonsmokers (34).

Conclusion The prospective studies that investigated recurrence of vascular disease and mortality (including mortality from vascular disease) observed a positive association with homocysteine levels. The studies that investigated special populations, such as the elderly, also found positive associations between homocysteine and risk of vascular disease. The seven prospective studies in Table 29.2 that observed no associations or weak ones were all among healthy populations and not high-risk populations. However, there appears to be too little evidence to conclude that elevated homocysteine is a risk factor among high-risk populations only. Moreover, the evidence on interac-

tion between conventional risk factors and homocysteine is still limited and inconclusive.

3. Elevated Homocysteine is Related to Thrombosis, but not to Atherosclerosis

The origin of this hypothesis probably lies in two observations. First, some studies of intermediate endpoints of atherosclerotic disease, such as stenosis of the coronary arteries or carotid artery intima-media wall thickness, found weak or no associations with homocysteine levels. Second, baseline homocysteine levels bear a strong relation to vascular death among patients with vascular disease. No reason exists currently to favor either an atherogenic or thrombogenic mechanism over the other, as many possible pathophysiological mechanisms have been postulated for each of them (73). We will evaluate current data to see whether a clear pattern emerges.

Atherosclerosis CORONARY ARTERY STENOSIS A thrombotic event such as a myocardial infarction is usually the result of the development of atherosclerosis and an acute process (i.e., clot formation). Homocysteine may be involved in both processes (73). With angiographically defined coronary atherosclerosis as the disease endpoint, several studies sought to determine whether elevated homocysteine levels have an atherogenic effect. This goal could also be reached by grading the disease (i.e., by investigating a possible dose-response relationship between plasma homocysteine and extent of arterial occlusion).

Inevitably, when choosing an angiographic endpoint, many patients will have had a history of myocardial infarction before the catheterization, which makes it difficult to separate between atherogenesis and thrombus formation. Nevertheless, in a case-control study (67), the mean plasma homocysteine level was similar for patients with and without a history of myocardial infarction, and there was a trend of increasing plasma homocysteine with an increasing number of occluded vessels. Other studies made similar observations (61, 70). Thus, these data support an atherogenic action of elevated homocysteine levels, independent of their possible thrombogenic effects. However, if homocysteine levels rise as a result of atherosclerosis (see the earlier discussion on homocysteine and C-reactive protein), this result could also be an artifact. Unlike the previously mentioned studies, a prospective study among coronary artery disease patients observed only a weak correlation between homocysteine levels and the extent of coronary artery disease (39). The relationship was much stronger for lipid-related factors.

CAROTID ARTERY INTIMA-MEDIA THICKENING AND STENOSIS Carotid artery intima-media thickening is assessed noninvasively with ultrasound techniques. The thickening is associated with atherosclerosis elsewhere in the arterial system and with risk factors for vascular disease, and it can predict future risk for stroke and myocardial infarction (10, 15, 41).

As discussed in Chapter 31, several cross-sectional studies have observed that elevated plasma levels of total homocysteine are associated with increased carotid artery intima-media thickening (12, 18, 34, 71), carotid artery stenosis (51), and carotid plaque area (54). However, a small study did not show evidence of increased carotid artery intima-media thickening or stenosis among homozygotes and heterozygotes for cystathionine β-synthase deficiency compared with control subjects (53). One prospective study observed that an elevated homocysteine level was associated with an increased rate of progression of carotid plaque area in patients with atherosclerosis (44), whereas another one observed no increased progression of carotid artery stenosis among those with elevated homocysteine levels (59). At present, the possibility that elevated homocysteine is a consequence of atherosclerosis cannot be excluded.

Thrombosis ARTERIAL THROMBOSIS The Physicians' Health Study examined both an atherosclerotic coronary endpoint (i.e., angina pectoris followed by coronary bypass surgery) (64), and an atherothrombotic endpoint (i.e., myocardial infarction) (55). Homocysteine levels were not associated with angina pectoris but were positively associated with myocardial infarction. Furthermore, the pronounced association with mortality from vascular disease among vascular patients (39, 59) strongly suggests that homocysteine may be a thrombotic agent, but it does not exclude the possibility that it is atherogenic as well.

VENOUS THROMBOSIS The pathology of venous thrombosis differs from that of arterial thrombosis because atherosclerosis is not involved (see Chapter 33). Furthermore, different hemostatic factors are related to venous thrombosis than to arterial thrombosis. Most epidemiological studies have found that elevated homocysteine levels increase the risk of venous thrombosis (7, 46).

Three prospective studies have been published (21, 45, 48). The study of patients with systemic lupus erythematosus observed no relationship between homocysteine and venous thrombotic disease, whereas the association was positive for arterial thrombosis (45) (see also Table 29.2). In the nested case-control study in the Physicians' Health Study, the association was absent for any venous thrombotic event but positive for idiopathic venous thrombosis (48). The study of recurrence of venous thrombotic disease observed a positive relationship (21).

Conclusion As an atherothrombotic endpoint, such as a myocardial infarction, is generally a result of both atherosclerosis and thrombus formation, it is difficult to draw conclusions about separate atherogenic and arterial thrombotic effects of homocysteine elevation. Prospective studies appear to provide sufficient evidence that homocysteine is related to acute arterial and venous thrombotic events. For a pure atherosclerotic endpoint, such as coronary narrowing and carotid artery intima-media thickening, the evidence is more limited. However, it appears premature to conclude that homocysteine is not related to atherosclerosis.

4. Elevated Total Homocysteine is a Marker of Low B-Vitamin Status, which Confers the True Elevation of Risk

Dietary intake or plasma levels of the vitamins are strong determinants of homocysteine; if vitamin levels are inversely related to vascular disease, one might consider this additional evidence that elevated homocysteine is a risk factor for vascular disease. However, because the risk of vascular disease associated with the MTHFR polymorphism was lower than that expected for the elevation in homocysteine, some have suggested that, apart from genetically increased levels, homocysteine elevations are mainly a marker of low B-vitamin status, which is the basic cause of the excess risk.

Several prospective studies investigated the relationship between the B vitamins (mainly folate and vitamin B_6) and risk of coronary heart disease. As patients may change their diet in response to vascular disease, we will consider prospective studies only. Clearly, observational studies (or even clinical trials) do not permit unraveling of independent effects between the vitamins and homocysteine, which are strongly interrelated. Some studies have controlled for homocysteine levels when studying relationships between vitamins and risk of vascular disease.

Prospective Studies on Folate, Vitamin B_6, and Risk of Vascular Disease Table 29.3 provides a list of prospective studies on folate, vitamin B_6, and risk of vascular disease (all coronary heart disease). Only two studies (16, 23) measured both homocysteine and vitamins and were able to compare the associations of these with risk of vascular disease.

All five studies summarized in Table 29.3 showed inverse associations between folate status or intake and risk of coronary heart disease, but the findings were statistically significant in only two studies (36, 50). Furthermore, only the studies by Rimm et al. (50) and Giles et al. (25) included alcohol intake as a covariate in the multivariate models. As previously explained, in beer drinking populations alcohol may

Table 29.3 Prospective Studies of Vitamins and the Risk of Vascular Disease

Year (ref)	Study, Country	Study Design; Follow-up	Outcome	Vitamin(s) Measured	# Cases/ Controls or Events	Age (yr) and Gender	Results
1995 (25)	NHANES I, US	Prospective cohort study (n = 2006); 13 years	Ischemic stroke	Serum folate	98 events 1908 no event	mean: 62 mean: 52 M & F	RR for ≤ 9.2 nmol/L vs. higher: 1.4 (0.8–2.3)
1996 (16)	PHS, US	Nested case-control; 7.5 years	MI	Plasma levels of folate and PLP	333 case-control pairs matched for age and smoking	40–84 M	OR bottom 20% vs. upper 80%: Folate: 1.4 (0.9–2.3) B$_6$: 1.5 (1.0–2.2)
1996 (36)	Nutrition Canada Survey, Canada	Retrospective cohort study (n = 5056); 15 years	CHD	Serum folate	165 events	35–79 M & F	RR for < 6.8 nmol/L vs. > 13.6 nmol/L: 1.7 (1.1–2.6)
1998 (23)	ARIC, US	Case-cohort (n = 15792); median 3.3 years	CHD	Plasma levels of folate and PLP	232 events 537 controls	45–64 M & F	OR upper 20% vs. bottom 20%: PLP: 0.3 (0.1–0.7) Folate: 0.7 (0.3–1.5)
1998 (50)	Nurses' Health Study, US	Prospective cohort study; (n = 80082); 14 years	Nonfatal MI and fatal CHD	Intake of folate and vitamin B$_6$	658 nonfatal 281 fatal	30–55 F	OR upper 20% vs. bottom 80%: Folate: 0.7 (0.6–0.9) B$_6$: 0.7 (0.5–0.9)

ARIC = Atherosclerosis Risk in Communities study; CHD = coronary heart disease; F = females; M = males; MI = myocardial infarction; NHANES = National Health and Nutrition Examination Survey; PHS = Physicians' Health Study; OR = odds ratio; PLP = pyridoxal 5′-phosphate; RR = relative risk

be a strong potential confounder. Furthermore, one could expect confounding by other factors, such as smoking or a healthy diet, which could be related both to folate status and risk of coronary heart disease.

In the study by Chasan-Taber et al. (16), the direct association between homocysteine and risk of myocardial infarction was as weak as the inverse association between folate or vitamin B$_6$ status and myocardial infarction. When all three variables were put into one logistic regression model, elevated homocysteine was still predictive of myocardial infarction risk, at least in the first half of the follow-up interval (a threefold increase in risk for men in the top 5% of homocysteine values). In the Atherosclerosis Risk in Communities study (23), among women only, homocysteine was associated positively and folate was associated negatively with coronary heart disease. Among men, no such associations occurred. The authors did not include homocysteine and plasma folate in one model. Furthermore, in both women and men, plasma vita-

min B$_6$ was strongly inversely associated with risk of coronary heart disease. This suggests that vitamin B$_6$ may be independently related to coronary heart disease. In general, however, low vitamin B$_6$ levels relate more strongly to postmethionine load homocysteine levels than fasting homocysteine levels, and only fasting homocysteine levels were measured.

Conclusion The available evidence does not permit any distinction between an independent effect of B vitamins and that of homocysteine. A truly homocysteine-independent effect of the vitamins can be derived only from clinical trials that use nonvitamin agents to lower homocysteine and compare their effects with those of vitamins.

REFERENCES

1. Alfthan, G, Pekkanen, J, Jauhiainen, M, Pitkaniemi, J, Karvonen, M, Tuomilehto, J, Salonen, JT, Ehnholm, C.

Relation of serum homocysteine and lipoprotein(a) concentrations to atherosclerotic disease in a prospective Finnish population based study. *Atherosclerosis* 1994; 106: 9–19.

2. Andersson, A, Brattström, L, Israelsson, B, Isaksson, A, Hamfelt, A, Hultberg, B. Plasma homocysteine before and after methionine loading with regard to age, gender and menopausal status. *Eur J Clin Invest* 1992; 22: 79–87.

3. Araki, A, Yoshiyasu, S, Fukushima, Y, Matsumoto, M, Asada, T, Kita, T. Plasma sulfhydryl-containing amino acids in patients with cerebral infarction and in hypertensive patients. *Atherosclerosis* 1989; 79: 139–46.

4. Armstrong, BK, White, E, Saracci, R. Exposure measurement error and its effect. In *Principles of Exposure Measurement in Epidemiology*. (Armstrong, BK, White, E, Saracci, R, eds.). Oxford University Press, Oxford, 1992; pp. 49–77.

5. Arnesen, E, Refsum, H, Bonaa, KH, Ueland, PM, Forde, OH, Nordrehaug, JE. Serum total homocysteine and coronary heart disease. *Int J Epidemiol* 1995; 24: 704–9.

6. Bagley, PJ, Selhub, J. A common mutation in the methylenetetrahydrofolate reductase gene is associated with an accumulation of formylated tetrahydrofolates in red blood cells. *Proc Natl Acad Sci U S A* 1998; 95: 13217–20.

7. Bos, GM, den Heijer, M. Hyperhomocysteinemia and venous thrombosis. *Semin Thromb Hemost* 1998; 24: 387–91.

8. Bostom, AG, Shemin, D, Lapane, KL, Miller, JW, Sutherland, P, Nadeau, M, Seyoum, E, Hartman, W, Prior, R, Wilson, PWF, Selhub, J. Hyperhomocysteinemia and traditional cardiovascular disease risk factors in end-stage renal disease patients on dialysis: A case-control study. *Atherosclerosis* 1995; 114: 93–103.

9. Bostom, AG, Silbershatz, H, Rosenberg, IH, Selhub, J, D'Agostino, RB, Wolf, PA, Jacques, PF, Wilson, PW. Nonfasting plasma total homocysteine levels and all-cause and cardiovascular disease mortality in elderly Framingham men and women. *Arch Intern Med* 1999; 159: 1077–80.

10. Bots, ML, Hoes, AW, Koudstaal, PJ, Hofman, A, Grobbee, DE. Common carotid intima-media thickness and risk of stroke and myocardial infarction: The Rotterdam Study. *Circulation* 1997; 96: 1432–37.

11. Bots, ML, Launer, LJ, Lindemans, J, Hoes, AW, Hofman, A, Witteman, JC, Koudstaal, PJ, Grobbee, DE. Homocysteine and short-term risk of myocardial infarction and stroke in the elderly: The Rotterdam Study. *Arch Intern Med* 1999; 159: 38–44.

12. Bots, ML, Launer, LJ, Lindemans, J, Hofman, A, Grobbee, DE. Homocysteine, atherosclerosis and prevalent cardiovascular disease in the elderly: The Rotterdam Study. *J Intern Med* 1997; 242: 339–47.

13. Boushey, CJ, Beresford, SAA, Omenn, GS, Motulsky, AG. A quantitative assessment of plasma homocysteine as a risk factor for vascular disease. Probable benefits of increasing folic acid intakes. *JAMA* 1995; 274: 1049–57.

14. Brattström, L, Wilcken, DEL, Öhrvik, J, Brudin, L. Common methylenetetrahydrofolate reductase gene mutation leads to hyperhomocysteinemia but not to vascular disease. The result of a meta-analysis. *Circulation* 1998; 98: 2520–26.

15. Chambless, LE, Heiss, G, Folsom, AR, Rosamond, W, Szklo, M, Sharrett, AR, Clegg, LX. Association of coronary heart disease incidence with carotid arterial wall thickness and major risk factors: The Atherosclerosis Risk in Communities (ARIC) Study, 1987–1993. *Am J Epidemiol* 1997; 146: 483–94.

16. Chasan-Taber, L, Selhub, J, Rosenberg, IH, Malinow, MR, Terry, P, Tishler, PV, Willett, W, Hennekens, CH, Stampfer, MJ. A prospective study of folate and vitamin B_6 and risk of myocardial infarction in US physicians. *J Am Coll Nutr* 1996; 15: 136–43.

17. Chen, J, Giovannucci, E, Hankinson, SE, Ma, J, Willett, WC, Spiegelman, D, Kelsey, KT, Hunter, DJ. A prospective study of methylenetetrahydrofolate reductase and methionine synthase gene polymorphisms, and risk of colorectal adenoma. *Carcinogenesis* 1998; 19: 2129–32.

18. Clarke, R, Fitzgerald, D, O'Brien, C, O'Farrell, C, Roche, G, Parker, RA, Graham, I. Hyperhomocysteinaemia: A risk factor for extracranial carotid artery atherosclerosis. *Ir J Med Sci* 1992; 161: 61–5.

19. Clarke, R, Woodhouse, P, Ulvik, A, Frost, C, Sherliker, P, Refsum, H, Ueland, PM, Khaw, KT. Variability and determinants of total homocysteine concentrations in plasma in an elderly population. *Clin Chem* 1998; 44: 102–7.

20. Egerton, W, Silberberg, J, Crooks, R, Ray, C, Xie, L, Dudman, N. Serial measures of plasma homocyst(e)ine after acute myocardial infarction. *Am J Cardiol* 1996; 77: 759–61.

21. Eichinger, S, Stumpflen, A, Hirschl, M, Bialonczyk, C, Herkner, K, Stain, M, Schneider, B, Pabinger, I, Lechner, K, Kyrle, PA. Hyperhomocysteinemia is a risk factor of recurrent venous thromboembolism. *Thromb Haemost* 1998; 80: 566–69.

22. Evans, RW, Shaten, BJ, Hempel, JD, Cutler, JA, Kuller, LH. Homocyst(e)ine and risk of cardiovascular disease in the Multiple Risk Factor Intervention Trial. *Arterioscler Thromb Vasc Biol* 1997; 17: 1947–53.

23. Folsom, AR, Nieto, FJ, McGovern, PG, Tsai, MY, Malinow, MR, Eckfeldt, JH, Hess, DL, Davis, CE. Prospective study of coronary heart disease incidence in relation to fasting total homocysteine, related genetic polymorphisms, and B vitamins. The Atherosclerosis Risk in Communities (ARIC) Study. *Circulation* 1998; 98: 204–10.

24. Frosst, P, Blom, HJ, Milos, R, Goyette, P, Sheppard, CA, Matthews, RG, Boers, GJ, den Heijer, M, Kluijtmans, LA, van den Heuvel, LP, Rozen, R. A candidate genetic risk factor for vascular disease: A common mutation in methylenetetrahydrofolate reductase. *Nat Genet* 1995; 10: 111–13.

25. Giles, WH, Kittner, SJ, Anda, RA, Croft, JB, Casper, ML. Serum folate and risk for ischemic stroke. First National Health and Nutrition Examination Survey Epidemiologic Follow-up Study. *Stroke* 1995; 26: 1166–70.

26. Graham, IH, Daly, LE, Refsum, HM, Robinson, K, Brattström, LE, Ueland, PM, Palma-Reis, RJ, Boers, GHJ, Sheahan, RG, Israelsson, B, Uiterwaal, CS, Meleady, R, McMaster, D, Verhoef, P, Witteman, J, Rubba, P, Bellet, H, Wautrecht, JC, de Valk, HW, Sales Luis, AC, Parrot-Roulaud, FM, Soon Tan, K, Higgins, I, Garcon, D, Medrano, MJ, Candito, M, Evans, AE, Andria, G. Plasma

homocysteine as a risk factor for vascular disease: The European Concerted Action Project. *JAMA* 1997; 277: 1775–81.

27. Herbert, V, Colman, N, Jacob, E. Folic acid and vitamin B₁₂. In *Modern Nutrition in Health and Disease.* (Goodhart, RS, Shils, ME, eds.). Lea and Febiger, Philadelphia, 1980; pp. 229–59.

28. Hultberg, B, Andersson, A, Lindgren, A. Marginal folate deficiency as a possible cause of hyperhomocystinaemia in stroke patients. *Eur J Clin Chem Clin Biochem* 1997; 35: 25–8.

29. Israelsson, B, Brattström, L, Refsum, H. Homocysteine in frozen blood samples. A short cut to establish hyperhomocysteinemia as a risk factor for coronary atherosclerosis? *Scand J Clin Lab Invest* 1993; 3: 465–69.

30. Kris-Etherton, PM, Miller, R, Remick, BA, Wilkinson, W. Modifications in food intake by myocardial infarct patients. *J Am Diet Assoc* 1983; 83: 39–43.

31. Landgren, F, Israelsson, B, Lindgren, A, Hultberg, B, Andersson, A, Brattström, L. Plasma homocysteine in acute myocardial infarction: Homocysteine-lowering effect of folic acid. *J Intern Med* 1995; 237: 381–88.

32. Lindgren, A, Brattström, L, Norrving, B, Hultberg, B, Andersson, A, Johansson, BP. Plasma homocysteine in the acute and convalescent phases after stroke. *Stroke* 1995; 26: 795–800.

33. Ma, J, Stampfer, MJ, Giovannucci, EL, Artigas, C, Hunter, DJ, Fuchs, C, Willett, WC, Selhub, J, Hennekens, CH, Rozen, R. Methylenetetrahydrofolate reductase polymorphism, dietary interactions, and risk of colorectal cancer. *Cancer Res* 1997; 57: 1098–102.

34. Malinow, MR, Nieto, FJ, Szklo, M, Chambless, LE, Bond, G. Carotid artery intimal-medial wall thickening and plasma homocyst(e)ine in asymptomatic adults. The Atherosclerosis Risk in Communities Study. *Circulation* 1993; 87: 1107–13.

35. Mereau-Richard, C, Muller, JP, Faivre, E, Ardouin, P, Rousseaux, J. Total plasma homocysteine determination in subjects with premature cerebral vascular disease. *Clin Chem* 1991; 37: 126.

36. Morrison, HI, Schaubel, D, Desmeules, M, Wigle, DT. Serum folate and risk of fatal coronary heart disease. *JAMA* 1996; 275: 1893–96.

37. Mudd, SH, Finkelstein, JD, Irreverre, F, Laster, L. Homocystinuria: An enzymatic defect. *Science* 1964; 143: 1443–45.

38. Newens, AJ, McColl, E, Bond, S. Changes in reported dietary habit and exercise levels after an uncomplicated first myocardial infarction in middle-aged men. *J Clin Nurs* 1997; 6: 153–60.

39. Nygård, O, Nordrehaug, JE, Refsum, H, Ueland, PM, Farstad, M, Vollset, SE. Plasma homocysteine levels and mortality in patients with coronary artery disease. *N Engl J Med* 1997; 337: 230–36.

40. Nygård, O, Vollset, SE, Refsum, HM, Stensvold, I, Tverdal, A, Nordrehaug, JE, Ueland, PM, Kvale, G. Total plasma homocysteine and cardiovascular risk profile: The Hordaland homocysteine study. *JAMA* 1995; 274: 1526–33.

41. O'Leary, DH, Polak, JF, Kronmal, RA, Manolio, TA, Burke, GL, Wolfson, SK Jr. Carotid-artery intima and

media thickness as a risk factor for myocardial infarction and stroke in older adults. Cardiovascular Health Study Collaborative Research Group. *N Engl J Med* 1999; 340: 14–22.

42. Pancharuniti, N, Lewis, CA, Sauberlich, HE, Perkins, LL, Go, RCP, Alvarez, JO, Macaluso, M, Acton, RT, Copeland, RB, Cousins, AL, Gore, TB, Cornwell, PE, Roseman, JM. Plasma homocyst(e)ine, folate, and vitamin B₁₂ concentrations and risk of early-onset coronary artery disease. *Am J Clin Nutr* 1994; 59: 940–48.

43. Perry, IJ, Refsum, H, Morris, RW, Ebrahim, SB, Ueland, PM, Shaper, AG. Prospective study of serum total homocysteine concentration and risk of stroke in middle-aged British men. *Lancet* 1995; 346: 1395–98.

44. Peterson, JC, Spence, JD. Vitamins and progression of atherosclerosis in hyperhomocyst(e)inaemia. *Lancet* 1998; 351: 263.

45. Petri, M, Roubenoff, R, Dallal, GE, Nadeau, MR, Selhub, J, Rosenberg, H. Plasma homocysteine as a risk factor for atherothrombotic events in systemic lupus erythematosus. *Lancet* 1996; 348: 1120–24.

46. Ray, JG. Meta-analysis of hyperhomocysteinemia as a risk factor for venous thromboembolic disease. *Arch Intern Med* 1998; 158: 2101–16.

47. Refsum, H, Ueland, PM, Nygård, O, Vollset, SE. Homocysteine and cardiovascular disease. *Annu Rev Med* 1998; 49: 31–62.

48. Ridker, PM, Hennekens, CH, Selhub, J, Miletich, JP, Malinow, MR, Stampfer, MJ. Interrelation of hyperhomocyst(e)inemia, factor V Leiden, and risk of future venous thromboembolism. *Circulation* 1997; 95: 1777–82.

49. Ridker, PM, Manson, JE, Buring, JE, Shih, J, Matias, M, Hennekens, CH. Homocysteine and risk of cardiovascular disease among postmenopausal women. *JAMA* 1999; 281: 1817–21.

50. Rimm, EB, Willett, WC, Hu, FB, Sampson, L, Colditz, GA, Manson, JE, Hennekens, C, Stampfer, MJ. Folate and vitamin B-6 from diet and supplements in relation to risk of coronary heart disease among women. *JAMA* 1998; 279: 359–64.

51. Selhub, J, Jacques, PF, Bostom, AG, D'Agostino, RB, Wilson, PW, Belanger, AJ, O'Leary, DH, Wolf, PA, Schaefer, EJ, Rosenberg, IH. Association between plasma homocysteine concentrations and extracranial carotid-artery stenosis. *N Engl J Med* 1995; 332: 286–91.

52. Skovby, F. Homocystinuria. Clinical, biochemical and genetic aspects of cystathionine β-synthase and its deficiency in man. *Acta Paediatr Scand* 1986; 321: 1–21.

53. Smilde, TJ, van den Berkmortel, FW, Boers, GH, Wollersheim, H, de Boo, T, van Langen, H, Stalenhoef, AF. Carotid and femoral artery wall thickness and stiffness in patients at risk for cardiovascular disease, with special emphasis on hyperhomocysteinemia. *Arterioscler Thromb Vasc Biol* 1998; 18: 1958–63.

54. Spence, JD, Malinow, MR, Barnett, PA, Marian, AJ, Freeman, D, Hegele, RA. Plasma homocyst(e)ine concentration, but not MTHFR genotype, is associated with variation in carotid plaque area. *Stroke* 1999; 30: 969–73.

55. Stampfer, MJ, Malinow, MR, Willett, WC, Newcomer, LM, Upson, B, Ullmann, D, Tishler, PV, Hennekens, CH.

A prospective study of plasma homocyst(e)ine and risk of myocardial infarction in US physicians. *JAMA* 1992; 268: 877–81.

56. Stehouwer, CD, Gall, MA, Hougaard, P, Jakobs, C, Parving, HH. Plasma homocysteine concentration predicts mortality in non-insulin-dependent diabetic patients with and without albuminuria. *Kidney Int* 1999; 55: 308–14.

57. Stehouwer, CD, Weijenberg, MP, van den Berg, M, Jakobs, C, Feskens, EJ, Kromhout, D. Serum homocysteine and risk of coronary heart disease and cerebrovascular disease in elderly men: A 10-year follow-up. *Arterioscler Thromb Vasc Biol* 1998; 18: 1895–901.

58. Taylor, LM Jr, DeFrang, RD, Harris, EJ Jr, Porter, JM. The association of elevated plasma homocyst(e)ine with progression of symptomatic peripheral arterial disease. *J Vasc Surg* 1991; 13: 128–36.

59. Taylor, LM Jr, Moneta, GL, Sexton, GJ, Schuff, RA, Porter, JM. Prospective blinded study of the relationship between plasma homocysteine and progression of symptomatic peripheral arterial disease. *J Vasc Surg* 1999; 29: 8–19.

60. Ubbink, JB, Fehily, AM, Pickering, J, Elwood, PC, Vermaak, WJ. Homocysteine and ischaemic heart disease in the Caerphilly cohort. *Atherosclerosis* 1998; 140: 349–56.

61. Ubbink, JB, Vermaak, WHJ, Bennett, JM, Becker, PJ, Van Staden, DA, Bissbort, S. The prevalence of homocysteinemia and hypercholesterolemia in angiographically defined coronary heart disease. *Klin Wochenschr* 1991; 69: 527–34.

62. Ueland, PM, Refsum, H, Stabler, SP, Malinow, MR, Andersson, A, Allen, RH. Total homocyst(e)ine in plasma or serum: Methods and clinical applications. *Clin Chem* 1993; 39: 1764–79.

63. Van der Put, NMJ, Steegers-Theunissen, RPM, Frosst, P, Trijbels, FJ, Eskes, TKAB, van den Heuvel, LP, Mariman, ECM, den Heijer, M, Rozen, R, Blom, HJ. Mutated methylenetetrahydrofolate reductase as a risk factor for spina bifida. *Lancet* 1995; 346: 1070–71.

64. Verhoef, P, Hennekens, CH, Allen, RH, Stabler, SP, Willett, WC, Stampfer, MJ. Plasma total homocysteine and risk of angina pectoris with subsequent coronary artery bypass surgery. *Am J Cardiol* 1997; 79: 799–801.

65. Verhoef, P, Hennekens, CH, Malinow, MR, Kok, FJ, Willett, WC, Stampfer, MJ. A prospective study of plasma homocyst(e)ine and risk of ischemic stroke. *Stroke* 1994; 25: 1924–30.

66. Verhoef, P, Kok, FJ, Kluijtmans, LA, Blom, HJ, Refsum, H, Ueland, PM, Kruyssen, DA. The 677C→T mutation in the methylenetetrahydrofolate reductase gene: Associations with plasma total homocysteine levels and risk of coronary atherosclerotic disease. *Atherosclerosis* 1997; 132: 105–13.

67. Verhoef, P, Kok, FJ, Kruyssen, DA, Schouten, EG, Witteman, JC, Grobbee, DE, Ueland, PM, Refsum, H. Plasma total homocysteine, B-vitamins and risk of coronary atherosclerosis. *Arterioscler Thromb Vasc Biol* 1997; 17: 989–95.

68. Verhoef, P, Stampfer, MJ, Buring, JE, Gaziano, JM, Allen, RH, Stabler, SP, Reynolds, RD, Kok, FJ, Hennekens, CH, Willett, WC. Homocysteine metabolism and risk of myocardial infarction: Relation with vitamins B$_6$, B$_{12}$, and folate. *Am J Epidemiol* 1996; 143: 845–59.

69. Verhoef, P. Hyperhomocysteinemia and risk of vascular disease in women. *Semin Thromb Hemost* 2000; 26: 325–34.

70. Von Eckardstein, A, Malinow, MR, Upson, B, Heinrich, J, Schulte, H, Schonfeld, R, Kohler, E, Assmann, G. Effects of age, lipoproteins, and hemostatic parameters on the role of homocyst(e)inemia as a cardiovascular risk factor in men. *Arterioscler Thromb* 1994; 14: 460–64.

71. Voutilainen, S, Alfthan, G, Nyyssonen, K, Salonen, R, Salonen, JT. Association between elevated plasma total homocysteine and increased common carotid artery wall thickness. *Ann Med* 1998; 30: 300–6.

72. Wald, NJ, Watt, HC, Law, MR, Weir, DG, McPartlin, J, Scott, JM. Homocysteine and ischemic heart disease: Results of a prospective study with implications regarding prevention. *Arch Intern Med* 1998; 158: 862–67.

73. Welch, GN, Loscalzo, J. Homocysteine and atherothrombosis. *N Engl J Med* 1998; 338: 1042–50.

74. Whincup, PH, Refsum, H, Perry, IJ, Morris, R, Walker, M, Lennon, L, Thomson, A, Ueland, PM, Ebrahim, SBJ. Serum total homocysteine and coronary heart disease: Prospective study in middle-aged men. *Heart* 1999; 82: 448–54.

75. Willett, WC. *Nutritional Epidemiology.* Oxford University Press, New York, 1989.

30

Homocysteine and Coronary Artery Disease

KILLIAN ROBINSON

An elevated plasma concentration of homocysteine has been linked to the development of coronary artery disease ever since the description of the long-term pathological sequelae of homocystinuria (33). The high frequency of coronary events in these patients was later shown in a pooled study by Mudd et al. (37) who demonstrated the propensity of these patients to develop coronary, peripheral, and cerebral vascular disease, as well as venous thrombosis. Coronary artery disease, however, occurred less frequently than other atherosclerotic complications of this rare disorder. Since then various studies have examined the possibility that an elevated homocysteine level might be a risk factor for conventional atherosclerosis. This chapter focuses on some of the landmark studies in this area, from the earlier case-control studies to the more recent prospective investigations and to therapeutic studies in this patient population.

Background to Clinical Studies of Homocysteine and Coronary Artery Disease

During 1982 and 1983, Mudd et al. (37) conducted an international questionnaire survey of 629 patients to define the natural history of homocystinuria resulting from cystathionine β-synthase deficiency. Time-to-event curves showed that the chance of initial clinically detected thromboembolic events at age 15 was about 15% to 20% and continued to rise thereafter. Of the 629 patients, 158 had 253 events. The principal type of event was peripheral venous thromboembolism, which accounted for 51% of these vascular episodes, although cerebrovascular accidents (32% of events), peripheral vascular disease events (11% of events), and myocardial infarction (4% of events) were also seen. A small number of events were related to other vascular beds. After 586 surgical procedures, 25 postoperative thromboembolic complications occurred, of which 6 were fatal. Thus, this large follow-up study confirmed the earlier observations of other investigators that patients with congenital homocystinuria were at risk of developing vascular disorders.

From the coronary perspective, it should be emphasized that this was a retrospective questionnaire study and recorded clinically apparent events. Thus, the true prevalence of coronary disease in patients with homocystinuria is likely to be greater. Indeed, autopsy studies frequently demonstrate pathological findings in the coronary arteries in those who have died from other causes. Pathological arterial changes have also been documented in other vascular beds without any apparent history of related clinical events, emphasizing the silent nature of much of this atherosclerotic burden.

It is tempting to think that the vascular complications of congenital homocystinuria are etiologically related to the high circulating levels of homocysteine so often seen in this condition. Both abnormalities, however, may simply stem from the common underlying genetic abnormality. Also, the pathological findings of fraying and splitting of vessels in homocystinuria are not typical of conventional atherosclerosis, in which the lipid laden plaque is so characteristic. Finally, the concentrations of homocysteine in patients with homocystinuria are usually far in excess of those seen in patients with coronary artery disease or other forms of conventional atherosclerosis. Therefore, although homocystinuria may be a valuable model for studying the relationship between homocysteine and vascular disease, there are important limitations to the notion that one is causally related to the other.

Hyperhomocysteinemia and Coronary Disease Risk

Case-Control Studies

The early observations on the natural history of homocystinuria and the hypothesis that homocysteine might be noxious to the vasculature were the inspiration for the first of the formal case-control studies in patients with coronary artery disease. Wilcken and Wilcken (59) studied methionine metabolism in 25 patients <50 years old with angiographically proved coronary artery disease and in 22 control subjects—17 with normal coronary arteries at angiography and 5 healthy volunteers. After an overnight fast, venous blood was drawn before and 4 hours after oral L-methionine, 100 mg/kg, and levels of both methionine and of homocysteine-cysteine mixed disulfide were measured in plasma. The concentration of methionine was similar in the two groups, but high levels of homocysteine-cysteine mixed disulfide were detected in 17 of 25 coronary patients and only 5 of 22 in the noncoronary group (Figure 30.1). Although age, weight, height, body mass index, glucose tolerance, fasting serum urate, and triglycerides were similar in both groups, serum cholesterol was higher in the coronary patients. The authors suggested a reduced ability to metabolize homocysteine in some patients with premature coronary artery disease.

Later, Boers et al. (6) studied the frequency of excessive homocysteine elevation in 75 patients with clinical signs of vascular disease before the age of 50 years. In all, 25 had occlusive peripheral arterial disease, 25 had occlusive cerebrovascular disease, and 25 had suffered a myocardial infarction. A standardized, methionine loading test demonstrated pathological elevation of homocysteine in seven patients in each of the first two groups,

but in none of the patients with myocardial infarction. This suggested that heterozygosity for homocystinuria could predispose to premature occlusive arterial disease, causing intermittent claudication, renovascular hypertension, and ischemic cerebrovascular disease but not myocardial infarction. Clarke et al. (16) performed a similar study and examined the strength of this association and its independence of other risk factors for cardiovascular disease using the methionine loading test. Hyperhomocysteinemia was detected in 16 of 38 patients with cerebrovascular disease (42%) and in 7 of 25 with peripheral vascular disease (28%). It was also seen in 18 of 60 with coronary vascular disease (30%). After adjusting for conventional risk factors, the lower 95% confidence limit for the odds ratio for vascular disease among those with hyperhomocysteinemia was greater than 3. These authors also emphasized the possible role of cystathionine β-synthase deficiency in the causation of hyperhomocysteinemia. They concluded that hyperhomocysteinemia was a risk factor for vascular disease, independent of other risk factors, including coronary disease, and was likely to be due to cystathionine β-synthase deficiency.

There were important differences in methodology between these studies. Definitions of vascular disease, methods of measuring the circulating homocysteine levels and analysis of the relationship with vascular disease, documentation of other risk factors, and conclusions in relation to the risk of coronary heart disease were notable. A later, larger multicenter case-control study, therefore, was designed to try to standardize some of these methodological problems and to examine the strength of the relationship between total plasma homocysteine and the risk of vascular disease of all types in both men and women (22). The study revealed useful information concerning the relationship between homocysteine concentrations and vascular disease both before and after a methionine loading test. Particular advantages of this study were the sample size, large enough to study interaction effects between plasma homocysteine level and conventional risk factors, and the availability of blood levels of the nutrients that modulate plasma homocysteine levels, including folate, cobalamin, and pyridoxal phosphate. Nineteen centers in nine countries recruited 750 cases with coronary, cerebral, and peripheral atherosclerosis and 800 control subjects younger than 60 years. The relative risk for vascular disease in the top quintile compared with the bottom four quintiles of the control fasting total homocysteine distribution was 2.2. Hyperhomocysteinemia following loading with methionine identified an additional 27% of at-risk individuals over and above the fasting level and a dose-response effect was noted between total homocysteine level and risk. Circulating folate,

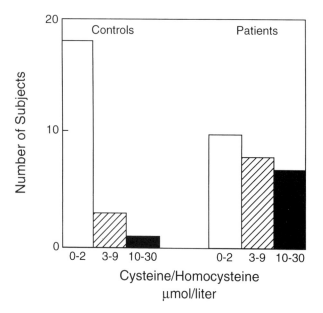

Fig. 30.1. The original case control study of Wilcken and Wilcken (59) showing the significantly greater frequency of higher homocysteine/cysteine mixed disulfide concentrations in 25 patients with coronary artery disease than in 22 controls. (Reproduced from Wilcken & Wilcken [59], with permission.)

cobalamin, and pyridoxal phosphate levels were inversely related to those of homocysteine.

In a large meta-analysis of 27 case-control and prospective studies, Boushey et al. (8) determined the risk of elevated total homocysteine levels for vascular disease. They also speculated on the potential reduction of coronary artery disease mortality by increasing folic acid intake. Three prospective, 5 cross-sectional, and 19 case-control studies, 6 of which were population-based, were included. The odds ratio for coronary disease of a 5 μmol/L increment in homocysteine was 1.6 for men and 1.8 for women with a highly significant 95% confidence interval of 1.3 to 1.9 overall. These authors suggested that some 10% of the risk of the population for coronary disease was attributable to elevated homocysteine levels.

Prospective Studies

The previous studies are only some of the many case-control studies of patients with coronary artery disease. In general, they have shown a reliable and reproducible relationship between hyperhomocysteinemia and atherosclerosis and thrombosis. Many prospective, or nested case-control studies have now been performed, with varying results however. In the US Physicians' Health Study, 14,916 male physicians, aged 40 to 84 years, with no history of myocardial infarction were monitored for 5 years (50). Homocysteine concentrations were measured in blood samples that had been collected before the development of myocardial infarction. The values of 271 men who suffered a myocardial infarction were compared with paired control subjects, matched by age and smoking. Levels of homocysteine were significantly greater in cases than in control subjects (11.1 ± 4.0 vs. 10.5 ± 2.8 μmol/L), and the difference was attributable to an excess of high values among men who later suffered a myocardial infarction. The relative risk for the highest 5% versus the bottom 90% of homocysteine levels was 3.4 after adjustment for other risk factors. The association of homocysteine with vascular disease was visible above a threshold level of homocysteine of about 15 μmol/L. In this study, however, there was almost complete overlap between cases and control subjects, and the higher mean levels in the cases were attributable to a small number in the upper decile. Indeed, with further follow-up evaluation and inclusion of folate and vitamin B_6 in statistical models, the relationship between elevated homocysteine levels and myocardial infarction in these patients no longer remained significant (14).

This original report from the US Physicians' Health Study was followed by a population study from Finland (1). During a 9-year follow-up period, the incidence of atherosclerotic disease was investigated among 7,424 men and women aged 40 to 64 years who had been free of atherosclerosis at baseline in 1977. In this study, serum, and not plasma, homocysteine was measured in 134 male and 131 female cases with either myocardial infarction or stroke as well as in control subjects of the same sex and 5-year age group. At baseline, the mean homocysteine concentrations were 9.99 μmol/L and 9.82 μmol/L in male cases and control subjects, respectively, and 9.58 μmol/L and 9.24 μmol/L in female cases and control subjects, respectively. There was no association between elevated homocysteine concentrations and myocardial infarction or stroke. Although the authors concluded that the lack of association between homocysteine and atherosclerosis may have been due to a low gene frequency predisposing to hyperhomocysteinemia in Finland, the levels of essential B vitamins in this population were not provided.

In the Tromsø Study (4), 21,826 community subjects, aged 12 to 61 years, were surveyed. Serum homocysteine levels were measured in 123 subjects initially free from myocardial infarction and in 4 control subjects selected for each case. Among those who later developed myocardial infarction, the mean homocysteine level was higher than in control subjects (12.7 ± 4.7 vs. 11.3 ± 3.7 μmol/L, $p = 0.002$). The relative risk for each 4 μmol/L increase adjusted for possible confounders was 1.32. Unlike the initial report of the US Physicians' Health Study, there was no threshold level above which circulating homocysteine was associated with coronary events.

Other prospective studies have appeared using similar nested case-control designs from large community studies. In the Multiple Risk Factor Intervention Trial, homocysteine was analyzed using stored serum in 712 men (19). The concentrations were analyzed in relation to the development of nonfatal myocardial infarction and death due to coronary heart disease after the time of the blood draw. Mean homocysteine concentrations, ranging from 12.6 to 13.1 μmol/L in patients and control subjects, did not differ significantly in relation to coronary endpoints between cases and control subjects.

In yet another prospective investigation, the Atherosclerosis Risk in Communities Study, plasma total homocysteine was related to incident coronary artery disease (20). This biracial sample of middle-aged men and women was followed for an average of more than 3 years. Coronary artery disease incidence was associated positively with homocysteine concentration in women only, although even this did not achieve significance after adjustment for other risk factors.

In another subinvestigation from the US Physicians' Health Study, the association between plasma total homocysteine and risk of angina pectoris with subsequent coronary artery bypass surgery was investigated (56). This endpoint was considered a surrogate for atherosclerotic disease enabling the authors to consider the importance of the possible atherogenicity, as opposed to thrombogenicity, of an elevated plasma total homocysteine level. Follow-up time in this study was 9 years, but the mean plasma total homocysteine concentrations were not statistically different in the 149 patients with angina pectoris than in matched control subjects (56).

In summary, unlike the case-control studies, the prospective investigations of coronary risk in persons apparently free of atherosclerosis have been conflicting and often negative, and the risk of development of vascular disease, at worst, seems modest. Some limitations of the nested case-control studies include underestimation of the presence of coronary atherosclerosis in control subjects with silent coronary artery disease (56). In some studies, a smaller proportion of subjects with other risk factors (e.g., smoking) could also have reduced the odds ratio for coronary disease (56), although this might suggest that homocysteine is a proxy rather than an independent risk factor. Other possible limitations of the nested case-control studies include small sample sizes, short follow-up time, and, possibly, effects of repeated thawing of stored samples. Plasma has been used in some studies (20, 56) and serum in others (1, 4, 19), and other methodological issues may also be important in obscuring risk associated with a high homocysteine level. Total homocysteine levels in the various studies (and possibly, therefore, also between populations) are also different, with concentrations in the cases ranging from 12 to 13 μmol/L in some studies (4, 19) to less than 10 μmol/L in another (1). Indeed, some populations such as physicians and nurses may not be ideal to study the homocysteine hypothesis, as their nutritional status is likely to be more satisfactory than that of the general population and case-control differences in homocysteine levels may be lessened. Variation in homocysteine concentrations within subjects over time could also conceivably attenuate the estimated relative risk effect (56).

The possibility also exists, of course, that an elevated plasma homocysteine is a consequence, not a cause, of cardiovascular disease. It could also be an unrelated epiphenomenon or simply a marker of worse disease. The latter is supported by a number of prospective cohort studies of patients with various disorders (including established vascular disease), which have shown that an elevated homocysteine concentration predicts an adverse outcome. Nygård et al. (40) investigated the relationship between plasma homocysteine levels and mortality in 587 patients with coronary artery disease and found a direct link between

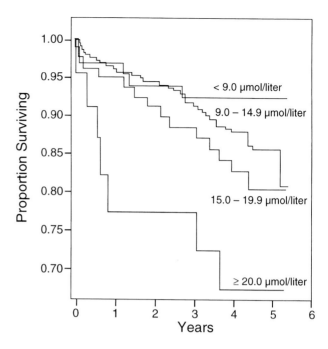

Fig. 30.2. The relationship between circulating homocysteine concentrations and prognosis in patients with coronary artery disease. Survival is shown for groups with varying total homocysteine concentrations. (Reproduced from Nygård et al. [40], with permission.)

plasma homocysteine levels and overall mortality. After 4 years, 3.8% of patients with homocysteine levels below 9 μmol/L had died compared with 24.7% of those with levels of 15 μmol/L or higher (Figure 30.2). Homocysteine levels were strongly related to other prognostic determinants such as a history of myocardial infarction, left ventricular ejection fraction, and serum creatinine levels; however, higher homocysteine levels remained a predictor of an increased mortality rate after adjustment for these and other potential confounders.

In another prospective study of patients with established vascular disease, the Homocysteine and Progression of Atherosclerosis Study, consecutive patients with stable symptomatic cerebrovascular or lower extremity vascular disease were monitored for a mean of 37 months, after having undergone baseline testing for homocysteine and other risk factors (52). Primary endpoints included ankle-brachial pressure index, carotid stenosis, and death. All-cause mortality, death from cardiovascular diseae, and clinical progression of coronary disease occurred significantly more frequently or more rapidly if homocysteine levels were elevated. After adjustment for other risk factors, each 1.0 μmol/L increase in the concentration of plasma homocysteine resulted in a 3.6% increase in the risk of all-cause mortality at 3 years and a 5.6% increase in the risk of death from cardiovascular disease.

In other disease populations, such as those with systemic lupus erythematosus, homocysteine has also been a potentially modifiable, independent risk factor for cardiovascular disease (45). Moustapha et al. (35) prospectively studied the association between total homocysteine and cardiovascular outcomes in 167 patients with end-stage renal disease who were monitored for a mean time of more than 17 months. Even after this relatively short follow-up period, the relative risk for cardiovascular events, including death, increased 1% for each 1 μmol/L rise in total homocysteine concentration, independent of other risk factors for cardiovascular morbidity and mortality. Similar observations were made by Bostom et al. (7), who studied 73 patients undergoing maintenance peritoneal dialysis or hemodialysis and determined the incidence of nonfatal and fatal vascular events, including coronary disease outcomes, during a follow-up time of 17 months. Homocysteine levels in the upper quartile were associated with a threefold to fourfold increase in relative risks of both nonfatal and fatal cardiovascular disease adjusted for confounding variables.

There are conflicting reports concerning outcomes in transplant patients, in whom hyperhomocysteinemia occurs frequently. In one study, an adverse cardiovascular disease outcome, although of only borderline statistical significance, was seen in male recipients monitored for a mean of 11 years after renal transplantation (31). The difference in homocysteine levels between women with and without cardiovascular disease did not achieve significance. Ambrosi et al. (2) found a higher homocysteine level in 18 cardiac transplant recipients with evidence of cardiac graft vasculopathy than in control subjects without graft disease. However, the findings of Nahlawi et al. (38), who followed 160 cardiac transplant recipients for a mean duration of about 28 months, differed. Mean homocysteine values were elevated at 18.4 μmol/L, with values ranging from 4.3 to 63.5 μmol/L. Levels greater than 15 μmol/L were seen in 62% of patients, but were no higher in those who died of cardiovascular causes. Further prospective studies are required to confirm the relationship between homocysteine levels and outcomes in the transplantation population. Although hyperhomocysteinemia may be common in such patients, it may have no causal role in their frequent atherothrombotic vascular complications.

Prevalence of High Homocysteine Levels in Patients with Coronary Artery Disease

Although hyperhomocysteinemia is often seen in patients with coronary artery disease, the exact prevalence varies owing to differing definitions of an elevated plasma concentration. For example, in the U.S.

Physicians' Health Study (50), values above the 95th percentile cutpoint were seen in 11% of cases. In the European Concerted Action Project (22), a homocysteine value greater than the 80th percentile for controls (fasting ≥12 μmol/L, postmethionine load ≥38 μmol/L) was used to define hyperhomocysteinemia. By using this value, 50% of patients with vascular disease had high homocysteine levels. Thus, depending on the value that is used to define normality, 10% to 50% of patients with vascular disease will have levels that are high. It is clear that the normal and abnormal ranges overlap considerably, and many patients with vascular disease have levels well within the range currently deemed acceptable.

Many patients with fasting values in the normal range may have abnormal levels after a methionine loading test, however. This test, which is discussed in Chapter 19, was used by Wilcken and Wilcken (59) to detect higher homocysteine levels in patients with coronary artery disease, and has been used by many other investigators in patients with vascular disorders.

Hyperhomocysteinemia and Conventional Risk Factors in Cardiovascular Disease

In the Hordaland study of community subjects, plasma homocysteine increased with the number of cigarettes smoked and also with total cholesterol level and blood pressure (41). Levels were inversely related to physical activity (see Chapter 28). In patients with vascular disease, homocysteine levels often correlate positively with cholesterol, blood pressure, and smoking (32, 46). An elevated concentration is still associated with vascular disease of all types, independent of these risk factors. In the European Concerted Action Study (22) interactions and risks of coronary artery disease for hyperhomocysteinemia, alone and combined with other risk factors, were studied (Figure 30.3). The relative risk of coronary artery disease associated with fasting hyperhomocysteinemia alone was 2.0, with a highly significant confidence interval of 1.4 to 2.8. The risks of coronary artery disease for postload hyperhomocysteinemia and for the difference between fasting and postload values were also significant at 2.0 and 1.4, respectively. There were substantial interaction effects between homocysteine and the other major cardiovascular risk factors of smoking, hypertension, and hypercholesterolemia. For example, the combination of elevated fasting total homocysteine and hypercholesterolemia conferred an overall relative risk of 2.1 for all forms of atherosclerosis, including coronary disease. The relative risks associated with an elevated fasting total homocysteine combined with smoking and hypertension were 4.6 and 11.3, respectively. In some of these analyses, especially in women, the interaction

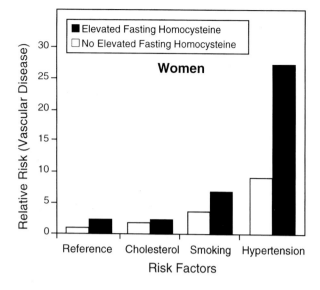

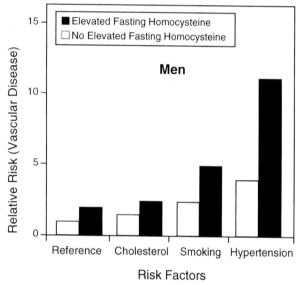

Fig. 30.3. Interaction effects of elevated fasting homocysteine concentrations and the traditional risk factors for vascular disease, including coronary artery disease, in women (top panel) and men (bottom panel). (Reproduced from Graham et al. [22], with permission.)

although some case-control studies suggest the possibility of significant risk factor interactions, further investigations are required to confirm the nature and intensity of these interrelationships.

In summary, in case-control studies, hyperhomocysteinemia is an independent risk factor for atherosclerosis including coronary artery disease. Interactions with, or modifications of, the effects of other risk factors are suggested by some investigations.

Factors Causing Hyperhomocysteinemia in Patients with Coronary Artery Disease

Genetic Mutations

Because of the observations of vascular complications and high homocysteine levels in homocystinuria, deficiency of cystathionine β-synthase was originally inferred in patients with vascular disease (6, 16, 59). Despite these early reports, mutations in cystathionine β-synthase have not been seen in patients with vascular disease. In the Atherosclerosis Risk in Communities Study, there was no association of coronary disease with three mutations of the cystathionine β-synthase gene (20). Intuitively, this would seem to be the case, given the disparity between the rarity of mutations in cystathionine β-synthase on the one hand and the frequency of hyperhomocysteinemia in patients with coronary disease on the other. Likewise, abnormalities of methionine synthase have not been seen in cases of vascular disease (54).

Since its original description (27), the thermolabile mutation of 5,10-methylenetetrahydrofolate reductase (MTHFR) has aroused considerable interest (see Chapter 22). Kang et al. (26) reported its prevalence to be 17% in patients with coronary artery disease but only 5% in control subjects. Since then, there have been conflicting reports on its prevalence in patients with coronary disease, and the relationship of this mutation to the pathogenesis of cardiovascular disease is controversial. In a recent meta-analysis, the thermolabile MTHFR variant was associated with elevated plasma homocysteine concentrations but not with an increased risk of vascular disease (11). Thus, no clear association between coronary artery disease and mutations in the major enzymes responsible for the metabolism of homocysteine has been seen. Higher homocysteine concentrations seen in patients with thermolabile MTHFR, however, may appear more frequently in the presence of lower folate levels (24).

The Nutritional Dimension

As reviewed extensively elsewhere in this book, concentrations of homocysteine rise as the levels of folate,

effects were intense, and it should be noted that the numbers were relatively small in some subsets. Thus, in women with hypertension and hyperhomocysteinemia, the odds ratio for vascular disease was more than 25. This effect was unlike that seen in men with the combination of these two risk factors. In addition, this risk was also far greater than that seen in women with the combination of hyperhomocysteinemia and other risk factors. Glueck et al. (21) showed that the risk of a myocardial infarction in hyperlipidemic patients was greatest in those with hyperhomocysteinemia and low concentrations of high-density lipoproteins. Thus,

cobalamin, and vitamin B_6 fall. Low levels of these vitamins appear to be common in the general population, especially the elderly (49), although folate deficiency appears to have become less prevalent in the United States as a consequence of the folic acid food-fortification plan (25) and increased use of supplements. The relationship between homocysteine and folate in patients with coronary artery disease has been assessed in several investigations. Not only have these studies showed an important role for folate in determining homocysteine concentrations in these patients, but it is now clear that low levels of the vitamins are themselves associated with an increased risk of vascular disease. In one case-control study, Pancharuniti et al. (43) showed an inverse association between homocysteine and folate in white men < 50 years of age with angiographic evidence of ≥ 50% occlusion of one or more major coronary arteries. There was also an association between lower folate levels and vascular disease, although this was attenuated by adjustment for homocysteine.

In the European Concerted Action Project (48), plasma total homocysteine was correlated with concentrations of red cell folate, cobalamin, and vitamin B_6. Lower concentrations of folate occurred more frequently in patients with vascular disease of all types, including coronary artery disease. In the prospective Atherosclerosis Risk in Communities Study (20), lower folate levels predicted incident coronary heart disease, but only in women. In addition, a low folate level may be associated with an increased death rate from vascular disease. A higher 15-year coronary mortality rate was reported in Canadians with lower folate concentrations (34), although no data were given on homocysteine levels.

Lower concentrations of vitamin B_6, also important in the metabolism of homocysteine, are often seen in patients with vascular disease including coronary heart disease. In the European Concerted Action Project, vitamin B_6 deficiency was commonplace with a 20% prevalence in cases (48). This was not due to confounding disorders such as cancer, renal disease, diabetes, or alcoholism, which may also reduce vitamin B_6 levels. Risk of vascular disease fell with rising vitamin B_6 concentrations and was independent of traditional risk factors. Furthermore, adjustment for fasting and postload homocysteine concentrations did not reduce this risk. In other investigations, an increase in coronary artery risk with lower vitamin B_6 concentrations has also been found. In the Nurses' Health Study, healthy women in the highest quintile for folate and vitamin B_6 intake had a lower risk for coronary disease than those in the lowest quintile (47) (Figure 30.4). In the Atherosclerosis Risk in Communities Study, lower vitamin B_6 levels independently predicted

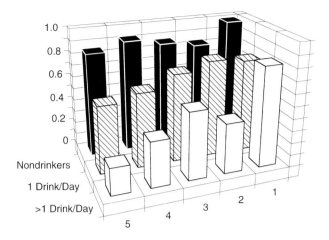

Fig. 30.4. The relationship between quintiles of folate intake, alcohol consumption, and coronary heart disease risk. Relative risk is indicated along the ordinate axis and quintile of folate intake along the abscissa. Compared with nondrinkers, the inverse association between a folate intake and coronary heart disease was strongest among women who consumed up to, or more than, one alcoholic beverage/day. Such data suggest that high folate and vitamin B_6 intake may be important in the primary prevention of coronary disease in women. (Reproduced from Rimm et al. [47], with permission.)

incident coronary heart disease in both men and women (20). The mechanism for the vascular damage is unclear but may be mediated through effects on coagulation, platelet function, or cholesterol concentrations as well as homocysteine concentrations (9, 10, 51). The adverse cardiovascular effect of a low vitamin B_6 level may also be seen in other patient populations. Nahlawi et al. (38) followed patients who had undergone cardiac transplantation. A low level of vitamin B_6 was seen in 32% of recipients with cardiovascular complications but in only 12% of those without complications ($p < 0.001$). The relative risk for vascular events, including death, increased 2.8 times for vitamin B_6 deficiency compared with those who had normal vitamin levels.

Therapeutic Studies in Patients with Coronary Artery Disease

Folic acid is the most important and effective agent in the treatment of hyperhomocysteinemia (see Chapter 23), as demonstrated many years ago in a study of twins with coronary artery disease (57). In a meta-analysis of 12 randomized trials, doses less than 0.5 mg/day were effective in reducing homocysteine concentrations (3). In a placebo-controlled study of approximately 100 patients with coronary artery disease, 5 mg of folic acid was directly compared with 1 and 0.4 mg/day (28). There was little difference in the effectiveness of the three doses (Figure 30.5), supporting the concept that low-dose folic acid reduces homocysteine concentrations by about 30% in patients with coronary artery disease.

Fortified cereals may be an alternative vehicle for the administration of folic acid. Malinow et al. (30) compared three levels of folic acid fortification, also containing the recommended dietary allowances of vitamins B_6 and cobalamin, in a randomized, double-blind, placebo-controlled, crossover trial in 75 men and women with coronary artery disease (Table 30.1). Cereal providing 127 μg of folic acid daily, approximating the increased intake resulting from the fortification policy of the Food & Drug Administration, decreased plasma homocysteine insignificantly, whereas more highly fortified cereals providing 499 and 665 μg of folic acid daily decreased plasma homocysteine by 11.0% and 14.0%, respectively. Folic acid fortification and supplementation issues and effects are discussed in more detail in Chapter 23.

Folic acid is the mainstay of treatment in the reduction of homocysteine levels in patients with coronary disease, but other alternatives also exist. Cobalamin may also be used, although its effect is slight and it appears to have only a modest independent homocysteine-lowering effect of about 10% to 15% (53).

Vitamin B_6 does not appear to have any effect on homocysteine concentrations in the fasting state but does reduce postload homocysteine concentrations after a methionine loading test (9). The benefit of this effect, if any, in patients with coronary artery disease, however, is unclear. Dudman et al. (18) used choline and betaine to reduce postload homocysteine levels in patients with vascular disease including coronary disease. Homocysteine levels fell by about 20% to 30% but the regimen's advantage, if any, over folic acid is unclear.

Low-dose folic acid lowers homocysteine by about 30% to 40% in most patients with coronary disease, but higher doses may be needed in some situations. Patients with coexisting renal failure, for example, may also have high homocysteine concentrations (15), which are an independent risk factor for cardiovascular morbidity and death (7, 35). Such patients' homocysteine levels can be reduced with folic acid, but requirements are higher and normal basal homocysteine concentrations may not be achieved (see Chapter 26).

Other situations in which folic acid requirements may increase in patients with coronary artery disease include the concomitant use of lipid-lowering agents. Blankenhorn et al. (5) reported increased homocysteine levels in patients taking the combination of colestipol and niacin. Recently, bezafibrate and fenofibrate, commonly used drugs in the treatment of hyperlipidemia, have been shown to increase homocysteine concentrations (17). In this study, vitamin concentrations remained unaltered, although a functional reduction in glomerular filtration was suggested by an

Fig. 30.5. A placebo-controlled study of the effect of 400 μg, 1 mg and 5 mg/day of folic acid, each combined with 12.5 mg of vitamin B_6 and 0.5 mg of cobalamin, on homocysteine concentrations in patients with coronary artery disease. (Reproduced from Lobo et al. [28], with permission.)

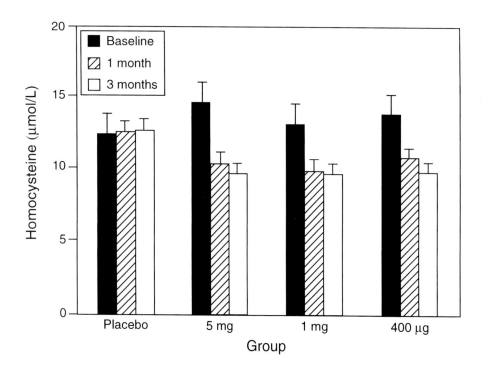

Table 30.1. Effect of Folic Acid-Fortified Cereal on Homocysteine Levels (μmol/L) in Patients with Coronary Artery Disease

Group	Mean Folic Acid Content (μg/30 g)	Homocysteine Level Basal	Homocysteine Level F/U	Mean Δ in Homocysteine Level	p
A (n = 24)					
Placebo phase	10	9.9 ± 3.1	10.1 ± 3.7		
Experimental phase	127	10.0 ± 3.0	9.5 ± 2.5	−3.7 (9.9 to 2.6)	0.24
B (n = 25)					
Placebo phase	10	10.7 ± 3.3	11.0 ± 14.1		
Experimental phase	499	11.4 ± 3.4	9.7 ± 2.3	−11.0 (−15.5 to −6.0)	< 0.001
C (n = 26)					
Placebo phase	10	13.4 ± 10.8	14.6 ± 12.0		
Experimental phase	665	14.6 ± 12.7	11.8 ± 7.3	−14.0 (−12.2 to −6.2)	< 0.001

F/U = follow-up; Δ = change, either positive or negative. Note that more than 127 μg of folic acid/30 g of cereal (group A) are required to produce a significant fall in homocysteine levels; group B received 499 μg and group C 665 μg of folic acid. (Reproduced from Malinow et al. [30] with permission.)
$p = 0.02$ for A vs. B; $p = 0.03$ for A vs. C; $p = 0.53$ for B vs. C.

increase in serum levels of creatinine and cystatin C. Other situations in which patients with coronary artery disease may experience a higher folic acid requirement are the post-transplantation state or the use of certain drugs, such as metformin for the treatment of diabetes (23) or antifolate drugs (32, 46) such as methotrexate.

Beneficial Effects of Treatment with Folic Acid

Folic acid improves endothelial function, possibly by a number of mechanisms. It lowers homocysteine levels, and improved endothelium-dependent vasodilatation may be a direct consequence of this effect. However, Verhaar et al. (55) found that impaired endothelium-dependent vasodilatation was reversed in hypercholesterolemic patients by 5-methyltetrahydrofolate; notably, folate levels increased significantly, but homocysteine levels did not change. These observations suggest that folic acid has beneficial effects on endothelium independent of its effect on homocysteine concentrations.

Conversely, some of the adverse effects associated with hyperhomocysteinemia may be prevented by the administration of antioxidants. Chambers et al. (13) examined the relationship between plasma homocysteine concentration and brachial artery diameter responses to endothelium-dependent hyperemic flow in healthy individuals after a methionine loading test. Pretreatment with vitamin C improved the reduction in flow-mediated dilatation seen after the methionine load without affecting rising homocysteine concentra-

tions. Nappo et al. (39) administered the methionine loading test to healthy volunteers, which resulted in hyperhomocysteinemia and an impaired vascular response to L-arginine. Pretreatment with vitamins C and E attenuated these responses associated with acute hyperhomocysteinemia.

Clinical Studies

Boushey et al. (8) calculated the effect of increased dietary folate, supplementation by tablets, and grain fortification on coronary mortality and proposed that 13,500 to 50,000 coronary deaths annually could be avoided by increasing folic acid intake. The homocysteine hypothesis, the epidemiological evidence, and ease of administration of folic acid have been the prelude to a number of secondary prevention studies. Folic acid, either alone or combined with vitamin B_6 or cobalamin, reduced the rate of progress of carotid plaque as assessed by ultrasound examination in a small, uncontrolled investigation (44). Several larger, randomized intervention studies in patients with vascular diseases, including coronary artery disease, are now in progress (see Chapter 39). Two other studies in progress, one in France and the other in the United States, are assessing the effect of high-dose folic acid therapy on cardiovascular outcomes in patients with end-stage renal disease. These investigations may provide more definitive answers concerning the contribution of homocysteine to the atherosclerotic process and to cardiovascular outcomes.

Folic acid is the most effective method to reduce fasting homocysteine concentrations, although vitamin B_6 treatment may reduce homocysteine after a methionine load. The effect of vitamin B_6 on the outcome of patients with vascular diseases, if any, is unknown, but it is notable that vitamin B_6 reduces the incidence of thromboembolic events in patients with homocystinuria (36, 58). The beneficial effects may be seen in patients with homocystinuria, even when homocysteine levels remain high, suggesting benefits of vitamin B_6 that are independent of homocysteine (42). Whether this intervention will help patients with coronary disease should become clearer after the completion of the Norwegian studies in which the effect of vitamin B_6 will be studied separately from folic acid.

What Should Current Practice Be?

What advice can be given to those involved in patient care who wish to lower homocysteine levels? Both the American Heart Association and the International Task Force for the Prevention of Cardiovascular Disease have issued position statements (29). According to the American view, "some consider it a reasonable approach to determine levels of fasting homocysteine in 'high risk patients,' i.e. in those with

a strong family history for or with arterial occlusive disease, as well as members of their family..." The European view is that "homocysteine should be measured in patients with a history of atherosclerotic and/or thromboembolic vessel disease. Individuals with a homocysteine level >12 μmol/L should increase and/or supplement the dietary intake of folic acid."

Based on these recommendations, an algorithm is proposed in Figure 30.6. Until the results of clinical trials are available, it should be emphasized that such an approach is speculative, although it is of theoretical benefit, is inexpensive, and is very unlikely to be harmful. In older patients given maintenance folic acid, it may be prudent to check cobalamin status before commencing treatment and perhaps also during the follow-up period, because borderline or clinically silent cobalamin deficiency often occurs in the elderly. Appropriate correction with oral or parenteral cobalamin supplements may then be given to prevent possible neurological complications of inappropriate treatment with folic acid.

For the future, the most eagerly awaited results are surely those of the clinical trials now in progress. Other questions, however, remain unanswered concerning the relationship of homocysteine to coronary disease. For example, is homocysteine a causal risk factor, an epiphenomenon, or a risk marker? Are there gender effects as suggested by the Atherosclerosis Risk in Communities Study? Is there any relationship with severity of coronary disease? Does homocysteine predict vascular risk in other populations, such as those who have undergone cardiac or renal transplantation or have connective tissue diseases or inflammatory bowel disease (12)? These areas all require further

Fig. 30.6. A proposed algorithm for approach to the management of hyperhomocysteinemia. A homocysteine level of 12 μmol/L has been mooted by some as a reasonable target level, but such an approach should be regarded as speculative until the results of randomized controlled trials become available. (Rx = treatment; MD = physician)

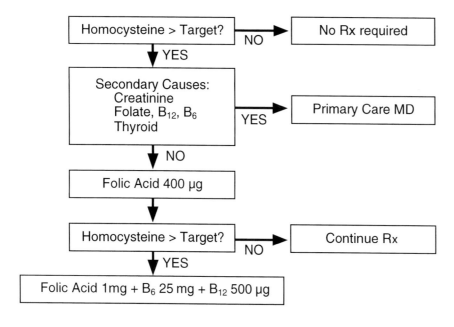

Treatment of Hyperhomocysteinemia

study and will help to clarify the role of an elevated homocysteine concentration in patients with, or at risk of, coronary artery disease in various clinical settings.

REFERENCES

1. Alfthan, G, Pekkanen, J, Jauhiainen, M, Pitkaniemi, J, Karvonen, M, Tuomilehto, J, Salonen, JT, Ehnholm, C. Relation of serum homocysteine and lipoprotein (a) concentrations to atherosclerotic disease in a prospective Finnish population based study. *Atherosclerosis* 1994; 106: 9–19.

2. Ambrosi, P, Garcon, D, Riberi, A, Habib, G, Barlatier, A, Kreitmann, B, Rolland, PH, Bouvenot, G, Luccioni, R, Metras, D. Association of mild hyperhomocysteinemia with cardiac graft vascular disease. *Atherosclerosis* 1998; 138: 347–50.

3. Anonymous. Lowering blood homocysteine with folic acid based supplements: Meta-analysis of randomised trials. Homocysteine Lowering Trialists' Collaboration. *Br Med J* 1998; 316: 894–98.

4. Arnesen, E, Refsum, H, Bonaa, KH, Ueland, PM, Forde, OH, Nordrehaug, JE. Serum total homocysteine and coronary heart disease. *Int J Epidemiol* 1995; 24: 704–9.

5. Blankenhorn, D, Malinow, R, Mack, W. Colestipol plus niacin therapy elevates plasma homocyst(e)ine levels. *Coron Artery Dis* 1991; 2: 357–60.

6. Boers, GH, Smals, AG, Trijbels, FJ, Fowler, B, Bakkeren, JA, Schoonderwaldt, HC, Kleijer, WJ, Kloppenborg, PW. Heterozygosity for homocystinuria in premature peripheral and cerebral occlusive arterial disease. *N Engl J Med* 1985; 313: 709–15.

7. Bostom, AG, Shemin, D, Verhoef, P, Nadeau, MR, Jacques, PF, Selhub, J, Dworkin, L, Rosenberg, IH. Elevated fasting total plasma homocysteine levels and cardiovascular disease outcomes in maintenance dialysis patients. A prospective study. *Arterioscler Thromb Vasc Biol* 1997; 17: 2554–58.

8. Boushey, CJ, Beresford, SA, Omenn, GS, Motulsky, AG. A quantitative assessment of plasma homocysteine as a risk factor for vascular disease. Probable benefits of increasing folic acid intakes. *JAMA* 1995; 274: 1049–57.

9. Brattström, L, Israelsson, B, Norrving, B, Bergqvist, D, Thorne, J, Hultberg, B, Hamfelt, A. Impaired homocysteine metabolism in early-onset cerebral and peripheral occlusive arterial disease. Effects of pyridoxine and folic acid treatment. *Atherosclerosis* 1990; 81: 51–60.

10. Brattström, L, Stavenow, L, Galvard, H. Pyridoxine reduces cholesterol and low-density lipoprotein and increases antithrombin III activity in 80-year-old men with low plasma pyridoxal 5-phosphate. *Scand J Clin Lab Invest* 1990; 50: 873–77.

11. Brattström, L, Wilcken, D, Öhrvick, J, Brudin, L. Common methylenetetrahydrofolate reductase gene mutation leads to hyperhomocysteinemia but not to vascular disease. The results of a meta-analysis. *Circulation* 1998; 98: 2520–26.

12. Cattaneo, M, Vecchi, M, Zighetti, M, Omodei, P, Martinelli, I, Saibeni, S, Mannucci, PM, de Franchis, R. High prevalence of hyperhomocysteinemia in patients with inflammatory bowel disease. *Neth Med J* 1998; 52: S35.

13. Chambers, JC, McGregor, A, Jean-Marie, J, Obeid, OA, Kooner, JS. Demonstration of rapid onset vascular endothelial dysfunction after hyperhomocysteinemia: An effect reversible with vitamin C therapy. *Circulation* 1999; 99: 1156–60.

14. Chasan-Taber, L, Selhub, J, Rosenberg, IH, Malinow, MR, Terry, P, Tishler, PV, Willett, W, Hennekens, CH, Stampfer, MJ. A prospective study of folate and vitamin B6 and risk of myocardial infarction in US physicians. *J Am Coll Nutr* 1996; 15: 136–43.

15. Chauveau, P, Chadefaux, B, Coude, M, Aupetit, J, Hannedouche, T, Kamoun, P, Jungers, P. Increased plasma homocysteine concentration in patients with chronic renal failure. *Miner Electrolyte Metab* 1992; 18: 196–98.

16. Clarke, R, Daly, L, Robinson, K, Naughten, E, Cahalane, S, Fowler, B, Graham, I. Hyperhomocysteinemia: An independent risk factor for vascular disease. *N Engl J Med* 1991; 324: 1149–55.

17. Dierkes, J, Westphal, S, Luley, C. Serum homocysteine increases after therapy with fenofibrate or bezafibrate [letter]. *Lancet* 1999; 354: 219–20.

18. Dudman, NP, Wilcken, DE, Wang, J, Lynch, JF, Macey, D, Lundberg, P. Disordered methionine/homocysteine metabolism in premature vascular disease. Its occurrence, cofactor therapy, and enzymology. *Arterioscl Thromb* 1993; 13: 1253–60.

19. Evans, RW, Shaten, BJ, Hempel, JD, Cutler, JA, Kuller, LH. Homocyst(e)ine and risk of cardiovascular disease in the Multiple Risk Factor Intervention Trial. *Arterioscl Thromb Vasc Biol* 1997; 17: 1947–53.

20. Folsom, AR, Nieto, FJ, McGovern, PG, Tsai, MY, Malinow, MR, Eckfeldt, JH, Hess, DL, Davis, CE. Prospective study of coronary heart disease incidence in relation to fasting total homocysteine, related genetic polymorphisms, and B vitamins: The Atherosclerosis Risk in Communities (ARIC) study. *Circulation* 1998; 98: 204–10.

21. Glueck, CJ, Shaw, P, Lang, JE, Tracy, T, Sieve-Smith, L, Wang, Y. Evidence that homocysteine is an independent risk factor for atherosclerosis in hyperlipidemic patients. *Am J Cardiol* 1995; 75: 132–36.

22. Graham, IM, Daly, LE, Refsum, HM, Robinson, K, Brattstrom, LE, Ueland, PM, Palma-Reis, RJ, Boers, GH, Sheahan, RG, Israelsson, B, Uiterwaal, CS, Meleady, R, McMaster, D, Verhoef, P, Witteman, J, Rubba, P, Bellet, H, Wautrecht, JC, de Valk, HW, Sales Luis, AC, Parrot-Rouland, FM, Tan, KS, Higgins, I, Garcon, D, Andria, G. Plasma homocysteine as a risk factor for vascular disease. The European Concerted Action Project. *JAMA* 1997; 277: 1775–81.

23. Hoogeveen, EK, Kostense, PJ, Jakobs, C, Bouter, LM, Heine, RJ, Stehouwer, CD. Does metformin increase the serum total homocysteine level in non-insulin-dependent diabetes mellitus? *J Intern Med* 1997; 242: 389–94.

24. Jacques, PF, Bostom, AG, Williams, RR, Ellison, RC, Eckfeldt, JH, Rosenberg, IH, Selhub, J, Rozen, R. Relation between folate status, a common mutation in methylenetetrahydrofolate reductase, and plasma homocysteine concentrations. *Circulation* 1996; 93: 7–9.

25. Jacques, PF, Selhub, J, Bostom, AG, Wilson, PWF, Rosenberg, IH. The effect of folic acid fortification on plasma folate levels and total homocysteine concentrations. *N Engl J Med* 1999; 340: 1449–54.

26. Kang, SS, Wong, PW, Susmano, A, Sora, J, Norusis, M, Ruggie, N. Thermolabile methylenetetrahydrofolate reductase: An inherited risk factor for coronary artery disease. *Am J Hum Genet* 1991; 48: 536–45.

27. Kang, SS, Zhou, J, Wong, PW, Kowalisyn, J, Strokosch, G. Intermediate homocysteinemia: A thermolabile variant of methylenetetrahydrofolate reductase. *Am J Hum Genet* 1988; 43: 414–21.

28. Lobo, A, Naso, A, Arheart, K, Kruger, WD, Abou-Ghazala, T, Alsous, F, Nahlawi, M, Gupta, A, Moustapha, A, van Lente, F, Jacobsen, DW, Robinson, K. Reduction of homocysteine levels in coronary artery disease by low-dose folic acid combined with vitamins B6 and B12. *Am J Cardiol* 1999; 83: 821–25.

29. Malinow, MR, Bostom, AG, Krauss, RM. Homocyst(e)ine, diet, and cardiovascular diseases: A statement for healthcare professionals from the Nutrition Committee, American Heart Association. *Circulation* 1999; 99: 178–82.

30. Malinow, MR, Duell, PB, Hess, DL, Anderson, PH, Kruger, WD, Phillipson, BE, Gluckman, RA, Block, PC, Upson, BM. Reduction of plasma homocyst(e)ine levels by breakfast cereal fortified with folic acid in patients with coronary heart disease. *N Engl J Med* 1998; 338: 1009–15.

31. Massy, ZA, Chadefaux-Vekemans, B, Chevalier, A, Bader, CA, Drueke, TB, Legendre, C, Lacour, B, Kamoun, P, Kreis, H. Hyperhomocysteinaemia: A significant risk factor for cardiovascular disease in renal transplant recipients. *Nephrol Dial Transpl* 1994; 9: 1103–8.

32. Mayer, EL, Jacobsen, DW, Robinson, K. Homocysteine and coronary atherosclerosis. *J Am Coll Cardiol* 1996; 27: 517–27.

33. McCully, KS. Vascular pathology of homocysteinemia: Implications for the pathogenesis of arteriosclerosis. *Am J Pathol* 1969; 56: 111–28.

34. Morrison, HI, Schaubel, D, Desmeules, M, Wigle, DT. Serum folate and risk of fatal coronary heart disease. *JAMA* 1996; 275: 1893–96.

35. Moustapha, A, Naso, A, Nahlawi, M, Gupta, A, Arheart, KL, Jacobsen, DW, Robinson, K, Dennis, VW. Prospective study of hyperhomocysteinemia as an adverse cardiovascular risk factor in end-stage renal disease [published erratum in *Circulation* 1998; 97: 711]. *Circulation* 1998; 97: 138–41.

36. Mudd, SH, Levy, HL, Skovby, F. Disorders of transsulfuration. In *The Metabolic Basis of Inherited Disease*, 7th ed. (Scriver, CR, Beaudet, AL, Sly, WS, Valle, D, eds.). McGraw Hill, New York, 1995; pp. 1279–1327.

37. Mudd, SH, Skovby, F, Levy, HL, Pettigrew, KD, Wilcken, B, Pyeritz, RE, Andria, G, Boers, GH, Bromberg, IL, Cerone, R, Fowler, B, Gröbe, H, Schmidt, H, Schweitzer, L. The natural history of homocystinuria due to cystathionine beta-synthase deficiency. *Am J Hum Genet* 1985; 37: 1–31.

38. Nahlawi, M, Naso, A, Boparai, N, Moustapha, A, Ko, D, Jacobsen, D, McCarthy, P, Robinson, K. Low vitamin B6: An independent predictor of cardiovascular morbidity and mortality in heart transplant recipients. *Circulation* 1998; 98 (Suppl I): 690.

39. Nappo, F, De Rosa, N, Marfella, R, De Lucia, D, Ingrosso, D, Perna, AF, Farzati, B, Giugliano, D. Impairment of endothelial functions by acute hyperhomocysteinemia and reversal by antioxidant vitamins. *JAMA* 1999; 281: 2113–18.

40. Nygård, O, Nordrehaug, JE, Refsum, H, Ueland, PM, Farstad, M, Vollset, SE. Plasma homocysteine levels and mortality in patients with coronary artery disease. *N Engl J Med* 1997; 337: 230–36.

41. Nygård, O, Vollset, SE, Refsum, H, Stensvold, I, Tverdal, A, Nordrehaug, JE, Ueland, PM, Kvale, G. Total plasma homocysteine and cardiovascular risk profile. The Hordaland Homocysteine Study. *JAMA* 1995; 274: 1526–33.

42. Palareti, G, Coccheri, S. Lowered antithrombin III activity and other clotting changes in homocystinuria: Effects of a pyridoxine-folate regimen. *Haemostasis* 1989; 19 (Suppl 1): 24–8.

43. Pancharuniti, N, Lewis, CA, Sauberlich, HE, Perkins, LL, Go, RC, Alvarez, JO, Macaluso, M, Acton, RT, Copeland, RB, Cousins, AL, Gore, TB, Cornwell, PE, Roseman, JM. Plasma homocyst(e)ine, folate, and vitamin B-12 concentrations and risk for early-onset coronary artery disease [erratum in *Am J Clin Nutr* 1996; 63: 609]. *Am J Clin Nutr* 1994; 59: 940–48.

44. Peterson, JC, Spence, JD. Vitamins and progression of atherosclerosis in hyper-homocyst(e)inaemia [letter]. *Lancet* 1998; 351: 263.

45. Petri, M, Roubenoff, R, Dallal, GE, Nadeau, MR, Selhub, J, Rosenberg, IH. Plasma homocysteine as a risk factor for atherothrombotic events in systemic lupus erythematosus. *Lancet* 1996; 348: 1120–24.

46. Refsum, H, Ueland, PM, Nygård, O, Vollset, SE. Homocysteine and cardiovascular disease. *Annu Rev Med* 1998; 49: 31–62.

47. Rimm, EB, Willett, WC, Hu, FB, Sampson, L, Colditz, GA, Manson, JE, Hennekens, C, Stampfer, MJ. Folate and vitamin B6 from diet and supplements in relation to risk of coronary heart disease among women. *JAMA* 1998; 279: 359–64.

48. Robinson, K, Arheart, K, Refsum, H, Brattstrom, L, Boers, G, Ueland, P, Rubba, P, Palma-Reis, R, Meleady, R, Daly, L, Witteman, J, Graham, I. Low circulating folate and vitamin B6 concentrations: Risk factors for stroke, peripheral vascular disease, and coronary artery disease. European COMAC Group. *Circulation* 1998; 97: 437–43.

49. Selhub, J, Jacques, PF, Wilson, PW, Rush, D, Rosenberg, IH. Vitamin status and intake as primary determinants of homocysteinemia in an elderly population. *JAMA* 1993; 270: 2693–98.

50. Stampfer, MJ, Malinow, MR, Willett, WC, Newcomer, LM, Upson, B, Ullmann, D, Tishler, PV, Hennekens, CH. A prospective study of plasma homocyst(e)ine and risk of myocardial infarction in US physicians. *JAMA* 1992; 268: 877–81.

51. Subbarao, K, Kuchibhotla, J, Kakkar, VV. Pyridoxal 5′-phosphate—A new physiological inhibitor of blood coag-

ulation and platelet function. *Biochem Pharmacol* 1979; 28: 531–34.

52. Taylor, LM Jr, Moneta, GL, Sexton, GJ, Schuff, RA, Porter, JM. Prospective blinded study of the relationship between plasma homocysteine and progression of symptomatic peripheral arterial disease. *J Vasc Surg* 1999; 29: 8–19.

53. Ubbink, JB, Vermaak, WJ, van der Merwe, A, Becker, PJ, Delport, R, Potgieter, HC. Vitamin requirements for the treatment of hyperhomocysteinemia in humans. *J Nutr* 1994; 124: 1927–33.

54. van der Put, NM, van der Molen, EF, Kluijtmans, LA, Heil, SG, Trijbels, JM, Eskes, TK, van Oppenraaij-Emmerzaal, D, Banerjee, R, Blom, HJ. Sequence analysis of the coding region of human methionine synthase: Relevance to hyperhomocysteinaemia in neural-tube defects and vascular disease. *Q J Med* 1997; 90: 511–17.

55. Verhaar, MC, Wever, RM, Kastelein, JJ, van Dam, T, Koomans, HA, Rabelink, TJ. 5-Methyltetrahydrofolate, the active form of folic acid, restores endothelial function in familial hypercholesterolemia. *Circulation* 1998; 97: 237–41.

56. Verhoef, P, Hennekens, CH, Allen, RH, Stabler, SP, Willett, WC, Stampfer, MJ. Plasma total homocysteine and risk of angina pectoris with subsequent coronary artery bypass surgery. *Am J Cardiol* 1997; 79: 799–801.

57. Wilcken, DE, Reddy, SG, Gupta, VJ. Homocysteinemia, ischemic heart disease, and the carrier state for homocystinuria. *Metabolism* 1983; 32: 363–70.

58. Wilcken, DE, Wilcken, B. The natural history of vascular disease in homocystinuria and the effects of treatment. *J Inherit Metabol Dis* 1997; 20: 295–300.

59. Wilcken, DE, Wilcken, B. The pathogenesis of coronary artery disease. A possible role for methionine metabolism. *J Clin Invest* 1976; 57: 1079–82.

31

Homocysteine and Cerebral Vascular Disease

J. DAVID SPENCE
JAMES F. TOOLE

The term *'stroke'* is deliberately nonspecific, chosen to avoid early overcommitment to a mistaken etiology at the time a patient presents. For that reason, the term *CVA*, for cerebrovascular accident, is to be deplored (it can be translated as "cursory vascular analysis"). About 15% of patients presenting to an emergency room have a nonvascular mimic of stroke. In its broadest sense, stroke means "sudden onset of a central nervous system deficit." Cerebral vascular events can broadly be divided into hemorrhages and infarctions; in this chapter we use the term *stroke* to mean *cerebral infarction*.

A common problem in the analysis of risk factors for stroke is failure to be clear about which type of stroke is being considered in relation to possible factors that could cause or aggravate stroke. For example, hypertension causes stroke because of its effect on the resistance vessels at the base of the brain; intracerebral hemorrhage resulting from hypertension and lacunar infarction are both due to hyaline degeneration or fibrinoid necrosis of arterioles or small resistance arteries. Lumping different kinds of stroke types together causes hypertension to be overemphasized as a risk factor for stroke, and dyslipidemia to be underemphasized. Failure to distinguish between strokes caused by hypertensive small vessel disease and strokes caused by atherosclerosis would obscure the role of atherosclerosis

risk factors, particularly when hypertensive strokes in the past accounted for nearly half the total. Thus, Hachinski et al. (25) were able to show that dyslipidemia was a risk factor for stroke in a community in which hypertensive stroke had largely been eliminated by effective control of blood pressure (59, 60).

Cerebral infarction can be caused by occlusion of small resistance vessels (lacunar infarction caused by hypertensive small-vessel disease) or large arteries such as the internal carotid or middle cerebral artery. Mechanisms of occlusion include dissection (often in the setting of minor trauma, particularly in the case of the vertebral arteries), an embolus, or a plaque event such as intraplaque hemorrhage. Emboli can consist of red thrombus (fibrin polymer with entrapped red cells) that forms in the setting of stasis, platelet aggregates that form in the setting of turbulence or vortex formation at the site of a proximal stenosis, or atheromatous debris (often including cholesterol crystals) (Table 31.1). Cardioembolic strokes are often due to underlying myocardial infarction, either recent (about 8% of ischemic stroke) or remote in time, with either atrial fibrillation or a ventricular aneurysm secondary to the previous myocardial infarction. Thus, risk factors for atherosclerotic stroke are the same as for myocardial infarction (age, male sex, smoking, high blood pressure, diabetes, and dyslipidemia); hypertension is the major risk factor for intracerebral hemorrhage. It appears likely that homocysteine is a risk factor for atherosclerotic causes of stroke, as well as lacunar infarctions, and for cardioembolic strokes resulting from myocardial infarction.

Homocysteine as a Risk Factor for Stroke

The association between high levels of homocysteine and cerebrovascular disease was first made in homozygous homocystinuria due to a deficiency of cystathionine β-synthase (9, 19). McCully (40) suggested in 1969 that more moderate levels of hyperhomocysteinemia might be associated with atherosclerosis. Subsequently, Boers et al. (3) reported that homocysteine levels greater than 14 μmol/L were present in about 30% of patients with premature peripheral and cerebrovascular disease, but not coronary artery disease. This finding was probably incorrectly attributed to heterozygosity for cystathionine β-synthase deficiency. Clarke et al. (14) confirmed that about 30% of patients with premature atherosclerosis had plasma homocysteine levels greater than 14 μmol/L.

Until recently, there has not been compelling evidence of a familial propensity to cerebrovascular episodes,

Table 31.1. Causes of Stroke

Hemorrhage	Infarction	Nonvascular Mimics of Stroke[a]
Intracerebral hemorrhage	Lacunar infarction	Postictal
Rupture of small resistance vessel	Occlusion of small resistance vessel due to	Tumor
due to hypertension	hypertension, diabetes	Subdural hematoma
Rupture of AVM	Large artery occlusion	Abscess
Rupture of cavernous angioma	Embolic	Migraine
	Red thrombus	
Subarachnoid hemorrhage	cardiac, venous origin (paradoxical)	
Rupture of berry aneurysm or AVM	White thrombus (platelet aggregates)	
Rupture of cavernous angioma	proximal stenosis	
	Atheromatous debris	
	Other emboli (fat, air, amniotic, etc.)	
	Atherosclerotic occlusion	
	Intraplaque hemorrhage, rupture	
	Venous infarction	
	Pregnancy, Crohn's disease, etc.	
	Diffuse microvascular obstruction	
	Macroglobulinemia, sickle cell disease,	
	malaria, etc.	
	Vasculitis	
	Giant cell arteritis, SLE, etc.	

AVM, arteriovenous malformation; SLE, systemic lupus erythematosus
[a]About 15% of cases presenting to emergency rooms.

except for cerebral autosomal dominant arteriopathy with stroke (CADASIL) and clusters of risk factors such as hypertension, diabetes, and homocystinuria. However, it is increasingly evident that both arterial and venous strokes can be the result of a genetic predisposition. For example, hyperhomocysteinemia and disorders of hypercoagulability, such as deficiencies of protein C and protein S and Factor V Leiden, have been recognized as risk factors for deep venous thrombosis with pulmonary embolism. The recent report of a youth and father who developed saggital sinus thrombosis owing to hyperhomocysteinemia and protein C deficiency type I is suggestive of a role for homocysteine in infarctions resulting from venous thrombosis (18). Homocysteine inhibits thrombomodulin expression on endothelial cells' surfaces and inactivates irreversibly both thrombomodulin and protein C (34) (see Chapter 34).

It is now clear, as discussed in Sections V and VI of this book, that there are many ways to develop high plasma levels of homocysteine. In some patients with stroke, a relationship has been shown between the 677C→T genotype of 5,10-methylenetetrahydrofolate reductase (MTHFR) and serum homocysteine concentration, with an interaction with serum folate concentration, which suggests that the genotype could be a risk factor in populations with low folic acid intake (39).

One cause for elevated homocysteine levels is a deficiency of folic acid, possibly indicated by serum folate concentrations that are even as high as 9.2 nmol/L (see Chapter 23). This excess may be especially evident in blacks (20). These authors determined in a later survey of the same population, that an elevated serum total homocysteine level is an independent risk factor for stroke. They also found serum cobalamin and folate concentrations to be significantly lower in those individuals in the highest quartile of plasma homocysteine levels. Such individuals were also older, had higher cholesterol levels and blood pressure levels, and were more likely to smoke (20, 21).

There is a steep dose-response curve for vascular risk in relation to homocysteine. Patients with plasma total homocysteine levels above 10.2 μmol/L have about double the risk of patients with lower levels (23), and levels above 20 μmol/L are associated with a 10-fold increase in vascular risk compared with levels below 9 μmol/L (46).

Brattström et al. (5) were among the first to report that greatly elevated concentrations of homocysteine are found in plasma and urine of patients who have inherited abnormalities of methionine metabolism and an excess incidence of vascular complications during childhood. In 1991, Coull et al. (15) reported that increased homocysteine levels were an independent risk factor for stroke.

Before 1994, most studies were case reports or retrospective studies. One of the first prospective studies reported a small but nonsignificant association between elevated plasma homocysteine and the risk of ischemic stroke (72). However, the sample size was small, so that a moderate increase in risk could not be excluded, particularly in sub-groups such as younger men and normotensive persons, who were otherwise at low risk. Another early prospective study, the Physicians' Health Study, which reported an association between elevated homocysteine levels and myocar-dial infarction, found no significant relationship between homocysteine and ischemic stroke (68).

Table 31.2.   Homocysteine as a Risk Factor for Stroke in Middle-aged British Men

	Cases	Controls	p Value
Plasma total homocysteine (μmol/L):			
mean	13.7	11.9	0.004
(95% confidence interval)	(12.7–14.8)	(11.3–12.6)	
Relative risk for stroke in:			
2nd quartile of homocysteine[a]	1.3		0.005[b]
3rd quartile of homocysteine[a]	1.9		
4th quartile of homocysteine[a]	2.8		

The data are from Perry et al. (50); n = 5,661 men, ages 40–59 years; 141 incident strokes between 1978–1980 and 1991.
[a] Compared against the 1st (lowest level) quartile of plasma total homocysteine levels.
[b] p for trend.

Soon thereafter, Perry et al. (50) suggested that the association with serum total homo-cysteine concentration in stroke victims was a strong, independent, and graded increase in the relative risk for stroke (Table 31.2). This association was not atten-uated by adjustment for age group, town, social class, body mass index, smoking, diabetes, and levels of high-density lipoprotein and serum creatinine. This confirmed previous suggestions (6, 7).

A Korean case-control study comparing 78 male stroke patients with 140 male control subjects found that the proportion of cases with moderate hyperhomo-cysteinemia (> 15.5 μmol/L) was significantly higher in cases than control subjects (16.7% vs. 5%; p = 0.0004) (74). Patients with stroke were 4.7 times more likely to have homocysteine levels in the top 5% (p = 0.002). Moreover, the plasma homocysteine levels of patients with three or two stenosed sites in their carotid arteries were significantly higher than in patients with one or no stenoses (14.6 ± 1.4 and 11.0 ± 1.4 μmol/L with three or two stenoses, respectively, vs. 7.8 ± 1.5 and 8.9 ± 1.4 μmol/L with no and one stenosis, respectively [p < 0.02]).

Homocysteine as a Risk Factor for Lacunar Stroke

As discussed earlier, lacunar stroke is due to occlusion of arterioles or small resistance arteries. It usually occurs in the setting of hypertension and/or diabetes. Thus, the pathophysiology and causes of lacunar infarc-tion differ from embolic or atheroocclusive infarctions.

Brattström et al. (7) subsequently studied the rela-tionship between plasma homocysteine and different stroke types in 147 survivors of stroke. They found that 40% of stroke patients had hyperhomocysteinemia ver-sus 6% of control subjects; this finding was indepen-dent of stroke type, being as true for hemorrhagic and lacunar stroke as for carotid stroke patients. Much of

the variation in plasma homocysteine levels was accounted for by serum cobalamin, folate, and creati-nine levels. It is possible that the relatively small sample size obscured differences between stroke types. It is also likely that severe hypertension associated with intrace-rebral hemorrhages and lacunar infarctions would be associated with hypertensive nephropathy and elevation of homocysteine levels caused by renal insufficiency.

It seems clear that homocysteine is involved in some way in atherosclerosis. The question of a relationship between homocysteine and small vessel disease that may lead to lacunar strokes might be assessed indirectly by studying the role of homocysteine in diabetic microvascular disease. Indeed, studies have shown an association between elevated levels of plasma homocys-teine and diabetic small vessel disease. Lanfredini et al. (32) described higher plasma homocysteine levels in patients with Type 2 diabetes and microalbuminuria (a marker for microvascular disease) compared with con-trol subjects. Chico et al. (13) found that plasma homo-cysteine was related to albumin excretion in diabetes. Hoogeveen et al. (28) also reported that homocysteine was associated with microalbuminuria; the odds ratio for microalbuminuria was 1.33 per 5 μmol/L increase in plasma homocysteine, after correcting for age, sex, cat-egory of glucose tolerance, dyslipidemia, and smoking. Hofmann et al. (27) found that, compared with control subjects, diabetics with hyperhomocysteinemia had more microalbuminuria, higher levels of thrombomod-ulin (a marker of endothelial dysfunction), and a higher prevalence of nephropathy (76% vs. 33%), retinopathy (65% vs. 51%), and neuropathy (57% vs. 41%).

Timing of Homocysteine Blood Samples

Part of the difficulty in ascertaining whether there is a direct relationship between homocysteine level and stroke is that it depends on the relationship in time between the determination of the homocysteine level and the event. Although no consistent patterns have yet emerged, homocysteine levels may vary with diet and may rise acutely after an animal protein meal (12). Fasting, too, may affect homocysteine levels, which may apply to patients soon after an event such as stroke.

There are currently no data in regard to homocysteine levels immediately before or during the index stroke (38). Furthermore, there are no substantial data in regard to correlation of homocysteine levels with the variety of stroke (i.e., embolism from the heart, lacunar stroke, atherosclerotic stenosis of the major vessels, venous occlusion, hemorrhage). Some have related the reduction in homocysteine following infarction of the brain to a decrease in albumin, which binds homocysteine and may sometimes affect homocysteine levels (see Chapter 18), or to the use of vitamins, particularly folic acid, which may reduce homocysteine levels. Moreover, position affects homocysteine concentrations and recumbency, which is expected in many patients after a stroke, can decrease homocysteine levels (see Chapter 18).

Lindgren et al. (35) found that plasma homocysteine levels averaged 11.4 μmol/L shortly after a stroke. After 2 to 3 years, plasma homocysteine was 14.5 μmol/L in the same 20 stroke patients, but there was no difference between baseline and repeat levels in control subjects. The likeliest reasons for the difference are the aforementioned hemodilution from recumbency at the time of the stroke (8) or an increase over time after the stroke owing to a deterioration in renal function. There was a higher risk of vascular events with increased creatinine levels in the North American Symptomatic Carotid Endarterectomy Trial (2) (Eliasziw, M, unpublished observation), and there is a higher proportion of patients with renovascular hypertension among patients with carotid stenosis (62). These observations may be explained by the association of renal failure with high plasma homocysteine levels (65).

Effect of Homocysteine on Carotid Arteries

Several studies have shown that plasma homocysteine levels are associated with increased thickness of the carotid intima and media (38, 42, 73). As intima-media thickness is associated with vascular risk (47, 54), this association has been regarded as important; however, there are problems with intima-media thickness as a surrogate for atherosclerosis. Adams et al. (1) found that intima-media thickness was only a weak predictor of coronary disease, and O'Leary et al. (48) found that Framingham risk factors predicted only 15% of internal carotid intima-media thickness and only 18% of common carotid intima-media thickness. In contrast, the R^2 for prediction of carotid plaque cross-sectional area with Framingham risk factors is 0.5 (61, 63, 64).

It is important, therefore, to distinguish between intima-media thickness, which is a marker of arterial end-organ damage closely associated with hypertension and left ventricular mass (36, 37, 41, 43), and atherosclerosis. It is also important to distinguish between stenosis, as a marker of atherosclerosis, and other measurements of the wall itself, such as plaque area or three-dimensional plaque volume (17, 58). The British Regional Heart Study found that intima-media thickness was a stronger predictor of stroke, whereas the presence of carotid plaque was a stronger predictor of coronary artery disease (16); this finding suggests that mainly hypertensive stroke was predicted by intima-media thickness.

Selhub et al. (57) found an association between plasma total homocysteine levels and carotid artery stenosis, defined by Doppler ultrasound. In the Framingham cohort of 1,041 persons in whom homocysteine and carotid artery wall thickness were measured, the adjusted odds ratio for stenosis greater than 25% and wall thickening was 2 for subjects with the highest versus the lowest quintile of homocysteine levels. Another study, however, produced what seem to be conflicting findings. Taylor et al. (69) showed, in a prospective follow-up study of patients with peripheral vascular disease, that high homocysteine levels were associated with increased mortality, but the study did not find a relationship with progression of the ankle-brachial index (the ratio of blood pressure in the lower leg to the arm, a marker of atherosclerosis) or ultrasonographic evidence of carotid stenosis. This apparent paradox may be explained by a combination of sample size and low sensitivity of the methods used, together with the phenomenon of compensatory enlargement.

Much of the misunderstanding of atherosclerosis is based on an angiographic perspective. Contrary to popular belief, plaque, in its early stages, does not cause stenosis *ab initio*. What actually happens is that the artery enlarges to accommodate the plaque; this process is called *remodeling*, or *compensatory enlargement* (61). Glagov et al. (22) hypothesized that compensatory enlargement occurs in order to maintain a constant shear rate at the intima. Angiography and ultrasound Doppler velocity measurements of stenosis depend on the diameter of the residual lumen, which changes relatively slowly at sites of stenosis with scarring. As atherosclerosis is in the wall rather than the lumen, measurements of plaque in the wall are more sensitive to change, as described later.

Mechanisms of Action of Homocysteine

Homocysteine may contribute to cerebral vascular disease by many mechanisms. These include increased production of hydrogen peroxide (66, 67), oxidative stress, and endothelial dysfunction (10, 11, 29, 70, 71), with increased oxidation of low-density lipoprotein and changes in lipoprotein(a) (33), and coagulation changes (44, 45). These and other mechanisms are reviewed in Chapters 4, 5, and 34–36.

Effect of Treatment with Vitamins

As reviewed in Chapters 23–25 and 38, folate and to a lesser extent cobalamin and perhaps vitamin B_6 therapy reduce plasma homocysteine levels (4, 71). Associations of acute increases in homocysteine levels, such as after methionine load or meals, with evidence of endothelial dysfunction have been described by some (10–12). Although antioxidant vitamin therapy appears to improve endothelial dysfunction (11), the effect of B vitamins on endothelium has been less clear. Effects have been reported on endothelium-related proteins (70). A preliminary report suggested that vitamin therapy also reduces plasma levels of fibrinogen and lipoprotein(a) in patients with renal failure and very high levels of homocysteine (31).

The first evidence of an effect of vitamin therapy on the progression of atherosclerosis in human beings was reported in 1998 by Peterson and Spence (51), who found that vitamin therapy halted progression of carotid atherosclerosis in 38 patients with carotid atherosclerosis and plasma homocysteine greater than 14 μmol/L. Hackam et al. (26) have extended those observations to 51 patients with plasma homocysteine levels above 14 μmol/L and 51 patients with levels below 14 μmol/L (Figure 31.1). Carotid artery plaque in both groups of patients progressed rapidly before treatment, but not after treatment. The change in rate of progression was –0.15 + 0.44 cm²/yr below 14 μmol/L (p = 0.022), and –0.265 + 0.46 cm²/yr above 14 μmol/L (p = 0.0001); there was no significant difference in the response rate between the two groups.

What is the Level to Treat?

This subject is discussed in Chapters 38 and 40. Given the apparent modification of carotid plaque progression by vitamin therapy in Figure 31.1, and given the epidemiological evidence, it appears likely that in the

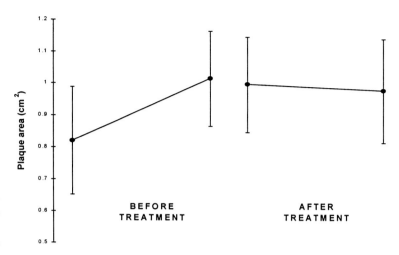

Homocyst(e)ine > 14

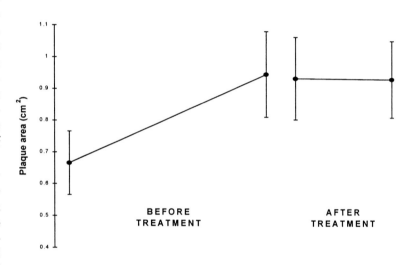

Homocyst(e)ine <14

Fig. 31.1. Rate of atherosclerosis progression before and after vitamin treatment in patients with plasma total homocysteine [Homocyst(e)ine] >14 μmol/L (top panel) and <14 μmol/L (bottom panel). **(Top panel)** The mean duration of treatment before initiation of vitamin therapy was 2.6 ± 1.4 years (range 0.9 to 6 years); the post-treatment period was 1.8 ± 0.7 years (0.8 to 3.3 years). Before initiation of vitamin therapy, the rate of carotid artery plaque progression was steeply upward, with a rate of progression of 0.21 ± 0.41 cm²/year before vitamin therapy, and the rate became negative at –0.049 ± 0.24 cm²/year after vitamin therapy (p^2 = 0.0001; paired t test). **(Bottom panel)** The duration of follow-up study before treatment was 2.7 ± 1.7 years (0.9 to 6.0); follow-up period after treatment was 1.6 ± 0.9 years (0.8 to 4.2 years). Before initiation of vitamin therapy, the rate of atherosclerosis progression was steeply upward, with a rate of progression of 0.13 ± 0.24 cm²/year before vitamin therapy, and the rate became negative at –0.024 ± 0.29 cm²/year after vitamin therapy (p^2 = 0.022, paired t-test). (Reproduced from Hackam et al. [26], with permission.)

future we may consider treating patients with vascular disease to a low target level of plasma homocysteine, such as below 9 μmol/L, rather than selecting patients for treatment on the basis of very high levels. Such an approach would be analogous to approaches now taken to treatment of low-density lipoprotein cholesterol in patients with vascular disease.

Future Directions

Some of the difficulties requiring resolution are the methods used to measure homocysteine and the time elapsed between the collection of the blood specimens and their measurements. One of the most important issues is the lack of information to date regarding fluctuations in homocysteine levels over time in the normal population. Is there a diurnal, seasonal, or other variation based on substantial changes in diet, renal function, blood pressure, or other confounding factors, including dietary supplements, that must be considered? Moreover, studies in large populations of women and minority groups are lacking and socioeconomic variables are unexplored.

Interventional studies under way are discussed in Chapter 39. The first of these was the Vitamin Intervention in Stroke Prevention Trial, a randomized, controlled trial of high-dose versus low-dose folate, vitamin B6 and cobalamin for secondary prevention of nondisabling stroke. In that trial, both fasting levels and methionine load studies are being performed. So far, the combination of fasting and postmethionine load measurements of total homocysteine seem to be more sensitive than those of the fasting total homocysteine level alone because fasting levels may be more sensitive to poor remethylation by MTHFR, methionine synthase, and betaine:homocysteine methyltransferase, whereas the postmethionine load levels might be related more to dysfunction of cystathione β-synthase (38, 56).

Epidemiological studies of homocysteine are still needed and normative data related to age, gender, race, geographical location, and customary diet are still lacking. Furthermore, alcohol, smoking, physical activity, and many environmental factors could all affect homocysteine levels (see Chapter 28). Most powerful among them are the use of medications for other diseases, such as methotrexate and antiepileptic therapy (24, 30, 49, 52, 55), many of which affect folate metabolism.

The fortification of grains and cereals with folic acid, which was introduced in the United States officially in January 1998, has apparently had an effect on reducing the levels of homocysteine in the population of patients with stroke in the Vitamin Intervention for Stroke Prevention trial. In that trial, the plasma homocysteine

level was set above the 25th percentile of plasma homocysteine levels. Based on pilot data, the 25th percentile was at 10.5 μmol/L for men and 9.5 μmol/L for women. Over time, with the addition of folate to the grain supply of North Americans, the 25th percentile has fallen to 9.5 μmol/L in men and 8.5 μmol/L in women (Malinow MR, personal communication).

In summary, high levels of plasma homocysteine are a significant independent risk factor for stroke. Potential mechanisms include acceleration of atherosclerosis, impaired endothelial function, and increased coagulation (see Chapters 4 and 34–36). Vitamin therapy reduces plasma homocysteine and may improve endothelial function and, in uncontrolled clinical practice, alter the progression of carotid plaque. Controlled clinical trials should determine whether vitamin therapy will prevent stroke in high-risk patients.

REFERENCES

1. Adams, MR, Nakagomi, A, Keech, A, Robinson, J, McCredie, R, Bailey, BP, Freedman, SB, Celermajer, DS. Carotid intimal-media thickness is only weakly correlated with the extent and severity of coronary artery disease. *Circulation* 1995; 92: 2127–34.
2. Barnett, HJ, Taylor, DW, Eliasziw, M, Fox, AJ, Ferguson, GG, Haynes, RB, Rankin, RN, Claggett, GP, Hachinski, VC, Sackett, DL, Thorpe, KE, Meldrum, HE. Benefit of carotid endarterectomy in patients with symptomatic moderate or severe stenosis. North American Symptomatic Carotid Endarterectomy Trial Collaborators. *N Engl J Med* 1998; 339: 1415–25.
3. Boers, GHJ, Smals, AG, Trijbels, FJM, Fowler, B, Bakkeren, JAJ, Schoonderwaldt, HC, Kleijer, WJ, Kloppenborg, PW. Heterozygosity for homocystinuria in premature peripheral and cerebral occlusive arterial disease. *N Engl J Med* 1985; 313: 709–15.
4. Brattström, LE. Vitamins as homocysteine-lowering agents. *J Nutr* 1996; 126: S1276–80.
5. Brattström, LE, Hardebo, JE, Hultberg, BL. Moderate hyper-homocyst(e)inemia—A possible risk factor for arteriosclerotic cerebrovascular disease. *Stroke* 1984; 15: 1012–16.
6. Brattström, LE, Lindgren, A, Israelsson, B, Andersson, A, Hultberg, B. Homocysteine and cysteine: determinants in plasma levels in middle aged and elderly subjects. *J Intern Med* 1994; 236: 633–41.
7. Brattström, L, Lindgren, A, Israelsson, B, Malinow, MR, Norrving, B, Upson, B, Hamfelt, A. Hyperhomocysteinemia in stroke: Prevalence, cause, and relationships to type of stroke and stroke risk factors. *Eur J Clin Invest* 1992; 22: 214–21.
8. Campbell, N, Brant, R, Stalts, H, Stone, JMH, Mahallati, H. Fluctuations in blood lipid levels during furosemide therapy: A randomized, double-blind, placebo-controlled crossover study. *Arch Intern Med* 1998; 158: 1461–63.

9. Carson, NA, Neill, DW. Metabolic abnormalities detected in a survey of mentally backward individuals in Northern Ireland. *Arch Dis Child* 1962; 37: 505–13.

10. Chambers, JC, McGregor, A, Jean-Marie, J, Kooner, JS. Acute hyperhomocysteinaemia and endothelial dysfunction. *Lancet* 1998; 351: 36–7.

11. Chambers, JC, McGregor, A, Jean-Marie, J, Obeid, OA, Kooner, JS. Demonstration of rapid onset vascular endothelial dysfunction after hyperhomocysteinemia: An effect reversible with vitamin C therapy. *Circulation* 1999; 99: 1156–60.

12. Chambers, JC, Obeid, OA, Kooner, JS. Physiological increments in plasma homocysteine induces vascular endothelial dysfunction in normal human subjects. *Arterioscler Thromb Vasc Biol* 1999; 19: 2922–27.

13. Chico, A, Perez, A, Cordoba, A, Arcelus, R, Carreras, G, de Leiva, A, Gonzalez-Sastre, F, Blanco-Vaca, F. Plasma homocysteine is related to albumin excretion rate in patients with diabetes mellitus: A new link between diabetic nephropathy and cardiovascular disease? *Diabetologia* 1998; 41: 684–93.

14. Clarke, R, Daly, L, Robinson, K, Naughten, E, Cahalane, S, Fowler, B, Graham, I. Hyperhomocysteinemia: An independent risk factor for vascular disease. *N Engl J Med* 1991; 324: 1149–55.

15. Coull, BM, Malinow, MR, Beamer, N, Sexton, G, Nordt, F, de Garmo, P. Elevated plasma homocyst(e)ine concentration as a possible independent risk factor for stroke. *Stroke* 1991; 21: 572–76.

16. Ebrahim, SB, Papacosta, O, Whincup, P, Wannamethee, G, Walker, M, Nicolaides, AN, Dhanjil, S, Griffin, M, Belcaro, G, Rumley, A, Lowe, GD. Carotid plaque, intima media thickness, cardiovascular risk factors, and prevalent cardiovascular disease in men and women. The British Regional Heart Study. *Stroke* 1999; 30: 841–50.

17. Fenster, A, Lee, D, Sherebrin, S, Rankin, R, Spence, D, Downey, D. Three-dimensional ultrasound imaging of carotid occlusive disease. In *New Trends in Cerebral Hemodynamics and Neurosonology* (Klingelhöfer, J, Bartels, E, Ringelstein, EB, eds.). Elsevier Science B.V., Amsterdam, 1997; pp. 17–24.

18. Franken, DG, Vreugdenhil, A, Boers, GHJ, Verrips, A, Blom, HJ, Novakova, IRO. Familial cerebrovascular accidents due to concomitant hyperhomocysteinemia and protein C deficiency type 1. *Stroke* 1993; 24: 1599–600.

19. Gerritsen, T, Vaughn, JG, Waisman, HA. The identification of homocystine in the urine. *Biochem Biophys Res Commun* 1962; 9: 493–96.

20. Giles, WH, Croft, JB, Greenlund, KJ, Ford, ES, Kittner, SJ. Total homocyst(e)ine concentration and the likelihood of nonfatal stroke: Results from the Third National Health and Nutrition Examination Survey, 1988–1994. *Stroke* 1998; 29: 2473–77.

21. Giles, WH, Kittner, SJ, Anda, RF, Croft, JB, Casper, ML. Serum folate and risk for ischemic stroke. First National Health and Nutrition Examination Survey epidemiologic follow-up study. *Stroke* 1995; 26: 1166–70.

22. Glagov, S, Weisenberg, E, Zarins, CK, Stankunavicius, R, Kolettis, GJ. Compensatory enlargement of human atherosclerotic coronary arteries. *N Engl J Med* 1987; 316: 1371–75.

23. Graham, IM, Daly, L, Refsum, H, Robinson, K, Brattström, LE, Ueland, PM, Palma-Reis, RJ, Boers, GH, Sheahan, RG, Israelsson, B, Uiterwaal, CS, Meleady, R, McMaster, D, Verhoef, P, Witteman, J, Rubba, P, Bellet, H, Wautrecht, JC, deValk, HW, Sales Luis, AC, Parratt-Rouland, FM, Tan, KS, Higgins, I, Garcon, D, Andria, G. Plasma homocysteine as a risk factor for vascular disease. *JAMA* 1997; 277: 1775–81.

24. Guttormsen, AB, Ueland, PM, Lonning, PE, Mella, O, Refsum, H. Kinetics of plasma total homocysteine in patients receiving high-dose methotrexate therapy. *Clin Chem* 1998; 44: 1987–89.

25. Hachinski, V, Graffagnino, C, Beaudry, M, Bernier, G, Buck, C, Donner, A, Spence, JD, Doig, G, Wolfe, BM. Lipids and stroke: A paradox resolved. *Arch Neurol* 1996; 53: 303–8.

26. Hackam, DG, Peterson, JC, Spence, JD. What level of plasma homocyst(e)ine should be treated? Effects of vitamin therapy on progression of carotid atherosclerosis in patients with homocyst(e)ine levels above and below 14 μmol/L. *Am J Hypertens* 2000; 13: 105–10.

27. Hofmann, MA, Kohl, B, Zumbach, MS, Borcea, V, Bierhaus, A, Henkels, M, Amiral, J, Fiehn, W, Ziegler, R, Wahl, P, Nawroth, PP. Hyperhomocyst(e)inemia and endothelial dysfunction in insulin-dependent diabetes mellitus. *Diabetes Care* 1997; 20: 1880–86.

28. Hoogeveen, EK, Kostense, PJ, Beks, PJ, Mackaay, AJ, Jakobs, C, Bouter, LM, Heine, RJ, Stehouwer, CD. Hyperhomocysteinemia is associated with an increased risk of cardiovascular disease, especially in non-insulin-dependent diabetes mellitus: A population-based study. *Arterioscler Thromb Vasc Biol* 1998; 18: 133–38.

29. Ikeda, U, Ikeda, M, Minota, S, Shimada, K. Homocysteine increases nitric oxide synthesis in cytokine-stimulated vascular smooth muscle cells. *Circulation* 1999; 99: 1230–35.

30. James, GK, Jones, MW, Pudek, MR. Homocyst(e)ine levels in patients on phenytoin therapy. *Clin Biochem* 1997; 30: 647–49.

31. Klinke, K, Dziewanowski, K, Staniewicz, A, Bukowska, H, Narusciewicz, M. Effect of vitamin therapy on homocyst(e)ine, fibrinogen and Lp(a) in dialysis patients. *Czynniki Ryzyka* 1998; Suppl. 4: 28.

32. Lanfredini, M, Fiorina, P, Peca, MG, Veronelli, A, Mello, A, Astorri, E, Dall'Aglio, P, Craveri, A. Fasting and post-methionine load homocyst(e)ine values are correlated with microalbuminuria and could contribute to worsening vascular damage in non-insulin-dependent diabetes mellitus patients. *Metabolism* 1998; 47: 915–21.

33. Leerink, CB, van Ham, AD, Heeres, A, Duif, PF, Bouma, BN, van Rijn, HJ. Sulfhydryl compounds influence immunoreactivity, structure and functional aspects of lipoprotein(a). *Thromb Res* 1994; 74: 219–32.

34. Lentz, SR, Sadler, JE. Inhibition of thrombomodulin surface expression and protein C activation by the thrombogenic agent, homocysteine. *J Clin Invest* 1991; 88: 1906–14.

35. Lindgren, A, Brattström, LE, Norrving, B, Hultberg, B, Andersson, A, Johansson, BB. Plasma homocysteine in the acute and convalescent phases after stroke. *Stroke* 1995; 26: 795–800.

36. Linhart, A, Gariepy, J, Giral, P, Levenson, J, Simon, A. Carotid artery and left ventricular structural relationship

in asymptomatic men at risk for cardiovascular diseases. *Atherosclerosis* 1996; 127: 103–12.

37. Lonati, L, Cuspidi, C, Sampieri, L. Left ventricular concentric remodeling in hypertensive patients is associated with carotid changes. *J Hypertens* 1996; 14(Suppl. 1):s104.

38. Malinow, MR, Nieto, FJ, Szklo, M, Chambless, LE, Bond, G. Carotid intimal-medial wall thickening and plasma hyper-homocyst(e)inemia in asymptomatic adults. The Atherosclerosis Risk in Communities Study. *Circulation* 1993; 87: 1107–13.

39. Markus, HS, Ali, N, Swaminathan, R, Sankaralingam, A, Molloy, J, Powell, J. A common polymorphism in the methylenetetrahydrofolate reductase gene, homocysteine, and ischemic cerebrovascular disease. *Stroke* 1997; 28: 1739–43.

40. McCully, KS. Vascular pathology of homocysteinemia: Implications for the pathogenesis of atherosclerosis. *Am J Pathol* 1969; 56: 111–28.

41. Megnien, JL, Gariepy, J, Denarie, N, Levenson, J, Simon, A. Large arteries intima-media thickness is not an independent predictor of coronary atherosclerosis in asymptomatic men. *J Hypertens* 1996; 14(Suppl. 1): S198.

42. Megnien, JL, Gariepy, J, Saudubray, JM, Nuoffer, JM, Denarie, N, Levenson, J, Simon, A. Evidence of carotid artery wall hypertrophy in homozygous homocystinuria. *Circulation* 1998; 98: 2276–81.

43. Mukai, M, Sumimoto, T, Matsuzaki, K. Left ventricular concentric geometric pattern and carotid artery structure in essential hypertensive patients. *J Hypertens* 1996; 14(Suppl. 1):s88.

44. Nishinaga, M, Ozawa, T, Shimada, K. Homocysteine, a thrombogenic agent, suppresses anticoagulant heparan sulfate expression in cultured porcine aortic endothelial cells. *J Clin Invest* 1993; 92: 1381–86.

45. Nishinaga, M, Shimada, K. [Heparan sulfate proteoglycan of endothelial cells: homocysteine suppresses anticoagulant active heparan sulfate in cultured endothelial cells]. *Rinsho Byori* 1994; 42: 340–45.

46. Nygård, O, Nordrehaug, JE, Refsum, H, Ueland, PM, Farstad, M, Vollset, SE. Plasma homocysteine levels and mortality in patients with coronary artery disease. *N Engl J Med* 1997; 337: 230–36.

47. O'Leary, DH, Polak, JF, Kronmal, RA, Manolio, TA, Burke, GL, Wolfson, SK Jr. Carotid artery intima and media thickness as a risk factor for myocardial infarction and stroke in older adults. Cardiovascular Health Study Collaborative Research Group. *N Engl J Med* 1999; 340: 14–22.

48. O'Leary, DH, Polak, JF, Kronmal, RA, Savage, PJ, Borhani, NO, Kittner, SJ, Tracy, R, Gardin, JM, Price, TR, Furberg, CD. Thickening of the carotid wall: A marker for atherosclerosis in the elderly? *Stroke* 1996; 27: 224–31.

49. Ono, H, Sakamoto, A, Eguchi, T, Fujita, N, Nomura, S, Ueda, H, Sakura, N, Ueda, K. Plasma total homocysteine concentrations in epileptic patients taking anticonvulsants. *Metabolism* 1997; 46: 959–62.

50. Perry, IJ, Refsum, H, Morris, RW, Ebrahim, SB, Ueland, PM, Shaper, AG. Prospective study of serum total homocysteine concentration and risk of stroke in middle-aged British men. *Lancet* 1995; 346: 1395–98.

51. Peterson, JC, Spence, JD. Vitamins and progression of atherosclerosis in patients with hyper-homocyst(e)inemia. *Lancet* 1998; 351: 263.

52. Refsum, H, Ueland, PM. Clinical significance of pharmacological modulation of homocysteine metabolism. *Trends Pharmacol Sci* 1990; 11: 411–16.

53. Reinhardt, D, Sigusch, HH, Vogt, SF, Farker, K, Muller, S, Hoffmann, A. Absence of association between a common mutation in the methylenetetrahydrofolate reductase gene and the risk of coronary artery disease. *Eur J Clin Invest* 1998; 28: 20–3.

54. Salonen, JT, Salonen, R. Ultrasound B-mode imaging in observational studies of atherosclerotic progression. *Stroke* 1993; 87(Suppl. 3): II56–65.

55. Schwaninger, M, Ringleb, P, Winter, R, Kohl, B, Fiehn, W, Rieser, PA, Walter-Sack, I. Elevated plasma concentrations of homocysteine in antiepileptic drug treatment. *Epilepsia* 1999; 40: 345–50.

56. Selhub, J, D'Angelo, A. Hyperhomocysteinemia and thrombosis: Acquired conditions. *Thromb Haemost* 1997; 78: 527–31.

57. Selhub, J, Jacques, PF, Bostom, AG, D'agostino, RB, Wilson, PWF, Belanger, AJ, O'Leary, DH, Wolf, PA, Schaefer, EJ, Rosenberg, IH. Association between plasma homocysteine concentrations and extracranial carotid-artery stenosis. *N Engl J Med* 1995; 332: 286–91.

58. Sherebrin, S, Fenster, A, Rankin, RN, Spence, JD. Freehand three-dimensional ultrasound: Implementation and applications. *S.P.I.E.* 1997; 2707: 296–303.

59. Spence, JD. Antihypertensive drugs and prevention of atherosclerotic stroke. *Stroke* 1986; 17: 808–10.

60. Spence, JD. Cerebral consequences of hypertension. In *Hypertension: Pathophysiology, Diagnosis, and Management.* (Laragh, JH, Brenner, B, eds.). Raven Press, New York, 1995; pp. 741–53.

61. Spence, JD. New approaches to atherosclerosis based on endothelial function. In *Current Review of Cerebrovascular Disease* (Fisher, M, Bogousslavsky, J, eds.). Churchill Livingstone, Philadelphia, 1998; pp. 1–13.

62. Spence, JD. High prevalence of renovascular hypertension in patients with carotid stenosis. *Stroke* 1999; 30: 269.

63. Spence, JD, Barnett, PA, Bulman, DE, Hegele, R. An approach to ascertain probands with a non-traditional risk factor for carotid atherosclerosis. *Atherosclerosis* 1999; 144: 429–34.

64. Spence, JD, Malinow, MR, Barnett, PA, Marian, AJ, Freeman, D, Hegele, RA. Plasma homocyst(e)ine concentration, but not MTHFR genotype, is associated with variation in carotid plaque area. *Stroke* 1999; 30: 969–73.

65. Spence, JD, Cordy, P, Kortas, C, Freeman, DJ. Effect of usual doses of folate supplementation on elevated plasma homocyst(e)ine in hemodialysis patients: No difference between 1 mg and 5 mg daily. *Am J Nephrol* 1999; 19: 405–10.

66. Stamler, JS, Osborne, JA, Jaraki, O, Rabbani, LE, Mullins, M, Singel, D, Loscalzo, J. Adverse vascular effects of homocysteine are modulated by endothelium-derived relaxing factor and related oxides of nitrogen. *J Clin Invest* 1993; 91: 308–18.

67. Stamler, JS, Slivka, A. Biological chemistry of thiols in the vasculature and in vascular-related disease. *Nutr Rev* 1996; 54: 1–30.

68. Stampfer, MJ, Malinow, MR, Willett, WC, Newcomer, LM, Upson, B, Ullmann, D, Tishler, PV, Hennekens, CH. A prospective study of plasma homocyst(e)ine and risk of myocardial infarction. *JAMA* 1992; 268: 887–91.

69. Taylor, LM Jr, Moneta, GL, Sexton, GJ, Schuff, RA, Porter, JM. Prospective blinded study of the relationship between plasma homocysteine and progression of symptomatic peripheral arterial disease. *J Vasc Surg* 1999; 29: 8–19.

70. van den Berg, M, Boers, GH, Franken, DG, Blom, HJ, van Kamp, GJ, Jakobs, C, Rauwerda, JA, Kluft, C, Stehouwert, CD. Hyperhomocysteinaemia and endothelial dysfunction in young patients with peripheral arterial occlusive disease. *Eur J Clin Invest* 1995; 25: 176–81.

71. van den Berg, M, Franken, DG, Boers, GH, Blom, HJ, Jakobs, C, Stehouwer, CDA, Rauwerda, JA. Combined vitamin B6 plus folic acid therapy in young patients with arteriosclerosis and hyperhomocysteinemia. *J Vasc Surg* 1994; 20: 933–40.

72. Verhoef, P, Hennekens, CH, Malinow, MR, Kok, FJ, Willett, WC, Stampfer, MJ. A prospective study of plasma homocyst(e)ine and risk of ischemic stroke. *Stroke* 1994; 25: 1924–30.

73. Voutilainen, S, Alfthan, G, Nyyssonen, K, Salonen, R, Salonen, JT. Association between elevated plasma total homocysteine and increased common carotid artery wall thickness. *Ann Med* 1998; 30: 300–6.

74. Yoo, JH, Chung, CS, Kang, SS. Relation of plasma homocyst(e)ine to cerebral infarction and cerebral atherosclerosis. *Stroke* 1998; 29: 2478–83.

32

Peripheral Arterial Disease

GODFRIED BOERS

Peripheral vascular disease can be very diverse if patients with intermittent claudication, aortic aneurysm, carotid stenosis, deep venous thrombosis, and pulmonary embolism are included. This chapter focuses on peripheral arterial disease caused by stenosis of large and medium-sized arteries in the legs. This stenosis may lead to intermittent claudication or even pain at rest, muscle and skin atrophy of the leg, and finally to necrosis. In general, the prevalence of intermittent claudication is approximately 2% for men under the age of 50 years, increasing to over 5% in those older than 70 years. Women reach these rates almost 10 years after men, although the gender difference decreases with advanced age (37).

In two of three patients with decreased blood flow to the legs, there are no complaints or symptoms (12), and patients can be identified only by the use of ankle-brachial index measurement or Doppler-signal technique. However, intermittent claudication as well as asymptomatic peripheral arterial disease, whose incidence is three to four times as high as intermittent claudication, are indicators of excess risk of fatal and nonfatal cardiovascular events (12, 18). Mortality in peripheral arterial disease is attributable in 75% of cases to vascular events involving coronary (50%), cerebrovascular (15%), or abdominal aortic (10%) atherosclerosis (10). Cardiovascular mortality in the Edinburgh Artery Study was twice as high in subjects with asymptomatic peripheral arterial disease and almost three times as high in symptomatic patients compared with persons free of those signs (12). In the Framingham study, the mortality rate in men with intermittent claudication was 39 per 1,000 over 14 years versus 10 per 1,000 in men without claudication (18). The life expectancy of patients suffering from claudication was about 10 years shorter than that of unaffected persons (23).

For peripheral arterial as well as coronary artery disease, the atherosclerosis becomes clinically manifest at a younger age and has a more severe course in the presence of risk factors, especially when several coexist, than in their absence. Therefore, screening for modifiable risk factors should have priority in cases of premature peripheral arterial disease (i.e., in males below the age of 50 years and in females below the age of 55 years), although cutoff points are arbitrary. It is mandatory to advise cessation of smoking, to control hypertension, and to treat elevated levels of total cholesterol, lowered high-density cholesterol levels, and high triglycerides or glucose concentrations in the blood if such conventional risk factors are present. Moderately and even mildly elevated total homocysteine levels, first reported in 1976 in patients with coronary artery disease (40), have also been recognized in the last 2 decades to be associated with increased risk of cardiovascular disease. In 1985, a significant association with peripheral arterial disease was also shown (4), and a series of subsequent studies confirmed this finding. As hyperhomocysteinemia can be normalized by safe, cheap and simple treatment with folic acid, vitamin B_6, and cobalamin, it might indeed be categorized as a modifiable factor. Whether it will achieve a status equivalent to that of the conventional risk factors for peripheral arterial disease remains to be explored and depends largely on ultimate proof of a causative role for homocysteine in cardiovascular disease.

Review of Studies on Hyperhomocysteinemia and Peripheral Arterial Disease (Table 32.1)

After their preliminary report (3), Boers et al. (4) reported a more extensive study in 1985 that showed that 7 of 25 patients (28%) presenting with clinical signs of intermittent claudication (n = 16), renal arterial occlusive disease (n = 7), or abdominal angina (n = 2) had elevated homocysteine concentrations in the blood after oral methionine loading that were comparable with levels in obligate carriers for classic homocystinuria caused by cystathionine β-synthase deficiency. Four of these seven patients had intermittent claudication as the predominant ischemic sign. Postload hyperhomocysteinemia was also found in 25 patients (28%) with occlusive cerebrovascular disease resulting in transient ischemic attacks or strokes. All patients and control subjects were younger than 50 years and had no conventional cardiovascular risk factors such as hyperlipidemia, diabetes, or hypertension. That study showed for the first time the possibility of normalization of the pathological homocysteine levels by B vitamins in hyperhomocysteinemic vascular patients. This finding suggested a practical reason for screening for mild hyperhomocysteinemia in young patients whose occlusive peripheral arterial disease produced common clinical syndromes such as intermittent claudication.

Malinow et al. (19) confirmed the high prevalence of hyperhomocysteinemia in 47 patients with peripheral arterial disease who had demonstrated stenosis of iliofemoral arteries ($n = 32$), aortic aneurysm ($n = 8$), carotid artery stenosis ($n = 7$), or a combination of these. In all, 22 of the 47 patients (47%) showed fasting blood levels of homocysteine more than 2 standard deviations above the mean of the control values. Age, hypercholesterolemia, and the prevalence of smoking and diabetes were similar in patients and control subjects, suggesting that elevated homocysteine was an independent risk factor for arterial disease.

A comparable prevalence of hyperhomocysteinemia was reported in 37 patients with occlusive arterial disease of aortoiliac vessels before the age of 55 years (6). The frequency of fasting homocysteine levels more than 2 standard deviations above the control mean was 32%, as was the frequency of postmethionine load hyperhomocysteinemia.

Clarke et al. (8) also established a prevalence of 28% for postmethionine load hyperhomocysteinemia in 25 patients with peripheral arterial disease before the age of 55 years. Taylor et al. (33), in the same year, reported elevated basal homocysteine levels in 39% of 214 patients. However, it is not clear how many of those patients specifically had symptomatic lower extremity arterial occlusions. Patients with cerebral vascular disease resulting in strokes or transient ischemic attacks, either as the sole arteriosclerotic manifestation or in combination with lower extremity

Table 32.1. Previous Case-Control Studies of Hyperhomocysteinemia and Peripheral Arterial Disease

Study (Ref.)	No. of Cases/ Controls	Age (years)	Definition of Hyperhomocystinemia	Prevalence of Hyperhomocysteinemia	
				Cases	Controls
Boers, 1985 (4)	16/40	<50	Peak postmethionine load level > 97.5 percentile of controls	25%	0%
Malinow, 1989 (19)	32/29	70/66[a]	Fasting level > 97.5 percentile of controls	47%[b]	0%
Brattström, 1990 (6)	37/46	<59/<63	Fasting level > 97.5 percentile of controls	32%	4%
Clarke, 1991 (8)	25/27	<55	Peak postmethionine load level ≥ 24 μmol/L[c]	28%	0%
Taylor, 1991 (33)[d]	214/29	65/>60	Basal level > 97.5 percentile of controls[e]	39%	NG
Mölgaard, 1992 (22)	78/98	45–69	Fasting level > 95 percentile of controls	23%	5%
Bergmark, 1993 (2)	58/65	<50	Fasting level > 97.5 percentile of controls	28%	6%
Dudman, 1993 (11)	18/56	<61	4-hour postmethionine load level > 97.5 percentile of controls	17%	4%
Franken, 1994 (13)	131/63	<56	Peak postmethionine level > 97.5 percentile of controls	33%	0%
van den Berg, 1994 (35)	143/91	<50	Peak postmethionine level > 97.5 percentile of controls	25%	3%
Cheng, 1997 (7)	100/100	67[f]	Fasting level > 90 percentile of controls	27%	9%
Graham, 1997 (15)	156/800	48/44	Fasting level > 80 percentile of controls	40%	20%
			Fasting level > 90 percentile of controls	26%	10%

[a] Mean ages were 70 ± 11 (standard deviation) and 66 ± 4 years in patients and control subjects, respectively.

[b] 47% of 47 patients, including cases with vascular disease other than peripheral arterial disease.

[c] This cutoff point was selected because it distinguished, with the highest sensitivity and specificity, a group of 25 obligate heterozygotes for homocystinuria from the control group.

[d] The study included an unknown proportion of cases of vascular disease other than peripheral arterial disease.

[e] Basal level means the level in a sample taken without regard to fasting.

[f] Mean age was 67 years, range 40 to 80 years.

disease, had been included as well. The frequencies of risk factors such as age, male sex, diabetes, hypertension, smoking, renal failure, and plasma cholesterol were identical in patients with and without hyperhomocysteinemia. Therefore, hyperhomocysteinemia as a risk factor for peripheral atherosclerosis appeared to be independent of the other factors analyzed, as had been suggested earlier (19).

In Linköping County, Sweden, Mölgaard et al. (22) screened 15,253 middle-aged men (ages 45 to 69 years) for intermittent claudication by means of a Rose questionnaire (29). The results showed that 1.2% of them had symptoms indicative of intermittent claudication. In 23% of randomly selected patients who showed an abnormal treadmill excercise test, fasting plasma homocysteine levels were above the 95th percentile for sex- and age-matched healthy control subjects. The difference in plasma levels—16.7 ± 5.5 μmol/L (mean ± standard deviation) in patients versus 13.8 ± 3.2 μmol/L in control subjects—was independent of the presence of smoking, hypertension, diabetes, hypercholesterolemia, hypertriglyceridemia, low high-density-lipoprotein cholesterol, and age. Remarkably, the elevation of plasma homocysteine was largely confined to subjects with serum folate concentrations lower than 11.0 nmol/L, a finding that may justify intervention with folic acid supplementation in hyperhomocysteinemic patients with intermittent claudication.

Bergmark et al. (2) measured fasting homocysteine levels in 58 patients who had had surgery for leg ischemia at a mean age of 44 years. In 28% of the patients, these levels exceeded the control mean by more than 2 standard deviations (i.e., above 18.6 μmol/L in that study). At the time of their surgery, all but two patients had been heavy smokers for 20 years. At follow-up evaluation, after a mean postsurgical interval of 5 years, 53% of the patients admitted to continued smoking, and their homocysteine levels were significantly higher than in patients who had stopped smoking (i.e., 18.8 μmol/L vs. 14.1 μmol/L). Homocysteine was not significantly influenced by smoking in the control subjects. Several studies have failed to prove an effect of smoking on homocysteine levels (6, 22), whereas others found a positive correlation (24, 41) (see also Chapter 28). Smoking has been reported to lower vitamin B_6 (32, 38) and folate levels (28) even in healthy subjects. Regression analysis in Bergmark's study, however, showed that these effects on vitamins could not fully explain the effect of smoking on homocysteine levels (2). The authors postulated the "allergy-to-smoke" hypothesis, that is, that some individuals have a low tolerance for smoking because of pathogenic mechanisms induced by smoking. One of these mechanisms could be hyperhomocysteinemia partially mediated by lowering of folate and vitamin

B_6 levels due to tobacco. Smoking therefore seems to be associated with increased homocysteine levels in patients with early atherosclerosis, which may constitute an additional reason for a younger atherosclerotic patient to stop smoking.

Three interventional studies of homocysteine-lowering regimens provided data on the prevalence of hyperhomocysteinemia among patients with symptomatic peripheral vascular disease as well. Dudman et al. (11) found that 3 of 18 patients (17%) were hyperhomocysteinemic after methionine loading. Two Dutch homocysteine-lowering studies (13, 35) reported that 33% of 131 patients and 25% of 143 patients, respectively, had postmethionine loading homocysteine levels more than 2 standard deviations above the mean control level. A regimen of 250 mg vitamin B_6 or 250 mg vitamin B_6 plus 5 mg folic acid daily normalized the pathological hyperhomocysteinemia in 56% and 90% of patients, respectively. The absolute decreases of the mean homocysteine levels in the treated hyperhomocysteinemic vascular patients were 40% and 50%, respectively. These studies showed for the first time in a substantial number of treated patients the possibility of nearly total control of high postmethionine load hyperhomocysteinemia by simple vitamin therapy.

More recently, Cheng et al. (7) established fasting hyperhomocysteinemia above the 90th percentile of the control range in 27% of 100 Hong Kong Chinese with a mean age of 67 years and suffering from symptomatic peripheral arterial insufficiency. The estimated relative risk of peripheral arterial atherosclerosis for such hyperhomocysteinemia was 3.7 ($p < 0.001$), which is comparable to the relative risks of other factors such as smoking, triglycerides, diabetes, and hypertension. Furthermore, the independence of hyperhomocysteinemia from those well-established risk factors was again confirmed.

Within the European Community Concerted Action structure, a large case-control study was designed to establish the strength of the relationship between plasma total homocysteine and vascular disease risk and to explore a possible interaction with conventional risk factors (15). Nineteen centers in nine European countries contributed 750 cases of atherosclerotic vascular disease and 800 control subjects of both sexes younger than 60 years. There were 156 claudicants with proven obstruction of one major peripheral artery to the legs. To provide an outcome with relevance to general health care, hyperhomocysteinemia was defined as a common factor in the normal population. Homocysteine levels in the top fifth of the control distribution, either in the fasting state or after methionine loading, were considered to be pathological. By this criterion, a rather low cutoff point for hyperhomocysteinemia was selected, (i.e., 12 µmol/L for fasting levels and 38 µmol/L for postload values). Hyperhomocysteinemia was identified in 40% of the 156 patients with peripheral arterial disease in the fasting state, and an identical percentage showed pathological postmethionine load levels.

Despite the low cutoff points, a relative risk for peripheral arterial disease of 2.0 (95% confidence interval, 1.2 to 3.1) for fasting hyperhomocysteinemia and 1.5 (1.0 to 2.4) for postload hyperhomocysteinemia was calculated. A higher cutoff set at the 90th percentile led to higher relative risks, such as 5.3 (3.2 to 8.7) for postload hyperhomocysteinemia in the entire group of vascular patients. Even the level of risk calculated at the 80th percentile was equivalent to that for hypercholesterolemia or smoking and did not differ significantly from the risks for other categories of vascular disease, such as coronary heart disease or cerebrovascular disease. Moreover, the risk estimate for hyperhomocysteinemia proved to be independent of the effects of hypercholesterolemia, smoking, and hypertension. However, interaction effects were noted between homocysteine and smoking or hypertension by which the risks associated with these conventional factors were powerfully increased by hyperhomocysteinemia. It seemed conceivable that homocysteine may enhance smoking- or hypertension-related effects on platelets, clotting, or the endothelium. Control of smoking and high blood pressure seemed particularly warranted in subjects with abnormal homocysteine levels.

Meta-Analysis

Boushey et al. (5) conducted a meta-analysis of data relating homocysteine to arteriosclerotic vascular disease in 27 case-control, cross-sectional, or prospective studies published before mid-1994. Nine of the reports being discussed here had been included in their analysis of the specific association with peripheral arterial disease (2, 4, 6, 8, 11, 15, 19, 22, 33). Although published in 1997, the outcome from the European Concerted Action Study (15) could have been incorporated because some of the preliminary data had been reported in 1994 (9, 14). Data on fasting homocysteine values from only three studies (2, 6, 22) were considered suitable for pooling, and the calculated summary odds ratio of fasting hyperhomocysteinemia, as defined in each study, appeared to be 6.8 (95% confidence interval, 2.9 to 15.8) for peripheral arterial disease specifically. Two studies provided estimates of the relative risk of postload hyperhomocysteinemia and these ranged from 5.3 (95% confidence interval, 3.2 to 8.7) to 22.3 (95% confidence interval, 1.9 to infinity) (8, 9, 14). Two other studies could not be used in the calculations because of

their inclusion of an unknown proportion of hyperhomocysteinemic cases with other than peripheral arterial disease (19, 33). Data from two other studies were considered insufficient for estimation of an odds ratio but supported homocysteine as a risk factor for peripheral arterial disease (3, 11). The meta-analysis also concluded that the studies had shown that the effect of homocysteine levels on vascular disease was independent of total cholesterol, low- or high-density cholesterol, diabetes, smoking, body mass index, age, and high blood pressure. Furthermore, although impaired renal function raises homocysteine levels in the blood, homocysteine persisted as a risk factor for vascular disease after adjustment for serum creatinine.

The outcome of this meta-analysis suggested a stronger association of hyperhomocysteinemia with peripheral arterial disease than with cerebrovascular or coronary artery disease. The odds ratios of fasting levels were 6.8 (95% confidence interval, 2.9 to 15.8), 2.3 (1.8 to 2.9), and 1.8 (1.6 to 2.0), respectively. However, the European Concerted Action Study, which contributed the largest group of patients with peripheral arterial disease (n = 156) to the meta-analysis, showed an equally strong association with cerebrovascular disease in 211 patients and with coronary artery disease in 383 patients in its definitive report in 1997 (15). In later studies not included in the meta-analysis, only the data by Franken et al. (13) showed a higher prevalence of hyperhomocysteinemia in patients with peripheral arterial disease compared with cerebrovascular disease (i.e., 33% of 131 vs. 20% of 290 patients). van den Berg et al. (35) found mild hyperhomocysteinemia in 36 of 143 patients with peripheral arterial disease (25%) versus 24 of 86 patients with cerebrovascular disease (28%), and 12 of 80 patients with coronary artery disease (15%). In a recent cross-sectional study of a large 50 to 75-year-old population in the Netherlands (n = 631), the association of hyperhomocysteinemia with cardiovascular disease was comparable to that with peripheral, cerebrovascular, and coronary artery diseases (17).

A rough meta-analysis of the results of all the studies published thus far is listed in Table 32.1. The studies by Malinow et al. (19) and Taylor et al. (33) cannot be incorporated in such an analysis for the reason given in Boushey's previous meta-analysis (5). The remaining data showed that 206 of 762 patients with peripheral arterial disease (27%) had hyperhomocysteinemia versus 101 of 1,386 control subjects (7%). Total homocysteine levels were measured in 429 of the patients and 1,109 of the control subjects in the fasting state, and postmethionine load values were used in the others. The cutoff points for hyperhomocysteinemia, however, varied: seven studies selected the 97.5th percentile (2 standard deviations above the mean), one the 95th percentile, and another the 90th percentile as cutoff points. The data from the European Concerted Action Study originally used an 80th percentile cutoff level but were recalculated for a cutoff level at the 90th percentile (i.e., 13.4 μmol/L) to be more in line with the other studies. A pooled odds ratio as an estimate of relative risk of hyperhomocysteinemia can be calculated by a Mantel-Haenszel method and confidence intervals according to the method of Robins (30). This odds ratio was 5.7 (95% confidence interval, 4.2 to 7.6) and proved to be in line with the summary odds ratio of fasting hyperhomocysteinemia established earlier by Boushey et al. (5) in no more than 173 patients with peripheral arterial disease and 209 control subjects.

Figure 32.1 shows the individual odds ratios in all the studies, except for three in which they could not be calculated because there were no subjects with hyperhomocysteinemia in the control groups. All studies had

point estimates of the odds ratio above 3.3, and the lower limit of the 95% confidence interval was below 1.0 in only one, rather small, study. The test for heterogeneity (16), which had to be restricted to the studies shown in Figure 32.1 for which an odds ratio could be calculated, did not reach significance ($\chi^2 = 3.8$; $p > 0.75$). The distribution of the effect measures in Figure 32.1 also does not point to heterogeneity of effect.

Relationship Between Total Homocysteine Levels and Severity of Atherosclerosis in Patients with Peripheral Arterial Disease

Taylor et al. (33) concluded that patients with hyperhomocysteinemia with symptomatic peripheral arterial disease showed significantly greater clinical progression of their lower extremity atheroclerotic lesions and developed more coronary artery disease, but not more cerebral vascular disease, than patients with normal homocysteine levels. The observed rate of progression of peripheral arterial disease was significantly more rapid in the hyperhomocysteinemic patients, both clinically ($p = 0.002$) and as assessed in the vascular laboratory ($p = 0.01$).

Fig. 32.1. The odds ratios (95% confidence intervals) for elevated total homocysteine levels in individual case-control studies of peripheral arterial disease.

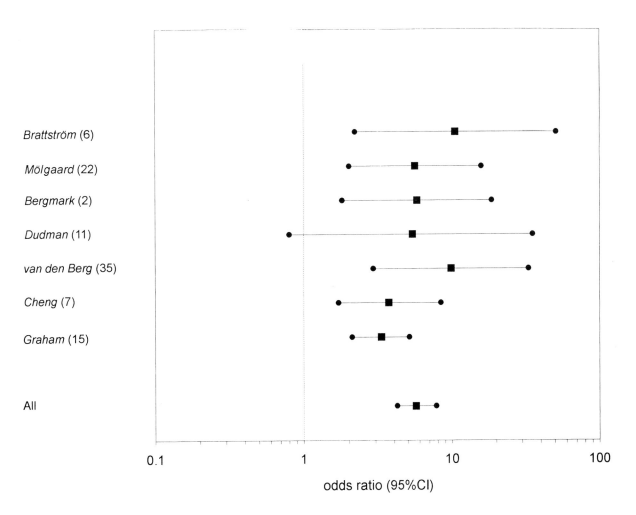

More recently, the same center reported results of a blinded prospective study of the influence of homocysteine levels on the progression of atherosclerotic disease in 351 patients with vascular disease (34). Lower limb disease was present in 296 of the patients (85%), cerebral vascular disease in 124 (35%), and both in 86 (25%). After 3 years of follow-up observation, patients with plasma total homocysteine levels in the upper quintile of the distribution showed more frequent clinical progression of their leg disease than patients with levels in the lowest quintile (i.e., in 15% vs. 7.3%), but the difference was not significant ($p = 0.31$), in contrast with the finding in the earlier retrospective study (33). A significant difference in progression of leg disease, as assessed by the ankle-brachial index, could not be established either. Those patients in the upper quintile, however, had demonstrated significantly greater clinical progression of concomitant coronary artery disease than patients with values in the lowest quintile ($p = 0.0068$). However, there was no difference in the clinical progression of cerebral arterial disease.

In the first 3 years of the follow-up period, deaths from any cause and from cardiovascular disease were significantly more likely in patients with elevated homocysteine levels (i.e., above 14 µmol/L in this study) than in those with lower levels (18.6% vs. 9.4% total deaths and 12.5% vs. 6.3% cardiovascular deaths; $p = 0.02$ and 0.05, respectively). For each 1.0 µmol/L increase of plasma homocysteine, there was a 3.6% increment ($p = 0.06$) in the risk of death from all causes at 3 years and a 5.6% increase ($p = 0.003$) in the risk of death from cardiovascular disease. A similar, graded relationship between increasing levels of homocysteine and mortality was found in Norwegian patients with coronary artery disease (25). The lack of significant differences in progression of lower extremity disease, clinically or measured by the ankle-brachial index, between patients with elevated homocysteine levels and those with normal values could have been due to earlier death in the former group, which may have mitigated detection of nonfatal progression in many cases.

A strong relationship between total homocysteine levels and the prevalence of concomitant coronary artery disease and cerebrovascular disease was reported in 171 Dutch patients with peripheral arterial disease under the age of 55 years (36). Values of homocysteine in the upper quartile showed a significant relative risk of about 3 for such comorbidity versus lower homocysteine levels. The extent of leg disease was defined angiographically, and the prevalence of occlusions at more than one level was significantly increased in the upper quartile of fasting homocysteine concentrations with an odds ratio of

4.0. The composite score for severity of lower limb atherosclerotic disease that was used ("total run-off resistance") also proved to be strongly related to the homocysteine levels, especially after methionine loading ($r = 0.25$, $p = 0.003$). These robust associations were independent of the classic risk factors for atherosclerosis.

These findings were in line with the earlier report by Bergmark et al. (2), who found the highest homocysteine levels in the subgroup of patients with multilevel disease among 58 patients suffering from peripheral arterial disease. Cheng et al. (7) in their study of 100 patients with intermittent claudication at the relatively old mean age of 67 years, compared patients with homocysteine values above 34 µmol/L (i.e., the 90th percentile of their control range) and lower concentrations. They could not confirm a significant differences either in disease pattern in the leg arteries or severity of claudication symptoms.

Thus, the literature to date indicates, albeit without unequivocal proof, a dose-response relationship between homocysteine levels and severity of peripheral arterial disease in affected patients. A similarly graded effect of increasing total homocysteine levels has been postulated in coronary disease (1, 5, 15, 21, 25, 26, 39), carotid artery intimal-medial thickening (20, 31), and stroke (27). Extended evidence of a dose-response relationship would help prove that hyperhomocysteinemia is indeed causally associated with atherosclerotic disease.

Current Status of the Evidence

Overall, the association between mild or moderate hyperhomocysteinemia and peripheral arterial disease appears to have been documented far less intensively than the association with coronary heart disease. Not more than 12 reports are available, all case-controlled and predominantly retrospective studies. Moreover, data from two studies (19, 33) are of limited value owing to the inclusion of an unknown proportion of hyperhomocysteinemic patients with other vascular disorders. Nevertheless, it can be concluded that of 762 patients with peripheral arterial disease pooled from the remaining 10 studies, 27% had hyperhomocysteinemia, in contrast with only 7% of 1,386 control subjects. A substantial pooled odds ratio of 5.7 for hyperhomocysteinemia can be calculated, which is in line with the odds ratio calculated in an earlier meta-analysis by Boushey et al. (5). The distribution of individual odds ratios of the seven studies in which these could be assessed suggests homogeneity of the effect (Figure 32.1).

Admittedly, calculations and conclusions from the pooled data are rather crude because the designs of the studies differed in important ways, such as definitions of hyperhomocysteinemia and use of fasting versus methionine-loaded homocysteine measurements. Notwithstanding these limitations, the conclusion that a robust association exists between hyperhomocysteinemia and peripheral arterial disease seems justified. This association proved to be independent of the presence of conventional risk factors for peripheral vascular disease such as hyperlipidemia, smoking, hypertension, and diabetes. The strength of those independent risk factors was comparable to that of hyperhomocysteinemia. Of interest, some studies detected a synergistic effect between hyperhomocysteinemia and smoking (2, 15) or hypertension (15).

The literature suggests, but does not yet prove solidly, a graded relationship between homocysteine levels in patients with peripheral arterial disease and severity of their leg abnormalities, as well as with signs of more generalized atherosclerosis. Such a dose-response relationship, previously shown in coronary and cerebrovascular disease, supports causality of hyperhomocysteinemia as a risk factor for vascular disease. Important and perhaps conclusive proof should be provided by the clinical homocysteine-lowering intervention studies now under way. Worldwide, trials involving about 60,000 patients with coronary artery or cerebrovascular disease are being undertaken. However, only one interventional study in about 350 patients with peripheral arterial disease with a follow-up period of 5 years has been announced (34). The latter entails a double-blinded, placebo-controlled trial of 4 mg folic acid daily. More extended clinical trials are needed for mild hyperhomocysteinemia to rank with conventional causal risk factors for peripheral arterial disease.

REFERENCES

1. Arnesen, E, Refsum, H, Ueland, PM, Forde, OH, Nordrehaug, JE. Serum total homocysteine and coronary heart disease. *Int J Epidemiol* 1995; 24: 704–9.
2. Bergmark, C, Mansoor, MA, Swedenborg, J, de Faire, U, Svardal, AM, Ueland, PM. Hyperhomocysteinemia in patients operated for lower extremity ischaemia below the age of 50. Effect of smoking and extent of disease. *Eur J Vasc Surg* 1993; 7: 391–96.
3. Boers, G, Smals, A, Trijbels, J, Kloppenborg, P. Homocystinuria in heterozygous form as a risk factor of premature arteriosclerosis. *Eur J Clin Invest* 1984; 14: no 2-II: 9.
4. Boers, GHJ, Smals, AGH, Trijbels, FJM, Fowler, B, Bakkeren, JA, Schoonderwaldt, HC, Kleijer, WJ. Heterozygosity for homocystinuria in premature peripheral and cerebral occlusive arterial disease. *N Engl J Med* 1985; 313: 709–15.
5. Boushey, CJ, Beresford, SAA, Omenn, GS, Motulsky, AG. A quantitative assessment of plasma homocysteine as a risk factor for vascular disease. *JAMA* 1995; 274: 1049–57.
6. Brattström, L, Israelsson, B, Norrving, B, Bergqvist, D, Thorne, J, Hultberg, B, Hamfelt, A. Impaired homocysteine metabolism in early-onset cerebral and peripheral occlusive arterial disease. *Atherosclerosis* 1990; 81: 51–60.
7. Cheng, SWK, Ting, ACW, Wong, J. Fasting total plasma homocysteine and atherosclerotic peripheral vascular disease. *Ann Vasc Surg* 1997; 11: 217–23.
8. Clarke, R, Daly, L, Robinson, K, Naughten, E, Cahalane, S, Fowler, B, Graham, I. Hyperhomocysteinemia: An independent risk factor for vascular disease. *N Engl J Med* 1991; 324: 1149–55.
9. Daly, L, Graham, I. Hyperhomocysteinaemia: A powerful risk factor for vascular disease. Presented at the Annual Scientific Meeting Working Group, Epidemiology and Prevention; April 25, 1994; Venice, Italy.
10. Dormandy, J, Mahir, M, Ascady, G, Balsano, F, De Leeuw, P, Blombery, P, Bousser, MG, Clement, D, Coffman, J, Deutshinoff, A. Fate of the patient with chronic leg ischaemia. *J Cardiovasc Surg* 1989; 30: 50–7.
11. Dudman, NPB, Wilcken, DEL, Wang, J, Lynch, JF, Macey, D, Lundberg, P. Disordered methionine/homocysteine metabolism in premature vascular disease. Its occurrence, cofactor therapy, and enzymology. *Arterioscler Thromb* 1993; 13: 1253–60.
12. Fowkes, FGR, Housley, E, Cawood, EHH, Macintyre, CC, Ruckley, CV, Prescott, RJ. Edinburgh Artery Study: prevalence of asymptomatic and symptomatic peripheral arterial disease in the general population. *Int J Epidemiol* 1991; 20: 384–92.
13. Franken, DG, Boers, GHJ, Blom, HJ, Trijbels, FJM, Kloppenborg, PWC. Treatment of mild hyperhomocysteinemia in vascular disease patients. *Arterioscler Thromb* 1994; 14: 465–70.
14. Graham, I. Interactions between homocysteinaemia and conventional risk factor in vascular disease. *Eur Heart J* 1994; 15 (suppl): 530.
15. Graham, IM, Daly, LE, Refsum, HM, Robinson, K, Brattström, LE, Ueland, PM, Palma-Reis, RJ, Boers, GH, Sheahan, RG, Israelsson, B, Uiterwaal, CS, Meleady, R, McMaster, D, Verhoef, P, Witteman, J, Rubba, P, Bellet, H, Wautrecht, JC, de Valk, HW, Sales Luis, AC, Parrot-Rouland, FM, Tan, KS, Higgins, I, Garcon, D, Andria, G. Plasma homocysteine as a risk factor for vascular disease. *JAMA* 1997; 277: 1775–81.
16. Greenland, S. Quantitative methods in the review of epidemiologic literature. *Epidemiol Rev* 1987; 9: 1–30.
17. Hoogeveen, EK, Kostense, PJ, Beks, PJ, Mackaay, AJ, Jakobs, C, Bouter, LM, Heine, RJ, Stehouwer, CD. Hyperhomocysteinemia is associated with an increased risk of cardiovascular disease, especially in non-insulin-dependent diabetes mellitus: a population-based study. *Arterioscler Thromb Vasc Biol* 1998; 18: 133–38.
18. Kannel, WB, Skinner, JJ, Schwartz, MJ, Shurtleff, D. Intermittent claudication incidence in the Framingham study. *Circulation* 1970; 41: 875–83.
19. Malinow, MR, Kang, SS, Taylor, LM, Wong, PWK, Coull, B, Inahara, T, Mukerjee, D, Sexton, G, Upson, B. Prevalence of hyperhomocyst(e)inemia in patients with

peripheral arterial occlusive disease. *Circulation* 1989; 79: 1180–88.

20. Malinow, MR, Nieto, FJ, Szklo, M, Chambless, LE, Bond, G. Carotid artery intimal-medial wall thickening and plasma homocyst(e)ine in asymptomatic adults. *Circulation* 1993; 87: 1107–13.

21. Malinow, MR, Ducimetiere, P, Luc, G, Evans, AE, Arveiler, D, Cambien, F, Upson, BM. Plasma homocyst(e)ine levels and graded risk for myocardial infarction: findings in two populations at contrasting risk for coronary heart disease. *Atherosclerosis* 1996; 126: 27–34.

22. Mölgaard, J, Malinow, MR, Lassvik, C, Holm, AC, Upson, B, Olsson, AG. Hyperhomocyst(e)inaemia: An independent risk factor for intermittent claudication. *J Intern Med* 1992; 231: 273–79.

23. Müller-Bühl, U, Diehm, C, Sieben, U, Berger, B, Schuler, G, Zimmermann, R, Scheuermann, W, Heuck, CC, Morl, H, Kubler, W. Prävalenz und Risikofaktoren von peripherer-arterieller Verschlusskrankheit und koronarer Herzkrankheit. *Vasa* 1987; 16 Suppl 21: 1–46.

24. Nygård, O, Vollset, SE, Refsum, H, Stensvold, I, Tverdal, A, Nordrehaug, JE, Ueland, PM, Kvale, G. Total plasma homocysteine and cardiovascular risk profile. Hordaland Homocysteine Study. *JAMA* 1995; 274: 1526–33.

25. Nygård, O, Nordrehaug, JE, Refsum, H, Ueland, PM, Farstad, M, Vollset, SE. Plasma homocysteine levels and mortality in patients with coronary artery disease. *N Engl J Med* 1997; 337: 230–6.

26. Pancharuniti, N, Lewis, CA, Sauberlich, HE, Perkins, LL, Go, RC, Alvarez, JO, Macaluso, M, Acton, RT, Copeland, RB, Cousins, AL. Plasma homocyst(e)ine, folate, and vitamin B12 concentrations and risk of early-onset coronary artery disease. *Am J Clin Nutr* 1994; 59: 940–48.

27. Perry, IJ, Refsum, H, Morris, RW, Ebrahim, SB, Ueland, PM, Shaper, AG. Prospective study of serum total homocysteine concentration and risk of stroke in middle-aged British men. *Lancet* 1995; 346: 1395–98.

28. Piyathilake, CJ, Hine, RJ, Dasanayake, AP, Richards, EW, Freeberg, LE, Vaughn, WH, Krumdieck, CL. Effect of smoking on folate levels in buccal mucosal cells. *Int J Cancer* 1992; 52: 566–69.

29. Rose, GA, Blackburn, H. *Cardiovascular Survey Methods.* World Health Organization, Geneva, Monograph Series No. 56, 1982.

30. Rothman, KJ. *Modern Epidemiology.* Little Brown, Boston/Toronto, 1986.

31. Selhub, J, Jacques, P, Bostom, AG, D'Agostino, RB, Wilson, PW, Belanger, AJ, O'Leary, DH, Wolf, PA, Schaefer, EJ, Rosenberg, IH. Association between plasma homocysteine concentrations and extracranial carotid-artery stenosis. *N Engl J Med* 1995; 332: 286–91.

32. Serfontein, W, Ubbink, J, De Villiers, L, Becker, P. Depressed plasma pyridoxal-5′-phosphate levels in tobacco-smoking men. *Atherosclerosis* 1986; 59: 341–46.

33. Taylor, LM, DeFrang, RD, Harris, EJ, Porter, JM. The association of elevated plasma homocyst(e)ine with progression of symptomatic peripheral arterial disease. *J Vasc Surg* 1991; 13: 128–36.

34. Taylor, LM, Moneta, GL, Sexton, GJ, Schuff, RA, Porter, JM. Prospective blinded study of the relationship between plasma homocysteine and progression of symptomatic peripheral arterial disease. *J Vasc Surg* 1999; 29: 8–21.

35. van den Berg, M, Franken, DG, Boers, GHJ, Blom, HJ, Jakobs, C, Stehouwer, CD, Rauwerda, JA. Combined vitamin B6 plus folic acid therapy in young patients with arteriosclerosis and hyperhomocysteinaemia. *J Vasc Surg* 1994; 20: 933–40.

36. van den Berg, M, Stehouwer, CDA, Bierdrager, E, Rauwerda, JA. Plasma homocysteine and severity of atherosclerosis in young patients with lower-limb atherosclerotic disease. *Arterioscler Thromb Vasc Biol* 1996; 16: 165–71.

37. Verhaeghe, R. Epidémiologie et pronostic de l'artériopathie oblitérante des membres inférieurs. *Drugs* 1998; 56 (Suppl. 3): 1–10.

38. Vermaak, WJ, Ubbink, JB, Barnard, HC, Potgieter, GM, van Jaarsveld, H, Groenewald, AJ. Vitamin B-6 nutrition status and cigarette smoking. *Am J Clin Nutr* 1990; 51: 1058–61.

39. von Eckardstein, A, Malinow, MR, Upson, B, Heinrich, J, Schulte, H, Schonfeld, R, Kohler, E, Assmann, G. Effects of age, lipoproteins, and hemostatic parameters on the role of homocyst(e)inemia as a cardiovascular risk factor in men. *Arterioscler Thromb* 1994; 14: 460–64.

40. Wilcken, DEL, Wilcken, B. The pathogenesis of artery disease: A possible role for methionine metabolism. *J Clin Invest* 1976; 57: 1079–82.

41. Williams, R, Malinow, MR, Hunt, SC, Upson, B, Wu, LL, Hopkins, PN, Stults, BN, Kuida, H. Hyperhomocysteinemia in Utah siblings with coronary disease. *Coron Artery Dis* 1990; 1: 681–85.

33

Venous Disease

ARMANDO D'ANGELO
CHIARA BELTRAMETTI

The venous thrombophilic state is characterized clinically by the occurrence of recurrent thrombosis, thrombosis occurring at a young age, idiopathic thrombosis, thrombosis after trivial provocation, and thrombosis in an unusual site (46). The predisposing biochemical abnormalities include congenital and acquired defects.

The earliest described congenital defects (deficiencies of antithrombin, protein C, and protein S) contributed a high risk of thrombotic events but were rare, thus explaining only a small part of the thrombophilic diathesis. The setting changed dramatically with the discovery of the factor V Leiden mutation, which is responsible for more than 90% of cases of the activated protein C resistance phenomenon,[1] and the prothrombin 20210G→A mutation. These two defects have a high prevalence, especially in the European population. Although they contribute a relatively moderate thrombotic risk (odds ratios between 2 and 6), they explain a large part of the thrombophilic state (54, 55). In addition, the discovery of common congenital defects has permitted the epidemiological evaluation of the thrombotic risk conferred by their coexistence in the same individual, which often produces a synergistic effect

---

[1] Because activated protein C resistance occasionally is not due to the factor V Leiden mutation, the two terms will be used separately depending on the study.

(77). In most cases, there is a close association between the genotype and the phenotype, which is consistently expressed in either the heterozygous or the homozygous state. Homozygosity implies a higher thrombotic risk, with the occurrence of thrombotic manifestations in infancy and the appearance of skin necrosis (54, 55). Acquired conditions predisposing to thrombosis in most instances have an autoimmune pathogenesis (20, 38, 39). In these cases, there is no familial history of thrombosis, and treatment may represent a serious problem (5, 18, 24, 48). With the exception of lupus anticoagulant antibodies, which are also implicated in arterial thrombosis, all the preceding abnormalities predispose largely to venous thromboembolic diseases.

Venous thromboembolism accounts for 50% of the vascular complications of congenital homocystinuria (64), but the potential involvement of less severe hyperhomocysteinemia in venous thromboembolic disease was overlooked until recently. Many homocystinuric patients with homozygous and/or compound heterozygous cystathionine β-synthase deficiency respond to the administration of vitamin B_6 (63). In most instances, the treatment transforms their severe hyperhomocysteinemia into moderate or mild hyperhomocysteinemia. Although the effectiveness of vitamin B_6 in preventing thromboembolism in pyridoxine-responsive patients was significant, the occurrence of thromboembolism was not abolished by vitamin supplementation; the chance of having a clinically detected thromboembolic event by the age of 15 years was 27% for pyridoxine-unresponsive individuals and 12% for pyridoxine-responsive individuals (63).

The natural history of homocystinuria had already set the stage for the recognition of hyperhomocysteinemia as a congenital thrombophilic diathesis (both arterial and venous), with a thrombotic risk that paralleled the plasma total homocysteine levels. Epidemiological evidence indicates a clear association of moderate hyperhomocysteinemia with venous thromboembolic diseases (21, 22, 68, 75, 76, 82). If there are doubts about a causal link (12), these reflect our relatively modest knowledge of the gene-environment interaction in the phenotypic expression of hyperhomocysteinemia and the uncertainty about the thrombogenic mechanisms of hyperhomocysteinemia (see Chapter 34).

Moderate Fasting Hyperhomocysteinemia and Venous Thromboembolic Disease

Brattström et al. (9) found no significant differences in plasma homocysteine concentrations between 42

patients with venous thromboembolism and healthy control subjects, although male patients showed a tendency to higher plasma homocysteine than male control subjects. Similarly, Amundsen et al. (2) studied 35 patients less than 56 years old with verified deep vein thrombosis and found no difference in fasting plasma homocysteine levels compared with age- and sex-matched healthy control subjects. However, the number of patients evaluated in these studies was relatively small. For the results to be statistically significant, crude odds ratios for hyperhomocysteinemia should have been > 5.0, which, based on the prevalence in control subjects, would have required frequencies of hyperhomocysteinemia between 20% and 30% in patients with venous thromboembolism. Such a high frequency was reported only in a single small series of patients who developed venous thrombosis before the age of 60 years (6).

Falcon et al. (36) studied 80 patients who had at least one verified episode of venous thromboembolism before the age of 40 years and were free of known predisposing hemostatic abnormalities. Fasting hyperhomocysteinemia was found in 8.8% of the patients and in none of the control subjects.

In a cross-sectional, 2-year evaluation of 157 consecutive, unrelated, cancer-free patients with a history of venous or arterial occlusive disease occurring before the age of 45 years or at unusual sites, moderate fasting hyperhomocysteinemia was detected in 9.3% and 8.0% of patients with venous and arterial diseases, respectively (37). Hyperhomocysteinemia was identified in 8 of 12 families, in agreement with Falcon et al. (36), who found a history of thrombosis and familial hyperhomocysteinemia in more than 50% of their families. Thrombophilic defects (deficiencies of protein C, protein S, and plasminogen and activated protein C resistance) were detected only in patients with venous occlusive disease, with an overall prevalence of 18.7%. After adjusting for circumstantial factors predisposing to thromboembolism (e.g., use of contraceptive drugs, pregnancy, surgery, prolonged bed rest) and for a family history of thrombosis, the age at first event for patients with moderate hyperhomocysteinemia was similar to that of patients with thrombophilic defects—mainly activated protein C resistance—and significantly lower than that of patients without defects (25.5 years vs. 31.0 years). Accordingly, event-free survival analysis showed that the relative risk for occlusive diseases in patients with moderate hyperhomocysteinemia or with the other defects was 1.7 times greater (95% confidence interval: 1.19 to 2.42)[2] than in patients without defects (37).

We have extended our cross-sectional observation of patients with early-onset venous thromboembolic dis-

eases to include 427 patients aged 44 ± 16.6 years and 298 control subjects aged 41.4 ± 15.8 years (23). Events included deep vein thrombosis and/or pulmonary embolism, thrombosis of the superficial veins, and venous thrombosis occurring at unusual sites, such as cerebral veins, central retinal veins, and internal veins. The prevalence of fasting hyperhomocysteinemia in patients and control subjects was 15.0% and 6.4%, respectively, with a crude odds ratio of 2.59 (1.47 to 4.59). After adjusting for sex and age, the relative risk contributed by moderate hyperhomocysteinemia was similar across the different sites of thromboembolism, irrespective of the presence of circumstantial risk factors. After excluding patients with other thrombophilic defects, the relative risk contributed by hyperhomocysteinemia was 3.18 (1.70 to 5.47). The risk of thrombosis increased from 1.8 for total homocysteine levels between the 95th and 97.5th percentile of the distribution in control subjects to 6.8 for total homocysteine levels exceeding the 99th percentile (23). These data strongly support the role of moderate and possibly familial (40) hyperhomocysteinemia in the development of premature venous thromboembolic disease.

High plasma homocysteine levels are also a risk factor for deep vein thrombosis in the general population. Fasting homocysteine concentrations were measured in 269 patients younger than 70 years old with no known cancer and a first episode of deep vein thrombosis (30). Hyperhomocysteinemia exceeding the 95th percentile of the matched control group was found in 10% of patients, with an odds ratio of 2.4 (1.17 to 5.02). The risk of thrombosis did not increase among subjects with homocysteine levels up to 18 μmol/L, but it was greatly increased above 22 μmol/L, suggesting a threshold effect rather than a continuous dose-response relation. The effect of hyperhomocysteinemia was independent of other risk factors for thrombosis, including protein C, protein S and antithrombin deficiencies, and the factor V Leiden mutation. Although the risk of thrombosis associated with hyperhomocysteinemia increased sharply in both sexes at increasing ages, the association was much stronger among women than among men. When calculating the 95th percentile of the distribution of homocysteine levels for control women (17.1 μmol/L) and men (20.0 μmol/L) separately, odds ratios for thrombosis were 3.8 (1.4 to 10.8) for women and 1.8 (0.6 to 5.4) for men (30). Because nutritional markers were not evaluated, it cannot be ruled out that vitamin status differences explain the stronger association observed in women.

That hyperhomocysteinemia is also associated with an increased risk of venous thromboembolism in men was shown in a prospective, nested, case-control study involving 14,916 apparently healthy men who provided baseline plasma samples and were prospectively moni-

---

[2] All relative risks and odds ratios are followed by 95% confidence intervals shown in parentheses.

tored for about 12 years (69). A total of 145 subjects who developed deep vein thrombosis or pulmonary embolism and had baseline plasma samples analyzed were matched with 646 subjects who remained free of vascular disease during the follow-up period. Venous thromboembolism was idiopathic in 73 subjects (50.3%) and was associated with cancer, recent surgery, or trauma in the others. Hyperhomocysteinemia, defined as total homocysteine levels exceeding the 95th percentile of the study distribution, was significantly associated with an increased risk of idiopathic venous thromboembolism (relative risk = 3.38; 1.6 to 7.3) but not all venous thromboembolism (relative risk = 1.58; 0.8 to 3.3). In comparison, the factor V Leiden mutation was associated with an increased risk of developing both (relative risks of 2.3 and 3.6, respectively). The crude relative risk of idiopathic thromboembolism increased from 0.77 (0.5 to 1.3) for homocysteine levels >10.1 μmol/L (50th percentile) to 1.64 (0.8 to 3.3) for levels >15.0 μmol/L (90th percentile) (69).

Simioni et al. (78) determined fasting levels in 208 consecutive outpatients who underwent phlebography because of a first episode of clinically suspected deep vein thrombosis of the legs, had no deficiencies of antithrombin, protein C, and protein S, and did not have activated protein C resistance, lupus anticoagulants, or active cancer. Thrombosis was diagnosed in 29% of the patients. Homocysteine levels greater than 18.5 μmol/L were detected in 25% of patients with thrombosis and in 11.5% of subjects without thrombosis (odds ratio = 2.6; 1.1 to 5.9). The prevalence of

hyperhomocysteinemia was slightly, but not significantly, higher in patients with idiopathic thrombosis than with deep vein thrombosis secondary to recent trauma or surgery, prolonged immobilization, estrogen pill use, or delivery.

Table 33.1 shows unadjusted odds ratios for moderate fasting hyperhomocysteinemia as a risk factor for venous thromboembolism. By pooling data from 11 studies, including 1,473 patients and 1,842 control subjects, an unadjusted odds ratio of 3.16 (2.44 to 4.10) can be estimated for moderate fasting hyperhomocysteinemia as a risk factor. This odds ratio is not different from the 2.5 (1.8 to 3.5) reported in a meta-analysis (32) of eight of the studies shown in Table 33.1. The issue of whether fasting hyperhomocysteinemia should or should not be considered a graded risk factor for thrombosis remains controversial, because some studies showed a clear trend for an increasing risk within the range of physiological total homocysteine concentrations.

Methionine Intolerance and Venous Thromboembolic Disease

Based on studies in vitamin-deficient animal models (reviewed in Selhub and D'Angelo [76]), fasting hyperhomocysteinemia is thought to reflect an impairment in the remethylation pathway resulting from inadequate status of either folate or cobalamin or to defects in the gene encoding for 5,10-methylenetetrahydrofo-

Table 33.1. Moderate Fasting Hyperhomocysteinemia and the Risk of Venous Thromboembolism

Author (ref)	tHcy Cut-off Value (μmol/L) Women/Men	High Fasting tHcy in Patients with Venous Thromboembolism		High Fasting tHcy in Controls		Odds Ratio (Crude)	95% Confidence Interval
		n/total n	%	n/total n	%		
Brattström et al., 1991 (9)	15.7/17.2	4/42	9.5	3/42	7.1	1.33	0.24–8.38
Ridker et al., 1997 (69)	–/17.3	10/145	6.9	29/646	4.5	1.58	0.70–3.47
Cattaneo et al., 1996 (13)	18.8	7/89	7.9	4/89	4.5	1.81	0.45–7.71
Fermo et al., 1995 (37)	15.0/19.5	10/107	9.3	3/60	5.0	1.96	0.47–12.7
Amundsen et al., 1995 (2)	15.5	2/35	5.7	1/39	2.5	2.30	0–∞
den Heijer et al., 1996 (30)	18.5	28/269	10.4	13/282	4.8	2.40	1.17–5.02
Simioni et al., 1996 (78)	18.5	15/60	25.0	17/148	11.5	2.57	1.11–5.95
D'Angelo et al., 1998 (23)	15.0/19.5	64/427	15.0	19/298	6.4	2.59	1.47–4.59
Bozic et al., 1998 (8)	11.8	22/157	14.0	6/138	4.4	3.59	1.32–10.2
Falcon et al., 1994 (36)	12.1	7/80	8.8	0/51	0	∞	0.57–61.1
Bienvenue et al., 1993 (6)	14.1	7/23	30.4	0/49	0	∞	2.26–138
All studies		216/1,474	14.7	95/1,842	5.2	3.16	2.44–4.10

tHcy, total homocysteine.

late reductase (MTHFR) (74). In contrast, mild impairment in the transsulfuration pathway will lead, at most, to a very slight increase in fasting homocysteine levels. This mild impairment, which may be due to heterozygous defects in the cystathionine β-synthase gene or inadequate levels of vitamin B_6, is normally identified by an abnormal increase in plasma homocysteine after a methionine loading test or a meal (61, 62, 74) (see Chapter 19).

Relatively few studies have evaluated postmethionine load total homocysteine levels in patients with venous thromboembolism. However, the accumulated evidence strongly suggests an increased risk of venous thromboembolic diseases in postmethionine load hyperhomocysteinemia (Table 33.2). Brattström et al. (9) found a higher prevalence of hyperhomocysteinemia in patients less than 50 years of age after a methionine load (odds ratio = 3.3) than in fasting conditions (odds ratio = 1.37). Two studies observed a significant association of elevated postmethionine load total homocysteine levels with venous thromboembolism (36, 37). However, others found no difference in the thrombotic risk conferred by either fasting or postmethionine load hyperhomocysteinemia (2, 13).

Although the available evidence does suggest that the thrombotic risk conferred by postmethionine load hyperhomocysteinemia is at least similar to that of fasting hyperhomocysteinemia, translation of these results into clinical practice is not straightforward. In the first place, patients defined as hyperhomocysteinemic based on absolute postmethionine load total homocysteine levels may differ from those patients defined on the basis of an abnormally great increment of postmethionine load levels over fasting levels (13, 21, 22). In the study of den Heijer et al. (29) 27 of the 46 patients with fasting hyperhomocysteinemia also had postload hyperhomocysteinemia, whereas 17 patients had isolated methionine intolerance. Hence, the overall prevalence of hyperhomocysteinemia in this patient population was 34.1%, possibly contributing a greater thrombotic risk than that reported by the authors for increased fasting (25.0%) and postmethionine load (24.0%) total homocysteine levels (see later). In a case-control study of 263 patients with early-onset venous thromboembolism or with venous thrombosis occurring at unusual sites (23), methionine intolerance—defined as an abnormally great difference between postmethionine load and fasting total homocysteine levels—was significantly associated with an increased risk of venous thromboembolism after adjusting for sex and age (odds ratio = 3.13; 1.35 to 7.28) in the absence of coexisting fasting hyperhomocysteinemia. Because the latter (in the absence or in the presence of methionine intolerance) provided an independent risk for venous thromboembolism (odds ratio = 2.62; 1.47 to 4.67), the odds ratio for venous thromboembolism in any form of hyperhomocysteinemia amounted to 4.60 (2.13 to 9.95). These data strongly

Table 33.2   Methionine Intolerance and the Risk of Venous Thromboembolism

Author (Ref)	PML/ΔPML (Time PML)[a]	tHcy Cutoff Value (μmol/L) Women/Men	Methionine Intolerance in Patients with Venous Thromboembolism		Methionine Intolerance in Control Subjects		Odds Ratio (Crude)	95% Confidence Interval
			n/total n	%	n/total n	%		
Amundsen et al., 1995 (2)	PML (6 hrs)	65.6	2/35	5.7	1/39	2.5	2.30	0–∞
den Heijer et al., 1995 (29)	PML (6 hrs)	58.8	44/185	23.8	20/220	9.1	3.12	1.70–5.75
Brattström et al., 1991 (9)	ΔPML (4 hrs)	36.4/30.6	6/42	14.3	2/42	4.8	3.33	0.55–27.7
Falcon et al., 1994 (36)	ΔPML (4 hrs)	15.1	14/79	17.7	1/40	2.5	8.40	1.08–63.0
Fermo et al., 1995 (37)	ΔPML (8 hrs)	30.0/35.0	11/58	19.0	3/60	5.0	4.45	1.06–18.4
Cattaneo et al., 1996 (13)	ΔPML (4 hrs)	29.9	7/89	7.9	4/89	4.5	1.81	0.45–7.71
D'Angelo et al., 1998 (23)	ΔPML (8 hrs)	30.0/35.0	33/263	12.6	8/143	5.6	2.42	1.03–5.87
PML studies			46/220	20.9	21/259	8.1	3.00	1.67–5.40
ΔPML studies			71/531	13.4	18/374	4.8	3.05	1.74–5.41
All the studies			127/761	16.7	39/633	6.2	3.05	2.06–4.52

tHcy = total homocysteine
[a] PML = absolute postmethionine load total homocysteine level; ΔPML = post-methionine load increment in total homocysteine over the fasting level; time PML = time interval between the oral methionine load and blood sampling.

indicate that, irrespective of the biochemical defects underlying fasting versus postmethionine load hyperhomocysteinemia (74), postload increments identify a greater number of hyperhomocysteinemic patients than do absolute total homocysteine levels (12).

Additional, potentially confounding factors in the interpretation of postmethionine load homocysteine levels are represented by the time of sampling after the oral methionine load, which is not consistent across the studies (Table 33.2), and by loading with L-methionine or with D,L-methionine (see Chapter 19).

Moderate Hyperhomocysteinemia and Recurrent Venous Thromboembolism

Fermo et al. (37) made the interesting observation that patients with mild hyperhomocysteinemia (either fasting or postmethionine load) had a recurrence rate twofold higher than those without defects (52% vs. 25%). A retrospective study measured plasma homocysteine concentrations before and after oral methionine loading in 185 patients with a history of recurrent venous thrombosis and 220 control subjects (29). Hyperhomocysteinemia, defined by a fasting or postmethionine value greater than that found for the 90th percentile of the control subjects, was observed in 25% (fasting) and 24% (postload) of patients. After adjustment for age, sex, and menopausal status, the odds ratios for fasting and postmethionine hyperhomocysteinemia were 2.0 (1.5 to 2.7) and 2.6 (1.9 to 3.5), respectively, leading to the conclusion that 17% of recurrent episodes of venous thrombosis may be due to hyperhomocysteinemia.

That moderate fasting hyperhomocysteinemia is a risk factor for recurrent venous thromboembolism after an originally idiopathic thrombosis was recently shown in a prospective study in Austria (35). The study included consecutive patients older than 18 years who had been treated with oral anticoagulants for at least 3 months after an objectively documented first episode of idiopathic deep vein thrombosis and/or pulmonary embolism. Of the 668 patients enrolled over 5 years, 404 were excluded because thromboembolism had occurred in association with circumstantial, congenital or acquired risk factors, or because patients required long-term anticoagulation for reasons other than venous thromboembolism. The diagnosis of recurrent venous thromboembolism was based on venography and/or a perfusion/ventilation lung scan. Of the remaining 264 patients, 25% had homocysteine levels above the 95th percentile (8.8 μmol/L in females, 11.6 μmol/L in males) of a control population. After discontinuation of oral anticoagulant therapy, 18.2% of patients with hyperhomocysteinemia and 8.1% of patients without hyperhomocysteinemia had recurrent deep vein thrombosis and/or pulmonary embolism. Probabilities of recurrence at 12 and 24 months were 12.6% and 19.2% in hyperhomocysteinemic patients and 3.5% and 6.3% in normohomocysteinemic patients (relative risk = 2.7; 1.3 to 5.8). In addition, the mean time until recurrence of venous thromboembolism was significantly shorter in patients with hyperhomocysteinemia (8.1 ± 8.6 months) than in the remaining patients (16.1 ± 9.9 months). Hyperhomocysteinemia remained an independent risk factor of recurrent venous thromboembolism after adjustment for age, sex, and factor V Leiden (relative risk = 2.6; 1.1 to 6.1). However, because 3 of 16 patients (19%) with a combination of factor V Leiden and hyperhomocysteinemia developed recurrent venous thromboembolism, this study does not rule out the possibility that presence of the two defects may actually increase the risk of recurrence (see later).

Because substantial normalization of elevated homocysteine levels is achieved by multivitamin treatment of patients with venous thromboembolism (31), two studies are currently underway in Europe to evaluate the effect of vitamin administration on the recurrence rate of venous thrombosis in patients with moderate hyperhomocysteinemia. The results may answer the question of the causal link between moderate hyperhomocysteinemia and venous thromboembolic diseases.

Gene Abnormalities and the Risk of Venous Thromboembolic Disease

In their study of hyperhomocysteinemia as a risk factor for recurrent venous thromboembolism, den Heijer et al. (29) observed higher folate and cobalamin levels in patients than in control subjects, despite lower use of vitamin supplements. In studies of patients with premature venous thromboembolic diseases (36, 37), excess hyperhomocysteinemia was again not explained on the basis of vitamin deficiency. Notwithstanding the importance of micronutrient status in hyperhomocysteinemia, this implicates possible gene abnormalities responsible for coding defective enzymes involved in homocysteine metabolism.

In 1988, Kang et al. (47) reported a thermolabile variant of MTHFR, later shown to be due to a homozygous 677C→T point mutation (41) (see Chapter 22). Because of the high frequency of this polymorphism in subjects of Caucasian descent (5% to 20%), MTHFR thermolability was initially thought to explain the hyperhomocysteinemia of patients with occlusive vascular disease (41, 49, 50). However, a meta-analysis of 13 studies (10) revealed no difference between patients and control subjects in either the allele frequency or the frequency of mutant homozygotes. The apparent paradox that the 677C→T genotype, a strong predictor of hyperhomocysteinemia in the general population (41, 43, 44), is not unequivocally associated with increased vascular risk has led to questioning of a causative role for hyperhomocysteinemia in the development of thrombotic events (12).

After an initial report in a small series of patients with premature venous and/or arterial thrombosis (26), MTHFR thermolability has been extensively investigated as a risk factor for venous thromboembolism (Table 33.3). In 5 studies where the mutant MTHFR was found to be a significant risk factor for venous thromboembolism, the prevalence of the homozygous variant in control subjects (4.1% to 18.1%) did not differ from that of 10 studies that had substantially negative results (8.0% to 22.7%). Pooling of the data from 3,190 venous thromboembolism patients and 4,438 control subjects (Table 33.3) results in an unadjusted odds ratio of 1.11 (0.98 to 1.27).

Although this finding may still be consistent with a small thrombotic risk contributed by the MTHFR gene abnormality, it opens the way to alternative possibilities. Kluijtmans et al. (53) raised the question of whether homocysteine itself, rather than another metabolite related to homocysteine metabolism, is the prime compound causing venous thrombosis. The thrombogenic effect of hyperhomocysteinemia could depend on the primary underlying cause of the moderate hyperhomocysteinemia, opening the possibility

that the latter is only a marker rather than an independent cause of venous thromboembolism. Such an explanation cannot be fully rejected at present. However, alternative hypotheses are equally valid.

First, by causing a redistribution of folate derivatives and a higher availability of one-carbon moieties for thymidine synthesis, MTHFR thermolability may have a concomitant beneficial effect on the vascular system. Normohomocysteinemic subjects homozygous for the mutation may thus be protected from other diseases, as suggested for colorectal cancer (16). A study of the carotid artery in subjects free of atherosclerotic lesions suggested that moderate hyperhomocysteinemia and the 677TT genotype are associated with opposite preclinical effects on the vessel wall (28).

Second, MTHFR thermolability by itself may explain only some of the elevation in homocysteine levels (43), possibly contributing only in part to the risk of venous thromboembolism. Few studies of venous thromboembolism have examined the phenotypic expression of the 677TT genotype. In one study, 39% of the patients versus 17% of the control subjects with thermolabile MTHFR were hyperhomocysteinemic (53). In another study (69), 43% of subjects defined as hyperhomocysteinemic were homozygous for the abnormal MTHFR polymorphism. Given the relatively moderate thrombotic risk ascertained for hyperhomocysteinemia in these studies (Table 33.1), it

Table 33.3. Thermolabile MTHFR Status and the Risk of Venous Thromboembolism

Author (ref)	MTHFR 677TT Genotype in Patients with Venous Thromboembolism		MTHFR 677TT Genotype in Control Subjects		Odd Ratio (Crude)	95% Confidence Interval
	n/total n	%	n/total n	%		
Brown et al., 1998 (11)	55/558	9.9	67/500	13.4	0.71	0.48–1.05
Von Depka et al., 1998 (83)	25/220	11.4	31/234	13.3	0.84	0.46–1.53
Cattaneo et al., 1997 (14)	16/77	20.8	35/154	22.7	0.89	0.43–1.20
Tosetto et al., 1997 (80)	8/65	12.3	17/130	13.1	0.93	0.34–2.47
Kluijtmans et al., 1998 (53)	47/471	10.0	47/474	9.9	1.01	0.64–1.58
Alhenc-Gelas et al., 1999 (1)	26/205	12.7	49/398	12.3	1.04	0.62–1.72
De Stefano et al., 1997 (33)	36/194	18.6	35/198	17.7	1.06	0.62–1.83
Salden et al., 1997 (72)	26/216	12.0	18/164	11.0	1.11	0.56–2.21
Perry et al., 1997 (65)	8/81	9.9	8/100	8.0	1.26	0.41–3.92
de Franchis et al., 1998 (27)	47/200	23.5	130/787	16.5	1.55	1.05–2.30
Hessner et al., 1999 (45)	49/330	14.9	19/192	9.9	1.59	0.88–2.90
Margaglione et al., 1998 (59)	60/222	27.0	78/431	18.1	1.68	1.12–2.51
Salomon et al., 1999 (73)	37/162	22.8	48/336	14.3	1.78	1.07–2.94
Arruda et al., 1997 (4)	14/121	11.6	12/296	4.1	3.10	1.30–7.41
Liebman et al., 1997 (57)	18/68	26.5	4/44	9.1	3.60	1.03–13.8
All studies	472/3,190	14.8	598/4,438	13.5	1.11	0.98–1.27

is not surprising that a potential pathogenic effect of the MTHFR mutation might have been missed.

Additional genetic determinants may be required for consistent phenotype expression of hyperhomocysteinemia in subjects with the MTHFR mutation. We evaluated fasting total homocysteine levels, homozygosity for the 677C→T mutation, and cobalamin and folate levels in 170 consecutive patients with documented early-onset venous and/or arterial thrombosis and in 182 age- and gender-matched, healthy control subjects (25). Elevated homocysteine levels were detected in 26.5% of patients and in 9.9% of control subjects (odds ratio = 3.28; 1.81 to 5.94). The 677TT genotype had comparable prevalences in patients (27.6%) and in control subjects (21.4%) (odds ratio = 1.42; 0.84 to 2.41), contributing a risk of hyperhomocysteinemia that was similar in patients and in control subjects (relative risk = 8.29; 4.61 to 14.9). Total homocysteine levels correlated inversely with folate and cobalamin levels in both patients and control subjects, with higher slopes of the regression lines relating total homocysteine to vitamin levels in subjects with the 677TT genotype than with the other MTHFR genotypes. However, the vitamin levels and the 677TT genotype contributed little to the higher prevalence of hyperhomocysteinemia in the patients. In a generalized linear model, 44.0% of the variation in total homocysteine levels was explained by folate and cobalamin levels, the MTHFR genotype, gender, and the interaction of the MTHFR genotype with folate. The interactions of cobalamin with the MTHFR genotype, gender, and patient status also contributed to the variation in total homocysteine levels. These data suggest that subjects carrying the 677TT genotype and patients with early-onset thrombosis have a higher cobalamin requirement, raising the possibility that yet unidentified abnormalities of methionine synthase or any of the enzymes, receptors, or carriers participating in the synthesis of methylcobalamin—alone or in association with thermolabile MTHFR—may play an important role in moderate hyperhomocysteinemia (25).

Early studies in vascular patients often concluded that an abnormal response to a methionine load was due to heterozygosity for cystathionine β-synthase deficiency (7, 17). However, obligate heterozygotes for cystathionine β-synthase deficiency apparently have no excess risk of vascular disease (34, 63), and genetic analyses indicate that the known cystathionine β-synthase mutations occur only sporadically in patients with vascular disease (49, 68). There is an urgent need for studies investigating the interaction of cystathionine β-synthase gene abnormalities with vitamin status in the frequent expression of postmethionine load hyperhomocysteinemia in patients with venous thromboembolic disease (Table 33.2).

The possibility that coexistence of mild enzyme abnormalities in both the remethylation and transsulfuration pathways may result in fasting hyperhomocysteinemia should not be overlooked. Recently, a 68 base pair insertion (844ins68) in the coding region of exon 8 of the cystathionine β-synthase gene was identified in 7.5% to 18.8% of normal individuals (51, 79, 81). Although this mutation does not apparently result in enzyme activity impairment or hyperhomocysteinemia (81), mRNA data have provided evidence for poor transcription of the allele carrying the insertion (79). The 844ins68 mutation produced conflicting results as a risk factor for arterial occlusive disease and hyperhomocysteinemia. In view of the relatively high prevalence of this mutation and of the thermolabile MTHFR mutation in the general population, the prevalence of the cystathionine β-synthase insertion was examined in 309 consecutive patients with premature venous and/or arterial occlusive disease genotyped for the 677C→T MTHFR mutation (27). Moderate fasting hyperhomocysteinemia was detected in 15.5% of the patients. The homozygous 677C→T mutation, the heterozygous 844ins68 insertion, and the combination of the two had respective frequencies of 16.5%, 7.8%, and 1.1% in 787 control subjects. Corresponding frequencies in the patient population were 19.4%, 6.9%, and 3.9%. Thus, only the combination of the two gene abnormalities was significantly associated with an increased risk of venous or arterial occlusive diseases (relative risk = 3.63; 1.48 to 8.91). When evaluated as a function of the genotype and of cobalamin and folate status, adjusted fasting homocysteine levels were 72% higher in patients with both gene abnormalities than in patients with thermolabile MTHFR only ($p = 0.004$), whereas the isolated cystathionine β-synthase insertion had no significant effect on homocysteine levels.

These data suggest that heterozygosity for the 844ins68 mutation is not per se a risk factor for premature arterial and/or venous occlusive diseases but may be one in combination with thermolabile MTHFR by increasing the risk and degree of fasting hyperhomocysteinemia (27). Association of thermolabile MTHFR with the heterozygous 844ins68 insertion of the cystathionine β-synthase gene was also observed in 7 of 69 subjects with intermediate hyperhomocysteinemia (10.1%) but in only 1 of 249 control subjects (0.4%) from the Hordaland Homocysteine Study (3). In a Danish study, coexistence of the 844ins68 mutation and thermolabile MTHFR was also more frequent among patients with thrombosis at intermediate or severe hyperhomocysteinemia (10.7%) than in the general population (1.7%) (42a).

Venous Thromboembolism as a Multigenic Disorder: Association of Hyperhomocysteinemia with Established Thrombophilic Defects

As with established thrombophilic defects, such as abnormalities of the protein C anticoagulant system (54, 55), not all patients with hyperhomocysteinemia develop thrombosis. The possibility that synergistic factors may be required for the development of thrombotic manifestations was first explored in 45 members of seven unrelated consanguineous kindreds in which at least one member was homozygous for homocystinuria (58). Thrombosis occurred in 6 of 11 patients with homocystinuria before the age of 8 years; all six patients also had activated protein C resistance. Conversely, of four patients with homocystinuria who did not have activated protein C resistance, none had thrombosis before the age of 17 years. These results were challenged by Quéré et al. (67), who reported the absence of such an interaction in 15 homocystinuric patients with genetically proven cystathionine β-synthase deficiency from 13 unrelated kindreds.

Kluijtmans et al. (52) studied 24 patients with homocystinuria caused by homozygous cystathionine β-synthase deficiency from 18 unrelated kindreds. Venous thrombotic complications were diagnosed in six patients, of whom only one was a carrier of factor V Leiden. However, thermolabile MTHFR was observed frequently among homocystinuric patients, especially among those with thrombotic complications. Three of six homocystinuric patients who had suffered from a thromboembolic event had thermolabile MTHFR, suggesting that this enzyme abnormality may be an important additional factor in the risk of thrombosis in homozygous cystathionine β-synthase-deficient patients (52). Yap et al. (84) evaluated the presence of factor V Leiden in 26 homocystinuric patients from 21 families who had received early treatment. Two subjects were carriers of the factor V abnormality, but thrombosis had occurred in only one patient who did not carry factor V Leiden.

Taken together, these results indicate that factor V Leiden is not an absolute prerequisite for venous thrombosis in homocystinuria. However, as factor V Leiden was detected in 50% of 18 patients with thrombosis and in 10.3% of 58 patients without thrombosis, it surely represents a synergistic factor, by markedly increasing the thrombotic risk of patients with homocystinuria (odds ratio = 8.7; 2.13 to 37.1).

The bulk of evidence now suggests that the thrombotic risk associated with moderate hyperhomocysteinemia is independent of the coexistence of abnormalities of the natural anticoagulant systems. Five reports showed that the association of moderate hyperhomocysteinemia and venous thrombosis persisted after exclusion of patients with known congenital risk factors, such as deficiencies of natural inhibitors of coagulation, activated protein C resistance, and/or factor V Leiden (30, 36, 37, 69, 78). However, based on the findings in congenital homocystinuria, it is anticipated that the coexistence of additional risk factors would also increase the thrombotic risk of individuals with moderate hyperhomocysteinemia.

Both activated protein C resistance and moderate hyperhomocysteinemia are highly prevalent in patients with early-onset venous thromboembolism. If the association of the two defects markedly increases the thrombotic risk, one would anticipate its prevalence to be significantly higher than expected based on the prevalence of the isolated defects. In a series of 307 patients with early-onset venous or arterial disease or with thrombosis occurring at unusual sites, the prevalence of isolated activated protein C resistance and moderate hyperhomocysteinemia (fasting or postmethionine load) were 10% and 27%, respectively. The combined defect was detected in 3.6% of the patients, a figure slightly, but not significantly, higher than the 2.7% prevalence expected assuming no synergistic effect of the association on the risk of thrombosis (19). However, data obtained in a larger population of patients with only venous thromboembolic disease indicate that the association of activated protein C resistance with any form of moderate hyperhomocysteinemia is about threefold greater than expected from the prevalence of the isolated abnormalities (23). The prospective data from the Physicians Health Study strongly support the evidence of a synergistic effect of the combination of factor V Leiden and moderate hyperhomocysteinemia in increasing the thrombotic risk (69). With respect to the relative risks of 3.2 attributed to isolated hyperhomocysteinemia and 3.6 to factor V Leiden, individuals with both disorders had a 20-fold risk of developing idiopathic venous thromboembolism. In addition, although isolated hyperhomocysteinemia was not proven a risk factor for all venous thromboembolism, it increased the relative risk contributed by the factor V Leiden mutation from 2.3 to 9.7 (69).

Data are also available on the thrombotic risk contributed by the association of the thermolabile MTHFR mutation with factor V Leiden. The thermolabile MTHFR mutation alone was associated with an increased thrombotic risk in only one (59) of eight case-control studies, whereas the relative risk contributed by the factor V Leiden mutation was significant in all studies (Table 33.4). The crude relative risks of venous thromboembolism calculated for each gene abnormality by pooling data from all studies (1,807 patients and 2,337 control subjects) were 1.00 and

Table 33.4. Interaction of Thermolabile MTHFR with Factor V Leiden and the Prothrombin 20210G→A mutation and the Risk of Venous Thromboembolism[a]

Author (ref)	Without Gene Abnormalities	MTHFR 677TT	F. V Leiden	Prothrombin 20210G→A Mutation	F. V Leiden + MTHFR 677TT	Prothrombin 20210G→A Mutation + MTHFR 677TT
Cattaneo et al., 1997 (14)	51/116	10/34 0.67 (0.28–1.54)	10/3 7.58 (1.82–27.3)	—	6/1 13.6 (1.56–95.3)	—
De Stefano et al., 1997 (33)	109/157	30/35 1.23 (0.69–2.21)	35/6 8.40 (3.23–23.1)	—	6/0 ∞ (1.01–73.2)	—
Liebman et al., 1997 (57)	39/38	14/4 3.41 (0.93–13.6)	11/2 5.36 (1.01–28.3)	—	4/0 ∞ (0.38–104.2)	—
Kluijtmans et al., 1998 (53)	342/416	37/44 1.02 (0.63–1.66)	82/11 9.10 (4.60–18.3)	—	10/3 4.05 (1.02–16.0)	—
D'Angelo et al., 1999 (unpublished)	65/136	23/38 1.27 (0.67–2.39)	11/7 3.29 (1.11–9.92)	—	2/1 4.18 (0.05–341)	—
Brown et al., 1998 (11)	396/408	42/64 0.68 (0.44–1.04)	83/14 6.11 (3.31–11.5)	24/11 2.25 (1.04–4.96)	9/1 9.27 (1.20–64.9)	4/2 2.06 (0.32–51.5)
Alhenc-Gelas et al., 1999 (1)	131/325	22/48 1.14 (0.63–2.02)	27/13 5.15 (2.46–10.9)	12/11 2.71 (1.08–6.78)	4/1 9.92 (1.04–92.8)	0/0
Margaglione et al., 1998 (59)	114/315	45/74 1.68 (1.07–2.63)	24/21 3.16 (1.62–6.16)	19/17 3.09 (1.47–6.48)	13/1 35.9 (4.84–142.4)	9/3 8.29 (2.01–28.4)
MTHFR 677TT-F. V Leiden interaction (all studies)	1,247/1,911	223/341 1.00 (0.83–1.21)	283/77 5.63 (4.30–7.38)	—	54/8 10.3 (4.72–23.6)	—
MTHFR 677TT-Prothrombin 20210G→A interaction (all studies)	641/1,048	109/186 0.96 (0.74–1.25)	—	55/39 2.31 (1.48–3.59)	—	13/5 4.25 (1.41–13.7)

[a]The results are shown as numbers of patients versus controls on the top line and relative risks with 95% confidence intervals in parentheses on the bottom line. F. V Leiden, factor V Leiden.

5.63, respectively. A pooled, crude relative risk of 10.3 was obtained for the association of thermolabile MTHFR with factor V Leiden, strongly suggesting a synergistic interaction of the two gene abnormalities, especially when considering that hyperhomocysteinemia is expressed only in a fraction of subjects with thermolabile MTHFR. A possible overrepresentation of the frequency of the coexistence of factor V Leiden with thermolabile MTHFR in a population of patients with venous thromboembolism compared with the expected frequency in healthy persons was also reported in a Danish study (42).

A similar scenario is apparent in the relative thrombotic risk conferred by the association of thermolabile MTHFR with the prothrombin 20210G→A mutation. In 818 patients and 1,278 control subjects from three studies, the crude relative risk of thrombosis in the presence of both abnormalities was twice that contributed by the isolated prothrombin mutation (Table 33.4). No studies are available on the association of the prothrombin 20210G→A mutation with moderate hyperhomocysteinemia.

Whenever hyperhomocysteinemia resulting from thermolabile MTHFR is more frequently expressed, one would expect a greater thrombotic risk contributed by the association of thermolabile MTHFR with other thrombophilic abnormalities. This was the case in an Italian study (59) (Table 33.4) and an Israeli study (73). In the latter case-control study, factor V Leiden, the prothrombin 20210G→A mutation, and thermolabile MTHFR were all found to be independent risk factors for venous thromboembolism, with odds ratios of 16.3, 3.6, and 2.1, respectively (73). Two or more polymorphisms were detected in 27 of 162 patients (16.7%) and in 3 of 336 control subjects (0.9%). Logistic regression analysis disclosed odds ratios of 35.0 (14.5 to 84.7) for the joint occurrence of factor V Leiden and thermolabile MTHFR and of 7.7 (3.0 to 19.6) for the joint occurrence of the prothrombin mutation and thermolabile MTHFR (73).

Taken together, these data are consistent with the notion that any form of moderate hyperhomocysteinemia by itself is an independent risk factor for venous thromboembolism, and that the combination of hyperhomocysteinemia with activated protein C resistance/factor V Leiden—and possibly the prothrombin mutation—increases the risk.

A different approach has been taken by other authors who tested for hyperhomocysteinemia and/or thermolabile MTHFR in relatives of index patients with thrombosis and one thrombophilic defect (33, 56, 70). These studies did not show a significant enhancement in the thrombotic risk by the association with either hyperhomocysteinemia or thermolabile MTHFR. This apparent contradiction may depend in part on the rela-

tively small number of subjects investigated and in part on the presumably selective pattern of cosegregation of thrombophilic defects with additional risk factors for thrombosis across the families studied.

In 337 patients with systemic lupus erythematosus that were studied prospectively for 1,619 person-years, baseline fasting homocysteine levels were independently associated with an increased risk for stroke (odds ratio = 2.44; 1.04 to 5.75) and arterial thromboses (odds ratio = 3.49; 0.97 to 12.54), but not venous thrombotic events (66). The apparent lack of association of raised total homocysteine levels with venous thromboembolism (34 events) should be interpreted critically. Only 26 patients (7.0%) were men and hyperhomocysteinemia, defined as total homocysteine values greater than 14.1 μmol/L, was observed in 15.0% of the entire population. In univariate analysis, venous thrombotic events were strongly associated with male sex (odds ratio = 3.03; 1.12 to 8.16, $p = 0.03$) and a prolonged Russell viper venom time (odds ratio = 1.04 for each second of prolongation; 1.00 to 1.08; $p = 0.02$). As expected, total homocysteine levels were about 30% higher in men than in women, and they were also about 30% higher in patients with systemic lupus erythematosus with an abnormal Russell viper venom time than in those with normal values. These findings complicate the interpretation of the results of multivariate analysis because of the gender dependency of hyperhomocysteinemia and the strong predictive value of lupus anticoagulants for venous thromboembolic events.

Preoperative homocysteine levels were not associated with venous thromboembolism in patients who underwent elective hip replacement surgery and were screened for postoperative deep vein thrombosis with bilateral phlebography (15). This finding is not surprising when considering the extremely high rate of postoperative thrombosis in these patients, which is strongly dependent on the surgical procedure. For comparison, the factor V Leiden genotype was also not associated with postoperative deep vein thrombosis in patients undergoing hip or knee replacement surgery (71). When the circumstantial risk factor for thrombosis is major, neither hyperhomocysteinemia nor other established thrombophilic defects may be strong enough to predict the event. As an example, venous thrombosis of the upper arm, for which strenuous physical exercise is a major pathogenic cause, was not associated with thrombophilic defects in one study (60).

REFERENCES

1. Alhenc-Gelas, M, Arnaud, E, Nicaud, V, Aubry, M-L, Fiessinger, J-N, Aiach, M, Emmerich, J. Venous thromboembolic disease and the prothrombin, methylenete-

trahydrofolate reductase and factor V genes. *Thromb Haemost* 1999; 81: 506–10.

2. Amundsen, T, Ueland, PM, Waage, A. Plasma homocysteine levels in patients with deep venous thrombosis. *Arterioscler Thromb Vasc Biol* 1995; 15: 1321–23.

3. Andria, G, Buoniconti, A, Sperandeo, MP, de Franchis, R, D'Angelo, A, Sebastio, G, Guttormsen, AB, Refsum, H, Ueland, PM. Intermediate hyperhomocysteinemia and the 844ins68 mutation of the cystathionine β-synthase gene. *Am J Hum Genet* 1998; 63(Suppl): A207.

4. Arruda, VR, von Zuben, PM, Chiaparini, LC, Annichino Bizzacchi, JM, Costa, FF. The mutation ALA677→VAL in the methylenetetrahydrofolate reductase gene: A risk factor for arterial disease and venous thrombosis. *Thromb Haemost* 1997; 77: 818–21.

5. Bergmann, F, D'Angelo, SV, Hoyer, PF, Oestereich, C, Mazzola, G, Barthels, M, D'Angelo, A. Severe autoimmune protein S deficiency in a boy with idiopathic purpura fulminans. *Br J Haematol* 1995; 89: 610–15.

6. Bienvenue, T, Ankri, A, Chadefauz, B, Montalescot, G, Kamoun, P. Elevated total plasma homocysteine, a risk factor for thrombosis: Relation to coagulation and fibrinolytic parameters. *Thromb Res* 1993; 70: 123–29.

7. Boers, GHJ, Smals, AGH, Trijbels, FJM, Fowler, B, Bakkeren, JAJM, Schoonderwaldt, HC, Klijer, WJ, Kloppenborg, PWC. Heterozygosity for homocystinuria in premature peripheral and cerebral occlusive arterial disease. *N Engl J Med* 1985; 313: 709–15.

8. Bozic, M, Fermo, I, Ritonja, A, D'Angelo, A, Peternel, P, Stegnar, M. Hyperhomocysteinemia and resistance to activated protein C in patients with history of venous thromboembolism. *Neth J Med* 1998; 52(Suppl): S19.

9. Brattström, L, Tengborn, L, Lagerstedt, C, Israelsson, B, Hultberg, B. Plasma homocysteine in venous thromboembolism. *Haemostasis* 1991; 21: 51–7.

10. Brattström, L. Common mutation in the methylenetetrahydrofolate reductase gene offers no support for mild hyperhomocysteinemia being a causal risk factor for cardiovascular disease. *Circulation* 1997; 96: 3805–6.

11. Brown, K, Luddington, R, Baglin, T. Effect of the MTHFR C677T variant on risk of venous thromboembolism: Interaction with factor V Leiden and prothrombin (F2G20210A) mutations. *Br J Haematol* 1998; 103: 42–4.

12. Cattaneo, M. Hyperhomocysteinemia, atherosclerosis and thrombosis. *Thromb Haemost* 1999; 81: 165–76.

13. Cattaneo, M, Martinelli, I, Mannucci, PM. Hyperhomocysteinemia as a risk factor for deep-vein thrombosis. *N Engl J Med* 1996; 335: 974–75.

14. Cattaneo, M, Tsai, MY, Bucciarelli, P, Taioli, E, Zighetti, ML, Bignell, M, Mannucci, PM. A common mutation of the methylene-tetrahydrofolate reductase gene (C677T) increases the risk for deep-vein thrombosis in patients with mutant factor V (factor V:Q506). *Arterioscl Thromb Vasc Biol* 1997; 17: 1662–66.

15. Cattaneo, M, Zighetti, ML, Turner, RM, Thompson, SG, Lowe, GDO, Haverkate, F, Bertina, RM, Turpie, AGG, Mannucci, PM, ECAT DVT Study Group. Fasting plasma homocysteine levels do not predict the occurrence of deep-vein thrombosis after elective hip replacement surgery. *Neth J Med* 1998; 52(Suppl): S21.

16. Chen, J, Giovannucci, E, Kelsey, K, Rimm, EB, Stampfer, MJ, Colditz, GA, Spiegelmann, D, Willett, WC, Hunter, DJ. A methylenetetrahydrofolate reductase polymorphism and the risk of colorectal cancer. *Cancer Res* 1996; 56: 4862–64.

17. Clarke, R, Daly, L, Robinson, K, Naughten, E, Cahalane, S, Fowler, B, Graham, I. Hyperhomocysteinemia: An independent risk factor for vascular disease. *N Engl J Med* 1991; 324: 1149–55.

18. D'Angelo, A, Della Valle, P, Crippa, L, Grimaldi, L, Pattarini, E, Vigano'D'Angelo, S. Autoimmune protein S deficiency in a boy with severe thromboembolic disease. *N Engl J Med* 1993; 328: 1753–57.

19. D'Angelo, A, Fermo, I, Vigano'D'Angelo, S. Thrombophilia, homocystinuria, and mutation of the factor V gene. *N Engl J Med* 1996; 335: 289.

20. D'Angelo, A, Della Valle, P, Garlando, AM, Pattarini, E, Crippa, L, Vigano'D'Angelo, S. Recurrent warfarin-induced skin necrosis associated with an autoantibody to protein C. *Blood* 1997; 90: 399a.

21. D'Angelo, A, Mazzola, G, Crippa, L, Fermo, I, Vigano' D'Angelo, S. Hyperhomocysteinemia and venous thromboembolic disease. *Haematologica* 1997; 82: 211–18.

22. D'Angelo, A, Selhub, J. Homocysteine and thrombotic disease. *Blood* 1997; 90: 1–11.

23. D'Angelo, A, Fermo, I, Mazzola, G, Paroni, R, Di Minno, G, Vigano'D'Angelo, S. Isolated methionine intolerance is a risk factor for early-onset venous thromboembolic disease. *Neth J Med* 1998; 52 (Suppl): S38.

24. D'Angelo, A, Della Valle, P, Crippa, L. Monitoring warfarin therapy in patients with lupus anticoagulants. *Ann Intern Med* 1998; 128: 504.

25. D'Angelo, A, Coppola, A, Madonna, P, Fermo, I, Pagano, A, Mazzola, G, Galli, L, Cerbone, AM. The role of vitamin B12 in fasting hyperhomocysteinemia and its interaction with the homozygous C677T mutation of the methylenetetrahydrofolate reductase (MTHFR) gene. A case-control study of patients with early-onset thrombotic events. *Thromb Haemost* 2000: 83: 563–70.

26. de Franchis, R, Mancini, FP, D'Angelo, A, Sebastio, G, Fermo, I, De Stefano, V, Margaglione, M, Mazzola, G, Di Minno, G, Andria, G. C667T mutation of the 5,10-methylenetetrahydrofolate reductase gene and hyperhomocysteinemia in thrombotic vascular disease. *Am J Hum Genet* 1996; 59: 262–63.

27. de Franchis, R, Fermo, I, Mazzola, G, Sebastio, G, Di Minno, G, Coppola, A, Andria, A, D'Angelo, A. Contribution of the cystathionine β-synthase gene (844ins68) polymorphism to the risk of early-onset venous and arterial occlusive disease and fasting hyperhomocysteinemia. *Thromb Haemost* 2000; 84: 576–82.

28. Demuth, K, Moatti, N, Hanon, O, Benoit, MO, Safar, M, Grirerd, X. Opposite effects of plasma homocysteine and the methylenetetrahydrofolate reductase C677T mutation on carotid artery geometry in asymptomatic adults. *Arterioscler Thromb Vasc Biol* 1998; 18: 1838–43.

29. den Heijer, M, Blom, HJ, Gerrits, WBJ, Rosendaal, FR, Haak, HL, Wijermans, PW, Bos, GMJ. Is hyperhomocys-

teinemia a risk factor for recurrent thrombosis? *Lancet* 1995; 345: 882–85.

30. den Heijer, M, Koster, T, Blom, HJ, Bos, GMJ, Briet, E, Reitsma, PH, Vandenbroucke, JP, Rosendaal, F. Hyperhomocysteinemia as a risk factor for deep vein thrombosis. *N Engl J Med* 1996; 334: 759–62.

31. den Heijer, M, Brower, IA, Bos, GM, Blom, HJ, van der Put, NM, Spaans, AP, Rosendaal, FR, Thomas, CM, Haak, HL, Wijermans, PW, Gerrits, WB. Vitamin supplementation reduces blood homocysteine levels. A controlled trial in patients with venous thrombosis and healthy volunteers. *Arterioscler Thromb Vasc Biol* 1998; 18: 356–61.

32. den Heijer, M, Rosendaal, FR, Blom, HJ, Gerrits, WBJ, Bos, GMJ. Hyperhomocysteinemia and venous thrombosis: a meta-analysis. *Thromb Haemost* 1998; 80: 874–77.

33. De Stefano, V, Chiusolo, P, Paciaroni, K, Casorelli, I, Serra, FG, Bizzi, B, Leone, G. Prevalence of factor V 1691G to A and methylenetetrahydrofolate reductase 677C to T mutated genes in patients with venous thrombosis. *Thromb Haemost* 1997; (Suppl): 569(PD-2330).

34. de Valk, HW, van Eeden, MKG, Banga, JD, van der Griend, R, de Groot, E, Haas, FJ, Meuwissen, OJ, Duran, M, Smeitimk, JA, Poll-The, BT, de Klerk, JB, Wittebol-Post, D, Rolland, MO. Evaluation of the presence of premature atherosclerosis in adults with heterozygosity for cystathionine β-synthase deficiency. *Stroke* 1996; 27: 1134–36.

35. Eichinger, S, Stumpfen, A, Hirschl, M, Blalonczyk, C, Herkner, K, Stain, M, Schneider, B, Pabinger, I, Lechner, K, Kyrle, PA. Hyperhomocysteinemia is a risk factor of recurrent venous thromboembolism. *Thromb Haemost* 1998; 80: 566–69.

36. Falcon, CR, Cattaneo, M, Panzeri, D, Martinelli, I, Mannucci, PM. High prevalence of hyperhomocysteinemia in patients with juvenile venous thrombosis. *Arterioscler Thromb* 1994; 14: 1080–83.

37. Fermo, I, D'Angelo, SV, Paroni, R, Mazzola, G, Calori, G, D'Angelo, A. Prevalence of moderate hyperhomocysteinemia in patients with early-onset venous and arterial occlusive disease. *Ann Intern Med* 1995; 123: 747–53.

38. Finazzi, G, Brancaccio, V, Moia, M, Ciavarella, N, Mazzucconi, MG, Schinco, PC, Ruggeri, M, Pogliani, EM, Gamba, G, Rossi, E, Baudo, F, Manotti, C, D'Angelo, A, Palareti, G, De Stefano, V, Berrettini, M, Barbui, T. Natural history and risk factors for thrombosis in 360 patients with antiphospholipid antibodies. A five-year prospective study from the Italian registry. *Am J Med* 1996; 100: 530–36.

39. Fiore, S, Mazzola, G, D'Angelo, SV, Bondel, M, Francois, D, Huber, A, Konrad, D, Hasselmann, D, Kreuz, W, Lenz, E, D'Angelo, A. High prevalence of severe, transient autoimmune protein S deficiency in young patients with purpura fulminans or extensive venous thromboembolism associated with varicella infection. *Thromb Res* 1998; 91: S97.

40. Franken, DG, Boers, GHJ, Blom, HJ, Cruysberg, JRM, Trijbels, FJM, Hamel, BCJ. Prevalence of familial mild hyperhomocysteinemia. *Atherosclerosis* 1996; 125: 71–80.

41. Frosst, P, Blom, HJ, Milos, R, Goyette, P, Sheppard, CA, Matthews, RG, Boers, GJH, den Heijer, M, Kluijtmans, LAJ, van den Heuvel, LP, Rozen, R. A candidate genetic risk factor for vascular disease: A common mutation in methylenetetrahydrofolate reductase. *Nat Genet* 1995; 10: 111–13.

42. Guastadnes, M, Larsen, TB, Norgard-Petersen, B, Madsen, M, Bihl, K, Rüdiger, N. Prevalence of the factor V Leiden mutation and the MTHFR C677T mutation in thrombophilic and healthy persons. *Thromb Haemost* 1997; (Suppl): 569 (PD-2327).

42a. Guastadnes, M, Rüdiger, N, Rasmussen, K, Ingerslev, J. Intermediate and severe hyperhomocysteinemia with thrombosis: A study of genetic determinants. *Thromb Haemost* 2000; 83: 554–58.

43. Gudnason, V, Stansbie, D, Scott, J, Bowron, A, Nicaud, V, Humphries, S, on behalf of the EARS Group. C677T (thermolabile alanine/valine) polymorphism in methylenetetrahydrofolate reductase (MTHFR): Its frequency and impact on plasma homocysteine concentration in different European populations. *Atherosclerosis* 1998; 136: 347–54.

44. Guttormsen, AB, Ueland, PM, Nesthus, I, Nygård, O, Schneede, J, Vollset, SE, Refsum, H. Determinants and vitamin responsiveness of intermediate hyperhomocysteinemia (>40 μmol/liter): The Hordaland Homocysteine Study. *J Clin Invest* 1996; 98: 2174–83.

45. Hessner, MJ, Luhm, RA, Pearson, SL, Endean, DJ, Friedman, KD, Montgomery, RR. Prevalence of prothrombin G20210A, Factor V G1691A (Leiden), and methylenetetrahydrofolate reductase (MTHFR) C677T in seven different populations determined by multiplex allele-specific PCR. *Thromb Haemost* 1999; 81: 733–38.

46. Hirsh, J, Prins, MH, Samama, M. Approach to the thrombophilic patient. In *Hemostasis and Thrombosis: Basic and Clinical Practice* (Colman, RW, Hirsh, J, Marder, VJ, Salzman, E, eds.). Lippincott Company, Philadelphia, 1994, pp.1543–61.

47. Kang, SS, Zhou, J, Wong, PWK, Kowalisyn, J, Strokosch, G. Intermediate homocysteinemia: A thermolabile variant of methylenetetrahydrofolate reductase. *Am J Hum Genet* 1988; 43: 414–21.

48. Khamashta, MA, Cuadrado, MJ, Mujic, F, Taub, NA, Hunt, BJ, Hughes, GRV. The management of thrombosis in the antiphospholipid-antibody syndrome. *N Engl J Med* 1995; 332: 993–97.

49. Kluijtmans, LAJ, van den Heuvel, LPWJ, Boers, GHJ, Frosst, P, Stevens, EMB, van Oost, BA, den Heijer, M, Trijbels, FJM, Rozen, R, Blom, HJ. Molecular genetic analysis in mild hyperhomocysteinemia: A common mutation in the methylenetetrahydrofolate reductase gene is a genetic risk factor for cardiovascular disease. *Am J Hum Genet* 1996; 58: 35–41.

50. Kluijtmans, LAJ, Kastelein, JJP, Lindemans, J, Boers, GHJ, Heil, SG, Bruschke, AVG, Jukema, JW, van den Heuvel, LPWJ, Trijbels, FJM, Boerma, GJM, Verheugt, FWA, Willems, F, Blom, HJ. Thermolabile methylenetetrahydrofolate reductase in coronary artery disease. *Circulation* 1997; 96: 2573–77.

51. Kluijtmans, LAJ, Boers, GHJ, Trijbels, FJM, van Lith-Zanders, HMA, van den Heuvel, LPWJ, Blom, HJ. A

common 844ins68 insertion variant in the cystathionine β synthase gene. *Biochem Mol Med J* 1997; 62: 23–25.

52. Kluijtmans, LAJ, Boers, GHJ, Verbruggen, B, Trijbels, FJM, Novakova, IRQ, Blom, HJ. Homozygous cystathionine β-synthase deficiency, combined with factor V Leiden or thermolabile methylenetetrahydrofolate reductase in the risk of venous thrombosis. *Blood* 1998; 91: 2015–18.

53. Kluijtmans, LAJ, den Heijer, M, Reitsma, PH, Heil, SG, Blom, HJ, Rosendaal, FR. Thermolabile methylenetetrahydrofolate reductase and factor V Leiden in the risk of deep vein thrombosis. *Thromb Haemost* 1998; 79: 254–58.

54. Lane, DA, Mannucci, PM, Bauer, KA, Bertina, RM, Bochkov, NP, Boulyjenkov, V, Chandy, M, Dahlback, B, Ginter, EK, Miletich, JP, Rosendaal, F, Seligsohn, U. Inherited thrombophilia. Part 1. *Thromb Haemost* 1996; 76: 651–62.

55. Lane, DA, Mannucci, PM, Bauer, KA, Bertina, RM, Bochkov, NP, Boulyjenkov, V, Chandy, M, Dahlback, B, Ginter, EK, Miletich, JP, Rosendaal, F, Seligsohn, U. Inherited thrombophilia. Part 2. *Thromb Haemost* 1996; 76: 824–34.

56. Legnani, C, Palareti, G, Grauso, F, Sassi, S, Grossi, G, Piazzi, S, Bernardi, F, Marchetti, G, Ferraresi, P, Coccheri, S. Hyperhomocysteinemia and a common methylenetetrahydrofolate reductase mutation (Ala223Val MTHFR) in patients with inherited thrombophilic coagulation defects. *Arteriosc Thromb Vasc Biol* 1997; 17: 2924–29.

57. Liebman, HA, Sutherland, D, McGehee, W. A common mutation in methylenetetrahydrofolate reductase is associated with an increased risk of venous thrombosis. *Thromb Haemost* 1997; (Suppl): 528(PS-2159).

58. Mandel, H, Brenner, B, Berant, M, Rosenberg, N, Lanir, N, Jakobs, C, Fowler, B, Seligsohn, U. Coexistence of hereditary homocystinuria and factor V Leiden. Effect on thrombosis. *N Engl J Med* 1996; 335: 763–68.

59. Margaglione, M, D'Andrea, G, d'Addedda, M, Giuliani, N, Cappucci, G, Iannaccone, L, Vecchione, G, Grandone, E, Brancaccio, V, Di Minno, G. The methylenetetrahydrofolate reductase TT677 genotype is associated with venous thrombosis independently of the coexistence of the FV Leiden and the prothrombin A^{20210} mutation. *Thromb Haemost* 1998; 79: 907–11.

60. Martinelli, I, Cattaneo, M, Panzeri, D, Taioli, E, Mannucci, PM. Risk factors for primary deep vein thrombosis of the upper extremities. *Ann Intern Med* 1997; 126: 707–11.

61. Miller, JW, Ribaya-Mercado, JD, Russell, RM, Shepard, DC, Morrow, FD, Cochary, EF, Szdowski, JA, Gershoff, SN, Selhub, J. Effect of vitamin B_6 deficiency on plasma homocysteine concentrations. *Am J Clin Nutr* 1992; 55: 1154–60.

62. Miller, JW, Nadeau, MR, Smith, D, Selhub, J. Vitamin B_6 deficiency vs. folate deficiency: Comparison of responses to methionine loading in rats. *Am J Clin Nutr* 1994; 59: 1033–39.

63. Mudd, SH, Levy, HL, Skovby, F. The natural history of homocystinuria due to cystathionine β-synthase deficiency. *Am J Hum Genet* 1985; 37: 1–31.

64. Mudd, SH, Levy, HL, Skovby, F. Disorders of transsulfuration. In *The Metabolic and Molecular Basis of Inherited Disease* (Scriver, CR, Beaudet, AL, Sly, WS, Valle, D, eds.). McGraw-Hill, New York, 1995; pp. 1279–327.

65. Perry, DJ, Riddell, AF, Pasi, KJ. TL-MTHFR and venous thromboembolic disease. *Thromb Haemost* 1997; (Suppl): 568(PD-2323).

66. Petri, M, Roubennoff, R, Dallal, GE, Nadeau, MR, Selhub, J, Rosenberg, IH. Plasma homocysteine as a risk factor for atherothrombotic events in systemic lupus erythematosus. *Lancet* 1996; 348: 1120–24.

67. Quéré, I, Lamarti, H, Chadefaux-Vekemans, B. Thrombophilia, homocystinuria, and mutation of the factor V gene. *N Engl J Med* 1996; 335: 289.

68. Refsum, H, Ueland, PM, Nygard, O, Vollset, SE. Homocysteine and cardiovascular disease. *Annu Rev Med* 1998; 49: 31–62.

69. Ridker, PM, Hennekens, CH, Selhub, J, Miletich, JP, Malinow, MR, Stampfer, MJ. Interrelation of hyperhomocyst(e)inemia, factor V Leiden, and risk of future venous thromboembolism. *Circulation* 1997; 95: 1777–82.

70. Rintelen, C, Pabinger, I, Lechner, K, Eichinger, S, Kyrle, PA, Mannhalter, C. No evidence for an increased risk of venous thrombosis in patients with factor V Leiden by the homozygous mutation in the methylenetetrahydrofolate reductase gene. *Thromb Haemost* 1997; (Suppl): 569(PD-2329).

71. Ryan, DH, Crowther, MA, Ginsberg, JS, Francis, CW. Relation of factor V Leiden genotype to risk for acute deep venous thrombosis after joint replacement surgery. *Ann Intern Med* 1998; 128: 270–76.

72. Salden, A, Keeney, S, Hay, CRM, Cumming, AM. The C677T MTHFR variant and the risk of venous thrombosis. *Br J Haematol* 1997; 99: 472.

73. Salomon, O, Steinberg, DM, Zivelin, A, Gitel, S, Dardik, R, Rosenberg, N, Berliner, S, Inbal, A, Many, A, Lubetski, A, Varon, D, Martinowitz, U, Seligsohn, U. Single and combined prothrombotic factors in patients with idiopathic venous thromboembolism. Prevalence and risk assessment. *Arteriosc Thromb Vasc Biol* 1999; 19: 511–18.

74. Selhub, J, Miller, JW. The pathogenesis of homocysteinemia: Interruption of the coordinate regulation by *S*-adenosylmethionine of the remethylation and transsulfuration of homocysteine. *Am J Clin Nutr* 1991; 55: 131–38.

75. Selhub, J, D'Angelo, A. Homocysteine and thrombosis: Acquired conditions. *Thromb Haemost* 1997; 78: 527–31.

76. Selhub, J, D'Angelo, A. Relationship between homocysteine and thrombotic disease. *Am J Med Sci* 1998; 316: 129–41.

77. Seligsohn, U, Zivelin, A. Thrombophilia as a multigenic disorder. *Thromb Haemost* 1997; 78: 297–301.

78. Simioni, P. Prandoni, P, Burlina, A, Tormene, D, Sardella, C, Ferrari, V, Beneditti, L, Girolami, A. Hyperhomocsyteinemia and deep-vein thrombosis. A case control study. *Thromb Haemost* 1996; 76: 883–86.

79. Sperandeo, MP, de Franchis, R, Andria, G, Sebastio, G. A 68bp insertion found in a homocystinuric patient is a

common variant and is skipped by alternative splicing of the cystathionine β-synthase mRNA. *Am J Hum Genet* 1996; 59: 1391–92.

80. Tosetto, A, Missiaglia, E, Frezzato, M, Rodeghiero, F. The VITA project: C677T mutation in the methylenetetrahydrofolate reductase gene and the risk of venous thromboembolism. *Br J Haematol* 1997; 97: 804–6.

81. Tsai, MY, Bignell, M, Schwichtenberg, K, Hanson, NQ. High prevalence of a mutation in the cystathionine β-synthase gene. *Am J Hum Genet* 1996; 59: 1262–64.

82. Vigano D'Angelo, S, Fermo, I, D'Angelo, A. The investigation of congenital thrombophilia: A critical evaluation. *J Int Fed Clin Chem* 1996; 8: 102–7.

83. Von Depka Prondzinski, M, Rutjes, J, Aschermann, G, Wermes, C, Barthels, M, Ganser, A. Coexpression of inherited risk factors of thrombophilia, lipoprotein(a) and homocysteine. *Blood* 1998; 92(Suppl 1): 559a.

84. Yap, S, O'Donnell, KA, O'Neill, C, Mayne, PD, Thornton, P, Naughten, E. Factor V Leiden (Arg506Gln), a confounding genetic risk factor but not mandatory for the occurrence of venous thromboembolism in homozygotes and obligate heterozygous for cystathionine β-synthase deficiency. *Thromb Haemost* 1999; 81: 502–5.

34

Homocysteine and Hemostasis

KATHERINE A. HAJJAR

Homocysteine and Hemostatic Balance

Hemostasis is a delicate balance that requires the participation of blood platelets, vascular endothelial cells, and plasma coagulation proteins. These three components act in concert to stem the flow of blood after vascular injury. Under some circumstances, however, unregulated hemostatic activity can lead to fibrin accumulation and blood vessel occlusion due to thrombosis. Factors that control the hemostatic process in vivo are only partly understood.

Both arterial and venous thromboses are common and frequently lethal complications of congenital homocystinuria (16, 55), and several prothrombotic effects have been reported in humans in association with homocysteine (Table 34.1). In addition, individuals with hyperhomocysteinemia show a strong propensity toward thrombotic disease involving both the arterial and venous circulation (7). However, because mice with cystathionine β-synthase deficiency do not have evidence of thrombotic disease (64), it is conceivable that homocysteine predisposes to thrombosis only in pathological contexts specific to humans. Although the mechanistic basis for this prethrombotic state is unknown, three theories have been advanced. First, activation of platelets may be enhanced in the presence of elevated homocysteine levels. Second, increased

generation of thrombin may predispose to fibrin deposition within vessels. Third, deficiencies in fibrinolytic surveillance may lead to the propagation of an existing microthrombus. This chapter considers the evidence for each of these hypotheses.

Homocysteine and Platelet Function

The development of the primary hemostatic plug is the initial physiological response to blood vessel injury (48) (Figure 34.1). This process requires platelet adhesion to subendothelial matrix, platelet activation and aggregation, and platelet recruitment to the growing thrombus. The notion that increased platelet "stickiness" might contribute to thrombosis in homocystinuria was first proposed by McDonald et al. (43) who noted increased adhesion of homocystinuric platelets adhering to a glass surface. These effects, however, have not been substantiated in later studies (57).

Traditional platelet aggregation studies appear to be normal in hyperhomocysteinemic states. When platelets from 11 homocystinuric patients were evaluated in vitro, aggregation in response to adenosine diphosphate (ADP), collagen, arachidonate, and epinephrine were all normal (8). In another study, four homocystinuric children with homocystine levels in the 60 to 150 μmol/L range had grossly normal platelet aggregation (45). Furthermore, a group of 17 patients with homocysteine levels in the 15 to 120 μmol/L range and three children with classic homocystinuria all had normal bleeding times (47, 60).

In addition, homocysteine appears to have little if any effect on platelet count or platelet survival (52). Platelet enumeration in patients with homocystinuria has been reported to be normal (29, 43, 47). In contrast, Harker et al. (29) initially reported that four individuals with homocystinuria had reduced platelet survival times (4.3 ± 0.6 vs. 9.5 ± 0.6 days, mean ± standard deviation [SD]), and enhanced platelet turnover rates (96,000 ± 12,000 vs. 35,000 ± 4,500 platelets/μL/day, mean ± SD) compared with normal control subjects. Two subsequent studies, however, showed no difference in survival of either [^{51}Cr] or [^{111}In]labeled autologous platelets infused into homocystinuric versus normal subjects (32, 59). In addition, the fate and distribution of infused platelets were unaltered (59).

Further studies suggest that individuals with homocystinuria may have subtle abnormalities of platelet metabolism. Di Minno et al. (8) showed that 11 patients with homocystinuria exhibited high urinary excretion of a breakdown product of the eicosanoid,

Table 34.1.   Reported Prothrombotic Effects of Homocysteine on Hemostasis in Humans

Effect	Reference
Platelet Function	
Increased thromboxane A_2 synthesis	Diminno et al. (8), Graeber et al. (17)
Procoagulant Activity	
Increased factor VIIIc	Freyburger et al. (12)
Increased vWF	Freyburger et al. (12)
Increased thrombin-antithrombin complexes	Undas et al. (60)
Increased prothrombin fragment 1+2	Kyrle et al. (35), Undas et al. (60)
Deficiency of factor VII	Brattström et al. (3), Merckx and Kuntz (44), Munnich et al. (45)
Reduced Natural Anticoagulant Activity	
Deficiency of antithrombin III	Brattström et al. (3), Giannini et al. (15), Maruyama et al. (42)
Deficiency of protein C antigen	Brattström et al. (3)

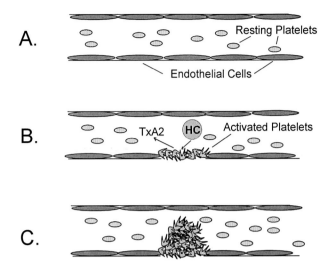

Fig. 34.1. Primary hemostatic plug formation and proposed effect of homocysteine (HC). (**A**). Normal vessel in which resting platelets circulate freely. (**B**). Injured vessel in which activated platelets adhere to subendothelial matrix on denudation of endothelial cells and secrete increased thromboxane A_2 in the presence of homocysteine. (**C**). Activated platelets recruit additional platelets to form the primary hemostatic plug.

thromboxane. In all subjects, 11-dehydro-thromboxane B_2 was elevated by more than 2 SD, suggesting enhanced production of thromboxane. The elevation in thromboxane metabolite could be reduced by ingestion of low-dose aspirin or by treatment with the antioxidant probucol. Although this study suggests that platelet reactivity may be modestly increased in the presence of hyperhomocysteinemia, the clinical significance of this finding remains to be established particularly since in vitro platelet aggregation studies were normal.

Similarly, elevations in plasma homocysteine induced by dietary manipulation in rats appear to influence platelet eicosanoid metabolism. Animals placed on a folate-deficient diet (250 μg/kg vs. 750 μg/kg) who had 32% reduction in erythrocyte folate levels showed an enhancement in platelet aggregation in response to thrombin (64%) (9). Moreover, thromboxane synthesis from arachidonate was increased by thrombin stimulation compared with normal control animals. Thromboxane represents a marker of platelet activation and a weak platelet agonist. In further studies, methionine loading, which led to a transient fourfold increase in plasma homocysteine levels, also potentiated platelet aggregation in response to thrombin and significantly enhanced thrombin-induced thromboxane synthesis (10). These studies parallel an earlier report in which homocysteine treatment of

platelet-rich plasma was associated with a modest (30% to 40%) increase in thromboxane A_2 production (17).

Endothelial cell elaboration of the platelet inhibitor, prostacyclin, furthermore, does not appear to be affected by homocysteine. Homocysteine treatment of umbilical artery rings (1 mmol/L, 20 minutes) had no effect on prostacyclin activity in a bioassay of platelet aggregation (17). In addition, neither treatment of cultured human umbilical vein endothelial cells with homocysteine in doses up to 1 mmol/L nor propagation of the cells in medium containing homocystinuric human serum had any significant effect on production of the prostacyclin metabolite, 6-keto-prostaglandin $F1_\alpha$ (63). Thus, the prothrombotic effect of homocysteine is not likely to relate to aberrations in platelet-inhibitory eicosanoids derived from endothelial cells.

Although its significance is unclear, a malfunction in trafficking of the procoagulant, von Willebrand factor, may also be seen in the presence of homocysteine (37). von Willebrand factor is a large protein composed of multiple subunits joined by covalent disulfide bonds. It is found in plasma, on basement membrane, in platelets, and in endothelial cells (62). Its major function is to promote platelet attachment to regions of blood vessel injury. von Willebrand factor forms a bridge between platelet glycoprotein I on the platelet surface and components of the basement membrane. von Willebrand factor exists as a series of multimers ranging in size from 500 to 20,000 kDa. Oligosacch-

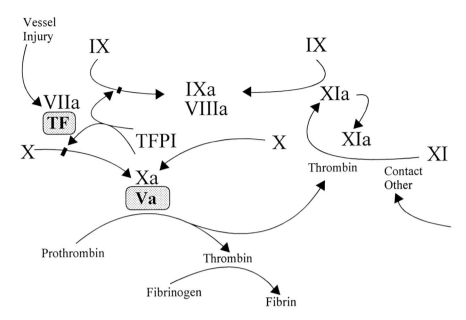

Fig. 34.2. Revised coagulation cascade and proposed effects of homocysteine. Blood vessel injury leads to expression of tissue factor (TF), which complexes with factor VIIa (extrinsic pathway). This complex activates factor X to Xa and factor IX to IXa. Factor Xa with factor Va converts prothrombin to its active form, thrombin, which then modifies fibrinogen, allowing it to polymerize, forming fibrin. Factor IXa with its cofactor VIIIa also activates factor X (intrinsic pathway). Thrombin or contact with certain surfaces activates factor XI to XIa, which can activate additional factor IX. Tissue factor pathway inhibitor (TFPI) inhibits activation of factor X and factor IX by TF-factor VIIa. Proteins thought to be affected by homocysteine are shaded. (Modified from Broze [4], with permission.)

aride processing, formation of multimers, and propeptide cleavage and secretion, which take place in the endoplasmic reticulum, Golgi, and post-Golgi secretory vesicles, respectively, are all inhibited by hyperhomocysteine (37). Studies on the structure and function of von Willebrand factor in patients with hyperhomocysteinemia, however, have not yet been reported.

Nitric oxide is a significant modulator of platelet reactivity (41). Several studies strongly suggest that homocysteine inhibits formation of nitric oxide by endothelial cells both in vivo and in vitro (see also Chapter 5). In the first, cynomolgus monkeys were made hyperhomocysteinemic (11 μmol/L) by placement on a diet high in methionine, depleted of folate, and devoid of choline (38). When platelet activation was induced by infusion of collagen, blood flow in the leg was decreased by 42% as opposed to 14% in control animals. Blood vessel response to endothelial cell-dependent vasodilators was markedly impaired. Similarly, production of nitric oxide by endothelial cells in vitro is significantly impaired in the presence of

homocysteine (57), possibly by a mechanism involving glutathione peroxidase (34).

Induction of Procoagulant Activity by Homocysteine

The primary hemostatic plug is a temporary entity that is rapidly replaced by a more stable, cross-linked, fibrin-containing clot (14). Fibrin is formed as the result of a series of proteolytic activation reactions that ultimately generate the serine protease, thrombin (Figure 34.2). Exposure of anionic phospholipids on the surface of activated platelets and injured endothelial cells promotes assembly of clotting factors and activation of the coagulation cascade (14). Activation of thrombin leads to enzymatic modification of fibrinogen and its polymerization to form fibrin, the major protein constituent of the thrombus.

The idea that homocysteine, or its derivatives, might stimulate thrombin generation was first suggested by Ratnoff (49). L-homocystine (10 mmol/L) added to normal whole blood decreased the clotting time from 34 to 10 minutes. In addition, coagulation of recalcified citrated human plasma was shortened from 845 seconds to 400 seconds in the presence of L-homocystine (25 mmol/L). It was postulated that homocystine crystals in tissues might provide a surface for ectopic activation of factor XII, the first component of the intrinsic arm of the coagulation pathway. The physiological role of factor XII in blood coagulation in vivo, however, has been questioned because patients lacking factor XII do not bleed (50).

In human hyperhomocysteinemia, thrombin generation may be enhanced. Freyburger et al. (12) noted that mildly increased fasting levels of homocysteine in a group of patients with arterial vascular disease were associated with significant elevations in factor VIIIc, von Willebrand factor, and thrombin-antithrombin III complexes. In another study, approximately 20% of patients with hyperhomocysteinemia and a history of venous thromboembolism had persistently elevated plasma levels of prothrombin fragment 1+2, a marker of thrombin activity, for up to 9 months after discontinuation of anticoagulant therapy (35). A third study revealed another marker of thrombin activity, thrombin-antithrombin complex level, as well as prothrombin fragment 1+2, to be elevated in patients whose homocysteine levels exceeded 60 μmol/L (60). Among subjects with classic homocystinuria, deficiencies of antithrombin III and factor VII have also been noted with some consistency (2, 15, 44, 45, 47). Nevertheless, it is not yet clear whether these perturbations in circulating hemostatic factors are sufficient to explain the tendency toward thrombosis observed in these individuals.

Several pieces of data indicate that homocysteine may induce the expression of abnormal procoagulant activity in vitro. Tissue factor is a 45 kDa integral membrane protein of endothelial cells that serves as a receptor for coagulation factor VII (56). Tissue factor represents the initiating molecule of the extrinsic arm of the coagulation pathway. Although tissue factor is expressed constitutively by many nonvascular cells, its expression on endothelial cells, monocytes, and macrophages requires certain specific stimuli (39). In rats treated with low-folate diets, peritoneal macrophages expressed 20 times more tissue factor activity than did control animals (9). In addition, homocysteine in micromolar concentrations (100 to 600 μmol/L) enhanced tissue factor activity in cultured human umbilical vein endothelial cells by 25% to 100% in a dose- and time-dependent manner (13). This effect peaked at 8 hours and was inhibited on pretreatment of homocysteine with a thiol-blocking reagent such as N-ethylmaleimide. Enhanced tissue factor activity was accompanied by increased steady-state levels of tissue factor mRNA that peaked at 3 hours. This time course is similar to that by which tissue factor gene expression is induced by endotoxin in monocytes (18).

Factor V is a 330 kDa glycoprotein that is constitutively expressed by endothelial cells and activated by thrombin (14). Factor Va serves as a cofactor that supports the activation of prothrombin by factor Xa in the presence of calcium ions and phospholipid. High doses of homocysteine (2 to 10 mmol/L) appear to induce a threefold to fourfold increase in factor Va activity with no increase in factor V antigen levels (53). Enhanced activation of factor V was associated with cleavage products distinct from those observed in the presence of thrombin or factor Xa. Interestingly, cysteine exhibited about 50% of the activity of homocysteine,

whereas homocystine, methionine, and cystine were all inactive. These data suggest that alternative pathways of thrombin activation may play a role in the hyperhomocysteinemic prothrombotic state.

The clinical risk of a thromboembolic event in patients with homocystinuria appears to increase significantly in the presence of hereditary resistance to activated protein C (40). When thrombin interacts with the endothelial cell protein, thrombomodulin, it acquires the ability to activate the circulating natural anticoagulant, protein C. Activated protein C can then inactivate the clotting cofactors VIIIa and Va. The most common known cause of familial thrombosis is a mutation in factor V, known as factor V Leiden, that renders it insensitive to inactivation by protein C. A recent study of patients with homocystinuria resulting from deficiency of cystathionine β-synthase, deficiency of methylenetetrahydrofolate reductase, or a defect in cytosolic metabolism of cobalamin, thrombotic events occurred only in those patients who were also homozygous or heterozygous for factor V Leiden (40).

Inhibition of Natural Anticoagulant Activity

Several lines of investigation suggest that homocysteine can dampen the activity of natural anticoagulants. The coagulation cascade is a series of proteolytic reactions mediated by serine proteases and subject to inhibition by several mechanisms (11). The three major anticoagulant mechanisms are the heparin-antithrombin III complex, which blocks vitamin K-dependent clotting factors (11); the thrombomodulin-protein C-protein S system, which inactivates clotting cofactors Va and VIIIa (11); and tissue factor pathway inhibitor (1) (Figure 34.3). The importance of the first two pathways is emphasized by the fact that patients with abnormalities of the protein C-thrombomodulin system or deficiencies in antithrombin III have thrombophilia, a tendency toward thrombosis that can be life-threatening (11). Patients deficient in tissue factor pathway inhibitor have not yet been reported (4).

Endothelial cells synthesize and express on their surface heparan sulfate, which binds circulating antithrombin III and renders it competent to inhibit the action of thrombin (11). Heparan sulfate expression in cultured endothelial cells appears to be sharply inhibited by homocysteine (46). Micromolar concentrations of homocysteine (100 to 1,000 μmol/L) reduced the capacity of the endothelial cell to bind antithrombin III by up to 80% in a dose-dependent manner. Maximal inhibition was observed after 12 hours of homocysteine exposure. This effect was completely blocked on coincubation with catalase, suggesting that it might reflect generation of hydrogen peroxide. Total cell surface-associated glycosaminoglycan was not reduced, but

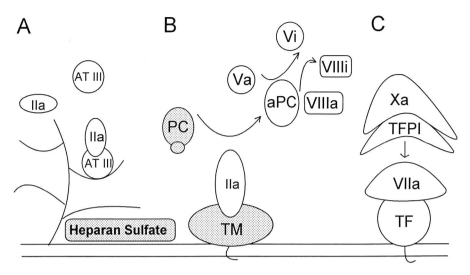

Fig. 34.3. Suggested effects of homocysteine on natural anticoagulant activity. (A). Antithrombin III system. Heparan sulfate proteoglycan is expressed on the endothelial cell surface and can bind antithrombin III (AT III), which circulates in plasma. This interaction renders antithrombin III competent to bind and inactivate circulating thrombin (IIa). Homocysteine appears to limit endothelial cell synthesis of heparan sulfate proteoglycan. (B). Thrombomodulin (TM) is an integral endothelial cell membrane protein that binds thrombin, thereby converting thrombin to a protein C (PC) activator. Activated protein C (aPC) can then inactivate factors Va and VIIIa to inactive Vi and VIIIi, respectively. Homocysteine appears to inhibit thrombin binding to TM and alter TM transport to the cell surface and may also reduce disulfide bonds within protein C itself, thereby inhibiting protein C activation. (C). Tissue factor pathway inhibitor (TFPI). Tissue factor (TF) is an integral membrane protein that is expressed on the surface of perturbed endothelial cells. TFPI binds to both factor VIIa and factor Xa, creating an inactive complex that modulates thrombin generation. At present, there are no known effects of homocysteine on the TFPI pathway.

sure to very high concentrations of homocysteine (0.6 to 1.25 mmol/L), 12% to 33% reductions in protein C activation were observed. Maximal decreases were seen at 7.5 to 10 mmol/L homocysteine, doses that are pharmacological and not seen in vivo in any known human condition. The K_d of the protein C reaction was affected much more dramatically than V_{max}. Diminished protein C activation after homocysteine treatment was accompanied by a decreased affinity of thrombomodulin for thrombin as homocysteine behaved as a competitive inhibitor to thrombin. Homocysteine may also block protein C activation by directly reducing critical disulfide bonds within epidermal growth factor domains of both thrombomodulin and protein C (36). Despite these data, there is no convincing evidence that protein C activation is impaired in hyperhomocysteinemic human subjects, although protein C antigen was reported to be low in two of three homocystinuric patients (3).

In the presence of homocysteine, intracellular transport of thrombomodulin appears to be abnormal. Incorporation of [^{35}S]sulfate into chondroitin sulfate glycosaminoglycan associated with thrombomodulin is decreased, and transport of thrombomodulin through the Golgi apparatus is also perturbed (36). In addition, homocysteine may inhibit the cofactor activity of thrombomodulin with respect to thrombin-mediated activation of anticoagulant protein C (31). The effect was maximal after a 3 to 11 hour incubation and was observed at doses in the millimolar range (1 to 10 mmol/L) that far exceed upper limits observed in human plasma. The amount of unreduced thrombomodulin on the surface of cultured human umbilical vein endothelial cells was reduced by up to 80%, and total cellular thrombomodulin was reduced by 25%. Kinetically similar reductions were observed in rates of thrombin binding to thrombomodulin and protein C activation. Of

synthesis of the anticoagulant heparan sulfate portion was specifically blocked. This study suggests a thiol-specific effect of homocysteine on synthesis of heparan sulfate core protein, on assembly of its oligosaccharide components, or on its transport to the cell surface via the endoplasmic reticulum–Golgi complex.

Homocysteine appears to have important inhibitory effects on the thrombomodulin-protein C anticoagulant system. Endothelial cells express thrombomodulin, an integral membrane protein that binds thrombin, redirecting its substrate specificity from fibrinogen to protein C. Protein C circulates and, once activated by thrombomodulin-associated thrombin, can cleave factors Va and VIIIa, rendering them inactive. Factors Va and VIIIa are key cofactors in activation of factors Xa and thrombin, respectively.

Protein C activation by both arterial and venous endothelial cells appears to be inhibited in the presence of homocysteine in vitro (54). After 1 hour of expo-

interest, steady-state thrombomodulin mRNA levels estimated under the same conditions were increased by twofold to threefold. These data suggest an inhibition of thrombomodulin function that may be partially compensated by an increase in the synthetic rate of the protein. However, the high concentrations of homocysteine required to induce these effects suggest that results be interpreted with caution.

Impairment of Fibrinolysis

The fibrinolytic system consists of a series of proteolytic reactions that culminate in the generation of the serine protease, plasmin (22) (Figure 34.4). Plasminogen is a 93 kDa glycoprotein that circulates in plasma at a concentration of about 1.5 μmol/L. Itself inactive, plasminogen is converted to the functional serine protease, plasmin, on cleavage of a single peptide bond at position 560 to 561 (Arg-Val). This hydrolysis can be carried out by either of two major plasminogen activators: tissue plasminogen activator, a product of some endothelial cells, or urokinase, a product of renal epithelial cells. Fibrin, the principal substrate of plasmin, is also the most potent known cofactor for tissue plasminogen activator-dependent activation of plas-

minogen, accelerating its catalytic efficiency by ∼ 500-fold. Further regulation of the system is provided by an array of circulating inhibitors such as plasminogen activator inhibitor-1 or α2-antiplasmin, which immediately neutralize freely circulating tissue plasminogen activator and urokinase or plasmin, respectively. Finally, fibrinolytic activity is localized to cell surfaces through the interaction of plasminogen and its activators with specific cell surface receptors (Figure 34.4B).

Circulating components of the fibrinolytic system appear to be present in normal quantities in the presence of elevated homocysteine concentrations. In patients with homocystinuria, turnover rates for both fibrinogen and plasminogen are only modestly, if at all, increased (29). Likewise, total fibrinolytic activity, tissue plasminogen activator antigen, and plasminogen activator inhibitor-1 antigen were all within normal limits both before and after 10 minutes of venous stasis (8). In patients with peripheral arterial occlusive disease and elevated homocysteine levels (20.7 ± 14.7 μmol/L, mean ± SD), plasma levels of tissue plasminogen activator were also normal (61). Similarly, no differences in circulating tissue plasminogen activator, plasminogen activator inhibitor-1 antigen levels, or euglobulin clot lysis times before and after venous occlusion were found in patients with fasting hyperhomocysteinemia (13 to 38 μmol/L) (12). Thus, it appears that global measures of fibrinolytic activity are not perturbed in the presence of elevated homocysteine in vivo.

Fibrinolysis is a surface-oriented process (22), and homocysteine may inhibit plasmin generation on the surface of a thrombus by blocking the assembly of fibrinolytic proteins (Figure 34.4A). Lipoprotein(a) is a low-density, lipoprotein-like particle that contains an apoprotein known as apolipoprotein(a) (26). Apolipoprotein(a) is genetically linked to plasminogen on chromosome 6, and these two loci probably arose from a common ancestral gene. Because apolipoprotein(a) contains multiple tandemly repeated copies of

Fig. 34.4. Postulated effects of homocysteine on fibrinolysis and fibrinolytic surveillance. (A) Tissue plasminogen activator (tPA) and plasminogen (PLG) assemble on the surface of a fibrin-containing thrombus. Normally, plasmin (PN) is efficiently activated and degrades fibrin (represented by broken lines). In the presence of homocysteine (HC), however, lipoprotein(a) [Lp(a)] may bind more avidly to fibrin, preventing its interaction with PLG, and inhibiting plasmin generation and thrombolysis. Urokinase (uPA) can also efficiently activate plasminogen in the vicinity of a fibrin-containing clot. (B) On the endothelial cell (EC) surface, tPA and PLG assemble via their binding domains on annexin II. Normally, plasmin is produced constitutively and can degrade fibrin that might form in response to endothelial cell perturbation or injury. HC prevents the binding of tPA to annexin II, thereby downregulating plasmin generation and blocking clearance of fibrin.

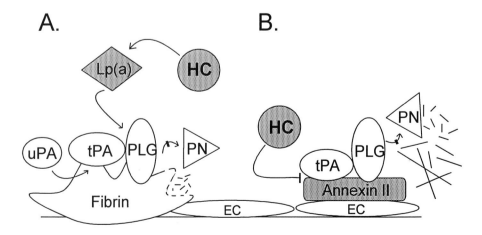

the "kringle" four domain of plasminogen, it may compete with plasminogen for binding to fibrin, thereby inhibiting clot lysis. Of interest, homocysteine in concentrations ranging from 8 to 400 µmol/L promotes binding of lipoprotein(a) to plasmin-modified fibrin in vitro (30). Lipoprotein(a) exposed to 500 µmol/L homocysteine (90 minutes, 37°C) demonstrated altered mobility by immunoblot analysis, suggesting that increased binding to fibrin was accompanied by reduction of one or more disulfide bonds. Thus, increased affinity of lipoprotein(a) for fibrin could block sites normally available to plasminogen and reduce plasminogen activation in the vicinity of a forming thrombus.

The fibrinolytic system can also assemble on cell surfaces through the expression of receptors for both plasminogen and plasminogen activators (22) (Figure 34.4B). Annexin II, for example, is a widely distributed, highly conserved, 36 kDa peripheral membrane protein expressed abundantly on endothelial cells, monocyte/macrophages, myeloid cells, and some tumor cells (22). All 20 known annexins consist of a conserved "core" domain (30 to 40 kDa), which imparts phospholipid-binding capacity, and a variable amino terminal "tail" domain (3 to 6 kDa) through which specialized functions are acquired (51, 58). Annexin II possesses the unique property of binding both plasminogen (K_d = 114 nmol/L) and tissue plasminogen activator (K_d = 30 nmol/L) (20, 23, 24), thereby stimulating the catalytic efficiency of tissue plasminogen activator-dependent plasminogen activation by 60-fold (5) (Figure 34.4). This "fibrin-like" cofactor activity is completely inhibited in the presence of lysine analogs or on removal of its basic carboxyl-terminal amino acids. Although it lacks a classic signal peptide, annexin II is constitutively translocated to the endothelial cell surface within 16 hours of its biosynthesis. It binds to cell surface phospholipid via core repeat 2 containing the linear sequence KGLGT and downstream aspartate residue (Asp161) (25). Annexin II heterotetramer, composed of two annexin monomers and two p11 subunits, may have even greater stimulatory effects on tissue plasminogen activator-dependent plasmin generation (33).

Homocysteine appears to profoundly impair the endothelial cell's ability to generate plasmin in vitro (27). Treatment of cultured endothelial cells with D,L-homocysteine is specifically associated with a 65% reduction in functional binding sites for tissue plasminogen activator, whereas no effect on plasminogen binding is observed (21). This finding was associated with a 60% reduction in cell-associated tissue plasminogen activator activity even though the intrinsic catalytic capability of tissue plasminogen activator is not altered by homocysteine. Binding of tissue plas-

minogen activator, but not plasminogen, to annexin II monomer is also markedly reduced by ligand blot analysis. These studies suggest that homocysteine might perturb the intrinsic fibrinolytic potential of the endothelial cell by selectively blocking the tissue plasminogen activator binding domain of annexin II (Figure 34.4B).

Tissue plasminogen activator binding to annexin II depends on a specific domain containing or closely associated with residues 8 to 13 (LCKLSL) within the receptor's amino terminal "tail" (28). Recombinant annexin II, from which the tail domain has been cleaved, fails to compete with immobilized intact annexin II for tissue plasminogen activator binding. In addition, the hexapeptide LCKLSL specifically blocks binding of tissue plasminogen activator to both intact recombinant annexin II and endothelial cell monolayers.

The effect of homocysteine on the tissue plasminogen activator-binding annexin II tail domain has been examined in physical biochemical studies (28). Electrospray ionization mass spectrometric analysis of recombinant annexin II indicated that homocysteine physically alters the receptor, increasing its mass by 135 ± 4 daltons. Tandem mass spectrometric analysis of a tryptic digest of homocysteine-treated annexin II revealed derivatization of a single cysteine residue (C9) within the amino terminal tissue plasminogen activator-binding domain. A disulfide-mediated complex between homocysteine and annexin II was also demonstrated in cultured endothelial cells that were metabolically labeled with [^{35}S]homocysteine. Modification of annexin II by homocysteine in the 10 to 50 µmol/L range was associated with a dose- and time-related reduction in tissue plasminogen activator binding. Interestingly, the I_{50} for inhibition of tissue plasminogen activator binding to annexin II was ~ 11 µmol/L, a value close to the upper limit of normal for homocysteine in plasma (~14 µmol/L). Thus, inhibition of tissue plasminogen activator–annexin II assembly on the endothelial cell, and subsequent reduction in plasmin generation, could underlie the prothrombotic/proatherogenic state associated with homocysteine in vivo.

Proteins that become derivatized by homocysteine may be subject to increased metabolic turnover, thus placing an increased synthetic demand on the cell. Endothelial cells exposed to homocysteine in vitro upregulate acute translational response genes that control the rate at which mRNA is translated into new protein (6). When mRNA transcripts from vascular endothelial cells treated for 6 to 42 hours with homocysteine were analyzed using differential display, a threefold to sevenfold, time-dependent induction of a 220-bp fragment was observed. This transcript showed complete sequence identity with elongation factor-1δ, a member of a multimeric complex regulating mRNA translation. Similar increases in steady state mRNA levels were observed for elongation factor-1α and β, as well as increased protein levels for elongation factor-1α, β and γ. Elongation factor-1 is a complex of polypeptides (α₂βγδ) that regulates the efficiency and fidelity of mRNA translation in eukaryotic cells. Of importance, fibroblasts from cystathionine β-synthase –/– individuals also showed increased levels of mRNA for elongation factor-1α, β, and δ compared with normal cells (6). Pulse-chase studies in homocysteine-treated endothelial cells revealed a doubling in the rate of appearance and disappearance of annexin II, but no change in synthesis or degradation of plasminogen activator inhibitor-1. These changes may represent an adaptive response to homocysteine-induced oxidative stress and protein degradation.

Although there is a clear epidemiological association between thrombosis and both homocystinuria and homocysteinemia, a precise causal mechanism has yet to be defined. The consequences of platelet exposure to homocysteine appear to be limited to a subtle shift in eicosanoid metabolism. Although there is some evidence for enhanced thrombin generation in hyperhomocysteinemic states, it is not yet clear which of several potential pathways implicated in vitro may apply in vivo. Both ectopic activation of procoagulant proteins and depression of natural anticoagulant systems have been reported. Fibrinolytic surveillance, finally, may be impaired owing to direct derivatization of the tissue plasminogen binding domain of annexin II. A clear understanding of the relevance of each of these potential mechanisms awaits confirmation in carefully designed in vivo studies.

REFERENCES

1. Bajaj, MS, Bajaj, SP. Tissue factor pathway inhibitor: Potential therapeutic applications. *Thromb Haemost* 1997; 78: 471–77.
2. Bienvenu, T, Chadefaux, B, Ankri, A, Leblond, V, Coude, M, Salehian, B, Binet, JL, Kamoun, P. Antithrombin III activity is not related to plasma homocysteine concentrations. *Hemostasis* 1991; 21: 65–7.
3. Brattström, L, Israelsson, B, Tengborn, L, Hultberg, B. Homocysteine, factor VII and antithrombin III in subjects with different gene dosage for cystathionine β-synthase 1. *J Inherit Metab Dis* 1989; 12: 475–82.
4. Broze, GJ. Tissue factor pathway inhibitor and the revised theory of coagulation. *Annu Rev Med* 1995; 46: 103–12.
5. Cesarman, GM, Guevara, CA, Hajjar, KA. An endothelial cell receptor for plasminogen/tissue plasminogen activator. II. Annexin II-mediated enhancement of t-PA-dependent plasminogen activation. *J Biol Chem* 1994; 269: 21198–203.
6. Chacko, G, Ling, Q, Hajjar, KA. Induction of acute translational response genes by homocysteine: Elongation factors EF-1 alpha, beta, and delta. *J Biol Chem* 1998; 273: 19840–46.
7. D'Angelo, A, Selhub, J. Homocysteine and thrombotic disease. *Blood* 1997; 90: 1–11.
8. Di Minno, G, Davi, G, Margaglione, M, Cirillo, F, Grandone, E, Ciabattoni, G, Catalano, I, Strisciuglio, P, Andria, G, Patrono, C, Mancini, M. Abnormally high thromboxane biosynthesis in homozygous homocystinuria: Evidence for platelet involvement and probucol-sensitive mechanism. *J Clin Invest* 1993; 92: 1400–6.
9. Durand, P, Prost, M, Blache, D. Pro-thrombotic effects of a folic acid deficient diet in rat platelets and macrophages related to elevated homocysteine and decreased n-3 polyunsaturated fatty acids. *Atherosclerosis* 1996; 121: 231–43.
10. Durand, P, Lussier-Cacan, S, Blache, D. Acute methionine load-induced hyperhomocysteinemia enhances platelet aggregation, thromboxane biosynthesis, and macrophage-derived tissue factor activity in rats. *FASEB J* 1997; 11: 1157–68.
11. Esmon, CT. Regulatory mechanisms in hemostasis: Natural anticoagulants. In *Hematology: Basic Principles and Practice.* 2nd ed. (Hoffman, R, Benz, EJ, Shattil, SJ, Furie, B, Cohen, HJ, Silberstein, LE, eds.). Churchill Livingstone, New York, 1995; pp. 1597–605.
12. Freyburger, G, Labrouche, S, Sassoust, G, Rouanet, F, Javorschi, S, Parrot, F. Mild hyperhomocysteinemia and hemostatic factors in patients with arterial vascular diseases. *Thromb Haemost* 1997; 77: 466–71.
13. Fryer, RH, Wilson, BD, Gubler, DB, Fitzgerald, LA, Rodgers, GM. Homocysteine, a risk factor for premature vascular disease and thrombosis, induces tissue factor activity in endothelial cells. *Arterioscler Thromb* 1993; 13: 1327–33.
14. Furie, B, Furie, BC. Molecular basis of blood coagulation. In *Hematology: Basic Principles and Practice.* 2nd ed. (Hoffman, R, Benz, EJ, Shattil, SJ, Furie, B, Cohen, HJ, Silberstein, LE, eds.). Churchill Livingstone, New York, 1995; pp. 1566–87.
15. Giannini, MJ, Coleman, M, Innerfield, I. Antithrombin activity in homocystinuria. *Lancet* 1975; 1: 1094.
16. Gibson, JB, Carson, NJ, Neill, DW. Pathologic findings in homocystinuria. *J Clin Pathol* 1964; 17: 427–37.
17. Graeber, JE, Slott, JH, Ulane, RE, Schulman, JD, Stuart, MJ. Effect of homocysteine and homocystine on platelet and vascular arachidonic acid metabolism. *Pediatr Res* 1982; 16: 490–93.
18. Gregory, SA, Morrissey, JH, Edgington, TS. Regulation of tissue factor gene expression in the monocyte procoagulant response to endotoxin. *Mol Cell Biol* 1989; 9: 2752–55.
19. Habben, JE, Moro, GL, Hunter, BG, Hamaker, BR, Larkins, BA. Elongation factor 1alpha concentration is highly correlated with the lysine content of maize endosperm. *Proc Natl Acad Sci USA* 1995; 92: 8640–44.
20. Hajjar, KA. The endothelial cell tissue plasminogen activator receptor: Specific interaction with plasminogen. *J Biol Chem* 1991; 266: 21962–70.
21. Hajjar, KA. Homocysteine-induced modulation of tissue plasminogen activator to its endothelial cell membrane receptor. *J Clin Invest* 1993; 91: 2873–79.

22. Hajjar, KA. The molecular basis of fibrinolysis. In *Hematology of Infancy and Childhood,* 5th ed. (Nathan, DG, Orkin, SH, eds.). WB Saunders, Philadelphia, 1998; pp. 1557–73.

23. Hajjar, KA, Hamel, NM. Identification and characterization of human endothelial cell membrane binding sites for tissue plasminogen activator and urokinase. *J Biol Chem* 1990; 265: 2908–16.

24. Hajjar, KA, Jacovina, AT, Chacko, J. An endothelial cell receptor for plasminogen and tissue plasminogen activator. I. Identity with annexin II. *J Biol Chem* 1994; 269: 21191–97.

25. Hajjar, KA, Guevara, CA, Lev, E, Dowling, K, Chacko, J. Interaction of the fibrinolytic receptor, annexin II, with the endothelial cell surface: essential role of endonexin repeat 2. *J Biol Chem* 1996; 271: 21652–59.

26. Hajjar, KA, Nachman, RL. The role of lipoprotein(a) in atherogenesis and thrombosis. *Annu Rev Med* 1996; 47: 423–42.

27. Hajjar, KA, Jacovina, AT. Modulation of annexin II by homocysteine: Implications for atherothrombosis. *J Invest Med* 1998; 46: 1–6.

28. Hajjar, KA, Mauri, L, Jacovina, AT, Zhong, F, Mirza, UA, Padovan, JC, Chait, BT. Tissue plasminogen activator binding to the annexin II tail domain: Direct modulation by homocysteine. *J Biol Chem* 1998; 273: 9987–93.

29. Harker, LA, Slichter, SJ, Scott, CD, Ross, R. Homocysteinemia: Vascular injury and arterial thrombosis. *N Engl J Med* 1974; 291: 537–43.

30. Harpel, PC, Chang, VT, Borth, W. Homocysteine and other sulfhydryl compounds enhance the binding of lipoprotein(a) to fibrin: A potential biochemical link between thrombosis, atherogenesis, and sulfhydryl compound metabolism. *Proc Natl Acad Sci USA* 1992; 89: 10193–97.

31. Hayashi, T, Honda, G, Suzuki, K. An atherogenic stimulus homocysteine inhibits cofactor activity of thrombomodulin and enhances thrombomodulin expression in human umbilical vein endothelial cells. *Blood* 1992; 79: 2930–36.

32. Hill-Zobel, R, Pyeritz, RE, Scheffel, U, Malpica, O, Engin, S, Camargo, EE, Abbott, M, Guilarte, TR, Hill, J, McIntyre, PA, Murphy, EA, Min-Fu, T. Kinetics and distribution of 111-indium-labeled platelets in patients with homocystinuria. *N Engl J Med* 1982; 307: 781–86.

33. Kassam, G, Choi, KS, Ghuman, J, Kang, HM, Fitzpatrick, SL, Zackson, T, Zackson, S, Toba, M, Shinomiya, A, Waisman, DM. The role of annexin II tetramer in the activation of plasminogen. *J Biol Chem* 1998; 273: 4790–99.

34. Keaney, JF, Loscalzo, J. Homocyst(e)ine decreases bioavailable nitric oxide by a mechanism involving glutathione peroxidase. *J Biol Chem* 1997; 272: 17012–17.

35. Kyrle, PA, Stumpflen, A, Hirschl, M, Bialonczyk, C, Herkner, K, Speiser, W, Weltermann, A, Kaider, A, Pabinger, I, Lechner, K, Eichinger, S. Levels of prothrombin fragment F1 + 2 in patients with hyperhomocysteinemia and a history of venous thromboembolism. *Thromb Haemost* 1997; 78: 1327–31.

36. Lentz, SR, Sadler, JE. Inhibition of thrombomodulin surface expression and protein C activation by the thrombogenic agent homocysteine. *J Clin Invest* 1991; 88: 1906–14.

37. Lentz, SR, Sadler, JE. Homocysteine inhibits von Willebrand factor processing and secretion by preventing transport from the endoplasmic reticulum. *Blood* 1993; 81: 683–89.

38. Lentz, SR, Sobey, CG, Piegers, DJ, Bhopatkar, MY, Faraci, FM, Malinow, MR, Heistad, DD. Vascular dysfunction in monkeys with diet-induced hyperhomocyst(e)inemia. *J Clin Invest* 1996; 98: 24–9.

39. Mackman, N. Regulation of the tissue factor gene. *Thromb Haemost* 1997; 78: 747–54.

40. Mandel, H, Brenner, B, Berant, M, Rosenberg, N, Lanir, N, Jakobs, C, Fowler, B, Seligsohn, U. Coexistence of hereditary homocystinuria and factor V Leiden: Effect on thrombosis. *N Engl J Med* 1996; 334: 763–68.

41. Marcus, AJ, Safier, LB, Broekman, MJ, Islam, N, Fliessbach, JH, Hajjar, KA, Kaminski, WE, Jendraschak, E, Silverstein, RL, von Schacky, C. Thrombosis and inflammation as multicellular processes: Significance of cell-cell interactions. *Thromb Haemost* 1995; 74: 213–17.

42. Maruyama, I, Fukuda, R, Kaszmama, M, Abe, T, Yoshida, Y, Igata, A. A case of homocystinuria with low antithrombin activity. *Acta Hem Jap* 1977; 40: 267–71.

43. McDonald, L, Bray, C, Field, C, Love, F, Davies, B. Homocystinuria, thrombosis, and blood-platelets. *Lancet* 1964; 1: 745–46.

44. Merckx, J, Kuntz, F. Deficit en facteur VII et homocystinurie: Association fortuite ou syndrome? *Nouv Presse Med* 1981; 10: 3796.

45. Munnich, A, Saudubray, JM, Dautzenberg, MD, Parvy, P, Ogier, H, Girot, R, Manigne, P, Frezal, J. Diet-responsive proconvertin (factor VII) deficiency in homocystinuria. *J Pediatr* 1983; 102: 730–34.

46. Nishinaga, M, Ozawa, T, Shimada, K. Homocysteine, a thrombogenic agent, suppresses anticoagulant heparan sulfate expression in cultured porcine aortic endothelial cells. *J Clin Invest* 1993; 92: 1381–86.

47. Palareti, G, Salardi, S, Piazzi, S, Legnani, C, Poggi, M, Grauso, F, Caniato, A, Coccheri, S, Cacciari, E. Blood coagulation changes in homocystinuria: Effects of pyridoxine and other specific therapy. *J Pediatr* 1986; 109: 1001–6.

48. Plow, EF, Ginsberg, MH. Molecular basis of platelet function. In *Hematology: Basic Principles and Practice,* 2nd ed. (Hoffman, R, Benz, EJ, Shattil, SJ, Furie, B, Cohen, HJ, Silberstein, LE, eds). Churchill Livingstone, New York, 1995; pp.1524–35.

49. Ratnoff, OD. Activation of Hageman factor by L-homocysteine. *Science* 1968; 162: 1007–9.

50. Ratnoff, OD, Calopy, JE. A familial hemorrhagic trait associated with a deficiency of a clot-promoting fraction of plasma. *J Clin Invest* 1955; 34: 602–13.

51. Raynal, P, Pollard, HB. Annexins: The problem of assessing the biologic role for a gene family of multifunctional calcium- and phospholipid-binding proteins. *Biochim Biophys Acta* 1994; 1197: 63–93.

52. Rees, MM, Rodgers, GM. Homocysteinemia: Association of a metabolic disorder with vascular disease and thrombosis. *Thromb Res* 1993; 71: 337–59.

53. Rodgers, GM, Kane, WH. Activation of endogenous factor V by a homocysteine-induced vascular endothelial cell activator. *J Clin Invest* 1986; 77: 1909–16.

54. Rodgers, GM, Conn, MT. Homocysteine, an atherogenic stimulus, reduces protein C activation by arterial and venous endothelial cells. *Blood* 1990; 75: 895–901.

55. Schimke, RN, McKusick, VA, Huang, T, Pollack, AD. Homocystinuria: Studies of 20 families with 38 affected members. *JAMA* 1965; 193: 711–19.

56. Semeraro, N, Colucci, M. Tissue factor in health and disease. *Thromb Haemost* 1997; 78: 759–64.

57. Stamler, JS, Osborne, JA, Jaraki, O, Rabbani, LE, Mullins, M, Singel, D, Loscalzo, J. Adverse vascular effects of homocysteine are modulated by endothelium-derived relaxing factor and related oxides of nitrogen. *J Clin Invest* 1993; 91: 308–18.

58. Swairjo, MA, Seaton, BA. Annexin structure and membrane interactions: A molecular perspective. *Annu Rev Biophys Biomol Struct* 1994; 23: 193–213.

59. Uhlemann, ER, TenPas, JH, Lucky, AW, Schulman, JD, Mudd, SH, Shulman, NR. Platelet survival and morphology in homocystinuria due to cystathionine synthase deficiency. *N Engl J Med* 1976; 295: 1283–86.

60. Undas, A, Domagala, TB, Jankowski, M, Szczeklik, A. Treatment of hyperhomocysteinemia with folic acid, vitamin B12, and B6 attenuates thrombin generation. *Thromb Res* 1999; 95: 281–88.

61. van der Berg, M, Boers, GHJ, Franken, DG, Blom, HJ, van Kamp, GJ, Jakobs, C, Rauwerda, JA, Kluft, C, Stehouwer, CDA. Hyperhomocysteinaemia and endothelial dysfunction in young patients with peripheral arterial occlusive disease. *Eur J Clin Invest* 1995; 25; 176–81.

62. Wagner, DD, Ginsburg, D. Structure, biology, and genetics of von Willebrand factor. In *Hematology: Basic Principles and Practice,* 2nd ed. (Hoffman, R, Benz, EJ, Shattil, SJ, Furie, B, Cohen, HJ, Silberstein, LE, eds.). Churchill Livingstone, New York, 1995; pp. 1717–25.

63. Wang, J, Dudman, NPB, Wilcken, DE. Effects of homocysteine and related compounds on prostacyclin production by cultured vascular endothelial cells. *Thromb Haemost* 1993; 6: 1047–52.

64. Watanabe, M, Osada, J, Aratani, Y, Kluckman, K, Reddick, R, Malinow, MR, Maeda, N. Mice deficient in cystathionine beta-synthase: Animal models for mild and severe homocyst(e)inemia. *Proc Natl Acad Sci USA* 1995; 92: 1585–89.

35

Cellular Mechanisms of Homocysteine Pathogenesis in Atherosclerosis

DONALD W. JACOBSEN

The vast majority of case-control studies and many, but not all, of the prospective studies reviewed in other chapters suggest that hyperhomocysteinemia is a major independent risk factor for cardiovascular disease. However, a causal role for homocysteine in atherothrombogenesis and/or progression of vascular disease has yet to be shown. Four decades of research with homocystinuric patients, animal models, cultured cells, and in vitro chemical systems have produced numerous suggestions on the potential roles that homocysteine could play. We now suspect that homocysteine has procoagulant activity toward platelets and the vascular endothelium, and that homocysteine has prooxidant activity and could serve as a source of reactive oxygen species during its autooxidation and oxidation with other thiols. Homocysteine may also induce gene expression, and a growing body of evidence suggests that homocysteine may interact with specific molecular targets such as membrane receptors, cell surface proteins, intracellular proteins, and small molecules such as nitric oxide. This chapter focuses on cellular mechanisms of homocysteine pathogenicity.

Early Observations on Mechanism in Humans and Animal Models

The earliest thoughts on the pathogenicity of homocysteine are coincidental with the discovery of homocystinuria by Carson and Neill (9) and by Gerritsen et al. (31). Gerritsen noted that "oxidation [of homocysteine] to homocystine must take place somewhere along this route [i.e., from plasma to urine], possibly in the kidneys." The suspicion that homocysteine was oxidized in the circulation was also supported by the observation that the liver of a homocystinuric patient had high levels of homocystine, which was undetectable in normal liver (86). By the mid 1960s, it was clear that homocystinuric patients had precocious cardiovascular and thromboembolic disease (8, 32).

That homocysteine might be involved in the cardiovascular diseases of very young patients with homocystinuria was investigated by McCully (59). Sections of cardiovascular tissues from an infant with cystathionine β-synthase (CBS) deficiency and a boy with a cobalamin *(Cbl)* mutation were examined. The cardiovascular lesions were similar in both cases and involved "numerous large, medium-sized, and small arteries in many organs." There was narrowing of the lumens owing to "focal intimal and medial fibrosis, often associated with fraying and discontinuity of the internal elastic membranes." McCully also observed "focal proliferation of perivascular connective tissue surrounding many small arteries, with an increase in the number of fibroblasts, collagen bundles, and small elastic fibers." There was also thickening of the media in some medium-sized and small arteries. However, there appeared to be an absence of venous involvement.

McCully (59) suggested that the vascular abnormalities in the two patients was due to their severe hyperhomocysteinemia. His observations led to the "homocysteine theory of arteriosclerosis" published in 1975 (65).

During the early and mid 1970s, investigators attempted to develop animal models of hyperhomocysteinemia. Using a pulsatile pump, Harker et al. (36) continuously infused L-homocystine[1] through a femoral arteriovenous shunt into male baboons over a 5-day period. Plasma concentrations of 110, 200, and 450 μmol/L L-homocystine, equivalent to 220, 400, and 900 μmol/L L-homocysteine, respectively, were achieved by varying the infusion rate. The investigators observed patchy desquamation of the vascular endothelium and

---

[1] In this chapter the precise form of homocysteine used in a study is indicated. Unfortunately, many investigators did not provide this information, and it was necessary to make an educated guess as to the precise form based on a knowledge of what has been available from commerical sources over the years.

platelet turnover that was dose-dependent for homocysteine. Two animals receiving extremely high levels of L-homocysteine, with plasma homocysteine concentrations reaching 1.4 to 1.9 mmol/L, experienced arterial thrombosis within a week. Harker et al. (35) also infused L-homocysteine thiolactone[2] into baboons over a 3-month period, resulting in L-homocysteine levels of 100 to 200 µmol/L.

Potential problems associated with the use of homocysteine thiolactone in vivo include acid formation as the thiolactone hydrolyzes and formation of insoluble diketopiperazine in concentrated solutions of thiolactone (27). Nevertheless, Harker et al. (35) observed patchy endothelial desquamation of the aorta along with a threefold increase in platelet turnover. The baboons developed "arteriosclerotic and preatherosclerotic intimal lesions composed of proliferating smooth muscle cells averaging 10 to 15 cell layers surrounded by large amounts of collagen, elastic fibers, glycosaminoglycans, and sometimes lipid." Interestingly, the antiplatelet drug, dipyridamole, prevented intimal lesion formation but had no effect on endothelial cell desquamation.

Although the Harker animal model demonstrates a causal role for homocysteine in the severe hyperhomocysteinemia seen in homocystinuric patients, by design it does not serve as a model for the mild hyperhomocysteinemia most often associated with cardiovascular disease. McCully and Ragsdale (63) and McCully and Wilson (65) developed a rabbit model of homocysteine-induced arteriosclerosis and atherosclerosis, but two other groups failed to reproduce the results (21, 56). Because of the possible cytotoxic effects of homocysteine thiolactone and the inability of some investigators to establish experimental arteriosclerosis in animal models, the relevance of the early animal studies in understanding homocysteine-induced vascular disease can be questioned.

Are All Forms of Homocysteine Atherogenic?

It is usually accepted that free reduced homocysteine is the form most likely to be atherogenic. Yet it makes up less than 2% of plasma total homocysteine (homocystinurics are the exception and have much higher levels [58]). Of course, a plasma total homocysteine level is a static marker and does not reflect chemical reactivity and turnover. Whether homocysteine alone or homocysteine and its oxidized counterparts are atherothrombogenic is unknown. Thus, the atherogenicity and atherogenic potential of homocystine,

homocysteine-cysteine mixed disulfide, and protein-bound homocysteine mixed disulfide remain to be determined (see Chapter 2 for details on circulating forms of homocysteine).

Homocysteine thiolactone, the condensed ring form of homocysteine, should also be considered as a potential atherogen, because it, too, is found endogenously. The elegant studies on the biosynthesis of homocysteine thiolactone through aminoacyl tRNA synthetase editing by Jakubowski are described in Chapter 3. This work establishes the possibility that homocysteine thiolactone could play a role in atherothrombogenesis through its unique chemical reactivity. Briefly, primary amines (e.g., the ε-amino group of lysine), can attack the "activated" carbonyl of homocysteine thiolactone to form a stable amide bond. The entry of homocysteine thiolactone into the circulation could result in the acylation of protein lysine residues ("amine homocysteinylation"). Because the amide bond is very stable, *homocystamide*-modified proteins would not lose their homocysteine by thiol/disulfide exchange. However, a homocystamide-modified protein might be recognized as "foreign" and eliminated by an immune response or subjected to more rapid degradation.

Homocysteine thiolactone, which does not undergo oxidation, in contrast to easily oxidizable homocysteine, was used extensively in the animal model studies cited previously (21, 35, 56, 63, 65). More recently, numerous reviews and editorials have suggested that homocysteine thiolactone is an important player in atherothrombogenesis (53, 61, 62, 102, 103, 105), although the evidence for this is scant.

That serum contains homocysteine thiolactone or homocystamide-modified protein is controversial. Olszewski and Szostak (72) reported that acid hydrolysates of plasma from 26 male survivors of myocardial infarction contained a mean of 958 ± 84 µmol/L homocysteine (measured as homocystine and homocysteine-cysteine mixed disulfide by ion-exchange amino acid analysis), which was 25 times higher than the homocysteine found in the control group. However, Dudman et al. (25) were unable to confirm this observation and found that the homocysteine content of acid-hydrolyzed plasma proteins was nearly identical in myocardial infarct patients and control subjects. Furthermore, electrophoretic studies were unable to confirm the presence of homocystamide-modified proteins in plasma from patients who had suffered a myocardial infarction (25). McCully and Vezeridis (64) reported that millimolar concentrations of homocysteine thiolactone could be extracted from human plasma or serum. However, Mudd et al. (68) were unable to show this, and McCully (60) later retracted his earlier report.

Additional studies are needed to determine if plasma contains homocysteine thiolactone or homo-

---

[2] Although Harker et al. (35) state that L-homocystine was used in this study, apparently L-homocysteine thiolactone was actually infused. See Harker's personal communication to Dudman et al. (24).

cystamide-modified proteins. The greatest likelihood for detecting these entities will be in severely hyperhomocysteinemic individuals (>100 µmol/L total homocysteine). Although the concentration of free reduced homocysteine in patients with congenital homocystinuria can approach 100 µmol/L (58), it does not readily cyclize to form the thiolactone (27). Cyclization occurs spontaneously only at acidic pH. Of course, this does not rule out the possibility of an energy-dependent, enzyme-mediated condensation reaction.

How stable is homocysteine thiolactone in circulation, and is it possible that it might not be found even in severely hyperhomocysteinemic serum? Dudman et al. (22) provided evidence that homocysteine thiolactone is very unstable in the circulation and is undetectable in the serum of patients with homocystinuria. Using cultured human endothelial cells from arteries dissected from umbilical cords, they found that homocysteine thiolactone was rapidly and quantitatively hydrolyzed by a cell-mediated process that showed saturation kinetics and was stereospecific for L-homocysteine thiolactone. Human serum alone was also capable of eliminating homocysteine thiolactone by a process appearing to involve both homocysteinylation of protein and hydrolysis. These studies suggest that the small amounts of homocysteine thiolactone produced during aminoacyl tRNA synthetase editing (see Chapter 3) and exported to the circulation would, in all likelihood, be hydrolyzed to free reduced homocysteine. Clearly, more studies are needed to establish whether homocysteine thiolactone or homocystamide-modified proteins are present intracellularly, or in the circulation of normal and hyperhomocysteinemic individuals.

Homocysteine and Endothelial Cell Dysfunction

A growing body of evidence indicates that mild elevations of plasma total homocysteine can adversely affect the endothelium. This finding has been seen in a primate animal model with diet-induced hyperhomocysteinemia (50) (see Chapter 36), in hyperhomocysteinemic individuals (88, 106), and in humans challenged with a methionine load to induce an acute transient hyperhomocysteinemia (2, 11–13, 42, 45) (see chapter 19 for greater detail). In the last named studies, subjects receive an oral dose of L-methionine in fruit juice (usually 100 mg/kg body weight). Plasma methionine rapidly rises and peaks usually within 1 hour, whereas plasma total homocysteine slowly rises to a maximum within 6 to 8 hours. Measurements are taken at baseline and usually 4 hours later, but well before the maximal increase in plasma total homocysteine is achieved. Between 4 and 8 hours postmethionine load, plasma total homocysteine concentrations usually increase by 200% to 300%, but in some subjects, the increase can

be much greater, and this may represent defective transsulfuration pathway activity. All of these studies showed impaired endothelium-dependent, flow-mediated vasodilatation. Chambers et al. (13) went on to show that the effect was methionine dose-dependent and could also be achieved by a high animal protein meal. Of interest mechanistically is the observation that impaired flow-mediated vasodilatation could be ameliorated by ascorbic acid (12, 42), which suggests that oxidative stress might be occurring during methionine-induced mild hyperhomocysteinemia.

Although these interesting in vivo studies point to the vascular endothelium as the target site affected by methionine-load induced transient hyperhomocysteinemia, the mechanism is by no means clear. Preceding the slowly rising peak of plasma total homocysteine is a rapidly rising and falling peak of methionine that occurs within 1 to 2 hours after ingestion. It seems reasonable to assume that vascular endothelial cells experience a "methionine load" during this time as well. Intracellular generation of homocysteine from the methionine load may have adverse effects on endothelial cell nitric oxide generation and bioavailability.

In Vitro Cytotoxicity Studies

It has long been suspected that homocysteine adversely effects endothelial cell function and viability. Early in vitro studies on cultured endothelial cells showed that homocysteine and/or homocysteine thiolactone were cytotoxic (19, 85, 99) and that the generation of hydrogen peroxide as a product of the autooxidation of homocysteine was partially responsible for the cytotoxicity (85, 99). Copper and other transition metals, which catalyze homocysteine autooxidation (85), may be required for the cytotoxic effect of homocysteine. Using human umbilical artery endothelial cells in culture, Dudman et al. (24) showed that both homocysteine and cysteine were capable of promoting cell detachment. In an in vitro model using monolayers of bovine aortic endothelial cells, homocysteine in the presence of copper increased albumin transfer across the monolayer, suggesting that a possible barrier dysfunction could occur in vivo (3). In the presence of catalase but not superoxide dismutase, increased albumin transfer was blocked. Hydrogen peroxide alone also caused barrier dysfunction suggesting that copper-catalyzed homocysteine autooxidation, which produces hydrogen peroxide as an endproduct, was responsible. Many of these early in vitro studies of cytotoxicity used supraphysiological concentrations of homocysteine and other thiols.

An important consideration for toxicity and endothelial dysfunction is the metabolic capacity for homocysteine metabolism in the vascular endothelium.

Not all tissues and organs, including rat heart, express an active transsulfuration pathway (30). Although it has been reported that extracts from cultured human umbilical vein endothelial cells have low levels of CBS activity (101), Chen et al. (15) found that human cardiovascular cells and tissues expressed neither functional CBS nor the alternate remethylation enzyme betaine:homocysteine methyltransferase. The same group reported that cultured human aortic endothelial cells also lacked functional CBS and betaine:homocysteine methyltransferase activities and thus had a limited capacity to metabolize homocysteine (40, 89). When normal human umbilical vein endothelial cells were compared with those from a patient with homozygous CBS deficiency, no differences were found in homocysteine export and in markers of endothelial dysfunction, suggesting that the two cell types had similar capacities for homocysteine metabolism (96). These observations suggest that the only metabolic route to detoxify intracellular homocysteine in the vascular endothelium is by folate- and cobalamin-dependent remethylation.

It is interesting to note that cultured vascular smooth muscle cells were extremely resistant to up to 40 mmol/L D,L-homocysteine thiolactone (99). This could be explained by the observation that induction of CBS expression and activity occurs when primary cultures of adult human aortic smooth muscle cells are established (15).

Folate or cobalamin deficiency may lead to inefficient homocysteine remethylation activity in endothelial cells. Coupled with its already limited capacity for homocysteine metabolism, the vascular endothelium may be particularly vulnerable to the elevated levels of plasma total homocysteine seen in systemic hyperhomocysteinemia.

A Caveat on In Vitro Mechanism Studies Many of the studies described below used massive concentrations, that is 5-10 mmol/L, of homocysteine, most often as the D,L-form. One has to interpret the results of these studies with caution. In cell culture medium, homocysteine undergoes rapid autooxidation and oxidation with other thiols to produce hydrogen peroxide and other reactive oxygen species. Thus, the effects observed could be due to the reactive oxygen species and not to homocysteine directly. When other thiols such as L-cysteine and glutathione elicit a response similar to that of homocysteine, it is likely that oxidative intermediates are playing a role. The use of catalase and superoxide dismutase can also be informative. Another problem associated with the use of D,L-homocysteine is the unnatural D-isomer and the ill effects it might have on cellular metabolism. In defense of the use of high concentrations of homocysteine is the

argument that homocysteine is poorly transported and high concentrations are needed to raise intracellular concentrations. Therefore, the relevance of a particular study depends on the concentration and form of homocysteine used, the use of antioxidant defense systems (e.g., catalase, superoxide dismutase, glutathione peroxidase), and the specificity of the response to homocysteine in contrast to other thiols.

Thromboresistance Many of the early in vitro studies on cultured endothelial cells examined the effect of homocysteine on coagulation factors. These studies are described in Chapter 34.

Nitric Oxide Production A growing body of evidence suggests that mild hyperhomocysteinemia and transient hyperhomocysteinemia associated with methionine loading impairs endothelium-dependent nitric oxide generation (2, 11, 13, 45, 69, 88, 106). Although antioxidants seem to protect against impaired flow-mediated vasodilatation during hyperhomocysteinemia (12, 42), the mechanism behind the putative endothelial dysfunction induced by homocysteine is poorly understood. A series of ex vivo and in vitro studies have attempted to gain some insight on mechanism.

D,L-Homocysteine (100 μmol/L) in the presence of copper (10 to 100 μmol/L) inhibited endothelium-dependent relaxation of isolated rat aorta segments (29). In the presence of catalase and/or superoxide dismutase, the inhibitory effect was reduced, suggesting that reactive oxygen species were involved. Because other thiols were not studied, the specificity for homocysteine-impaired relaxation is unknown. Similar results were obtained for isolated rabbit aorta segments (46) and for rat pancreatic vascular beds (77). Isolated skeletal muscle arterioles from rats with diet-induced hyperhomocysteinemia had impaired acetylcholine-induced vasodilatation and enhanced norepinephrine-induced constriction (93). The impaired vasodilatation response by acetylcholine in hyperhomocysteinemic arterioles was unaffected by catalase and superoxide dismutase. These ex vivo studies suggest that homocysteine can interfere with nitric oxide-dependent responses, but the mechanism is far from clear.

Evidence that homocysteine might impair nitric oxide production in cultured endothelial cells came from Stamler et al. (84). Bovine aortic endothelial cells were grown on carrier beads and treated with 5.0 mmol/L D,L-homocysteine for 6 hours. The homocysteine-treated endothelial cells were unable to inhibit adenosine diphosphate (ADP)-induced platelet aggregation compared with control cells, suggesting that nitric oxide production had been suppressed.

In contrast, D,L-homocysteine (0.05 to 5.0 mmol/L) actually enhanced the production of nitrosothiols in cultured bovine aorta endothelial cells stimulated to produce nitric oxide by either bradykinin or the calcium ionophore A23187 (95). L-Cysteine or glutathione (5.0 mmol/L) had no effect on nitrosothiol production in bradykinin-stimulated cells, suggesting that the observed stimulation of nitric oxide was specific for homocysteine. Cells that had been pretreated with homocysteine for 4 hours and then washed also showed a homocysteine dose-dependent enhancement of nitrosothiol production after bradykinin stimulation. Treatment of cells with 5.0 mmol/L homocysteine for 4 hours resulted in a 58% increase in steady-state mRNA levels for nitric oxide synthase 3 (95).

The same group reported that homocysteine in a dose-dependent manner actually decreased the bioavailability of nitric oxide independent of its enzymatic production by synthase (94). In this study, 5.0 mmol/L D,L-homocysteine treatment of cultured bovine aortic endothelial cells had no effect on nitric oxide synthase 3 mRNA levels or enzyme activity. However, treatment of cells with 0.05 to 1.0 mmol/L homocysteine for 4 hours led to a dose-dependent inhibition of intracellular glutathione peroxidase activity. Steady-state levels of mRNA for glutathione peroxidase decreased by 90% in cells treated with 5.0 mmol/L homocysteine but not with 5.0 mmol/L L-cysteine. This study suggests that homocysteine inhibits the expression of an important antioxidant defense system, namely glutathione peroxidase, resulting in decreased bioavailability of nitric oxide (94). Decreased bioavailability of nitric oxide was also observed by Demuth et al. (20) when the endothelial cell line, EA.hy 926, was treated with homocysteine. The major focus of this study was on the vasoconstrictor, endothelin-1. D,L-Homocysteine, L-cysteine and N-acetylcysteine caused a dose-dependent decrease in steady-state levels of endothelin-1 mRNA and secretion of the protein by EA.hy 926 cells. These in vitro studies show that very large concentrations of homocysteine can interfere with the production and bioavailability of nitric oxide, but shed little light on the mechanism.

Homocysteine and Endothelial Cell proliferation

Although homocysteine is mitogenic to smooth muscle cells *(vide infra)*, it appears to inhibit proliferation of vascular endothelial cells. ³H-Thymidine incorporation was inhibited by D,L-homocysteine in a dose-dependent manner in cultured human umbilical vein endothelial cells (90). The mechanism of growth inhibition may be related to the formation of S-adenosylhomocysteine (AdoHcy), a potent endproduct inhibitor of S-adenosylmethionine (AdoMet)-dependent methyltransferases. Wang et al. (100) found that 10 to 50 μmol/L D,L-homocysteine, in the presence of 50 μmol/L adenosine and an adenosine deaminase inhibitor, suppressed DNA synthesis and arrested vas-

cular endothelial cells in the G_1 phase of the cell cycle. Under these conditions, the intracellular concentration of AdoHcy increased owing to the reversibility of AdoHcy hydrolase (Metabolic Diagram, Reaction 3). There was no increase in AdoHcy if L-cysteine replaced D,L-homocysteine, and L-cysteine had no effect on DNA synthesis. The increase in AdoHcy affected the AdoHcy/AdoMet ratio and hypomethylation potential, resulting in decreased carboxyl methylation of the p21ras carboxy terminus. In the absence of carboxyl methylation, p21ras is unable to associate with the plasma membrane. The inability of p21ras to immobilize on the membrane may have been responsible for decreased mitogen-activated protein kinase ERK1/2 activity, which is involved in cell proliferation. Homocysteine and adenosine had no effect on vascular smooth muscle cell proliferation (100), possibly owing to the removal of homocysteine by CBS activity in cultured smooth muscle cells (15). Although this is a novel in vitro mechanism for endothelial cell dysfunction, it is unknown if a combination of high intracellular homocysteine plus adenosine can exist under in vivo conditions.

Homocysteine and Gene Expression Using Differential Displays

Recent investigations have utilized differential display to study the effect of homocysteine on gene expression in cultured endothelial cells (10, 44, 73, 74). Kokame et al. (44) treated human umbilical vein endothelial cells with 10.0 mmol/L D,L-homocysteine for 4 hours and found that six genes were upregulated and one gene was downregulated. The upregulated genes included the stress protein GRP78/BiP, the bifunctional enzyme methylenetetrahydrofolate dehydrogenase/methenyltetrahydrofolate cyclohydrolase and activating transcription factor 4. GRP78/BiP is an endoplasmic reticulum molecular chaperone that is upregulated when misfolding of endoplasmic reticulum proteins occurs. Some evidence exists that homocysteine causes misfolding and entrapment of proteins in the endoplasmic reticulum (48, 49). However, in the study by Kokame et al. (44), cysteine and 2-mercaptoethanol also induced gene expression. The possibility that reactive oxygen species, produced during thiol autooxidation, were responsible for gene induction was not investigated.

Treatment of human umbilical vein endothelial cells with 5.0 mmol/L D,L-homocysteine produced a twofold to fourfold, time-dependent induction of mRNA for elongation factors 1α, β, and δ (10). Elongation factor 1 is a 5-member multimeric protein complex ($\alpha_2\beta\gamma\delta$) that regulates the efficiency and fidelity of mRNA translation in mammalian cells. Upregulation of mRNA elongation factors 1α, β, and δ was observed with as little as 15 μmol/L homocysteine, and L-cysteine had no effect. In addition, all four proteins of the complex increased after homocysteine treatment. Although it was suggested that homocysteine-induced oxidative stress was responsible for the upregulation of elongation factor 1, no evidence to document this was presented.

Outinen et al. (73) found that 1.0 and 5.0 mmol/L D,L-homocysteine upregulated the expression of mRNA for GRP78, as reported earlier (44). A > 20-fold induction was observed with 5.0 mmol/L homocysteine at 8 hours, whereas 5.0 mmol/L L-cysteine or L-methionine had no effect. Heat shock induced a twofold expression of GRP78 but did not block the enhanced expression observed with 5.0 mmol/L homocysteine. Homocysteine had no effect on the expression of mRNA for heat shock protein HSP70. Interestingly, 5.0 mmol/L hydrogen peroxide alone induced a twofold induction of GRP78 mRNA at 4 and 8 hours, and the combination of 5.0 mmol/L hydrogen peroxide and 5.0 mmol/L homocysteine induced a 10- and 20-fold induction at 4 and 8 hours, respectively, suggesting that homocysteine may be acting directly. GRP78 protein levels were increased twofold and fivefold after 18 hours by 1.0 and 5.0 mmol/L homocysteine, respectively, whereas homocysteine had no effect on HSP70 protein levels, which is consistent with the mRNA data.

To study the relevance of these observations in vivo, total RNA was extracted from the livers of wild-type and heterozygous and homozygous CBS-deficient mice and subjected to Northern blot analysis (73). GRP78 mRNA was markedly upregulated in the homozygous CBS-deficient animals compared with wild-type and heterozygous animals. HSP70 mRNA was unaffected. Finally, a human cDNA microarray was screened with radiolabeled cDNA derived from poly(A)+ RNA from control and 5.0 mmol/L-treated human umbilical vein endothelial cells. Homocysteine upregulated the expression of GADD153, a member of the C/EBP family of transcription factors inducible by thiols and endoplasmic reticulum stress, and downregulated the expression of the antioxidant enzymes, glutathione peroxidase and natural killer-enhancing factor β. Although 1.0 and 5.0 mmol/L homocysteine exceed even pathophysiological levels of plasma total homocysteine (let alone free reduced homocysteine), the cumulative data presented in this study tend to argue against oxidative stress as a mechanism for induction of GRP78 and suggest that homocysteine may have a direct, adverse effect ("reductive stress") on the endoplasmic reticulum.

In an extension of their earlier study, Outinen et al. (74) used cDNA microarrays to show that 5.0 mmol/L D,L-homocysteine upregulated genes responsive to endoplasmic reticulum stress (GADD45, GADD153, ATF-4, YY1) and downregulated antioxidant genes (glutathione peroxidase, proliferation-associated glycoprotein, natural killer-enhancing factor β, superoxide dismutase).

Homocysteine and Leukocyte Recruitment to the Vascular Endothelium The "response to injury" hypothesis states that the vascular endothelium becomes "activated" in response to an injurious event such as viral or bacterial infection, exposure to oxidized low-density lipoprotein or exposure to thrombin, and it may apply to homocysteine as well (81). As depicted in Figure 35.1, the injurious event serves as an activation signal to which the endothelium responds in a variety of ways. In early atherogenesis, monocytes firmly attach to sites of endothelial cell injury using cellular adhesion molecules and then undergo diapedesis across the vascular endothelium into the subendothelial space at or near sites of endothelial injury. Here, they transform into macrophages and engulf large amounts of lipid, becoming foam cells in the process. Monocyte recruitment as a response to injury is shown in Figure 35.2. The arrival of monocytes in the subendothelial space is orchestrated by a repertoire of cytokines, which play critical roles in atherosclerosis and inflammatory diseases in general. Dysregulation of cytokine expression in vascular cells may contribute to the atherosclerotic process.

Endothelial cell activation is characterized by the release of proinflammatory cytokines (80, 81). Some of these cytokines, in particular monocyte chemoattractant factor 1 (MCP-1) and interleukin-8, serve as chemokines for the recruitment of monocytes and neutrophils, respectively, to the site of injury. Relatively low concentrations of D,L-homocysteine (25 to 50 μmol/L) induce the expression of mRNAs for MCP-1 and interleukin-8 in cultured human aortic endothelial cells in a dose–dependent manner (75). L-cysteine, L-homocystine, and L-methionine were unable to induce expression. Expression of other cytokines, including tumor necrosis factor, granulocyte-macrophage colony stimulating factor, interleukin-1β and transforming growth factor-β, was not affected by homocysteine. D,L-Homocysteine also triggered the release of MCP-1 and interleukin-8 into the culture medium. Conditioned medium from homocysteine-treated human aortic endothelial cells was chemotactic for U937 monocytic cells. However, if the conditioned medium was first treated with anti-recombinant MCP-1 antibody, U937 cell migration was blocked (75). The mechanism whereby homocysteine modulates expression of MCP-1 and interleukin-8 is unknown. L-homocysteine (50 to 200 μmol/L) and L-homocystine (25 to 100 μmol/L) stimulated the

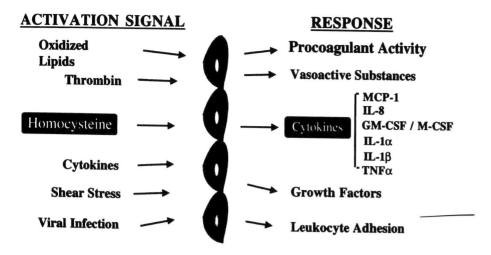

ACTIVATION SIGNAL

Oxidized Lipids

Thrombin

Homocysteine

Cytokines

Shear Stress

Viral Infection

RESPONSE

Procoagulant Activity

Vasoactive Substances

Cytokines
- MCP-1
- IL-8
- GM-CSF / M-CSF
- IL-1α
- IL-1β
- TNFα

Growth Factors

Leukocyte Adhesion

Fig. 35.1. The response of the vascular endothelium to injury. Injurious agents can serve as activation signals to the vascular endothelium. The homocysteine-activated endothelium can respond by changing from an anticoagulant to procoagulant phenotype, by releasing vasoactive substances, by secreting cytokines such as monocyte chemoattractant factor 1 (MCP-1), interleukin 8 (IL-8), granulocyte/macrophage colony stimulating factor (GM-CSF), macrophage colony stimulating factor (M-CSF), interleukin 1α (IL-1α), interleukin 1β (IL-1β), and tumor necrosis factor α (TNFα), and by becoming more adhesive to leukocytes.

Fig. 35.2. Recruitment of monocytes to the vascular endothelium. Through a process of random contact, rolling, and sticking, monocytes cross the endothelial barrier by diapedesis and migrate into the subendothelial space where they transform into macrophages and foam cells. Homocysteine (Hcy) may activate the vascular endothelium by promoting adhesion of leukocytes and by stimulating the production of chemokines such as monocyte chemoattractant protein 1 and interleukin-8. The transformation of macrophages to foam cells is, in part, thought to be mediated by oxidized low-density lipoprotein (oxLDL).

production of interleukin-6 by monocytic Mono Mac 6 cells in a thiol-specific manner, but they had no effect on the production of MCP-1 and interleukin-8 by these cells (95a).

Adhesion and migration of human neutrophils were stimulated when the cells were cocultured with human umbilical vein endothelial cells that had been first treated with L-homocysteine (26). Adhesion and migration occurred in a dose-dependent fashion over the concentration range of 50 to 400 μmol/L L-homocysteine. In contrast, L-cysteine over the same concentration range had practically no effect on adhesion and migration. Human neutrophils, treated with as little as 10 μmol/L L-homocysteine, were much more adhesive to non-homocysteine-treated human umbilical vein endothelial cell monolayers (23). These studies suggest that homocysteine can enhance leukocyte recruitment to the vascular endothelium by "activation" of both leukocytes and endothelial cells.

Random → Rolling → Sticking → Chemotaxis → Diapedesis
Contact

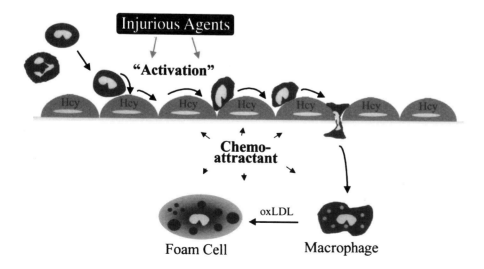

Injurious Agents

"Activation"

Chemo-attractant

oxLDL

Foam Cell

Macrophage

Homocysteine and Smooth Muscle Cell Dysfunction

Vascular smooth muscle cells play important roles in atherogenesis as shown by their ability to migrate out of the media and into the intima at sites of endothelial cell injury (82). After reaching the intima, vascular smooth muscle cells proliferate and produce a variety of proinflammatory cytokines. Perhaps the most important, but often overlooked, activity that vascular smooth muscle cells carry out while residing in the intima is the production of collagen and other matrix proteins. In classic homocystinuria, fibrous matrix deposition is a hallmark of atherosclerotic plaques, an observation made by McCully more than 30 years ago (59).

In Vitro Cytotoxicity Studies

Vascular smooth muscle cells appear to be resistant to the damaging effects of homocysteine in vitro. Using ^{51}Cr-release to assess cell damage and viability, Wall et al. (99) found that cultured human vascular smooth muscle cells from umbilical vein and renal artery were unaffected by 25 mmol/L D,L-homocysteine thiolactone treatment for 24 hours. When the concentration was increased to 40 mmol/L, there was a small but significant release of ^{51}Cr. The ability of cultured smooth muscle cells to withstand high concentrations of homocysteine could be related to poor transport or to an enhanced capacity to metabolize homocysteine via the transsulfuration pathway (15).

Nitric Oxide Production Although there is substantial evidence, both in vivo and in vitro, that homocysteine impairs the production and bioavailability of nitric oxide in endothelial cells, investigations on the effect of homocysteine on nitric oxide production by vascular smooth muscle cells are limited. Welch et al. (104) reported that D,L-homocysteine (5 to 500 µmol/L) stimulated cytokine-induced release of nitric oxide in the media using the Saville reaction (nitrite plus nitrosothiols) by cultured rat aortic smooth muscle cells. Homocysteine also enhanced steady-state levels of mRNA for inducible nitric oxide synthase (NOS2) and increased protein levels of the enzyme as well. Interestingly, homocysteine also activated the transcription factor NF-κB and potentiated the activation of NF-κB by cytokines (104). Although thiol specificity was not reported in this study, upregulation of the *NOS2* gene and gene products by homocysteine could potentiate the inflammatory response in atherogenesis.

In a similar study, 0.1 to 1.0 mmol/L homocysteine (D,L or L not reported) stimulated nitrite production by cultured rat aortic smooth muscle cells treated with interleukin-1β (37). Both mRNA and protein for inducible nitric oxide synthase were elevated by homo-

cysteine as well. However, cysteine, glutathione, and hydrogen peroxide also stimulated nitrite production, suggesting a general thiol effect. Moreover, in the presence of superoxide dismutase or catalase, homocysteine-induced nitrite production was inhibited. This study suggests that the mechanism of enhanced nitric oxide production involves the generation of reactive oxygen species as a result of thiol autooxidation.

Homocysteine and Smooth Muscle Cell Proliferation

Smooth muscle cells migrate to the intimal subendothelial space at sites of vascular injury in early atherogenesis where they can proliferate (82). Induction of smooth muscle cellular proliferation in the intima can be mediated by platelet-derived growth factor, fibroblast growth factor 2, and transforming growth factor β. Tsai et al. (90, 91) suggested that elevated homocysteine may also stimulate smooth muscle cell proliferation. Using cultured rat aortic smooth muscle cells, they found that 0.1 to 1.0 mmol/L D,L-homocysteine stimulated ^{3}H-thymidine incorporation, induced expression of mRNAs for cyclin D1 and cyclin A, and acted synergistically with serum to promote proliferation in quiescent cells (90). D,L-homocysteine (1.0 mmol/L) and 2% calf serum each stimulated mRNA levels for cyclin A by 8- and 14-fold, respectively. However, when homocysteine and calf serum were combined, a 40-fold synergistic stimulation was observed (91). Nuclear run-on experiments suggested that the rate of transcription of cyclin A mRNA, and not its half-life, was the cause of the induction. Homocysteine also stimulated promoter activity of the cyclin A gene and increased levels of the transcription factor ATF in cultured rat aortic smooth muscle cells. However, there is some question concerning thiol specificity in these studies because cysteine and glutathione were equally effective in promoting thymidine uptake in quiescent cells. It is possible that effects observed with homocysteine were due to the generation of reactive oxygen species during thiol autooxidation.

Tang et al. (87) found that homocysteine-stimulated thymidine incorporation in cultured human smooth muscle cells from saphenous vein and internal mammary artery was biphasic. There was modest stimulation (24% to 34%) with D,L-homocysteine up to 1.0 mmol/L, but incorporation was significantly inhibited at higher concentrations (up to 10 mmol/L) compared with nontreated control cells. Other thiols were not tested.

Majors et al. (55) found that L-homocysteine (50 to 500 µmol/L) and L-cysteine (600 µmol/L) stimulated proliferation in long-term cultured rabbit smooth muscle cells. Evidence that homocysteine may stimulate vascular smooth muscle cell proliferation by generating reactive oxygen species has been provided by Nishio and

Watanabe (70). They observed an interesting synergistic effect between D,L-homocysteine (500 μmol/L) and platelet-derived growth factor (1 nmol/L) in stimulating the proliferation of cultured rat aortic smooth muscle cells. However, the synergistic effect was completely blocked in the presence of catalase or N-acetylcysteine.

The inability to show thiol specificity and a possible oxidative stress response in these studies throw some doubt on the physiological relevance of homocysteine-stimulated proliferation of cultured vascular smooth muscle cells. One should be aware that the concentration of plasma total cysteine is 20 to 30 times that of plasma total homocysteine, even in mild to moderate hyperhomocysteinemia.

Homocysteine and the Vascular Matrix Soon after the discovery of homocystinuria (9, 31), it was suspected that elevated homocysteine might produce abnormalities in the extracellular matrix (reviewed by Pyeritz [76]). McCully (59) recognized the similarities of the arterial fibroproliferative lesions in patients with CBS and methionine synthase deficiencies. McKusick (66) proposed that homocysteine might interfere with the cross-linking of collagen, and, indeed, there is evidence for this proposal (38, 43, 52, 54). Is there any evidence that homocysteine affects collagen biosynthesis and posttranslational processing at the cellular level?

Majors et al. (55) reported that L-homocysteine (50 to 500 μmol/L) enhanced collagen synthesis and accumulation in cultured rabbit aortic smooth muscle cells. L-Cysteine had a similar effect but at much higher concentrations (approximately 600 μmol/L). Analysis of the hydroxyproline content of the cell layers showed that the newly synthesized collagen was actually deposited and not simply degraded. It has also been reported that L-homocystine (5 to 10 μmol/L) can upregulate the expression of collagen (I) mRNA in cultured human vascular smooth muscle cells (92). Although the mechanism of homocysteine-induced collagen synthesis in vascular smooth muscle cells is unknown, Mujumder et al. (68a) have shown that 0.1 to 10 μmol/L D,L-homocysteine, in a thiol-specific manner, can mobilize calcium from intracellular stores, which may activate multiple signalling pathways.

Homocysteine may also affect matrix architecture by stimulating or inhibiting the degradation of specific matrix protein components. The diet-induced hyperhomocysteinemic minipig model has provided evidence for "intense focal deterioration of the arterial elastic structure" due to increased elastolytic activity (1, 14, 79). Elastolytic prometalloproteinase 2 could be activated by D,L-homocysteine (homocysteine/proteinase molar ratio = 10:1) but was inhibited at higher molar ratios (> 1,000:1) (4). In contrast, L-cysteine and glutathione could not activate prometalloproteinase 2, nor could L-methionine or L-homocystine. These observations suggest that homocysteine is attacking

Fig. 35.3. The cysteine-switch mechanism for activation of metalloproteinases. Homocysteine (Hcy) displaces the propeptide cysteine from the active-site zinc, allowing water to coordinate. In the presence of excess homocysteine, the catalytic site is inactivated by the coordination of homocysteine to zinc. (Reproduced from Bescond et al. [4], with permission).

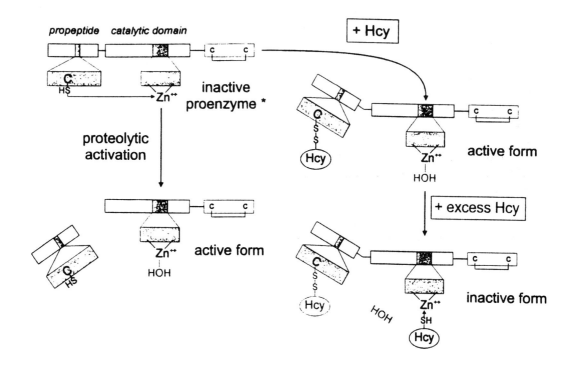

and forming a mixed disulfide with a propeptide cysteine residue, which activates the zinc-containing catalytic domain (Figure 35.3). This is consistent with the "cysteine switch" mechanism in which a cysteine-zinc coordinate bond is disrupted, allowing zinc to interact with a water molecule that is required for catalysis (83, 97). Homocysteine was inhibitory at molar ratios, presumably by coordinating to the active site zinc. These observations support the molecular target hypothesis of homocysteine pathogenesis *(vide infra)*.

Do Vascular Smooth Muscle Cells Have "Receptors" for Homocysteine?

Signal transduction pathways are activated when specific ligands bind to membrane receptors such as those associated with tyrosine kinases, G-coupled proteins and the N-methyl-D-aspartate (NMDA) ligand-gated ion channel. A common point of convergence for these pathways is mitogen-activated protein (MAP) kinase. It was of interest then when Brown et al. (7) found that D,L-homocysteine transiently activated the extracellular signal-regulated kinase isoform 2 (ERK2) of MAP kinase in cultured vascular smooth muscle cells from chick embryos. The activation response of ERK2, which requires phosphorylation of a tyrosine and threonine residue, to homocysteine was dose-dependent (0.1 to 100 µmol/L) with a half-maximal dose response of approximately 500 nmol/L. Activation by homocysteine was blocked by PD98059, a specific inhibitor of the kinase that phosphorylates ERK2. MK801, a specific inhibitor of the NMDA receptor channel, also blocked homocysteine activation of the ERK2. Previously, this group had shown that MK801 blocked homocysteine-mediated mitogenesis of vascular smooth muscle cells derived from the neural crest of chick embryos (17). These observations suggest that vascular smooth muscle cells may express a NMDA-like receptor that is activated by homocysteine. Studies using L-cysteine and other sulfur compounds were not reported, so the question of thiol specificity remains. If a NMDA-like receptor is involved, then it could be responsive to several homocysteine-related compounds, including homocysteine sulfinic acid, homocysteic acid, cysteine, cysteine sulfinic acid, and cysteic acid (51, 71).

We are only now beginning to understand the effect of homocysteine on smooth muscle cell metabolism and function. In cultured smooth muscle cells, it appears that homocysteine can modulate the production of nitric oxide, inhibit cell proliferation, and stimulate the synthesis and accumulation of collagen. However, a word of caution is necessary. Cultured smooth muscle cells express functional CBS, whereas cells from aortic tissue appear not to have a functional enzyme (15). This is similar to the situation with skin fibroblasts. Cultured skin fibroblasts express functional CBS, but the active enzyme is not found in skin punch biopsy extracts. However, the inability of vascular smooth muscle cells to metabolize homocysteine through the transsulfuration pathway in vivo is likely to potentiate the effects of exogenous homocysteine.

Mechanisms of Homocysteine-Induced Vascular Pathology

There is currently no unifying mechanism to explain the pathophysiology associated with hyperhomocysteinemia and cardiovascular diseases and more recent associations between hyperhomocysteinemia and neural tube defects and cognitive dysfunction. Although possible, it seems unlikely that homocysteine will turn out to be just a passive marker for these diseases. If homocysteine plays a causal role in any of these conditions, what are the possible mechanisms?

Oxidative Stress Hypothesis

The oxidant stress hypothesis is frequently invoked to explain the damaging effects of homocysteine on vascular cells and tissues because homocysteine and other thiols have prooxidant activity (53, 61). Recent use of antioxidants to block endothelial dysfunction during transient hyperhomocysteinemia induced by methionine loading is also cited as additional evidence for the involvement of oxidative stress in the mechanism (12, 42, 69). Oxidative stress is often cited as the mechanism responsible for the effects of homocysteine on cultured endothelial and smooth muscle cells. As depicted in Figure 35.4, homocysteine undergoes autooxidation in the presence of molecular oxygen. This can occur in the circulation or intracellularly. Reactive oxygen species can attack membranes, platelets, lipoprotein, and leukocytes. Intracellular target sites include the endoplasmic reticulum, Golgi apparatus, and nitric oxide.

Many of these studies, however, used supraphysiological concentrations (1 to 10 mmol/L) of homocysteine or homocysteine thiolactone, which hydrolyzes to homocysteine in the culture medium under conditions that more than likely led to the generation of reactive oxygen species. It should be realized that in vitro tissue culture conditions usually lack the elaborate antioxidant defense systems that are found in vivo, particularly in blood.

Homocysteine with its reactive sulfhydryl group (–SH), like most thiols (RSH), undergoes oxidation to the disulfide (RSSR) at physiological pH in the presence of O_2:

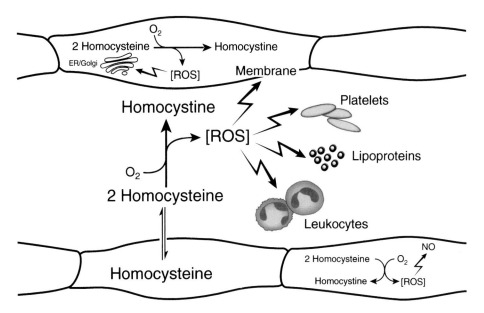

Fig. 35.4. The oxidative stress hypothesis of homocysteine pathogenesis. Homocysteine can undergo intracellular and extracellular autooxidation in the presence of molecular oxygen to generate reactive oxygen species (ROS). The ROS, in turn, do the actual damage by reacting with cellular constituents, including organelles, such as the endoplasmic reticulum (ER) and Golgi apparatus, and small molecules, such as nitric oxide (NO).

$$2 \text{ Homocysteine (RSH)} + O_2 \rightarrow$$
$$\text{Homocystine (RSSR)} + [O_2^{\bullet-}] \rightarrow H_2O_2$$

The reaction is catalyzed by transition metals (85) and a variety of reactive oxygen species are produced including superoxide anion radical, hydrogen peroxide, and under some circumstances hydroxyl radical (41, 67). Thiol oxidation occurs in the circulation because >98% of plasma total homocysteine in normal (5 to 12 μmol/L) and mildly hyperhomocysteinemic plasma (>12 to 25 μmol/L) is oxidized (see Chapter 2). In severe hyperhomocysteinemia, where plasma total homocysteine ranges from 100 to 500 μmol/L, is there evidence that free reduced homocysteine accounts for a substantially greater portion (up to 20%) of plasma total homocysteine (58).

The daily flux of plasma homocysteine in a healthy adult weighing 70 kg and having a total homocysteine level of 10 μmol/L is approximately 1.3 mmol/day (33). Assuming that all of the homocysteine entering circulation is reduced and that it undergoes rapid oxidation to homocystine and mixed disulfides, 0.65 mmol/day of hydrogen peroxide would be generated. This is equivalent to 94 pmol/min/mL blood in the 70 kg subject (blood volume = ~70 mL/kg). An individual with mild hyperhomocysteinemia (plasma total homocysteine = 20 μmol/L) would generate twice the level of hydrogen peroxide, or 188 pmol/min/mL. Transient hyperhomocysteinemia, observed 4 to 8 hours after methionine loading and 12 hours after an animal protein meal (13), may contribute to hydrogen peroxide flux as well.

However, the potential oxidative stress resulting from cysteine flux is much greater. The concentration of total cysteine in normal plasma is 25 to 30 times higher than that of total homocysteine, and oxidized forms of cysteine account for 94% to 95% of total plasma cysteine (57). Generating oxidative stress through the daily flux of cysteine (78) would appear to be much greater than with homocysteine, yet cysteine is not usually considered to be a significant risk factor of cardiovascular disease (however, see Jacob et al. [39]). Moreover, the blood is not without its potent, built-in, antioxidant defense system that includes antioxidants (e.g., ascorbate, tocopherols), glutathione peroxidase, superoxide dismutase, and catalase.

If oxidative stress resulting from hyperhomocysteinemia (or for that matter, thiol oxidation in general) causes vascular damage, then one might expect to detect oxidant stress markers in the blood. However, older studies have been unable to document markers of oxidative stress in serum from subjects with homocystinuria (5, 6, 16, 28). Voutilainen et al. (98), using a more sensitive indicator of oxidative stress, measured plasma F_2-isoprostanes as an in vivo indicator of lipid peroxidation in 100 men. F_2-isoprostanes, which are derived from free radical-mediated lipid peroxidation reactions of arachidonic acid, increased linearly across plasma total homocysteine quintiles. In a linear regression model, homocysteine had the strongest association with F_2-isoprostanes. Perhaps it is now time to reinvestigate the status of oxidative stress markers in hyperhomocysteinemic subjects with cardiovascular disease using more sensitive techniques to assess lipid and protein oxidation (18, 47).

Molecular Target Hypothesis

An alternative to the oxidative stress hypothesis is the molecular target hypothesis. Homocysteine itself may be interacting with specific molecular targets, either extracellularly or intracellularly, and modulating their activity. Nishio and Watanabe (70) showed that glutathione peroxidase activity decreased after treatment of rat aorta smooth muscle cells with D,L-homocysteine (0 to 500 μmol/L). In contrast, superoxide dismutase activity increased in a dose-dependent manner, but there was no effect on catalase activity. They also found that homocysteine inactivated purified bovine liver glutathione peroxidase, again in a dose-depen-

dent manner. Upchurch et al. (94) found that 50 to 250 μmol/L D,L-homocysteine inhibited glutathione peroxidase activity in cultured bovine aortic endothelial cells, but they did not obtain evidence for direct inactivation of the enzyme. They did observe that 5.0 mmol/L homocysteine (but not cysteine) decreased steady-state mRNA for glutathione peroxidase by 90%. These studies suggest that "oxidative stress" may be generated within vascular cells, but not necessarily as a result of thiol oxidation.

Other studies support the molecular target hypothesis as well. Homocysteine forms a mixed disulfide with Cys9 on annexin II, thereby inhibiting the binding of tissue plasminogen activator and limiting the conversion of plasminogen to plasmin (see Chapter 34) (34). As described previously, homocysteine appears to form a mixed disulfide with prometalloprotease 2, thereby activating the protease via a cysteine switch mechanism (4). Homocysteine also reacts with nitric oxide in the presence of transition metals, and, although this could limit the bioavailabilty of nitric oxide if trapped as a nitrosothiol intracellularly, there are probably insufficient molar equivalents of homocysteine to react with catalytically generated nitric oxide. As shown in Figure 35.5, homocysteine in the circulation can interact with membrane components of the vascular endothelium such as annexin II. It can also react with nitric oxide to form nitrosothiols. Through oxidative and thiol/disulfide exchange reactions, homocysteine is converted to oxidized forms such as protein-bound homocysteine (see Chapter 2) and low-molecular-weight disulfides. Entry of these oxidized forms into cells would generate free homocysteine owing to the reducing environment of the cell.

Fig. 35.5. The molecular target hypothesis of homocysteine pathogenesis. Intracellular and extracellular homocysteine (Hcy) can interact and modulate the activity of molecular targets directly. Most of the homocysteine in circulation undergoes oxidation and thiol/disulfide exchange reactions to form protein-bound homocysteine (protein-S-S-Hcy) and low-molecular-weight disulfides. The oxidized forms of homocysteine, on entering the reducing environment of the cell, are converted back to homocysteine. Homocysteine impairs the binding of tissue plasminogen activator (tPA) to annexin II, alters the redox potential of the endoplasmic reticulum (ER) and Golgi apparatus, thus inhibiting the surface expression and secretion of proteins, and reacts with both extracellular and intracellular nitric oxide (NO), generated by endothelial cell NO synthase, to form homocysteine nitrosothiol (HcySNO). It is possible that intracellular HcySNO decreases the bioavailability of NO.

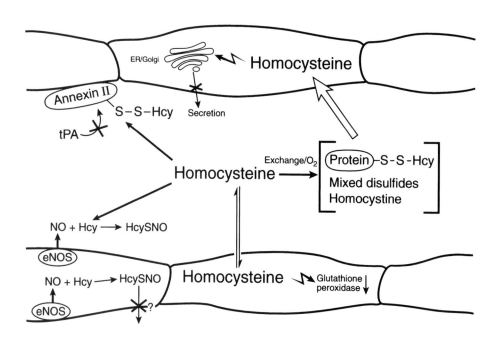

Homocysteine could then attack intracellular targets as well. Homocysteine thiolactone, with its activated carbonyl, may also be capable of inactivating specific molecular targets (see Chapter 3).

The interest in homocysteine as a risk factor for cardiovascular disease will no doubt be heightened if any of the ongoing homocysteine-lowering clinical trials are positive (15a). In the meantime, investigations continue on oxidative stress and molecular targeting as working hypotheses to explain the mechanisms of homocysteine pathogenesis in atherosclerosis.

REFERENCES

1. Augier, T, Charpiot, P, Chareyre, C, Remusat, M, Rolland, PH, Garçon, D. Medial elastic structural alterations in atherosclerotic arteries in minipigs: Plaque proximity and arterial site specificity. *Matrix Biol* 1996; 15: 455–67.
2. Bellamy, MF, McDowell, IFW, Ramsey, MW, Brownlee, M, Bones, C, Newcombe, RG, Lewis, MJ. Hyperhomocysteinemia after an oral methionine load acutely impairs endothelial function in healthy adults. *Circulation* 1998; 98: 1848–52.
3. Berman, RS, Martin, W. Arterial endothelial barrier dysfunction: Actions of homocysteine and the hypoxanthine-oxidase free radical generating system. *Br J Pharmacol* 1993; 108: 920–26.
4. Bescond, A, Augier, T, Chareyre, C, Garçon, D, Hornebeck, W, Charpiot, P. Influence of homocysteine on matrix metalloproteinase-2: Activation and activity. *Biochem Biophys Res Commun* 1999; 263: 498–503.
5. Blom, HJ, Engelen, DPE, Boers, GHJ, Stadhouders, AM, Sengers, RCA, de Abreu, R, TePoele-Pothoff, MTWB, Trijbels, JMF. Lipid peroxidation in homocysteinaemia. *J Inherit Metab Dis* 1992; 15: 419–22.
6. Blom, HJ, Kleinveld, HA, Boers, GHJ, Demacker, PNM, Hak-Lemmers, HLM, TePoele-Pothoff, MTWB, Trijbels, JMF. Lipid peroxidation and susceptibility of low-density lipoprotein to *in vitro* oxidation in hyperhomocysteinaemia. *Eur J Clin Invest* 1995; 25: 149–54.
7. Brown, JC III, Rosenquist, TH, Monaghan, DT. ERK2 activation by homocysteine in vascular smooth muscle cells. *Biochem Biophys Res Commun* 1998; 251: 669–76.
8. Carson, NAJ, Dent, CE, Field, CMB, Gaull, GE. Homocystinuria: Clinical and pathological review of ten cases. *J Pediatr* 1965; 66: 565–83.
9. Carson, NAJ, Neill, DW. Metabolic abnormalities detected in a survey of mentally backward individuals in Northern Ireland. *Arch Dis Child* 1962; 37: 505–13.
10. Chacko, G, Ling, Q, Hajjar, KA. Induction of acute translational response genes by homocysteine: Elongation factors-1α, -β, and -δ. *J Biol Chem* 1998; 273: 19840–46.
11. Chambers, JC, McGregor, A, Jean-Marie, J, Kooner, JS. Acute hyperhomocysteinaemia and endothelial dysfunction. *Lancet* 1998; 351: 36–7.
12. Chambers, JC, McGregor, A, Jean-Marie, J, Obeid, OA, Kooner, JS. Demonstration of rapid onset vascular endothelial dysfunction after hyperhomocysteinemia: An effect reversible with vitamin C therapy. *Circulation* 1999; 99: 1156–60.
13. Chambers, JC, Obeid, OA, Kooner, JS. Physiological increments in plasma homocysteine induce vascular endothelial dysfunction in normal human subjects. *Arterioscler Thromb Vasc Biol* 1999; 19: 2922–27.
14. Charpiot, P, Bescond, A, Augier, T, Chareyre, C, Fraterno, M, Rolland, PH, Garçon, D. Hyperhomocysteinemia induces elastolysis in minipig arteries: Structural consequences, arterial site specificity and effect of captopril-hydrochlorothiazide. *Matrix Biol* 1998; 17: 559–74.
15. Chen, P, Poddar, R, Tipa, EV, DiBello, PM, Moravec, CD, Robinson, K, Green, R, Kruger, WD, Garrow, TA, Jacobsen, DW. Homocysteine metabolism in cardiovascular cells and tissues: Implications for hyperhomocysteinemia and cardiovascular disease. *Adv Enzymol Regul* 1999; 39: 93–109.
15a. Clarke, R, Collins, R. Can dietary supplements with folic acid or vitamin B$_6$ reduce cardiovascular risk? Design of clinical trials to test the homocysteine hypothesis of vascular disease. *J Cardiovasc Risk* 1998; 5: 249–55.
16. Córdoba-Porras, A, Sánchez-Quesada, JL, González-Sastre, F, Ordóñez-Llanos, J, Blanco-Vaca, F. Susceptibility of plasma low- and high-density lipoproteins to oxidation in patients with severe hyperhomocysteinemia. *J Mol Med* 1996; 74: 771–76.
17. Dalton, ML, Gadson, PF Jr, Wrenn, RW, Rosenquist, TH. Homocysteine signal cascade: Production of phospholipids, activation of protein kinase C, and the induction of *c-fos* and *c-myb* in smooth muscle cells. *FASEB J* 1997; 11: 703–11.
18. Davies, MJ, Fu, S, Wang, H, Dean, RT. Stable markers of oxidant damage to proteins and their application in the study of human disease. *Free Radic Biol Med* 1999; 27: 1151–63.
19. De Groot, PG, Willems, C, Boers, GHJ, Gonsalves, MD, van Aken, WG, van Mourik, JA. Endothelial cell dysfunction in homocystinuria. *Eur J Clin Invest* 1983; 13: 405–10.
20. Demuth, K, Atger, V, Borderie, D, Benoit, MO, Sauvaget, D, Loterzstajn, S, Moatti, N. Homocysteine decreases endothelin-1 production by cultured human endothelial cells. *Eur J Biochem* 1999; 263: 367–76.
21. Donahue, S, Sturman, JA, Gaull, G. Arteriosclerosis due to homocyst(e)inemia. *Am J Pathol* 1974; 77: 167–74.
22. Dudman, NPB, Hicks, C, Lynch, JF, Wilcken, DEL, Wang, J. Homocysteine thiolactone disposal by human arterial endothelial cells and serum in vitro. *Arterioscler Thromb* 1991; 11: 663–70.
23. Dudman, NPB, Hale, SET. Endothelial- and leukocyte-mediated mechanisms in homocysteine-associated occlusive vascular disease. In *Homocysteine Metabolism: From Basic Science to Clinical Medicine* (Graham, I, Refsum, H, Rosenberg, IH, Ueland, PM, eds.). Kluwer Academic, Boston, 1997; pp. 267–71.
24. Dudman, NPB, Hicks, C, Wang, J, Wilcken, DEL. Human arterial endothelial cell detachment in vitro: Its promotion by homocysteine and cysteine. *Atherosclerosis* 1991; 91: 77–83.

25. Dudman, NPB, Lynch, J, Wang, J, Wilcken, DEL. Failure to detect homocysteine in the acid-hydrolyzed plasmas of recent myocardial infarct patients. *Atherosclerosis* 1991; 86: 201–9.

26. Dudman, NPB, Temple, SE, Guo, XW, Fu, WY, Perry, MA. Homocysteine enhances neutrophil-endothelial interactions in both cultured human cells and rats in vivo. *Circ Res* 1999; 84: 409–16.

27. Dudman, NPB, Wilcken, DEL. Homocysteine thiolactone and experimental homocysteinemia. *Biochem Med* 1982; 27: 244–53.

28. Dudman, NPB, Wilcken, DEL, Stocker, R. Circulating lipid hydroperoxide levels in human hyperhomocysteinemia. Relevance to development of arteriosclerosis. *Arterioscler Thromb* 1993; 13: 512–16.

29. Emsley, AM, Jeremy, JY, Gomes, GN, Angelini, GD, Plane, F. Investigation of the inhibitory effects of homocysteine and copper on nitric oxide-mediated relaxation of rat isolated aorta. *Br J Pharmacol* 1999; 126: 1034–40.

30. Finkelstein, JD. Methionine metabolism in mammals. *J Nutr Biochem* 1990; 1: 228–37.

31. Gerritsen, T, Vaughn, JG, Waisman, HA. The identification of homocystine in the urine. *Biochem Biophys Res Commun* 1962; 9: 493–96.

32. Gibson, JB, Carson, NAJ, Neill, DW. Pathological findings in homocystinuria. *J Clin Pathol* 1964; 17: 427–37.

33. Guttormsen, AB, Ueland, PM, Svarstad, E, Refsum, H. Kinetic basis of hyperhomocysteinemia in patients with chronic renal failure. *Kidney Int* 1997; 52: 495–502.

34. Hajjar, KA, Mauri, L, Jacovina, AT, Zhong, FM, Mirza, UA, Padovan, JC, Chait, BT. Tissue plasminogen activator binding to the annexin II tail domain: Direct modulation by homocysteine. *J Biol Chem* 1998; 273: 9987–93.

35. Harker, LA, Ross, R, Slichter, SJ, Scott, RC. Homocystine-induced arteriosclerosis. The role of endothelial cell injury and platelet response in its genesis. *J Clin Invest* 1976; 58: 731–41.

36. Harker, LA, Slichter, SJ, Scott, CR, Ross, R. Homocystinemia. Vascular injury and arterial thrombosis. *N Engl J Med* 1974; 291: 537–43.

37. Ikeda, U, Ikeda, M, Minota, S, Shimada, K. Homocysteine increases nitric oxide synthesis in cytokine-stimulated vascular smooth muscle cells. *Circulation* 1999; 99: 1230–35.

38. Jackson, SH. The reaction of homocysteine with aldehyde; an explanation of the collagen defects in homocystinuria. *Clin Chim Acta* 1973; 45: 215–17.

39. Jacob, N, Bruckert, E, Giral, P, Foglietti, MJ, Turpin, G. Cysteine is a cardiovascular risk factor in hyperlipidemic patients. *Atherosclerosis* 1999; 146: 53–9.

40. Jacobsen, DW, Savon, SR, Stewart, RW, Robinson, K, Green, R, Kottke-Marchant, K, DiCorleto, PE. Limited capacity for homocysteine catabolism in vascular cells and tissues: A pathophysiologic mechanism for arterial damage in hyperhomocysteinemia? *Circulation* 1995; 91: 29.

41. Jacobsen, DW, Troxell, LS, Brown, KL. Catalysis of thiol oxidation by cobalamins and cobinamides: Reaction products and kinetics. *Biochemistry* 1984; 23: 2017–25.

42. Kanani, PM, Sinkey, CA, Browning, RL, Allaman, M, Knapp, HR, Haynes, WG. Role of oxidant stress in endothelial dysfunction produced by experimental hyperhomocyst(e)inemia in humans. *Circulation* 1999; 100: 1161–68.

43. Kang, AH, Trelstad, RL. A collagen defect in homocystinuria. *J Clin Invest* 1973; 52: 2571–78.

44. Kokame, K, Kato, H, Miyata, T. Homocysteine-respondent genes in vascular endothelial cells identified by differential display analysis: GRP78/BiP and novel genes. *J Biol Chem* 1996; 271: 29659–65.

45. Lambert, J, van den Berg, M, Steyn, M, Rauwerda, JA, Donker, AJM, Stehouwer, CDA. Familial hyperhomocysteinaemia and endothelium-dependent vasodilatation and arterial distensibility of large arteries. *Cardiovasc Res* 1999; 42: 743–51.

46. Lang, D, Hussain, SA, Lewis, MJ. Homocysteine inhibits endothelium-dependent relaxation in isolated rabbit aortic rings. *Br J Pharmacol* 1997; 120: 145P.

47. Lawson, JA, Rokach, J, FitzGerald, GA. Isoprostanes: Formation, analysis and use as indices of lipid peroxidation *in vivo*. *J Biol Chem* 1999; 274: 24441–44.

48. Lentz, SR, Sadler, JE. Inhibition of thrombomodulin surface expression and protein C activation by the thrombogenic agent homocysteine. *J Clin Invest* 1991; 88: 1906–14.

49. Lentz, SR, Sadler, JE. Homocysteine inhibits von Willebrand factor processing and secretion by preventing transport from the endoplasmic reticulum. *Blood* 1993; 81: 683–89.

50. Lentz, SR, Sobey, CG, Piegors, DJ, Bhopatkar, MY, Faraci, FM, Malinow, MR, Heistad, DD. Vascular dysfunction in monkeys with diet-induced hyperhomocyst(e)inemia. *J Clin Invest* 1996; 98: 24–9.

51. Lipton, SA, Kim, WK, Choi, YB, Kumar, S, D'Emilia, DM, Rayudu, PV, Arnelle, DR, Stamler, JS. Neurotoxicity associated with dual actions of homocysteine at the N-methyl-D-aspartate receptor. *Proc Natl Acad Sci USA* 1997; 94: 5923–28.

52. Liu, GM, Nellaiappan, K, Kagan, HM. Irreversible inhibition of lysyl oxidase by homocysteine thiolactone and its selenium and oxygen analogues: Implications for homocystinuria. *J Biol Chem* 1997; 272: 32370–77.

53. Loscalzo, J. The oxidant stress of hyperhomocyst(e)inemia. *J Clin Invest* 1996; 98: 5–7.

54. Lubec, B, Arbeiter, K, Hoeger, H, Lubec, G. Increased cyclin dependent kinase in aortic tissue of rats fed homocysteine. *Thromb Haemost* 1996; 75: 542–45.

55. Majors, A, Ehrhart, LA, Pezacka, EH. Homocysteine as a risk factor for vascular disease: Enhanced collagen production and accumulation by smooth muscle cells. *Arterioscler Thromb Vasc Biol* 1997; 17: 2074–81.

56. Makheja, AN, Bombard, RL, Randazzo, RL, Bailey, JM. Anti-inflamatory drugs in experimental atherosclerosis. Part 3. Evaluation of the atherogenicity of homocystine in rabbits. *Atherosclerosis* 1978; 29: 105–12.

57. Mansoor, MA, Bergmark, C, Svardal, AM, Lonning, PE, Ueland, PM. Redox status and protein binding of plasma homocysteine and other aminothiols in patients with early-onset peripheral vascular disease. Homocysteine and peripheral vascular disease. *Arterioscler Thromb Vasc Biol* 1995; 15: 232–40.

58. Mansoor, MA, Ueland, PM, Aarsland, A, Svardal, AM. Redox status and protein binding of plasma homocysteine and other aminothiols in patients with homocystinuria. *Metabolism* 1993; 42: 1481–85.

59. McCully, KS. Vascular pathology of homocysteinemia: Implications for the pathogenesis of arteriosclerosis. *Am J Pathol* 1969; 56: 111–28.

60. McCully, KS. Homocysteinemia and arteriosclerosis: Failure to isolate homocysteine thiolactone from plasma and lipoproteins. *Res Commun Chem Pathol Pharmacol* 1989; 63: 301–4.

61. McCully, KS. Homocysteine and vascular disease. *Nature Med* 1996; 2: 386–89.

62. McCully, KS. Homocysteine, folate, vitamin B6, and cardiovascular disease. *JAMA* 1998; 279: 392–93.

63. McCully, KS, Ragsdale, BD. Production of arteriosclerosis by homocysteinemia. *Am J Pathol* 1970; 61: 1–8.

64. McCully, KS, Vezeridis, MP. Homocysteine thiolactone in arteriosclerosis and cancer. *Res Commun Chem Pathol Pharmacol* 1988; 59: 107–19.

65. McCully, KS, Wilson, RB. Homocysteine theory of arteriosclerosis. *Atherosclerosis* 1975; 22: 215–27.

66. McKusick, VA. *Heritable Disorders of Connective Tissue.* CV Mosby, St. Louis, 1966; p. 155.

67. Misra, HP. Generation of superoxide free radical during the autoxidation of thiols. *J Biol Chem* 1974; 249: 2151–55.

68. Mudd, SH, Matorin, AI, Levy, HL. Homocysteine thiolactone: Failure to detect in human serum or plasma. *Res Commun Chem Pathol Pharmacol* 1989; 63: 297–300.

68a. Mujumdar, VS, Hayden, MR, Tyagi, SC. Homocyste(e)ine induces calcium second messenger in vascular smooth muscle cells. *J Cell Physiol* 2000; 183: 28–36.

69. Nappo, F, De Rosa, N, Marfella, R, De Lucia, D, Ingrosso, D, Perna, AF, Farzati, B, Giugliano, D. Impairment of endothelial functions by acute hyperhomocysteinemia and reversal by antioxidant vitamins. *JAMA* 1999; 281: 2113–18.

70. Nishio, E, Watanabe, Y. Homocysteine as a modulator of platelet-derived growth factor action in vascular smooth muscle cells: A possible role for hydrogen peroxide. *Br J Pharmacol* 1997; 122: 269–74.

71. Olney, JW, Price, MT, Salles, KS, Labruyere, J, Ryerson, R, Mahan, K, Frierdich, G, Samson, L. L-homocysteic acid: An endogenous excitotoxic ligand of the NMDA receptor. *Brain Res Bull* 1987; 19: 597–602.

72. Olszewski, AJ, Szostak, WB. Homocysteine content of plasma proteins in ischemic heart disease. *Atherosclerosis* 1988; 69: 109–113.

73. Outinen, PA, Sood, SK, Liaw, PCY, Sarge, KD, Maeda, N, Hirsh, J, Ribau, J, Podor, TJ, Weitz, JI, Austin, RC. Characterization of the stress-inducing effects of homocysteine. *Biochem J* 1998; 332: 213–21.

74. Outinen, PA, Sood, SK, Pfeifer, SI, Pamidi, S, Podor, TJ, Li, J, Weitz, JI, Austin, RC. Homocysteine-induced endoplasmic reticulum stress and growth arrest leads to specific changes in gene expression in human vascular endothelial cells. *Blood* 1999; 94: 959–67.

75. Poddar, R, Sivasubramanian, N, DiBello, PM, Robinson, K, Jacobsen, DW. Homocysteine induces the expression and secretion of MCP-1 and IL-8 in human aortic endothelial cells: Implications for vascular disease. *Circulation* 2001; in press.

76. Pyeritz, RE. Homocystinuria. In *McKusick's Heritable Disorders of Connective Tissue* (Breighton, P, ed.). CV Mosby, St. Louis, 1993; pp. 137–78.

77. Quéré, I, Hillaire-Buys, D, Brunschwig, C, Chapal, J, Janbon, C, Blayac, JP, Petit, P, Loubatières-Mariani, MM. Effects of homocysteine on acetylcholine- and adenosine-induced vasodilatation of pancreatic vascular bed in rats. *Br J Pharmacol* 1997; 122: 351–57.

78. Raguso, CA, Regan, MM, Young, VR. Cysteine kinetics and oxidation at different intakes of methionine and cystine in young adults. *Am J Clin Nutr* 2000; 71: 491–99.

79. Rolland, PH, Friggi, A, Barlatier, A, Piquet, P, Latrille, V, Faye, MM, Guillou, J, Charpiot, P, Bodard, H, Ghiringhelli, O, Calaf, R, Luccioni, R, Garçon, D. Hyperhomocysteinemia-induced vascular damage in the minipig: Captopril-hydrochlorothiazide combination prevents elastic alterations. *Circulation* 1995; 91: 1161–74.

80. Rollins, BJ. Chemokines. *Blood* 1997; 90: 909–28.

81. Ross, R. The pathogenesis of atherosclerosis: A perspective for the 1990s. *Nature* 1993; 362: 801–9.

82. Ross, R. Atherosclerosis—An inflammatory disease. *N Engl J Med* 1999; 340: 115–26.

83. Springman, EB, Angleton, EL, Birkedal-Hansen, H, van Wart, HE. Multiple modes of activation of latent fibroblast collagenase: Evidence for the role of a Cys^{73} active-site zinc complex in latency and a "cysteine switch" mechanism for activation. *Proc Natl Acad Sci U S A* 1990; 87: 364–68.

84. Stamler, JS, Osborne, JA, Jaraki, O, Rabbani, LE, Mullins, M, Singel, D, Loscalzo, J. Adverse vascular effects of homocysteine are modulated by endothelium-derived relaxing factor and related oxides of nitrogen. *J Clin Invest* 1993; 91: 308–18.

85. Starkebaum, G, Harlan, JM. Endothelial cell injury due to copper-catalyzed hydrogen peroxide generation from homocysteine. *J Clin Invest* 1986; 77: 1370–76.

86. Tada, K, Yoshida, T, Hirono, H, Arakawa, T. Homocystinuria: Amino acid pattern of the liver. *Tohoku J Exp Med* 1967; 92: 325–32.

87. Tang, LL, Mamotte, CDS, Van Bockxmeer, FM, Taylor, RR. The effect of homocysteine on DNA synthesis in cultured human vascular smooth muscle. *Atherosclerosis* 1998; 136: 169–73.

88. Tawakol, A, Omland, T, Gerhard, M, Wu, JT, Creager, MA. Hyperhomocyst(e)inemia is associated with impaired endothelium-dependent vasodilation in humans. *Circulation* 1997; 95: 1119–21.

89. Tipa, EV, Chen, P, Majors, AK, Robinson, K, Jacobsen, DW. Failure of homocysteine to restore the glutathione (GSH) pool in cysteine-starved human aortic endothelial cells (HAEC). *FASEB J* 2000; 14: A460.

90. Tsai, J-C, Perrella, MA, Yoshizumi, M, Hsieh, C-M, Haber, E, Schlegel, R, Lee, M-E. Promotion of vascular smooth muscle growth by homocysteine: A link to atherosclerosis. *Proc Natl Acad Sci USA* 1994; 91: 6369–73.

91. Tsai, J-C, Wang, H, Perrella, MA, Yoshizumi, M, Sibinga, NES, Tan, LC, Haber, E, Chang, T H-T,

Schlegel, R, Lee, M-E. Induction of cyclin A gene expression by homocysteine in vascular smooth muscle cells. *J Clin Invest* 1996; 97: 146–53.

92. Tyagi, SC. Homocysteine redox receptor and regulation of extracellular matrix components in vascular cells. *Am J Physiol Cell Physiol* 1998; 274: C396–C405.

93. Ungvari, Z, Pacher, P, Rischák, K, Szollár, L, Koller, A. Dysfunction of nitric oxide mediation in isolated rat arterioles with methionine diet-induced hyperhomocysteinemia. *Arterioscler Thromb Vasc Biol* 1999; 19: 1899–1904.

94. Upchurch, GR Jr, Welch, GN, Fabian, AJ, Freedman, JE, Johnson, JL, Keaney, JF Jr, Loscalzo, J. Homocyst(e)ine decreases bioavailable nitric oxide by a mechanism involving glutathione peroxidase. *J Biol Chem* 1997; 272: 17012–17.

95. Upchurch, GR Jr, Welch, GN, Fabian, AJ, Pigazzi, A, Keaney, JF Jr, Loscalzo, J. Stimulation of endothelial nitric oxide production by homocyst(e)ine. *Atherosclerosis* 1997; 132: 177–85.

95a. van Aken, BE, Jansen, J, van Deventer, SJH, Reitsma, PH. Elevated levels of homocysteine increase IL-6 production in monocytic Mono Mac 6 cells. *Blood Coagul Fibrinolysis* 2000; 11: 159–64.

96. van der Molen, EF, Hiipakka, MJ, van Lith-Zanders, H, Boers, GHJ, van den Heuvel, LPWJ, Monnens, LAH, Blom, HJ. Homocysteine metabolism in endothelial cells of a patient homozygous for cystathionine β-synthase (CS) deficiency. *Thromb Haemost* 1997; 78: 827–33.

97. van Wart, HE, Birkedal-Hansen, H. The cysteine switch: A principle of regulation of metalloproteinase activity with potential applicability to the entire matrix metalloproteinase gene family. *Proc Natl Acad Sci USA* 1990; 87: 5578–82.

98. Voutilainen, S, Morrow, JD, Roberts, LJ II, Alfthan, G, Alho, H, Nyyssönen, K, Salonen, JT. Enhanced in vivo lipid peroxidation at elevated plasma total homocysteine levels. *Arterioscler Thromb Vasc Biol* 1999; 19: 1263–66.

99. Wall, RT, Harlan, JM, Harker, LA, Striker, GE. Homocysteine-induced endothelial cell injury in vitro: A model for the study of vascular injury. *Thromb Res* 1980; 18: 113–21.

100. Wang, H, Yoshizumi, M, Lai, K, Tsai, J-C, Perrella, MA, Haber, E, Lee, M-E. Inhibition of growth and p21[ras] methylation in vascular endothelial cells by homocysteine but not cysteine. *J Biol Chem* 1997; 272: 25380–85.

101. Wang, J, Dudman, NPB, Wilcken, DEL, Lynch, JF. Homocysteine catabolism: Levels of 3 enzymes in cultured human vascular endothelium and their relevance to vascular disease. *Atherosclerosis* 1992; 97: 97–106.

102. Welch, GN, Loscalzo, J. Homocysteine and atherothrombosis. *N Engl J Med* 1998; 338: 1042–50.

103. Welch, GN, Upchurch, G Jr, Loscalzo, J. Hyperhomocyst(e)inemia and atherothrombosis. *Ann NY Acad Sci* 1997; 811: 48–59.

104. Welch, GN, Upchurch, GR Jr, Farivar, RS, Pigazzi, A, Vu, K, Brecher, P, Keaney, JF Jr, Loscalzo, J. Homocysteine-induced nitric oxide production in vascular smooth-muscle cells of NF-κB-dependent transcriptional activation of *Nos2*. *Proc Assoc Am Physicians* 1998; 110: 22–31.

105. Welch, GN, Upchurch, GR Jr, Loscalzo, J. Homocysteine, oxidative stress, and vascular disease. *Hosp Pract* 1997; 32: 81–92.

106. Woo, KS, Chook, P, Lolin, YI, Cheung, BN, Chan, RN, Sun, YY, Sanderson, JE, Metreweili, C, Celermajer, DS. Hyperhomocyst(e)inemia is a risk factor for arterial endothelial dysfunction in humans. *Circulation* 1997; 96: 2542–44.

36

Homocysteine and Cambridge University Physiology

Homocysteine and
Cardiovascular Physiology

STEVEN R. LENTZ

A large number of epidemiological studies indicate that hyperhomocysteinemia is a common risk factor for myocardial infarction, stroke, peripheral arterial disease, and venous thrombosis (see Chapters 29–33). In contrast to a relative wealth of clinical epidemiological data, the mechanisms by which hyperhomocysteinemia predisposes to cardiovascular events are just beginning to become understood. It is still uncertain whether homocysteine itself causes vascular dysfunction, or whether elevated total plasma homocysteine concentration is a marker for another factor that increases cardiovascular risk. Part of the uncertainty stems from the fact that hyperhomocysteinemia is caused by several distinct genetic and dietary factors, and it is not known which of these factors confers a risk of cardiovascular disease.

Many studies have been performed in an effort to identify adverse cardiovascular effects of homocysteine (see Chapter 34 and 35). The approach of most of these studies has been to examine effects of exogenous homocysteine on functional properties of cultured endothelial cells or vascular smooth muscle cells. For example, exposure of cultured endothelial cells to exogenous homocysteine inhibits endothelium-dependent anticoagulant reactions (40, 50, 65), induces the expression of procoagulants (31, 66), decreases interactions between endothelial cells and plasminogen activators (32, 33),

and impairs the bioavailability of endothelium-derived nitric oxide (72). Exogenous homocysteine stimulates proliferation of cultured vascular smooth muscle cells (18, 61, 75, 76) and increases production of collagen by smooth muscle cells (55).

Because exogenous homocysteine has many potentially adverse effects on vascular cells in culture, it has been suggested that elevated plasma levels of homocysteine may directly predispose to thrombosis and vascular occlusion (5, 47, 83). A direct pathological role for homocysteine has not been shown in a clinically relevant model of hyperhomocysteinemia, however, and the studies that have examined effects of homocysteine on vascular cells in culture have some important limitations. Although experiments performed with cultured cells can identify plausible mechanisms of cardiovascular injury and dysfunction, it is not possible to determine with certainty whether similar mechanisms are important in the pathophysiology of hyperhomocysteinemia in vivo. One concern about many of the studies that have examined effects of exogenous homocysteine on cultured cells is that the concentration of homocysteine required to produce adverse effects generally was in the range of 0.1 to 1.0 mmol/L or higher, which is much higher than the plasma concentration of total homocysteine in patients with mild or moderate hyperhomocysteinemia (usually 15 to 50 µmol/L). Another concern is that, with a few exceptions, adverse effects on cultured cells are observed only with the free thiol form of homocysteine, which represents only a small fraction of plasma total homocysteine. Recognition of the limitations of in vitro studies has led to renewed interest in the development of experimental models of hyperhomocysteinemia in animals and humans.

Experimental Hyperhomocysteinemia in Animals

Several experimental approaches have been developed to produce hyperhomocysteinemia in animals (Figure 36.1). These include oral or parenteral administration of L-homocysteine or L-methionine, diet-induced deficiency of vitamin B_6 and/or folate, and administration of drugs that interfere with homocysteine remethylation or transsulfuration. In addition to these dietary and pharmacological approaches, genetic manipulation of key enzymes involved in homocysteine metabolism has led to the development of new experimental models of hyperhomocysteinemia in mice. The main advantage of using experimental animals to study the

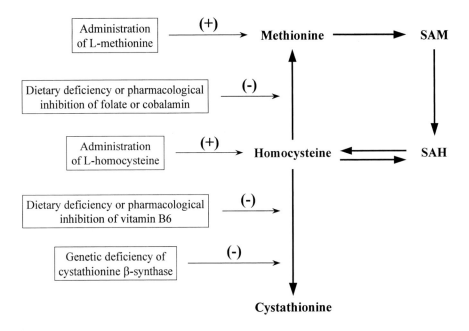

Fig. 36.1. Experimental approaches to produce hyperhomocys-teinemia. Hyperhomocysteinemia can be produced by oral or parenteral administration of L-homocysteine or L-methionine, or by diets that are deficient in B vitamins. Dietary deficiency of folate or cobalamin produces hyperhomocysteinemia by limiting homocysteine remethylation, whereas deficiency of vitamin B_6 produces hyperhomocysteinemia by interfering with homocys-teine transsulfuration. Alternatively, hyperhomocysteinemia can be produced pharmacologically by the administration of drugs that inhibit the bioavailability of vitamin B_6 (theophylline), cobalamin (nitrous oxide), or folate (methotrexate). Mice with genetic deficiency of cystathionine β-synthase have been pro-duced by gene targeting, and it is likely that genetic manipulation of other enzymes of homocysteine metabolism will soon lead to additional new animal models of hyperhomocysteinemia. (+) denotes that the intervention increases the plasma concentration of the indicated amino acid; (–) denotes that the intervention decreases the rate of the indicated reaction. (SAM = S-adenosyl-methionine; SAH = S-adenosylhomocysteine)

cardiovascular effects of hyperhomocysteinemia is that mechanisms of vascular dysfunction can be tested under physiological conditions.

Early evidence supporting the hypothesis that homocysteine may cause structural abnormalities of blood vessels was obtained from studies in rabbits (58, 59), baboons (35–37), and rats (43). In these studies, parenteral injection of homocysteine or homocysteine thiolactone led to desquamation of endothelium and an increase in circulating endothelial cells, and pro-duced structural changes in arteries that resembled early atherosclerotic lesions. These observations were not consistently reproduced in subsequent studies (20, 64), however, and concern was raised that some of the structural abnormalities may have been caused by hydrolysis of the thiolactone ring rather than by

homocysteine itself (22). Another limitation of these early animal studies was that they mainly examined effects of hyperhomocysteinemia on vascular struc-ture, with little assessment of functional properties of blood vessels. Nevertheless, these pioneering stud-ies clearly demonstrated the utility of experimental animals for examining pathophysiological effects of hyperhomocysteinemia.

In a landmark study published in 1995, Rolland et al. (67) reported that minipigs fed a methionine-rich caseinate diet developed mild elevation of plasma homocysteine (mean fasting plasma total homocysteine was 10 μmol/L vs. 5 μmol/L in animals fed control diet). After 4 months, animals fed the methionine-rich diet exhibited marked structural abnormalities of the abdominal aorta, left coronary artery, and common carotid artery. Histological examination of these ves-sels showed fragmentation of the internal elastic lam-ina, disruption of elastic fibers, and focal areas of smooth muscle hyperplasia. This study also was among the first to show hemodynamic abnormalities associated with hyperhomocysteinemia in an animal model. Compared with minipigs fed the control diet, minipigs fed the methionine-rich diet had tachycardia and hypertension, and they exhibited prolonged reac-tive hyperemia after transient vascular occlusion. In a subsequent study using the same animal model, mini-pigs fed the methionine-rich diet had a decreased level of elastin in the media of large arteries that was associ-ated with increased metalloproteinase activity (15). Similar abnormalities, including erosion of the internal elastic lamina and degeneration of medial smooth muscle cells, were observed in the aortas of rats after oral administration of methionine for up to 7 weeks (56). These studies show that specific structural abnormalities of large arteries can be produced by experimental hyperhomocysteinemia in animals, and they also indicate that mild hyperhomocysteinemia is associated with abnormal hemodynamic function.

More convincing evidence that hyperhomocysteinemia is associated with abnormal cardiovascular function was obtained from a study performed with cynomolgus monkeys (51). In this randomized, crossover study, mild hyperhomocysteinemia was produced by feeding monkeys a diet that was enriched in methionine, deficient in folate, and free of choline. The mean fasting plasma total homocysteine concentration was 11 μmol/L when monkeys were fed the experimental diet for 4 weeks, compared with 4 μmol/L when the same monkeys were fed the control diet for 4 weeks. This reversible 2.7-fold elevation in plasma total homocysteine concentration was associated with impaired responses to endothelium-dependent vasodilators, which were detected by measuring changes in hindlimb blood flow. Impaired endothelium-dependent relaxation also was observed when carotid artery rings from monkeys fed the hyperhomocysteinemic diet were studied ex vivo (Figure 36.2A). Because nitric oxide is a major mediator of endothelium-dependent vasodilatation (16, 38), these findings are consistent with the observation that homocysteine decreases bioavailability of nitric oxide in cultured endothelial cells (72, 78). Decreased bioavailability of nitric oxide is a credible candidate for mediation of

increased risk of cardiovascular disease in hyperhomocysteinemia, because endothelium-derived nitric oxide inhibits platelet aggregation and leukocyte adhesion, and prevents vasoconstriction (83). The finding that diet-induced hyperhomocysteinemia is associated with abnormal cardiovascular function in monkeys (51) strongly predicted that similar abnormalities may occur in humans with hyperhomocysteinemia. This prediction was confirmed in subsequent studies in which impairment of endothelium-dependent vasodilatation was observed in humans with acute or chronic hyperhomocysteinemia (see later).

In addition to exhibiting impaired responses to endothelium-dependent vasodilators, monkeys with diet-induced hyperhomocysteinemia also had evidence for impaired endothelium-dependent activation of protein C (51). This finding is consistent with earlier studies in which activation of protein C was found to be inhibited by exogenous homocysteine in cultured endothelial cells (40, 50, 65). Because protein C is a clinically important anticoagulant, particularly in the venous system (86), this effect may contribute to the increased risk of venous thrombosis in patients with hyperhomocysteinemia (see Chapters 33 and 34). However, abnormalities of protein C activation associated with hyperhomocysteinemia have not been observed in humans (11).

The development of an experimental model of hyperhomocysteinemia in cynomolgus monkeys provides an opportunity to examine interactions between hyperhomocysteinemia and hypercholesterolemia. When fed a high-fat diet, cynomolgus monkeys spontaneously develop atherosclerotic lesions in large arteries that are structurally similar to those seen in humans with hypercholesterolemia (2). Diet-induced atherosclerosis in monkeys is associated with impairment of endothelium-dependent vasodilatation (3, 30, 52), and endothelial function improves when atherosclerotic monkeys are placed on a low-fat regression diet (4, 7, 39). Interestingly, when cynomolgus monkeys are fed a high-fat, atherogenic diet for 17 months (49), they develop mild hyperhomocysteinemia

Fig. 36.2. Effects of hyperhomocysteinemia and atherosclerosis on endothelium-dependent relaxation of carotid artery in monkeys. (A) Relaxation response to the endothelium-dependent vasodilator, acetylcholine, was impaired in monkeys fed a hyperhomocysteinemic diet (open circles) compared with a control diet (filled circles). (B) Relaxation response to acetylcholine also was impaired in monkeys fed an atherogenic diet that produces both hyperhomocysteinemia and hypercholesterolemia (filled squares). When the atherogenic diet was supplemented with B vitamins for 6 months, plasma homocysteine concentration normalized, but relaxation responses to acetylcholine remained impaired (open squares). *$p < 0.05$. (Reproduced from Lentz et al. [49, 51], with permission.)

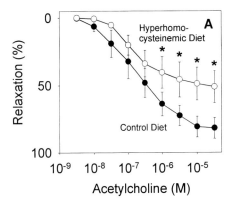
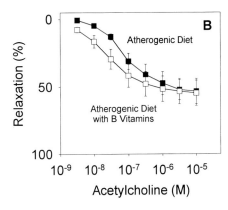

(plasma total homocysteine > 10 μmol/L) as well as hypercholesterolemia (plasma total cholesterol > 400 mg/dL). The hyperhomocysteinemia probably is caused by a relative deficiency of B vitamins in the atherogenic diet, because supplementation with large doses of folic acid, cyanocobalamin, and pyridoxine hydrochloride led to a significant decrease in plasma total homocysteine to < 4 μmol/L (49). These incidental observations suggested that treatment of hyperhomocysteinemia by dietary supplementation with B vitamins might improve endothelial function in atherosclerotic monkeys. Despite normalization of plasma total homocysteine, however, endothelium-dependent regulation of vasomotor function remained abnormal after 6 months of vitamin supplementation (Figure 36.2B). Vitamin supplementation also failed to prevent the progressive development of atherosclerotic lesions in the carotid artery (49). These findings indicate that dietary intervention to correct hyperhomocysteinemia is insufficient to normalize cardiovascular function or prevent progression of arterial lesions in the presence of persistent hypercholesterolemia in nonhuman primates. This result raises concern about the potential clinical benefit of dietary vitamin supplementation for the prevention of cardiovascular disease in patients with hyperhomocysteinemia and other risk factors. It is likely that interventions directed toward lowering both cholesterol and total homocysteine will be necessary to effectively prevent cardiovascular events in such patients.

In addition to the informative experimental models of hyperhomocysteinemia in minipigs and monkeys discussed previously, a growing number of alternative animal models of hyperhomocysteinemia have been developed. Essentially all of the experimental approaches illustrated in Figure 36.1 have been used to produce hyperhomocysteinemia in animals. Studies of experimental hyperhomocysteinemia in small animals (rats and rabbits) have demonstrated induction of procoagulant tissue factor (24, 25), increased proliferation of vascular smooth muscle (54, 71), and enhanced leukocyte-endothelial interactions (21). Other studies have indicated a possible association between experimental hyperhomocysteinemia in animals and elevation of plasma cholesterol or triglycerides (29, 87).

Perhaps the most interesting of the animal models are those that have been developed using genetic approaches to produce hyperhomocysteinemia in mice. The first well-characterized genetic model of hyperhomocysteinemia was developed by engineering a targeted deletion of the cystathionine β-synthase gene in mice (82). When fed a standard laboratory diet, control mice have plasma total homocysteine levels of < 5 μmol/L. In contrast, heterozygous cystathio-

nine β-synthase-deficient mice have moderately elevated plasma total homocysteine levels (6 to 15 μmol/L), and homozygous cystathionine β-synthase-deficient mice develop more marked hyperhomocysteinemia (plasma total homocysteine > 200 μmol/L) (82). These concentrations of plasma total homocysteine are similar to those seen in humans with heterozygous or homozygous cystathionine β-synthase deficiency, respectively (see Chapter 20). These observations suggest that impairment of homocysteine transsulfuration produces similar effects on homocysteine metabolism in humans and mice. Cystathionine β-synthase-deficient mice have not been observed to develop spontaneous atherosclerotic lesions in the aorta or other conduit arteries, but two recent reports indicate that such mice do have impaired endothelial regulation of vasomotor function (26, 48).

It is anticipated that several additional genetic models of hyperhomocysteinemia may become available in the near future, including mice with targeted deletions of genes involved in the homocysteine remethylation pathway. These genetic models should be useful for examining mechanisms of cardiovascular dysfunction in hyperhomocysteinemia. Possible experimental approaches might include combining genetic and dietary models of hyperhomocysteinemia in mice, and cross-breeding hyperhomocysteinemic mice with other genetically altered strains of mice to address specific mechanisms by which hyperhomocysteinemia produces cardiovascular dysfunction. In the next few years, we will likely learn much more about the causes and consequences of altered homocysteine metabolism in mice.

Cardiovascular Dysfunction in Human Hyperhomocysteinemia

As mentioned previously, impaired endothelial regulation of vasomotor function has been demonstrated recently in humans with hyperhomocysteinemia. Endothelial function related to nitric oxide release can be assessed noninvasively in human subjects by measuring flow-mediated dilatation of the brachial artery after transient vascular occlusion (1, 69). An association between hyperhomocysteinemia and impaired flow-mediated dilatation was first observed in children with hereditary homocystinuria owing to homozygous cystathionine β-synthase deficiency (12). Two subsequent studies in selected adult subjects with moderate hyperhomocysteinemia (mean plasma total homocysteine concentration 19 to 35 μmol/L) showed impaired flow-mediated dilatation compared with control subjects without hyperhomocysteinemia (mean plasma total homocysteine concentration 8 to 10 μmol/L) (74, 84). Because these subjects presumably had chronic hyperhomocysteinemia with some degree of atherosclerosis, however, it could not be determined whether impaired endothelial function was caused by hyperhomocysteinemia itself or by secondary effects of atherosclerosis.

More recently, several groups have observed impaired endothelium-dependent dilatation of conduit or resistance vessels in human subjects after acute oral methionine loading (6, 13, 14, 41, 46, 79). In each of these studies, acute impairment of endothelial function was detected within 2 to 8 hours after ingestion of methionine, which increased mean plasma total homocysteine concentration to 20 to 30 μmol/L. These findings suggest that it is either homocysteine itself or a factor that is directly related to plasma homocysteine concentration, rather than a secondary effect of atherosclerosis, that causes endothelial dysfunction in hyperhomocysteinemia.

Mechanisms of Endothelial Dysfunction

As outlined previously, it has become clear from recent studies in experimental animals and humans that endothelial vasomotor dysfunction is a consistent and reproducible consequence of hyperhomocysteinemia. One potential mechanism for endothelial dysfunction in hyperhomocysteinemia that has received considerable attention is vascular damage caused by increased oxidative stress (53, 57). Because it contains a reactive thiol group, homocysteine can undergo autooxidation and directly generate hydrogen peroxide and other reactive oxygen species (60, 68). Homocysteine-induced reactive oxygen species have been shown to directly inactivate nitric oxide derived from endothelial cells in vitro (72). Therefore, if autooxidation of homocysteine occurs in vivo, increased generation of reactive oxygen species may be one mechanism for decreased bioavailability of endothelial nitric oxide. Homocysteine-derived reactive oxygen species also may contribute to other adverse cardiovascular effects of hyperhomocysteinemia, including induction of procoagulant tissue factor and proliferation of vascular smooth muscle (24, 25, 54, 71). In addition, hyperhomocysteinemia also may indirectly potentiate the vascular toxicity of reactive oxygen species by decreasing the activity of certain antioxidant enzymes (61, 78). The oxidative stress mechanism is attractive because it has the potential to account for many adverse vascular effects of hyperhomocysteinemia, and because of the accepted importance of oxidant mechanisms in atherosclerosis (53).

Experimental evidence supporting the oxidative stress mechanism has been obtained mostly from studies performed in vitro, including the observation that endothelial cell injury correlates with generation of hydrogen peroxide from homocysteine (73) and the finding that homocysteine promotes oxidation of low-density lipoprotein (34, 42, 45, 62). Several groups have reported that addition of exogenous homocysteine inhibits endothelium-dependent relaxation of arterial rings in vitro (27, 44, 63), and one recent study found that exogenous homocysteine induced constriction of human coronary arteries in vitro (77). It is likely that reactive oxygen species derived from the autooxidation of homocysteine contributed to these pathological responses, because addition of catalase or superoxide dismutase was found to attenuate the effects of homocysteine (27, 44). These observations are consistent with the hypothesis that homocysteine may directly inhibit nitric oxide-mediated vasodilatation through oxidative mechanisms. The physiological relevance of these experiments is questionable, however, because very high concentrations of homocysteine were used. Moreover, the effects of exogenous homocysteine on nitric oxide-mediated relaxation of arterial rings appear to be highly dependent on buffer conditions, including the concentration of copper, which promotes autooxidation of homocysteine (27).

Relatively few studies have been performed in animals or humans to test the hypothesis that increased oxidative stress is an important mechanism for the development of vascular dysfunction in hyperhomocysteinemia. Attempts to show increased levels of oxidation products in humans with chronic hyperhomocysteinemia have been largely unsuccessful (8, 17, 23). Two groups of investigators have found that the susceptibility of low-density lipoprotein from hyperhomocysteinemic subjects to oxidative modification did not differ from that of low-density lipoprotein from control subjects (9, 17). In contrast to these negative findings, increased levels of lipid peroxidation products have been detected in some animal models of hyperhomocysteinemia (24, 25, 85), and one recent study showed increased plasma levels of thiobarbituric acid-reactive substances after methionine loading in human volunteers (19). Additional support for the oxidative stress mechanism was obtained from human studies in which acute impairment of flow-mediated brachial artery dilatation after methionine loading was prevented or reversed by large doses of vitamin C (14, 46). It is not known whether this protective effect of vitamin C is mediated by its antioxidant properties. Coadministration of large doses of folic acid also protects from endothelial dysfunction caused by acute methionine loading, without attenuating the increased plasma levels of total homocysteine (79). Again, the mechanism of this effect of folic acid and its relationship to oxidative stress are unknown. A similar protective effect of folates on endothelium-dependent vasodilatation has been observed in familial hypercho-

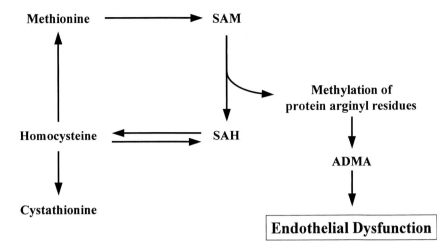

lesterolemia (81). A major goal of future studies will be to define the relative importance of oxidative mechanisms in the development of cardiovascular dysfunction in hyperhomocysteinemia in vivo.

An alternative potential mechanism by which hyperhomocysteinemia may decrease the bioavailability of endothelial nitric oxide is suggested by the metabolic relationship between homocysteine and methyl transfer reactions (Figure 36.3). Metabolism of homocysteine is coupled tightly to cellular levels of *S*-adenosylmethionine and *S*-adenosylhomocysteine, which are allosteric regulators of homocysteine transsulfuration and homocysteine remethylation (28, 70) (see Chapter 9). In addition to regulating homocysteine metabolism, *S*-adenosylmethionine functions as a major donor for methylation of DNA, proteins, phospholipids, and biogenic amines. The tight metabolic linkage between homocysteine, *S*-adenosylmethionine, and *S*-adenosylhomocysteine suggests that altered cellular methylation may account for some of the adverse effects of hyperhomocysteinemia on cardiovascular function. In hyperhomocysteinemia resulting from excess dietary methionine, for example, an increased *S*-adenosylmethionine/*S*-adenosylhomocysteine ratio may lead to increased production of asymmetrical dimethylarginine. Asymmetrical dimethylarginine is an endogenous competitive inhibitor of nitric oxide synthase that is formed from degradation of methylated proteins (80). Elevated plasma levels of asymmetrical dimethylarginine were detected in cynomolgus monkeys fed a hyperhomocysteinemic diet that is enriched in methionine (10). Plasma levels of asymmetrical dimethylarginine correlated with impairment of endothelium-dependent relaxation of the carotid artery in the hyperhomocysteinemic monkeys. These observations are consistent with the hypothesis that methionine loading may produce increased *S*-adenosylmethionine-dependent generation of asymmetrical dimethylarginine, which in turn may inhibit synthesis of nitric oxide by endothelial nitric oxide synthase (Figure 36.3).

Fig. 36.3. A potential mechanism for endothelial dysfunction based on the relationship between homocysteine metabolism and methyl transfer reactions. Methyl transferase activity is regulated by cellular levels of *S*-adenosylmethionine (SAM) and *S*-adenosylhomocysteine (SAH). In certain clinical situations, such as methionine loading or excess methionine in the diet, hyperhomocysteinemia may be associated with an increased SAM/SAH ratio resulting in increased methylation of protein arginyl residues. Proteins containing methylated arginyl residues appear to be a major source of asymmetrical dimethylarginine (ADMA), which may produce endothelial dysfunction by inhibiting nitric oxide synthase.

Emerging Themes and Future Directions

Clinical epidemiological studies have shown that hyperhomocysteinemia is associated with increased risk for cardiovascular events, but the precise mechanisms by which hyperhomocysteinemia alters cardiovascular physiology are incompletely understood. Studies performed with cultured cells in vitro have suggested that homocysteine has a wide variety of adverse effects that may contribute to increased cardiovascular risk. Until relatively recently, however, most of these potential mechanisms for cardiovascular dysfunction in hyperhomocysteinemia had not been examined using physiologically relevant approaches in experimental animals or human subjects.

Within the last 5 years, several promising new experimental models of hyperhomocysteinemia have been developed in minipigs, cynomolgus monkeys, rats, and mice. Elegant new approaches to measure cardiovascular function in human subjects with chronic or experimental hyperhomocysteinemia also have become available recently. Using these new in vivo approaches, investigators are beginning to clarify some of the mechanisms that may be most relevant to the pathophysiology of cardiovascular disease in hyperhomocysteinemia (Figure 36.4). One of the most consistent abnormalities of cardiovascular physiology that has been observed in studies of hyperhomocys-

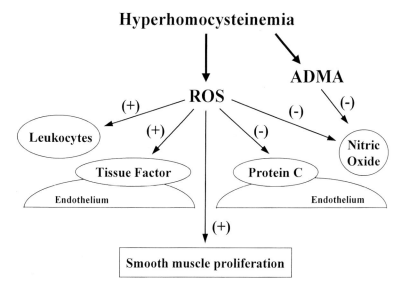

Fig. 36.4. Some adverse cardiovascular effects of hyperhomocysteinemia. Recent studies performed in experimental animals and humans have provided support for the hypothesis that hyperhomocysteinemia has atherogenic and prothrombotic effects on vascular cells in vivo. Experimental hyperhomocysteinemia enhances leukocyte-endothelial interactions, induces expression of procoagulant tissue factor by endothelial cells and leukocytes, decreases endothelium-dependent activation of the anticoagulant, protein C, and promotes proliferation of vascular smooth muscle. One of the most reproducible findings that has been observed in studies of hyperhomocysteinemia in animals and humans is impairment of endothelium-dependent vasodilatation, which is thought to be caused by decreased bioavailability of endothelium-derived nitric oxide. Current models propose that many of these adverse effects of hyperhomocysteinemia may be mediated through increased production of reactive oxygen species (ROS) or asymmetrical dimethylarginine (ADMA). (+) denotes that the indicated effect is increased in hyperhomocysteinemia; (–) denotes that the indicated effect is decreased in hyperhomocysteinemia.

teinemia in animals and humans is impairment of endothelium-dependent vasodilatation. This abnormality appears to be related to impaired bioavailability of endothelium-derived nitric oxide, which may be caused by either increased oxidative inactivation of nitric oxide or decreased synthesis of nitric oxide. Other abnormalities that have been shown in animal models of hyperhomocysteinemia include endothelial anticoagulant dysfunction, enhanced proliferation of vascular smooth muscle, and alterations of structural components of the arterial wall such as collagen and elastin. Some, but not all, of these abnormalities also have been detected in human subjects with hyperhomocysteinemia. Recent advances in molecular genetics promise to generate additional experimental models of hyperhomocysteinemia that should allow investigators to define the effects of hyperhomocysteinemia on cardiovascular function more precisely.

REFERENCES

1. Anderson, EA, Mark, AL. Flow-mediated and reflex changes in large peripheral artery tone in humans. *Circulation* 1989; 79: 93–100.
2. Armstrong, ML, Heistad, DD. Animal models of atherosclerosis. *Atherosclerosis* 1990; 85: 15–23.
3. Armstrong, ML, Heistad, DD, Marcus, ML, Megan, MB, Piegors, DJ. Structural and hemodynamic responses of peripheral arteries of macaque monkeys to atherogenic diet. *Arteriosclerosis* 1985; 5: 336–46.
4. Armstrong, ML, Heistad, DD, Marcus, ML, Piegors, DJ, Abboud, FM. Hemodynamic sequelae of regression of experimental atherosclerosis. *J Clin Invest* 1983; 71: 104–13.
5. Bellamy, MF, McDowell, IFW. Putative mechanisms for vascular damage by homocysteine. *J Inherit Metab Dis* 1997; 20: 307–15.
6. Bellamy, MF, McDowell, IFW, Ramsey, MW, Brownlee, M, Bones, C, Newcombe, RG, Lewis, MJ. Hyperhomocysteinemia after an oral methionine load acutely impairs endothelial function in healthy adults. *Circulation* 1998; 98: 1848–52.
7. Benzuly, KH, Padgett, RC, Kaul, S, Piegors, DJ, Armstrong, ML, Heistad, DD. Functional improvement precedes structural regression of atherosclerosis. *Circulation* 1994; 89: 1810–18.
8. Blom, HJ, Engelen, DP, Boers, GH, Stadhouders, AM, Sengers, RC, de Abreu, R, TePoele-Pothoff, MT, Trijbels, JM. Lipid peroxidation in homocysteinaemia. *J Inherit Metab Dis* 1992; 15: 419–22.
9. Blom, HJ, Kleinveld, HA, Boers, GH, Demacker, PN, Hak-Lemmers, HL, TePoele-Pothoff, MT, Trijbels, JM. Lipid peroxidation and susceptibility of low-density lipoprotein to in vitro oxidation in hyperhomocysteinaemia. *Eur J Clin Invest* 1995; 25: 149–54.
10. Böger, RH, Bode-Böger, SM, Sydow, K, Heistad, DD, Lentz, SR. Plasma concentration of asymmetric dimethylarginine, an endogenous inhibitor of nitric oxide synthase, is elevated in monkeys with hyperhomocyst(e)inemia or hypercholesterolemia. *Arterioscler Thromb Vasc Biol* 2000; 20: 1557–64.

11. Cattaneo, M, Franchi, F, Zighetti, ML, Martinelli, I, Asti, D, Mannucci, PM. Plasma levels of activated protein C in healthy subjects and patients with previous venous thromboembolism: Relationships with plasma homocysteine levels. *Arterioscler Thromb Vasc Biol* 1998; 18: 1371–75.

12. Celermajer, DS, Sorensen, K, Ryalls, M, Robinson, J, Thomas, O, Leonard, JV, Deanfield, JE. Impaired endothelial function occurs in the systemic arteries of children with homozygous homocystinuria but not in their heterozygous parents. *J Am Coll Cardiol* 1993; 22: 854–58.

13. Chambers, JC, McGregor, A, Jean-Marie, J, Kooner, JS. Acute hyperhomocysteinemia and endothelial dysfunction. *Lancet* 1998; 351: 36–7.

14. Chambers, JC, McGregor, A, Jean-Marie, J, Obeid, OA, Kooner, JS. Demonstration of rapid onset vascular endothelial dysfunction after hyperhomocysteinemia. An effect reversible with vitamin C therapy. *Circulation* 1999; 99: 1156–60.

15. Charpiot, P, Bescond, A, Augier, T, Chareyre, C, Fraterno, M, Rolland, PH, Garçon, D. Hyperhomocysteinemia induces elastolysis in minipig arteries: Structural consequences, arterial site specificity and effect of captopril-hydrochlorothiazide. *Matrix Biol* 1998; 17: 559–74.

16. Cooke, JP, Dzau, VJ. Nitric oxide synthase: Role in the genesis of vascular disease. *Annu Rev Med* 1997; 48: 489–509.

17. Cordoba-Porras, A, Sanchez-Quesada, JL, Gonzalez-Sastre, F, Ordonez-Llanos, J, Blanco-Vaca, F. Susceptibility of plasma low- and high-density lipoproteins to oxidation in patients with severe hyperhomocysteinemia. *J Mol Med* 1996; 74: 771–76.

18. Dalton, ML, Gadson, PF, Wrenn, RW, Rosenquist, TH. Homocysteine signal cascade: Production of phospholipids, activation of protein kinase C, and the induction of c-fos and c- myb in smooth muscle cells. *FASEB J* 1997; 11: 703–11.

19. Domagala, TB, Libura, M, Szczeklik, A. Hyperhomocysteinemia following oral methionine load is associated with increased lipid peroxidation. *Thromb Res* 1997; 87: 411–16.

20. Donohue, S, Sturman, JA, Gaull, G. Arteriosclerosis due to homocyst(e)inemia. Failure to reproduce the model in weanling rabbits. *Am J Pathol* 1974; 77: 167–74.

21. Dudman, NPB, Temple, SE, Guo, XW, Fu, WY, Perry, MA. Homocysteine enhances neutrophil-endothelial interactions in both cultured human cells and rats in vivo. *Circ Res* 1999; 84: 409–16.

22. Dudman, NPB, Wilcken, DEL. Homocysteine thiolactone and experimental hyperhomocysteinemia. *Biochem Med* 1982; 27: 244–53.

23. Dudman, NPB, Wilcken, DEL, Stocker, R. Circulating lipid hydroperoxide levels in human hyperhomocysteinemia. Relevance to development of arteriosclerosis. *Arterioscler Thromb* 1993; 13: 512–16.

24. Durand, P, Lussier-Cacan, S, Blache, D. Acute methionine load-induced hyperhomocysteinemia enhances platelet aggregation, thromboxane biosynthesis, and macrophage-derived tissue factor activity in rats. *FASEB J* 1997; 11: 1157–68.

25. Durand, P, Prost, M, Blache, D. Pro-thrombotic effects of a folic acid deficient diet in rat platelets and macrophages related to elevated homocysteine and decreased n-3 polyunsaturated fatty acids. *Atherosclerosis* 1996; 121: 231–43.

26. Eberhardt, RT, Forgione, MA, Cap, A, Leopold, JA, Rudd, MA, Tolliet, M, Heyrick, S, Stark, R, Klings, ES, Moldovan, NI, Yaghoubi, M, Goldschmidt-Clermont, PJ, Farber, HW, Cohen, R, Loscalzo, J. Endothelial dysfunction in a murine model of mild hyperhomocyst(e)inemia. *J Clin Invest* 2000; 106: 483–91.

27. Emsley, AM, Jeremy, JY, Gomes, GN, Angelini, GD, Plane, F. Investigation of the inhibitory effects of homocysteine and copper on nitric oxide-mediated relaxation of rat isolated aorta. *Br J Pharmacol* 1999; 126: 1034–40.

28. Finkelstein, JD, Martin, JJ. Methionine metabolism in mammals. Adaptation to methionine excess. *J Biol Chem* 1986; 261: 1582–87.

29. Frauscher, G, Karnaukhova, E, Muehl, A, Hoeger, H, Lubec, B. Oral administration of homocysteine leads to increased plasma triglycerides and homocysteic acid: Additional mechanisms in homocysteine induced endothelial damage? *Life Sci* 1995; 57: 813–17.

30. Freiman, PC, Mitchell, GG, Heistad, DD, Armstrong, ML, Harrison, DG. Atherosclerosis impairs endothelium-dependent vascular relaxation to acetylcholine and thrombin in primates. *Circ Res* 1986; 58: 783–89.

31. Fryer, RH, Wilson, BD, Gubler, DB, Fitzgerald, LA, Rodgers, GM. Homocysteine, a risk factor for premature vascular disease and thrombosis, induces tissue factor activity in endothelial cells. *Arterioscler Thromb* 1993; 13: 1327–33.

32. Hajjar, KA. Homocysteine-induced modulation of tissue plasminogen activator binding to its endothelial cell membrane receptor. *J Clin Invest* 1993; 91: 2873–79.

33. Hajjar, KA, Mauri, L, Jacovina, AT, Zhong, FM, Mirza, UA, Padovan, JC, Chait, BT. Tissue plasminogen activator binding to the annexin II tail domain: Direct modulation by homocysteine. *J Biol Chem* 1998; 273: 9987–93.

34. Halvorsen, B, Brude, I, Drevon, CA, Nysom, J, Ose, L, Christiansen, EN, Nenseter, MS. Effect of homocysteine on copper ion-catalyzed, azo compound-initiated, and mononuclear cell-mediated oxidative modification of low density lipoprotein. *J Lipid Res* 1996; 37: 1591–600.

35. Harker, LA, Harlan, JM, Ross, R. Effect of sulfinpyrazone on homocysteine-induced endothelial injury and arteriosclerosis in baboons. *Circ Res* 1983; 53: 731–39.

36. Harker, LA, Ross, R, Slichter, SJ, Scott, CR. Homocysteine-induced arteriosclerosis: The role of endothelial cell injury and platelet response in its genesis. *J Clin Invest* 1976; 58: 731–41.

37. Harker, LA, Slichter, SJ, Scott, CR, Ross, R. Homocysteinemia. Vascular injury and arterial thrombosis. *N Engl J Med* 1974; 291: 537–43.

38. Harrison, DG. Cellular and molecular mechanisms of endothelial cell dysfunction. *J Clin Invest* 1997; 100: 2153–57.

39. Harrison, DG, Armstrong, ML, Freiman, PC, Heistad, DD. Restoration of endothelium-dependent relaxation by

dietary treatment of atherosclerosis. *J Clin Invest* 1987; 80: 1808–11.

40. Hayashi, T, Honda, G, Suzuki, K. An atherogenic stimulus homocysteine inhibits cofactor activity of thrombomodulin and enhances thrombomodulin expression in human umbilical vein endothelial cells. *Blood* 1992; 79: 2930–36.

41. Haynes, WG, Sinkey, CA, Kanani, P. Acute methionine loading produces endothelial dysfunction in humans. *J Invest Med* 1997; 45: 210A.

42. Heinecke, JW, Rosen, H, Suzuki, LA, Chait, A. The role of sulfur-containing amino acids in superoxide production and modification of low density lipoprotein by arterial smooth muscle cells. *J Biol Chem* 1987; 262: 10098–103.

43. Hladovec, J. Experimental homocystinemia, endothelial lesions, and thrombosis. *Blood Vessels* 1979; 16: 202–5.

44. Jia, Li, Liu, XJ, Furchgott, RF. Blockade of nitric oxide-induced relaxation of rabbit aorta by cysteine and homocysteine. *Acta Pharmacologica Sinica* 1997; 18: 11–20.

45. Jones, BG, Rose, FA, Tudball, N. Lipid peroxidation and homocysteine induced toxicity. *Atherosclerosis* 1994; 105: 165–70.

46. Kanani, P, Sinkey, CA, Knapp, HR, Haynes, WG. Endothelial dysfunction caused by experimental hyperhomocyst(e)inemia is rapidly normalized by anti-oxidant therapy. *J Am Coll Cardiol* 1998; 31: 178A.

47. Lentz, SR. Mechanisms of thrombosis in hyperhomocysteinemia. *Curr Opin Hematol* 1998; 5: 343–49.

48. Lentz, SR, Erger, RA, Dayal, S, Maeda, N, Malinow, MR, Heistad, DD, Faraci, FM. Folate dependence of hyperhomocysteinemia and endothelial dysfunction in cystathionine β-synthase-deficient mice. *Am J Physiol* 2000; 278: H970–75.

49. Lentz, SR, Malinow, MR, Piegors, DJ, Bhopatkar-Teredesai, M, Faraci, FM, Heistad, DD. Consequences of hyperhomocyst(e)inemia on vascular function in atherosclerotic monkeys. *Arterioscler Thromb Vasc Biol* 1997; 17: 2930–34.

50. Lentz, SR, Sadler, JE. Inhibition of thrombomodulin surface expression and protein C activation by the thrombogenic agent homocysteine. *J Clin Invest* 1991; 88: 1906–14.

51. Lentz, SR, Sobey, CG, Piegors, DJ, Bhopatkar, MY, Faraci, FM, Malinow, MR, Heistad, DD. Vascular dysfunction in monkeys with diet-induced hyperhomocyst(e)inemia. *J Clin Invest* 1996; 98: 24–9.

52. Lopez, JAG, Armstrong, ML, Piegors, DJ, Heistad, DD. Effect of early and advanced atherosclerosis on vascular responses to serotonin, thromboxane A2, and ADP. *Circulation* 1989; 79: 698–705.

53. Loscalzo, J. The oxidant stress of hyperhomocyst(e)inemia. *J Clin Invest* 1996; 98: 5–7.

54. Lubec, B, Labudova, O, Hoeger, H, Muehl, A, Fang-Kircher, S, Marx, M, Mosgoeller, W, Gialamas, J. Homocysteine increases cyclin-dependent kinase in aortic rat tissue. *Circulation* 1996; 94: 2620–25.

55. Majors, A, Ehrhart, LA, Pezacka, EH. Homocysteine as a risk factor for vascular disease: Enhanced collagen production and accumulation by smooth muscle cells. *Arterioscler Thromb Vasc Biol* 1997; 17: 2074–81.

56. Matthias, D, Becker, CH, Riezler, R, Kindling, PH. Homocysteine induced arteriosclerosis-like alterations of the aorta in normotensive and hypertensive rats following application of high doses of methionine. *Atherosclerosis* 1996; 122: 201–16.

57. McCully, KS. Homocysteine and vascular disease. *Nat Med* 1996; 2: 386–89.

58. McCully, KS, Ragsdale, BD. Production of arteriosclerosis by homocysteinemia. *Am J Pathol* 1970; 61: 1–11.

59. McCully, KS, Wilson, RD. Homocysteine theory of arteriosclerosis. *Atherosclerosis* 1975; 22: 215–27.

60. Misra, HP. Generation of superoxide free radical during the autoxidation of thiols. *J Biol Chem* 1974; 249: 2151–55.

61. Nishio, E, Watanabe, Y. Homocysteine as a modulator of platelet-derived growth factor action in vascular smooth muscle cells: A possible role for hydrogen peroxide. *Br J Pharmacol* 1997; 122: 269–74.

62. Parthasarathy, S. Oxidation of low density lipoprotein by thiol compounds leads to its recognition by the acetyl LDL receptor. *Biochim Biophys Acta* 1987; 917: 337–40.

63. Quere, I, Hillaire-Buys, D, Brunschwig, C, Chapal, J, Janbon, C, Blayac, JP, Petit, P, Loubatieres-Mariani, MM. Effects of homocysteine on acetylcholine- and adenosine-induced vasodilatation of pancreatic vascular bed in rats. *Br J Pharmacol* 1997; 122: 351–57.

64. Reddy, GSR, Wilcken, DEL. Experimental homocysteinemia in pigs: Comparison with studies in sixteen homocystinuric patients. *Metabolism* 1982; 31: 778–83.

65. Rodgers, GM, Conn, MT. Homocysteine, an atherogenic stimulus, reduces protein C activation by arterial and venous endothelial cells. *Blood* 1990; 75: 895–901.

66. Rodgers, GM, Kane, WH. Activation of endogenous factor V by a homocysteine-induced vascular endothelial cell activator. *J Clin Invest* 1986; 77: 1909–16.

67. Rolland, PH, Friggi, A, Barlatier, A, Piquet, P, Latrille, V, Faye, MM, Guillou, J, Charpiot, P, Bodard, H, Ghiringhelli, O, Calaf, R, Luccioni, R, Garçon, D. Hyperhomocysteinemia-induced vascular damage in the minipig: Captopril-hydrochlorothiazide combination prevents elastic alterations. *Circulation* 1995; 91: 1161–74.

68. Rowley, DA, Halliwell, B. Superoxide-dependent formation of hydroxyl radicals in the presence of thiol compounds. *FEBS Lett* 1982; 138: 33–6.

69. Rubanyi, GM, Romero, C, Vanhoutte, PM. Flow-induced release of endothelium-derived relaxing factor. *Am J Physiol* 1986; 250: 1115–19.

70. Selhub, J, Miller, JW. The pathogenesis of homocysteinemia: interruption of the coordinate regulation by *S*-adenosylmethionine of the remethylation and transsulfuration of homocysteine. *Am J Clin Nutr* 1992; 55: 131–38.

71. Southern, FN, Cruz, N, Fink, LM, Cooney, CA, Barone, GW, Eidt, JF, Moursi, MM. Hyperhomocysteinemia increases intimal hyperplasia in a rat carotid endarterectomy model. *J Vasc Surg* 1998; 28: 909–18.

72. Stamler, JS, Osborne, JA, Jaraki, O, Rabbani, LE, Mullins, M, Singel, D, Loscalzo, J. Adverse vascular effects of homocysteine are modulated by endothelium-derived relaxing factor and related oxides of nitrogen. *J Clin Invest* 1993; 91: 308–18.

73. Starkebaum, G, Harlan, JM. Endothelial cell injury due to copper-catalyzed hydrogen peroxide generation from homocysteine. *J Clin Invest* 1986; 77: 1370–76.

74. Tawakol, A, Omland, P, Gerhard, M, Wu, JT, Creager, MA. Hyperhomocyst(e)inemia is associated with impaired endothelium-dependent vasodilation in humans. *Circulation* 1997; 95: 1119–21.

75. Tsai, JC, Perrella, MA, Yoshizumi, M, Hsieh, CM, Haber, E, Schlegel, R, Lee, ME. Promotion of vascular smooth muscle cell growth by homocysteine: A link to atherosclerosis. *Proc Natl Acad Sci USA* 1994; 91: 6369–73.

76. Tsai, JC, Wang, H, Perrella, MA, Yoshizumi, M, Sibinga, NES, Tan, LC, Haber, E, Chang, THT, Schlegel, R, Lee, ME. Induction of cyclin A gene expression by homocysteine in vascular smooth muscle cells. *J Clin Invest* 1996; 97: 146–53.

77. Tyagi, SC, Smiley, LM, Mujumdar, VS, Clonts, B, Parker, JL. Reduction-oxidation (redox) and vascular tissue level of homocyst(e)ine in human coronary atherosclerotic lesions and role in extracellular matrix remodeling and vascular tone. *Mol Cell Biochem* 1998; 181: 107–16.

78. Upchurch, GR, Welch, GN, Fabian, AJ, Freedman, JE, Johnson, JL, Keaney, JF, Loscalzo, J. Homocyst(e)ine decreases bioavailable nitric oxide by a mechanism involving glutathione peroxidase. *J Biol Chem* 1997; 272: 17012–17.

79. Usui, M, Matsuoka, H, Miyazaki, H, Ueda, S, Okuda, S, Imaizumi, T. Endothelial dysfunction by acute hyperhomocyst(e)inemia: restoration by folic acid. *Clin Sci* 1999; 96: 235–39.

80. Vallance, P, Leone, A, Calver, A, Collier, J, Moncada, S. Endogenous dimethylarginine as an inhibitor of nitric oxide synthesis. *J Cardiovasc Pharmacol* 1992; 20 (Suppl 12): S60–2.

81. Verhaar, MC, Wever, RM, Kastelein, JJ, van Dam, T, Koomans, HA, Rabelink, TJ. 5-Methyltetrahydrofolate, the active form of folic acid, restores endothelial function in familial hypercholesterolemia. *Circulation* 1998; 97: 237–41.

82. Watanabe, M, Osada, J, Aratani, Y, Kluckman, K, Reddick, R, Malinow, MR, Maeda, N. Mice deficient in cystathionine beta-synthase: Animal models for mild and severe homocyst(e)inemia. *Proc Natl Acad Sci USA* 1995; 92: 1585–89.

83. Welch, GN, Loscalzo, J. Homocysteine and atherothrombosis. *N Engl J Med* 1998; 338: 1042–50.

84. Woo, KS, Chook, P, Lolin, YI, Cheung, ASP, Chan, LT, Sun, YY, Sanderson, JE, Metreweli, C, Celermajer, DS. Hyperhomocyst(e)inemia is a risk factor for arterial endothelial dysfunction in humans. *Circulation* 1997; 96: 2542–44.

85. Young, PB, Kennedy, S, Molloy, AM, Scott, JM, Weir, DG, Kennedy, DG. Lipid peroxidation induced in vivo by hyperhomocysteinaemia in pigs. *Atherosclerosis* 1997; 129: 67–71.

86. Zöller, B, Hillarp, A, Berntorp, E, Dahlbäck, B. Activated protein C resistance due to a common factor V gene mutation is a major risk factor for venous thrombosis. *Annu Rev Med* 1997; 48: 45–58.

87. Zulli, A, Buxton, B, Doolan, L, Liu, JJ. Effect of homocysteine and cholesterol in raising plasma homocysteine, cholesterol and triglyceride levels. *Life Sci* 1998; 62: 2191–94.

37

Homocysteine and Human Reproduction

T.K.A.B. ESKES

The role of mild hyperhomocysteinemia, a risk factor for arterial disease and venous thrombosis, assumed importance in obstetrics and gynecology with publication of the large, randomized clinical trials on the protective effect of folic acid on the occurrence and recurrence of neural tube defects and the involvement of homocysteine. Birth defects other than neural tube defects, vascular diseases such as placental vasculopathy, and preeclampsia, and the postmenopausal state were also investigated. Information about the possibility of preventing birth defects and possibly also major vascular problems before or during pregnancy by simple means such as nutrition and/or vitamins deserves wide dissemination to all who care for women and their reproductive problems. Because the evidence is strong that homocysteine metabolism is involved in these processes, evidence on the role of homocysteine and the related B vitamins in human reproduction is discussed.

Homocysteine, the Menstrual Cycle, and Oral Contraceptives

The menstrual cycle begins at approximately 11 to 13 years (menarche) and ends at approximately 50 years (menopause). The intervals of the menstrual cycle are most regular between the ages of 20 and 30 years.

Hormonal fluctuations in the blood at various periods of the menstrual cycle are characteristic: a steady increase of estrogens owing to the development of graafian follicles followed by the addition of progesterone after ovulation produced by the corpus luteum. The decrease of these steroids at the end of the secretory phase of the cycle results in withdrawal bleeding (menstruation). About 10% to 20% of women have clinical problems associated with the menstrual cycle such as dysmenorrhea, menorrhagia, and metrorrhagia.

To avoid pregnancy, 75 million women around the world use oral contraceptives. Oral contraceptives contain synthetic steroids, ethinylestradiol or mestranol, and various progestational agents. These steroids inhibit the release of hypothalamic-pituitary gonadotrophins resulting in inhibition of ovarian follicles and ovulation. Oral contraceptives also avoid the strong fluctuations of naturally produced steroids. Side effects of the use of oral contraceptives do occur. Thromboembolic events, although rare in young women, are still of concern.

Reproductive Steroids Lower Homocysteine

Silverberg et al. (93) stressed the general need for gender-specific reference ranges for laboratory values, which applies to fasting homocysteine levels as well. In premenopausal women, fasting and postmethionine-load serum homocysteine levels are significantly lower than in postmenopausal women (7). This finding suggests that premenopausal women remethylate homocysteine to methionine better or that their transsulfuration rate or renal excretion differs from postmenopausal women.

Methionine metabolism, as judged by urinary excretion, was reported not to be influenced by the use of (high-dose) oral contraceptives (69). The homocysteine-lowering effect of steroid hormones was confirmed in cortisol- and estradiol-treated rats (54).

It seems quite plausible that reproductive steroids such as estrogens and progesterone are responsible for the unique difference in the efficiency of homocysteine-methionine metabolism. Detectable amounts of homocysteine and methionine are found in follicular fluid in women undergoing an in vitro fertilization program. There was a significant correlation between the corresponding serum and follicular concentrations of homocysteine, folate, and cobalamin (101). It is also interesting to note that the variance of the menstrual cycle is lower during the use of multivitamins including folic acid (32).

Oral Contraceptives Produce Cyclically Recurrent Periods of Hyperhomocysteinemia

Estrogens and progesterone are present in oral contraceptives in the form of synthetic steroids such as ethinylestradiol and various progestational agents. As in the ovulatory menstrual cycle, the blood levels of reproductive steroids are highest in the second phase of the cycle, around day 23, and lowest during menstruation or withdrawal bleeding.

Early studies on contraceptives containing high levels of estrogens suggested an adverse effect on folate status. Later surveys reported no influence on folate metabolism. Nevertheless, oral contraceptives containing less than 50 μg of estrogens alter folate kinetics. After oral folate loading, significantly lower serum folate and cobalamin concentrations were found in pill users versus control subjects (102).

Steegers–Theunissen et al. (100) showed that serum homocysteine levels were significantly higher in the low-hormonal phase of the contraceptive cycle than in the high-hormonal phase. The levels were comparable to those of heterozygotes for homocystinuria. Brattström et al. (11) found no difference in fasting plasma homocysteine concentrations in women taking oral estrogen-containing contraceptives. The day of blood sampling was not reported however.

In women who used oral contraceptives and had documented vascular occlusion, higher levels of homocysteine were reported compared with control subjects. (3). An interesting observation was a decrease in methionine tolerance and an increase of detached endothelial cells in the blood in young women using oral contraceptives (46). This phenomenon could be prevented by using vitamin B_6.

Summary

Plasma homocysteine values are lower in the second half of the menstrual cycle than in the first. The same is true for the days that oral contraceptives are used compared with the period of withdrawal bleeding. This suggests an inverse correlation between plasma homocysteine and the blood levels of natural or synthetic reproductive steroids.

Homocysteine and the Menopausal Transition

The menopause is defined as the moment of the last vaginal bleeding. Because of the loss of production of ovarian estrogens and progesterone, the levels of gonadotrophins (follicle-stimulating hormone and luteinizing hormone) rise markedly. When the gonadotrophin levels exceed 10 IU/L or when vaginal bleeding does not return in 1 year, the period of the postmenopause has begun. The menopausal transition creates climacteric complaints in 10% to 20% of women, and estrogen-dependent flushes predominate among the complaints.

Loss of Ovarian Function is a Major Risk Factor for Coronary Artery Disease

Coronary artery disease strongly increases in women older than 50 years. The evidence supporting the hypothesis that loss of ovarian function, inducing estrogen loss, is a major risk factor for the development of coronary artery disease has been reviewed (97).

Homocysteine and Vascular Disease Risk in Postmenopausal Women

Homocysteine is an independent risk factor among the known risk factors for arterial disease, such as smoking, cholesterol, body weight, and familial occurrence (18). Hyperhomocysteinemia is an independent risk factor for atherosclerosis and thromboembolic disease (9) even when the homocysteine concentrations are only moderately elevated (98). A strong, graded association between plasma homocysteine concentrations and overall mortality has been reported in patients with coronary artery disease (80).

Postmenopausal women have significantly higher plasma homocysteine values than premenopausal women (130). This holds for both the fasting and postmethionine load values.

Homocysteine levels are negatively correlated with estrogen levels (130). It was suggested that a unique efficiency of methionine metabolism in premenopausal women may protect them against vascular disease (7). Differences in methionine catabolism may also be present, owing to a high degradation rate via the transamination pathway (5).

Estrogens, Estrogen Agonists, Folate, and Homocysteine

Estrogens and agonists lower plasma homocysteine levels in postmenopausal women (Table 37.1). Women with the highest pretreatment homocysteine levels show the largest absolute decrease in homocysteine.

Tamoxifen is a nonsteroidal estrogen agonist and antagonist that is used for the treatment of advanced breast cancer. Tested in postmenopausal women with breast cancer, tamoxifen lowered plasma homocysteine values by 25% to 30% (2). Raloxifene, a novel nonsteroidal compound, binds to a unique area of DNA and produces tissue-specific estrogen-agonistic and antagonistic effects. This drug is now under investigation for the treatment of climacteric complaints and osteoporo-

Table 37.1. Studies on the Homocysteine-Lowering Effect of Estrogens and Agonists in Postmenopausal Women

Authors (Ref.)	Population	Exposure	Methods	Homocysteine Change	Remarks
Anker et al. (2)	$n = 31$ Norway	Tamoxifen 30 mg/d	Observational	−29.8% after 9–12 mo.	Median age 65 years
van der Mooren et al. (115)	$n = 2$ (healthy) Netherlands	17β estradiol 2 mg/d dydrogesterone 10 mg/d 14 d/28 d cycle, 2 years	Prospective, observational	−10.9% lasting decrease after 6 mo.	FSH > 40 IU/L; no previous folate supplementation
van der Mooren et al. (116)	$n = 39$ (healthy) Netherlands	Conjugated estradiol 0.625 mg/d, medrogeston 10 mg/d, 14 d/28 d cycle 1 year treatment	Prospective, longitudinal, open	−12.3% lasting decrease after 6 mo.	FSH > 36 IU/L; no previous folate supplementation
Mijatovic et al. (66)	$n = 27$ (healthy) Netherlands	Estradiol 1 mg/d dydrogesterone 10 mg/d 14 d/28 d cycle controls, 15 months	Randomly assigned, controlled	−12.6%	FSH > 35 IU/L; no previous hormones or folate
Mijatovic et al. (67)	$n = 135$ (healthy) Netherlands	Micronized 17 β estradiol 2 mg dydrogesterone 2.5, 5.0, 10, and 15 mg/d, 6 months	Uncontrolled	−13.5% lasting decrease after 3 mo.	FSH > 35 IU/L; no previous hormones or folate
Mijatovic et al. (68)	$n = 52$ (hysterectomized)	Raloxifene 60 mg/d, 150 mg/d conjugated estrogen 0.625 mg/d	Randomized, double-blind placebo controlled	−16.0% for raloxifene after 12 mo; −13.0% for raloxifene and −10.0% for estrogen after 24 mo.	FSH > 40 IU/L; estradiol < 73 pmol/L; no previous folate supplementation

FSH, follicle-stimulating hormone; d, day.

sis. Raloxifene significantly reduces plasma homocysteine concentrations in postmenopausal women (68, 123b). The mechanisms underlying the estrogen-lowering effect of homocysteine are currently under investigation.

As discussed in other chapters, data on B vitamins as potent homocysteine-lowering agents are promising (85). Folic acid administration (5 mg/day) reduced homocysteine concentrations before and after methionine loading in postmenopausal women (10). Moderate folate depletion increases plasma homocysteine. It also results in decreased lymphocyte DNA methylation, as demonstrated in postmenopausal women (49). Folate deficiency can lead to misincorporation of uracil into DNA, requiring increased DNA repair. The clinical consequences could be an increased vascular risk, chromosomal damage, and preneoplastic lesions. The DNA hypomethylation may be reversed by folate repletion.

Summary

Plasma homocysteine values increase postmenopausally, perhaps because of the loss of ovarian production of estrogens. Estrogens and estrogen agonists lower plasma homocysteine values. However longitudinal studies in women comparing plasma homocysteine values with the endocrine profile are lacking. The cardiovascular risk increases postmenopausally. A challenging hypothesis is that homocysteine is an independent risk factor for vascular disease for postmenopausal women.

Homocysteine and Pregnancy

Pregnancy is characterized by a rapid increase of virtually all hormone levels, blood volume, cardiac output, peripheral vasodilatation, renal clearance, and body weight. Resetting of the hormonal balance takes place after delivery to initiate and maintain lactation. All these changes occur within 1 year, after which the menstrual cycle recurs. In that regard, pregnancy is a unique longitudinal "study model" during which physiological and endocrine changes can be studied and when each woman serves as her own control. Worldwide, 200 million women become pregnant each year.

Plasma Homocysteine Concentrations During Pregnancy

Homocysteine concentrations in the plasma of normal pregnant women are 50% to 60% lower than in nonpregnant subjects (1, 8, 51). Possible explanations include hemodilution, an increased production of steroids, or a higher utilization of methionine and homocysteine by the fetus.

When folates and other vitamins are measured longitudinally in the course of pregnancy, all the values are also far below the recommended values (14). In addition to well-known alterations in pregnancy, such as hemodilution, an accelerated breakdown has been suggested (64).

Active Transport of Methionine to the Coelomic Cavity and Amniotic Fluid During Early Pregnancy

Steegers–Theunissen et al. (105) sampled extraembryonic and amniotic fluid by transvaginal ultrasound guidance. Total homocysteine concentrations were very low in the embryonic fluid compartments compared with maternal serum. In contrast, the levels of methionine were four times higher in the extraembryonic coelomic fluid and twice as high in the amniotic fluid compared with maternal serum.

The presence of homocysteine in ovarian follicular fluid (101) supports the hypothesis that the ovum might be exposed to high homocysteine or low methionine concentrations and/or a lack of vitamins that are important for fertilization and early embryogenesis.

Methionine is essential for cell proliferation and DNA and tRNA methylation. After conversion to S-adenosylmethionine, methionine can function as a universal methyl donor. The low total homocysteine concentrations in embryonic fluids, together with a high methionine concentration, suggests that the remethylation pathway is important for the growth and development of the embryo. Because folate and cobalamin are essential for the remethylation of homocysteine to methionine, demonstration of high levels of cobalamin in the extraembryonic and amniotic cavity support this hypothesis (15, 16). The gradient of methionine levels may also indicate an active transport of methionine from maternal serum to the coelomic cavity followed by active transport or diffusion into the amniotic cavity. It must be emphasized that the "intervillous space" at this early stage of pregnancy is virtually devoid of blood and consists merely of a small pool of maternal serum (48).

Homocysteine and the Fetal Metabolic Cycle

Malinow et al. (63) determined the concentration of homocysteine in peripheral venous plasma and umbilical cord blood from 35 healthy women during labor. A descending concentration gradient of 1 μmol/L of homocysteine from maternal blood to the umbilical vein and artery was found. Homocysteine seems to be incorporated into the fetal metabolic cycle and might have a potential nutritional role.

Summary

The few studies that have been performed indicate that plasma homocysteine concentrations are lower during pregnancy than in the nonpregnant state. During early pregnancy, active transport of methionine takes place from the mother to the coelomic cavity and amniotic fluid of the embryo. Studies late in pregnancy suggest that homocysteine is incorporated in the fetal metabolic cycle.

Homocysteine and Neural Tube Defects

The neural tube is formed in the human embryo by a neurulation process of the ectodermal neural plate. Closure of the tube occurs from day 21 until day 28 after conception. This is a period when women only begin to think that they are pregnant, as their menstrual periods are 1 week overdue. If closure fails rostrally, anencephaly occurs; when closure fails caudally, spina bifida is the end result.

Most neural tube defects are caused by interaction of the environment with a genetic susceptibility of the embryo. Only a minority of neural tube defects are due to chromosomal or single gene defects. The prevalence of neural tube defects varies among different countries and ethnic groups, ranging from 2 per 1,000 infants in Mexico and Ireland to 0.2 per 1,000 infants in Finland and Japan. The recurrence rate in subsequent pregnancies is 2%. Although the prevalence rate is low, spina bifida is a disabling disease and is the most frequent birth defect in general. Worldwide, 400,000 children are born each year with a neural tube defect. Furthermore, women carrying an affected fetus are confronted with the many issues of prenatal diagnosis, including the medicoethical question of pregnancy interruption.

Factors establishing a genetic role in neural tube defects include a preponderance in females, ethnic differences persisting after migration, parental consanguinity, increased rate of concordance in monozygotic twin pairs, and an increased incidence in siblings and children of affected patients (21, 41). Environmental influences include diabetes mellitus, hyperthermia, the use of valproic acid and other anticonvulsants, alcohol abuse, and a family history of neural tube defects. Geography, the month of conception, maternal age, birth order, socioeconomic class, and maternal diet also contribute to an increased risk (16).

The History of Homocysteine Research and Neural Tube Defects

Neural tube defects were known to the ancient Egyptians and drew continuous attention over the centuries because of the enigma of birth defects. One of the first detailed pictures of spina bifida was made in 1641 by Nicholas Tulp, a disciple of Rembrandt (Figure 37.1). The history of research on the neural tube is also an example of serendipity, such as the finding that homocysteine is involved (35). Nutrition was one of the first causal factors for spina bifida to be identified. Stein et al. (106) reported a high incidence of spina bifida among 18-year-old Dutch males drafted for military service who were conceived during the famine at the end of World War II. Further refinement of a nutritional connection was made by Hibbard (44) and Hibbard and Smithells (45). They observed vitamin deficiencies in women who had offspring with an open neural tube defect. After multivitamin supplementation containing folic acid, the recurrence rate of neural tube defects was markedly reduced (94).

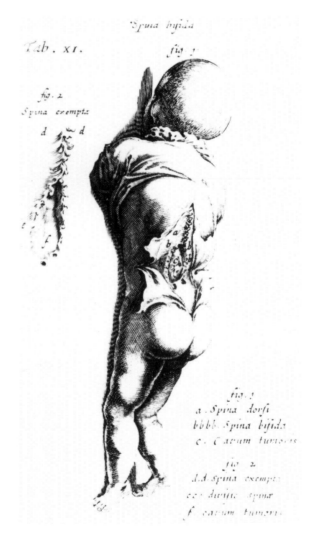

Fig. 37.1. Child with spina bifida. Copy of copperplate made by Nicolaas Tulp, a disciple of Rembrandt. This engraving was published in 1641 by Apud Ludovicum Elzevrium, Amsterdam, currently called Elsevier. (Reproduced with permission of the publisher.)

Credit must be given to the first attempt to perform a randomized trial by Laurence et al. (60) and the pioneering work of Smithells et al. (95) in Leeds. It is also interesting to note that the protocol of the Leeds group containing a placebo, double-blind controlled study was rejected by three hospital research ethics committees.

Folic Acid, Alone or in a Multivitamin Preparation, Prevents Neural Tube Defects

The considerable evidence from observational and intervention studies, that the periconceptional administration of multivitamins or of folic acid alone prevents both the occurrence and recurrence of neural tube defects, has been critically reviewed (25).

Fortunately, the Medical Research Council in the United Kingdom mounted a multicenter, double-blind, randomized trial to investigate the possible effect of multivitamins and folic acid on the recurrence rate of neural tube defects (76). This study fulfilled all the criteria for an excellent randomized investigation involving several arms: daily supplementation with folic acid (4 mg/day) alone, folic acid (4 mg/day) with other vitamins, vitamins without folic acid, and placebo. The results showed a 72% reduction in the recurrence rate in the groups given folic acid. The rationale for the choice of such a high dose of folic acid was to avoid the risk of an ineffective low dose, given the low possibility of repeating such a long-lasting, costly study. The trial was closed early when significant differences became apparent.

The Hungarian randomized trial (23) provided evidence that the occurrence of neural tube defects could be prevented as well. Subjects took a daily multivitamin containing 800 μg folic acid. The control group used a placebo containing only trace elements and vitamin C. It could not be determined if the significant effect was due to folic acid alone or to folic acid embedded within the multivitamin preparation.

It is important to recognize that both the British and the Hungarian studies were performed in populations with a rather high prevalence of neural tube defects.

Studies of maternal folate status, using serum, plasma, or red blood cells, as a possible predictor for neural tube defects were not conclusive (55, 74). The negative findings stimulated a search for new leads in the field of prevention of these serious birth defects.

Derangement of Homocysteine Metabolism as a Possible Basis for Neural Tube Defects

Steegers–Theunissen et al. (99) were the first to report on a possible derangement of folate-dependent homocysteine metabolism in women who had offspring with neural tube defects (odds ratio, 6.8; 95% confidence interval, 1.2–48.7). This finding was extended and confirmed (70, 103, 120), showing that the risk of spina bifida was increased at the 75th percentile of homocysteine values and at the 5th and 25th percentile of cobalamin levels in mothers with affected offspring.

Mills et al. (71) further showed that mothers of children with a neural tube defect had higher homocysteine values than did cobalamin-matched control subjects. The difference was highly significant ($p = 0.04$) in the lower half of the distribution after adjusting for plasma folate. Elevated methylmalonic acid levels were not observed, indicating that methylmalonyl-CoA mutase functioned normally in both groups. Despite their normal cobalamin status, affected mothers nevertheless had more difficulty metabolizing homocysteine compared with control subjects who had similar cobalamin levels. The authors raised the possibility of adding cobalamin to fortified food to enhance methionine synthase activity, allowing the amount of folic acid fortification to be reduced.

Many controlled studies have shown that plasma homocysteine concentrations rise when folate intake is inadequate (see Chapter 23). Plasma homocysteine concentrations are inversely associated with red blood cell and serum folate concentrations (81) and are a sensitive indicator of folate status. Dietary intake patterns also relate to plasma homocysteine concentrations, as shown in the Framingham study (109). As discussed in Chapter 23, folic acid supplements are clearly capable of lowering plasma homocysteine concentrations (9, 19, 25). The studies were performed in cardiovascular patients, volunteers, and elderly people. It is interesting to note that the use of folic acid leads to a decrease in plasma homocysteine concentrations even in healthy volunteers (13, 30, 31, 124).

Homocysteine and the Embryo: Lack of Methylation

Almost all evidence for the influence of homocysteine on the embryo comes from animal studies (36). Methionine can prevent neural tube defects in rat embryos cultured in bovine or human serum (20). van Aerts et al. (111) found evidence for a lack of methyl group donation and, therefore, impaired DNA synthesis and DNA and tRNA methylation, which is involved in gene expression. An important step in the closing process of the neural tube is the methylation of contractile proteins in the cells of the neural epithelium (72). Homocysteine and folic acid have a direct role in the closing mechanism of the neural tube in the chicken embryo (91).

Homocysteine and the Fetus

Amniotic fluid is the mirror image of the composition of the early embryo because of the transparent and totally permeable skin. As pregnancy advances, the amniotic pool reflects its own composition derived from the mother, her fetus, and the placental membranes.

Steegers–Theunissen et al. (104) found elevated homocysteine levels in the amniotic fluid of 27 fetuses with neural tube defects, compared with 31 control samples. The gestational ages of the groups differed, however, with median ages of 22 versus 16 weeks, respectively. The total homocysteine concentration in the amniotic fluid of both groups was significantly lower than in plasma (by a factor of 3 to 4) as shown previously in normal pregnancies (51). The report of Kurczynski et al. (58), who first described an untreated homocystinuric pregnant woman with dramatically increased homocysteine concentrations, is in accordance with this observation. Methionine levels were reported to be low in amniotic fluid in neural tube-affected pregnancies (24).

Homocysteine and the Child: Disturbance of Folate-Dependent Homocysteine Metabolism in Children with Neural Tube Defects

Folate and homocysteine metabolism is disturbed in children with spina bifida (117). A strong correlation was found between plasma homocysteine, B vitamins, and age in 70 children with spina bifida and 185 control subjects. This strong dependence of homocysteine and vitamin levels on age in children necessitates accounting for age before applying statistical analysis. After adjustment for age, homocysteine levels above the 95th percentile showed an odds ratio of 6.4 (95% confidence interval, 2.7–15.2), and folate levels in the 5th percentile showed an odds ratio of 6.0 (95% confidence interval, 2.5–14.5) for neural tube defect. Adjustment for plasma folate resulted in a folate-independent odds ratio of 4.1 (95% confidence interval, 1.6–10.5) for neural tube defect. This indicates that elevated homocysteine and decreased plasma folate levels are partly independent risk factors for neural tube defects. Vitamin B_6 levels were also decreased in affected patients with elevated homocysteine levels. The association with vitamin B_6 suggests that cystathionine-β-synthase might be a factor. In addition, plasma folate levels were decreased in children with neural tube defects independently of homocysteine, compared with control subjects. This implies that folate metabolism unrelated to homocysteine may be impaired in these patients.

The attributable risk percentages of elevated homocysteine and decreased plasma folate concentrations on neural tube defects can be determined by calculating the etiological fractions of these metabolites (9). The determined etiological fractions of homocysteine levels above the 95th percentile and plasma folate levels below the 5th percentile were 30.7% and 25.7%, respectively. The etiological fraction of elevated homocysteine levels not associated with plasma folate was 0.6%.

There is not complete agreement, however. A major role for homocysteine and folate in the etiology of neural tube defect was not found in some studies (4, 39). Those studies were small, however, and were not adjusted for age, which is a crucial factor in judging homocysteine values in children. No indication was found for a major role of methionine synthase or cystathionine-β-synthase (89, 122) or 5,10-methylenetetrahydrofolate reductase in the etiology of neural tube defects. No polymorphism was found for folate receptors in patients with spina bifida (43).

Summary

Folic acid alone or embedded in a multivitamin prevents the occurrence and recurrence of neural tube defects in many cases. Vitamin profiles are not suitable to identify women at risk for offspring with neural tube defects, however. A derangement of homocysteine metabolism seems to be the basis in about 30% of these women. Homocysteine is a sensitive indicator for folate status, and plasma homocysteine values can be improved by increased folate intake. Based on studies in whole rat embryo cultures, the common denominator for the effect of homocysteine on the developing embryo may be inadequate methylation of DNA or tRNA or impairment of their respective synthetic pathways.

Methylenetetrahydrofolate Reductase and Neural Tube Defects

When it became clear that a derangement of homocysteine metabolism was one of the possibilities for the pathogenesis of neural tube defects, research efforts focused on possible enzyme deficiencies and underlying polymorphisms in the remethylation pathway, in which folic acid and cobalamin play an essential role. Kang et al. (52) had already reported that thermolability of the 5,10-methylenetetrahydrofolate reductase (MTHFR) enzyme may be a risk factor for coronary heart disease. One common polymorphism, 677C→T (37), which decreases the activity of MTHFR by 35% (33), predisposes to mild hyperhomocysteinemia in the presence of a poor folate status (42, 56). However 5% to 15% of the general population is homozygous for the 677C→T variant. Red cell folate and plasma folate are significantly lower in these homozygous individuals. Therefore, a substantial minority of people may have increased folate needs (73). There is a close relationship between the common 677C→T mutation, low folate status, and hyperhomocysteinemia. When folate status is normalized, plasma homocysteine concentrations decrease and the adverse effects of the mutation are hidden (50, 62, 79, 120). MTHFR defects are discussed in detail in Chapter 22.

MTHFR Deficiency in Families with Neural Tube Defects

van der Put et al. (119) found mildly impaired MTHFR activity due to the 677C→T mutation in Dutch families with neural tube defects. The mutation was present in 16% of mothers, 10% of fathers, and 13% of children with spina bifida compared with 5% of control subjects. This finding was confirmed in Irish mothers of offspring with neural tube defects (126), affected Irish fetuses (82), affected Irish families (92) and affected Canadian families (17).

It can be concluded that the mutation occurs in about 10% of white populations (127) and between 2.3% and 16.6% in different ethnic groups (26, 27, 84, 121). This finding might explain the geographical and racial differences in the risk for neural tube defect.

van der Put et al. (118) pulled together three pieces of the etiological jigsaw puzzle: the proven protective effect of periconceptional folic acid supplementation, the familial clustering, and the increased risk of neural tube defects in the presence of elevated maternal homocysteine levels. The B-vitamin status of these women was not deficient, although folate levels were in the lower range of the control values (55, 119–121).

Meta-analysis of studies on the MTHFR mutation resulted in odds ratios of 1.7 (95% confidence interval, 1.2–2.6) for spina bifida patients, 1.8 (95% confidence interval, 1.1–3.1) for mothers and 1.9 (95% confidence interval, 1.3–2.8) for fathers. International controls were used for this calculation (121). The 677C→T mutation was associated with a sevenfold risk if both the mother and the child were homozygous. This finding suggested that defective homocysteine metabolism might also be present in the affected children themselves.

However, studies from France (75), Turkey (6), China (65), and South Africa (110) failed to show an association between homozygosity and an increased risk of neural tube defect. This controversy stresses the need for studies that include examination of the variations of dietary sources of folate, which modulate the effect of the 677C→T mutation. A recent meta-analysis (26) concluded that homozygosity for the 677C→T mutation is a moderate risk factor for spina bifida in Europe and that other genes should be investigated.

Interaction with Other Mutations

Another mutation of MTHFR has been found, 1298A→C (123, 125). This mutation reduces MTHFR activity to a lesser extent than does the 677C→T mutation. The risk for neural tube defects for the two mutations together had an odds ratio of 2.5 (95% confidence interval, 1.1–5.5). A combined heterozygosity for the 677C→T or the 1298A→C mutation was associated with reduced MTHFR specific activity (119), higher plasma homocysteine, and decreased plasma folate levels. This combined heterozygosity was observed in 28% of 86 patients with neural tube defects compared with 20% of 403 control subjects (odds ratio 2.04; 95% confidence interval, 0.9–4.7). Both mutations may explain 35% to 50% of the clinical effect of folic acid (117).

Associations of neural tube defects with other mutations or enzymes have not been found thus far, at least for methionine synthase (122) and cystathionine β-synthase (89).

The 677C→T Mutation, Hyperhomocysteinemia, and Other Birth Defects

Some evidence is developing that folic acid, homocysteine, and the MTHFR mutation are involved in the pathogenesis and/or prevention of congenital heart disease (53), orofacial abnormalities (128) and Down syndrome (50a). Hyperhomocysteinemia (22, 77, 129) and the 677C→T mutation (79) increase the risk of early pregnancy loss threefold.

Summary

The derangement of homocysteine metabolism in mothers with offspring affected by neural tube defects is based on the 677C→T and 1298A→C mutations of MTHFR. Both defects can interact and may explain 35% to 50% of the preventive effect on neural tube defects of the periconceptional use of folic acid. The 677C→T mutation doubles the risk of having offspring with neural tube defects. The prevalence of the 677C→T mutation varies in different ethnic groups. Because about 10% of people carry this mutation, a substantial minority of people may have increased folate needs. Early evidence now suggests that homocysteine metabolism is also involved in other birth defects.

Homocysteine and Obstetric Vascular Disease

Preeclampsia and Placental Abruption

Preeclampsia is defined as the occurrence of hypertension (diastolic blood pressure > 90 mm Hg over 24 hours). The prevalence is about 10% in the pregnant population, with a recurrence rate of 1% to 2%. The risk factors are primigravidity, pathological enlargement such as a hydatid mole or a multiple pregnancy, and hypertensive renal disease. Endothelial dysfunction seems to be the basic pathological factor (90).

Preeclampsia occurs mainly in primigravidas without previous hypertensive disease (i.e., pregnancy-induced hypertension) or in multigravidas with previous hypertensive disease (i.e., pregnancy-aggravated hypertension). The mother is at risk for renal and liver dysfunction, placental abruption, or even eclampsia (convulsions) and death. The fetus is at risk for fetal growth retardation, preterm birth, and increased mortality and morbidity.

Homocysteine and Endothelial Dysfuncton in Preeclampsia Rajkovic et al. (88) reported elevated homocysteine levels at the time of delivery in pregnant nulliparous American women with preeclampsia. The hematocrit values did not differ between preeclamptic women and control subjects, which excluded hemoconcentration. Folic acid concentrations also did not differ. Powers et al. (86) confirmed these observations and found evidence for endothelial activation as shown by an increase of cellular fibronectin, a marker of oxidative stress. Vollset et al. (123a) reported a 32% increased risk for preeclampsia in the highest quartile of homocysteine levels.

Laivuori et al. (59) found that the elevated plasma homocysteine levels in preeclampsia were inversely related to insulin sensitivity. Hemostatic and metabolic disturbances associated with a tendency to vascular thrombosis were found in 79 women with severe, early-onset preeclampsia; these included protein S deficiency (24.7% of the patients), activated protein C resistance (16.0%), and both fasting and postmethionine load hyperhomocysteinemia (17%) (28).

MTHFR Polymorphism and Preeclampsia The prevalence of the 677C→T mutation was significantly increased in Japanese preeclamptic women (24%) compared with normal pregnant women (11%) and healthy adults (11%) (96). The odds ratio was 2.5 (95% confidence interval, 1.3–4.8) for the homozygous genotype. An Italian study reported 677C→T homozygosity in 29.8% of cases versus 18.6% of control subjects (odds ratio 1.8; 95% confidence interval, 1.0–3.5) (40). The study also found that the effect of the MTHFR polymorphism and the genetic susceptibility to preeclampsia may be attenuated by the presence of the factor V Leiden mutation. However, Powers et al. (87) found that the 677C→T mutation was not a risk factor for preeclampsia in a nulliparous American population.

Folic acid and vitamin B$_6$ supplementation lowered postmethionine load homocysteine values in patients with preeclampsia, fetal growth restriction, and hyperhomocysteinemia (61).

Placental Abruption Placental abruption is a classic vascular problem in obstetrics with great risks for both mother and child (34). The clinical syndrome involves separation of the placenta from the uterine wall by retroplacental bleeding and clotting. Usually placental infarcts are present, as well as fetal growth retardation due to placental vasculopathy. Because of severe abdominal pain and blood loss, hypovolemic shock can occur, sometimes resulting in multisystem failure, involving the coagulation and renal systems. Fetal death occurs when the placenta separates completely; when there is partial separation, there is high risk for fetal brain damage. Remarkably, the incidence of congenital defects of the fetal heart is high.

The prevalence of this severe syndrome is reported to approximate 3%; the recurrence rate is 6% to 10%. Known risk factors are maternal hypertension, smoking, cocaine use, "old age," a history of fetal death/growth retardation, premature rupture of membranes, and the supine position, which induces a high vena caval pressure.

Maternal Hyperhomocysteinemia and Placental Abruption (Vasculopathy) Goddijn-Wessel et al. (38) found hyperhomocysteinemia in 26 of 84 Dutch patients (31.0%) who experienced placental abruption, placental infarcts, and fetal growth retardation—all summarized as placental vasculopathy—compared with 9% of 46 control subjects. This difference had an odds ratio of 4.7 (95% confidence interval, 1.4–17.3). Serum and red cell folate, serum cobalamin, and vitamin B$_6$ levels were significantly lower in the study group compared with the control subjects. This finding was confirmed in a small study from South Africa, but without the differences in vitamin profiles (83).

Extended studies on placental abruption in the Dutch population found significantly higher homocysteine levels in 175 women with placental vasculopathy than in 141 matched control subjects (odds ratio 3.3; 95% confidence interval, 1.4–7.9) (113). The odds ratio for low folic acid levels was 2.1 (95% confidence interval, 1.1–4.0) and for low cobalamin levels 2.6 (95% confidence interval, 1.3–4.9). Vollset et al. (123a) reported a higher risk for placental abruption with hyperhomocysteinemia (odds ratio 3.1; 95% confidence interval, 1.6–6.0).

The 677C→T MTHFR Mutation and Placental Abruption The 677C→T mutation was found in 19 of 165 Dutch women with vasculopathy (12.0%) compared with 7 of 135 matched control subjects (5%) (odds ratio 2.5; 95% confidence interval, 1.0–6.0) and 106 of 250 population-based control subjects (8.5%) (odds ratio 1.4; 95% confidence interval, 0.8–2.4) (114). The homocysteine-related expression of the MTHFR mutation depends on the subject's folate status (62). Therefore it may not be surprising that a meta-analysis of the clinical effect of the MTHFR mutation did not find an increased risk for coronary vascular disease (12).

Reduction of fasting and postmethionine load plasma homocysteine values can be achieved by the daily administration of 250 mg vitamin B_6 and 5 mg folic acid for 6 weeks (29). This opens possibilities for the prevention of recurrence of placental abruption, which will require validation with randomized, placebo-controlled trials of vitamins.

Endothelial Cells and Homocysteine In Vitro

Homocysteine metabolism in endothelial cells depends on folic acid. When cultured human umbilical vein endothelial cells are studied in vitro, homocysteine concentrations rise under standard culture conditions. Folic acid supplementation lowers this homocysteine export in a dose-dependent manner. 5-Methyltetrahydrofolate and folinic acid are 10 times more active than folic acid. Addition of vitamin B_6 or cobalamin does not affect the in vitro homocysteine cellular export (112). Among the many hypotheses for the atherosclerotic action of homocysteine, the demonstrated dual action of homocysteine in promoting growth of smooth muscle cells of blood vessels while inhibiting endothelial cell growth is particularly attractive (107, 108).

The Combination of Hyperhomocysteinemia and Thrombotic Disorders and the Risk for Placental Vasculopathy

Inherited thrombophilia is associated with early onset preeclampsia, fetal growth retardation, fetal demise, and placental abruption. Kupferminc et al. (57) found inherited thrombophilia in 22 of 48 patients (46%) with the aforementioned obstetrical complications. Thirteen patients (27%) carried the factor V Leiden mutation and 9 (19%) were homozygous for the 677C→T MTHFR mutation. Thus testing is relevant for prognostic and possibly therapeutic reasons. The combination of thrombotic risk factors (such as hyperhomocysteinemia, MTHFR mutation, factor V Leiden, and protein C deficiency) raised the odds ratio for two risk factors to 3.40 (95% confidence interval, 1.80–6.42) and for three risk factors to 6.83 (95% confidence interval, 1.52–30.7) (van der Molen et al., personal communication).

Summary

Homocysteine is also an independent factor for obstetrical vascular disease, which can manifest itself in mater-

nal arteries (preeclampsia) or spiral arteries supplying the placenta (placental abruption). Low vitamin status (folic acid, vitamin B_6, and cobalamin), hyperhomocysteinemia, and the MTHFR 677C→T mutation may combine with thrombotic factors such as deficiencies of protein C, protein S, or antithrombin III and factor V Leiden as risk factors for obstetrical vascular disease. The discrepant findings in the literature on the presence and impact of the 677C→T mutation may be resolved by taking into account the clinical differences between preeclampsia in nulliparous and multiparous patients.

REFERENCES

1. Andersson, A, Hultberg, B, Brattström, L, Isaksson, A. Decreased serum homocysteine in pregnancy. *Eur J Clin Chem Clin Biochem* 1992; 30: 377–79.
2. Anker, G, Lønning, PE, Ueland, PM, Refsum, H, Lien, EA. Plasma levels of the atherogenic amino acid homocysteine in post-menopausal women with breast cancer treated with tamoxifen. *Int J Cancer* 1995; 60: 365–68.
3. Beaumont, V, Malinow, MR, Sexton, G, Wilson, D, Lemort, N, Upson, B, Beaumont, JL. Hyperhomocyst(e)inemia, anti-estrogen antibodies and other risk factors for thrombosis in women on oral contraceptives. *Atherosclerosis* 1992; 94: 147–52.
4. Bjørke-Monsen, AL, Ueland, PM, Schneede, J, Vollset, SE, Refsum, H. Elevated plasma total homocysteine and C677T mutation of the methylenetetrahydrofolate reductase gene in patients with spina bifida. *Q J Med* 1997; 90: 593–96.
5. Blom, HJ, Boers, GHJ, Elzen, JPAM, van Roessel, JJM, Trijbels, JMF, Tangerman, A. Difference between premenopausal women and young men in the transamination pathway of methionine catabolism and the protection against vascular disease. *Eur J Clin Invest* 1988; 18: 633–38.
6. Boduroglu, K, Alikasifoglu, M, Anar, B, Tuncbilek, E. Association of the 677 C-T mutation on the methylenetrahydrofolate reductase gene in Turkish patients with neural tube defects. *J Child Neurol* 1999; 14: 159–61.
7. Boers, G, Smals, A, Trijbels, J, Leermakers, AI, Kloppenborg, PW. Unique efficiency of methionine metabolism in premenopausal women may protect against vascular disease in the reproductive years. *J Clin Invest* 1983; 72: 1971–76.
8. Bonnette, RE, Caudii, MA, Boddie, AM, Hutson, AD, Kauwell, GPA, Bailey, LB. Plasma homocyst(e)ine concentrations in pregnant and non pregnant women with controlled folate intake. *Obstet Gynecol* 1998; 92: 167–70.
9. Boushey, CJ, Beresford, SAA, Omenn, GS, Motulsky, AG. A quantitative assessment of plasma homocysteine as a risk factor for vascular disease: probable benefits of increasing folic acid intakes. *JAMA* 1995; 274: 1049–57.
10. Brattström, LE, Hultberg, BL, Hardebo, JE. Folic acid responsive postmenopausal homocysteinemia. *Metabolism* 1985; 35: 1073–77.

11. Brattström, L, Israelsson, B, Olsson, A, Andersson, A, Hultberg, B. Plasma homocysteine in women on oral contraceptives and in men with oestrogen-treated prostatic carcinoma. *Scand J Clin Lab Invest* 1992; 52: 283–87.

12. Brattström, L, Wilcken, DEL, Öhrvik, J, Brudin, L. Common methylenetetrahydrofolate gene mutation leads to hyperhomocysteinemia but not to vascular disease. *Circulation* 1998; 98: 2520–26.

13. Brouwer, IA, van Dusseldorp, M, Thomas, CMG. Low-dose folic acid supplementation decreases plasma homocysteine concentration: A randomized trial. *Am J Clin Nutr* 1999; 69: 99–104.

14. Bruinse, HW, van den Berg, H, Haspels, AA. Maternal serum folacin levels during and after normal pregnancy. *Eur J Obstet Gynecol Reprod Biol* 1985; 20: 153–58.

15. Campbell, J, Wathen, N, Perry, G, Soneji, S, Sourial, N, Chard, T. The coelomic cavity: An important site of materno-fetal nutrient exchange in the first trimester of pregnancy. *Br J Obstet Gynaecol* 1993; 100: 765–67.

16. Campbell, RP, Dayton, DH, Sohal, GS. Neural tube defects: A review of human and animal studies on the etiology of neural tube defects. *Teratology* 1986; 34: 171–87.

17. Christensen, B, Arbour, L, Tran, P, Leclerc, D, Sabbaghian, N, Platt, R, Gilfix, BM, Rosenblatt, DS, Gravel, RA, Forbes, P, Rozen, R. Genetic polymorphisms in methylenetetrahydrofolate reductase and methionine synthase, folate levels in red blood cells and risk for neural tube defects. *Am J Med Genet* 1999; 84: 151–57.

18. Clarke, R, Daly, L, Robinson, K, Naughten, E, Cahalane, S, Fowler, B, Graham, I. Hyperhomocysteinemia: an independent risk factor for vascular disease. *N Engl J Med* 1991; 324: 1149–55.

19. Clarke, R, Frost, C, Leroy, V, Collins, R. Lowering blood homocysteine with folic acid based supplements: meta-analysis of randomised trials. *Br Med J* 1998; 316: 894–98.

20. Coelho, ND, Klein, NW. Methionine and neural tube closure in cultured rat embryos: morphological and biochemical analyses. *Teratology* 1990; 42: 437–51.

21. Copp, AJ, Brook, FA, Estibeiro, JP, Shum, ASW, Cockroft, DL. The embryonic development of mammalian neural tube defects. *Prog Neurobiol* 1990; 35: 363–403.

22. Coumans, ABC, Huijgens, PC, Jakobs, C, Schats, R, de Vries, JIP, Van Pampus, MG, Dekker, GA. Haemostatic and metabolic abnormalities in women with unexplained recurrent abortion. *Hum Reprod* 1999; 14: 211–14.

23. Czeizel, AE, Dudás, I. Prevention of the first occurrence of neural-tube defects by periconceptional vitamin supplementation. *N Engl J Med* 1992; 327: 1832–35.

24. Dawson, EB, Harris, WA, Evans, DR, van Hook, JW. Amniotic fluid amino and nucleic acid in normal and neural tube defect pregnancies: A comparison. *J Reprod Med* 1999; 44: 28–32.

25. De Bree, A, van Dusseldorp, M, Brouwer, IA, van het Hof, KH, Steegers–Theunissen, RPM. Folate intake in Europe: Recommended, actual and desired intake. *Eur J Clin Nutr* 1997; 51: 643–60.

26. de Franchis, R, Buoniconti, A, Mandato, C, Pepe, A, Sperandeo, MP, del Gado, R, Capra, V, Salvaggio, E, Andria, G, Mastroiacovo, P. The C677T mutation of the 5,10-methylenetetrahydrofolate reductase gene is a moderate risk factor for spina bifida in Italy. *J Med Genet* 1998; 35: 1009–13.

27. Franco, RF, Araujo, AG, Guerreiro, JF, Elion, J, Zago, M. Analysis of the 677C-T mutation of the methylenetetrahydrofolate reductase gene in different ethnic groups. *Thromb Haemost* 1998; 79: 119–21.

28. Dekker, GA, De Vries, JL, Doelitzsch, PM, Huijgens, PC, von Blomberg, BME, Jakobs, C, van Geijn, HP. Underlying disorders associated with severe early-onset preeclampsia. *Am J Obstet Gynecol* 1995; 173: 1042–48.

29. De Vries, JIP, Dekker, GA, Huijgens, PC, Jakobs, C, Blomberg, BME, van Geijn, HP. Hyperhomocysteinemia and protein-S deficiency in complicated pregnancies. *Br J Obstet Gynaecol* 1997; 104: 1248–54.

30. den Heijer, M, Brouwer, IA, Bos, GMJ, Blom, HJ, van der Put, NMJ, Spaans, AP, Rosendaal, FR, Thomas, CMG, Haak, HL, Wijermans, PW, Gerrits, WB. Vitamin supplementation reduces blood homocysteine levels. A controlled trial in patients with venous thrombosis and healthy volunteers. *Arterioscler Thromb Vasc Biol* 1998; 18: 356–61.

31. Dierkes, J, Kroesen, M, Pietrzik, K. Folic acid and vitamin B_6 supplementation and plasma homocysteine concentrations in healthy young women. *Int J Vitam Nutr Res* 1998; 82: 98–103.

32. Dudás, I, Rockenbauer, M, Czeizel, AE. The effect of preconceptional multivitamin supplementation on the menstrual cycle. *Arch Gynecol Obstet* 1995; 256: 115–23.

33. Engbersen, AMT, Franken, DG, Boers, GHJ, Stevens, EMB, Trijbels, FJM, Blom HJ. Thermolabile 5,10-methylenetetrahydrofolate reductase as a cause of mild hyperhomocysteinemia. *Am J Hum Genet* 1995; 56: 142–150.

34. Eskes, TKAB. Abruptio placentae: A "classic" dedicated to Elizabeth Ramsey. *Eur J Obstet Gynecol Reprod Biol* 1997; 75: 63–71.

35. Eskes, TKAB. Open or closed? A world of difference: A history of homocysteine research. *Nutr Rev* 1998; 56: 236–44.

36. Fleming, A, Gerrelli, D, Greene, NDE, Copp, AJ. Mechanisms of normal and abnormal neurulation: Evidence from embryo culture studies. *Int J Dev Biol* 1997; 41: 100–12.

37. Frosst, P, Blom, HJ, Milos, R, Goyette, P, Sheppard, CA, Matthews, RG, Boers, GHJ, den Heijer, M, Kluijtmans, LAJ, van den Heuvel, LP, Rozen, R. A candidate genetic risk factor for vascular disease: a common mutation in methylenetetrahydrofolate reductase. *Nature Genet* 1995; 10: 111–13.

38. Goddijn-Wessel, TAW, Wouters, MGAJ, van der Molen, EF, Spuijbroek, MDEH, Steegers–Theunissen, RPM, Blom, HJ, Boers, GHJ, Eskes, TKAB.

Hyperhomocysteinemia: A risk factor for placental abruption or infarction. *Eur J Obstet Gynecol Reprod Biol* 1996; 66: 23–9.

39. Graf, WD, Oleinik, OE, Jack, RM, Eder, DN, Shurtleff, DB. Plasma homocysteine and methionine concentrations in children with neural tube defects. *Eur J Pediatr Surg* 1996; 6(Suppl 1): 7–9.

40. Grandone, E, Margaglione, M, Colaizzo, G, Cappucci, G, Paladini, D, Martinelli, P, Montanaro, S, Pavone, G, Di Minno, G. Factor V Leiden, C> T MTHFR polymorphism and genetic susceptibility to pre-eclampsia. *Thromb Haemostat* 1997; 77: 1052–54.

41. Hall, JG, Friedman, JM, Kenna, BA, Popkin, J, Jawanda, M, Arnold, W. Clinical genetic and epidemiological factors in neural tube defects. *Am J Hum Genet* 1988; 43: 827–37.

42. Harmon, DL, Woodside, JV, Yarnell, JWG, McMaster, D, Young, IS, McCrum, EE, Gey, KF, Whitehead, AS, Evans, AE. The common 'thermolabile' variant of methylenetetrahydrofolate reductase is a major determinant of mild hyperhomocysteinemia. *Q J Med* 1996; 9: 571–77.

43. Heil, SG, van der Put, NMJ, Trijbels, FJM, Gabreëls, FJM, Blom, HJ. Molecular genetic analysis of human folate receptors in neural tube defects. *Eur J Hum Genet* 1999; 7: 393–96.

44. Hibbard, BM. The role of folic acid in pregnancy with particular reference to anaemia, abruption and abortion. *J Obstet Gynaecol Br Common* 1964; 1: 529–42.

45. Hibbard, BM, Smithells, RW. Folic acid metabolism and human embryopathy. *Lancet* 1965; 1: 1254.

46. Hladovec, J, Koutský, J, Prérovský, Dvořak, V, Novotný, A. Oral contraceptives, methionine and endothelial lesion. *Vasa* 1983; 12: 117–20.

47. Hol, FA, van der Put, NMJ, Geurds, MPA, Heil, SG, Trijbels, FJM, Hamel, BCJ, Mariman, ECM, Blom, HJ. Molecular genetic analysis of the gene encoding the trifunctional enzyme MTHFD (methyltetrahydrofolate-dehydrogenase, methenyltetrahydrofolate-cyclohydrolase, formyl-tetrahydrofolate synthetase) in patients with neural tube defects. *Clin Genet* 1998; 53: 119–25.

48. Hustin, J, Schaaps, JP. Echocardiographic and anatomic studies of the maternotrophoblastic border during the first trimester of pregnancy. *Am J Obstet Gynecol* 1987; 157: 162–68.

49. Jacob, RA, Gretz, DM, Taylor, PC, James, SJ, Pogribny, IP, Miller, BJ, Henning, SM, Swenseid, ME. Moderate folate depletion increases plasma homocysteine and decreases lymphocyte DNA methylation in postmenopausal women. *J Nutr* 1998; 128: 1204–12.

50. Jacques, PF, Bostom, AG, Williams, RR, Ellison, RC, Eckfelt, JH, Rosenberg, IH, Selhub, J, Rozen, R. Relation between folate status, a common mutation in methylenetetrahydrofolate reductase, and plasma homocysteine concentrations. *Circulation* 1996; 93: 7–9.

50a. James, SJ, Pogribna, M, Pogribny, IP, Melnyk, S, Hine, RJ, Gibson, JB, Yi, P, Tafoya, DL, Swenson, DH, Wilson, VL, Gaylor, DW. Abnormal folate metabolism and mutation in the methylenetetrahydrofolate reduc-

tase gene may be maternal risk factors for Down syndrome. *Am J Clin Nutr* 1999; 70: 495–501.

51. Kang, SS, Wong, PWK, Zhou, JM, Cook, HY. Total homocyst(e)ine in plasma and amniotic fluid of pregnant women. *Metabolism* 1986; 35: 889–91.

52. Kang, SS, Wong, PWK, Susmano, A, Sora, Y, Nurusis, M, Ruggie, N. Thermolabile methylenetetrahydrofolate reductase: an inherited risk factor for coronary disease. *Am J Hum Genet* 1991; 48: 536–45.

53. Kapusta, L, Haagmans, MLM, Steegers, EAP, Cuypers, MHM, Blom, HJ, Eskes, TKAB. Congenital heart defects and derangement of homocysteine metabolism. *J Pediatr* 1999; 135: 773–74.

54. Kim, MH, Kim, E, Passen, EL, Meyer, J, Kang, SS. Cortisol and estradiol: Nongenetic factors for hyperhomocysteinemia. *Metabolism* 1997; 46: 247–49.

55. Kirke, PN, Molloy, AM, Daly, LE, Burke, H, Weir, DG, Scott, JM. Maternal plasma folate and vitamin B_{12} are independent risk factors for neural tube defects. *Q J Med* 1993; 86: 703–8.

56. Kluijtmans, LAJ, van den Heuvel, LPWJ, Boers, GHJ, Frosst, P, van Oost, BA, den Heijer, M, Stevens, EMB, Trijbels, JMF, Rozen, R, Blom, H. Molecular genetic analysis in mild hyperhomocysteinemia: A common mutation in the methylenetetrahydrofolate reductase gene is a genetic risk factor for cardiovascular disease. *Am J Hum Genet* 1996; 58: 35–41.

57. Kupferminc, MJ, Steinman, N, Eldor, A, Many, A, Fait, G, Baram, A, Daniel, J, Gull, I, Shenhav, M, Pausner, D, Yaffa, A, Lessing, JB. Inherited thrombophilia is associated with early onset pre-eclampsia, fetal growth restriction, fetal demise and abruptio placentae. *J Soc Gynecol Invest* 1998; 5: 137A.

58. Kurczynski, TW, Muir, WA, Fleisher, LD, Palomaki, JF, Gaull, GE, Rassin, DK, Abramowsky, C. Maternal homocystinuria: studies of an untreated mother and fetus. *Arch Dis Child* 1980; 55: 721–23.

59. Laivuori, H, Kaaja, R, Turpeinen, U, Viinikka, L, Ylikorkala, O. Plasma homocysteine levels elevated and inversely related to insulin sensitivity in pre-eclampsia. *Obstet Gynecol* 1999; 93: 489–93.

60. Laurence, KM, James, N, Miller, MH, Tennant, GB, Campbell, H. Double-blind randomised control trial of folate treatment before conception to prevent recurrence of neural-tube defects. *Br Med J* 1981; 282: 1509–11.

61. Leeda, M, Riyazi, N, De Vries, JI, Jakobs, C, van Geijn, HP, Dekker, GA. Effects of folic acid on women with hyperhomocysteinemia and a history of pre-eclampsia and fetal growth retardation. *Am J Obstet Gynecol* 1998; 179: 135–39.

62. Malinow, MR, Nieto, FJ, Kruger, WD, Duell, PB, Hess, DL, Gluckman, RA, Block, P, Holzganger, CR, Anderson, PH, Seltzer, D, Upson, B, Lin QRI. The effects of folic acid supplementation on plasma homocysteine are modulated by multivitamin use and methylenetetrahydrofolate reductase genotypes. *Arterioscler Thromb Vasc Biol* 1997; 17: 1157–62.

63. Malinow, MR, Rajkowic, A, Duell, PB, Hess, DL, Upson, BM. The relationship between maternal and

neonatal umbilical cord plasma homocyst(e)ine suggests a potential role for maternal homocyst(e)ine in fetal metabolism. *Am J Obstet Gynecol* 1998; 178: 228–33.

64. McPartlin, J, Halligan, A, Scott, JM, Darling, M, Weir, DG. Accelerated folate breakdown in pregnancy. *Lancet* 1993; 341: 148–49.

65. Melwick, M, Marazita, ML. Neural tube defects, methylenetetrahydrofolate reductase mutation, and north/south dietary differences in China. *J Craniofac Genet Dev Biol* 1998; 18: 233–35.

66. Mijatovic, V, Kenemans, P, Jakobs, C, van Baal, WM, Peters-Muller, ERA, van der Mooren, MJ. A randomized controlled study of the effects of 17β-estradiol-dydrogesterone on plasma homocyseine in postmenopausal women. *Obstet Gynecol* 1998; 91: 432–36.

67. Mijatovic, V, Kenemans, P, Netelenbos, JC, Jakobs, C, Popp-Snijders, C, Peters-Muller, ERA, van der Mooren, MJ. Postmenopausal oral 17β-estradiol continuously combined with dydrogesterone reduces fasting serum homocysteine levels. *Fertil Steril* 1998; 69: 876–82.

68. Mijatovic, V, Netelenbos, C, van der Mooren, MJ, de Valk-de Roo, GW, Jakobs, C, Kenemans, P. Randomized, double-blind, placebo-controlled study of the effects of raloxifene and conjugated equine estrogen on plasma homocysteine in healthy postmenopausal women. *Fertil Steril* 1998; 70: 1085–89.

69. Miller, LT, Dow, MJ, Kokkeler, SC. Methionine metabolism and vitamin B_6 status in women using oral contraceptives. *Am J Clin Nutr* 1978; 31: 619–25.

70. Mills, JL, McPartlin, JM, Kirke, PN, Lee, YJ, Conley, MR, Weir, DG, Scott, JM. Homocysteine metabolism in pregnancies complicated by neural-tube defects. *Lancet* 1995; 345: 149–51.

71. Mills, JL, Scott, JM, Kirke, PN, McPartlin, JM, Conley, MR, Weir, DG, Molloy, AM, Lee, YJ. Homocysteine and neural tube defects. *J Nutr* 1996; 126: 756S–760S.

72. Moephuli, SR, Klein, NW, Baldwin, MT, Krider, HM. Effects of methionine on the cytoplasmatic distribution of actin and tubulin during neural tube closure in rat embryos. *Proc Natl Acad Sci USA* 1997; 94: 543–48.

73. Molloy, AM, Daly, S, Mills, JL. Thermolabile variant of 5,10-methylenetetrahydrofolate reductase associated with low red-cell folates: Implications for folate intake recommendations. *Lancet* 1997; 349: 1591–93.

74. Mooij, PNM, Steegers–Theunissen, RPM, Thomas, CMG. Periconceptional vitamin profiles are not suitable for identifying women at risk for neural tube defects. *J Nutr* 1993; 123: 197–203.

75. Mornet, E, Muller, F, Lenvoise-Furet, A, Delezoide, AL, Col, JY, Simon-Bouy, B, Serre, JL. Screening of the C677T mutation on the methylenetetrahydrofolate reductase gene in French patients with neural tube defects. *Hum Genet* 1997; 100: 512–14.

76. MRC Vitamin Study Research Group. Prevention of neural tube defects: results of the Medical Research Council Vitamin Study. *Lancet* 1991; 338: 131–37.

77. Nelen, WLDM, Steegers, EAP, Eskes, TKAB, Blom, HJ. Genetic risk factor for unexplained recurrent early pregnancy loss. *Lancet* 1997; 350: 861.

78. Nelen, WLDM, van der Molen, EF, Blom, HJ, Heil, SG, Steegers, EA, Eskes, TKAB. Recurrent early pregnancy

loss and genetic-related disturbances in folate and homocysteine metabolism. *Br J Hosp Med* 1997; 58: 511–13.

79. Nelen, WLDM, Blom, HJ, Thomas, CMG, Steegers, EAP, Boers, GHJ, Eskes TKAB. Methylenetetrahydrofolate reductase polymorphism affects the change in homocysteine and folate concentrations resulting from low dose folic acid supplementation in women with unexplained recurrent miscarriages. *J Nutr* 1998; 128: 1336–41.

80. Nygård, O, Nordrehaug, EJ, Refsum, H, Ueland, PM, Farstad, M, Vollset, SE. Plasma homocysteine levels and mortality in patients with coronary artery disease. *N Engl J Med* 1997; 337: 230–36.

81. O'Keefe, CA, Bailey, LB, Thomas, EA, Hofler, SA, Davis, BA, Cerda, JJ, Gregory, JF III. Controlled dietary folate affects folate status in nonpregnant women. *J Nutr* 1995; 125: 2717–25.

82. Ou, CY, Stevenson, RE, Brown, VK, Schwartz, CE, Allen, WP, Khoury, MJ, Rozen, R, Oakley, GP Jr, Adams, MJ Jr. 5,10-Methylenetetrahydrofolate reductase genetic polymorphism as a risk factor for neural tube defects. *Am J Med Genet* 1996; 63: 610–14.

83. Owen, EP, Human, L, Carolissen, AA, Harley, EH, Odendaal, HJ. Hyperhomocysteinemia—a risk factor for abruptio placentae. *J Inherit Metab Dis* 1997; 20: 359–62.

84. Papapetrou, C, Lynch, SA, Burn, J, Edwards, YH. Methylenetetrahydrofolate reductase and neural tube defects. *Lancet* 1996; 348: 58.

85. Peterson, JC, Spence, JD. Vitamins and progression of atherosclerosis in hyper-homocyst(e)inaemia. *Lancet* 1998; 351: 550–53.

86. Powers, RW, Evans, RW, Majors, AK, Ojimba, JI, Ness, RB, Crombleholme, WR, Roberts, JM. Plasma homocysteine concentration is increased in pre-eclampsia and is associated with evidence of endothelial activation. *Am J Obstet Gynecol* 1998; 179: 1605–11.

87. Powers, RW, Minich, LA, Lykins, DL, Ness, RB, Crombleholme, WR, Roberts, JM. Methylenetetrahydrofolate reductase polymorphism, folate, and susceptibility to pre-eclampsia. *J Soc Gynecol Invest* 1999; 6: 74–9.

88. Rajkovic, A, Catalano, PM, Malinow, MR. Elevated homocyst(e)ine levels with pre-eclampsia. *Obstet Gynecol* 1997; 90: 168–71.

89. Ramsbottom, D, Scott, JM, Weir, DG, Kirke, PN, Mills, JL, Gallagher, PM, Whitehead, AS. Are common mutations of cystathionine beta synthase involved in the aetiology of neural tube defects? *Clin Genet* 1997; 51: 39–42.

90. Roberts, JM, Taylor, RN, Musci, TJ. Pre-eclampsia: An endothelial cancer. *Am J Obstet Gynecol* 1989; 161: 1200–4.

91. Rosenquist, TH, Ratashak, SA, Selhub, J. Homocysteine induces congenital defects of the heart and neural tube: Effect of folic acid. *Proc Natl Acad Sci USA* 1996; 93: 15227–32.

92. Shields, DC, Kirke, PN, Mills, JL, Ramsbottom, D, Molloy, AM, Burke, H, Weir, DG, Scott, JM,

Whitehead, AS. The "thermolabile" variant of methylenetetrahydrofolate reductase and neural tube defects: An evaluation of genetic risk and the relative importance of the genotypes of the embryo and the mother. *Am J Hum Genet* 1999; 64: 1045–55.

93. Silberberg, J, Crooks, R, Fryer, J, Wlodarczyk, J, Nair, B, Guo, XW, Xie, LJ, Dudman, N. Gender differences and other determinants of the rise in plasma homocysteine after L-methionine loading. *Atherosclerosis* 1997; 133: 105–10.

94. Smithells, RW, Sheppard, S, Schorah, CJ, Seller, MJ, Nevin, NC, Harris, R, Read, AP, Fielding, DW. Possible prevention of neural tube defects by periconceptional vitamin supplementation. *Lancet* 1980; 1: 339–40.

95. Smithells, RW, Nevin, NC, Seller, MJ, Sheppard, S, Harris, R, Read, AP, Fielding, DW, Walker, S, Schorah, CJ, Wild, J. Further experience of vitamin supplementation for prevention of neural-tube defect recurrences. *Lancet* 1983; 1: 1027–31.

96. Sohda, S, Arinami, T, Hamada, H. Methylenetetrahydrofolate reductase polymorphism and pre-eclampsia. *J Med Genet* 1997; 34: 525–26.

97. Stampfer, MJ, Colditz, JA, Willett, WC. Menopause and heart disease: A review. *Ann NY Acad Sci* 1990; 592: 193–203.

98. Stampfer, MJ, Malinow, MR, Willett, WC, Newcomer, LM, Upson, B, Ullman, D, Tishler, PV, Hennekens, CH. A prospective study of plasma homocyst(e)ine and risk of myocardial infarction in US physicians. *JAMA* 1992; 268: 877–81.

99. Steegers–Theunissen, RPM, Boers, GHJ, Trijbels, FJM, Eskes, TKAB. Neural-tube defects and derangement of homocysteine metabolism. *N Engl J Med* 1991; 324: 199–200.

100. Steegers–Theunissen, RPM, Boers, GHJ, Steegers, EAP, Trijbels, JMF, Thomas, CMG, Eskes, TKAB. Effects of sub-50 oral contraceptives on homocysteine metabolism: A preliminary study. *Contraception* 1992; 45: 129–39.

101. Steegers–Theunissen, RPM, Steegers, EAP, Thomas, CMG, Hollanders, HMS, Peereboom–Stegeman, JH, Trijbels, FJ, Eskes, TKAB. Study on the presence of homocysteine in ovarian follicular fluid. *Fertil Steril* 1993; 60: 1006–10.

102. Steegers–Theunissen, RPM, van Rossum, JM, Steegers, EAP, Thomas, CMG, Eskes, TKAB. Sub-50 oral contraceptives affect folate kinetics. *Gynecol Obstet Invest* 1993; 36: 230–33.

103. Steegers–Theunissen, RPM, Boers, GHJ, Trijbels, FJM, Finkelstein, JD, Blom, HJ, Thomas, CMG, Borm, GF, Wouters, MGAJ, Eskes, TKAB. Maternal hyperhomocysteinemia: A risk factor for neural-tube defects. *Metabolism* 1994; 43: 1475–80.

104. Steegers–Theunissen, RPM, Boers, GH, Blom, HJ. Neural tube defects and elevated homocysteine levels in amniotic fluid. *Am J Obstet Gynecol* 1995; 172: 1436–41.

105. Steegers–Theunissen, RPM, Wathen, NC, Eskes, TKAB, van Raaij–Selten, B, Chard, T. Maternal and fetal levels of methionine and homocysteine in early

human pregnancy. *Br J Obstet Gynaecol* 1997; 104: 20–4.

106. Stein, Z, Susser, M, Saenper, G, Marolla, F (eds.). *Famine and Human Development: the Dutch Hunger Winter of 1944–1945.* Oxford University Press, New York, 1975.

107. Tsai, JC, Perrella, MA, Yoshizumi, M, Hsieh, CM, Haber, E, Schlehel, R, Lee, ME. Promotion of vascular smooth muscle cell growth by homocysteine: A link to atherosclerosis. *Proc Natl Acad Sci USA* 1994; 91: 6369–73.

108. Tsai, JC, Wang, H, Perrella, MA, Yoshizumi, M, Sibinga, NES, Tan, LC, Haber, E, Chang, TTH, Schlegel, R, Lee, ME. Induction of cyclin A gene expression by homocysteine in vascular smooth muscle cells. *J Clin Invest* 1996; 97: 146–53.

109. Tucker, KL, Selhub, J, Wilson, PWF, Rosenberg, IH. Dietary intake pattern related to plasma folate and homocysteine concentrations in the Framingham study. *J Nutr* 1996; 126: 3025–31.

110. Ubbink, JB, Christianson, A, Bester, MJ, van Allen, MI, Venter, PA, Delport, R, Blom, HJ, van der Merwe, A, Potgieter, H, Vermaak, WJ. Folate status, homocysteine metabolism and methylenetetrahydrofolate reductase genotype in rural South African blacks with a history of pregnancy complicated by neural tube defects. *Metabolism* 1999; 48: 269–74.

111. van Aerts, LAGJM, Blom, HJ, De Abreu, RA, Trijbels, FJM, Eskes, TKAB, Peereboom–Stegeman, JHJC, Noordhoek, J. Prevention of neural tube defects by and toxicity of L-homocysteine in cultured postimplantation rat embryos. *Teratology* 1994; 50: 348–60.

112. van der Molen, EF, van den Heuvel, LP, TePoele-Pothof, MT, Monnens, LH, Eskes, TKAB, Blom, HJ. The effect of folic acid on the homocysteine metabolism of human umbilical vein endothelial cells (HUVEC's). *Eur J Clin Invest* 1996; 26: 304–9.

113. van der Molen, EF, Verbruggen, B, Nováková, I, Eskes, TKAB, Monnens, LAH, Blom, HJ. Hyperhomocysteinemia and other thrombotic risk factors in women with placental vasculopathy. *Brit J Obstet Gynaecol* 2000; 107: 785–91.

114. van der Molen, EF, Arends, GE, Nelen, WLDM, van der Put, NMJ, Heil, SG, Eskes, TKAB, Blom, HJ. A common mutation in the methylenetetrahydrofolate reductase gene as a new risk factor for placental vasculopathy. *Am J Obstet Gynecol* 2000; 182: 1258–63.

115. van der Mooren, MJ, Wouters, MGAJ, Blom, HJ, Schellekens, LA, Eskes, TKAB. Hormone replacement therapy may reduce high serum homocysteine in postmenopausal women. *J Clin Invest* 1994; 24: 733–36.

116. van der Mooren, MJ, Demacker, PNM, Blom, HJ, de Rijke, YB, Rolland, R. The effect of sequential threemonthly hormone replacement therapy on several cardiovascular risk estimators in postmenopausal women. *Fertil Steril* 1997; 67: 67–73.

117. van der Put, N. Homocysteine, folate and neural tube defects; biochemical and molecular genetic analysis. PhD Thesis, University of Nijmegen, 1999.

118. van der Put, NMJ, Steegers–Theunissen, RPM, Frosst, P, Trijbels, FJM, Eskes, TKAB, van den Heuvel, LP,

Mariman, ECM, den Heijer, M, Rozen, R, Blom, HJ. Mutated methylenetetrahydrofolate reductase as a risk factor for spina bifida. *Lancet* 1995; 346: 1070–71.

119. van der Put, NMJ, van den Heuvel, LP, Steegers–Theunissen, RPM, Trijbels, FJM, Eskes, TKAB, Mariman, EC, den Heijer, M, Blom, HJ. Decreased methylenetetrahydrofolate reductase activity due to the 677 C-T mutation in families with spina bifida offspring. *J Mol Med* 1996; 74: 691–94.

120. van der Put, NMJ, Thomas, CMG, Eskes, TKAB, Trijbels, FJM, Steegers–Theunissen, RPM, Mariman, ECM, De Graaf–Hess, A, Smeitink, JAM, Blom, HJ. Altered folate and vitamin B_{12} metabolism in families with spina bifida offspring. *Q J Med* 1997; 90: 505–10.

121. van der Put, NMJ, Eskes, TKAB, Blom, HJ. Is the common 677 C-T mutation in the methylenetetrahydrofolate reductase gene a risk factor for neural tube defects? A meta-analysis. *Q J Med* 1997; 90: 111–15.

122. van der Put, NMJ, van der Molen, EF, Kluijtmans, LAJ, Heil, SG, Trijbels, FJM, Eskes, TKAB, van Oppenraaij–Emmerzaal, D, Banerjee, R, Blom, HJ. Sequence analysis of the coding region of human methionine synthase: Relevance to hyperhomocysteinaemia in neural-tube defects and vascular disease. *Q J Med* 1997; 90: 511–17.

123. van der Put, NMJ, Gabreëls, F, Stevens, EMB, Smeitink, JAM, Trijbels, FJM, Eskes, TKAB, van den Heuvel, LP, Blom, HJ. A second common mutation in the methylenetetrahydrofolate reductase gene: a risk factor for neural-tube defects? *Am J Hum Genet* 1998; 62: 1044–51.

123a. Vollset, SE, Refsum, H, Irgens, LM, Emblem, BM, Tverdal, A, Gjessing, HK, Monsen, ALB, Ueland, PM. Plasma total homocysteine, pregnancy complications, and adverse pregnancy outcomes: the Hordaland Homocysteine Study. *Am J Clin Nutr* 2000; 71: 962–68.

123b. Walsh, BW, Paul, S, Wild, RA, Dean, RA, Tracy, RW, Cox, DA, Anderson, PW. The effects of hormone replacement therapy and raloxifene on C-reactive protein and homocysteine in healthy postmenopausal women: a randomized, controlled trial. *J Clin Endocrinol Metabol* 2000; 85: 214–18.

124. Ward, M, McNulty, H, McPartlin, J, Strain, JJ, Weir, DG, Scott, JM. Plasma homocysteine, a risk factor for cardiovascular disease, is lowered by physiological doses of folic acid. *Q J Med* 1997; 90: 519–24.

125. Weisberg, I, Tran, P, Christensen, B, Sibani, S, Rozen, R. A second genetic polymorphism in methylenetetrahydrofolate reductase (MTHFR) associated with decreased enzyme activity. *Mol Genet Metab* 1998; 64: 169–72.

126. Whitehead, AS, Gallagher, P, Mills, JL, Kirke, PN, Burke, H, Molloy, AM, Weir, DG, Shields, DC, Scott, JM. A genetic defect in 5,10-methylenetetrahydrofolate reductase in neural tube defects. *Q J Med* 1995; 88: 763–66.

127. Wilcken, DEL, Wang, XL. Relevance to spina bifida of mutated methylenetetrahydrofolate reductase. *Lancet* 1996; 347: 340.

128. Wong, WY, Eskes, TKAB, Kuijpers–Jagtman, A, Spauwen, PHM, Steegers, EAP, Thomas, CM, Hamel, BC, Blom, HJ, Steegers–Theunissen, RPM. Non-syndromic orofacial clefts: Association with maternal hyperhomocysteinaemia. *Teratology* 1999; 60: 253–57.

129. Wouters, MGAJ, Boers, GHJ, Blom, HJ, Trijbels, FJM, Thomas, CMG, Borm, GF, Steegers–Theunissen, RPM, Eskes, TKAB. Hyperhomocysteinemia: A risk factor in women with unexplained recurrent early pregnancy loss. *Fertil Steril* 1993; 60: 820–25.

130. Wouters, MGAJ, Moorrees, MTEC, van der Mooren, MJ, Blom, HJ, Boers, GHJ, Schellekens, LA. Plasma homocysteine and menopausal status. *Eur J Clin Invest* 1995; 25: 801–5.

38

Modification of Hyperhomocysteinemia

JOHN M. SCOTT

Homocysteine may be elevated in the plasma if for any reason any one of the three enzymes that controls its metabolism has impaired function. As discussed in other chapters, reduced function can arise where there is a reduced status of any one of the three nutrients, folate, cobalamin, or vitamin B_6. Reduced folate status impairs the activity of methionine synthase and 5,10-methylenetetrahydrofolate reductase. Reduced cobalamin status also impairs the function of methionine synthase, and reduced vitamin B_6 status impairs the function of cystathionine β-synthase.

The two active forms of riboflavin, flavin mononucleotide (FMN) and flavin adenine dinucleotide (FAD), are also involved in homocysteine metabolism. FMN is required for the enzymatic activation of vitamin B_6 to its coenzyme form, pyridoxal 5′-phosphate. As such, FMN is indirectly necessary for the activity of cystathionine β-synthase, which uses pyridoxal 5′-phosphate as a coenzyme. FAD is a prosthetic group in the active site of methylenetetrahydrofolate reductase (MTHFR). It seems that in communities where the diet is not fortified with riboflavin (as it is in the United States) there may be deficiency of riboflavin, at least in elderly persons, as determined by an enzyme marker for riboflavin status.

In addition, another enzyme exists in liver and kidney of humans (34) that metabolizes homocysteine, namely betaine:homocysteine methyltransferase, which requires zinc as a cofactor (see Chapter 13). It also requires betaine, the degradation product of choline, as a substrate. In theory, dietary deficiency of either zinc or choline could thus give rise to elevated plasma homocysteine. Reduced status or overt deficiency of any of these five micronutrients or choline could arise from a dietary intake insufficient to maintain normal status, a clinical condition causing malabsorption or increased demand, such as the need for extra folate in late pregnancy.

Finally, certain clinical conditions, mainly associated with impaired renal function, are accompanied by elevation of plasma homocysteine (see Chapters 26 and 27).

A completely separate set of circumstances also gives rise to hyperhomocystenemia, namely where there is a genetically inherited impairment of one of the enzymes discussed above. Such genetic mutations have been identified for two of the three key enzymes, cystathionine β-synthase and MTHFR (see Chapters 20 and 21). In addition several mutations of the enzymes and other proteins associated with cobalamin activation and transport have been identified (see Chapter 21).

In all of these mutations, studies have documented the treatment of the hyperhomocysteinemia. There is also one recognized common variant of MTHFR that, in the homozygous state and to some extent in the heterozygous state, is associated with reduced enzyme activity (20) (see Chapter 22). This variant gives rise to some, although not a profound, elevation of plasma homocysteine. Folate requirement is also increased in individuals homozygous for this variant (37).

It is probable that other variants of this enzyme or the other enzymes involved directly or even indirectly in homocysteine metabolism will be identified that will have associated with them impaired (or even enhanced) ability to regulate the level of homocysteine in cells and thus ultimately in plasma. Genetic polymorphisms giving rise to such variants may turn out to have a high prevalence. Even though their effect on homocysteine metabolism may be very small, they may be important clinically for two reasons. Small alterations in plasma homocysteine may be associated with much more profound reductions in cellular functions, which may in turn be associated with various increased risks of disease. In addition, most diseases probably have genetic variants that increase risk.

Some variants that may be perfectly tolerable in one circumstance may pose a high risk in other circumstances (e.g., they are a risk only if folate status is low).

Finally, a polymorphism that, even in the homozygous state, is not associated with an increased risk might show an increased risk if accompanied by another polymorphism in the same or another folate-related gene. Such other variants are as yet unidentified, which forces us to consider, when dealing with "normal people," that genetically and functionally this concept of normality may turn out to be a less and less valuable characterization.

The approach in this chapter is to consider intervention with nutrients and betaine under three categories: I) genetic mutations, which are rare and have associated with them a severely abnormal phenotype; II) clinical conditions where there is abnormal metabolism of homocysteine, such as renal disease; and III) normal subjects, among whom are included the general population.

Also included in the third category are subjects in whom a specific and separate condition, such as pernicious anemia, causes malabsorption of one of the nutrients. This occurs because when this condition is corrected, metabolism with respect to the other nutrients is probably the same as in normal people. The third category also includes subjects heterozygous or homozygous for the common 677C→T variant of MTHFR; in many communities nearly half the population is heterozygous for this variant, and the homozygous prevalence varies from 6% to 20%. Many additional variants probably exist. Finally, the third category also includes those with cardiovascular disease, even though they might not be considered by some to be normal subjects. Any differences in response between subjects with and without cardiovascular disease are of interest, because among the former, one expects to find as yet undetected and possibly less responsive variants to nutrient intervention.

A further consideration is the varying amounts of nutrients that have been used in studies to date. This factor becomes important when one considers the larger public health objective of lowering plasma homocysteine in populations rather than individuals. The experience with the use of folic acid to lower the prevalence of neural tube defects will probably be repeated if homocysteine is found to affect cardiovascular disease. If a reduction in cardiovascular risk were established, individuals with elevated homocysteine levels would presumably take a supplement. They might wish to know the lowest level of supplement that would be effective in all circumstances, although such supplements, even at twice the Recommended Dietary Allowance, would be unlikely to pose a serious risk compared with the potential benefit.

However, if one wished to carry out such intervention to effect a general change in public health, determining the lowest effective dose becomes crucial because such intervention could be achieved only through general fortification of the diet. When the lowest effective amount is added to a staple such as flour, trying to ensure that those with low flour intake receive the target amount will mean that those with high intake receive several times the target amount. For example, if the minimum target figure to optimally lower homocysteine levels was an extra 400 µg/day folic acid and folic acid was added to flour in sufficient quantities to ensure that most people received this amount, sectors of the community on higher intakes of flour would receive much more than this amount, with many being exposed to more than 1 mg/day. Such large amounts of folic acid may mask cobalamin deficiency in elderly people (55) (see Chapter 24). In addition, introducing large amounts of unaltered folic acid in the nervous system could be undesirable (26), and there may be other unknown risks. By contrast, if 100 µg of folic acid per day optimally reduced plasma homocysteine when given long-term in a staple such as flour, exposure for those with high intake of flour might be associated with minimal risk.

The most important public health issue is not how much of these various nutrients are needed to lower plasma homocysteine in those with severe genetic mutations or with clinical conditions such as renal failure that are associated with hyperhomocysteinemia. Those cases will be relatively rare and generally easily identified, and the amount to be used in a supplement is not really a critical issue. Of far greater public health interest are the amounts that will be effective in general populations and in the common genetic variants, especially if the particular nutrients are to be given perhaps for decades to completely normal subjects or to subjects with a mild variant. It would be important to use the lowest effective supplement for such chronic treatment.

Category I. Genetic Mutations

Cystathionine β-Synthase

Several different mutations have a similar phenotype, but two types can be distinguished with respect to intervention, namely vitamin B_6 unresponsive and vitamin B_6-responsive cystathionine β-synthase deficiency (see Chapter 20). Mudd et al. (39) have reviewed the literature. In many subjects with different cystathionine β-synthase mutations, significant reduction in plasma homocysteine can be achieved by daily doses of oral vitamin B_6. Typically, homozygotes have shown varying ranges of responses (4, 5, 40, 56). In some studies, other related nutrients such as folic acid and cobalamin (38) and betaine (57) have been used in conjunction with vitamin B_6 with apparent enhanced effect, at least in some cases.

Methionine Synthase-Related Mutations

Several different mutations, all rare, affect the activity of methionine synthase (see Chapter 12). As with cobalamin deficiency, they lead to anemia (2) and neuropathy (46). Many of them respond partially to large and frequent doses of cobalamin. Betaine has had no apparent benefit (1).

Methylenetetrahydrofolate Reductase

Patients have been recognized with different mutations of the gene coding for this enzyme (17) (see Chapter 22). The most common variant involves the 677 C→T MTHFR.

Category II. Clinical Conditions

Renal Disease

Uremic patients (11, 60), even when undergoing dialysis, have elevated plasma homocysteine (25, 59), as do recipients of renal transplants with mildly reduced renal function (58) (see Chapter 26). Wilcken et al (58) found that vitamin B_6 did not lower plasma homocysteine in renal transplant recipients. Nevertheless, vitamin B_6 supplements of 10 mg/day are thought to be advisable to maintain other functions such as erythrocyte glutamic pyruvic transaminase activity.

The use of folic acid to lower plasma homocysteine was initially questioned (13, 29, 30). Arnadottir et al. (3) compared vitamin B_6 and folic acid regimens in 18 patients. The vitamin B_6 regimen, if anything, increased the plasma homocysteine. The folic acid regimen significantly reduced it by 30%, as had previously been reported (58).

Category III. Normal Subjects

As discussed previously, this category represents the vast majority of the population who will have varying levels of plasma homocysteine depending on the status of the three key nutrients, folate, cobalamin, and vitamin B_6. Some of these subjects, who are apparently normal with respect to the metabolism of these three nutrients, may have underlying as yet unidentified genetic variants. Some may have diseases thought to be, but not proven to be, associated with elevated plasma homocysteine such as cardiovascular disease and stroke. Some subjects may also have malabsorptive conditions that produce deficiency of one of the key nutrients (e.g., cobalamin) but are included to determine the response to another nutrient (e.g., folate).

Folic Acid (see also Chapter 23)

Initial studies that used folic acid to lower plasma homocysteine all used pharmacological doses. In some studies, patients were shown to be folate deficient by measurement of their plasma and red cell folate levels. Other studies concerned themselves only with the reduction of homocysteine that was achieved, without ascertaining whether the underlying increase in homocysteine had been due to folate deficiency.

One early study found that folic acid supplements (5 mg/day) administered for 4 weeks lowered homocysteine-cysteine mixed disulfide in postmenopausal women with apparently normal folate status (7). The same group subsequently treated 13 apparently normal subjects with 5 mg/day folic acid for 2 weeks and obtained about a 50% reduction in total plasma homocysteine levels (8). The greatest reduction was observed in those who happened to have the highest starting homocysteine levels. Stabler et al. (47) reported a significant drop in plasma homocysteine in a single alcoholic with nutritional folate deficiency given 1 mg/day folic acid for 9 days, with most of the reduction being in place after the first day. Ubbink et al. (49), who earlier used supplements containing folic acid combined with cobalamin and vitamin B_6 (see later), showed that 19 subjects given folic acid alone as a daily supplement of 0.65 mg for 6 weeks had a significant reduction in plasma homocysteine. Nilsson et al. (42) found that 10 mg/day of folic acid for 1 to 1.5 weeks significantly lowered plasma homocysteine levels in 13 subjects from a psychogeriatric population.

Jacob et al. (23) kept 10 healthy males on a folate-deficient diet containing 25 µg of food folate per day for 30 days. The subjects' homocysteine levels rose. When 74 µg of folic acid was added daily for an additional 15 days, the plasma folate level returned to near the starting value. However, plasma homocysteine levels remained elevated. When the subjects were returned to their baseline diet that contained 440 µg of food folate and no added folic acid, the plasma homocysteine quickly returned to baseline values. If one assumes that food folate is about half as bioavailable as folic acid, this study implies that 200 µg of folic acid equivalent is sufficient to optimally lower homocysteine, whereas 87 µg/day (74 plus half of 25) is insufficient.

Landgren et al. (28) measured plasma homocysteine in the acute phase of myocardial infarction (24 to 36 hours) and compared it with the levels present 6 weeks later. Plasma homocysteine increased from 13.1 ± 4.6 to 14.8 ± 4.8 µmol/L ($p < 0.001$). The patients were then assigned to three groups receiving zero (n = 20), 2.5 mg (n = 17), or 10 mg/day (n = 16) folic acid. The untreated group showed a small increase in plasma homocysteine, and the latter two groups showed a significant decrease. There was no greater decrease at the higher doses.

O'Keefe et al. (43) maintained 17 young women on low-folate diets that contained 30 µg of natural folate to which they added 200, 300 or 400 µg/day of folic acid. The starting homocysteine levels were comparable in all three groups, but after 70 days those taking only 200 µg in supplements had a highly significant increase in plasma homocysteine over those taking 400 µg ($p = 0.009$); the differences between the 200 µg and 300 µg groups approached significance ($p = 0.067$). Dierkes et al. (16) examined the effect of 400 µg of folic acid for 4 weeks on a group of young women and found significant lowering of homocysteine levels.

den Heijer et al. (15) randomized healthy volunteers, classified as normohomocysteinemic because their homocysteine values were less than 16 µmol/L, into a placebo (n = 36), 5 mg/day folic acid (n = 35), or 0.5 mg/day folic acid (n = 36) group for 56 days. There was a reduction of 26% (range, 2% to 52%) and 25% (range, 5% to 40%) for the higher dose and lower dose folic acid interventions, respectively. Both were significantly better than placebo ($p < 0.001$), and no extra benefit seemed to be achieved by the higher supplement.

Clarke et al. (12) carried out an important meta-analysis of most of the randomized trials available at that time on the effect of folic acid on lowering plasma homocysteine. They excluded studies of less than 3 weeks of intervention or studies in which values had been determined after methionine loading. The eight studies used folic acid supplements in the range of 0.4 to 5.0 mg/day. A clear pattern emerged. The degree of homocysteine lowering was predominantly determined by the starting homocysteine and plasma folate values. The higher the former and the lower the latter, the greater the effect. Higher doses of folic acid did not appear to be more effective than lower doses. Doses below 1 mg/day (mean dose 0.5 mg/day; p value for heterogeneity = 0.15) compared with 1 to 3 mg/day (mean dose 1.2 mg/day; $p = 0.05$) or more than 3 mg/day (mean dose 5.7 mg/day; $p = 0.69$) showed similar effects on homocysteine. If one looked at the magnitude of the effect after standardization to pretreatment levels of homocysteine of 12.0 µmol/L and plasma folate of 12.0 nmol/L, intervention with folic acid at the three levels indicated here reduced homocysteine levels by 25% (95% confidence interval, 23% to 28%; $p < 0.001$). The analysis suggests that doses lower than 1 mg/day were as effective as higher doses. However, the data were insufficient to discriminate between doses of less than 1 mg/day. The addition of cobalamin (mean dose 0.5 mg/day) had a small but significant effect of an additional 7% lowering (3% to 10%), whereas vitamin B_6 (mean dose 16.5 mg/day) had no significant additional effect.

Guttormsen et al. (21) screened more than 18,000 subjects and selected 67 cases with elevated homocys-

teine levels $\geq$ 40 µmol/L. The prevalence of the 677C→T variant of MTHFR was 73.1% in the study cases and 10.2% in the 329 selected control cases. Seven of the cases had cobalamin deficiency. Two years later, 59 of the subjects were reinvestigated; 41 had homocysteine levels > 20 µmol/L; of these, 37 were given folic acid (200 µg/day). Almost all of these subjects (34, or 92%) were homozygous for the 677C→T mutation. In all but two subjects, there was a significant reduction in plasma homocysteine during a 7-month daily folic acid intervention period. However, there seemed to be two patterns of response. Homocysteine levels declined rapidly into the normal range in 21 subjects. The other 16 subjects did not show a rapid and appropriate response, although 12 did respond to 5 mg of folic acid/day.

It must be borne in mind that most of the subjects had the MTHFR variant. Also, they had originally been derived from a preselection of people with elevated plasma homocysteine, most of whom were homozygous for this variant. Thus, this study really measured responsiveness to folic acid in this 677C→T MTHFR variant (i.e., it was not a study of normal subjects but of subjects with an apparent defect in folate metabolism). It has since been established that having this variant impairs folate status (37). This study thus examined the effectiveness of 200 µg/day of folic acid in overcoming this known metabolic block. The regimen appeared to be sufficient in 21 (57%), but insufficient in 16 (43%) subjects with this variant.

D'Angelo et al. (14) treated subjects homozygous for the 677C→T mutation with 15 mg of 5-methyltetrahydrofolate daily for 4 weeks. Not surprisingly, this pharmacological dose normalized elevations of plasma homocysteine. Malinow et al. (33) treated subjects with the same mutation with 1 or 2 mg/day of folic acid for 3 weeks. They, too, found a significant reduction in plasma homocysteine. Nelen et al. (41) used the lower dose of 0.5 mg/day folic acid for 2 months for different MTHFR genotypes. Those homozygous (n = 8) had the highest starting total homocysteine level of 14.9 µmol/L, compared with those heterozygous (n = 23) and wild-type (n = 18), whose combined mean level was 12.8 µmol/L. The former group showed the largest reduction in homocysteine of 41% ($p < 0.01$), probably because of their high starting level of homocysteine rather than greater responsiveness.

Ward et al. (54) determined the effect of different low doses of folic acid in lowering plasma homocysteine in 30 normal males. The study was not placebo-controlled but monitored subjects who were placed sequentially on the following amounts of daily folic acid (for the weeks indicated): 100 µg (6 weeks), 200 µg (6 weeks), and 400 µg (14 weeks). The duration chosen had previously been shown to be the time required for plasma folate levels to plateau. In the group as a whole, homocysteine levels decreased on 100 μg doses, with a further decrease at 200 μg but no further reduction at 400 μg. When supplements were withdrawn, the individuals returned to their baseline homocysteine values. Dividing the group by tertiles according to their starting homocysteine levels showed that the highest tertile underwent the greatest reduction, with an intermediate reduction in the middle tertile and no change in the lowest tertile.

Thus, most of these apparently normal men had plasma homocysteine levels that could be improved by small physiological doses of folic acid. The group was not assessed for 677C→T mutation. However, because they were not preselected, less than 10% were probably homozygous, which is the norm for that community.

Brönstrup et al. (9) treated 41 normal women with placebo for 4 weeks followed by another 4 weeks of 400 μg/day of folic acid. Homocysteine levels did not change after placebo treatment but decreased significantly after folic acid treatment. Schorah et al. (45) treated 33 normal adults with breakfast cereals delivering 200 μg of folic acid per serving. Compared with the placebo group, there was a significant reduction in homocysteine levels after 4 weeks, with a further reduction after 24 weeks. As with many of the studies discussed previously, the largest reductions were in those with the highest starting levels of plasma homocysteine.

Malinow et al. (32) gave three groups of 24 to 26 normal women breakfast cereals fortified with different levels of folic acid, 127 μg, 499 μg, and 885 μg. Half of each treatment group initially received folic acid and half received a placebo for 6 weeks; a 4-week washout period was followed by a cross-over of placebo and folic acid intervention. Significant reductions in plasma homocysteine were achieved by the two highest treatment regimens, 499 and 885 μg/day. The prevalences of homozygosity for the 677C→T variant were 6 of 24, 1 of 25, and 3 of 25 for the three groups, respectively. Brouwer et al. (10) randomized 144 healthy women into three groups receiving placebo (n = 49), 500 μg/day folic acid (n = 45), and 500 μg folic acid every second day (n = 50). Plasma homocysteine decreased significantly in the two treatment groups compared with the placebo group.

Since the beginning of 1998, and often for 1 or 2 years before that, manufacturers in the United States fortified flour with 140 μg of folic acid per 100 g. Jacques et al. (24) recently determined the effect of this intervention in the Framingham Offspring Cohort. They compared plasma folate levels in two subcohorts from baseline values in 1991 to 1994 to either follow-up values at January 1995 to September 1996 (control

group) or September 1997 to March 1998 (study group). The study group, which was exposed to the effect of fortification of flour with folic acid, had a significant increase in plasma folate level from 11 to 23 nmol/L (p < 0.001); the proportion of subjects with values below 7 nmol/L declined from 22% to 1.7%. There was also an impressive reduction in plasma homocysteine from 10.1 to 9.4 μmol/L (p < 0.001), with those with values higher than 13 μmol/L decreasing from 18.7% to 9.8%. The predicted postfortification increase in intake from dietary intake models would have been 70 to 120 μg/day for this group.

Comment Folic acid, when used in pharmacological amounts, clearly lowers plasma homocysteine levels (7, 8, 28, 42, 47, 49). However, when one considers the effect of lower, more physiological amounts of folic acid, the picture is less clear. Because of the impact of fortification on folate intake by consumers of high levels of a staple such as flour, it becomes critical to try to determine lower or the lowest effective dose. Ward et al. (54) found 200 μg/day as a supplement to be as effective as 400 μg/day, with 100 μg/day for 6 weeks only partly effective. Later studies also found 400 μg/day of folic acid to be effective (10, 16), and 500 μg/day was just as effective as 5 mg/day (15). The meta-analysis by Clarke et al. (12) indicates that less than 1 mg/day provides optimum lowering of homocysteine. Folic acid in breakfast cereals at 200 μg/day was apparently effective.

However, not all studies support the conclusion that these lower doses are optimal. O'Keefe et al. (43) found 200 μg/day to be ineffective compared with 400 μg/day. Likewise, Jacob et al. (23) found that the equivalent of 87 μg/day of folic acid was ineffective compared with 400 μg/day. Malinow et al. (32) found that when delivered in breakfast cereals, an extra 127 μg/day significantly raised plasma folate levels but did not significantly reduce plasma homocysteine levels; a significant response was elicited equally from higher intakes of 459 or 885 μg/day. Jacques et al. (24) found that the fortification of flour that should have increased intake from 70 to 120 μg/day in the United States caused a significant decrease in plasma homocysteine levels.

Considering the 677C→T MTHFR variant, it appears that milligram amounts of folic acid optimally lower homocysteine levels even in homozygotes (21, 33); even 500 μg/day was effective (41). However, Guttormsen et al. (21) found that the response to 200 μg/day was effective in some, but not in others who ultimately responded to 5 mg/day. It is unclear if the conclusion of this study is that 200 μg/day is ineffective in some subjects with this variant and, if so, why. It seems that 200 μg/day of folic acid given long-term may be optimally effective in apparently normal people, but perhaps not in those with this MTHFR variant.

Cobalamin

Cobalamin deficiency, such as occurs in pernicious anemia (22), has been associated with increased plasma homocysteine levels (1). It is clear that treating with cobalamin reduces the plasma homocysteine of patients with cobalamin deficiency (5). Of greater public health interest, in view of the possible association of homocysteine with cardiovascular disease (53), is whether many people in the apparently normal population have a component of their plasma homocysteine level that can be lowered by cobalamin. This question was first addressed by Brattstrom et al. (8), who examined the effect of 1 mg of cobalamin taken orally for 14 days in 14 apparently normal adults. These subjects, who were not deficient to begin with, showed no homocysteine lowering.

Ubbink et al. (49) assigned 100 men with hyperhomocysteinemia to groups receiving folic acid, cobalamin, vitamin B_6, all three vitamins, or placebo. After 6 weeks, reduction of homocysteine levels in those given cobalamin was not significantly different from the placebo group, although homocysteine levels decreased by 15%.

den Heijer et al. (15) examined the effect of intervention with hydroxocobalamin at 0.4 mg/day for 56 days in 36 "normohomocysteinemic" (<16 µmol/L) subjects compared with a placebo group. The modest reduction in homocysteine levels in the treated group was not significant ($p = 0.14$). Rasmussen et al. (44) found that high doses of oral cobalamin (1 mg twice daily) for 1 to 2 weeks had a small but nonsignificant lowering effect in a nonrandomized study of 235 subjects.

Comment Oral cobalamin clearly lowers homocysteine in those who are deficient. There also appears to be some lowering in apparently normal subjects, but it is small compared with that achieved with folic acid (see also Chapters 23 and 24).

Vitamin B_6

Vitamin B_6, used frequently to treat patients with cystathionine β-synthase deficiency (see Chapter 20), has also been used to attempt to lower plasma homocysteine in apparently unaffected subjects. Brattström et al. (8) treated 15 normal subjects with 33 mg/day of vitamin B_6 for 2 weeks, with no significant effect. Brattström et al. (6) also used 198 mg/day of vitamin B_6 in 20 patients with arterial disease for 2 weeks. These supplements had no effect on fasting homocysteine but did lower the postmethionine load homocysteine level.

Miller et al. (36) used a depletion period design to examine the effect of oral vitamin B_6 on plasma homocysteine. The depletion period on a vitamin B_6-deficient diet lasted for 20 days followed by progressive reintroduction of vitamin B_6 into the diet. There was no significant effect on the plasma homocysteine. The depletion period may not have been long enough to cause any overt signs of vitamin B_6 deficiency or to raise the plasma homocysteine level. However, the lack of response to vitamin B_6 even after depletion suggests that vitamin B_6 had no significant effect on plasma homocysteine in these normal subjects.

Ubbink et al. (49) carried out a placebo-controlled intervention with the three vitamins individually and in combination. Although folic acid and cobalamin, alone or together, significantly reduced homocysteine compared with the starting baseline values, vitamin B_6 intervention caused no significant reduction.

Franken et al. (19) selected from patients with vascular disease a group who had mild hyperhomocysteinemia established by means of a standardized methionine loading test. Their fasting state and postmethionine loading homocysteine determinations were repeated after 6 weeks of intervention with either 50 or 250 mg/day of vitamin B_6. The intervention with 50 mg/day produced a slight increase in mean fasting homocysteine levels (from 15.1 to 16.3 µmol/L, $p > 0.05$) and the 250 mg/day intervention produced a slight but nonsignificant decrease (from 17.1 to 14.8 µmol/L). Because a placebo group was not included, it is difficult to interpret these changes, except to say that they were clearly not dramatic; however, there was a significant reduction in the postmethionine load level for both treatments. The 50 mg/day group reduced their postload homocysteine level by 21% (from 59.6 to 46.9 µmol/L, $p < 0.02$), with 6 of the 10 patients now showing a normal response. The reduction for the 250 mg/day group was 25% (from 69.7 to 51.1 µmol/L, $p < 0.0006$), with 7 of 10 patients now having a normal response to methionine loading.

Franken et al. (18) screened 421 patients with arterial disease, using methionine loading to identify mild hyperhomocysteinemia. They found that 33% of those with peripheral arterial and 20% of those with cerebral arterial disease had an abnormal methionine loading test. Of 82 of these subjects with an abnormal loading test response, 46 (56%) showed a normal response after treatment with 250 mg/day of vitamin B_6 for 6 weeks. Another 16 patients (20%) gave an intermediate response and 20 (24%) a poor or no response. Whereas the study by Franken et al. (19) measured total homocysteine, this study (18) reported on "free homocysteine," measured as "homocystine and homocysteine-cysteine mixed disulfide."

Comment Vitamin B_6 has little if any effect on basal homocysteine levels in normal subjects. It may have some effect on the postmethionine load homocysteine level in some people.

Riboflavin

As mentioned earlier, evidence of inadequate riboflavin status has been seen, at least in elderly people. Such status can be determined by the erythrocyte glutathione reductase activation coefficient. One study found abnormal activation coefficient levels in 49% of 92 subjects older than 65 years (31). In a pilot study, the ability of riboflavin intervention to decrease plasma homocysteine levels was studied in a placebo-controlled, double-blind, 12-week trial in which subjects more than 65 years old were assigned to daily placebo (n = 6) or 1.6 mg (n = 7) or 25 mg riboflavin (n = 3) (35). Even though there was evidence of a response in the activation coefficient as a result of riboflavin intervention, there was no significant change in plasma homocysteine. The numbers of subjects were small, however, and an effect could have been missed. In another study, riboflavin supplements (10 mg/day for 15 days) failed to alter homocysteine levels in 10 women (27).

Folic Acid, Vitamin B_6, Cobalamin, and Betaine Combinations

Several studies have used folic acid, vitamin B_6, cobalamin, and betaine combination in the same study. These studies were carried out in three distinct ways. Response was compared with 1) placebo and/or baseline, or 2) baseline with no placebo, or 3) combinations of different nutrients. These studies are valuable because they compare the relative effectiveness of the different nutrients in lowering plasma homocysteine in various groups.

Response Compared with Placebo and/or Baseline In a double-blind, placebo-controlled intervention, Ubbink et al. (49) compared placebo with daily oral folic acid (0.65 mg), cobalamin (0.4 mg), or vitamin B_6 (10 mg) for 6 weeks. As discussed for the individual vitamins, folic acid reduced plasma homocysteine to nearly half the base line ($p < 0.001$) or placebo ($p < 0.01$) levels, with cobalamin causing a small but significant reduction against baseline ($p < 0.05$) but not the placebo group. Vitamin B_6 had no significant lowering effect. These subjects had been recruited by screening 2,788 subjects to identify those with hyperhomocysteinemia (> 16.3 µmol/L). The study did not evaluate the presence of the 677C→T MTHFR variant. Based on the later experience of Guttormsen et al. (21), it

seems probable that those 91 men selected by Ubbink et al. (49), because they had elevated plasma homocysteine levels, included a large number of subjects who were homozygous for the MTHFR variant. Bearing this in mind, as little as 0.65 mg/day of folic acid was nevertheless quite effective.

Response Compared with Baseline with No Placebo An early study compared the relative effectiveness of daily high doses of folic acid (5 mg), cobalamin (1 mg), or vitamin B_6 (33 mg) in three different groups of normal subjects (n = 15, 14, and 13, respectively) (8). Despite the lack of placebo control subjects, folic acid decreased the baseline homocysteine level by more than half; the other two nutrients had no effect.

Allen et al. (2) studied five patients with proven cobalamin deficiency who had been inappropriately treated with folic acid. Three patients were given 1 mg folic acid orally for 1 to 2.5 months; in two of them, there was an increase in plasma homocysteine and, in the third, there was a small decrease. In two other cobalamin-deficient patients given 150 to 200 µg of folic acid intramuscularly for nearly 2 weeks, one showed an increase in plasma homocysteine level and one a significant decrease. The homocysteine levels in all five cases later decreased to normal after intramuscular cobalamin treatment. Although the results are variable, they showed in general that elevated plasma homocysteine due to cobalamin deficiency does not respond to folic acid even in large amounts.

Combined Therapies The value of combinations of these nutrients is diminished by the obvious problem that one cannot distinguish which nutrient is having the greater effect or indeed if a particular nutrient is effective at all. In some studies, a combination was used only after an individual nutrient had been tried, and these studies are of value in determining if a further reduction was induced. Brattström et al. (6) used a high dose of folic acid (10 mg/day) combined with an even higher supplement of vitamin B_6 (198 mg/day) for 2 weeks. They found a significant reduction in homocysteine levels with the combined supplement, whereas vitamin B_6 on its own, although it lowered postmethionine load homocysteine levels, had no effect on fasting homocysteine. Ubbink et al. (48) used a combination of folic acid (1 mg), cobalamin (0.05 mg), and vitamin B_6 (12.2 mg) for 6 weeks. In 22 subjects with hyperhomocysteinemia (> 16.3 µmol/L), a greater than 50% reduction from baseline levels was found. A similar combined regimen compared with a placebo group again showed a greater than 50% reduction (50).

In their placebo-controlled trial, as discussed earlier, Ubbink et al. (49) found that a combination of the three nutrients was slightly more effective than folic acid alone when compared with the placebo group ($p < 0.01$), although both regimens showed equivalent reductions from baseline levels ($p = 0.001$). van den Berg et al. (52) used a combined daily supplement of folic acid (5.0 mg) and vitamin B_6 (250 mg) for 6 weeks in 72 patients with vascular disease, all of whom had an abnormal methionine loading test. They found a significant reduction in both fasting and postmethionine load plasma homocysteine. van den Berg et al. (51) then carried out a similar study in 48 patients with arterial disease given supplements for 6 to 12 weeks. Again there was a significant reduction in both fasting and postmethionine load homocysteine.

Franken et al. (19), while comparing the effect of 50 to 250 mg of vitamin B_6, used the latter in combination with 5 mg of folic acid. Vitamin B_6 had no effect on the basal homocysteine level but significantly lowered the postmethionine load level. When folic acid was included with vitamin B_6, the basal homocysteine level also decreased by 53%, from 19.9 to 9.4 µmol/L ($p < 0.006$). The postload level decreased by 49%, from 66.3 to 33.7 µmol/L ($p < 0.006$), in contrast with a smaller decrease with vitamin B_6 alone (from 69.7 to 51.1 µmol/L). It thus appears that, in a group of subjects selected because they had an abnormal result of a methionine loading test, folic acid has some additional benefit in lowering the elevated plasma homocysteine that follows a methionine load. There was also evidence that addition of folic acid had an extra increment of effect in lowering the basal level not found with vitamin B_6. This study appears to consign vitamin B_6 mostly to reducing extreme elevations of plasma homocysteine found after methionine loading, with folic acid again the principal player in controlling basal levels.

Franken et al. (18) used 250 mg/day of vitamin B_6 to treat 82 patients with vascular disease who had an abnormal methionine loading test. The postmethionine elevation in plasma homocysteine returned to normal in 46 subjects (56%). The nonresponders or partial responders were then given 5 mg/day of folic acid in addition, and all but one of them now showed normal methionine loading test results. This study indicates that the homocysteine status of many subjects does not respond to vitamin B_6 unless a high dose of folic acid is used concurrently.

Rasmussen et al. (44) kept 235 normal subjects on high-dose cobalamin (2 mg/day) for 2 weeks, with daily folic acid (10 mg) added in combination for another 2 weeks. The cobalamin intervention caused only a modest reduction in homocysteine levels, from 9.24 ± 2.64 to 8.79 ± 2.54 µmol/L. However the addition of folic acid induced a further, significant reduction from 8.79 ± 2.54 to 6.88 ± 1.64 µmol/L.

Dierkes et al. (16) compared the homocysteine-lowering effect of a daily supplement containing a combination of folic acid (0.4 mg) and vitamin B_6 (2 mg) to each vitamin given alone at the same dose. Homocysteine level reduction was similar with the combined regimen and with folic acid alone. No apparent benefit was seen when vitamin B_6 was included in the regimen.

den Heijer et al. (15) compared the homocysteine-lowering effect of a multivitamin containing high doses of folic acid (5 mg), cobalamin (0.4 mg), and vitamin B_6 (50 mg). This multivitamin was compared with high (5.0 mg) and low (0.5 mg) folic acid alone or with cobalamin (0.4 mg) alone. Either dose of folic acid had almost as great a lowering effect on plasma homocysteine after 56 days of administration as did the multivitamin. The same study compared this higher dose of multivitamin with placebo in patients with a history of venous thrombosis and healthy volunteers. The reduction achieved in homocysteine levels was greater in those patients and volunteers who had the highest initial levels of homocysteine. There was no evidence of a difference in effect between cases and normal volunteers; both seemed to respond equally.

Comment Combination or sequential therapies bear out the picture that emerged from each vitamin used individually. Folic acid lowers homocysteine levels in most people, with cobalamin having a small but significant additional effect, but with no such additional effect for vitamin B_6.

REFERENCES

1. Allen, RH, Stabler, SP, Lindenbaum, J. Serum betaine, N, N-dimethylglycine and N-methylglycine levels in patients with cobalamin and folate deficiency and related inborn errors of metabolism. *Metabolism* 1993; 42: 1448–60.
2. Allen, RH, Stabler, SP, Savage, DG, Lindenbaum, J. Diagnosis of cobalamin deficiency. I. Usefulness of serum methylmalonic acid and total homocysteine concentrations. *Am J Hematol* 1990; 34: 90–8.
3. Arnadottir, M, Brattström, L, Simonsen, O, Thysell, H, Hultberg, B, Andersson, A, Nilsson-Ehle, P. The effect of high-dose pyridoxine and folic acid supplementation on serum lipid and plasma homocysteine concentrations in dialysis patients. *Clin Nephrol* 1993; 40: 236–40.
4. Boers, GHJ, Smals, AGH, Drayer, JIM, Trijbels, FJM, Leermakers, AI, Kloppenborg, PW. Pyridoxal treatment does not prevent homocystinemia after methionine loading in adult homocystinuria patients. *Metabolism* 1983; 32: 390–97.
5. Brattström, L, Israelsson, B, Lindgärde, F, Hultberg, B. Higher total plasma homocysteine in vitamin B12 deficiency than in heterozygosity for homocystinuria due to cystathionine β-synthase deficiency. *Metabolism* 1988; 37: 175–78.

6. Brattström, L, Israelsson, B, Norrving, B, Bergquist, D, Thörne, J, Hultberg, B, Hamfelt, A. Impaired homocysteine metabolism in early-onset cerebral and peripheral occlusive arterial disease. Effect of pyridoxine and folic acid treatment. *Atherosclerosis* 1990; 81: 51–60.

7. Brattström, LE, Hultberg, BL, Hardebo, JE. Folic acid responsive postmenopausal homocysteinemia. *Metabolism* 1985; 34: 1073–77.

8. Brattström, LE, Israelsson, B, Jeppsson, JO, Hultberg, BL. Folic acid: An innocuous means to reduce plasma homocysteine. *Scand J Clin Lab Invest* 1988; 48: 215–21.

9. Brönstrup, A, Hages, M, Prinz-Langenohl, R, Pietrzik, K. Effects of folic acid and combinations of folic acid and vitamin B-12 on plasma homocysteine concentrations in healthy, young women. *Am J Clin Nutr* 1998; 68: 1104–10.

10. Brouwer, IA, van Dusseldorp, M, Thomas, CMG, Duran, M, Hautvast, JGAJ, Eskes, TKAB, Steegers-Theunissen, RPM. Low-dose folic acid supplementation decreases plasma homocysteine concentrations: a randomized trial. *Am J Clin Nutr* 1999; 69: 99–104.

11. Chauveau, P, Chadefaux, B, Coudé, M, Aupetit, J, Hannedouche, T, Kamoun, P, Jungers, P. Increased plasma homocysteine concentration in patients with chronic renal failure. *Miner Electrolyte Metab* 1992; 18: 196–98.

12. Clarke, R, Frost, C, Leroy, V, Collins, R, for the Homocysteine Lowering Trialists' Collaboration. Lowering blood homocysteine with folic acid based supplements: Meta-analysis of randomised trials. *Br Med J* 1998; 316: 894–98.

13. Cunningham, J, Sharman, VI, Goodwin, FJ, Marsh, EP. Do patients receiving haemodialysis need folic acid supplements? *Br Med J* 1981; 282: 1582.

14. D'Angelo, A, Coppola, A, Fermo, I, Pagano, A, Mazzole, G, Guiotto, G, Paroni, R, Cerbone, AM, Crippa, L, Di Minno, G. Persistent total homocysteine reduction and folate accumulation following one month course of methyltetrahydrofolate (Prefolic) administration in thrombophilic patients with moderate hyperhomocysteinemia and/or homozygosity for the thermolabile variant of MTHFR. *Neth J Med* 1998; 52: S50.

15. den Heijer, M, Brouwer, IA, Bos, GMJ, Blom, HJ, van der Put, NMJ, Spaans, AP, Rosendaal, FR, Thomas, CMG, Hoak, PWW, Gerrits, WBJ. Vitamin supplementation reduces blood homocysteine levels. A controlled trial in patients with venous thrombosis and healthy volunteers. *Arterioscler Thromb Vasc Biol* 1998; 18: 356–61.

16. Dierkes, J, Kroesen, M, Pietrzik, K. Folic acid and vitamin B6 supplementation and plasma homocysteine concentrations in healthy young women. *Internat J Vitam Nutr Res* 1998; 68: 98–103.

17. Erbe, RW. Inborn errors of folate metabolism. In *Folates and Pterins: Nutritional, Pharmacological and Physiological Aspects*. (Blakely, RL, Whitehead, VM, eds.). Wiley, New York, 1986; pp. 413–65.

18. Franken, DG, Boers, GHJ, Blom, HJ, Trijbels, FJM, Kloppenborg, PWC. Treatment of mild hyperhomocysteinemia in vascular disease patients. *Arterioscler Thromb* 1994; 14: 465–70.

19. Franken, DG, Boers, GHJ, Blom, HJ, Trijbels, JMF. Effect of various regimens of vitamin B6 and folic acid on mild hyperhomocysteinaemia in vascular patients. *J Inher Metab Dis* 1994; 17: 159–62.

20. Goyette, P, Sumner, JS, Milos, R, Duncan, AM, Rosenblatt, DS, Mathews, RG, Rozen, R. Human methylenetetrahydrofolate reductase: Isolation of cDNA, mapping and mutation identification. *Nature Genet* 1994; 7: 551–55.

21. Guttormsen, AB, Ueland, PM, Nesthus, I, Nygård, O, Schneede, J, Vollset, SE, Refsum, H. Determinants and vitamin responsiveness of intermediate hyperhomocysteinemia (≥ 40 µmol/liter). *J Clin Invest* 1996; 273: 9987–93.

22. Herbert, V, Zalusky, R. Interrelation of vitamin B_{12} and folic acid metabolism: Folic acid clearance studies. *J Clin Invest* 1962; 41: 1263–76.

23. Jacob, RA, Wu, MM, Henning, SM, Swendseid, ME. Homocysteine increases as folate decreases in plasma of healthy men during short-term dietary folate and methyl group restriction. *J Nutr* 1994; 124: 1072–80.

24. Jacques, PF, Selhub, J, Bostom, AG, Wilson, PW, Rosenberg, IH. The effect of folic acid fortification on plasma folate and total homocysteine concentrations. *N Engl J Med* 1999; 340: 1449–54.

25. Kang, SS, Wong, PWK, Bidani, A, Milanez, S. Plasma protein-bound homocyst(e)ine in patients requiring chronic haemodialysis. *Clin Sci* 1983; 65: 335–36.

26. Kelly, P, McPartlin, J, Goggins, M, Weir, DG, Scott, JM. Unmetabolized folic acid in serum: Acute studies in subjects consuming fortified food and supplements. *Am J Clin Nutr* 1997; 65: 1790–95.

27. Lakshmi, AV, Ramalakshmi, BA. Effect of pyridoxine or riboflavin supplementation on plasma homocysteine levels in women with oral lesions. *Natl Med J India* 1998; 11: 171–72.

28. Landgren, F, Israelsson, B, Lindgren, A, Hultberg, B, Andersson, A, Brattström, L. Plasma homocystcinc in acute myocardial infarction: homocysteine-lowering effect of folic acid. *J Intern Med* 1995; 237: 381–88.

29. Lash, J, Smith, EC. Is folate supplementation necessary in dialysis patients? *Int J Artif Organs* 1990; 13: 785–86.

30. Lindner, A, Charra, B, Sherrard, DJ, Scribner, BH. Accelerated atherosclerosis in prolonged maintenance hemodialysis. *N Engl J Med* 1974; 290: 697–701.

31. Madigan, SM, Tracey, F, McNulty, H, Eaton-Evans, J, Coulter, J, McCartney, H, Strain, JJ. Riboflavin and vitamin B6 intakes and status and biochemical response to riboflavin supplementation in free-living elderly people. *Am J Clin Nutr* 1998; 68: 389–95.

32. Malinow, MR, Duell, PB, Hess, DL, Anderson, PH, Kruger, WD, Phillipson, BE, Gluckman, RA, Block, PC, Upson, BM. Reduction of plasma homocyst(e)ine levels by breakfast cereal fortified with folic acid in patients with coronary heart disease. *N Engl J Med* 1998; 338: 1009–15.

33. Malinow, MR, Nieto, FJ, Kruger, WD, Duell, PB, Hess, DL, Gluckman, RA, Block, PC, Holzgand, CR, Anderson, PH, Seltzer, D, Upson, B, Lin, QR. The effects of folic acid supplementation on plasma total homocysteine are modulated by multivitamin use and methylenetetrahydrofolate reductase genotypes. *Arterioscler Thromb Vasc Biol* 1997; 17: 1157–62.

34. McKeever, MP, Weir, DG, Molloy, A, Scott, JM. Betaine-homocysteine methyltransferase organ distribution in man, pig and rat and subcellular distribution in the rat. *Clin Sci* 1991; 82: 551–56.

35. McKinley, MC, McNulty, H, McPartlin, J, Strain, JJ, Madigan, S, Weir, DG, Scott, JM. Effect of low dose and high dose riboflavin (RBF) supplementation on plasma homocysteine (hcy) levels: A pilot study. *Neth J Med* 1998; 52: S42.

36. Miller, JW, Ribaya-Mercado, JD, Russell, RM, Shepard, DC, Morrow, FD, Cochary, EF, Sadowski, JA, Gershoff, SN, Selhub, J. Effect of vitamin B$_6$ deficiency on fasting plasma homocysteine concentrations. *Am J Clin Nutr* 1992; 55: 1154–60.

37. Molloy, AM, Daly, S, Mills, JL, Kirke, PN, Whitehead, AS, Ramsbottom, D, Conley, M, Weir, DG, Scott, JM. Thermolabile variant of 5,10-methylenetetrahydrofolate reductase associated with low red cell folates: Implications for folate intake recommendations. *Lancet* 1997; 349: 1591–93.

38. Morrow, G III, Barness, L. Combined vitamin responsiveness in homocystinuria. *J Pediatr* 1972; 81: 946–54.

39. Mudd, SH, Levy, HL, Skovby, F. Disorders of transsulfuration. In *The Metabolic Basis of Inherited Diseases,* 6th ed. (Scriver, CR, Beaudet, AL, Sly, WS, Valle, D, eds.). McGraw-Hill, New York, 1989; pp. 693–734.

40. Mudd, SH, Skovby, F, Levy, HL, Pettigrew, KD, Wilcken, B, Pyeritz, RE, Andria, G, Boers, GHJ, Bromberg, IL, Cerone, R, Fowler, B, Grobe, H, Schmidt, H, Schweitzer, L. The natural history of homocystinuria due to cystathionine-β-synthase deficiency. *Am J Hum Genet* 1985; 37: 1–31.

41. Nelen, WLDM, Blom, HJ, Thomas, CMG, Boers, GHJ, Steegers, EAP, Eskes, TKAB. Are the effects of low-dose folic acid on homocysteine (tHcy) and folate concentrations methylenetetrahydrofolate reductase (MTHFR)-genotype related? *Neth J Med* 1998; 52: S28.

42. Nilsson, K, Gustafson, L, Fäldt, R, Andersson, A, Hultberg, B. Plasma homocysteine in relation to serum cobalamin and blood folate in a psychogeriatric population. *Eur J Clin Invest* 1994; 24: 600–6.

43. O'Keefe, CA, Bailey, LB, Thomas, EA, Holfer, SA, Davis, BA, Cerda, JJ, Gregory, JF. Controlled dietary folate affects folate status in nonpregnant women. *J Nutr* 1995; 125: 2717–25.

44. Rasmussen, K, Moller, J, Lyngbak, M, Holm Pedersen, A-M, Dybkjaer, L. Age- and gender-specific reference intervals for total homocysteine and methylmalonic acid in plasma before and after vitamin supplementation. *Clin Chem* 1996; 42: 630–36.

45. Schorah, CJ, Devitt, H, Lucock, M, Dowell, AC. The responsiveness of plasma homocysteine to small increases in dietary folic acid: A primary care study. *Eur J Clin Nutr* 1998; 52: 407–11.

46. Scott, JM, Dinn, JJ, Wilson, P, Weir, DG. Pathogenesis of subacute combined degeneration. A result of methyl group deficiency. *Lancet* 1981; ii: 334–37.

47. Stabler, SP, Marcell, PD, Podell, ER, Allen, RH, Savage, DG, Lindenbaum, J. Elevation of total homocysteine in the serum of patients with cobalamin or folate deficiency detected by capillary gas chromatography-mass spectrometry. *J Clin Invest* 1988; 81: 466–74.

48. Ubbink, JB, van der Merwe, A, Vermaak, WJH, Delport, R. Hyperhomocysteinemia and the response to vitamin supplementation. *Clin Invest* 1993; 71: 993–98.

49. Ubbink, JB, Vermaak, WJH, van der Merwe, A, Becker, PJ, Delport, R, Potgieter, HC. Vitamin requirements for the treatment of hyperhomocysteinemia in humans. *J Nutr* 1994; 124: 1927–33.

50. Ubbink, JB, Vermaak, WJH, van der Merwe, A, Becker, PJ. Vitamin B-6, and folate nutritional status in men with hyperhomocysteinemia. *Am J Clin Nutr* 1993; 57: 47–53.

51. van den Berg, M, Boers, GHJ, Franken, DG, Blom, HJ, van Kamp, GT, Jacobs, C, Rauwerda JA, Kluft, C, Stehouwer, CDA. Hyperhomocystenemia and endothelial dysfunction in young patients with peripheral arterial occlusion disease. *Eur J Clin Invest* 1995; 25: 176–81.

52. van den Berg, M, Franken, DG, Boers, GHJ, Blom, HJ, Jacobs, C, Stehouwer, CDA, Rauwerda, JA. Combined vitamin B6 plus folic acid therapy in young patients with arteriosclerosis and hyperhomocysteinemia. *J Vasc Surg* 1994; 20: 933–40.

53. Wald, NJ, Watt, HC, Law, MR, Weir, DG, McPartlin, J, Scott, JM. Homocysteine and ischemic heart disease: Results of a prospective study with implications on prevention. *Arch Intern Med* 1998; 158: 862–67.

54. Ward, M, McNulty, H, McPartlin, J, Strain, JJ, Weir, DG, Scott, JM. Plasma homocysteine, a risk factor for cardiovascular disease, is lowered by physiological doses of folic acid. *Q J Med* 1997; 90: 519–24.

55. Weir, DG, Scott, JM. The biochemical basis of the neuropathy in cobalamin deficiency. In *Bailliere's Clinical Haematology,* Vol. 8 (Wickramasinghe, SM, ed.). Bailliere Tindall, London, 1995; pp. 479–97.

56. Wilcken, B, Turner, B. Homocystinuria:reduced folate levels during pyridoxine treatment. *Arch Dis Child* 1973; 48: 58–62.

57. Wilcken, DEL, Dudman, NPB, Tyrell, PA. Homocystinuria due to cystathionine β-synthase deficiency: The effects of betaine treatment in pyridoxine-responsive patients. *Metabolism* 1985; 34: 115–21.

58. Wilcken, DEL, Gupta, VJ, Betts, AK. Homocysteine in the plasma of renal transplant recipients: Effects of cofactors for methionine metabolism. *Clin Sci* 1981; 61: 743–49.

59. Wilcken, DEL, Gupta, VJ, Reddy, SG. Accumulation of sulphur-containing amino acids including cysteine-homocysteine in patients on maintenance haemodialysis. *Clin Sci* 1980; 58: 427–30.

60. Wilcken, DEL, Gupta, VJ. Sulphur-containing amino acids in chronic renal failure with particular reference to homocysteine and cysteine-homocysteine mixed disulphide. *Eur J Clin Invest* 1979; 9: 301–7.

39

Design of Clinical Trials to Test the Homocysteine Hypothesis of Vascular Disease

ROBERT CLARKE

Moderately elevated levels of blood total homocysteine have been identified as a potentially important modifiable risk factor for cardiovascular disease (6). Many studies conducted in various settings have reported that patients with coronary heart disease (1, 2, 4, 16, 18, 20, 22, 23, 27–29, 31, 35, 48, 56–59), stroke (7, 10, 17, 26, 36, 37, 55), and peripheral vascular disease (3, 9, 30, 32, 50, 54) have higher homocysteine levels than control subjects. The initial studies were case-control (or retrospective) studies that compared homocysteine levels in samples from cases, collected after the onset of disease, with those in control cases. Weaker associations have been reported in some prospective studies in which blood was taken some years before vascular disease was diagnosed (2, 48, 59), and no association was reported in others (1, 16). In an updated meta-analysis of the published epidemiological studies of homocysteine and coronary heart disease, it was estimated that the odds ratio of coronary heart disease for a 5 μmol/L higher blood total homocysteine level was 1.3 (95% confidence interval, 1.1–1.5) in prospective studies, 1.6 (95% confidence interval, 1.4–1.7) in retrospective studies with population control subjects, and 1.9 (95% confidence interval, 1.6–2.3) in retrospective studies with other control subjects (13). In addition, elevated homocysteine levels have been associated with an increased risk

of mortality among patients with established coronary disease (34).

It is unclear to what extent the discrepant results of different study designs are a result of random error, bias (resulting from the effects of illness on blood homocysteine levels), or incomplete adjustment for confounding factors (such as blood pressure, smoking, and cholesterol). Furthermore, substantial uncertainty persists about the strength of the relationship between homocysteine and vascular disease in age- and sex-specific groups, and about the graded nature of increasing risk with increasing homocysteine levels across the distribution found in the general population. This has prompted a meta-analysis of individual participant data from all the observational studies to address these issues.

Clinical trials in which patients are allocated randomly to either homocysteine-lowering therapy or placebo are not constrained by bias or confounding factors that limit the interpretation of observational epidemiology. Because blood homocysteine levels are easily reduced by folic acid treatment, there have been many calls for clinical trials to determine whether vitamin supplements to lower blood homocysteine levels could reduce the risk of vascular disease (19, 49). However, clinical trials of these vitamin supplements need to be large, to be performed in populations at high risk of events, and to include an adequate dose and duration of therapy, in order to detect small but worthwhile differences in risk. This review examines the evidence available for the proportional and absolute reductions in homocysteine levels that might be expected from dietary supplementation with folic acid, cobalamin, and vitamin B_6 and considers the issues involved in the design of large-scale clinical trials to test this hypothesis.

Effects of Vitamin Supplements on Blood Homocysteine Levels

Until recently, there was substantial uncertainty about the proportional and absolute reductions in blood total homocysteine levels that could be achieved by varying doses of folic acid or other B vitamins, partly because the nonrandomized studies were unreliable and partly because the previous randomized trials of vitamin supplements were either too small or were carried out in unrepresentative populations.

A meta-analysis of 12 randomized trials (21) involving individual data from 1,114 participants was carried out to address these issues. There was substantial heterogeneity in the blood concentrations of homocysteine and the reductions in absolute levels achieved in the individual trials (Table 39.1) (11, 14,

Table 39.1.   Blood Concentrations of Homocysteine in the Individual Trials

Author of Primary Report (Ref.)	Treatment Comparisons with Doses of Vitamins (mg)	N	Mean Homocysteine (µmol/L)			
			Pre-treat.	Post-treat.	Difference (& SD)	Ratio (& SD) of Post: Pre-treat. Homocysteine
Landgren et al. (24)	C	20	14.5	15.1	0.6 (1.2)	1.0 (0.1)
	2.5 F	16	16.9	12.0	–4.9 (3.9)	0.7 (0.2)
	10 F	17	15.8	11.3	–4.5 (3.5)	0.7 (0.1)
den Heijer et al. I (14)	P	27	18.9	17.8	–1.1 (5.6)	1.0 (0.2)
	5 F, 0.4 B$_{12}$, 50 B$_6$	25	18.7	11.3	–7.0 (7.0)	0.7 (0.2)
den Heijer et al. II (14)	P	36	11.9	11.4	–0.6 (2.7)	1.0 (0.2)
	0.5 F	36	12.4	9.7	–2.8 (2.4)	0.8 (0.2)
	5 F	35	12.1	8.9	–3.2 (2.2)	0.8 (0.1)
	0.4 B$_{12}$	36	12.6	11.3	–1.3 (2.0)	0.9 (0.2)
	5 F, 0.4 B$_{12}$, 50 B$_6$	35	12.1	8.3	–3.8 (3.9)	0.7 (0.2)
den Heijer et al. III (14)	P	46	14.0	14.5	0.5 (5.6)	1.0 (0.4)
	5 F, 0.4 B$_{12}$, 50 B$_6$	46	15.9	10.3	–5.7 (9.7)	0.7 (0.2)
Ubbink et al. I (53)	P	17	30.0	30.7	–0.7 (9.1)	1.0 (0.3)
	0.6 F	19	28.4	16.8	–11.6 (6.2)	0.6 (0.2)
	10 B$_6$	17	28.2	27.9	–0.3 (9.6)	1.0 (0.4)
	0.4 B$_{12}$	18	30.6	26.0	–4.6 (9.1)	0.9 (0.3)
	0.6 F, 0.4 B$_{12}$, 10 B$_6$	20	26.9	13.6	–13.3 (7.3)	0.5 (0.2)
Ubbink et al. II (51)	P	13	23.5	22.1	–1.4 (4.8)	1.0 (0.2)
	1 F, 0.4 B$_{12}$, 10 B$_6$	13	29.3	11.5	–17.8 (13.8)	0.5 (0.2)
Naurath et al. (33)	P	142	13.9	13.4	–0.5 (2.7)	1.0 (0.2)
	1.1 F, 1 B$_{12}$, 5 B$_6$	143	12.7	8.4	–4.4 (3.5)	0.7 (0.2)
Pietrzik, I (cited in 15)	P	37	8.1	8.7	0.6 (1.2)	1.1 (0.1)
	0.4 F, 0.1 B$_{12}$, 2 B$_6$	33	7.2	5.8	–1.4 (1.3)	0.8 (0.2)
Pietrzik, II (cited in 15)	P	86	8.1	8.2	0.2 (1.4)	1.0 (0.2)
	0.4 F, 2 B$_6$	42	7.8	6.6	–1.2 (1.2)	0.9 (0.1)
Woodside et al. (60)	P	55	9.9	9.0	–0.9 (1.8)	0.9 (0.2)
	1 F, 0.02 B$_{12}$, 7.2 B$_6$	57	11.9	7.8	–4.3 (3.4)	0.7 (0.1)
Cuskelly et al. (11)	C	8	7.0	6.7	–0.2 (0.7)	1.1 (0.1)
	0.4 F	9	5.8	5.0	–0.8 (1.0)	0.9 (0.2)
Saltzman et al. (42)	P	5	11.5	12.2	0.7 (1.5)	1.1 (0.1)
	2 F	5	19.6	15.0	–4.6 (3.5)	0.8 (0.1)

F, folic acid; B$_{12}$, cobalamin (vitamin B$_{12}$); B$_6$, vitamin B$_6$; C, untreated open control; P, placebo control group; SD, standard deviation.

15, 24, 25, 33, 42, 43, 47, 51, 53, 60). The proportional and absolute reductions in blood homocysteine produced by folic acid supplements were greater at higher pretreatment blood homocysteine levels and at lower pretreatment blood folate levels (Figure 39.1). After standardizing pretreatment blood levels of homocysteine to 12 µmol/L and folate levels to 12 nmol/L (i.e., approximate average levels for Western populations prior to the introduction of folate fortification), there was no longer any heterogeneity in the proportional reductions in homocysteine levels achieved in the individual trials (Figure 39.2). Under these circumstances, the meta-analysis estimated that dietary supplementation with folic acid reduced blood homocysteine levels by 25% (95% confidence inter-val, 23–28), with similar effects in the range of 0.5 to 5 mg/day folic acid. Cobalamin (mean dose, 0.5 mg/day) produced an additional 7% (95% confidence interval, 3–10) reduction in blood homocysteine, whereas vitamin B$_6$ (mean dose, 16.5 mg/day) had no additional effects on fasting or basal homocysteine levels.

Hence, the meta-analysis suggested that in typical Western populations, daily supplementation with both 0.5 to 5 mg folic acid and about 0.5 mg cobalamin would be expected to reduce blood homocysteine levels by about one fourth to one third (21). Studies in most Western populations prior to the introduction of folate fortification indicate that the average concentration of blood homocysteine is about 12 µmol/L, and so a reduction of about one fourth to one third might corre-

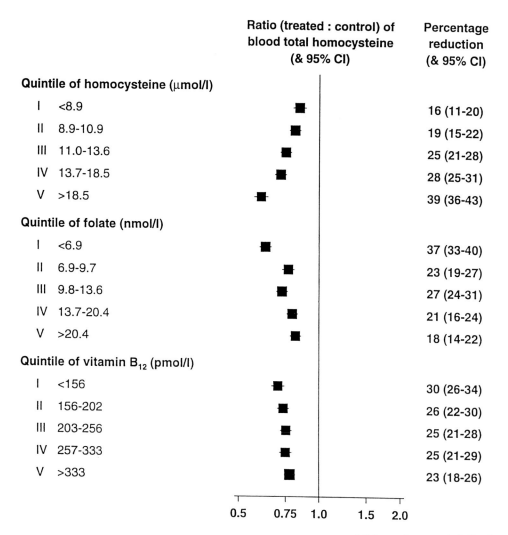

Ratio (treated : control) of blood total homocysteine (& 95% CI)

Percentage reduction (& 95% CI)

Quintile of homocysteine (μmol/l)

I	<8.9	16 (11-20)
II	8.9-10.9	19 (15-22)
III	11.0-13.6	25 (21-28)
IV	13.7-18.5	28 (25-31)
V	>18.5	39 (36-43)

Quintile of folate (nmol/l)

I	<6.9	37 (33-40)
II	6.9-9.7	23 (19-27)
III	9.8-13.6	27 (24-31)
IV	13.7-20.4	21 (16-24)
V	>20.4	18 (14-22)

Quintile of vitamin B$_{12}$ (pmol/l)

I	<156	30 (26-34)
II	156-202	26 (22-30)
III	203-256	25 (21-28)
IV	257-333	25 (21-29)
V	>333	23 (18-26)

0.5   0.75   1.0   1.5   2.0

Fig. 39.1. Reductions in blood homocysteine concentrations with folic acid supplements according to pretreatment blood concentrations of homocysteine, folate, and cobalamin (vitamin B$_{12}$). Squares indicate the ratios of post-treatment blood homocysteine concentrations among subjects allocated folic acid to those of control subjects. The size of each square is proportional to the number of individuals studied, and the horizontal line through the square indicates the 95% confidence interval (CI) for the ratio. (Reproduced from Homocysteine Lowering Trialists Collaboration [21], with permission.)

spond to an absolute reduction of about 3 to 4 μmol/L (e.g., from about 12 μmol/L to about 8 to 9 μmol/L).

Assessment of the Independent Effects of Folic Acid and of Vitamin B$_6$ Supplements

Among the vitamins studied, folic acid has had the dominant homocysteine-lowering effect, with the addition of cobalamin to folic acid having only a small additional homocysteine-lowering effect. Because cobalamin deficiency is common in elderly people and is not always detected by the standard screening tests, however, the addition of an oral daily dose of 1 mg cobalamin may simplify treatment regimens by avoiding the theoretical risk of neuropathy resulting from unopposed folic acid therapy in cobalamin-deficient patients (even those with intrinsic factor deficiency or malabsorption states) (8, 25, 43, 47). By contrast, vitamin B$_6$ did not appear to have any significant effect on fasting homocysteine levels. However, these trials did not assess the effects of homocysteine lowering after methionine loading, where post-load homocysteine concentrations are influenced by vitamin B$_6$ (5). Because vitamin B$_6$ levels are associated with cardiovascular risk, independent of their association with homocysteine levels, maximum reduction in risk may be achieved with the optimum intake of both vitamins (38–40). In view of the independent effects of folic acid and vitamin B$_6$ in observational epidemiology, clinical trials with factorial designs—in which participants are randomly allocated to receive either folic acid (probably with cobalamin) or placebo, and are separately randomized to receive either vitamin B$_6$ or placebo—would allow assessment of the separate and combined effects of both vitamins, without materially increasing the required number of patients.

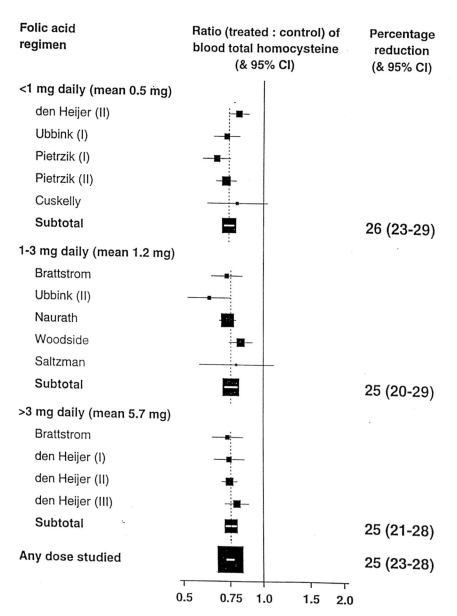

Folic acid regimen	Ratio (treated : control) of blood total homocysteine (& 95% CI)	Percentage reduction (& 95% CI)
<1 mg daily (mean 0.5 mg)		
den Heijer (II)		
Ubbink (I)		
Pietrzik (I)		
Pietrzik (II)		
Cuskelly		
Subtotal		26 (23–29)
1–3 mg daily (mean 1.2 mg)		
Brattstrom		
Ubbink (II)		
Naurath		
Woodside		
Saltzman		
Subtotal		25 (20–29)
>3 mg daily (mean 5.7 mg)		
Brattstrom		
den Heijer (I)		
den Heijer (II)		
den Heijer (III)		
Subtotal		25 (21–28)
Any dose studied		25 (23–28)

0.5   0.75   1.0   1.5   2.0

Fig. 39.2. Predicted proportional reductions (%) in blood homocysteine levels with folic acid supplementation (0.5 to 5 mg/day) after standardization for a pretreatment folate level of 12 nmol/L and a homocysteine level of 12 μmol/L. The squares indicate the ratios of post-treatment blood homocysteine among individuals receiving folic acid supplements to control individuals. The size of each square is proportional to the number of individuals studied, and the horizontal line through the square indicates the 95% confidence interval (CI) for the ratio. (Reproduced from Homocysteine Lowering Trialists Collaboration [21], with permission.)

Target Population, Sample Size, and Predicted Number of Events

The meta-analysis of the published epidemiological studies of homocysteine and coronary heart disease sug-

gests that a prolonged absolute difference of 3 to 4 μmol/L in usual blood total homocysteine levels may be associated with about 30% less coronary heart disease (13). If, as seems to be the case with total cholesterol (41, 44, 46), about half of the epidemiologically predicted reduction is achieved within a few years, an absolute difference of 3 to 4 μmol/L in usual blood homocysteine levels may be associated with about 10% to 15% less coronary heart disease. Reliable demonstration that dietary supplementation with folic acid and/or other B vitamins produced such reductions in the risk of vascular disease would be of substantial public health importance. This demonstration is likely to require large-scale clinical trials conducted in high-risk populations that adopt regimens and procedures that maximize the difference in homocysteine levels between the treatment groups for an adequate duration.

Ongoing or Planned Trials of Homocysteine-Lowering Therapy

Current and planned large-scale trials to assess the effects of vitamin supplements on risk of vascular disease should provide randomized evidence for the effects of these vitamins on risk of vascular disease in about 40,000 patients with prior coronary heart disease. Details of the target populations, sample trial size, and treatment regimens in these studies are shown in Table 39.2. All of the trials aim to compare the effects of folic acid and no supplement in populations at high risk of vascular disease, but some will also assess cobalamin and vitamin B_6. Although combined therapy with folic acid and vitamin B_6 might be expected to produce a greater reduction in vascular risk than folic acid, trials of combined therapy would be unable to distinguish the relative importance of either vitamin on its own.

Two US trials and a Canadian trial plan to compare a multivitamin combination of folic acid, cobalamin, and vitamin B_6 administered together versus placebo. Two Norwegian trials, the Western Norway B-Vitamin Trial (WENBIT) and the Norwegian Study of Homocysteine Lowering with B-Vitamins in Myocardial Infarction (NORVIT), using identical treatment regimens in different clinical settings will assess the independent effects on cardiovascular risk of folic acid and vitamin B_6 separately by using a 2×2 factorial design. The United Kingdom-based Study of the Effectiveness of Additional Reductions in Cholesterol and Homocysteine (SEARCH) is a 2×2 factorial design trial that will assess the effects of blood homocysteine reductions with folic acid (2 mg) and cobalamin (1 mg) versus placebo, and of standard versus larger cholesterol reductions with "statin" therapy (80 mg vs. 20 mg/day of simvastatin) in 12,000 patients with a history of a prior myocardial infarction.

The results of the Australian Prevention with a Combined Inhibitor and Folate in Coronary Heart Disease pilot trial (PACIFIC) should be particularly informative, as the lower dose of folic acid (0.2 mg) approximates the upper limit of what could be achieved through dietary folate or food fortification. If the magnitude of the homocysteine reduction achieved with the lower dose is equivalent to that with the higher dose, the organizers plan to adopt this regimen in a trial of 10,000 such patients.

Observational studies cannot exclude the influence of confounding due to other dietary or nondietary factors, and this influence could explain much of the

Table 39.2. Ongoing and Planned Large-Scale Clinical Trials to Address the Effect of Homocysteine-Lowering Vitamin Supplements on Vascular Risk

Study	Sample Size	Homocysteine-Lowering Regimen
Vitamin Intervention for Stroke Prevention (VISP), Wake Forest University, US	3,600	Folic acid (2.5 mg) + B-6 (25 mg) + B-12 (0.4 mg) vs. Folic acid (0.02 mg) + B-6 (0.2 mg) + B-12 (0.006 mg)
Women's Antioxidant and Cardiovascular Disease Study (WACS), Harvard Medical School, US	6,000–8,000	Folic acid (2.5 mg) + B-6 (50 mg) + B-12 (1 mg) vs. placebo
Study of the Effectiveness of Additional Reductions in Cholesterol and Homocysteine (SEARCH), University of Oxford, England	12,000	Folic acid (2 mg) + B-12 (1 mg) vs. placebo in a 2×2 factorial design with Simvastatin (80 mg vs. 20 mg)
Cambridge Heart Antioxidant Study (CHAOS-2), University of Cambridge, England	4,000	Folic acid (5 mg) vs. placebo
Norwegian Study of Homocysteine Lowering with B-vitamins in Myocardial Infarction (NORVIT), University of Tromsø, Norway	3,000	Folic acid (5 mg × 2 weeks + 0.8 mg) + B-12 (0.4 mg) vs. placebo in a 2×2 factorial design with B-6 (40 mg) vs. placebo
Western Norway B vitamin Trial (WENBIT), University of Bergen, Norway	2,000	Folic acid (5 mg × 2 weeks + 0.8 mg) + B-12 (0.4 mg) vs. placebo in a 2×2 factorial design trial with B-6 (40 mg) vs. placebo
Prevention with A Combined Inhibitor and Folate in Coronary heart disease (PACIFIC), University of Sydney, Australia	10,000	Folic acid (0.2 mg or 2 mg) vs. placebo in a 2×2 factorial trial with Omapatrilat. (Doses to be chosen after results of the pilot study.)
Heart Outcomes Prevention Evaluation-2 Study (HOPE-2), McMaster University, Canada	5,000	Folic acid (2.5 mg) + B-12 (1 mg) + B-6 (50 mg) vs. placebo

B-12, cobalamin (vitamin B_{12}).

moderate relative differences observed in such studies. Long-term, large-scale clinical trials of such vitamins in appropriate populations are required to address these questions. All of these large-scale trials will be carried out in patients with prior vascular disease or other factors that make them at high risk for such events. The individual trials differ somewhat in the choice of vitamin regimens adopted for lowering blood homocysteine levels, but all of the trials have adopted similar endpoints, which should enable the principal investigators to combine data from each study in a collaborative overview of their separate results.

Such a meta-analysis of all trials of folic acid-based therapy would provide randomized evidence of any benefits (or hazards) of lowering homocysteine levels in about 40,000 patients with coronary heart disease and several thousand patients with prior cerebrovascular disease. It could compare the relative importance of folic acid and vitamin B_6 on vascular risk, as well as provide reliable evidence of the effects of these vitamins in age-specific subgroups, in different disease categories, and across a wide range of blood homocysteine levels. These trials will provide the necessary evidence to guide policy on the use of screening for homocysteine levels, advocating the use of vitamin supplements in high-risk individuals, or changing the population mean levels of folate (by fortification of flour) for the prevention of cardiovascular diseases. The introduction of folate fortification of all cereal grain products in the United States during the course of trials conducted in that population will affect the statistical power of such trials to test the hypothesis that homocysteine lowering will reduce the risk of cardiovascular disease. This fact reinforces the need to assess the totality of evidence on this hypothesis in a meta-analysis of all such randomized trials in due course.

REFERENCES

1. Alfthan, G, Pekkanen, J, Jauhiainen, M, Pitkaniemi, J, Karvonen, M, Tuomilehto, J, Salonen, JT, Ehnholm, C. Relation of serum homocysteine and lipoprotein(a) concentrations to atherosclerotic disease in a prospective Finnish population based study. *Atherosclerosis* 1994; 106: 9–19.
2. Arnesen, E, Refsum, H, Bonaa, KH, Ueland, PM, Forde, OH, Nordrehaug, JE. Serum total homocysteine and coronary heart disease. *Int J Epidemiol* 1995; 24: 704–9.
3. Bergmark, C, Mansoor, MA, Swedenborg, J, deFaire, U, Svardal, AM, Ueland, PM. Hyperhomocyst(e)inemia in patients operated for lower extremity ischaemia below the age of 50-effect of smoking and extent of disease. *Eur J Vasc Surg* 1993; 7: 391–96.
4. Blacher, J, Montalescot, G, Ankri, A, Chadefaux-Vekemans, B, Benzidia, R, Grosgogeat, Y, Kamoun, P, Thomas, D. [Hyperhomocysteinemia in coronary artery diseases.

Apropos of a study on 102 patients]. *Arch Mal Coeur Vaiss* 1996; 89: 1241–46.
5. Bostom, AG, Jacques, PF, Nadeau, MR, Williams, RR, Elliston, RC, Selhub, J. Postmethionine load hyperhomocysteinemia in persons with normal fasting total plasma homocysteine: Initial results from the NHLBI Family Heart Study. *Atherosclerosis* 1995; 116: 147–51.
6. Boushey, C, Beresford, SAA, Omenn, GS, Motulsky, AG. A quantitative assessment of plasma homocysteine as a risk factor for vascular disease: Probable benefits of increasing folic acid intakes. *JAMA* 1995; 274: 1049–57.
7. Brattström, L, Israelsson, B, Norrving, B, Bergquist, D, Thorne, J, Hultberg, B, Hamfelt, A. Impaired homocysteine metabolism in early-onset cerebral and peripheral occlusive arterial disease. Effects of pyridoxine and folic acid treatment. *Atherosclerosis* 1990; 81: 51–60.
8. Cambell, NRC. How safe are folic acid supplements? *Arch Intern Med* 1996; 156: 1638–44.
9. Cheng, SW, Ting, AC, Wong, J. Fasting total plasma homocysteine and atherosclerotic peripheral vascular disease. *Ann Vasc Surg* 1997; 11: 217–23.
10. Coull, BM, Malinow, MR, Beamer, N, Sexton, G, Nordt, F, deGarmo, P. Elevated plasma homocyst(e)ine concentration as a possible independent risk factor for stroke. *Stroke* 1990; 21: 572–76.
11. Cuskelly, G, McNulty, W, McPartlin, J, Strain, JJ, Scott, JM. Plasma homocysteine response to folate intervention in young women. *Ir J Med Sci* 1995; 164: 3.
12. Dalery, K, Lussier Cacan, S, Selhub, J, Davignon, J, Latour, Y, Genest, J Jr. Homocysteine and coronary artery disease in French Canadian subjects: Relation with vitamins B12, B6, pyridoxal phosphate, and folate. *Am J Cardiol* 1995; 75: 1107–11.
13. Danesh, J, Lewington, S. Plasma homocysteine and coronary heart disease: Systematic review of published epidemiological studies. *J Cardiovasc Risk* 1998; 5: 229–32.
14. den Heijer, M, Brouwer, IA, Bos, GMJ, Blom, HJ, Spaans, AP, Rosendaal, FR, Thomas, CMG, Haak, HL, Wijermans, PW, Gerrits, WBJ. Vitamin supplementation reduces blood homocysteine levels: A controlled trial in patients with venous thrombosis and healthy volunteers. *Arterioscler Thromb Vasc Biol* 1998; 18: 356–61.
15. Dierkes, J. Vitamin requirements for the reduction of homocysteine blood levels in healthy young women. PhD thesis, University of Bonn, 1995.
16. Evans, RW, Shaten, BJ, Hempel, JD, Cutler, JA, Kuller, LH. Homocyst(e)ine and risk of cardiovascular disease in the Multiple Risk Factor Intervention Trial. *Arterioscler Thromb Vasc Biol* 1997; 17: 1947–53.
17. Evers, S, Koch, HG, Grotemeyer, KH, Lange, B, Deufel, T, Ringelstein, EB. Features, symptoms, and neurophysiological findings in stroke associated with hyperhomocysteinemia. *Arch Neurol* 1997; 54: 1276–82.
18. Genest, JJ Jr, McNamara, JR, Salem, DN, Wilson, PW, Schaefer, EJ, Malinow, MR. Plasma homocyst(e)ine levels in men with premature coronary artery disease. Impaired homocysteine metabolism in early-onset cerebral and peripheral occlusive arterial disease. *J Am Coll Cardiol* 1990; 16: 1114–19.

19. Graham, I, Meleady, R. Heart attacks and homocysteine. *Br Med J* 1996; 313: 1419–20.

20. Graham, IM, Daly, LE, Refsum, HM, Robinson, K, Brattström, LE, Ueland, PM, Palma-Reis, RJ, Boers, GH, Sheahan, RG, Israelsson, B, Uiterwaal, CS, Meleady, R, McMaster, D, Verhoef, P, Witteman, J, Rubba, P, Bellet, H, Wautrecht, JC, de Valk, HW, Sales Luis, AC, Parrot-Rouland, FM, Tan, KS, Higgins, I, Garçon, D, Medrano, MJ, Candito, M, Evans, AE, Andria, G. Plasma homocysteine as a risk factor for vascular disease: The European Concerted Action Project. *JAMA* 1997; 277: 1775–81.

21. Homocysteine Lowering Trialists' Collaboration. Lowering blood homocysteine with folic acid based supplements: Meta-analysis of randomised trials. *Br Med J* 1998; 316: 894–98.

22. Hopkins, PN, Wu, LL, Wu, J, Hunt, SC, James, BC, Vincent, GM, Williams, RR. Higher plasma homocyst(e)ine and increased susceptibility to adverse effects of low folate in early familial coronary artery disease. *Arterioscler Thromb Vasc Biol* 1995; 15: 1314–20.

23. Israelsson, B, Brattström, LE, Hultberg, BL. Homocysteine and myocardial infarction. *Atherosclerosis* 1988; 71: 227–33.

24. Landgren, F, Israelsson, B, Lindgren, A, Hultberg, B, Andersson, A, Brattström, L. Plasma homocysteine in acute myocardial infarction: homocysteine-lowering effect of folic acid. *J Intern Med* 1995; 237: 381–88.

25. Lindenbaum, J, Healton, EB, Savage, DG, Brust, JCM, Garrett, TJ, Podell, ER, Marcell, PD, Stabler, SP, Allen, RH. Neuropsychiatric disorders caused by cobalamin deficiency in the absence of anemia or macrocytosis. *N Engl J Med* 1988; 318: 1720–28.

26. Lindgren, A, Brattström, L, Norrving, B, Hultberg, B, Andersson, A, Johansson, BB. Plasma homocysteine in the acute and convalescent phases after stroke. *Stroke* 1995; 26: 795–800.

27. Loehrer, FM, Angst, CP, Haefeli, WE, Jordan, PP, Ritz, R, Fowler, B. Low whole-blood *S*-adenosylmethionine and correlation between 5-methyltetrahydrofolate and homocysteine in coronary artery disease. *Arterioscler Thromb Vasc Biol* 1996; 16: 727–33.

28. Lolin, YI, Sanderson, JE, Cheng, SK, Chan, CF, Pang, CP, Woo, KS, Masarei, JR. Hyperhomocysteinaemia and premature coronary artery disease in the Chinese. *Heart* 1996; 76: 117–22.

29. Malinow, MR, Ducimetiere, P, Luc, G, Evans, AE, Arvelier, D, Cambien, F, Upson, BM. Plasma homocyst(e)ine levels and graded risk for myocardial infarction: Findings in two populations at contrasting risk for coronary heart disease. *Atherosclerosis* 1996; 126: 27–34.

30. Malinow, MR, Kang, SS, Taylor, LM, Coull, B, Inahara, T, Mukerjee, D, Sexton, G, Upson, B. Prevalence of hyperhomocyst(e)inemia in patients with peripheral occlusive disease. *Circulation* 1989; 79: 1180–88.

31. Malinow, MR, Sexton, G, Auerbach, M, Grossman, M, Wilson, D, Upson, B. Homocyst(e)inemia in daily practice. *Coron Artery Dis* 1990; 1: 215–20.

32. Molgaard, J, Malinow, MR, Lassvik, C, Holm, AC, Upson, B, Olsson, AG. Hyperhomocyst(e)inemia: An independent risk factor for intermittent claudication. *J Intern Med* 1992; 231: 273–79.

33. Naurath, HJ, Joosten, E, Riezler, R, Stabler, SP, Allen, RH, Lindenbaum, J. Effects of vitamin B_{12}, folate, and vitamin B_6 supplements in elderly people with normal serum vitamin concentrations. *Lancet* 1995; 346: 85–9.

34. Nygård, O, Nordrehaug, JE, Refsum, H, Ueland, PM, Farstad, M, Vollset, SE. Plasma homocysteine levels and mortality in patients with coronary artery disease. *N Engl J Med* 1997; 337: 230–36.

35. Pancharuniti, N, Lewis, CA, Sauberlich, HE, Perkins, LL, Go, RC, Alvarez, JO, Macaluso, M, Acton, RT, Copeland, RB, Cousins, AL, Gore, TB, Corwell, PE, Roseman, JM. Plasma homocyst(e)ine, folate, and vitamin B-12 concentrations and risk for early-onset coronary artery disease. *Am J Clin Nutr* 1994; 59: 940–48.

36. Perry, IJ, Refsum, H, Morris, RW, Ebrahim, SB, Ueland, PM, Shaper, AG. Prospective study of serum total homocysteine and risk of stroke in middle-aged British men. *Lancet* 1995; 346: 1395–98.

37. Petri, M, Roubenoff, R, Dallal, GE, Nadeau, MR, Selhub, J, Rosenberg, IH. Plasma homocysteine as a risk factor for atherothrombotic events in systemic lupus erythematosus. *Lancet* 1996; 348: 1120–24.

38. Rimm, EB, Willett, WC, Hu, FB, Sampson, L, Colditz, GA, Manson, JE, Hennekens, C, Stampfer, MJ. Folate and vitamin B-6 from diet and supplements in relation to risk of coronary heart disease among women. *JAMA* 1998; 279: 359–64.

39. Robinson, K, Arheart, K, Refsum, H, Brattström, L, Boers, G, Ueland, P, Rubba, P, Palma-Reis, R, Meleady, R, Daly, L, Witteman, J, Graham, I. Low circulating folate and vitamin B6 concentrations: Risk factors for stroke, peripheral vascular disease, and coronary artery disease. *Circulation* 1998; 97: 437–43.

40. Robinson, K, Mayer, EL, Miller, DP, Green, R, van Lente, F, Gupta, A, Kotte-Marchant, K, Savan, SR, Selhub, J, Nissen, SE, Kutner, M, Topol, EJ, Jacobsen, DW. Hyperhomocysteinemia and low pyridoxal phosphate. Common and independent reversible risk factors for coronary artery disease. *Circulation* 1995; 92: 2825–30.

41. Sacks, FM, Pfeffer, MA, Moye, LA, Rouleau, JL, Rutherford, JD, Cole, TG, Brown, L, Warnica, W, Arnold, JM, Wun, CC, Davis, BR, Braunwald, E, for the Cholesterol and Recurrent Events Trials Investigators. The effects of pravastatin on coronary events after myocardial infarction in patients with average cholesterol levels. *N Engl J Med* 1996; 335: 1001–9.

42. Saltzman, E, Mason, JB, Jacques, PF, Selhub, J, Salem, D, Schaefer, EJ, Tursissini, C, Berdich, A, Rosenberg, IH. B vitamin supplementation lowers homocysteine levels in heart disease. *Clin Res* 1994; 42: 172A.

43. Savage, DG, Lindenbaum, J. Folate-cobalamin interactions. In *Folate in Health and Disease.* (Bailey, LB ed.). Marcel Dekker Inc, New York, 1995; pp. 237–85.

44. Scandinavian Simvastatin Survival Study Group. Randomised trial of cholesterol lowering in 4,444 patients with coronary heart disease: The Scandinavian Simvastatin Study (4S). *Lancet* 1994; 344: 1383–89.

45. Schwartz, SM, Siscovick, DS, Malinow, MR, Rosendaal, FR, Beverly, RK, Hess, DL, Psaty, BM, Longstreth, WT Jr, Koepsell, TD, Raghunathan, TE, Reitsma, PH. Myocardial infarction in young women in relation to plasma total homocysteine, folate, and a common variant in the methyl-enetetrahydrofolate reductase gene. *Circulation* 1997; 96: 412–17.

46. Shepherd, J, Cobbe, SM, Ford, I, Isles, CG, Lorimer, AR, Macfarlane, PW, McKillop, JH, Packard, CJ, for the West of Scotland Coronary Prevention Study Group. Prevention of coronary heart disease with pravastatin in men with hypercholesterolemia. *N Engl J Med* 1995; 333: 1301–7.

47. Stabler, SP, Allen, RH, Savage, DG, Lindenbaum, J. Clinical spectrum and diagnosis of cobalamin deficiency. *Blood* 1990; 76: 871–81.

48. Stampfer, MJ, Malinow, MR, Willett, WC, Newcomer, LM, Upson, B, Ullmann, D, Tishler, PV, Hennekens, CH. A prospective study of plasma homocyst(e)ine and risk of myocardial infarction in US physicians. *JAMA* 1992; 268: 877–81.

49. Stampfer, MJ, Malinow, MR, Can homocysteine lowering reduce cardiovascular risk? *N Engl J Med* 1995; 332: 328–29.

50. Taylor, LM, DeFrang, RD, Harris, EJ, Porter, JM. The association of elevated plasma homocysteine with progression of peripheral vascular disease. *J Vasc Surg* 1991; 13: 129–36.

51. Ubbink, JB, van der Merwe, A, Vermaak, WJH, Delport, R. Hyperhomocysteinemia and the response to vitamin supplementation. *Clin Invest* 1993; 71: 993–98.

52. Ubbink, JB, Vermaak, WJH, Bennett, PJ, van Staden, DA, Bisbort, S. The prevalence of hyperhomocysteinaemia and hypercholesterolaemia in angiographically defined coronary heart disease. *Klin Wochenschr* 1991; 69: 527–34.

53. Ubbink, JB, Vermaak, WJH, van der Merwe, A, Becker, PJ, Delport, R, Potgieter, HC. Vitamin requirements for the treatment of hyperhomocysteinemia in humans. *J Nutr* 1994; 124: 1927–33.

54. Valentine, RJ, Kaplan, HS, Green, R, Jacobsen, DW, Myers, SI, Clagett, GP. Lipoprotein(a), homocysteine and hypercoagulable states in young men with premature peripheral atherosclerosis: A prospective controlled analysis. *J Vasc Surg* 1996; 23: 53–61.

55. Verhoef, P, Hennekens, CH, Malinow, MR, Kok, FJ, Willett, WC, Stampfer, MJ. A prospective study of plasma homocyst(e)ine and risk of ischemic stroke. *Stroke* 1994; 10: 1924–30.

56. Verhoef, P, Kok, FJ, Kruyssen, DA, Schouten, EG, Witteman, JC, Grobbee, DE, Ueland, PM, Refsum, H. Plasma total homocysteine, B vitamins, and risk of coronary atherosclerosis. *Arterioscler Thromb Vasc Biol* 1997; 17: 989–95.

57. Verhoef, P, Stampfer, MJ, Buring, JE, Gaziano, JM, Allen, RH, Stabler, SP, Reynolds, RD, Hennekens, CH, Willett, WC. Homocysteine metabolism and risk of myocardial infarction: Relation with vitamins B-6, B-12 and folate. *Am J Epidemiol* 1996; 143: 845–59.

58. von Eckardstein, A, Malinow, MR, Upson, B, Heinrich, J, Schulte, H, Schonfeld, R, Köhler, E, Assmann, G. Effects of age, lipoproteins, and hemostatic parameters on the role of homocyst(e)inemia as a cardiovascular risk factor in men. *Arterioscler Thromb* 1994; 14: 460–64.

59. Wald, NJ, Watt, HC, Law, MR, Weir, DG, McPartlin, J, Scott, J. Homocysteine and ischemic heart disease: Results of a prospective study with implications regarding prevention. *Arch Intern Med* 1988; 158: 862–67.

60. Woodside, JV, Yarnell, JW, McMaster, D, Harmon, DL, McCrum, EE, Patterson, CC, Gey, KF, Whitehead, AS, Evans, A. Effect of B-group vitamins and antioxidant vitamins on hyperhomocysteinemia: a double-blind randomized, factorial-design, controlled trial. *Am J Clin Nutr* 1998; 67: 858–66.

40

What Is a Desirable Homocysteine Level?

JOHAN B. UBBINK

Clinicians often assume that a desirable level of any plasma component equals a concentration within the 95% reference interval for that specific component. In principle, there should be nothing wrong with this assumption; after all, reference intervals are being constructed to give an idea of normality and to provide a basis with which the patient's result may be compared.

Indeed, for many metabolites this assumption is true (e.g., for the plasma glucose determination). In our laboratory, the 95% statistical reference interval for plasma fasting glucose concentrations is 3.9 to 5.8 mmol/L (70 to 105 mg/dL). Detrimental long-term effects of consistent, long-term hyperglycemia (retinopathy, vasculopathy, nephropathy) develop with plasma fasting glucose concentrations higher than 7.0 mmol/L (2). Therefore, the American Diabetes Association recommends a diagnosis of diabetes mellitus if two successive fasting plasma glucose concentrations exceed 7.0 mmol/L (2). The definition of a desirable plasma fasting glucose concentration is thus straightforward and is simply a plasma glucose concentration within the statistically derived 95% reference interval. Plasma fasting glucose concentrations higher than 5.8 mmol/L would be undesirable, reflecting a state of "impaired fasting glucose," and fasting plasma glucose concentration above 7.0 mmol/L is consistent with the diagnosis of diabetes mellitus (2).

Not all plasma components are at desirable levels, even if they are within the statistically derived reference interval. A well-known example of a statistically derived reference interval that does not reflect desirable levels is found in plasma total cholesterol concentrations. A typical statistical reference interval, determined as mean serum cholesterol concentration ± 2 standard deviations of the mean, is 3.80 to 7.01 mmol/L (146 to 270 mg/dL) for men aged 30 to 39 years (15). However, follow-up data from a group of 361,662 men screened as part of the Multiple Risk Factor Intervention Trial (11) showed that coronary heart disease mortality increased progressively with serum cholesterol concentrations higher than 4.7 mmol/L (181 mg/dL).

Figure 40.1 shows the relation between the statistical reference interval for serum total cholesterol concentrations and mortality from coronary heart disease, and it is clear that serum cholesterol concentrations that confer a higher-than-basal risk for coronary heart disease start well below the upper limit of the statistical reference interval. Therefore, desirable values for serum cholesterol associated with good health have been derived from cholesterol concentrations in populations with a low incidence of coronary heart disease and from serum cholesterol concentrations in the lowest-risk segment of populations with a high incidence of coronary heart disease (6). This resulted in the well-known guidelines of the National Cholesterol Education Program, which considers a desirable serum cholesterol concentration to be below 5.1 mmol/L (17).

The chapter addresses whether the statistical 95% reference interval for plasma homocysteine concentrations reflects desirable levels, or whether there is reason to believe that desirable levels will be different from the 95% reference interval derived from data obtained from apparently healthy populations.

Desirable Plasma Homocysteine Concentrations

Perspective from Patients with Cystathionine β-Synthase Deficiency

A desirable plasma homocysteine concentration may be defined as one that is innocuous and not related to harmful clinical manifestations for the patient. Patients with cystathionine β-synthase deficiency often have plasma free homocysteine concentrations exceeding 200 μmol/L (13), resulting in homocystinuria and various clinical abnormalities including ectopia lentis, mental retardation, osteoporosis, and thromboembolism

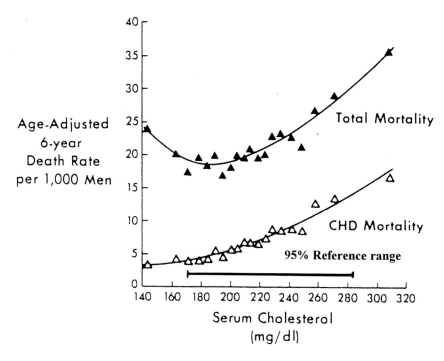

Fig. 40.1. The correlation between coronary heart disease (CHD) mortality and serum cholesterol concentrations in the Multiple Risk Factor Intervention Trial. There is a graded increase in coronary heart disease risk with increasing serum cholesterol concentrations within the 95% reference interval for serum cholesterol levels. (Reproduced from Martin et al. [11], with permission. The 95% reference interval for serum cholesterol concentrations [15] has been added to the figure.)

(13). Treatment of these patients with pyridoxine, folic acid, cobalamin, and, in some cases also with betaine, resulted in a 74% decrease in circulating free homocysteine concentrations and a considerable decrease in the number of thromboembolic events (26). Although vitamin and/or betaine therapy caused substantial reductions in circulating plasma free homocysteine concentrations, free homocysteine concentrations remained substantially elevated at about 20 μmol/L (26), which is approximately equal to a total homocysteine concentration of 100 μmol/L (12). Free plasma homocysteine concentrations, defined as the concentration of homocysteine-cysteine mixed disulfide plus twice the homocystine concentration, normally range between 3.0 and 3.8 μmol/L (27). Based on these observations, it may be concluded that a high plasma homocysteine concentration (> 100 μmol/L) resulting in homocystinuria may have harmful clinical sequelae and is thus undesirable.

When plasma total homocysteine concentrations are below 100 μmol/L, vascular derangements in the cystathionine β-synthase-deficient patient population seem to be prevented. Does this imply that a plasma homocysteine concentration up to 100 μmol/L is harmless? May we therefore conclude that 100 μmol/L is to be used as the cutoff point for desirable plasma total homocysteine concentrations in the general population?

Perspective from Patients with Folate or Cobalamin Deficiency

A second group of patients that offers a perspective on an undesirable plasma homocysteine concentration are those that suffer from a folic acid or cobalamin deficiency. Homocysteine metabolism is dependent on an adequate folic acid, vitamin B_6, and cobalamin status (see Metabolic Diagram). Stabler et al. (19) showed that 77 of 78 patients with cobalamin deficiency—as defined by low plasma cobalamin levels, megaloblastic bone marrow morphology, appropriate hematological or neurological abnormalities, and a significant response to parenteral cobalamin—had serum total homocysteine concentrations greater than 22 μmol/L. A later study by this group found that 94% of cobalamin-deficient patients had serum total homocysteine concentrations greater than 30 μmol/L (20). Similarly, 18 of 19 patients with clinical symptoms of a folic acid deficiency showed serum total homocysteine concentrations above 22 μmol/L (18). Considering that the upper limits of normal of statistically derived reference intervals for plasma total homocysteine have been reported to range between 15 and 30 μmol/L (21), it may be concluded that a plasma homocysteine concentration above the upper limit of normal suggests a vitamin deficiency and is thus undesirable.

It is important to note that these high homocysteine levels are not per se undesirable, but they are associated with the undesirable and potentially harmful effects of a folic acid and/or cobalamin deficiency. Conversely, a plasma homocysteine concentration within the statistically derived reference interval may be considered to reflect an adequate vitamin status and may be considered desirable, but only if the population for which the 95% statistical reference range has been obtained has an adequate vitamin nutritional status (see later).

Perspective from Vitamin Supplementation Studies

Plasma homocysteine concentrations above the 95% statistical reference range are easily lowered to concentrations within the reference range by folic acid supplementation (22). However, even plasma homocysteine concentrations within the reference range are readily modulated by folate supplementation (4), indicating that a 95% reference range obtained in any population is a function of the vitamin status of that population. A 95% reference range determined for a population with a compromised vitamin status, therefore, may be expected to have a higher upper limit of normal than that for a population with an adequate status. This suggests that a 95% reference range is not equal to desirable homocysteine levels in population groups with a suboptimal vitamin status.

Perspective from Patients with Cardiovascular Disease

Studies with regard to the possible role of homocysteine in cardiovascular disease indicate that a statistically derived reference interval for plasma homocysteine concentrations may be inadequate to describe desirable plasma homocysteine levels. However, it is still not proven that homocysteine is causally involved in cardiovascular diseases; in fact, the data in this regard remain controversial. A brief overview of these data is required before their implications for the definition of a desirable plasma homocysteine concentration can be considered.

Plasma homocysteine concentrations may be related to cardiovascular diseases in one of the following ways:

1. Elevated plasma homocysteine concentrations constitute an enhanced cardiovascular disease risk, but there is a threshold plasma homocysteine concentration above which homocysteine increases vascular disease risk. Data from the US Physicians' Health Study (21) suggest that vascular disease risk increases only if the plasma total homocysteine concentration exceeds the 95th percentile of the plasma homocysteine concentration frequency distribution.

Table 40.1. Plasma Homocysteine Concentrations and the Risk for Cardiovascular Disease

Study	Study Design	Group	1	2	3	4	5
Framingham Heart Study[a] (17)	Cross-sectional	Hcy	<9.1	9.2–11.3	11.4–14.3	>14.4	
		OR	1.0	1.1	1.6[d]	2.0[d]	
Angiographically confirmed CAD patients, Bergen, Norway[b] (14)	Prospective, cohort	Hcy	<9.0	9.0–14.9	15.0–19.9	>20.0	
		OR	1.0	1.92	2.78	4.51[d]	
Multiple Risk Factor Intervention Trial (5)	Prospective, nested case-control	Hcy	3.7–9.5	9.6–11.8	11.9–14.9	15.0–80.4	
		OR	1.0	1.03	0.84	0.82	
Caerphilly Prospective Study of Cardiac and Cerebral Ischaemia[c] (24)	Prospective, cohort	Hcy	<8.4	10.0	11.5	13.2	>16.7
		OR	1.0	1.1	1.2	1.1	1.4

Plasma Homocysteine (Hcy) Concentration in μmol/L and Odds Ratio (OR) for Cardiovascular Disease per Equal Group of the Study Population

The first two studies are examples of studies reporting a graded risk of cardiovascular disease with increasing plasma total homocysteine concentrations. The next two studies are examples of studies showing no significant cardiovascular disease risk associated with hyperhomocysteinemia.

[a] Data were adjusted for sex, age, total high-density lipoprotein/cholesterol ratio, smoking status, and systolic blood pressure.

[b] The endpoint in this study was mortality from cardiovascular disease. Mortality ratios were adjusted for sex, age, serum total cholesterol concentrations, treatment for hypertension, history of diabetes mellitus, smoking status, platelet count, and use of aspirin.

[c] Relative odds were adjusted for age, social class, body mass index, smoking, prevalent ischemic heart disease, diastolic blood pressure, diabetes and high-density lipoprotein cholesterol level.

[d] $p < 0.05$.

2. There is a graded risk of cardiovascular disease with increasing plasma levels of homocysteine. Many studies have reported data supporting this possibility (3, 7–9, 14, 16, 18), and data from two of these are summarized in Table 40.1.

3. There is no causal relation between premature cardiovascular disease and elevated plasma total homocysteine concentrations. Although virtually all retrospective case-control studies showed elevated plasma homocysteine concentrations in cardiovascular disease, several prospective studies failed to confirm this (1, 5, 24). Data from two prospective studies with negative results are summarized in Table 40.1. Therefore, it has been postulated that an elevated plasma homocysteine concentration is the result, and not the cause, of myocardial or cerebrovascular infarction (5).

The definition of the desirable plasma homocysteine range depends on which of these three possibilities will eventually be proved correct.

On one hand, if controlled intervention trials with vitamin supplementation and lowering of plasma total homocysteine concentrations fail to demonstrate any effect on cardiovascular disease incidence, it would be appropriate to view the statistically derived reference interval as desirable. A homocysteine concentration above the upper limit of normal would be undesirable for the sole reason that it reflects a vitamin deficiency that may be detrimental to the patient. Homocysteine per se would then be undesirable only if plasma total homocysteine concentrations exceed 100 to 200 μmol/L (i.e., in the genetic cases of homocystinuria).

On the other hand, if controlled clinical trials demonstrate a causal association between hyperhomocysteinemia and cardiovascular disease, the statistically derived reference interval may be inappropriate to define desirable plasma homocysteine concentrations. Current data supportive of a role for elevated plasma homocysteine concentrations in cardiovascular disease indicate that there is a considerable overlap between plasma homocysteine concentrations of patients with cardiovascular disease and control subjects (3, 8).

Figure 40.2 depicts the degree of overlap observed in these studies. There are several reasons for this overlap. Cardiovascular disease is multifactorial; thus many patients may have developed this disease through exposure to other risk factors. A further contributory factor to this overlap may be that an unknown number of subjects from the control (reference) population may already have subclinical cardiovascular disease. The recognition that an unknown number of participants contributing to reference data may have subclinical cardiovascular disease is one of the reasons why conventionally derived reference

intervals for serum cholesterol levels were abolished (6). The same approach may be required to define desirable plasma total homocysteine concentrations.

Let us assume that a graded risk for premature cardiovascular disease exists with increasing plasma total homocysteine concentrations, and that this association is causal. Furthermore, let us also assume that a controlled clinical trial has demonstrated a reduced incidence of cardiovascular disease following vitamin supplementation. Under these assumed circumstances, a plasma homocysteine level below the 25th percentile could be considered desirable. The first two studies quoted in Table 40.1 indicate that the lowest risk for cardiovascular disease was found in people with a plasma total homocysteine concentration below the 25th percentile. The 25th percentile is approximately equal to a plasma total homocysteine concentration of 9 μmol/L.

Is a Desirable Plasma Homocysteine Concentration Below 9 μmol/L Attainable?

It will be of little use to define a desirable homocysteine concentration below 9 μmol/L if this level is not attainable in the general population. Note that approximately 75% of a Western population may be expected to have plasma total homocysteine concentrations above 9 μmol/L. Fortunately, as discussed elsewhere in this book, plasma homocysteine concentrations may be easily reduced by daily, low-dose vitamin supplementation.

We recently used a mathematical prediction model to calculate the expected distribution of plasma total homocysteine concentrations in a population sample supplemented with daily vitamins (23). This model predicts that population plasma total homocysteine concentrations will approach a normal frequency distribution, with a 95% reference interval of 4.9 to 11.7 μmol/L, provided that the folate/cobalamin status of the population is optimized by vitamin supplementation (23). For this specific model, a plasma total homocysteine concentration of 9 μmol/L lies on the 80th percentile of the population frequency distribution. Therefore, most individuals will be able to maintain desirable plasma homocysteine concentrations when using a daily, modest, folate-containing vitamin supplement.

It is possible that the majority of the population will attain desirable plasma homocysteine concentrations if staple food is fortified with folate. Recent evidence, however, suggests that the current US flour folate fortification scheme may be insufficient to reduce population plasma homocysteine concentrations substantially (22), and higher levels of fortification may be required.

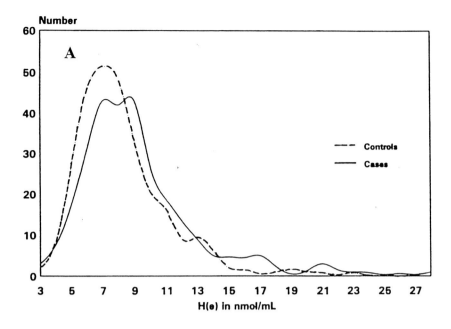

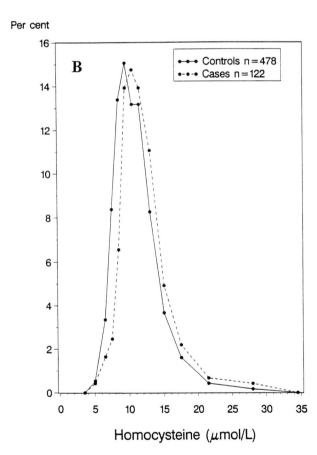

Fig. 40.2. Plasma total homocysteine [H(e)] concentrations in patients with cardiovascular disease (cases and controls). Note the considerable overlap in the frequency distributions of cases and controls in number of subjects (A) and proportions of subjects (B). (Figure A, from Malinow et al. [8], with permission. Figure B from Arnesen et al. [3], with permission.)

Overview

As discussed in this chapter, the definition of desirable plasma homocysteine concentrations depends on the pathogenic role of homocysteine in cardiovascular disease. Note that cardiovascular disease has been used as an example; similar arguments may be used in the definition of desirable homocysteine concentrations in any condition in which homocysteine may play a pathogenic role (e.g., neural tube defects). The contribution of elevated plasma total homocysteine concentrations to cardiovascular diseases is still controversial, and it is premature to define desirable plasma homocysteine concentrations that will reduce cardiovascular disease risk.

If controlled clinical trials show that a lowering of plasma total homocysteine concentrations reduces the incidence of cardiovascular disease, a plasma homocysteine concentration below 9 μmol/L would seem desirable. However, if controlled clinical trials fail to show any clinical benefit of homocysteine-lowering vitamin supplementation, a more lenient definition of desirable homocysteine concentrations may be adopted. The conventionally derived reference interval for plasma total homocysteine concentrations would then be synonymous with desirable levels. In this latter scenario, elevated plasma total homocysteine concentrations may not be undesirable per se, but may be associated with undesirable clinical effects resulting from a folate or cobalamin deficiency.

REFERENCES

1. Alfthan, G, Pekkanen, J, Jauhiainen, M, Pitkaniemi, J, Karvonen, M, Tuomilehto, J, Salonen, JT, Ehnholm, C.

Relation of serum homocysteine and lipoprotein(a) concentrations to atherosclerotic disease in a prospective Finnish population based study. *Atherosclerosis* 1994; 106: 9–19.

2. American Diabetes Association. Report of the Expert Committee on the Diagnosis and Classification of Diabetes Mellitus. *Diabetes Care* 1997; 78: 809A–F.

3. Arnesen, E, Refsum, H, Bonaa, KH, Ueland, PM, Forde, OH, Nordrehaug, JE. Serum total homocysteine and coronary heart disease. *Int J Epidemiol* 1995; 24: 704–9.

4. Bronstrup, A, Hages, M, Prinz-Langenohl, R, Pietzrik, D. Effects of folic acid and combinations of folic acid and vitamin B-12 on plasma homocysteine concentrations in healthy, young women. *Am J Clin Nutr* 1998; 68: 1104–10.

5. Evans, RW, Shaten, BJ, Hempel, JD, Cutler, JA, Kuller, LH. Homocyst(e)ine and Risk of Cardiovascular Disease in the Multiple Risk Factor Intervention Trial. *Arterioscler Thromb Vasc Biol* 1997; 17: 1947–53.

6. Expert Panel. Report of the National Cholesterol Education Program Expert Panel on detection, evaluation, and treatment of high blood cholesterol in adults. *Arch Intern Med* 1988; 148: 36–69.

7. Graham, IM, Daly, LE, Refsum, HM, Robinson, K, Brattström, LE, Ueland, PM, Palma-Reis, RJ, Boers, GH, Sheahan, RG, Israelsson, B, Uiterwaal, CS, Meleady, R, McMaster, D, Verhoef, P, Witteman, J, Rubba, P, Bellet, H, Wautrecht, JC, de Valk, HW, Sales Luis, AC, Parrot-Rouland, FM, Tan, KS, Higgins, I, Garcon, D, Medrano, MJ, Candito, M, Evans, AE, Andria, G. Plasma homocysteine as a risk factor for vascular disease. The European Concerted Action Project. *JAMA* 1997; 277: 1775–81.

8. Malinow, MR, Nieto, J, Szklo, M, Chambless, LE, Bond, G. Carotid artery intimal-medial wall thickening and plasma homocysteine in asymptomatic adults. *Circulation* 1993; 87: 1107–13.

9. Malinow, MR, Ducimetiere, P, Luc, G, Evans, AE, Arveiler, D, Cambien, F, Upson, BM. Plasma homocyst(e)ine levels and graded risk for myocardial infarction: Findings in two populations at contrasting risk for coronary heart disease. *Atherosclerosis* 1996; 126: 27–34.

10. Malinow, MR, Duell, PB, Hess, DL, Anderson, PH, Kruger, WD, Phillipson, BE, Gluckman, RA, Block, PC, Upson, BM. Reduction of plasma homocyst(e)ine levels by breakfast cereal fortified with folic acid in patients with coronary heart disease. *N Engl J Med* 1998; 338: 1009–15.

11. Martin, MJ, Hulley, SB, Browner, WS, Kuller, LH, Wentworth, D. Serum cholesterol, blood pressure, and mortality: Implications from a cohort of 361,662 men. *Lancet* 1986; ii: 933–36.

12. Moat, SJ, Bonham, JR, Tanner, MS, Allen, JC, Powers, HJ. Recommended approaches for the laboratory measurement of homocysteine in the diagnosis and monitoring of patients with hyperhomocysteinaemia. *Ann Clin Biochem* 1999; 36: 372–79.

13. Mudd, SH, Levy, HL, Skovby, F. Disorders of transulfuration. In *The Metabolic Basis of Inherited Disease*, 6th edition. (Scriver, CS, Beaudet, AL, Sly, WL, Valle, D, eds.). McGraw-Hill International Book Co, New York, 1989; pp. 693–734.

14. Nygård, O, Nordrehaug, JE, Refsum, H, Ueland, PM, Farstad, M, Vollset, SE. Plasma homocysteine levels and mortality in patients with coronary artery disease. *N Engl J Med* 1997; 337: 230–36.

15. Richterich, R, Colombo, JP. *Clinical Chemistry. Theory Practice and Interpretation*. John Wiley & Sons, New York, 1981; pp. 434–35.

16. Robinson, K, Mayer, EL, Miller, DP, Green, R, van Lente, F, Gupta, A, Kottke-Marchant, K, Savon, SR, Selhub, J, Nissen, SJ, Kutner, M, Topol, E, Jacobsen, DW. Hyperhomocysteinemia and low pyridoxal phosphate. Common and independent reversible risk factors for coronary artery disease. *Circulation* 1995; 92: 2825–30.

17. Second Expert Panel. Detection, evaluation and treatment of high blood cholesterol in adults (Adult Treatment Panel II). *Circulation* 1994; 89: 1329–1445.

18. Selhub, J, Jacques, PF, Bostom, AG, D'Agostino, RB, Wilson, PWF, Belanger, AJ, O'Leary, DH, Wolf, PA. Association between plasma homocysteine concentrations and extracranial carotid-artery stenosis. *N Engl J Med* 1995; 332: 286–91.

19. Stabler, SP, Marcell, PD, Podell, ER, Allen, RH, Savage, DG, Lindenbaum, J. Elevation of total homocysteine in the serum of patients with cobalamin or folate deficiency detected by capillary gas chromatography-mass spectrometry. *J Clin Invest* 1988; 81: 466–74.

20. Stabler, SP, Allen, RH, Savage, DG, Lindenbaum, J. Clinical spectrum and diagnosis of cobalamin deficiency. *Blood* 1990; 76: 871–81.

21. Stampfer, MJ, Malinow, R, Willet, WC, Newcomer, LM, Upson, B, Ullmann, D, Tishler, PV, Hennekens, CH. A prospective study of plasma homocyst(e)ine and risk of myocardial infarction in US physicians. *JAMA* 1992; 268: 877–81.

22. Ubbink, JB, Vermaak, WJH, Van der Merwe, A, Becker, PJ, Delport, R, Potgieter, HC. Vitamin requirements for the treatment of hyperhomocysteinemia in humans. *J Nutr* 1994; 124: 1927–33.

23. Ubbink, JB, Becker, PJ, Vermaak, WJH, Delport, R. Results of B-vitamin supplementation study used in a prediction model to define a reference range for plasma homocysteine. *Clin Chem* 1995; 41: 1033–37.

24. Ubbink, JB, Fehily, AM, Pickering, J, Elwood, PC, Vermaak, WJH. Homocysteine and ischaemic heart disease in the Caerphilly cohort. *Atherosclerosis* 1998; 140: 349–56.

25. Ubbink, JB, Delport, R. Reference ranges for homocysteine concentrations. In *Homocysteine and Vascular Disease*. (Robinson, K, ed.). Kluwer Academic Publishers, Boston, 2000; pp. 41–57.

26. Wilcken, DEL, Wilcken, B. The long-term outcome in homocystinuria. In *Homocysteine Metabolism: From Basic Science to Clinical Medicine*. (Graham, I, Refsum, H, Rosenberg, IH, Ueland, PM, eds.). Kluwer Academic Publishers, Boston, 1997; pp. 51–6.

27. Wiley, VC, Dudman, NPB, Wilcken, DEL. Free and protein-bound homocysteine in cystathionine beta-synthase deficiency: Interrelations during short- and long-term changes in plasma concentrations. *Metabolism* 1989; 38: 734–39.

Index

N-Acetylcysteine
    acidic dissociation constant, 14
    affecting homocysteine levels,
        334–335
N-Acetyl-lysine reaction with
        homocysteine thiolactone, 28
Acidic dissociation constants for
        thiols, 14
Adenosine
    analogs as inhibitors of
        S-adenosylhomocysteine
        hydrolase, 82–84
    and methionine metabolism, 63, 92
Adenosine-5′-carboxaldehyde as
        inhibitor of
        S-adenosylhomocysteine
        hydrolase, 83
Adenosine deaminase deficiency,
        S-adenosylhomocysteine
        hydrolase levels in, 80
Adenosine triphosphate in
        S-adenosylmethionine
        formation, 47
Adenosylcobalamin, 289
    deficiency, 248–249
        methylcobalamin deficiency with,
        249–250
S-Adenosylhomocysteine (AdoHcy),
    41
    abnormalities in homocysteine-
        related disorders, 190–193
    in cystathionine β-synthase
        deficiency, 234, 235, 236

inhibiting methyltransferase
    enzymes, 184
intracellular levels related to plasma
    total homocysteine, 63, 73
kinetic properties in methionine
    metabolism, 95–97
metabolic relationship to
    S-adenosylmethionine, 63
and methyltransferase inhibition,
    42, 64
    susceptibility of specific
        methyltransferases, 70–73
nitrous oxide affecting, 188
ratio to AdoMet
    AdoHcy hydrolase inhibitors
        affecting, 85, 86
    in renal failure, 64, 80, 324
    in regulation of methionine
        metabolism, 96
tissue distribution, 169–170
transport and uptake, 170–171
S-Adenosylhomocysteine hydrolase,
    63, 79–87
    activity in methionine metabolism
        age affecting, 94
        dietary protein affecting, 95
        hormones affecting, 95
    activity modulation, 80
    elevated levels in plasma and tissue,
        80
    forms, 79–80
    genes, 80–81
    inhibitors, 79, 82–87

antiparasitic effects, 85
antiviral effects, 84
apoptotic effects, 85–86
and cellular differentiation,
    84–85
and gene expression activation,
    85
inhibiting phospholipid
    methylation, 85
resistance to, 86–87
and sodium transport, 86
reaction mechanism, 79
structure, 81–82
tissue distribution, 163
S-Adenosylmethionine (AdoMet), 41
    abnormalities in homocysteine-
        related disorders, 190–193
    binding by methionine synthase,
        108
    in brain, 184
    in cerebrospinal fluid and plasma,
        in cystathionine β-synthase
        deficiency, 185–186
    clinical uses in liver disease, 55–57
    and cystathionine β-synthase
        activity, 156, 225
    in cystathionine β-synthase
        deficiency, 185–186, 234, 235
    decarboxylation of, 119
    deficiency of, neurologic disorders
        in, 185
    dependent methyltransferases,
        63–74

Diabetes mellitus *(continued)*
  microalbuminuria and
      hyperhomocysteinemia in,
      386
Dialysis patients. *See also* Renal
      failure
  folate deficiency in, 279
  homocysteine levels in, 321,
      323–325, 375, 469
    after methionine loading, 215
4′,5′-Didehydro-5′-deoxy-5′-
      fluoroadenosine as inhibitor
      of S-adenosylhomocysteine
      hydrolase, 83
Diet
  affecting methionine loading test,
      213
  and betaine:homocysteine
      methyltransferase activity,
      149–150
  choline intake affecting
      homocysteine remethylation,
      146
  and cobalamin deficiency, 294
  cobalamin sources in, 289–290
  in cystathionine β-synthase
      deficiency, 238
  folate deficiency in, 277
  folate sources in, 271
  folic acid supplements in, 280
  and homocysteine levels, 346–348,
      358
  in homocystinuria treatment,
      150–151
  omega-3 fatty acids in, 349
  protein in
    and enzyme activities in
        methionine metabolism,
        94–95
    and transsulfuration rate, 94
  vitamin B6 sources in, 309
Dietary Folate Equivalents, 271
Dihydrofolate
  production of, 113, 122
  subcellular distribution in rat, 119
Dihydrofolate reductase, 122
  drugs inhibiting, 278
  inhibition causing
      hyperhomocysteinemia, 333
Dimethylarginine, asymmetrical,
      homocysteine affecting, 446
Dimethylglycine dehydrogenase, 122
  in choline oxidation pathway, 146
  tetrahydrofolate binding to, 128
Diphthine synthase, 66, 70
Discovery of homocysteine, 1, 9
Dissociation constants for thiols, 14
Disulfides, 10, 32
  bond complexes, 10
  exchange with thiolate, 15–17

formation of, 10, 40
  mixed, 10, 32
  radial disulfide anion, 33
1,4-Dithioerythritol, acidic
      dissociation constant for, 14
1,4-Dithiothreitol, acidic dissociation
      constant for, 14
DNA
  (cytosine-5-)-methyltransferase 1,
      65, 69
    susceptibility to inhibition by S-
        adenosylhomocysteine, 71
  homocysteine affecting synthesis of,
      42
  strand breaks in megaloblastic
      anemia, 275
DNase I reaction with homocysteine
      thiolactone, 28
L-Dopa affecting homocysteine levels,
      335
Dopamine
  methyltransferases affecting, 69
  as vitamin B6 antagonist, 314
Down syndrome, methylenetetra-
      hydrofolate reductase variant
      in, 262, 458
Drug-induced conditions
  changes in homocysteine levels, 358
  folate deficiency, 278, 333
  hyperhomocysteinemia, 332–336
  vitamin B6 deficiency, 313–314

Electrophoresis, capillary, 204–205
Elongation factors
  EF-1α lysine N-methyltransferase,
      68
  in endothelial cells, homocysteine
      affecting, 429–430
Encephalitis in HIV infection,
      abnormalities of AdoMet
      and AdoHcy in, 192
Endothelial cells
  activation in response to injury,
      430–431
  cystathionine β-synthase in, 428
  dysfunction
    in hyperhomocysteinemia, 4, 36,
        40–41, 42
    in nitric oxide deficiency, 40–41
    in preeclampsia, 459
  gene expression affected by
      homocysteine, 429–430
  homocysteine affecting, 416–417,
      421, 427–431, 443,
      444–446
  homocysteine thiolactone in, 24
    from conversion of endogenous
        and exogenous
        homocysteine, 26

homocysteine toxicity, 33, 427–428
  homocysteine transport in, 166
  nitric oxide production affected by
      homocysteine, 417,
      428–429, 432
  pathways for low-density
      lipoprotein oxidation, 34–35
  proliferation affected by
      homocysteine, 429
Epidemiology of vascular disorders
      related to homocysteine,
      357–367
  blood sampling and handling in,
      358, 359
  case-control studies, 357–358
  confounders in, 359–360
  exposure measurement error in, 359
  and four popular hypotheses,
      360–367
  methodological issues in, 357–360
  preexisting diseases in, 358
  prolonged follow-up intervals in,
      358–359
  prospective studies, 358–359,
      361–363
  single measurements in, 359
Epileptic mice, S-adenosylhomocysteine
      hydrolase accumulation in
      brain, 80
Epinephrine, methyltransferases
      affecting, 69
Erythrocytes
  S-adenosylhomocysteine in, 169,
      170
  S-adenosylmethionine in, 169, 170
  causes of macrocytosis, 274
  folate content, 273–274
  homocysteine in, 164, 168
Escherichia coli
  AdoMet synthetase in, 47
  enzymes in microbial modeling of
      human disease, 100–110
    methionine synthase, 107–110
    methylenetetrahydrofolate
        reductase, 102–107
  folylpolyglutamate synthetase
      activity in, 121
  homocysteine thiolactone in,
      24–25
    from conversion of endogenous
        and exogenous
        homocysteine, 26
  methionine synthase in, 135–136
Estradiol, and enzyme activities in
      methionine metabolism, 96
Estrogen
  affecting homocysteine levels,
      332
  in postmenopausal women,
      452–454

protein intake, 347
smoking, 342–345
studies of, 342–344
vitamin intake and other nutrients, 346–347
B-vitamins, 346
weight reduction, 349
Lipid-lowering drugs affecting homocysteine levels, 334
Lipoprotein
high-density, association with homocysteine thiolactonase, 27–29
low-density
homocysteine thiolactone reaction with, 39
homocysteinylated, 27
oxidation of
and atherogenesis, 33–34
cellular pathways in, 34–35
promotion by thiols, 35–36
reaction with homocysteine thiolactone, 28
Liquid chromatography
and electrospray tandem mass spectrometry, 203
high-performance assays of homocysteine, 203–204
Liver
AdoMet and AdoHcy in, 169
AdoMet synthetase in, 48–49
activity regulation, 52–54
deficiency of, 54–55
gene expression regulation, 49–52
diseases of, AdoMet therapy in, 55–57. See also Cirrhosis
folate binding proteins in
cytosolic, 117
mitochondrial, 118
homocysteine levels in mice and rats, 165
subcellular folate pool distribution, 118
vitamin B6 metabolism, 308–309
Lungs, homocysteine levels in mice and rats, 165
Lupus erythematosus, homocysteine levels in
and cardiovascular disease, 375
and thrombosis, 366, 410
Lymphoblasts, AdoMet and AdoHcy in, 169
Lysine
affecting protein homocysteinylation, 27
reaction with homocysteine thiolactone, 28
Lysyl oxidase, homocysteine affecting, 42

Lysyl-tRNA synthetase in homocysteine thiolactone formation, 23

Macrocytosis
causes of, 274
in cobalamin deficiency, 292
α_2-Macroglobulin reaction with homocysteine thiolactone, 28
Magnesium intake affecting homocysteine levels, 347
Malabsorption
cobalamin deficiency in, 293
folate deficiency in, 277–278
food-cobalamin, 293, 295, 296
vitamin B6 deficiency in, 313
Malaria parasites, S-adenosylhomocysteine hydrolase inhibitors affecting, 85
Mass spectrometry
and capillary gas chromatography, 202
and liquid chromatography electrospray, 203
Megaloblastic anemia, 244, 247, 251, 274–275
in cobalamin deficiency, 292
in folate deficiency, 274–275
and folate levels in liver, 271
Melatonin, methyltransferases affecting, 69
Menopause, homocysteine levels in, 452–454
Menstrual cycle, steroid fluctuations in, 451
Mental status
in cystathionine β-synthase deficiency, 228, 230, 236
in folate deficiency, 275–276
Mercaptalbumin, and protein-bound homocysteine formation, 16
2-Mercaptoethanol, acidic dissociation constant for, 14
6-Mercaptopurine affecting homocysteine levels, 335
Metabolism of homocysteine, 1, 92–98
age affecting, 94
alternate and minor pathways, 93–94
in brain, 183–184
disorders affecting brain function, 184–187
in children with spina bifida, 457
clearance rates
after oral L-homocysteine, 166–167
after oral methionine, 215–216

concentrations of metabolic effectors and substrates affecting, 97
dietary protein affecting, 94–95
genetic defects in, 185–186
hormones affecting, 95, 96
and kidney and liver enzymes in humans and rats, 180
in kidneys, 179–180, 322–323
in methionine loading test, 215
kinetic properties of enzymes in, 95–97
methionine cycle, 92–93
and microbial modeling of human disease, 100–110
oxidation/reduction state affecting, 97–98
regulation of, 94–98
remethylation, 1, 12
betaine-dependent, 145–151
cobalamin-dependent, 135–141
tissue enzyme patterns affecting, 94–95
transsulfuration pathway, 1, 9, 12, 93–94, 135, 153–159
Metabolism of homocysteine thiolactone in cell cultures and serum, 25–26
Metal ions
oxidizing thiols, 14, 33
promoting low-density lipoprotein oxidation, 34
Metalloproteinase activation affected by homocysteine, 433–434
Metformin affecting homocysteine levels, 334
5,10-Methenyl cyclohydrolase
cytosolic, 122
mitochondrial, 123, 124
5,10-Methenyltetrahydrofolate, 114, 122
mitochondrial, 123
Methenyltetrahydrofolate synthetase in 5Y neuroblastoma cell line, 127
Methionine
in amniotic fluid, 454, 457
competition with homocysteine, 22
dietary
affecting homocysteine metabolism, 97
in cystathionine β-synthase deficiency, 238
intolerance as risk for venous thromboembolism, 403–405
loading test, 212–218
absolute rise in, 213
affecting homocysteine levels, 3, 13, 167
age affecting, 214

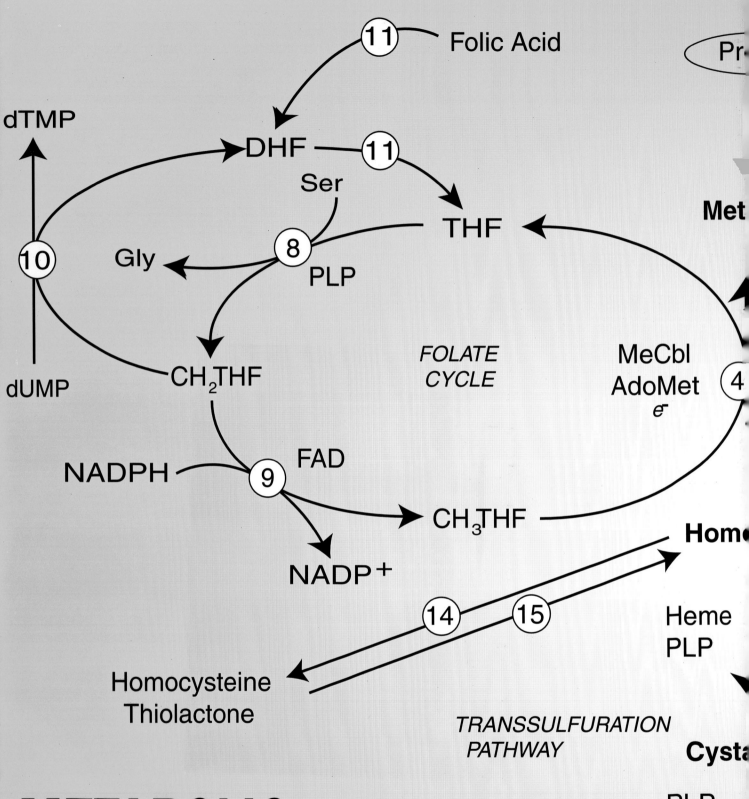

dTMP

⑪ — Folic Acid

Pr

⑪

DHF

Ser

Met

THF

Gly

⑧

PLP

⑩

FOLATE CYCLE

MeCbl
AdoMet
e⁻

④

dUMP

CH₂THF

NADPH

⑨

FAD

CH₃THF

Hom

NADP⁺

⑭ ⑮

Heme
PLP

Homocysteine
Thiolactone

TRANSSULFURATION PATHWAY

Cysta

PLP

METABOLIC

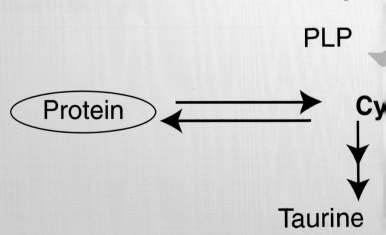

Protein — Cy

DIAGRAM

Taurine

Design by Jaine Liveson